D0842163

PERSPECTIVES IN CLINICAL PHARMACY

EDITED BY

Donald E. Francke

M.Sc., D.Sc. (H.C.)

Coordinator, Education and Research in Clinical Pharmacy
Veterans Administration, Washington, D.C. 20420
and Editor, *Drug Intelligence & Clinical Pharmacy*

AND

Harvey A. K. Whitney, Jr.

M.Sc. (Hospital Pharmacy)

Associate Professor of Clinical Pharmacy
and Director, Pharmacy Service
University of Cincinnati Medical Center
Cincinnati, Ohio 45229

PERSPECTIVES IN CLINICAL PHARMACY

first edition

a textbook for the clinically-oriented pharmacist wherever he may practice

DRUG INTELLIGENCE PUBLICATIONS
HAMILTON, ILLINOIS 62341

Library of Congress Catalog Number 74-177913

Printed in the United States of America by Hamilton Press, Inc., Hamilton, Illinois 62341

preface to first edition

In essence, clinical pharmacy represents a revolt by a group young in years and in spirit against the way the profession has developed, the manner in which it has been practiced, the nonrelevant isolation in which it has been taught, the exclusion of a clinical by a scientific faculty, the student's almost complete lack of contact with patients, physicians and other health practitioners during his educational process, the emphasis of the economic over the social sciences, the tasks customarily assigned to the pharmacist upon the completion of five or six years of college level studies and the setting in which he performs them. Whether or not the concept of clinical pharmacy will result in a successful revolution, or fizzle out as an aborted rebellion as it did some years ago remains a judgment for the future.

Fortunately, no one has yet succeeded in defining clinical pharmacy and it thus remains an evolving concept with great promise. When the concept finally matures, we believe that the clinical pharmacist will perhaps best be described as an applied pharmacology generalist. In this development, strong courses in pharmacology, biopharmaceutics, pharmacokinetics and biostatistics will serve as a sturdy bridge between the clinical pharmacist's studies in the basic sciences and his clinical clerkship. Additional courses in the social and behavioral sciences will help him as he gains clinical experience in association with other health professionals while serving the needs of patients.

Three objectives have guided the selection of the subject matter for this book. One is to give the reader an orientation to the health-care system of which he is a part. A second is to acquaint him with some of the still evolving concepts and practices of clinical pharmacy and to point out their relationship to various systems of drug distribution. The major portion of the book, however, is concerned with presenting the type of information the clinical pharmacist will use in his daily effort to promote the safe and effective use of drugs in patients working in close association with physicians as a part of the health-care team. The clinical pharmacist must be a special kind of drug expert in his own right if he is to serve the needs of patients and physicians. He must carry to the patient's bedside a range of specialized knowledge not possessed by other members of the health team. Only a limited few academic programs today prepare him for this role. Until many more colleges undertake to meet this objective, the new clinical pharmacist will not differ significantly from the traditional pharmacist. He will be "more of the same" with but a change in name.

We wish to acknowledge the splendid cooperation and dedicated work done by the authors of the various chapters. To them and to many who read this the editors owe a word of apology for the delay in publishing this first edition of *Perspectives in Clinical Pharmacy.* Change of positions by both editors during the past few months has been the principal reason. We also acknowledge some variations in type style in a few of the chapters. For the most part these were occasioned by haste in an effort to overcome delay.

In addition to the authors of the several chapters, the editors are particularly indebted to Miss Joanne B. Branson for her painstaking work with the original manuscript and her careful proofreading and checking of corrections for the final copy. We want to acknowledge the contributions of Gloria N. Francke whose capable, devoted and unselfish "work by the side of work" helped to move the final task more rapidly toward completion. We are also most appreciative to her for preparing the index to the work as well as for her help in many phases of the project.

There are many others without whose effort this book would have encountered further delay. Candace K. Brettschneider, who has served as a Doctor of Pharmacy degree student under both of the editors, labored untold hours with dedicated interest reading and re-reading manuscripts and proof copy. Another student and a current pharmacy resident at the University of Cincinnati Medical Center to whom we are indebted is Mr. Anthony S. Inglott, whose checking of many items relative to the study moved it along more rapidly than it would have otherwise progressed. We want also to express our thanks to Miss Doris Johnson whose work with the final stages of this book has been most helpful.

Finally, while it is unknown what the gestation period is for a book of this type, as previously indicated, it certainly was not born prematurely. As it is during most pregnancies, there are always those who suffer the agonies of supporting their loved ones. While normally it is the husband and children, in this circumstance we want to thank Mrs. Tina Whitney and daughters, Lisa Kay and Kim Ellen for bearing with us through the many months of tribulation. Without their understanding the book might have been a complete abortion.

DONALD E. FRANCKE
Washington, D.C. 20008

and

HARVEY A. K. WHITNEY, JR.
Cincinnati, Ohio 45229

February 20, 1972

contributors

Bell, J. Edward, B.S., Pharm.D.

is Director, Drug Information Services, Mercy Hospital; Clinical Instructor, Department of Clinical Pharmacy, Duquesne University, Pittsburgh, Pennsylvania 15219

Berman, Alex, Ph.D.

is Professor of Historical and Social Studies in Pharmacy, College of Pharmacy, and Professor of History, University of Cincinnati, Cincinnati, Ohio 45221

Bouchard, Vincent E., B.S., M.S.

is Associate Professor and Chairman, Department of Clinical Pharmacy, Duquesne University and Coordinator, Hospital Pharmacy Program, Mercy Hospital, Pittsburgh, Pennsylvania 15219

Buncher, Charles Ralph, Sc.D.

is Chief Biostatistician, Merrell-National Laboratories, Division of Richardson-Merrell Inc., Cincinnati, Ohio 45215; Adjunct Assistant Professor of Biostatistics, University of Cincinnati College of Medicine, Cincinnati, Ohio 45229

Canada, Andrew T. Jr., B.S., M.S., Pharm.D.

is head, Department of Pharmacy, Sunnybrook Hospital of the University of Toronto; Assistant Professor of Clinical Pharmacy, University of Toronto, Toronto, Ontario, Canada

Chudzik, Gregory M., Pharm. D.

is Assistant Professor of Pharmacy, State University of New York at Buffalo, School of Pharmacy, Buffalo, New York; Pediatric Clinical Pharmacist, Buffalo Children's Hospital, Buffalo, New York 14222

Cluxton, Robert J. Jr., B.S., Pharm.D. Candidate

is Pharmacy Resident, University of Cincinnati Medical Center, Cincinnati, Ohio 45229

Covington, Tim R., M.S., Pharm.D.

is Assistant Professor of Clinical Pharmacy, College of Pharmacy, University of Oklahoma, Norman, Oklahoma 73069

Dresback, David

is Research Associate, University of Michigan, College of Pharmacy, Ann Arbor, Michigan 48104

Eckel, Fred M., M.S.

is Director of Pharmacy Services, North Carolina Memorial Hospital and Assistant Professor of Hospital Pharmacy, University of North Carolina, Chapel Hill, North Carolina 27514

Francke, Gloria N., Pharm.D.

is Chief, Program Evaluation, Alcoholism and Drug Dependence Service, Veterans Administration, Washington, D.C. 20420

Hartshorn, Edward A., Ph.D.

is Pharmacologist, Attending Staff, and Director, Pharmacy Services, Evanston Hospital, Evanston, Illinois 60201; Associate, Department of Nursing Education, Northwestern University, Chicago, Illinois

Hirschman, Joseph L., Pharm.D.

is Assistant Clinical Professor of Pharmacy, School of Pharmacy, University of California, San Francisco; Supervisor, Drug Information Analysis Service, University of California Hospitals, San Francisco, California 94122

Ho, Norman F. H., Ph.D.

is Assistant Professor of Pharmacy, University of Michigan, College of Pharmacy, Ann Arbor, Michigan 48104

Inglott, Anthony S., B.S., Pharm.D. Candidate

is Pharmacy Resident, University of Cincinnati Medical Center, Cincinnati, Ohio 45229

Kramer, Warren R., M.S.

is Director of Pharmacy Service, Saint Francis Hospital, Evanston, Illinois 60202

Lofholm, Paul W., Pharm.D.

is Director of Pharmacy, Ross Valley Pharmacy, Ross Valley Medical Clinic, Greenbrae, California 94904; Assistant Clinical Professor of Pharmacy, University of California at San Francisco, California.

Mackewicz, Dennis W., Pharm.D.

is Assistant Director of Pharmacy and Central Services, Memorial Hospital Medical Center, Long Beach, California 90801; Assistant Clinical Professor of Pharmacy, University of Southern California, Los Angeles, California

McLeod, Donald C., M.S.

is Assistant Director of Pharmacy Services, Duke University Medical Center, Durham; Instructor in Clinical Pharmacy, School of Pharmacy, University of North Carolina, Chapel Hill, North Carolina 27514

Oliver, John A., M.S.

is Hospital Pharmacy Consultant, San Diego, California 92041

Piecoro, John J. Jr., M.S.

is Assistant Professor of Clinical Pharmacy, University of Kentucky College of Pharmacy, Lexington, Kentucky; Pediatric Clinical Pharmacist, A. B. Chandler Medical Center, Lexington, Kentucky 40506

Pierpaoli, Paul G., M.S.

is Director of Pharmacy Services, University of Connecticut Health Center, Hartford, Connecticut 06112; Assistant Clinical Professor, School of Pharmacy, University of Connecticut, Storrs, Connecticut

Ravin, Robert L., M.S.

is Director of Pharmaceutical Services, St. Joseph Mercy Hospital, Ann Arbor, Michigan 48104; Associate Professor of Hospital Pharmacy, Wayne State University, Detroit, Michigan

Ritschel, Wolfgang A., Ph.D., Pharm.D.

is Associate Professor of Biopharmaceutics, College of Pharmacy, University of Cincinnati; Assistant Director of Pharmacy Service, University of Cincinnati Medical Center, Cincinnati, Ohio 45229

Schreiner, George E., M.D.

is Editor, *Transactions,* American Society for Artificial Internal Organs, Professor of Medicine, Georgetown University School of Medicine, Washington, D.C. 20007.

Schumacher, Gerald E., Ph.D., Pharm.D.

is Associate Professor of Pharmacy, College of Pharmacy, The University of Toledo, Toledo, Ohio 43606

Simonelli, Anthony P., Ph.D.

is Associate Professor of Pharmacy, University of Michigan, College of Pharmacy, Ann Arbor, Michigan 48104

Smith, Dorothy L., B.S.P., Pharm.D. Candidate

is Clinical Instructor of Pharmacy, University of Cincinnati Medical Center, Cincinnati, Ohio 45229

Smith, William E., Pharm.D

is Director of Pharmacy and Central Services, Memorial Hospital Medical Center, Long Beach, California 90801; Assistant Clinical Professor of Pharmacy, University of Southern California, Los Angeles, California

Tester, William W., M.S.

is Associate Professor and Director Pharmaceutical Services, University of Iowa College of Pharmacy, Iowa City, Iowa 52240

contents

PERSPECTIVES IN CLINICAL PHARMACY

foreword

Impact of clinical pharmacy on the profession

by Alex Berman

We are presently witnessing in America a burgeoning movement designated "clinical pharmacy" which seeks to promote much stronger pharmacist-patient relationships and closer interaction with physicians and other professional health personnel. This movement defies strict definition, but its attitudinal and philosophical underpinnings are as important as its operational goals, which are to provide and integrate a significant number of patient-oriented services. These range from monitoring drug interactions and predicting drug stability of parenteral admixtures to providing patient drug surveillance and interviewing and advising the patient; from setting up a drug information service to directing pharmacy services in smaller hospitals, extended care facilities and nursing homes.

For this movement to succeed, it is essential that the tradition-bound patterns of pharmacy practice in this country be altered. To begin with, this requires, as D. E. Francke and Dorothy Smith point out, a fundamental understanding of the social and psychological needs of the sick person who is undergoing drug therapy. This awareness would also encompass patient relationships with physicians and reactions of the sick to the hospital environment; it would include a sufficient grasp by the pharmacist of behavioral sciences related to health care. The authors argue correctly that, in general, colleges of pharmacy and preceptors have not imbued students with this attitude and have not provided clinical models analogous to those found in medical education. "The clinical pharmacist," write Francke and Smith, "should partially replace the physician in fulfilling the psychological needs of the patient yet at the same time being supportive of the physician's therapeutic aims." In so doing, the pharmacist must practice with dignity in a strictly professional setting, offering expertise, drug information and consultation to patient and physician.

Can this social psychological role as described in detail by Francke and Smith be fostered in American pharmacy under present conditions? The authors consider the preponderance of community and chain drugstores, as opposed to the relatively few professional pharmacies, the greatest deterrent to such a role. Historically, the rigid economic structure of American pharmacy practice has resisted creative innovation; elsewhere I have observed that "basically there has been no significant change in the narrow entrepreneurial orientation of the community pharmacist in the last century. To be sure, he now dispenses revolutionary therapeutic agents never dreamed by his forbears and he is now required to complete five years of university education, but the schizoid character of his calling remains the same."[1] Francke and Smith offer a bold and imaginative recommendation:

> There must be a concerted, nationwide effort on the part of the college to train pharmacists in clinical practice under ideal conditions in an establishment operated, controlled and supervised by the college and preferably part of a health-care group practice. The pharmacy should be designed and constructed for teaching and research purposes and should be operated by professional practitioners holding appointments on the faculty.

In the meantime, another challenge confronts American Pharmacy: adaptation to imminent sweeping changes in the delivery of health care in the United States. The pent-up demand for restructuring health care in the United States and the rapid developments in this field are ably discussed by Whitney in the opening chapter of this book.

For those readers who are curious about how clinical pharmacy evolved into a concept and into an incipient movement, no better essay is available than that presented by Gloria Francke, who examines old and new ideas and practices which have been incorporated into this concept. She concludes: "Practicing in the patient care environment does call for new skills from the pharmacist and perhaps these are the newest things about clinical pharmacy." These new skills are expertly reviewed by various authors in this book: skill and knowledge to understand and implement interprofessional relationships (Oliver); the impressive range of services and activities involved in providing a comprehensve clinical pharmacy program in the hospital (Smith and Mackewicz); the evaluation and initiation of drug distribution systems (Tester); launching a clinically-oriented drug information service (Hirschman); techniques of interviewing and advising the patient (Covington); and clinical pediatric pharmacy (Piecoro and Chudzik). A careful reading of the chapters dealing with pharmacy services in smaller institutions (Eckel and McLeod) and with the clinical pharmacist in the context of an interprofessional group practice (Lofholm), should dispel the notion that clinical pharmacy cannot be practiced in a meaningful way by the community pharmacist. Utilizing his training in the pharmaceutical sciences and technology, the clinical pharmacist can also perform essential services as described in the chapters covering drug interactions (Hartshorn); the interference of drugs with diagnostic tests (Bouchard and Bell); the relation of drug therapy and diet (Pierpaoli); monitoring drugs for patient safety (Canada); and the more familiar technological and scientific tasks: parenteral admixtures (Ravin), predicting the drug stability of these solutions (Ho) and their chemical incompatibilities (Kramer, Inglott and Cluxton); formulated nonsterile dosage forms (Schumacher) and sterile dosage forms (Simonelli and Dresback). In recent years the newest of the pharmaceutical sciences, biopharmaceutics, has emerged as an important and indispensable tool for the pharmacist. The significance of biopharmaceutics in clinical pharmacy practice is shown in two chapters by Ritschel in his treatment of biological half-lives and pKa values. Buncher demonstrates how good clinical drug studies are designed, Schreiner discusses the dialysis of poisons and drugs, and Dorothy Smith provides some valuable information on significant laboratory tests.

If the perspectives in clinical pharmacy revealed in this work become widely accepted in American pharmacy, can anyone doubt that this would have a profound impact on the profession and that it would grow enormously in social esteem? But such an acceptance will require a conscious change of direction and goals as well as a planned restructuring of economic and institutional aspects of pharmacy.

---

1. Berman, Alex: Influence of Medicare on the Profession of Pharmacy, *Am. J. Hosp. Pharm.* 23:182 (Apr.) 1966.

1

Newer dimensions in health care systems

by Harvey A. K. Whitney, Jr.

The health care of this nation's people has been of primary concern more in the last five years than at any other time in history. It became a public issue in the past decade with the resultant passage of Medicare and Medicaid. That it will continue to be an important social issue for the 1970's is well illustrated by the ever-increasing quantity of articles in the professional and lay press and the number of bills presented to Congress. Congressional and public discussion will focus attention on this subject until the dominant thesis accepted by the majority—that health care is a *right* of everyone—has become a visible reality.

Pharmacists, along with other health professionals, must take an active interest in discussions on health care so that they may contribute to the development of impending changes. Clinical pharmacists are those pharmacists who have had an intensive education and training and who are prepared as full-fledged partners to work continuously with physicians in direct patient care. Because of their intensive and constant involvement with physicians and patients, clinical pharmacists will be vastly affected by the newer dimensions arising on the health care scene. Those pharmacists who choose to be involved today in planning the health care system for tomorrow will be an integral part rather than an appendage of the final product. With this thought in mind it is the purpose of this chapter to review current discussions by looking at the problems and suggested solutions for organized delivery of a total health care system. Because at present there are numerous schemes proposed for financing health care and because of the uncertain direction they will take, it is considered impractical to include a discussion of them in this chapter.

There must be an appreciation of the breadth of *modern* medicine in order to adequately comprehend the need for changes in medical care. It has been stated that "the scope of medicine now encompasses the health (1) of individual citizens, (2) of communities of citizens whether rural, urban or regional, (3) of the physical and social environment of human beings, and even (4) the biological health and survival of the human species."[1]

Failure of the Nonsystem

Health care delivery in the United States has been so haphazard in origin that it is frequently referred to as a "nonsystem." As a former Secretary of Health, Education, and Welfare put it: "American health care is not really a 'system' but is essentially a mosaic of public and private health programs—one that has grown piecemeal to meet needs as they arose."[2] The problem has largely centered around the inept methods of financing health care, the lack of organization and the inability of health professionals to modify the method of delivery rapidly enough. Today the complexity of medical practice and health care is such that it cannot be delivered by the traditionally accepted methods. "The situation seems like that which once existed in telephone communication. Each town, each city had its own telephone company, sometimes more than one. Each did a reasonably good job, but the demand for uniform and widespread service forced amalgamation. The independent company could not provide the integrated service that the new technology made possible and public demand required."[3] So it is that "the medical profession is no longer *the* determinant of its destiny . . . In short, medicine is looked upon as a public necessity—a public utility."[3]

Barometers of Failure

Morbidity and Mortality. It has been pointed

Figure 1

THE UNITED STATES RANKS 18TH IN MALE LIFE EXPECTANCY

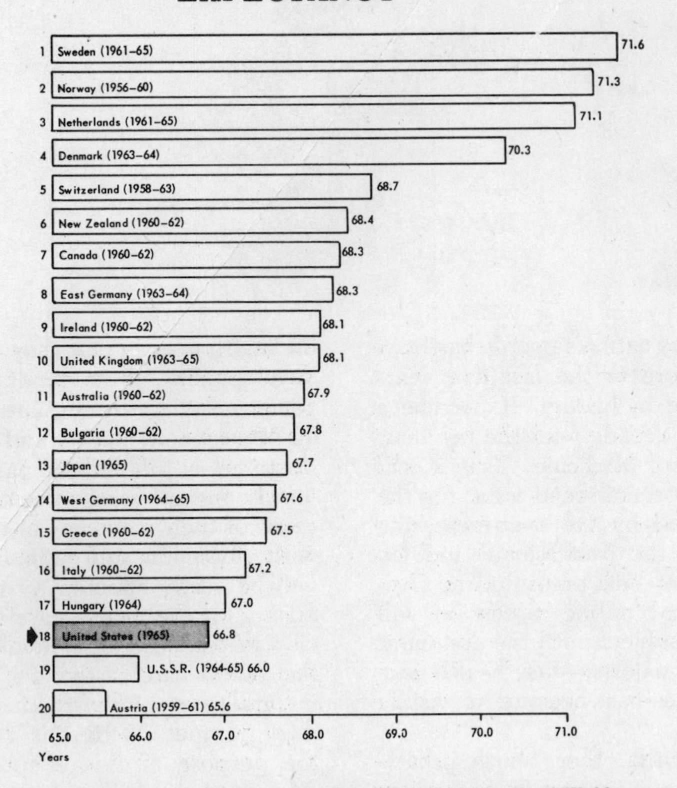

Source: U.S. Department of Health, Education, and Welfare.

out by many demographers that the United States has failed to maintain proper standards of health care. To support this contention, morbidity and mortality data from the U.S. have been compared with other countries. The following figures are given as examples. The United States ranks:

1. Thirteenth in maternal mortality rate,
2. Eighteenth in male life expectancy (Figure 1),
3. Eleventh in female life expectancy,
4. Eighteenth in percentage of male deaths between ages of 40 and 50, and
5. Fourteenth in infant mortality rate (Figure 2).[4]

While one may not wish to question the authenticity of these oftquoted statistics, it is prudent to recognize that direct comparisons such as these omit certain explanations which may be pertinent and may prevent the occurrence of false assumptions. For example, one might believe because the U.S. ranks fourteenth in infant mortality that the root cause of this is a quality of medical care inferior to those countries ranking higher. But is *medical* care to be faulted when a child is not wanted and abortions are illegal thus provoking infanticide? It is known that a society with a larger population of nonwhites and non-northern Europeans has a higher infant mortality rate partly because it produces a higher percentage of unwanted children, and partly because the mother and child are generally in a poorer nutritional state. Infant mortality rates in the U.S. are two times as great for nonwhites as for whites (Figure 3).[5] In addition to the differences in medical care statistics between the United States and other countries, there is also a notable disparity within our country when the city slums are compared with the rest of the nation. The slums have three times as much heart disease, five times as much high blood pressure, and four times the number of deaths before age thirty-five.[5] While many of these problems are sociological in nature and may not be considered the result of improper *medical* care, they can be attributed to our nonsystem of *health* care and certainly fall within the modern scope of medicine as previously defined.

High Cost and Financial Barriers. Appalling

Figure 2

THE UNITED STATES RANKS 14TH IN INFANT MORTALITY

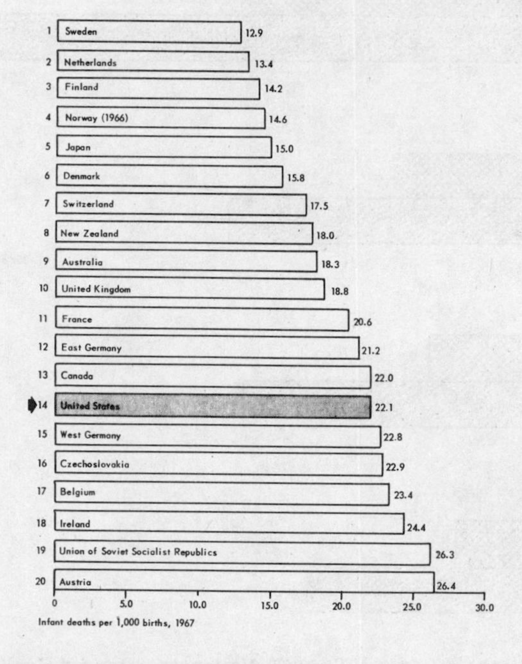

Source: *Population and Vital Statistics Report.* Series A, Volume XXI, No. 1, January 1, 1969 and No. 2, April 1, 1969. United Nations.

as these mortality figures are, it also must be noted that the amount spent per capita to achieve this abject status is considered by many as being unduly high. The $324 per person in 1970 (Figure 4) is more than any country in the world spends for health and medical care.[6] This represented 7 percent of our gross national product, a significant increase from 3.6 percent in 1929, 4.7 percent in 1955, and 6 percent in 1965.[7] The high cost of medical care has become prohibitive for people with low incomes while it is these people, not those with high incomes, who need the protection of health insurance (Figure 5). "Yet the extent of health insurance coverage varies in reverse degree (Figure 6). In 1967 only 35 percent of persons under the age of 65 with family incomes under $3,000 had some hospital insurance, and 57 percent of those with incomes between $3,000 and $5,000, as compared with 90 percent among those with incomes of $10,000 or more."[2]

The shortcomings of Medicare and Medicaid are well-known. Medicare is not comprehensive (it does not cover outpatient drugs, dental care or preventive medicine) and yet it is already costing the taxpayer over $6.75 billion a year. Medicare needs more tax money to meet a twenty-five year projected deficit of $236 billion just for Part A (hospital related benefits) and the trust fund for Part B (voluntary doctor-payment plan) is down almost to nothing. Compounding all this is the fact that currently "Medicare covers less than half the health expenses of the elderly population, at least one-third of whom are at or near the poverty line."[8] Medicaid reaches only fifteen million of the thirty to forty million people who potentially should be covered. This is despite the fact that "state and local expenditures for medical assistance rose from $764 million in 1965 to $2.3 billion in 1969."[9] There are some who contend the reason Medicaid costs are increasing is because the program is growing in accordance with the original legislative plan. Most authorities agree, though, that the structure of Medicaid has made it inefficient and subject to monetary abuses. The rate of increase in cost due to Medicare and Medicaid may be better appreciated from the following comments: "Med-

Figure 3

THE INFANT MORTALITY RATE OF NONWHITES IS DOUBLE THAT OF WHITES

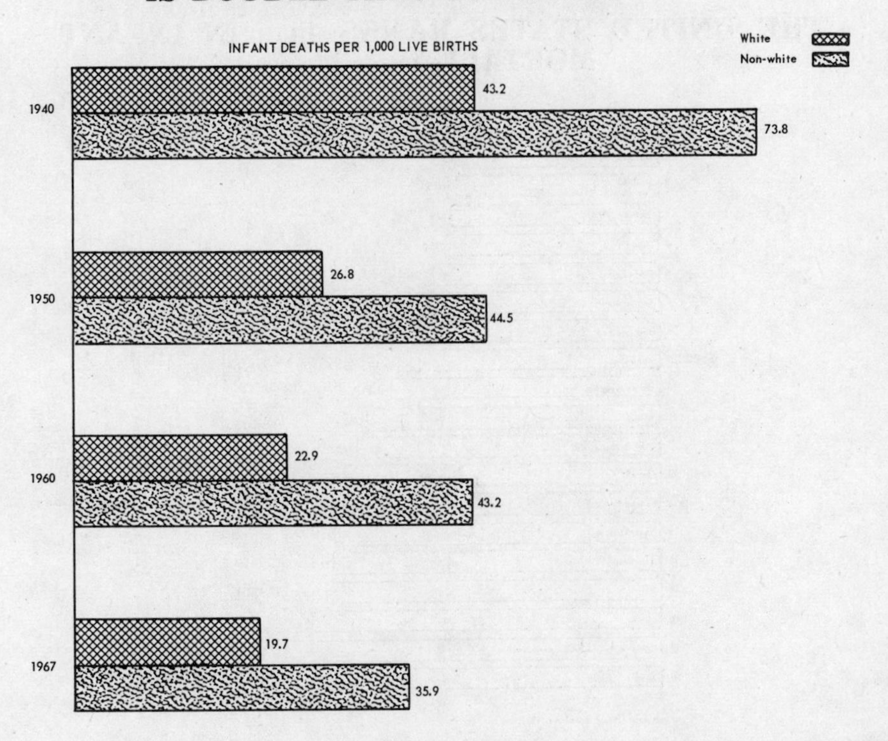

Source: *Vital Statistics of the U.S., 1967*. National Center for Health Statistics, U.S. Department of Health, Education, and Welfare.

ical costs were already increasing at twice the rate of increase in the Consumer Price Index when Medicaid and Medicare went into effect. But in that year physicians' fees shot up at almost three times the rate of general prices, while hospital charges, incredibly, increased at five times the rate of general prices."[5]

(Other indicators illustrating the high cost of medical care are provided in Figures 7, 8 and 9.)

Manpower Problems. Another failure has been in the adequacy and proper distribution of manpower—over which the government exerts little control (Figure 10). A 1965 survey of 1,500 cities and towns in the upper Midwest showed that 1,000 had no doctor at all and 200 had only one. In addition to rural areas there is also a shortage of manpower in our inner cities and highly populated areas. In Rochester, N. Y., the county medical society receives thirty to fifty calls every day from people looking for a physician.[4] There are those who contend these "shortages" are due to a maldistribution of medical manpower and are not really shortages at all. The 1970 ratio of one physician to 632 patients in the U.S.[10] when compared to other countries having an organized and effective system of health care (*e.g.*, Sweden, 1:860; U.K., 1:900),[11] is quite low and certainly conducive to better medical care than our non-system is producing. The maldistribution of physicians is further exemplified from 1967 statistics in which New York State had 200 doctors per 100,000 population while Mississippi had only 69.[12] (While exact figures are not important to this discussion, one must be careful about citing manpower information. It has been pointed out that for one year "the number of physicians per 100,000 civil population could be taken as 97, 118, 133, 140, or 148, depending on one's purpose."[13]) The shortage of doctors in certain areas of the country has had its greatest effect on 30 to 40 million indigent who "receive inadequate or no medical care until they are moribund."[13] (Figure 11).

Some examiners of the nation's health care crisis maintain the physician shortage, if in fact there is one, is a result of the "population control" exerted by organized medicine. This has been done by placing strict limitations on the number

Figure 4

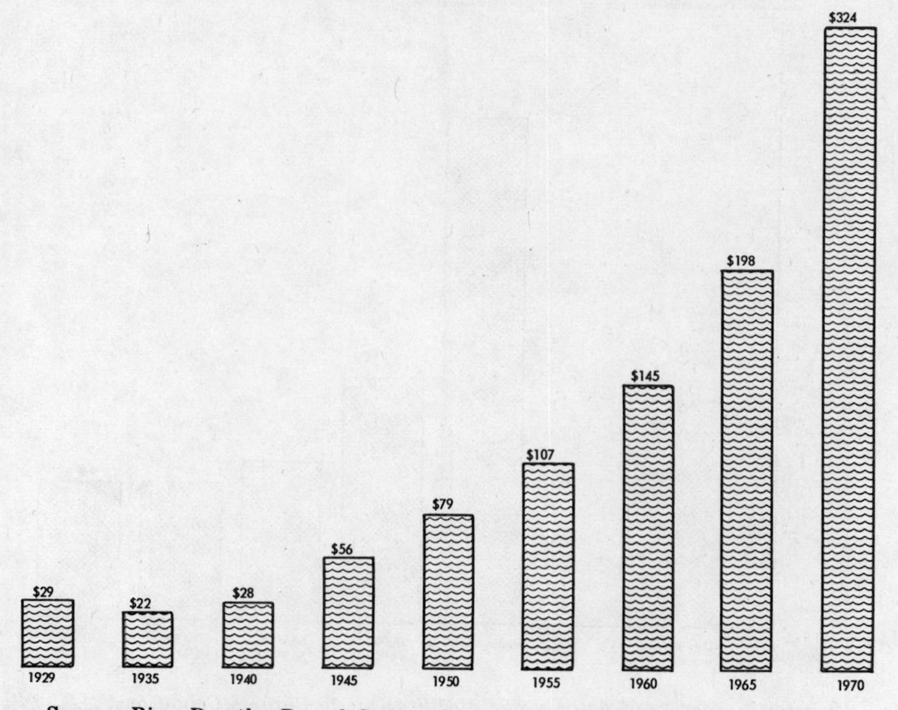

Source: Rice, Dorothy P. and Cooper, Barbara S. "National Health Expenditures, 1929–70," *Social Security Bulletin*, January 1971, U.S. Department of Health, Education, and Welfare.

of students entering and thus graduating from medical school. In 1970, about 60 percent (15,000) of the *qualified* applicants were not accepted to the nation's medical schools.[4] In the period from 1955-1965 the nation's output of physicians increased only slightly more than the population growth (22 percent and 17 percent, respectively). But the number of physicians who entered practice (direct patient care) increased by only 12 percent, and thus did not keep up with population growth at a time when the demand for medical services was rising significantly due to the introduction of Medicare.[5] Furthermore, organized medicine's lack of control over the number of doctors entering any certain specialty has resulted, for example, in surgeons being produced out of proportion to their need [14] (Figure 12).

Other forces also have had a definite effect on the manpower crisis. Federal research spending has greatly advanced scientific knowledge. The knowledge explosion has led to increased specialization among physicians which, in turn, has stimulated the growth of new information.[15] The combination of these and other factors has led many observers to conclude that there is currently a shortage of 50,000 physicians in the United States. If this figure is accepted, then the dilemma facing the nation is how to provide enough physicians to meet current and future needs when only 8,367 were graduated in 1970. A report of the Surgeon General's Consultant Group on Medical Education concluded "that it would be necessary to double the output of physicians by 1975 in order to maintain the 1959 ratio of physicians to population."[15] To even double this number within the next ten years seems unrealistic when one considers the number of graduates has not doubled in over 40 years.[16] "The achievement of this goal would require the establishment of 20 to 24 new medical schools, and this would necessitate massive federal financial support."[15] Other problems such as additional teaching manpower and laboratory space, make a 10 percent immediate increase in enrollment more likely. However, this "would add only 7,800 extra physicians to the national pool by 1990."[14] It has been concluded, therefore,

Figure 5

PERSONS WITH HIGHER INCOMES ARE HEALTHIER THAN THE POOR

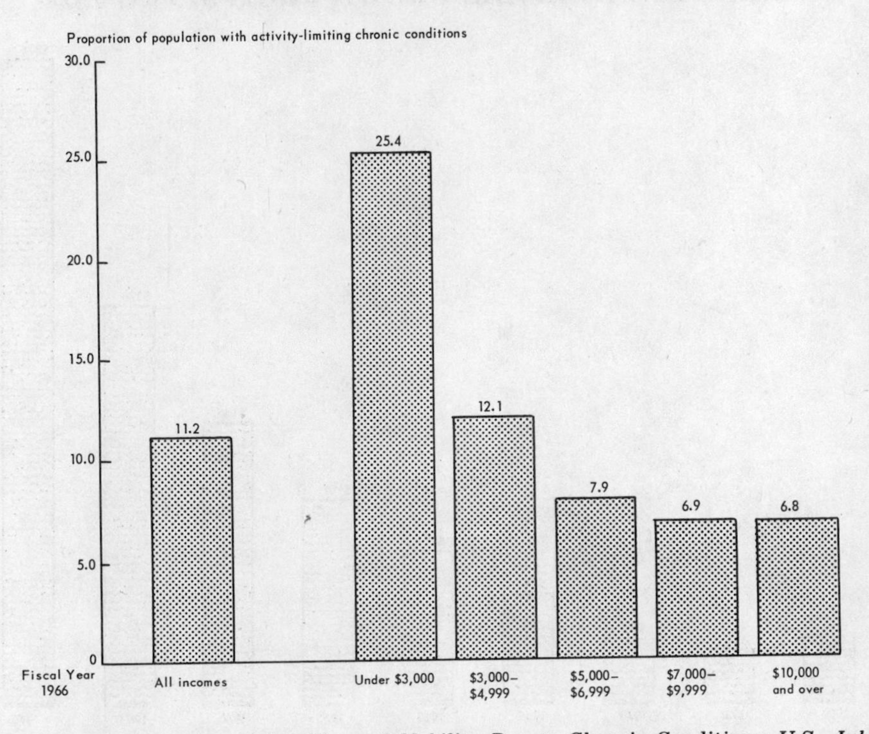

Source: ***Limitation of Activity and Mobility Due to Chronic Conditions, U.S., July 1965–June 1966.*** **Vital and Health Statistics, Series 10, No. 45. National Center for Health Statistics, U.S. Department of Health, Education, and Welfare.**

that it is not possible to sufficiently increase the number of physicians to meet the required needs within the next 20 to 30 years either by increasing the number of schools or by expanding enrollments.[13] In fact "the Association of American Medical Colleges released a report stating that it was 'essential that physician productivity be increased through delegation of specific tasks to others,' because not enough physicians *ever* (author's italics) would be produced to meet national requirements"[15] (Figure 13).

Lack of Responsive Leadership

Physician Failures. Is the failure of our method of providing health care directly attributable to the leader of the health team—the physician? Certainly as the captain, the physician must shoulder a large amount of the responsibility. His problem may be due to the fact that despite radical technological and societal change, the public's concept remains rooted in the nineteenth century model.

What precisely *is* a physician today, and what must he become? . . . . The very *concept* of a physician in our society — what and who he is, and how he functions — is obsolete. . . . The obsolescence of the American physician today is manifold, a product of his archaic education, his inappropriate orientation to disease and to people, the economic (fee-for-service) and societal (one-to-one) framework of the "physician-patient relationship," the traditional notion of a patient-centered rather than a community-centered responsibility. But the most dangerous aspect of the obsolescence is its established pattern of *physician primacy* in medical care. For centuries the doctor has been considered, and has considered himself, the absolute central figure in patient care, all-knowing and all-powerful. Despite the fact that advances in medical technology have significantly complicated the physician-patient relationship, doctors have retained their monopoly of control over patient care to the exclusion of nurses, technicians, administrators and paramedical personnel, without which the practitioner of modern medicine cannot function. . . . Our medical care mechanism is run by and for the physician rather than by and for the patient, and the practitioner is in no way *accountable* to the people that he "serves" . . . . . . The accountability of the physician must extend beyond the *micro*scopic concern for the particular patient to the *macro*scopic concern for the entire community of patients and (even more important) potential patients.[17]

Figure 6

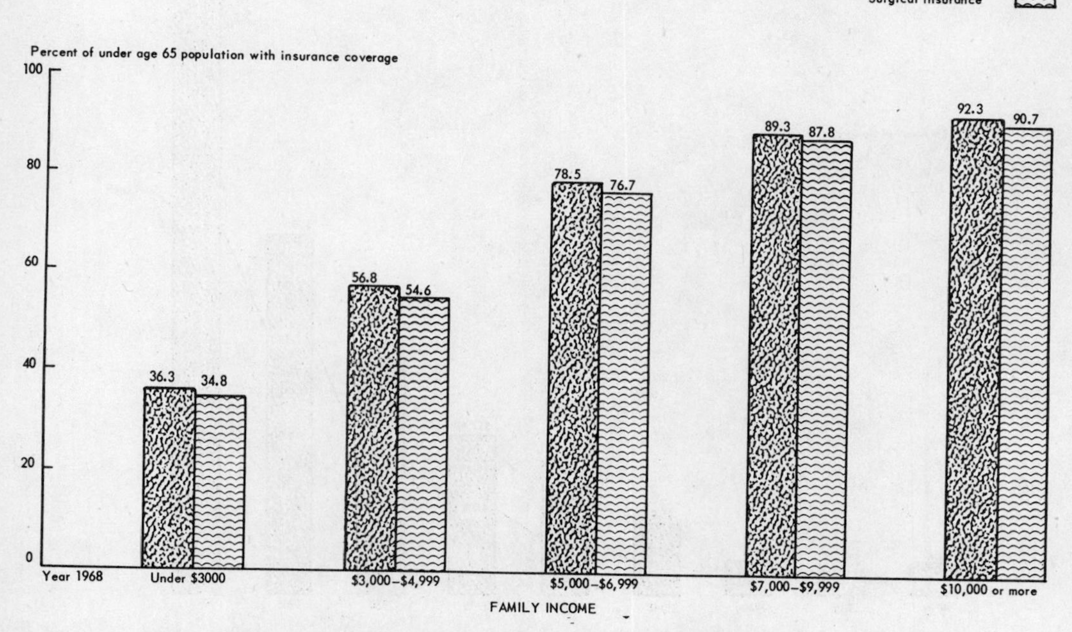

Source: *Monthly Vital Statistics Report*, February 2, 1970. National Center for Health Statistics, U.S. Department of Health, Education, and Welfare.

Physicians as a whole have not done well in considering the economic in addition to the medical consequences of their decisions. "Good decision making in health, as in any field, requires the weighing of additional (economists call them marginal) benefits against the additional (marginal) costs . . . The American people are clearly not intent on improving health to the exclusion of all other goals."[18]

Hospital Mismanagement. The medical care rendered patients by physicians cannot be considered separately from the management of medical institutions for one cannot exist without the other. The leadership in the management and operation of our nation's hospitals has suffered considerably over the years and has resulted in an adverse contribution to the costs and delivery of health care. While hospitals are organized to be run by professionally educated and trained administrators, the leadership is the *de facto* responsibility of physicians as well. However, physicians by and large do not have the authority granted through the management process commensurate with their responsibility and therein lies the problem. If the hospital suffers economic loss, for example, there is no direct effect on the physician. Consequently physicians have been accused of being "indifferent to economic considerations, opposing moves to save money— including even such arrangements as using operating rooms on Sundays."[19] At the same time the hospital trustees, the people with final administrative authority, have been taken to task as people who "are often chosen purely for their prestige and money-raising capabilities," and who "seem to permit inefficiencies that they would never tolerate in their own businesses."[19] While hospital administrators have been trained to operate the hospital, supervise the personnel and maintain proper relations with the community, it has been said they have not been "trained to formulate organizational strategy, assess risks, develop multimillion dollar financial projects and methodically transform plans into desired results."[20]

The victim of these truths about physicians, trustees and hospital administrators has been, of course, the patient—the consumer. The abuse has been felt in the consumer's pocketbook

Figure 7

HEALTH SPENDING TODAY—$67.2 BILLION—IS FIVE TIMES THE SPENDING OF 20 YEARS AGO

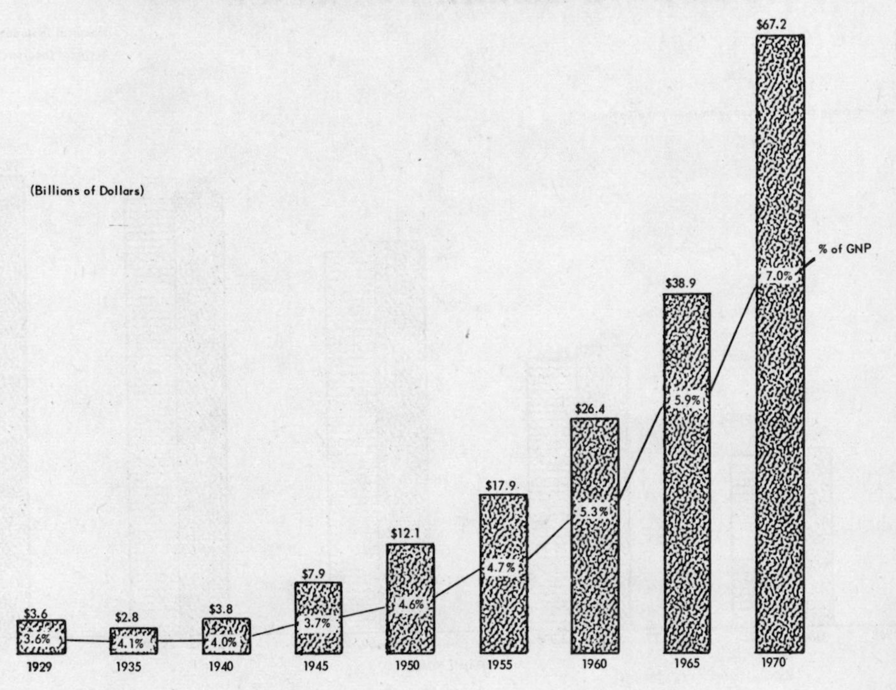

Source: Rice, Dorothy P. and Cooper, Barbara S. "National Health Expenditures, 1929–70" *Social Security Bulletin*, January 1971, U.S. Department of Health, Education, and Welfare.

through increased prices for services, higher room charges, and increased insurance premiums to name a few examples. The consumer ultimately even pays for the expensive and needless duplication of hospital facilities, personnel and equipment that exists around the country today. It has been stated that "in some cases the number of personnel providing inpatient care exceeds the legitimate need of communities for such services."[21] Furthermore, inefficiencies and uneconomic use of resources such as "excess of certain types of medical services leads to wasteful utilization—for example, unnecessary hospitalizations."[21] It has been said, "if we immediately discharge all hospitalized patients whose condition would not deteriorate because they did not sleep in the hospital tonight, the number of empty beds would be startling in most communities!"[21]

Neglect of the Poor

While all of the public has endured to some extent the failure to organize and deliver health care efficiently, it has been the lower income groups that have suffered the most. The poor and near poor, particularly those of various ethnic groups, have been deprived not only of medical care but of almost every benefit of society. This, of course, compounds the problem of medical care and clearly indicates the need to include it in the broadest context of health care. The ramifications of lack of new housing, decaying present housing, crowding, poor quality public services, over-population, inadequate education, pollution, under-employment, drug abuse and so on, and the interrelationships of these problems with each other as well as their impingement on health care must be understood by all health professionals. Many of the poor have a basic inability to cope with modern living. The poor are in a sense captives of their own culture and are being encircled by a culture of deprivation. The extent of the problem for the lower income groups can be summed up in a single statistic—the number of patients not having access to a primary care physician; in the urban ghettos it has been estimated at 25 million, while in the rural areas the figure

Figure 8

IN THE 1960's MEDICAL PRICES JUMPED ALMOST TWICE AS FAST AS PRICES FOR ALL CONSUMER ITEMS

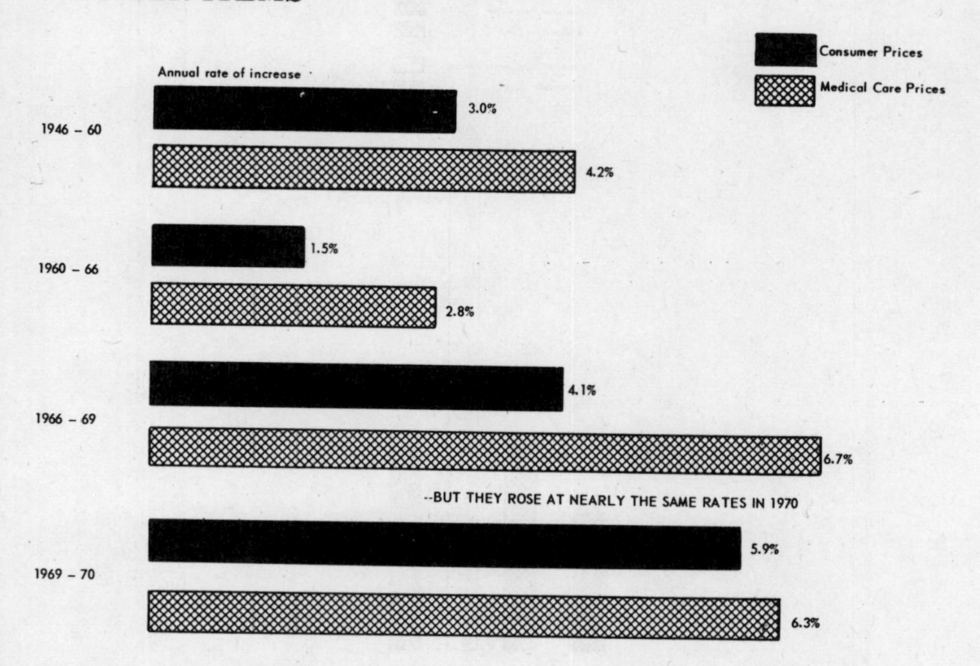

Source: ***Consumer Price Index*, Bureau of Labor Statistics, U.S. Department of Labor.**

approaches 40 million people.[22]

In any examination of the poor and their health problems, it is well to have a clear understanding of the facts which identify the 15-18 percent of the people below the poverty line. A clear majority of our poor work, most of them full time. Two-thirds are white. Only 25 percent of those eligible for welfare receive any aid and of the 8 million on the relief rolls, all but 50,000 (0.6 percent) are unable to work. One half are children, the rest are over 65 years old, are seriously ill or blind, or are the mothers of young children.[23]

What are some of the more specific problems facing the poor—problems that typify the neglect of our present scheme of health care? One readily recognizable problem is that these individuals are isolated from society and are unable to transport themselves to hospitals and clinics. Medical services are not readily accessible to them. Also, they do not know how to get medical care. They cannot cope with large hospitals, outpatient clinics, and emergency rooms. It seems if one is poor, one must be subjected to long lines and waiting periods, unattractive and uncomfortable waiting rooms, and be otherwise demeaned and denigrated. The poor, especially those belonging to a different ethnic group, are too infrequently treated as human beings with equal rights in our theoretically egalitarian society. Their medical care has been described as episodic, fragmented and anonymous. The barrier against effective care is frequently due to a breakdown in communications between the health professional and the patient. Consider the following example of Mrs. P., a woman of very limited intelligence, who lives alone in the core city with her five-year-old daughter.

Telephone conversation:

Mrs. P.: Sally has a terrible cough, dearie.

M.D.: How long has she been sick?

Mrs. P.: She's not six, she's only five.

M.D.: (With some exasperation) I think you had better bring her into the office to see me this afternoon.

Figure 9

MEDICAL CARE PRICES HAVE JUMPED 29 PERCENT IN 4 YEARS

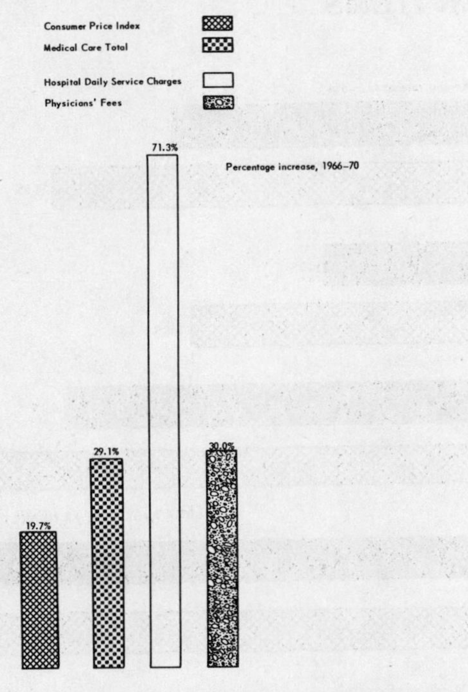

Source: *Consumer Price Index*, Bureau of Labor Statistics, U.S. Department of Labor.

Later in the office:

M.D.: (Automatically) How long has Sally been sick, Mrs. P.?

Mrs. P.: Oh, she's not six, doctor, she's only five.[24]

This inability to communicate has led to numerous misunderstandings by both parties, not the least of which is an attitude often acquired by the undereducated poor that physicians don't help much and "they'll mess you up, a lot of the time they will."[25] This, of course, explains in part the reluctance of many poor people to seek medical assistance.

The poor living in rural areas are generally more isolated than those in the core city. In addition, the rural areas have population densities that range from low to sparse, which usually results in a limited tax base, and scarce and widely dispersed health facilities.[26] Physicians tend to shy away from rural practice for a multitude of reasons. With more physicians in specialty practice, their expertise is in greater demand in larger cities. The lack of fellow physicians in the same town creates undesirable factors such as long hours and professional isolation. Often the most interesting cases must be referred to a larger city thus making it difficult for the rural physician to treat much more than colds, sore throats and arthritis. Furthermore, it is difficult to keep up with new medical techniques. All of these factors and others serve to deter physicians from living in rural areas despite seemingly attractive offers (Figure 14).

While this nation philosophically has adopted a national policy to give the poor equal rights to health care, the period of time until all of the poor benefit from this policy is many years away. The problem is best characterized by the situation which exists in municipal hospitals and care of the inner city poor. There has been a prevalent misconception that Medicare and Medicaid would eliminate public hospitals. This, in fact, has not happened nor is it happening; however, within a decade or so their character most certainly will change particularly with the passage of a national health insurance scheme. Until then (and perhaps thereafter, depending on the design of the health plan) the public hospital

Figure 10

THE NUMBER OF PHYSICIANS PER 100,000 PERSONS VARIES FROM 63 IN ALASKA TO 160 IN CALIFORNIA

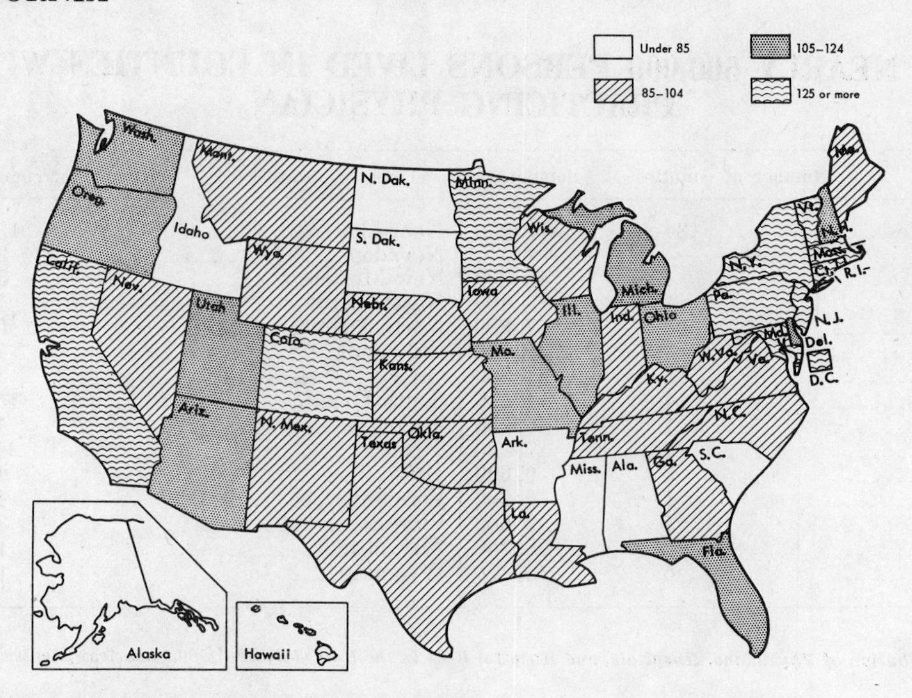

Source: *Reference Data on Socioeconomic Issues of Health*, **1971 Revised Edition, American Medical Association.**

will continue to serve as the "hospital that rounds out the eccentricities of the voluntary hospitals and that has ultimate responsibility to ensure that all the hospital needs of all members of the city's populations are met."[27] Largely this means the city must subsidize those services not provided by voluntary hospitals. Under current health plans, the patient with mental illness who can afford a "hotel suite" in a private hospital can get the best treatment and care. On the other hand, the poor patient has to use the public hospital. Furthermore, "as social policy transfers the care of alcoholics and drug addicts from the police to health institutions the public hospital for many reasons necessarily will be the first to assume the responsibility for their rehabilitation."[28] The public hospital today, and particularly the municipal hospital serving the core city, is struggling for continued existence. As always, it must compete with other city services for the tax dollar; unfortunately tax-support in many cities now is rapidly eroding. Many city hospitals have received even less financial support with the advent of Medicare and Medicaid while in the eyes of the general public this was to solve the hospitals' financial distress. The local politician knows the patient has a *right* to hospital care, therefore there is no political gain. Since "there is no longer a political payoff to the politician from the public hospital. . . . he is not anxious to support it."[27] Certainly the lack of a sound financial base has been the single factor most responsible for the deterioration of public hospitals. Like a disease, financial distress has spread its blight in the poor quality and lack of adequate equipment, personnel, facilities and services in many municipal hospitals to the extent that the Joint Commission on Accreditation of Hospitals has had to withhold accreditation from some. Most managers of public hospitals agree that ownership and control of these institutions must be removed from the hands of local governments in order to eliminate the excessive red tape that inhibits sound and progressive management. Such action might permit many public hospitals to regain their former eminence as medical centers.[29]

Figure 11

IN 1969, NEARLY 500,000 PERSONS LIVED IN COUNTIES WITH NO PRACTICING PHYSICIAN

State	Number of counties	Population	State	Number of counties	Population
United States	134	477, 800	Nebraska	13	15, 800
			Nevada	3	3, 300
Alaska	1	18, 800	New Mexico	3	24, 900
California	1	400	North Carolina	1	8, 600
Colorado	5	7, 800	North Dakota	5	12, 400
Florida	4	15, 000	Oklahoma	1	6, 100
Georgia	12	53, 200	Oregon	3	7, 500
Idaho	4	11, 500	South Dakota	15	46, 700
Indiana	1	6, 200	Tennessee	1	5, 000
Kansas	2	7, 200	Texas	24	60, 500
Michigan	2	6, 600	Utah	4	5, 100
Minnesota	1	6, 200	Vermont	1	2, 900
Mississippi	1	2, 600	Virginia	3	33, 700
Missouri	15	96, 300	Wisconsin	1	2, 700
Montana	6	10, 400	Wyoming	1	400

Source: *Distribution of Physicians, Hospitals, and Hospital Beds in the United States, 1969.* American Medical Association.

A System of Delivering Comprehensive Health Care

The numerous failures of the government and the private sector to provide the "patchwork" necessary to adequately solve the multitude of problems in organizing and delivering satisfactory health care has created the climate for a major reform in this area. Health care legislation and programs have been characterized as predominantly categorical in scope and intended for a selected few (*e.g.*, Medicare was designed for limited categories of service and only covered the aged). In the future the ideal model for health care must be comprehensive and available to all, *i.e.*, the general public. In striving for the ideal there will be a mix such that categorical programs are provided for the general public at the same time comprehensive health services are available to a selected few (Figure 15).[30]

A comprehensive method for the delivery of health care must include the following three elements: (1) primary health care, (2) health maintenance organizations, and (3) professional and public controls. Because there may be some question as to what is meant by *comprehensive* health care, it is defined here as the form of health care to the public which provides preventive care, hospital, medical and surgical care, nursing home care, ambulatory care, home health care, social services and any other care or service that is related to the total health of the individual.

Primary Health Care and Neighborhood Health Centers

The primary level of medical care traditionally has been recognized as being provided by the outpatient clinics (including the emergency room) of hospitals or by the physician in his private office. The private practitioner has generally administered care himself or referred the patient to another physician or admitted him to a hospital. While this is still quite true today, there are modifications occurring in the system that have a bearing on what primary health care will be like in the future.

Figure 12

THE UNITED STATES HAS TWICE THE NUMBER OF SURGEONS AND TWICE THE NUMBER OF OPERATIONS PER PERSON COMPARED WITH ENGLAND

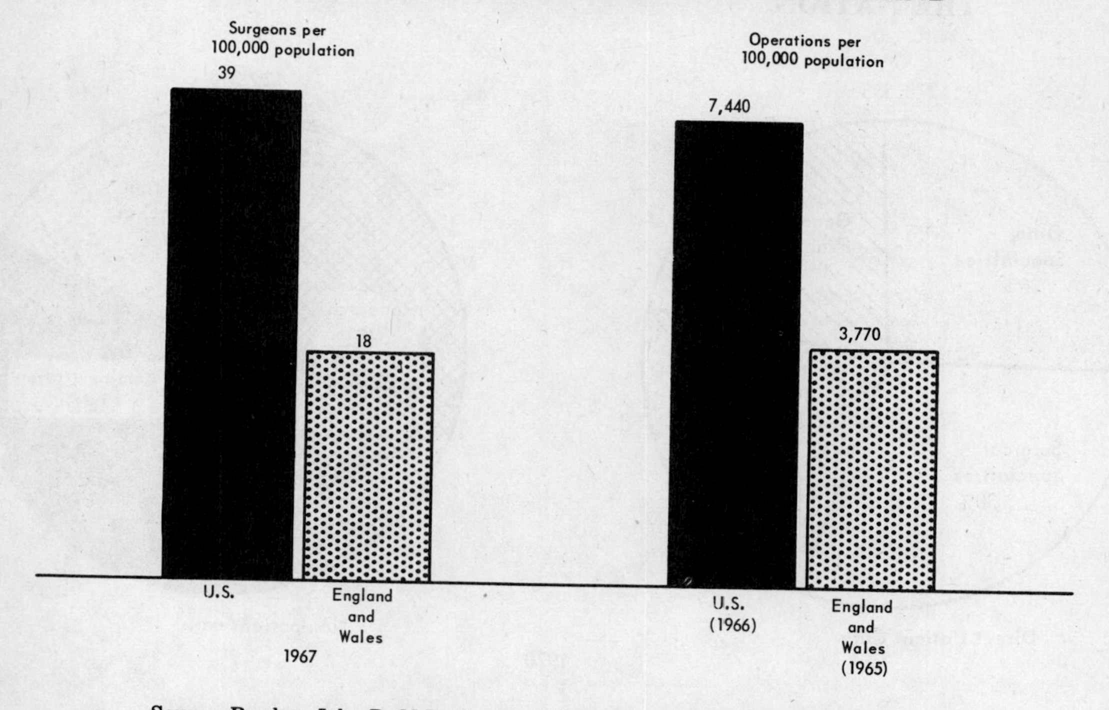

Source: Bunker, John P., M.D. "Surgical Manpower – A Comparison of Operations and Surgeons in the United States and England and Wales." *New England Journal of Medicine*, January 15, 1970.

In recent times it has been the tendency for physicians to cluster in and around hospitals—especially medical centers—where the latest in equipment and medical knowledge is available. This concurrently has caused a drain on the primary care offered the immobile poor in the rural areas and the inner cities. However, the role of the hospital of providing medical care strictly within its physical confines is changing. The tentacles of health resources available to the hospital are reaching out into the community to provide the individual in his environment with the services of an organized health care team. The mechanism by which this is being done varies with hospitals. Some hospitals are establishing satellite or branch hospitals in order to expand their services to a greater segment of the community.[31] Many hospitals are merging or affiliating with extended care facilities. (Although not considered primary care, the hospital's alignment with extended care facilities demonstrates how the services of the hospital are reaching out to respond to the needs of the individual.) Another way of extending the hospital's resources is to redefine the hospital's patient population and its means of obtaining patients. Instead of the traditional method of accepting those patients who are either referred by a physician or who simply choose of their own will to come in the door, the hospital may "seek out those who do not come for care, which is best called patient pursuit."[32] Learning to define patient populations and learning methods of patient pursuit are clinical skills which have been cited as some of the goals of education for primary health care.[32]

Origin of Neighborhood Clinics

The best example of hospitals extending their services into the community may be through the establishment of neighborhood health centers. While most hospitals do not have administrative authority over neighborhood clinics, it is quite common for members of the hospital's medical staff to be the primary physicians in these centers and, in fact, quite often they are the organizers behind the development of neighborhood health

Figure 13

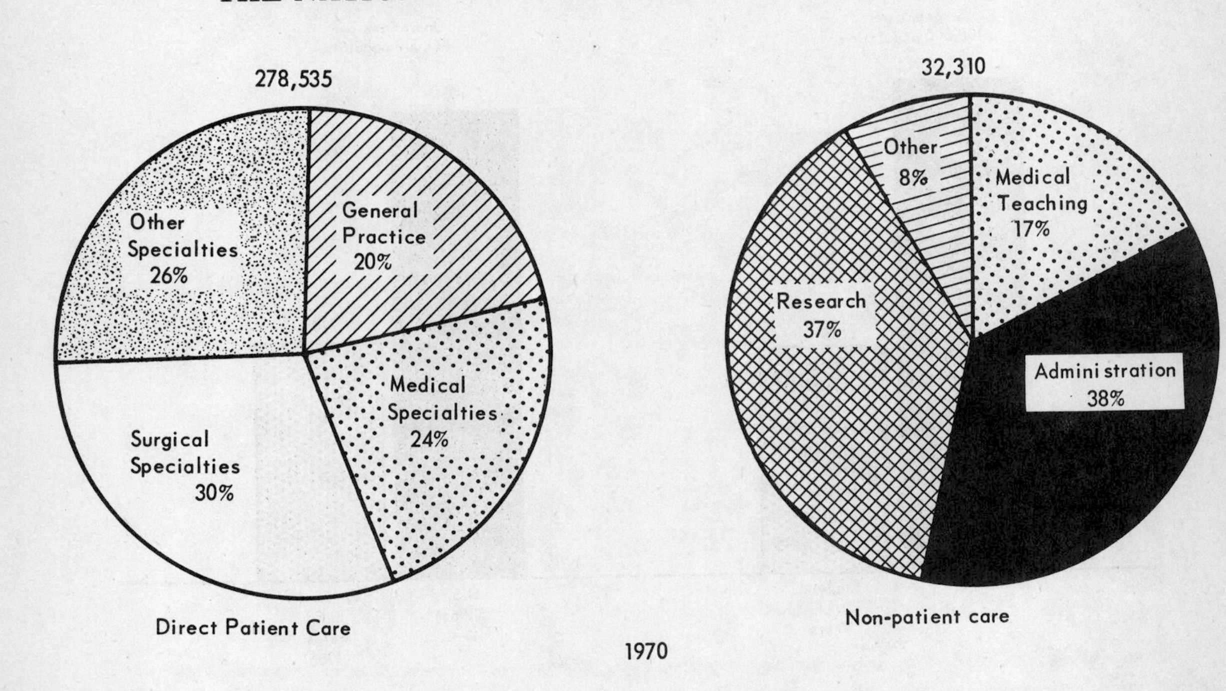

Source: *Reference Data on Socioeconomic Issues of Health*, 1971 Revised Edition, American Medical Association.

centers. Sponsors also include medical societies, citizen groups, medical schools and health departments.

The health center movement actually began in the early part of the twentieth century. The early health centers of 1910-15 were organized by voluntary agencies or municipal health departments with the intent of bringing health services closer to the residential life of the urban poor. Then, just as now, there was a great indifference of many slum dwellers to municipal health services located in city hall and in city hospital outpatient departments. It was believed that the staff of the neighborhood center could also serve to make home care visits to those people in the vicinity who either could not or would not go to the center. The early functions of these health centers were to treat infectious disease and infant malnutrition and to provide immunization and infant feeding. For the most part, the centers were considered as complementing the curative work of private physicians and thus were primarily involved with preventive medicine. Some centers went beyond prevention and treatment to include such activities as recreation and day care of children. These programs took the broader view of health care as a way of living—not simply freedom from disease. The early centers also acted for the triage of patients to hospitals.[33] It is perhaps unfortunate that the health centers did not evolve in the manner in which they were conceived by one early organizer. The founder of a health center in Pittsburgh proposed that health care ought to be like public schooling and similarly financed, organized and controlled.[33-34]

Many of the current ideas being implemented in neighborhood clinics had their antecedence in the centers established early in this century. One program enlisted neighborhood residents as assistants to recruit patients, to take household surveys and to participate in the governance of the center.[33,35] In Cincinnati in 1915 a plan was conceived to have neighborhood residents chosen on the basis of the block in which they lived to serve on the governing board of the health center. This idea failed because it aroused public suspicions and lacked political support.[33,36] Al-

Figure 14

THE WALL STREET JOURNAL, Tuesday, July 20, 1971

DOCTOR

LIVE— BRING UP YOUR FAMILY
IN A QUIET, PEACEFUL, FRIENDLY MIDWEST TOWN

Yet keep your income at the level of a big city doctor.
We want two to three general practitioners.
COME LIVE WITH US IN SAFETY AND HAPINESS . . .
SHENANDOAH, IOWA (Population 7,000. Trade area 20,000.)
Fully accredited 58 bed hospital adjoined by new, modern, 48 bed extended care unit. Best of facilities. Two fine resident surgeons. Plenty of stores, new schools, many churches, large municipal swimming pool, fine golf course, active flying club. Contact:

CY RAPP, Chairman Doctor Procurement Committee
HAND COMMUNITY HOSPITAL
Shenandoah

though many of the innovations died along with the neighborhood health center movement in the late 1930's, today they are back with more ideas and a stronger force.

A Modern Neighborhood Clinic

One new objective of today's neighborhood health center is to rehabilitate the poor. In the past, services were taken by the clinics to the indigent which permitted them to become healthy but still remain poor. Now health centers offer jobs, training, and the opportunity for the indigent to direct their own destiny.[33] Another new objective cited for neighborhood clinics is to reduce the use of hospital emergency rooms. Emergency care is episodic and expensive whereas the neighborhood centers offer comprehensive and continuous care.[37]

The forerunner of the new centers was established in 1965 by the Tufts University School of Medicine and funded by the U.S. Office of Economic Opportunity. The Tufts-Columbia Point Health Center is defined as a comprehensive facility providing or definitively arranging continuous family-centered preventive and curative services under one roof through one door for those of a defined community who wish to use it.[38-39] The services of the Tufts-Columbia Point Health Center are provided through three family health care groups (FHCG) *each* consisting of an internist, a pediatrician, and several community health nurses, social workers, and indigenous community residents. The community residents are trained as home health aides, social work assistants, and medical assistants. Each FHCG has available to it the part-time services of specialty practices (*e.g.*, obstetrics-gynecology) and the supporting services in the Health Center of pharmacy, x-ray, clinical lab and so

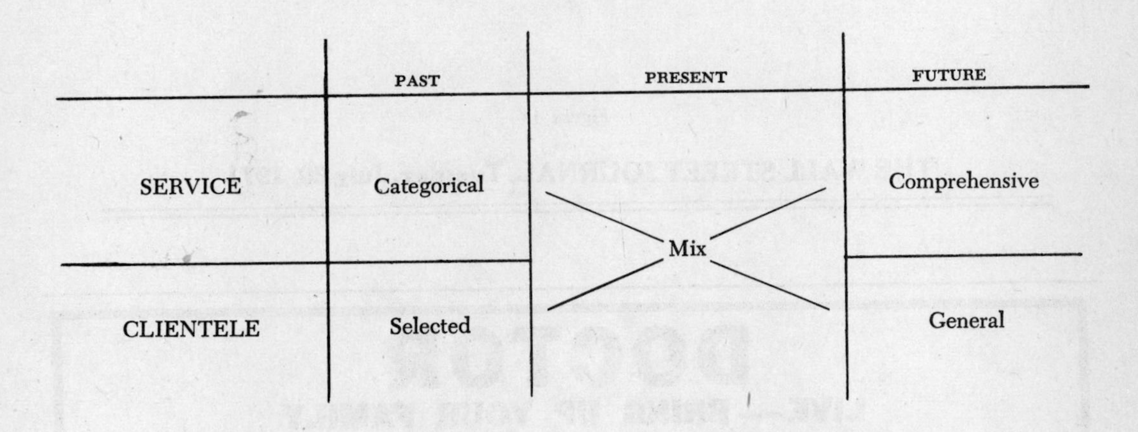

Figure 15. Health Care Legislation and Programs

on. Columbia Point is a low-income public housing development with about 5,500 residents.[39-40] This community is geographically isolated from alternative sources of health care with the closest hospital (Boston City Hospital) located an hour's trip from the housing project. The Health Center facilitates the ability of the Columbia Point residents to obtain not only medical care but immediate medical attention even for signs and symptoms, such as a sore throat or persistent cough which may seem inconsequential. Not only is the distance barrier removed for the poor, but so is the financial one as there is no fee charged since most of the residents have incomes below the poverty guidelines or are eligible for Medicare or Medicaid. One of the seemingly attractive features of the Tufts program is the continuity of care offered by the FHCG. "Although continuous and personal care of patients by *one* physician seems to be desirable," . . . the FHCG "provides a whole set of health professionals and aides, working together, with whom a continuous and personal relationship is maintained. If a change in one professional or one physician does occur, the patient still has five or six other familiar sources of care to continue with in the other members of the group."[40] By having three FHCG, the Tufts-Columbia Point Health Center permits patients to select the group of physicians they want, and also to change groups if they become dissatisfied with a physician; however, the entire family must change groups.[39] A multitude of neighborhood health centers have been established since the founding of the Tufts-Columbia Point Health Center. Some of these such as the ones in Philadelphia,[30,41] Rochester, N. Y.,[37] St. Louis,[42] Chicago,[43] Newark,[43] Martindale, Indiana,[44] Kansas City[45] and New York City[46] are cited as examples for further study.

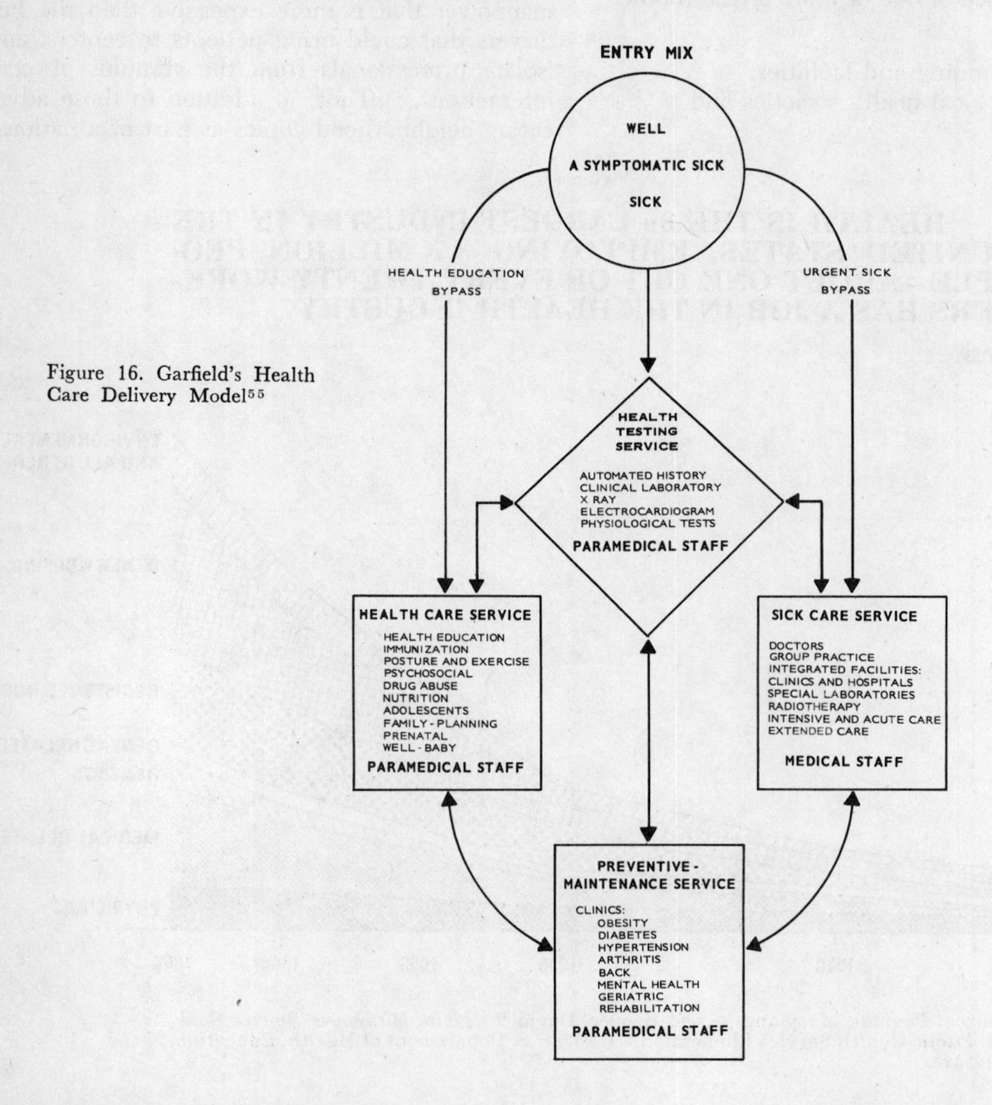

Figure 16. Garfield's Health Care Delivery Model[55]

Problems with Neighborhood Clinics

For all their virtues neighborhood clinics are not without problems. In many cases, the hospital or hospitals supporting the health centers by providing a staff and accepting referrals is not as magnanimous as appearances indicate. The support hospital will admit patients, if beds are empty, but it "assumes little if any responsibility for the clinic's operation or for cost and quality controls."[47] Another problem is that the neighborhood centers may develop into a clinic for the poor fraught with all the problems of hospital outpatient clinics: crowding, long waiting periods and numerous other physical discomforts and indignities. So long as these centers foster segregation of the very poor, they are regressive by nature and eventually may be the cause of their own demise. The lack of success of neighborhood health centers has been summed up as due to the absence of one or more of the following ingredients:

1. adequate funding and facilities;
2. support by local health societies and agencies;
3. inclusion of members of the neighborhood community in the organizational structure on a policy making level;
4. job training and employment opportunities for members of the community;
5. a qualified and concerned staff; and
6. adequate back-up hospital facilities.[48]

Whether neighborhood health centers should be included in the overall scheme of comprehensive health care is still an unresolved issue. "Neighborhood centers do have current political and emotional appeal, but they are based on the fallacy of a stable community in a nation with a notoriously mobile population."[49] This appeal is based, in part, on the theory that complex problems will not be treated in the clinic but referred to an affiliated hospital.[50] "Such centers perpetuate the myth that community medicine is separate from the rest of health care, further fragment an already sundered system, disperse manpower that is more expensive than the bus drivers that could bring patients to centers, and isolate professionals from the stimulus of peer interactions."[49] Thus, in addition to those advocating neighborhood clinics as part of a national

Figure 17.

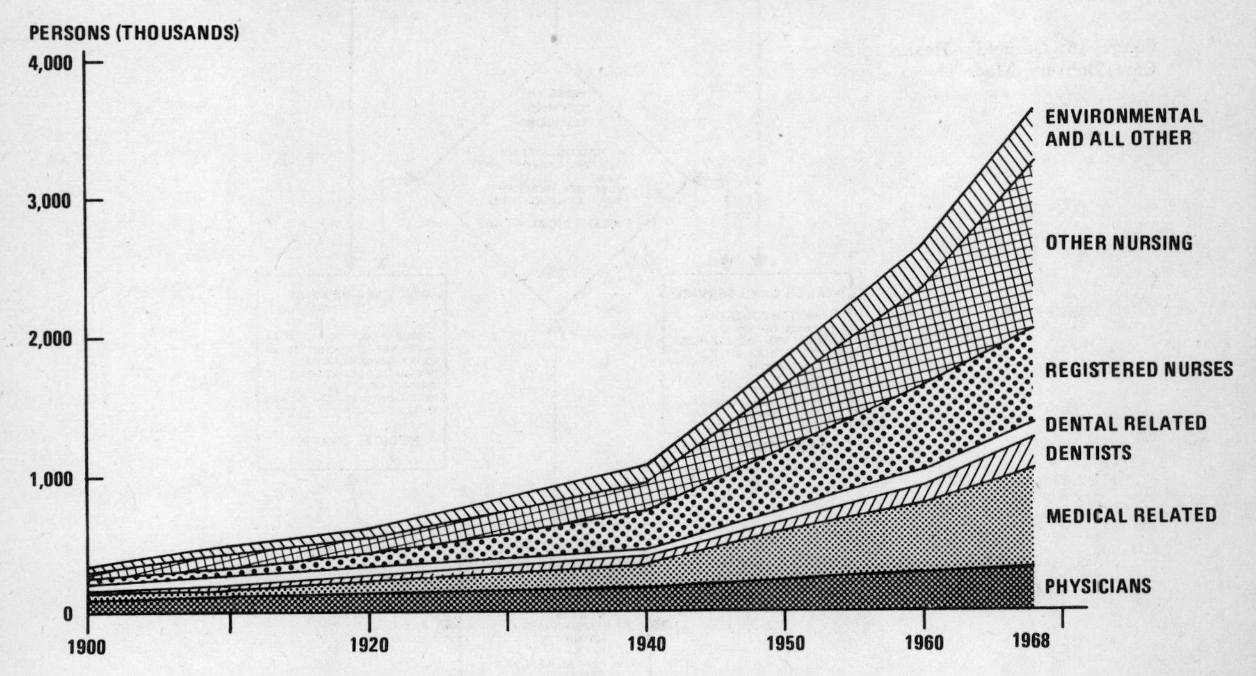

Source: Pennell, Maryland Y. and Hoover, David B. *Health Manpower Source Book*, Sec. 21, Public Health Service Publication No. 263. U.S. Department of Health, Education, and Welfare.

comprehensive plan for health care, there are those who believe the hospital can serve both as a crisis center and as a community health center.[50] Various proposals for health maintenance organizations, with and without neighborhood clinics serving as the focus of primary health care, will be considered. However, the present trend is to fund them and this will continue as long as there are those who believe "primary health care must be optimally rendered in a primary location."[40] It may be simply a question of where is the center of the health care universe: in the hospital or in the community? If this is the case, the answer may be dependent upon who is responding—the professional or the consumer.[41] Or, more likely, there is actually a sociologic difference in organization between the hospital and neighborhood health center which makes it more feasible for the center to relate to the community.[40] The community in order to relate must feel a sense of participation in the organization serving it and must be able to exert some control over the providers of service. "A health center is a possible vehicle for such consumer participation; as even the middle class knows well, a hospital is an unlikely one."[41]

Health Maintenance Organizations

The term health maintenance organization (HMO) has been used legislatively for an organization which:

1. provides a per capita prepayment health plan for insured members;
2. offers members comprehensive health coverage including inpatient hospital, ambulatory, emergency, and other services plus preventive care such as periodic health check-ups and immunizations;
3. provides continuity of medical care; and
4. provides services of physicians who may be employees or partners of the HMO or organized on a group practice basis under contract with the HMO.[51]

As with many new terms there is a degree of vagueness as to what precisely constitutes an HMO. For example, some state an HMO should have a "defined population" of members,[51] while others maintain that "the HMO doesn't have a defined population base."[52] For purposes of this chapter, an HMO will be used in its broadest context to include the criteria stated above so that essentially it is an organized group of physicians and allied health care workers providing comprehensive prepaid medical and preventive care for those choosing to enroll as members in the health maintenance plan. Although the delivery and financing of health care must be interlocked in HMO's, health insurance is not to be considered because of its current state of flux. Only the means of providing health care through various proposed systems involving HMO's and primary health care (*e.g.*, neighborhood health centers) is considered here.

The Kaiser Program—An HMO Model. The oldest, largest and most efficient group practice prepayment plan is the Kaiser Foundation Health Plan and Permanente Medical Group located in California and a few other states. The health plan and the hospitals are organized as nonprofit operations and the medical groups in each location are autonomous partnerships. The Kaiser Foundation Health Plan functions both as a marketing agency and as a prime contractor. It contracts with *members,* as groups or individuals, to arrange for their health care services in return for dues paid on a monthly basis, with subscribers paying the same rates for a given coverage, regardless of use. It also contracts with *physicians* organized as independent Permanente Medical Groups to provide professional services. The medical groups are responsible for their own personnel management. Finally the Kaiser Plan contracts with the Kaiser Foundation *Hospitals,* a nonprofit community service corporation, to provide inpatient and outpatient services. Six separate corporations, collectively called Permanente Service Organizations, perform centralized business and administrative services on a regional basis for the health plan, hospitals and medical groups, and also operate prescription pharmacies at nonhospital locations. The definition given previously for an HMO fits the Kaiser-Permanente medical care program so well that one might think the Kaiser plan was used to construct the definition. The Kaiser Foundation Health Plan offers the subscriber the following services:

1. Comprehensive care for every member of a *defined population* is available through hospital and clinic facilities and home visits.
2. The patient has free choice of physician and continuity of medical care. The patient may be referred by the primary physician he has selected to other specialists in the medical group as required and his medical record is available as a single unit to all physicians responsible for his care.
3. Benefits are adjusted to suit special requirements of the consumer group and are prepaid on a per capita basis.[53]

One of the problems reported with the Kaiser-Permanente type of system results from the elimination of the fee-for-service which in traditional practice acts as a barrier to health care for the poor. Conversion to a prepayment program in effect opens the flood gates to the well, worried-well, asymptomatic sick and sick people without regard to priority of illness being considered in relation to the physician's time. Thus the people who are extremely sick find themselves competing for the physician's time with those who are relatively well or asymptomatic.[54,55] As plausible as this would seem, it is argued that there are no data to support this contention and studies have revealed no significant abuse in the Kaiser system or other prepaid group practice plans.[53,56] A partial explanation may be found in the fact that preventive care is an option for the consumer. Even though, for example, annual health check-ups are about twice as high under the Kaiser plan (15 percent) as compared to the whole nation (8.4 percent) it appears this option is not exercised to the extent it should be by the Kaiser plan members.[53] (The percentages are given as a rough comparison, but cannot be considered precise due to indeterminable constants.) However, Permanente physicians, for the most part, are skeptical about disease prevention in that they doubt the general effectiveness of health examinations to reduce morbidity, mortality and disability. Moreover, it is felt that it would be "both a strategic and logistical mistake to promote annual health check-ups as a benefit . . . as long as serious shortages of primary care manpower persist, and the country is so strikingly lacking in capacity for comprehensive care of the sick."[53] At the present time Kaiser plan members must wait three to six weeks for a routine appointment and in some cases as long as two to three months. In the opinion of the executive director of the northern California Permanente Medical Group, "one of our big problems is developing an appointment system that will screen members so the sick can get in for service and yet the well and 'worried-well' can be appropriately taken care of without swamping our physicians."[57] In spite of this controversy, the elimination of the fee-for-service has the claimed advantage of reducing unnecessary hospital utilization. For instance, surgeons in group practice are not paid by the operation; whereas, in the case of surgeons paid a fee, the fee-for-service may be "a powerful, if subliminal, influence in the decision to operate"[53] and therefore result in unnecessary hospital utilization. The hospital admissions and days of hospitalization per 1000 members under the Kaiser system are reported much lower than state and national rates.[53]

Mechanisms for the Delivery System

Numerous proposals have been put forth incorporating the various elements of health care delivery systems in an attempt to provide a mechanism for a smoothly functioning system.[58] As previously stated, there are some who recommend neighborhood health centers as the entry point for primary care while others propose the hospital. Some of the plans fall short in their description but they still provide concepts worthy of consideration.

The Garfield Plan. Dr. Sidney R. Garfield was the founder and chief administrative officer of the Permanente Medical Group. His experience in the Kaiser-Permanente system has led him to the conclusion that the traditional fee-for-service, which serves as a barrier to health care for many people, must be replaced by a new regulator "more sensitive to real medical need than to the ability to pay and that can help to separate the well from the sick and establish entry priorities for the sick."[54] The central feature of Garfield's plan involves *automated multiphasic screening,* also referred to as health evaluation, health testing, health maintenance service or other combinations of these terms. Health testing techniques were developed by Garfield about twenty years ago for the major purpose of screening those patients demanding a health check-up who were sick from those who were well. The impetus for this was from the heavy burden placed on physicians' time to provide check-ups. It was then found that a sequence of tests and procedures and the use of paramedical personnel helped to relieve the physician to make optimum use of his services. In recent years computer technology has been applied to automate health testing. Data are retained in a computer to facilitate evaluation for determining the health status of a patient. Multiphasic health testing provides a detailed medical history, a preliminary work-up and a comprehensive series of biochemical, physiological, and psychological tests and measurements. Further, it establishes a health profile for continuing health care and saves days of hospitalization for routine and diagnostic studies.

It is Garfield's hypothesis that a *sick-care delivery system* has evolved under the conventional fee-for-service by which patients who are well and sick alike enter the system simultaneously. Such a system involves physicians at the point of entry and in each step of the delivery process, wasting doctor time and impairing services. The use of multiphasic health testing separates the entry mix of patients into the *well,* the *asymtomatic sick* and the *sick.* Garfield proposes the establishment of a new "health-care service" for the well and worried-well, a new "preventive maintenance service" for the asymtomatic sick and chronically ill, and a "sick-care service" for the sick (Figure 16). The two new services, health-care and preventive maintenance, along with the multiphasic health testing depend mostly on paramedical personnel with varying degrees of physician supervision—least in health testing and most in preventive maintenance. This frees physician time to concentrate on sick-care service. The health-care service has as its purpose to keep people well through lectures, health exhibits, audio-visual techniques, counseling and other services. The preventive-maintenance service serves to prevent chronic illnesses from progressing, to be alert to and prevent complications, and generally to improve the patient's condition.[54,55,59] "In the system being proposed a central medical center, well staffed and equipped, would provide sick care. It could have four or five 'outreach' neighborhood clinics, each providing the three primarily paramedical services: health testing, health care and preventive maintenance."[54]

Regional Health Plan. Another proposal which could be used in the application of Garfield's plan involves the regionalization of health-care units. A health-care unit is defined as a group of physicians and allied health workers in integrated practice consisting of a minimum of an internist, a general surgeon, an obstetrician and gynecologist, a pediatrician, and a psychiatrist. There would be sufficient nurses and their assistants, allied health scientists and administrative assistants to aid each physician at a ratio of about twenty to one. The physicians would have offices in a clinic building next to a community hospital. The health-care unit could be adequate for an area of 100 city blocks or 100 rural miles depending on such things as the population density, and would be responsible for the primary health care of all patients living within the defined community. A region would consist of many health-care units and one or more major health centers all commonly linked by a network of transportation and comunication. The major health center would serve the surrounding health-care units and community through: (1) support in the delivery of health care; (2) provision and evaluation of new knowledge from basic and applied research; and (3) education for all health care students and practitioners. A defined region then would have an organized system of transportation and communication linking a network of health-care units to a major health center all strategically located to provide the delivery of medical care to the sick, prevention of illness for the healthy, health education for students, trainees and the public, continuing education for practitioners, and new information through research for the entire system.[3]

Plan for Government Regulated Corporations. There has been at least one proposal that health delivery systems be organized and controlled analogous to commercial airlines. One of the objectives set forth is to establish local, regional and national competing health-services systems. These public utilities would be franchised, subsidized and regulated by the government. Each system would consist of multiple sources of primary care, a community hospital, home care and nursing-home services, laboratory services, a multiphasic screening clinic and a major medical center. The *primary care* unit would have no fewer than two physicians (a general internist and a pediatrician) and two physician assistants or nurse practitioners who could care for about 5,000 persons. The group could provide adequate care for about 20,000 people if expanded to four internists, two pediatricians, an obstetrician, two nurse midwives, six or more physician assistants or nurse practitioners, some laboratory technicians, a social worker and some secretaries. Such a group should be located in or adjacent to a community hospital with a home-care service and a nursing home and supported by a major medical center and a multiphasic screening clinic. "The patient, having enrolled himself and presumably his family in one of several available competing health-services systems, would be assured of a continuously available source of primary care and access to a complete health-services system employing a unit record, automatic data handling, responsible referral and communication systems, and assured access to the advantages of contemporary scientific medicine."[60]

Autonomous Corporations—The Massachusetts Model. An independent, nonprofit corporation affiliated with numerous hospitals and private businesses in Massachusetts has been established and is designed to fulfill the health care needs of a population group of 500,000 people. All modalities of care are under a single management and include: primary care centers, hospitals, nursing homes, extended care facilities, rehabilitation centers, chronic care facilities and home care programs. The advantages of a unified management are cited as proper planning, rational capital outlay, and more efficient use of resources leading to economies in operation. The management of the corporation is broadly based and includes the medical, governmental, business and community sectors. The medical representation is concerned with the methods and program of care, the government representation provides a channel for federal funds, the community representation participates in the development and guidance of the program, and the business representation provides management talents and permits centralization of such things as purchasing, payroll, billing, and medical records. In conjunction with the service corporation, an educational institution is planned to assist the various health care components in training health professionals in the delivery of comprehensive health care. While for the time being it is intended for the corporation to be fully financed by those paying for the service through prepaid insurance, it is believed that the final solution for financing this program is through some form of National Health Insurance.[61-62]

Affiliated Corporations — The Northbridge Model. A solution for the medical care problems of Northbridge, a city of 28,000 people, has been advanced as a model for other communities. Northbridge, like many cities its size, has relatively few primary physicians (1 per 4,700) and as a result many patients receive inadequate or no medical care. Others must travel at considerable expense to the outpatient clinics of the closest teaching hospital in a nearby city. Northbridge has its own community hospital of 75 beds but it is underutilized. A nonprofit corporation is to be established which will have working agreements with the community hospital, the teaching hospital and other facilities such as ambulatory-care clinics, nursing homes, and chronic disease hospitals. The corporation would enroll a large population group on a prepaid comprehensive basis. Fee-for-service would be permitted but not encouraged. Physicians could be either salaried employees of the corporation or could form a group practice and establish a contract with the corporation. Health workers would be trained to serve as physician expanders and would act as the portal of entry to the primary physician for all patients. The health worker would interview the patient to obtain the details of the illness and arrange for the necessary tests and procedures. When indicated the health worker would prescribe palliative measures and make an appointment for the patient to see a physician. The patient would have freedom of choice of health worker and primary physician. Most patients in need of hospitalization would enter Northbridge Community Hospital with the teaching hospital furnishing rotating resident physicians and consultants. While the community has had difficulty in obtaining enough physicians, it is believed that the new corporation would be able to attract physicians who are desirous of participating in group practice and who at the same time wish to be associated with a teaching institution.[63]

Mechanisms for Control

In recent years there has been an increased emphasis on two types of health care controls: those by professionals exerting a degree of self-regulation, and those by consumers seeking more power in the governance of the health team. Physicians practicing in hospitals have had the means to control themselves for many years through such committees as credentials, tissue, and medical records. Since Medicare the utilization review committee has been added to the list. Local medical societies have their insurance review and grievance committees. Even though these controlling bodies are effective, particularly in the area of professional standards of quality, they were not successful in preventing a mounting number of malpractice suits and abuses by some physicians of third party payers. The public and its representatives, whether third party payer or the government, want to be assured economies are effected. Consumers are seeking a more representative voice while physicians are taking action through peer review.

Peer Review. As mentioned, the review of physicians by their peers became law with the Medicare requirement for hospital utilization committees. In 1970 an attempt was made to change the Social Security Amendments to establish a national network of professional standards review organizations (PSRO). The group of physicians constituting the PSRO would decide whether Medicare and Medicaid beneficiaries should be admitted to hospitals and could decide the length of patient stay. The PSRO would evaluate health care in the physician's office as well as in the hospital. It now appears doubtful that the PSRO network will be established for awhile. Experimentation with various mechanisms of peer review will continue and the expanding technological possibilities will improve the controls over health workers. Utilizing computer technology, a gross review of a physician's practice can be achieved by auditing claims for such things as the number of visits per day, per patient and per diagnosis, the number of various tests per visit and so forth.[64]

Consumer Control. Although the words *patient*

and *consumer* are frequently used to identify the same person, a distinction should be recognized since the user (patient) and the buyer (consumer) of health care are increasingly becoming separate parties. The concern of consumers is broad and includes the cost, quality, safety, availability, efficiency, efficacy and responsibility of medical care. The consumer (patient) is interested in becoming involved in the planning of health programs and wants to exercise control over the final decisions.[65] In fact, because of increased knowledge about health care, the patient is rapidly becoming a *de facto* member of the health team. It has been asserted that "unless the professional members of that team become better organized and better oriented—both to each other and to the patient—the latter may end up, by default, as 'captain' of the team, the one who has to make the choices, however uninformed, among various specialties and modalities."[66]

The mechanisms of regulation by consumers have become manifest in many forms. Medicare requires a minimum of one representative of the general public on the Health Insurance Benefits Advisory Committee, the primary advisory committee to those government officials administering the program.

> There are several major current organizational patterns for consumer participation in health services. The most traditional and least disturbing to the medical establishment is the community advisory committee. . . . It is no exaggeration to state that poor and minority groups have almost totally rejected this approach as a sham . . . Another pattern may be called an amorphous or transitional group. The model is when a community group describes itself by some such name as a "Health Council" and tries to arrogate power to itself . . . . A third organizational pattern is the community-selected Board of Directors . . . . A fourth . . . is a board of trustees composed of providers and consumers of care.[67]

With the trend developing toward increased group practices, consumer control and peer review should become easier to implement and consequently more readily accepted.

Summary

The problems of providing health care to all have been highlighted and some new methods of organizing the delivery of health services are presented. Because of the dynamic status of health care, it is difficult to forecast what new system or systems will evolve. It is evident though that the physician's primacy is being diffused to allied health associates as he yields his dominance along with many of the tasks he delegates. This leads to closer relationships in the health team and will foster interprofessional group practices. While consumer control is becoming more evident, it is still imperative that health professionals concern themselves with the moral consequences of the technological and societal changes they introduce. The current methods of health care delivery in the U.S. could be compared to many cadavers interred in a necropolis: they should not be used to create a Frankenstein's monster.

References

1. Watts, M. S. M., ed.: The Scope and Responsibilities of Medicine, *California Med. 109*:509-514 (Dec.) 1968; abstracted, *Med. Care Rev. 27*:808-809 (Aug.) 1970.

2. Cohen, W. S.: Current Problems in Health Care, *New Engl. J. Med. 281*:193-197 (July 24) 1969.

3. Code, C. F.: Determinants of Medical Care—A Plan for the Future, *New Engl. J. Med. 283*:679-685 (Sept. 24) 1970.

4. Ribicoff, A.: The "Healthiest Nation" Myth, *Saturday Rev. 53*:18-20 (Aug. 22) 1970.

5. Anderson, F.: The Growing Pains of Medical Care. I. Paying More, Getting Less, *New Republic 162*:15-18 (Jan. 17) 1970.

6. Monroe, K. E., ed.: *Reference Data on Socioeconomic Issues of Health,* American Medical Association, Chicago, Ill. 1971, p. 68.

7. Darley, W. and Somers, A. R.: Medicine, Money, and Manpower—The Challenge to Professional Education. I. The Affluent New Health-Care Economy, *New Engl. J. Med. 276*:1234-1238 (June 1) 1967.

8. Schechter, M.: Medicare on Its Fourth Birthday—Alive But Not Well, *New Republic 163*:15-17 (July 11) 1970.

9. Lewis, I. J.: Government Investment in Health Care, *Sci. Am. 224*:17-25 (Apr.) 1971.

10. Monroe, K. E., *op. cit.,* p. 24.

11. Werko, L.: Swedish Medical Care in Transition, *New Engl. J. Med. 284*:360-366 (Feb. 18) 1971.

12. Cordtz, D.: Change Begins in the Doctor's Office, *Fortune 81*:84-89, 130-134 (Jan.) 1970.

13. Moore, F. J.: Information Technologies and Health Care, *Arch. Internal Med. 125*:351-355 (Feb.) 1970.

14. Cobb, C. M.: Solving the Doctor Shortage, *Saturday Rev. 53*:24-26, 64 (Aug. 22) 1970.

15. Miller, J. D. and Ferber, B.: Health Manpower in the 1960's, *Hospitals 45*:66-71 (Feb. 16) 1971.

16. Monroe, K. E., *op. cit.,* p. 100.

17. Michaelson, M. G.: The Failure of American Medicine, *Am. Scholar 39*:694-706 (Autumn) 1970.

18. Fuchs, V. R.: The Growing Demand for Medical Care, *New Engl. J. Med. 279*:190-195 (July 25) 1968.

19. Mecklin, J. M.: Hospitals Need Management Even More Than Money, *Fortune 81*:96-99, 150-151 (Jan.) 1970.

20. Wasyluka, R. G.: New Blood for Tired Hospitals, *Harvard Business Rev. 48*:65-74 (Sept.-Oct.) 1970.

21. Garrison, G. E. (editorial): Primary Medical Care—Its Attractiveness to Physicians Should Be Improved, *New Engl. J. Med. 282*:1267-1268 (May 28) 1970.

22. Holloman, J. L. S.: Medical Care and the Black Community, *Arch. Internal Med. 127*:51-56 (Jan.) 1971.

23. Wershow, H. J.: Pathogenesis of Urban Slums, *J. Am. Med. Assoc. 215*:1959-1962 (Mar. 22) 1971.

24. Heagarty, M. C. and Robertson, L. S.: Slave Doctors and Free Doctors—A Participant Observer Study of the Physician-Patient Relation in a Low-Income Comprehensive-Care Program, *New Engl. J. Med. 284*:636-641 (Mar. 25) 1971.

25. Coles, R.: The Doctor and the Newcomers to the Ghetto, *Am. Scholar 40*:66-80 (Winter) 1971.

26. Wilson, V. E.: Rural Health Care Systems, *J. Am. Med. Assoc. 216*:1623-1626 (June 7) 1971.

27. Brown, R. E.: The Public Hospital, *Hospitals 44*:40-43 (July 1) 1970.

28. Breslow, L.: Role of the Public Hospital, *Hospitals 44*:44-46 (July 1) 1970.

29. Elwood, P. M.: Problems of the Public Hospital, *Hospitals 44*:47-52 (July 1) 1970.

30. Gardner, E. A. and Snipe, J. N.: Toward the Co-ordination and Integration of Personal Health Services, *Am. J. Public Health 60*:2068-2078 (Nov.) 1970.

31. Crosby, E. L.: Improving the Delivery of Health Care Services, *Hospitals 41*:53-58 (Sept. 1) 1967.

32. Haggerty, R. J.: The University and Primary Medical Care, *New Engl. J. Med. 281*:416-422 (Aug. 21) 1969.

33. Stoeckle, J. D. and Candib, L. M.: The Neighborhood Health Center—Reform Ideas of Yesterday and Today, *New Engl. J. Med. 280*:1385-1391 (June 19) 1969.

34. White, W. C.: The Official Responsibility of the State in the Tuberculosis Problem, *J. Am. Med. Assoc. 65*:512-514 (Aug. 7) 1915.

35. Phillips, W. C.: *Adventuring for Democracy,* Social Unit Press, New York, 1940, p. 46.

36. Devine, E. T.: Social Unit in Cincinnati—Experiment in Organization, *Survey 42*:115-226 (Nov. 15) 1919.

37. Hochheiser, L. I., Woodward, K. and Charney, E.: Effect of the Neighborhood Health Center on the Use of Pediatric Emergency Departments in Rochester, New York, *New Engl. J. Med. 285*:148-152 (July 15) 1971.

38. Geiger, H. J.: The Neighborhood Health Center, *Arch. Environ. Health 18*:912 (June) 1967.

39. Gibson, C. D., Jr.: The Neighborhood Health Center—The Primary Unit of Health Care, *Am. J. Public Health 58*:1188-1191 (July) 1968.

40. Bellin, S. S. and Geiger, H. J.: Actual Public Acceptance of the Neighborhood Health Center by the Urban Poor, *J. Am. Med. Assoc. 214*:2147-2153 (Dec. 21) 1970.

41. Ingraham, N. R. and Lear, W. J.: A Big City Strives for Relevance in Its Community Health Services, *Am. J. Public Health 60*:804-810 (May) 1970.

42. Freidin, R., Levy, R. and Harmon, R.: A Student-Community Planned Health Project for the Poor, *New Engl. J. Med. 283*:1142-1147 (Nov. 19) 1970.

43. Anon.: Neighborhood Clinics—City People Help Themselves, *Mod. Hosp. 115*:69-75 (Aug.) 1970.

44. Liberman, A. and Fougerousse, J. G.: Community-Based Outpatient Clinic and Transportation Service, *Hosp. Topics 48*:73, 76-80, 124 (Apr.) 1970.

45. Dumouchel, J. R.: Urban Planning—Area Revitalizes Itself Through Hospital-Neighborhood Cooperation, *Hospitals 43*:59-62 (Nov. 1) 1969.

46. Kovner, A. R. *et al.*: Relating a Neighborhood Health Center to a General Hospital—A Case History, *Med. Care 7*:118-123 (Mar.-Apr.) 1969; abstracted, *Med. Care Rev. 28*:111-112 (Jan.) 1971.

47. Baehr, G.: Some Popular Delusions About Health and Medical Care, *Am. J. Public Health 61*:582-585 (Mar.) 1971.

48. Greene, C. R.: Medical Care for Underprivileged Populations, *New Engl. J. Med. 282*:1187-1193 (May 21) 1970.
49. Freymann, J. G. (editorial): Of Health Care, Hospitals and SST's, *New Engl. J. Med. 284*:272-273 (Feb. 4) 1971.
50. Freymann, J. G. (letter): Organization of Health Services, *New Engl. J. Med. 284*:921 (Apr. 22) 1971.
51. Anon.: HMO's Past and Present, *California Med. Assoc. News 16*:1 (May 7) 1971; reprinted, *Med. Care Rev. 28*:591-598 (June) 1971.
52. Anon.: Dr. Crosby Sees HMO's Turning into HCC's, *Mod. Hosp. 116*:36 (Feb.) 1971.
53. Williams, G.: Kaiser—What is It? How Does It Work? Why Does It Work?, *Mod. Hosp. 116*:67-85, 88-95 (Feb.) 1971.
54. Garfield, S. R.: The Delivery of Medical Care, *Sci. Am. 222*:15-23 (Apr.) 1970.
55. Garfield, S. R.: Multiphasic Health Testing and Medical Care as a Right, *New Engl. J. Med. 283*:1087-1089 (Nov. 12) 1970.
56. Donabedian, A.: An Evaluation of Prepaid Group Practices, *Inquiry 6*: (Sept.) 1969.
57. Marshall, T.: The Patient's View—What They Like and Don't Like, *Mod. Hosp. 116*:86-87 (Feb.) 1971.
58. Somers, A. R.: *Health Care in Transition—Directions for the Future*, Hospital Research and Educational Trust, 840 North Lake Shore Drive, Chicago, Ill., 1971, p. 99-126.
59. Garfield, S. R. (letters): Multiphasic Screening, *New Engl. J. Med. 284*:277-278 (Feb. 4) 1971.
60. White, K. L.: Primary Medical Care for Families—Organization and Evaluation, *New Engl. J. Med. 277*:847-852 (Oct. 19) 1967.
61. Cronkhite, L. W., Jr., Alpert, J. J. and Weiner, D. S.: A Health Care System for Massachusetts, *New Engl. J. Med. 284*:240-243 (Feb. 4) 1971.
62. Cronkhite, L. W., Jr.: Health, Inc., *Hospitals 45*: 71-72 (Mar. 16) 1971.
63. Hiatt, H. H.: Medical Care for Northbridge, *New Engl. J. Med. 284*:593-602 (Mar. 18) 1971.
64. Sanazaro, P. J. and Slosberg, B.: Patient Care Evaluation, *Hospitals 45*:131-136 (Apr. 1) 1971.
65. Hochbaum, G. M.: Consumer Participation in Health Planning—Toward Conceptual Clarification, *Am. J. Public Health 59*:1698-1705 (Sept.) 1969.
66. Somers, *op. cit.*, p. 81.
67. Notkin, H. and Notkin, M. S.: Community Participation in Health Services—A Review Article, *Med. Care Rev. 27*:1178-1201 (Dec.) 1970.

Additional References

1. Anon.: *Report of the Task Force on Medicaid and Related Programs*, U.S. Dept. HEW, pub. 398-052, Supt. of Documents, U.S. Govt. Printing Office, June 1970.
2. Anon.: *Basic Facts on the Health Industry*, Committee on Ways and Means, pub. 5270-1108, Supt. of Documents, U.S. Govt. Printing Office, June 1971.
3. Anon.: *Policy Statement on Provision of Health Services*, American Hospital Association, Chicago, Ill., 1971.
4. Anon.: *Higher Education and the Nation's Health*, A Special Report and Recommendations by the Carnegie Commission on Higher Education, McGraw-Hill Book Co., New York, NY, 1970.
5. Jones, B. (ed.): *The Health of Americans*, Prentice-Hall, Inc., Englewood Cliffs, N.J., 1970.
6. Kidder, S. W. and Isack, A. G.: Health Maintenance Organizations and Pharmaceutical Services, *J. Am. Pharm. Assoc. NS12*:8-12, 14-15 (Jan.) 1972.
7. Nixon, R.: *Message from the President of the United States Relative to Building a National Health Strategy*, H.R. document no. 92-49, Supt. of Documents, U.S. Govt. Printing Office, Feb. 18, 1971.

2

Evolvement of clinical pharmacy

by Gloria N. Francke

One of the most dramatic changes affecting pharmaceutical education and the future of pharmaceutical practice is the emerging concept of clinical pharmacy. This concept has emerged in different guises since the late fifties or early sixties, although its roots lie deeply ingrained in many facets of the profession. As we move into the next decade, it is evident that clinical pharmacy will be one of the important aspects in the practice of the profession. Thus, pharmaceutical educators and practitioners alike are reorienting their thinking in developing curricula which will prepare pharmacists to fill this new role.

Development of a new role for the pharmacist came about gradually with the many social and economic changes related to providing medical care. The "idea" of the new role referred to as "clinical pharmacy" evolved in several parts of the country and often with quite different concepts—all of which in 1969 appeared to emerge as one broad concept which connotes those activities which are related to the patient—often referred to as "patient-oriented." This of course results in more direct contact with other members of the medical care team, especially the physician and nurse. Though all segments of the profession may not accept this broad concept, at least some are convinced that clinical pharmacy may be the "savior" of the profession. At the Second Clinical Midyear Meeting of the American Society of Hospital Pharmacists in 1967, Paul Parker commented on the lack of an adequate definition for the term "clinical pharmacy." He said:

> The term, "clinical pharmacy," is grossly overused, misused and poorly defined; but, the concepts it expresses may be either the salvation or the 'Waterloo' for all of Pharmacy depending upon what we do about it.

He further suggested that:

> "Clinical pharmacy" is a concept or a philosophy emphasizing the safe and appropriate use of drugs in patients. It places the emphasis of drugs on the patient not on the product. It is achieved only by interacting responsibly for drugs with all the health disciplines which are in any way concerned with drugs.[1]

The concept of clinical pharmacy is further amplified by Parker in his Whitney Award Lecture in 1967.

> The following points are offered by which pharmacy can act responsibly to society: (1) pharmacy should involve itself in the total concept of drugs in health care; (2) pharmacists should be socially responsible individuals who are patient- and drug-oriented; (3) pharmacists should function as integral members of the health team; (4) pharmacists should be encouraged to specialize functionally.[2]

It is impossible, if not dangerous, to pinpoint absolute priorities; however, mention of some of the earlier references to this may bring forth further amplification and a clearer view of the concept.

The purpose here then is: (1) to look at the chronological evolvement of the concept "clinical pharmacy," (2) to analyze the concept "clinical pharmacy" as it was being used in 1969 and (3) to provide a workable definition for the term. Analysis of the use of the term and an acceptance of a definition will aid pharmacists and pharmaceutical educators in communicating their ideas. Further, pharmacists must be able to communicate the meaning of clinical pharmacy and its implications to other members of the health team, especially physicians and nurses, who will play important roles in educating and training the clinical pharmacist.

Chronological Evolvement of Term

Use of the term "clinical pharmacy" is usually thought of as having developed in the early sixties. However, one of the first uses of the term was by Heber W. Youngken, Jr., who in 1953 wrote an article entitled "The Washington Experiment—Clinical Pharmacy" published in the *American Journal of Pharmaceutical Education.*[3] Youngken, then on the faculty of the University of Washington, recounts how Professor L. Wait Rising of Washington had begun an imaginative research program in teaching pharmacy students, utilizing some of the numerous professional prescription pharmacies at hand in Seattle. The course provided three credits for one lecture, one laboratory period spent in the prescription pharmacies followed by one discussion period led by the professor. This experiment brought forth a storm of protest generated principally by one letter from a member of a Washington faculty to the American Association of Colleges of Pharmacy and the American Council on Pharmaceutical Education. As a result, both organizations passed resolutions disapproving of the experiment and causing it to be discontinued.[4] The resolutions were passed without permitting the professor who originated the plan, the students taking part in the experiment, nor the pharmacists participating in it, an opportunity to be heard.

In describing his program earlier, in 1945, Professor Rising pointed out that clinical experience for academic credit is the keystone of modern education and noted its use in medicine. He was, he said, "attempting to develop the pharmaceutical counterpart." Describing it, he noted, "It is analagous to the cadet training seniors get in hospital pharmacies attached to university medical schools, and is more broadly practical."[5] Rising explained "The Washington Experiment" more completely in 1946 at the convention and answered the objections to the course, raised in the letter, as the result of which his program was disapproved by the two organizations as mentioned previously. The disapproval caused the experimental program to be discontinued. Thus, the pharmaceutical educational "Establishment" killed an imaginative research program in teaching methods which then lay dormant for about a quarter of a century. Although Youngken again brought the concept of clinical pharmacy to the attention of educators in 1953, the concept did not meet with favor until groups of hospital practitioners began to develop it.

Whether or not the term as used in the early sixties or before was taken seriously, what it may have conveyed to the listener or whether it was acceptable to pharmacists are dubious. Leading pharmaceutical textbooks and journals published in the interim period, 1960 to 1967, do not mention or index* "Clinical Pharmacy" or "Clinical Pharmacist." First references, to any significant

*Checking an index as a criteria for use of a term may be questionable, especially if a term is not already in general use. Also, indexes for pharmaceutical publications (journals and texts) may often be inadequate.

degree, appear in 1967 and 1968. One exception to this is the text *Clinical Pharmacy* published by Jenkins, Sperandio and Latiolais in 1966.[6]

The fact that the book entitled, *Clinical Pharmacy* with the subtitle *A Text for Dispensing Pharmacy,* was intended to supplant the time-honored Scoville's *The Art of Compounding* leads one to believe that the concept is expressed in title only. Though it is possible to relate the subject matter of any chapter to clinical pharmacy, the authors' concepts do not appear to be as clear as those which have evolved since publication of the book. Exception to this is a rather clear concept expressed in the Preface which relates pharmaceutical services "to the patient in a clinical situation" and to other medical disciplines.

Antedating publication of the text, one of the authors, Dr. Glenn Sperandio, mentioned clinical pharmacy when beginning the series, *Hospital Pharmacy Notes,* Number 1, which appeared as an advertisement in the *American Journal of Hospital Pharmacy* in 1961.[7]

Here, in the introduction to the series which includes Dr. Sperandio's credentials, it is stated that he "directs graduate research in the areas of *clinical* (author's italics) pharmacy and product formulation." Whether or not Dr. Sperandio was relating "clinical" to the concept we speak about today is not clear.

Another point can be raised regarding a later reference (1965) to "clinical pharmacy" by Sperandio. This relates to the concept expressed at that time, again in contrast to the concept as it has evolved in 1968. On a chart which he presents, pharmacy is divided into three areas—clinical pharmacy, industrial pharmacy, and pharmaceutical sciences. Clinical pharmacy includes community practice, hospital practice and public health practice. Here he defines clinical pharmacy as:

> . . . that area which embraces the acquisition and preparation of medications and their distribution to the public. This is an accurate and appropriate description of the activities of the community pharmacist or the hospital pharmacist.[8]

In a further comment on use of the term, Dr. Sperandio says:

> Dictionary definitions of the word "clinical" differ in their complete interpretation of its meaning, yet all of them agree that direct contact with a person or persons is basic. Thus, we have clinical medicine, clinical psychology, clinical pharmacology, and clinical investigations —all specifically denoting a professional service or activity involving living human subjects. Certainly, the transfer of a physician's order for medication from pharmacist to patient is a clinical situation. The pharmacist's products and use of drugs, as well as the other health services which he performs daily, are best described as clinical activities. In this age of specialization, every progressive vocation has specialized divisions. Pharmacy has for some time been recognized as having these divisions. The name "clinical pharmacy" identifies one such area.[8]

There seems little question that this definition and concept as expressed then is inadequate for today's applications. Whereas the term as defined by Sperandio covered a broad aspect of pharmacy practice, it may be difficult to accept the all-embracing idea covering community, hospital and public health practice. But, if one can accept the "patient-oriented" aspect in each of these areas of practice, then we can define these as clinical pharmacy. As we may see later, it is hardly conceivable that *all* elements of either community practice or hospital practice could clearly be clinical pharmacy.

These references unquestionably had some influence on use of the term, especially among pharmaceutical educators. Certainly the idea of accepting a new meaning for the well-worn "hard-to-change" dispensing concept gave rise to some thought among pharmaceutical educators and may have shattered their complacency regarding curriculum changes.

There were other factors which may have influenced use of the term. Almost simultaneously educators were being prodded to "think about" this new role. An early reference to "clinical pharmacy" appears in a paper by Dr. John Autian entitled "Fourth or Terminal Course in Pharmacy," presented at the Teachers' Seminar in Pharmacy held at the University of Wisconsin in 1961. In rather glowing words he suggested the term "clinical pharmacy." At the same time, he did not appear convinced of its acceptance in stating that he would ". . . permit those much wiser . . . to coin a more useful name." Under the subheading, "Need for New Name For 'Compounding and Dispensing' Course," Dr. Autian stated:

> "A rose by any other name," or so it goes, "smells just as sweet." This undoubtedly, is quite true, but to many the aroma from the term 'compounding or dispensing' does not fill the nostrils with fragrance of enchanted lands. There is a definite need to replace this title in the future with a more suitable name. I believe that a new name such as *Clinical Pharmacy* may bring much responsibility and perhaps even a little glamour to this terminal pharmacy course. I will, however, for the present refer to this course only as the *Terminal Pharmacy Course* and permit those much wiser than I to coin a more useful name.[9]

Recognition of and actual use of the term "clinical pharmacy" came from educators. This may have had considerable impact since few pharmaceutical educators, until that time, could conceive of the hospital environment serving as a laboratory for the teaching of pharmacists. Nevertheless, recognition of Autian's suggestion has come about with time. Six years later Dr. Stanley V. Susina writing on "The Scope of the Terminal Course in Pharmacy" said:

> Dr. John Autian made some very valuable and pertinent suggestions concerning the terminal course in pharmacy. At that time there were some present who thought that many of the suggestions made might not be too germane to the course known as dispensing pharmacy. In the past few weeks I have had occasion to reread this paper and I recommend it to you as a most rewarding and profitable discussion of the terminal course in pharmacy.
>
> There were many observations which were made by Autian, and today, some five years later, it appears that he was an excellent prognosticator. Autian defined the role of the pharmacist of the future as a professional whose function would be to advise the medical practitioner or other paramedical personnel in the selection of drug products.[10]

Placed in time, another significant reference is made to "*Clinical* (author's italics) Professional Practice," in the recommendations of the *Audit of Pharmaceutical Service in Hospitals,* published in 1964.[11] The recommendation reads:

> *Clinical Professional Practice.* It is recommended that colleges of pharmacy be encouraged to utilize the facilities of the hospital pharmacy to expand their "dispensing" courses to a broader course encompassing clinical professional practice.

Here the recommendation under the section on "Education and Training" is directly related to the fact that more than half of all chief pharmacists felt "the need for more education in the biological sciences, including biochemistry and pharmacology." In response to a related question, 79 percent of chief pharmacists felt that they could be more helpful to physicians and nurses in supplying information on actions, uses, side effects, etc., of drugs if they had received a well planned sequence of courses in the biological sciences.

Clinical pharmacy has been related to various functions of the practitioner. As an example, let us look at one of these functions—decentralized pharmacy—and trace its beginnings. Perhaps this function, more than others, does connote "clinical pharmacy" in its purest state because, in the case of decentralized pharmacy, the pharmacist is brought into the patient environment where, in fact, he functions as a "clinical pharmacist."

Clinical pharmacy then is often related to decentralized pharmacy service. Probably the first approach to this concept was at the Seaside Memorial Hospital in Long Beach, California. When this hospital was built in 1959, it is believed that there was an attempt to employ one pharmacist for each one hundred units. Hospital Administrator Donald C. Carner, writing in *Hospital Pharmacy Notes* (1960), projected plans for the pharmacy service in the new hospital.[12] The decentralized pharmacy at Memorial Hospital of Long Beach is now one of several in the United States.

The concept was there although it is believed that the original plan for decentralized service did not originate with pharmacists but rather with the administrator. In fact, according to minutes of the Pharmacy and Therapeutics Committee of the hospital, pharmacists objected to the plan and, during the early period, refused to be assigned to the decentralized area.[13]

The concept of clinical pharmacy has evolved to the highest degree in the decentralized pharmacy located on a patient care unit where the pharmacist practices in close association with physicians, nurses and patients. The pharmacist in charge of the patient-unit pharmacy appears to fulfill the role as visualized by several leaders throughout the country.[14,15,16]

Numerous other events (speeches, papers, meetings) during more recent years have kindled the fire leading to use of the term clinical pharmacy. There are also numerous references to the fact that the pharmacist (and the pharmacy student) must be "clinically oriented." Not in the least among these is the fact that the American Society of Hospital Pharmacists in 1966 began its Annual Clinical Midyear Meetings. A perusal of papers presented at the 1968 meeting indicates the intent to be "clinical." Among titles of papers presented were, "Nursing Faculty Members Participate in a Clinical Pharmacy Course," "Clinical Orientation as an Innovation," and "Pharmaceutical Communications in the Clinical Environment."[17]

Factors Influencing Development of Clinical Pharmacy

Also recognized is the fact that many developments in hospital pharmacy practice, some apparent and others not, contribute to the need for and acceptance of clinical pharmacy. The acute shortage of nurses and other health personnel may also be related to the need for pharmaceutical services in the patient environment. Some of these developments predate reference to the term clinical pharmacy but undoubtedly relate to emergence of the concept. Among these are:

1. *Drug Information.* The role of the pharmacist as a consultant and the development of drug information centers in hospital pharmacy are not new. Reference to the pharmacist as a consultant and his approach to utilizing drug information has appeared in the literature often but has become a more clearly defined role in the past few years.[18] Also, the importance of the literature as a source of drug information was recognized early by the American Society of Hospital Pharmacists. In the *Minimum Standard for Pharmacies in Hospitals* the need for a library and information sources is recognized. As early as 1952, the Society published the *Comprehensive Bibliography on Hospital Pharmacy.*[19]

Later, in 1955, the Literature Number of the *American Journal of Hospital Pharmacy* appeared and was brought up-to-date in 1961.[20]

In more recent years the evolvement of drug information centers in hospitals and the trend toward educating pharmacists to serve as drug information specialists has resulted in the American Society of Hospital Pharmacists' establishing a Committee on Drug Information Services and publishing a statement on "The Hospital Pharmacist and Drug Information Services."[21] Certainly the pharmacist in the clinical setting can contribute little without a thorough background regarding sources of drug information and the facility for communicating with members of the health team.

2. *Medication Errors.* Studies pointing out the problems of detecting medication errors were reported by Barker and McConnell in 1962.[22] A follow-up study entitled "A Study of Medication Errors in a Hospital" by Barker, Kimbrough and Heller was reported in 1966 (though preliminary reports appeared earlier).[23]

The Study, conducted at the University of Arkansas Medical Center, Little Rock, under a grant from the Hartford Foundation, drew national attention to medication errors not only by hospital pharmacists but by other hospital and medical people as well. Recognition that medication errors occur and that such errors may involve the pharmacist, the physician and/or the nurse brought together members of the health team in the interest of the *patient.* Possibly for the first time, to any great extent, pharmacists began thinking about the need for working more closely with the nurse and the physician in providing and controlling medications—from the time of procurement to the time of administration. This is another factor in the evolvement of clinical pharmacy.

3. *Drug Distribution.* Changing patterns in drug distribution, the need for pharmacists to interpret the physician's original orders and the trend toward adoption of unit dose packaging, along with the emergence of computer applications in drug distribution systems, represent other aspects which have been influential in bringing about the concept of clinical pharmacy.

Research in drug distribution systems at several centers throughout the United States has given impetus to an acceptance of changing patterns. Studies at the University of Iowa and at the University of Arkansas relating to Centralized Unit Dose Dispensing (CUDD) and Decentralized Unit Dose Dispensing (DUDD) have also made an impact on clinical pharmacy.[24,25]

4. *Monitoring Adverse Effects of Drugs.* The increasing potency of drugs as well as possible drug interactions have resulted in concern for adverse effects. As a result, pharmacists have become involved in identifying and monitoring adverse reactions.[26]

5. *The Pharmacist in the Patient Environment.* In some instances the role of the clinical pharmacist is closely allied to his being in the patient environment in more direct contact with the patient, whether this be in a decentralized pharmacy or simply on the patient unit along with other members of the health team. Whatever his role may be in this capacity, it must not be as an observer. If the clinical pharmacist is going to make a contribution, he must become involved. Although it is easy to accept the pharmacist in the role, his contributions have not yet been clearly defined. Both educators and practitioners are giving a great deal of thought to the pharmacist who is serving on the patient unit. Educators are approaching the problem from the standpoint of development of a patient awareness in students. According to Carlin,

> Clinical education for pharmacy undergraduate students is needed for the development of a patient awareness and should assist the student in bringing together all of the scientific and professional skills and knowledge he has received and relating them to the patient, to the disease state, and to the practice of his profession. It may also enable him to adapt to changes in health care which are being and will be faced by the pharmaceutical profession in the near future.[27]

Others in hospital pharmacy have placed strong emphasis on the need for pharmacists to be patient-oriented and several schools of pharmacy have established courses in clinical

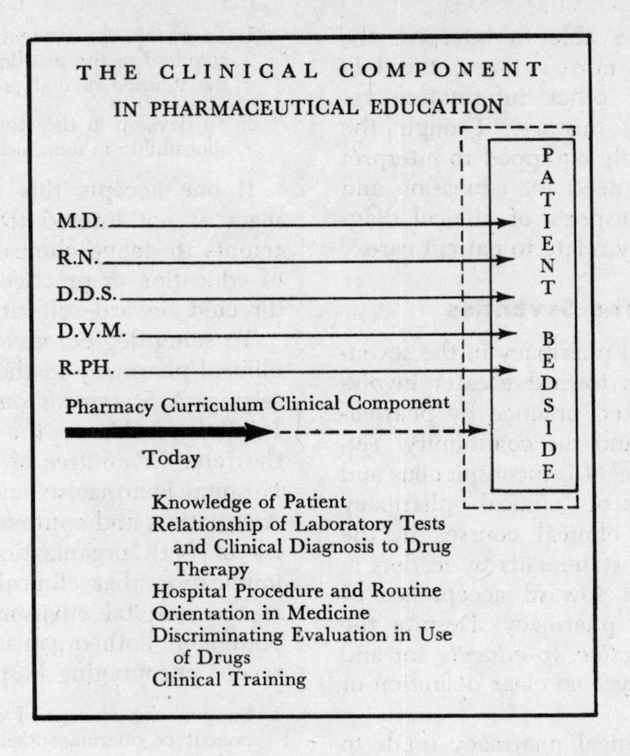

Figure 1. The clinical component in pharmaceutical education

pharmacy—though again the concept and the teaching of courses titled Clinical Pharmacy vary greatly from school to school.

One concept which emphasizes the clinical environment is that suggested by Sister Emmanuel in the outline of a course in clinical pharmacy being offered at Wayne State University.[28]

In referring to the clinical environment, Sister Emmanuel emphasizes the fact that:

> The student's observations stimulate a process of self-evaluation wherein he compares his own attitude and aspirations with those he witnesses and admires in action in the clinical situation. From this process of self-evaluation there is nurtured a concern and desire that he, too, may become more completely involved in patient-centered service.

The one common denominator in all aspects of that to which we refer as "clinical," whether it be pharmacy or a pharmacist, is the *patient*, and perhaps more correctly the *patient environment*. Brodie, speaking at the Conference on Health Education (University of Michigan, 1967), had this to say about the clinical environment.

> The gap between the termination of our present curriculum and the bedside is a new frontier—a new dimension—in pharmacy education. To bridge this gap, educationally-speaking, the development of a clinical component in pharmaceutical education will be required. The clue to the development of the clinical component lies in the fact that in the environment of the bedside the pharmacist functions as a biologist, because here the language of communication is the language of biology.[29]

The diagram (above) adapted from and supplementing Brodie's comments shows the extent of clinical contact by members of the health team with emphasis on knowledge of the patient.

6. *Patient Drug Profiles.* Use of the medical record or taking the patient's drug history by pharmacists is another aspect related to the role of the the clinical pharmacist. The importance of the patient's drug history is evident. Here

the pharmacist must be able to interpret the physician's orders, the nurse's notes, the laboratory tests and any other information relating to the patient's history. Though the pharmacist is undoubtedly equipped to interpret drug orders, there is a need for education and training in the overall aspects of clinical diagnosis and therapy as they relate to patient care.[30]

Clinical Pharmacy—The Seventies

Evolvement of clinical pharmacy in the seventies appears to progress toward greater involvment in a patient-oriented practice by pharmacists in both hospitals and the community. Yet, the pace of this involvement is inconspicuous and slow. Editorials, reports of "clinical" pharmacy practices, inclusion of clinical courses in the pharmacy curricula and statements by leaders in the profession all point toward acceptance of the concept of clinical pharmacy. Despite the continued efforts to *practice*, to *educate* for and to *write* about, there is yet no clear definition of "clinical pharmacy."

The concept of clinical pharmacy tends to bend—depending on whether one refers to education or to practice—to its applications in the institutional setting or in the community. From one vantage point, educators see clinical pharmacy applied to all areas of practice and with it goes the broad connotation that if it relates primarily to patient care and drug therapy, it is indeed "clinical pharmacy." This has been brought out on several occasions and specifically by a definition suggested in a 1968 report by the Committee on Curriculum of the American Association of Colleges of Pharmacy. This definition reads as follows:[31]

> Clinical pharmacy is that area within the pharmacy curriculum which deals with patient care with emphasis on drug therapy. Clinical pharmacy seeks to develop a patient-oriented attitude. The acquisition of new knowledge is secondary to the attainment of skills in interprofessional and patient communications.

As further clarification and enlargement of the above definition, the following objectives for instruction in clinical pharmacy were given:

1. To acquaint the student with clinical applications of pharmacological and pharmaceutical principles;
2. To help make the student more aware of the general methods of diagnosis and patient care specifically as they relate to drug therapy;
3. To develop in the student a facility for effective interaction with the patient and with practitioners of other health professions;
4. To help the student develop a patient awareness in providing pharmaceutical services;
5. To enable the student to integrate the knowledge acquired in the preclinical years and to apply it to the solution of real problems; and
6. To develop in the student an awareness of his responsibility in monitoring drug utilization.

If one accepts this definition, clinical pharmacy is not limited to hospital pharmacy. Attempts to define clinical pharmacy on the basis of education or practice appear futile and often directed toward self-interests.

To some degree, greater emphasis is given to clinical pharmacy in the institutional or hospital setting. A *Statement on Clinical Pharmacy and Its Relationship to the Hospital,* developed by the Joint Committee of the American Society of Hospital Pharmacists and the American Hospital Association, and approved by the governing bodies of both organizations in 1970, carries the implication that clinical pharmacy is practiced in the hospital environment. In approving the Statement both organizations officially went on record encouraging hospitals to:[32]

1. Support the concept of clinical pharmacy as a component of pharmaceutical services and drug control; and
2. Make their facilities available to schools of pharmacy for clinical preparation of future pharmacy practitioners.

Editorializing in the *American Journal of Hospital Pharmacy* in early 1971, Provost suggests that clinical pharmacy does extend beyond the hospital, especially if one looks to the practice of hospital pharmacy in the future when the system of the delivery of health care may be quite different. He notes that:[33]

> . . . hospital pharmacy as we know it today, may have already reached or passed its peak. Pharmacy of tomorrow, although it might be institution-based, may be practiced largely in a different type of controlled, multidisciplinary environment in which patients are offered compresensive health maintenance services on an outpatient basis.

Significantly, he concludes:

> If pharmacy embraces the opportunity to offer services that we now consider necessary to label as "clinical," the adjectives "clinical," "hospital," "institutional" and "community" can be dropped from the vocabulary of the profession and pharmacy can take its true place in health care without the need for academic exercises to define terms.

Among significant events during the past few years emphasizing increasing interest in the pharmacist's clinical role is establishment of the Drug-Related Studies Program at the National Center for Health Services Research and Development. Although the program's mission is broad, the first Task Force was appointed to develop a set of working criteria for a clinical role for the pharmacist, considered a preliminary step toward evaluating the effectiveness and cost feasibility of a clinical role.[34]

The Report of Task Force on Pharmacists' Clinical Role first appeared in *HSRD Briefs* in 1971[35] and is reprinted in the *Journal of the American Pharmaceutical Association* in September 1971.

Placing emphasis on the pharmacist's role in the delivery of health care and the professional functions that a pharmacist would perform in a clinical role, the report discussed these functions under the following classifications: prescribing drugs, dispensing and administering drugs, documenting professional activities, direct patient involvement, reviewing drug utilization, education and consultation. The following summary of the Task Force's findings recognizes the fact that the present clinical role of the pharmacist is associated more easily today with hospital than with non-hospital practice:

> The pharmacist's usefulness as a specialist in his own field can be enhanced by his assuming an attitude that will lead to an active concern for direct patient welfare. In addition, the pharmacist's usefulness as a professional health worker will likewise be enhanced through active participation in patient care with other health professionals. The present clinical role of the pharmacist is associated more easily today with hospital than non-hospital practice. However, the opportunity for clinical experience in the care of ambulant patients does exist. One difficulty at the present time is the fragmentation of the out-of-hospital delivery system. The role will become more uniform as the medical care delivery system is standardized in group medical practice, health education centers, and other systems. Furthermore, much of community pharmacy practice remains rooted in traditional patterns in which the pharmacist appears to be more or less apathetic to direct patient care needs. When pharmacists become identified actively with group medical practice or perhaps modify their own traditional practice arrangements, the true clinical nature of community pharmacy practice will emerge.

Concern and interest on the part of both educators and practitioners were expressed in 1969 when the American Association of Colleges of Pharmacy and the American Society of Hospital Pharmacists resolved to sponsor a joint invitational workshop. This became a reality in August 1971 when educators and hospital pharmacists joined "to provide a forum for the exchange of experiences and viewpoints among educators and practitioners relating to the clinical aspects of pharmaceutical practice." The forum used as its baseline the AACP definition and objectives of clinical pharmacy. The expressed objectives of the workshop were outlined as follows:[36]

1. To explore the most effective means of educating the patient-oriented pharmacists:
   a. Course versus program (didactic versus laboratory)
   b. Undergraduate and graduate education and training
2. To determine the necessary clinical pharmacy laboratory facilities for effective educational programs.
3. To establish criteria for clinical pharmacy educators.

Complete proceedings of the Workshop appear in the November (1971) issue of the *American Journal of Hospital Pharmacy.*[36]

Although it is too early to evaluate its long-term effects, the Workshop did bear fruit by bringing together leaders from two vitally concerned groups for frank discussions about their concepts of clinical practice, its place in the education of pharmacists and, more important, in the delivery of health care. Assuming that the AACP's definition of clinical pharmacy were followed, the Workshop more clearly delineated the curriculum needs in order to adequately prepare pharmacists to function in the patient care environment. Statements by representatives of the sponsoring organizations summarize the Workshop. Varro Tyler, Past-President of AACP, commented on the value of the meeting:

> I believe the conference served a valuable purpose in giving a large group of pharmacists and educators a real understanding of the emerging discipline of clinical pharmacy. Naturally, agreement was not obtained on all of the details of clinical pharmacy programs or their implementation. However, the participants were in complete agreement that, in the future, all pharmacy students should receive adequate exposure to the patient-oriented practice of pharmacy.

ASHP President R. David Anderson evaluated the Invitational Workshop this way:

> One of the complaints often voiced about colleges of pharmacy and pharmacy curricula is that practitioners seldom have an opportunity to influence them in any meaningful way. This conference proved that educators, practitioners and students can reach agreement on many topics that will have a profound influence on the future practice of the profession. It is pleasing that we were able to reach a consensus on so many areas of vital importance. I believe that when the history of the clinical pharmacy movement in this country is detailed, this conference will be recorded as having contributed significantly to infusing a new vitality into the profession.

Worthy of note at the Conference were the numerous viewpoints among practitioners and educators, along with admonitions from a hospital administrator, a nurse and a physician regarding the pharmacist's role "on the team" and the need to establish interplay with members of the health team. Need for a definition of clinical pharmacy became increasingly clear. Possibly the point which brings the profession more nearly to a definition relates to deciding the criteria to become a *safe* clinical pharmacist. It could be concluded from the Workshop that a scientific, professional and social background plus knowledge of the tools to perform effectively in the patient environment are essential. Yet, the ultimate is to assure the physician, the nurse and the patient that the drugs prescribed, dispensed and administered are safe and effective. The ability to do this brings into focus clinical pharmacy practice as it will present itself in the seventies.

Not dealt with in depth at the Workshop are at least three critical points referred to by Provost in an editorial, "Considerations in Clinical Pharmacy Education and Practice," appearing along with the Proceedings.[37] These include: (1) the immediate need for pharmacy to critically evaluate, via the scientific method, the effectiveness of its practitioners in new roles which are encompassed by "clinical pharmacy"; (2) the need to convince the public, other health practitioners, health planners, administrators and legislators that the clinical component is essential but will increase the cost of pharmacy education significantly; and (3) that restructuring pharmaceutical education is likely to have little future impact unless education of the pharmacist is integrated and coordinated with that of physicians, nurses and other health professions.

Also, during 1971, a Task Force representing seven national specialty groups in pharmacy framed a "Statement on Pharmacy Practice."[38] This Statement, quoted below, appears to indicate that the pharmaceutical Establishment is not anxious for the terms "clinical pharmacist" or "clinical pharmacy" to develop despite the continued evolvement of a new dimension of professional practice.

> Pharmacy Practice is defined as that personal health service that assures safety and efficacy in the procuring, storing, prescribing, compounding, dispensing, delivering, administering and use of drugs and related articles. The aspect of pharmacy practice that can be considered "clinical" is the assurance of safety and efficacy in the prescribing, administering and use of drugs and related articles.
>
> Clinical experience is a part of pharmacy practice, regardless of environment. However, the environment in which a pharmacist practices may determine some of the functions performed by him and may affect his degree of clinical involvement.
>
> Most practitioners exercise some degree of clinical involvement in their practice. All practitioners should involve themselves in the clinical functions of pharmacy that will result in increased patient-oriented pharmacy practice.
>
> Because the term "clinical" describes those functions of pharmacy practice in which evaluations and sound judgments are made regarding a patient's drug therapy, pharmacy should not be identified as "clinical pharmacy" and pharmacists should not be identified as "clinical pharmacists." While clinical functions of pharmacy practice do not constitute a specialty at this time, continued involvement of the pharmacist in patient-oriented activities may eventually lead to the development and recognition of a specialized area.

Another facet of clinical pharmacy practice relates to the political and legal considerations, which have been only occasionally referred to.

In a paper entitled "On a Political and Legal Foundation for Clinical Pharmacy Practice," Barker and Valentino give an in-depth look at these considerations.[39] "The advancement of the clinical pharmacy concept, particularly in the area of counseling the patient," they note, "may be seriously impeded by the pharmacist's legal vulnerability when he does counsel his patients." Barker and Valentino also bring out the possible need to change existing state pharmacy practice laws and the fact that the concept of clinical pharmacy as a pattern of practice needs a stronger foundation of political support than it now has.

To overcome, or as an alternative to major changes in laws, the authors suggest inclusion in the official compendia selected items of information about each drug. Such information could be transmitted to the patient by the pharmacists, without prior approval by the physician. Because of the unique legal status of the compendia, it is believed that with the support of the national organizations, this activity could be identified as *the* central activity of clinical pharmacy practice. Although the suggestion may have a place in clinical practice, providing drug information set down in official compendia is but a minute part of clinical pharmacy practice and could never substitute for judgments which the pharmacist would make based on his education and experience. The legal standards have a contribution to make to clinical practice but it would be disastrous to conclude that by merely relying on information set down in legal compendia, one establishes himself as a clinical pharmacist.

It is difficult to assess the extent of actual clinical practice by any definition. Numerous reports under the term "clinical pharmacy" continue to be presented at meetings and published in the profession's leading journals. However, more often than not, clinical pharmacy may be a new term attached to old roles. Nevertheless, those pharmacists who have taken on new roles, whether it be in a community or in an institutional setting, have found a mission in which is deeply rooted a professional service role intrinsic to the delivery of health care and the needs of the patient.

Conclusions and Definitions

Many functions now being performed by pharmacists are related to the concept of clinical pharmacy. Clinical pharmacy is not a completely new concept but admittedly the emphasis has changed during recent years. This is due, in part, to loss of the function of preparing medicines which formerly was a forte of all pharmacists. As this has been taken over by the industry, the profession has sought to replace it with a "new" thing—and today clinical pharmacy is the "thing." But its roots lie deeply enmeshed in the past of the profession. Hospital pharmacists in France, for example, have made medical rounds with physicians since 1815. After the internship in hospital pharmacy for the municipal hospitals of Paris had become effective in 1815, the pharmacy interns were expected to make hospital rounds with physicians and surgeons. By 1829, this responsibility of the pharmacy intern was explicitly stipulated in the regulations of Parisian hospitals.[40]

Kenneth Fitch, a former Editor of the *Journal Mondial de Pharmacie* and a contempory and associate of Martindale—the world famous author of *Martindale's Extra Pharmacopoeia*—went to the hospital to examine patients with amebic dysentery to note the effects of drugs synthesized by Martindale on their disease. Each of these and many other practices of pharmacists have had large components of what is now called "clinical pharmacy.[41]

There are numerous ways in which clinical pharmacy may be defined. Educationally, clinical pharmacy may be defined as a concept which considers the treatment and care of patients by members of the health team in the presence of pharmacy students, with particular emphasis on the safe and appropriate use of drugs.

The practice of clinical pharmacy maintains the same principal concept but here the pharmacist replaces the student and utilizes his professional judgment based on his theoretical knowledge while working with the members of the health-care team to foster the safe and appropriate use of drugs in patients.

The term "clinical" is an ancient term meaning "reclining in bed." A clinic is medical practice at the sickbed, or a class of medical instruction in a hospital held at the bedside of patients or a group of selected patients serving as case studies. Clinical involves or depends on the observation of the living patient; a clinician examines or observes the patient. As an adjective applied to pharmacy, *clinical* implies the practice of pharmacy in the presence of hospitalized patients.[42]

Practicing in the patient care environment does call for new skills from the pharmacist and perhaps these are the newest things about clinical pharmacy. It calls upon the pharmacist for a far better vocabulary so that he can understand the physician and talk to him, "communication" some people term it; it calls for the ability to verbalize, to recall more rapidly and to associate and relate facts more clearly. These skills are new to some pharmacists, but not to others. It also calls for a much better theoretical knowledge of the biological and physical sciences because in the practice of clinical pharmacy, the pharmacist is called upon often to use it. Formerly, when the pharmacist was safely isolated and insulated by his four walls, he had little opportunity to use his knowledge to demonstrate to others that he too is a university graduate, to know that his counsel can contribute to patient care and welfare, to gain understanding that the pharmacist's function is not limited to the dispensing of a drug product—these are some of the factors attracting so many pharmacists today to the concept of clinical pharmacy.

References

1. Parker, P. F.: The Hospital Pharmacist in the Clinical Setting. I. The Hospital Pharmacist's Viewpoint. Paper presented at Second Annual Clinical Midyear Meeting of the American Society of Hospital Pharmacists, December 4, 1967. (Not published)

2. Parker, P. F.: Drugs and the People, *Am. J. Hosp. Pharm. 24*:350-355 (July) 1967.

3. Youngken, H. W., Jr.: The Washington Experiment—Clinical Pharmacy, *Am. J. Pharm. Educ. 17*:64-70, 1953.

4. Johnson, H. S. (Chairman): Report of the Committee on Educational and Membership Standards, *Am. J. Pharm. Educ. 10*:80-90, 1946.

5. Rising, L. W.: Theory and Practice Can Be Combined, *Am. J. Pharm. Educ. 9*:557-559, 1945.

6. Jenkins, G. L., Sperandio, G. J. and Latiolais, C. L.: *Clinical Pharmacy, A Text for Dispensing Pharmacy,* McGraw-Hill Inc., New York, N. Y., 1966, p. 379.

7. Sperandio, G. J. (editor): *Hospital Pharmacy Notes* (advertisement), *Am. J. Hosp. Pharm. 18*: opp. 32 (Mar.) 1961.

8. Sperandio, G. J.: *Hospital Pharmacy Notes* (advertisement, Lilly) No. 1. (Jan.-Apr.) 1965.

9. Autian, J.: *Proceedings of the American Association of Colleges of Pharmacy Teachers' Seminar 13*:52 (July 9-15) 1961.

10. Susina, S. V.: The Scope of the Terminal Course in Pharmacy, *Am. J. Pharm. Educ. 31*:231-236 (May) 1967.

11. Francke, D. E. *et al.*: *Mirror to Hospital Pharmacy,* American Society of Hospital Pharmacists, 1964, p. 28, 164.

12. Carner, D.: A New Concept in Hospital Pharmacies, *Hospital Pharmacy Notes* (advertisement, Lilly) (Mar.-Apr.) 1960.

13. Personal conversation with William Smith, Director, Pharmacy Service, Memorial Hospital of Long Beach, California, January 1969.

14. Smith, W. E.: Future Role of the Hospital Pharmacist in the Patient Care Area, *Am. J. Hosp. Pharm. 24*:228-231 (Apr.) 1967.

15. Oliver, J. A.: An Improved Concept for Hospital Pharmacy Service. Memorial Hospital of Long Beach, *Drug Intelligence 1*:72-75 (Feb.) 1967.

16. Oliver, J. A.: New Concept for Hospital Pharmacy Practice, *Hosp. Management 103*:78-82 (June) 1967.

17. American Society of Hospital Pharmacists: Program, 1968 Annual Clinical Midyear Meeting, Washington, D.C., December 1968.

18. Brodie, D. C. and Meyers, F. H.: Role of the Pharmacist as Drug Consultant, *Am. J. Hosp. Pharm. 18*:11-13 (Jan.) 1961.

19. Niemeyer, G. F.: Comprehensive Bibliography on Hospital Pharmacy, *Bull. Am. Soc. Hosp. Pharmacists 8*:27-63 (Jan.-Feb.) 1951.

20. American Society of Hospital Pharmacists: Special Literature Number, *Am. J. Hosp. Pharm. 18*:1-106 (Jan.) 1961.

21. American Society of Hospital Pharmacists: The Hospital Pharmacist and Drug Information Services, *Am. J. Hosp. Pharm. 25*:381-382 (July) 1968.

22. Barker, K. and McConnell, W. E.: The Problems of Detecting Medication Errors in Hospitals, *Am. J. Hosp. Pharm. 19*:361-369 (Aug.) 1962.

23. Barker, K., Kimbrough, W. and Heller, W. M.: *A Study of Medication Errors in a Hospital,* University of Arkansas, Fayetteville, Arkansas, 1966.

24. Barker, K. N. and Heller, W. M.: The Development of a Centralized Unit Dose Dispensing System, Part One. Description of the UAMC Experimental System, *Am. J. Hosp. Pharm. 20*:568-579 (Nov.) 1963.

25. Black, H. J. and Tester, W. W.: Decentralized Pharmacy Operations Utilizing the Unit Dose Concept, *Am. J. Hosp. Pharm. 21*:345-350 (Aug.) 1964.

26. Smith, J. E. and Canada, A. T., Jr.: An Epidemiological Study of Adverse Drug Reactions—A Preliminary Report, *Am. J. Hosp. Pharm. 24*:268-272 (May) 1967.

27. Carlin, H. S.: The Impact of Clinical Pharmacy on Pharmaceutical Education, *Am. J. Pharm. Educ. 32*:587-592 (Nov.) 1968.

28. Sister Emmanuel: Experience with a Course in Clinical Pharmacy. Part One: The Preliminary Planning Stage, *Am. J. Hosp. Pharm. 25*:551-558 (Oct.) 1968.

29. Brodie, D. C.: "Emerging Patterns of Education and Practice in the Health Professions—Pharmacy," in Deno, R. A. (ed.): *Proceedings Pharmacy—Medicine—Nursing Conference on Health Education,* University of Michigan Press, Ann Arbor, Mich., 1967.

30. Berry, C. C.: The Use of the Medical Record by the Clinical Pharmacist, *Bull. Ohio Soc. Hosp. Pharm.* (Oct.) 1968.

31. Anon.: Report of the Committee on Curriculum of the American Association of Colleges of Pharmacy, presented at the 69th Annual Meeting of the AACP, Miami Beach, Florida, May 2-3, 1968.

32. Anon.: Statement on Clinical Pharmacy and Its Relationship to the Hospital, *Am. J. Hosp. Pharm. 28*:357 (May) 1971.

33. Provost, G. P.: Clinical Pharmacy and Hospital Pharmacy (editorial), *Am. J. Hosp. Pharm. 28*:17 (Jan.) 1971.

34. Anon.: HEW—Office of Drug Related Studies, *Focus 7*:8 (Winter) 1971. National Services Research and Development, Health Services and Mental Health Administration, Department of Health, Education and Welfare, Washington, D.C.

35. Anon.: Report of Task Force on the Pharmacist's Clinical Role, *HSRD Briefs 4*:1-9 (Spring) 1971.

36. Anon.: Proceedings of the ASHP-AACP Invitational Workshop on Clinical Pharmaceutical Practice and Education, *Am. J. Hosp. Pharm. 28*:841-906 (Nov.) 1971.

37. Provost, G. P.: Considerations in Clinical Pharmacy Education and Practice (editorial), *Am. J. Hosp. Pharm. 28*: 841 (Nov.) 1971.

38. Anon.: Report of the Task Force on the Definition of "Clinical Pharmacy," "Institutional Pharmacy," and "Group Practice," 1971.

39. Barker, K. N. and Valentino, J. G.: On a Political and Legal Foundation for Clinical Pharmacy Practice. Presented to the American Society of Hospital Pharmacists Annual Meeting, March 30, 1971, San Francisco, California (not published).

40. Goris, A. *et al.*: *Centenaire de l'internat en pharmacie des hôpitaux et hospices civils de Paris*, Paris: Imprimerie de la Cour d'Appel, 1920, p. 54.

41. Personal Communication.

42. Moore, F. D.: Therapeutic Innovation: Ethical Boundaries in the Initial Clinical Trials of New Drugs and Surgical Procedures, *Daedalus 98*:502-522 (Spring) 1969.

3

The social psychological role of the pharmacist in drug usage

by Donald E. Francke and Dorothy L. Smith

Most of the problems of illness which people face are due to a combination of social, behavioral and biologic causes of which the pharmacist has little understanding, partly because the strengths of his educational preparation have lain primarily in the physical sciences while his period of apprenticeship has tended to concentrate almost exclusively on the merchandising aspects of a business. The product of an educational system which until recently had no clinical component, the pharmacist has been ill-prepared to function as a member of the health-care team. Due to a number of reasons, this deficiency is slowly being corrected and several colleges of pharmacy have developed significant clinical faculties which use health-care institutions as laboratories for their students, thus permitting them contact with patients, nurses, physicians and other members of the health-care team in an appropriate setting. This could lead to the development of a new attitude of social interdependence on the part of students of the health professions with each recognizing more fully the capabilities and strengths of the others in the health-care delivery system. In turn, this recognition could hopefully lead to the development of a greater health role for the pharmacist and his pharmacy as part of the community's subsystem of health-care facilities, greater than that described by Sanders who cites only the functions of filling prescriptions written by physicians and selling nonprescription drugs as he presides over his mercantile emporium.[1] Before any significant advancement can take place, however, the pharmacist must practice not in an emporium but as a part of a health-related system in close association with the patient and members of the other health professions. It is in this context then that the social psychological role of the pharmacist must be examined.

The social psychological role is a new and important one for pharmacy in terms of both its purpose and its fulfillment. The purpose of the pharmacist is to serve the health needs of the public for health-related commodities and health-related information. He accomplishes this by dispensing medication prescribed by physicians and other practitioners, by furnishing prescription-free over-the-counter (OTC) medication selected by the patient himself, sometimes but not often enough in consultation with the pharmacist, and by supplying related health commodities. In addition, he also furnishes health and drug related information to patients, to the general public and to members of the other health professions.

The role of the pharmacist in supplying medication to the public is, in general, well performed. However, when he limits his performance to this function his purpose lacks fulfillment. This is a function carried out by pharmacy technicians in many countries, and one which will surely be done more efficiently by machines in the years to come. Unfortunately, pharmacists have been conditioned by a limited conception of the role of the pharmacist in society, first by colleges of pharmacy which have until recently almost completely lacked a clinical faculty or a clinical component, and reinforced later by the traditional community standard of practice with its greatest emphasis on non-health-related matters. Once the act of preparing the medicines the pharmacist dispenses was taken over by the large manufacturing establishments during the nineteenth century, it became necessary for the profession to develop new functions related to the public health in order to sustain and reinforce its purpose for being. In this, the profession has made only a small beginning.

Pharmacists must concentrate on perfecting new skills to satisfy their purpose. The pharmacist of tomorrow must broaden his horizons, widen his skills, deepen his knowledge and know much more than he does today about such subjects as the sociology of illness, principles of disease prevention and public health issues in general. He must serve not only the patient who is sick, but he must also advise the person who is well about his health needs. He is poorly prepared to do this by his present education which is so lacking in the social and behavioral sciences.[2] Pharmacy practice requires an understanding of the cultural and social forces which influence the patient's recognition that he needs help, his decision to seek medical care, and his response to it. The pharmacist must be aware not only of the pharmacological and pharmaceutical aspects of drug response but also of the social and psychological factors involved. The social psychological perspective is concerned with the ways individuals interact, communicate and influence each other. It illuminates the manner in which individuals affect the social process and how their intra-psychic states and personalities are molded within the context of social processes.[3]

The significance of the social and psychological role of the pharmacist has been lost in the evolution of pharmacy from the days of the apothecary shop to those of the present chain drugstores. Pharmacy will continue to make grave errors unless its importance is recaptured and utilized in the education of pharmacy students, in communicating with patients and health practitioners, and in designing socially oriented and patient oriented services.

Development of a Professional Self-Image

The development of a professional self-image is extremely important for the clinical pharmacist. History has demonstrated that when great social changes occur in a profession they do not alter the attitude and values of its members until a significant number of them assume new roles and perform successfully in them for two or three generations. Thus, it will require considerable time for pharmacy to transform itself and to change its pattern of practice. Only recently have there been developing conditions favorable to a change.

Pharmacy students have heretofore lacked good professional models to follow. Those who wanted to become pharmaceutical scientists could, of course, follow the model set by their professor. But those who wished to become professional practitioners found their professors inappropriate models because they themselves almost never engaged in the practice of pharmacy. Thus while they may have served as excellent models for the student preparing for research, they were unsuitable models for those preparing for a career in professional practice. The few deans of pharmacy schools who attempted to create model community pharmacies were thwarted by local and state pharmaceutical associations so that the only models students had to follow were those projected by pharmacists in a wide diversity of community pharmacies, in chain drugstores, and in a few scattered prescription pharmacies. The vast majority of these models are quite unsuitable for a professional person who plans to serve the public health.

A few years ago hospital practitioners decided that advanced education and training were desirable for specialization in a hospital-based practice. As a result, a number of colleges and teaching hospitals combined resources and offered advanced academic training either at the Master's or Pharm.D. level accompanied by an accredited internship or residency program. We are now in the process of training the third generation of practitioners and there are now in practice several hundred good models for a new generation of hospital pharmacists to follow. Students desiring to enter community practice still suffer from a paucity of good professional models and this deficit appears to grow rapidly as the number of community pharmacies decrease while the number of chain drugstores expand.

Pharmacy students should be able to develop a professional self-image in a manner similar to that used by physicians and nurses.[4,5] Medical students develop a self-image as a doctor early because of their social interaction with medical school faculty, medical residents, interns, fellows, nurses, dieticians, patients, classmates and others. These contacts are established in the student's first year of medical school and they grow and develop until by his third or fourth year he has developed a strong self-image of himself as a physician and tends to live up to the role expectation of others. One of the strongest influences in the medical student's development of a self-image are the patients to whom he is assigned, initially as an observer and later as an advisor on health problems. Pharmacy students do not have the opportunity to form a public health oriented self-image because they are not in contact with those who can help them until their course is almost over and then it is almost too late. Pharmacists need the right type of contact early in their educational process. Students learn not only from didactic instruction of their professors and from the precepts of practitioners; they learn perhaps more enduringly from their sustained involvement with the patient, physicians, nurses, dieticians and other members of the health-care team in an institution devoted to the care of the sick guided by the model of a clinically oriented pharmacist with whom they can readily identify.

In becoming a professional, a student "internalizes and makes his own the attitudes and values which will largely determine his future professional role."[6] Professionalization is thus "a growth concept which pictures the development in human individuals of a professional self, an identity in the role of doctor."[6] There is a professional culture that determines how the young professional will think and act. The values that it inculcates will create attitudes, or attitudinal predispositions, in the light of which experience will be evaluated and by which behavior will be judged.

Accelerate Research in Community Practice

Now that pharmaceutical education is beginning to adopt a clinical component to give the student a better understanding of the patient and to enhance his ability to communicate with the physician, it should turn its attention toward establishing community prescription pharmacies for the education and training of professional practitioners. We are not talking about a college-operated student health service pharmacy, but rather, one that serves the population of a town or city and thus would be a pharmacy servicing a representative population. There must be a concerted, nationwide effort on the part of the colleges to train pharmacists in clinical practice under ideal conditions in an establishment operated, controlled and supervised by the college and preferably part of a health-care group practice. The pharmacy should be designed and constructed for teaching and research purposes and should be operated by professional practitioners holding appointments on the faculty.

Such a pharmacy would reflect the best in pharmaceutical practice for students to emulate. It would establish patterns, explore new possibilities, conduct research, investigate unmet health needs and test new potential roles for pharmacists. It would be a living, viable, dynamic part of the college's instructional program with which the prospective community pharmacist could identify, in a manner similar to the way in which hospital pharmacists identify with the hospital in which they serve their residency. The pharmaceutical center could provide a model for all undergraduate students and would be an essential tool for the training of Doctor of Pharmacy candidates. We know the arguments against colleges engaging in activities of this type, but those in favor of it are so overwhelming that it could gain strong support from community pharmacists if properly explained. Community pharmacists who oppose the undertaking of such a project by the colleges for fear of losing prescription business are sowing the seeds of their own destruction. While they expend their energy in opposing the opening of one pharmacy by a college of pharmacy, a corporation may open ten or more units in the same city and pharmacists are powerless to do anything about it. In many cases, pressures from local and state pharmaceutical associations and pharmacy owners make it impossible for the colleges to move in this direction.[7] In these cases, we suggest that it would be entirely appropriate for the clinical faculty of the college to establish a nonprofit corporation whose tripartite objectives would be patient service, education and research into new roles for the pharmacist in group practice situations. These proposals would be similar in nature to those group practices now established by the faculties of 38 schools of medicine.[8]

THE PATIENT'S RELATIONSHIP WITH HIS PHYSICIAN

Every society has its healer. The medicine man, the witch doctor and the physician are closely related because the origin of disease was at one time thought to be supernatural, religious or mystical. The medicine man or witch doctor treated these ailments by means of various rites, ceremonies and incantations, often augmented by herbs and other medicine to relieve or cure the patient.[9] Later, as disease came to be increasingly regarded as more biological than supernatural or religious in nature, its treatment fell into the hands of the physician whose training in the biological sciences replaced the religious training of his counterpart. Even today, however, the magical connotations of the physician's power have not disappeared completely.

As the biological sciences unfolded and as new knowledge developed, the physician began to concern himself more with specific organs, tissues and cells and to develop greater specificity in his work with patients. As knowledge in the medical sciences increased, the physician tended to turn away from the patient as a whole person and to concentrate on the pathology of the disease process itself. This process finally led to specialization in the practice of medicine and a greater complexity in the physician-patient relationship.

The decline in the number of family doctors has been correlated with the increase in the number and the demand for services of specialists in psychiatry, pediatrics and internal medicine who treat psychophysiologic illness and who claim to be the "only" physicians who treat the "whole person".[9]

Affecting the patient's relationship with his physician has been the shift in the place where they ordinarily meet. The early practice of medicine was conducted almost exclusively in the home where the patient was often confined to bed surrounded by his family which afforded him great emotional support, showed its concern for him and was available at his beck and call to serve his needs. In this setting the patient-physician relationship was close, warm and supportive.

At that time, the physician's office was a secondary place for seeing the patient but, as the technology of medicine continued to increase, it soon became the primary place of treatment as the need to possess and to concentrate complex medical equipment grew. Later, as technology developed more rapidly and as instruments became more expensive, the hospital rapidly came into the forefront as the place to receive medical treatment. The use of the hospital as a treatment center was accelerated by the rapid rise in specialization of physicians and their need for expensive, sophisticated instrumentation, equipment and supportive services.[10]

The change in the treatment site from the patient's home, to the physician's office and then to the hospital in which neither usually had proprietary rights has affected fundamentally the patient's relationship with his physician. In the patient's home, the physician was welcomed by the family as a healer and a close personal relationship was established among the physician, the patient and members of the family. When the patient went to the physician's office the relationship between the two became more formal but still retained certain elements of their relationship in the home. However, when the patient went to the hospital his relationship with his physician was altered almost beyond recognition. Here the patient finds himself a stranger in an unknown land. His treatment setting includes many total strangers who take his pulse, temperature, x-rays, urine, blood, bring his meals, administer medications, ask personal questions and too often dehumanize and depersonalize him. In addition to his own physician, a number of other people come to see, observe, manipulate, question, and in other ways establish contact with him. These include medical interns and residents, other medical specialists called as consultants by his physician, nurses, pharmacists, dieticians, technicians of various sorts and in some hospitals a whole bevy of students of the health professions who examine, probe, question, awaken and interrupt him in an effort to determine some biological or physical factor contributing to his illness.

Many patients, however, have functional ailments without apparent physical etiology. These the health professions are generally poorly equipped to treat and the hospital setting does not seem an ideal place to carry out the treatment because the patient's relationships with his physician and other health professionals are so segmentalized. This is one of the reasons the behavioral sciences including sociology, cultural anthropology and social psychology are assuming more and more importance in health care and why those trained in clinical pharmacy need them for a better understanding of the whole patient and his problems. Today, the patient is often treated by a specialist he has never seen before. He is sometimes referred to several specialists for consultation. In many outpatient clinics, the patient seldom sees the same physician the second time. He is cared for by people who are strangers to him, who too often regard him as a "case" and know nothing of his social, psychological or cultural needs. Thus the old pattern of relationship between the physician and the patient is broken. The development of multiple specialties in medicine tends to accelerate this process.

The pattern of the patient's relationship to the physician is in certain ways the reflection of the pattern of medical education. Prior to the Flexner report, the medical trainee served an apprenticeship during which he saw patients in their home environment and studied disease first hand at the bedside. Later, proprietary schools were established where students were taught primarily by the didactic method in which the lecture and the book replaced direct observation and the student was removed from the living patient. The inadequacy of this method led to the Flexner report with its resultant reforms. The student returned to the patient but as Flexner stated so well "relying no longer altogether on the senses with which nature endowed him, but those senses made infinitely more acute, more accurate, and more helpful by the processes and instruments which the . . . (previous) half century's progress . . . placed at his disposal."[11] The students' return to the patient took, however, a completely new turn. It was not to the whole patient he returned, but to the patient's disease. The new instrumentation, the new methods of diagnosis, the many new discoveries in the basic sciences all tended to focus the attention of the student and the physician on the patient's disease rather than on his needs. This produced a dehumanizing effect about which so many patients complain today.

Illness Behavior of Patients

The manner in which different people respond to the same disease condition may vary markedly. One person may become unduly worried over very mild symptoms and display profound social and psychological reactions. He readily seeks medical attention and has a great tendency to become dependent on others. Another person may attempt to ignore the symptoms of the disease and avoid seeking medical care. Thus, the study of illness behavior involves not only those people who seek medical care but also those people who do not, and the response to illness determines the utilization of health care facilities in the community.

What factors influence the person's decision as to whether or not he will seek medical advice? Many patients first attempt to rationalize the problem and to cope with it within the boundaries of their intellectual, social and cultural backgrounds.[12] This "first line of defense" is not always rational from a medical point of view. If the symptoms persist, the person may casually discuss them with a relative, friend or work associate and explore the various possibilities for the cause of his illness. He may visit the community pharmacy and purchase some patent medicines "which worked" when he did not feel well a few months ago. Or the person may discuss his symptoms with the pharmacist and seek his professional opinion. The outcome of this discussion will depend very much on the ability of the pharmacist to understand the various forces motivating human behavior and to communicate effectively with the patient. The ill person may also seek the advice of clergymen, lawyers, chiropractors, etc. as to whether he should see a physician, and if so, which one. He may even make an appointment with a doctor in order to compare the physician's diagnosis with his own.[12] In summary, the seeking of professional help commonly occurs through a process which has been described as a "lay referral system":

> The whole process of seeking help involves a network of potential consultants, from the intimate and informal confines of the nuclear family through successively more select, distant, authoritative laymen, until the "professional" is reached. This network of consultants, which is part of the structure of the local lay community and which imposes form on the seeking of help, might be called the "lay referral structure." Taken together with the cultural understandings involved in the process, we may speak of it as the "lay referral system."[12]

The lay referral system is but one factor which influences the response to illness. The person must first experience symptoms which deviate from his normal state of health. The intensity and persistence of these symptoms and the degree of discomfort they cause are critical in the help-seeking process. Rheumatoid arthritis is an example of a disease which varies widely in chronicity and frequency of exacerbations. The more frequent and severe the exacerbations, the more likely the individual will seek medical advice. There are many insidious diseases *i.e.* gonorrhea, rheumatic heart disease, pulmonary tuberculosis and cancer, which progress while the patient appears asymptomatic.

The seriousness of the symptom as perceived by the person is another important consideration. It is highly unlikely that a mother who discovers that her three-year old child has just swallowed a bottle of aspirin tablets will not seek medical assistance. In contrast, if the child is complaining of "stomach ache" or a sore throat, it is less likely that the mother will telephone the physician. The same argument can be applied to the adult population. Regardless of how stoical a person is, an acute pulmonary embolism or a fractured limb will usually force him to seek medical care. Mere shortness of breath, however, is not an alarming signal to every person. The significance of anxiety and fear in the seeking of care is not definitely established. Some anxiety about illness may lead to a shorter delay in seeking care whereas a high level of fear may lead to denial of symptoms and reluctance to seek medical attention.[13]

Pain may be the most important initial symptom which alerts the individual to the fact that something is wrong.[14] People vary greatly in the amount of pain they are able to tolerate. One study is reported in which equal numbers of Christians and Jews were subjected to pain produced by a modified blood pressure cuff which was fitted with hard rubber projections that pressed into the subject's arm when inflated. The volunteers were told after the first session that the study was designed to evaluate some research that stated their particular group (Christians or Jews) could not tolerate as much pain as the other group. During the second trial, both the Jewish and Christian subjects tolerated a significantly greater degree of pain than they had before they were aware of the fictitious purpose of the trial. It was concluded that the amount of pain people are willing to tolerate depends partly upon the significance and meaning attached to the pain and also upon the amount of pain the patient is normally accustomed to. Because of this factor, many people commonly ignore minor physical complaints and only a small percentage of human ailments are ever brought to the attention of a physician.

The tolerance threshold for pain varies from one culture to another. Specific cultures have definite attitudes toward pain and parents teach their children, either directly or indirectly, the manner in which they are expected to react toward pain.[15] "Old Americans" tend to be highly stoic and the Irish deny pain frequently.[12] Members of both Italian and Jewish cultures are very sensitive to pain and commonly exhibit highly emotional responses.[15] Although the reactions between these two groups to pain appear similar, the underlying attitudes differ. Patients of Italian origin appear to be worried about the effects of the pain upon their immediate situation. They seek relief from pain and are satisfied once relief is obtained. In contrast, patients of Jewish origin are primarily concerned with the meaning and significance of their pain on their future welfare.

Jewish and Italian patients also demonstrate different attitudes toward the physician.[15] Italian patients usually display more confidence in the doctor and this confidence is reinforced once the physician relieves the pain. Jewish patients are more skeptical and even when the pain is relieved by some drug, they often consult other physicians in order to check the original physician's diagnosis.

Sociocultural features of the family environment are often very important. Mexican-American families have strong kinship bonds; the family authority is centralized in the husband-father; and the patient commonly displays great resistance to separation from the family.[16] A high degree of psychological dependency develops within the family unit. As a result, many Mexican-Americans are reluctant to accept medical treatment regimens and it is psychologically difficult for the family members to "let go" of the member who is sick.

The significance of cultural factors is valuable in understanding the great differences in behavioral trends among various groups. One must remember that no two people are exactly alike. Each individual in a particular culture does not share the same reactions and attitudes toward illness. Age, sex, religion, education, and socio-economic background are other variables which play a role in molding individual variations within each group. In a study of illness behavior of children, age and sex were the most prominent factors. Boys were more stoic than girls, and older children were more stoic than younger children. This finding correlates with the observation that women utilize health facilities more than do men.[12] Religion may have a large influence on the pervading concept of illness.[17] For example, the Christian Scientist believes that illness is an error which can be cleared up with the assistance of a religious practitioner. The Jehovah's Witness believes that there will be no death for the faithful believers. In this respect, medical interference may be a sign of lack of faith for the believer who expects to be made perfect when the world is scheduled to end.

Some physicians place heavy emphasis on the patient's knowledge of illness as a determining factor in the initial decision to seek medical care and cooperate later in the prescribed medical regimen.[18] The public is becoming more sophisticated about medical matters and great variations have been found between the highest and lowest social classes in the recognition that certain symptoms *i.e.* chest pain, lumps in the breast or abdomen, blood in stools, require medical attention.[12,14] The public knows more about arthritis, birth defects, and cancer because these are the most fearful diseases.[12] Tagliacozzo and Ima[18] found that knowledge played a significant role in the behavior of patients who had very limited experience with illness and who viewed their illnesses as interfering with their daily activities. However, patients with a low level of knowledge but with substantial experience with their illness were as likely to seek medical care as those patients with a high level of knowledge. Patients with a high degree of medical knowledge *i.e.* nurses, medical students, and pharmacists often spend a great deal of time attempting to treat themselves, but they usually go directly from self-treatment to a physician. Knowledge of illness is an important aspect of the help-seeking process and, thus, is a determining factor in preventive health care.

People are more likely to become concerned about their health if their symptoms interfere with social, family or work activities. For example, the crippling deformities of the hands associated with rheumatoid arthritis may pose a threat to the psychological security of a housewife. The manner in which a person interprets his symptoms also depends on the nature of his life and work situation. A person who performs heavy manual labor all day expects to be tired and will less likely consider fatigue as being indicative of illness. Students studying for exams are more likely to consider headache a result of eyestrain rather than an alarming symptom. In contrast, strep throats and fevers are symptoms which cannot easily be rationalized. In general, psychosomatic complaints can often be rationalized within frames of reference according to the individual rather than to illness.

A final and important factor in the orientation of society to seek medical care is the accessibility of health facilities. The physical proximity of the health center, the hours of operation, the receptive atmosphere of the health personnel, the lack of embarrassment and stigma resulting from his disease, and the cost of the treatments clearly influence the use of medical facilities. The existence of a relationship between socio-economic status and the seeking of medical assistance has also been established.[12,19] Persons of higher socio-economic status are more likely to buy health insurance, to eat balanced meals, and to receive annual medical check-ups. Cultural beliefs may be a link between socio-economic status and health care utilization.[19] Mechanic[20] has demonstrated that an attitude of fatalism is more prevalent in the lower socio-economic levels and less stigma is attached to medical ailments. Poverty may also produce an attitude of discontent which may lead to discontinuity in the use of health care facilities. In the United States, both physician and dentist utilization is positively correlated with the socio-economic status of the patient. In contrast, there is no such correlation in Great Britain where medical services are available without cost.[12] Therefore, the impact upon the family finances

Table 1. Rates of Noncompliance with Drug Recommendations

Investigator and Diagnosis	Measure Used	Drug	No. of Patients	Percentage of Noncompliance
Bergman and Werner streptococcal infections	Pill count	Penicillin	59	56 by 3rd day 71 by 6th day 82 by 9th day
	Urine test	Penicillin	41 of above 59	54 by 3rd day 69 by 6th day 92 by 9th day
Berry *et al.* tuberculosis	Urine test	INH PAS	26 26	6 8
Bonnar *et al.* pregnancy	Blood hemoglobin & stool specimen	Iron tablets	60	32 (after 2 mos.)
Brette tuberculosis	Urine test	PAS	76	65
Charney *et al.* streptococcal infections	Urine test	Penicillin	459	19% of 107 children on 5th day 44% of 352 children on 9th day
Chaves tuberculosis	Urine test	PAS	2622	39
Dixon *et al.* tuberculosis	Urine test	PAS	151	50
Feinstein *et al.* rheumatic fever	Patient report	Penicillin	113	27
	Pill count	Penicillin	109 of above 113	45
	Patient report	Sulfadiazine	126	33
	Pill count	Sulfadiazine	120 of above 126	67
Fox tuberculosis	Urine test	PAS	79	4
Gordis *et al.* rheumatic fever	Urine test Child or parent report	Penicillin Penicillin	103 same 103	20-35 9-15
Gordis *et al.* rheumatic fever	Urine test	Penicillin	136	36
Ireland tuberculosis	Patient report and whether returned for drugs	PAS, INH, and Streptomycin	87	74
Jenkins miscellaneous	Pill count	Various	22	50
Johnson myocardial infarction	Patient report	Various	162	23
Joyce arthritis	Urine test	Phenylbutazone C20410	38	65% of 108 samples
	Return of extra pills	Placebo	78	38
Leggat tuberculosis	Urine test	PAS	50	22
Leistyna and Macaulay streptococcal infections	Combination of urine test and return of remaining medication	Penicillin	144	11
Lipman *et al.* psychiatric	Pill count	Meprobamate Placebo	125 129	42 49
Luntz and Austin tuberculosis	Urine test	PAS	705	34
Maddock tuberculosis	Urine test	INH PAS	50 33	30 42
Mohler *et al.* streptococcal infections	Patient report	Penicillin	161	34
Morrow and Rabin tuberculosis	Urine test	INH	350	32
Neely and Patrick miscellaneous (elderly ambulatory)	Patient report	Various	236	59
Nugent *et al.* arthritis	Pill count	Prednisolone	20	25
Park and Lipman psychiatric	Pill count Patient report	Imipramine Placebo	36 (same)	51% of 117 samples 15% of 117 samples
Parkes *et al.* psychiatric	Patient report	Tranquilizers	100	44
Pitman *et al.* tuberculosis	Urine test	PAS	61	41

INVESTIGATOR AND DIAGNOSIS	MEASURE USED	DRUG	NO. OF PATIENTS	PERCENTAGE OF NONCOMPLIANCE
Preston and Miller tuberculosis	Urine test	PAS and INH	25	28
Roth and Berger ulcer and other gastric	Measured amount remaining in bottle	Antacid	75 85	43 (ulcer patients) 62 (other gastric patients)
Simpson tuberculosis	Urine test	PAS	100	24
Watkins *et al.* diabetes	Observation of patient and patient report	Insulin	115	35
	Patient report	Oral hypoglycemic drugs	47	23
Willcox *et al.* psychiatric	Urine test	Chlorpromazine and Imipramine	125	48
Wynn-Williams and Arris tuberculosis	Urine test	PAS	153	49

[a]Based on 145 urine samples from 26 patients
[b]Data on which these figures are based are unclear

may be a deciding factor in obtaining medical care.

In summary, the various ways in which patients respond to symptoms of sickness are products of their social and cultural environments. In order to understand the process of illness, one must appreciate the patient's perspective. Illness behavior is a dynamic response of the individual to control his environment and to overcome obstacles which interfere with his normal living pattern.

Patient's Compliance with Physician's Directions

Studies have shown that from 15 to 93 percent of all unsupervised patients are noncompliant with the physician's instructions relative to their use of medication.[21,22] If a patient does not adhere to the drug schedule, it is impossible for the physician to accurately assess the efficacy of the drugs prescribed. If the patient shows no response to a usually effective regimen, the physician may needlessly redesign the drug regimen or may even question the accuracy of his diagnosis. The most common types of medication errors made by patients include omission of doses, self-medication, incorrect dosages, and incorrect dosage schedules.[23] If the patient does not take his medications correctly, the entire efforts of the health team may be rendered futile. It is essential that the physician and the pharmacist recognize the variables involved in drug defaulting. Compliance is not a major problem in the treatment of hospitalized patients; however, the ambulatory patient is not under the constant supervision of a doctor and nurse and he is responsible for his own drug therapy. Table 1 shows the rates of noncompliance tabulated after a review of the literature.[22]

Human behavior varies from those patients who require a great deal of supervision in their drug therapy to those who are very reliable and require very little supervision. The literature is inconclusive with respect to the demographic attributes that characterize a noncompliant patient.[24-28] The significance of age, sex, ethnic background, duration of illness, marital status, and religious attitude on patient cooperation remains to be determined. The extent to which the suggested drug regimen interferes with the normal living pattern of the individual is an important feature of compliance. Patients on a once-daily dosage tend to have a higher compliance ratio than those on divided dosages.[27,29] As the number of medications prescribed for a patient increases, the number of medication errors does not always rise proportionately.[23] This may be explained by the fact that patients with complicated regimens usually receive special assistance in adapting the drug schedule to their daily routine of life. Family discord is closely associated with noncompliance while family cohesiveness during crises reinforces the doctor's recommendations.[30] Many patients do not understand the importance of following the physician's instructions or the reasons a particular drug has been prescribed. Inaccurate and incomplete knowledge can lead to dangerous repercussions. Teamwork between the physician and the pharmacist could have prevented the following incident:

> He (the doctor) explained it so carefully and the nurse went over them too before I left the clinic. He even said "now three of these are medicines which you'll only have to take for a little while. But this one is very important: you're going to have to remember to take this every day or you're

> going to be in trouble." He even folded the prescription differently for the important medicine. But I don't think he knows that you turn them all in together at the pharmacy and wait. And when you get them there's no way to know which one was the folded prescription. And the heart medicine doesn't look as important as the other kind does.[23]

Some patients discontinue their drug therapy if they experience certain side effects or if they feel the medication is not helping them.[31] The patient may be alerted to the consequences of irregular self-administration of his drugs if unpleasant symptoms result. Two examples are the treatment of epilepsy with anticonvulsants and the treatment of auricular fibrillation with digitalis. However, the consequences of omission of doses are not immediately apparent to the patient suffering from such quiescent diseases as pulmonary tuberculosis and rheumatic heart disease. It is this type of patient who is highly susceptible to drug defaulting.

It has been suggested that the patient who is satisfied with his physician will be more likely to comply with the medical advice than the patient who feels his needs were not met by the medical visit.[24] No plan of treatment which the patient rejects or does not fully accept can be of complete benefit to him. The cooperation of the patient depends not only upon his reaction to the entire social system but also upon the infringement his drug schedule will have on his daily life. It is, therefore, essential that the patient's reaction to medical advice and his degree of acceptance of it are considered in planning any drug regimen.[32] It must also be remembered that there will always be a small number of uncooperative patients who will resist medical advice regardless of the amount of exhortation of the physician and the pharmacist.

Factors Influencing Patient's Response to Drugs

The drug response which a patient experiences after receiving a particular medication is not solely due to the pharmacological and biopharmaceutical parameters inherent in the drug product. Non-drug variables which contribute to the clinical response include:

1. Attitude of the patient
2. Cultural and familial influences
3. Compliance with the drug regimen
4. Placebo effect.

Just as attitudes towards illness vary not only among social systems but also within each social system, human values and attitudes toward the use of drugs vary notably. Some people practice "TV medicine" and believe that drugs will provide almost instantaneous relief from physical, mental, emotional and social problems of illness. Still other people consider drugs as a "crutch" and an unnecessary luxury in modern society. Environmental and personal experiences are influential in the response of the patient to medical care. His feelings about therapy are often as critical to successful therapy as his feelings about illness are to the seeking of medical care.

Cultural differences exist in the attitudes toward drugs. Jewish and Italian patients have been reported to respond differently toward pain-relieving drugs.[15] The Italian patient readily requests and accepts an analgesic to relieve his immediate suffering and forgets his suffering once the pain is relieved. However, the Jewish patient is more reluctant to accept an analgesic because he is concerned with the long-term effects of the drug upon his general health and the habit-forming risks of the drugs. In addition, he feels that the drug will only relieve his pain and will not cure the disease which is causing the discomfort. Therefore, with many Jewish patients it is important to relieve the anxieties they have about the source of their pain before any drugs are prescribed.

The family is influential in the patient's reactions to drug therapy. For example, when a physician prescribes insulin for a patient suffering from diabetes mellitus, the attitude of the family to daily injections is important to the success of the therapy. After the patient has finally accepted the diagnosis, his family may react by saying, "It's terrible, you will look like a pin-cushion" or "Are you sure there is not a tablet or something you could take instead?" It is in this situation that the physician, nurse, and pharmacist can explain to the family that insulin is a natural substance of the body and is not a means of punishment but rather is necessary for the patient to live. The patient is also influenced by previous experiences members of his family or friends have had with drugs. If one of his acquaintances had a severe allergic reaction to Telepaque tablets, it is quite probable that the patient with gall bladder problems will fear that his physician will prescribe these tablets. Because of this one basic fear, the entire response of the patient to medical care and to hospitalization could be adversely affected. The cost of drugs to the family is another important aspect of drug therapy. In spite of the desire of the patient to follow the physician's instructions, the impact of drug treatment on the family finances may be the deciding factor which will prevent the purchase of the medication.

The Placebo

It is estimated that from 50 to 80 percent of patients consulting a physician have symptoms which are emotional rather than physical in origin. This percentage has changed little since the time of Galen who judged that about 60 percent of his patients had emotional rather than physical problems.[33] For thousands of years physicians have prescribed what we know now to have been ineffective and useless medications. Still, for thousands of years physicians have helped patients and despite scientific advances, the placebo still remains an important component in treatment of the patient.

Shapiro[33] has defined a placebo as follows:

> A placebo is any therapy, or component of therapy, that is deliberately or knowingly used for its nonspecific psychophysiologic effect, or that is used unknowingly for its presumed or believed specific effect on a patient, symptom, or illness, but which, unknown to the patient and therapist, is without specific activity for the condition being treated.

Thus, placebos may be either active or inactive drugs. For example, subtherapeutic doses of phenothiazine tranquilizers are active placebos while lactose is an inactive one.

The placebo effect is thus the nonspecific psychologic or psychophysiologic response produced by placebos. The placebo effect of drugs should never be underestimated. It may explain why two individuals receiving the same drug sometimes show completely different clinical responses. The placebo effect is especially significant in the response to drugs which act on the central nervous system. Age, sex, marital status, education, occupation and personality of the patient may be related to the placebo response.[34] In addition, a patient's prior experience with a given form of chemotherapy may influence his response to subsequent drug treatment.[35] Physical characteristics of the drug product may be an important determinant.[36] The expectations of the patient as well as the enthusiasm of the physician are also capable of altering the therapeutic response.[37] This physician-patient relationship has been referred to as "transference", a process whereby feelings such as love, hate, trust and distrust which the patients attached to significant persons such as his parents in the past are shifted to the physician in the present.[33] Those who expect comfort and help despite fright and discomfort are probably one group of positive placebo reactors. The patient's transference relationship to his physician and the physician's countertransference relationship with the patient are highly important in placebo reactions and in their direction—positive, negative or absent. The physician contributes to the placebo reaction by his interest in the patient and by his interest in the treatment.

Some of the less controversial indications for the use of placebos cited by Shapiro[33] include: (1) for patients with degenerative, malignant, or incurable diseases for which there is no specific treatment available; (2) for patients hospitalized for prolonged investigation who become impatient while undergoing tests; (3) for patients with a confusing clinical course, as a substitution for drugs which may contribute obfuscating symptoms; (4) for weening postoperative patients from opiates to prevent habituation; and (5) for elderly or chronic patients who have become accustomed to taking medication of questionable value, to differentiate

Table 2. Effectiveness of Placebos in Relieving Pain of Pathological Origin

Study Identification	Number of Subjects	Percentage Satisfactorily Relieved by Placebo
Severe Postoperative Wound		
A	118	21
B	29	31
C	34	26
D*	52	40
	36	26
	44	34
	40	32
E**	14	50
	20	37
	15	53
	21	40
	15	40
	15	15
Pain from Angina Pectoris		
F	66	38
G	19	26
H	27	38
Pain from Metastatic Disease		
I	67	42
Headache		
J	199	52
Totals (10 studies)	831	34.6±2.9

*Average percentage relieved by placebo was 33 percent
**Average percentage relieved by placebo was 39 percent

psychologic from nonpsychologic side effects in psychochemotherapy.

Least controversial is the use of placebos as a control in research in the evaluation of therapy.

The attitudes of health personnel toward drugs are often demonstrated in their verbal communications with the patient and may contribute significantly to the placebo effect.[22] For example, some physicians tell their patients: "This drug I am prescribing is going to help you feel better" or "This medication has helped many people who have had your same illness." Other physicians make the following comment when handing the prescription to the patient: "Get this prescription filled and come back to see me in a week to see if the drug has worked!" The effectiveness of placebos in relieving pain of pathological origin of various types is shown in Table 2.[60] In summary, a patient's response to a medication is influenced by the interaction of the drug and situational setting with the patient. Patients are not treated in a vacuum. They respond to the social forces of the hospital and medical clinic and the psychological forces of the various people they come in contact with during the illness cycle.

PATIENT'S RELATIONSHIP TO HIS PHARMACIST

Although the increase in medical specialization has tended to weaken the physician-patient relationship, it has not altered its fundamental form. The patient is a sick person or one who believes he is ill. He consults the physician who remains the same type of authoritarian figure as the ancient medicine man in other societies. The patient comes to the physician with faith in his competence to relieve his pain, restore his health, or arrest or cure his disease. He comes to the physician seeking help by all available means including cure by the use of instruments, procedures and medication. The patient also approaches the physician with a characteristic set of personality and cultural values to which the physician must respond. The patient craves health, security and self-esteem yet at the same time his illness makes him anxious and dependent. He needs psychological support badly and today's specialist rarely supplies it in sufficient quantity. The aim of the clinical pharmacist must be to take up where the physician leaves off and to supply to the patient some of his psychological needs in a humanitarian and compassionate manner.

The objective of the clinical pharmacist should be to transfer to himself the idealized attitude and relationship of the patient to his physician. This transfer should carry with it a portion of the confidence, respect, dependency and other desirable attributes felt by the patient toward his physician. The clinical pharmacist should partially replace the physician in fulfilling the psychological needs of the patient yet at the same time be supportive of the physician's therapeutic aims.[39] This role implies several conditions and needs for the clinical pharmacist among which are: (1) appropriately dignified manner, attitude, conduct and manner of dress, (2) a professional setting in which to function, (3) discrimination in the selection of tasks to be performed, (4) a knowledge not only of drug actions and usage but also of many aspects of public health, and (5) a knowledge of illness behavior, social and psychological factors influencing health and disease and factors influencing the use and abuse of drugs by society, some of which have been discussed previously.

Attitude, Dress and Conduct of the Pharmacist

In order for the patient to transfer some of his feelings for the physician to the pharmacist, he must not see the pharmacist as an anonymous person without any interest in him or his complaints. On the contrary, the pharmacist must conduct himself in such a manner as to evoke from the patient feelings of confidence, respect and dependency toward him. These will develop as the pharmacist talks with the patient in a sympathetic, understanding and friendly manner. In doing this, the pharmacist must place himself in the same position relative to the patient as the physician does, that is in the dominant role. Smečka has discussed the relative roles of the pharmacist and patient in various types of situations.[39] He points out that the pharmacist must maintain the same relative position as the physician *vis a vis* the patient, that is the pharmacist must be the dominant partner while the patient remains the submissive partner. In his role as the dominant partner, the pharmacist accepts a portion of the trust, confidence and dependency transferred by the patient from his physician. In return, the pharmacist gives the patient advice regarding his medication, explains how he should take it, cautions him relative to possible side effects, listens to the patient's questions, answers them with knowledge and understanding and compassion and thus becomes, in reality, an independent professional practitioner who, nevertheless, is supportive of the physician's therapeutic aims.

As regards the appearance of the pharmacist, we shall make only one comment: If one seeks a professional role, one must prepare for it. Part of this preparation is a recognition that his appearance influences the confidence the patient will place in him and in his profession. The patient cannot believe that a person who fails to take care of his appearance will take good care of him. Thus, he finds it difficult to transfer his attiturde and feeling toward the physician to the uncomely pharmacist.

The Setting

The character of the pharmacy can do much to motivate the transfer of some of the patient's feelings toward his physician to the pharmacist. The ideal setting is a separate consultation room or a private area where the pharmacist can discuss the patient's needs with him. Here the pharmacist ideally engages in a type of consultation ceremony which establishes a personal, confidential relationship with the patient whose objective is to reinforce the therapeutic objectives of the physician.

The pharmacist is in a position to supervise the physician's instructions on the use of the drug, to examine the patient's memory and to reinforce the patient's faith in both his physician and the drug. Times are changing. Patients are asking pharmacists to assure them that the drugs which have been prescribed for them are *safe* whereas, a few years ago the public sought assurance from the pharmacist that the drug was 100 percent effective.[40] The psychodynamic relationship between the patient and the pharmacist is based upon interpersonal communication. The manner in which the pharmacist receives the prescription and hands the dispensed drug back to the patient is important. The comments made by each party during this professional ceremony influence not only the drug response of the patient but also the opinion of the patient toward the profession. The entire process must be conducted in a dignified manner exemplifying professional expertise. The personal appearance of the pharmacist and the professional milieu also contribute to the patient's response. The pharmacist is the last person of the health team to have contact with the ambulatory patient before he receives the prescribed medication. It is logical to assume that

Figure 1. It is difficult for the patient to transfer some of his feelings toward the physician to the pharmacist in this typical drugstore setting

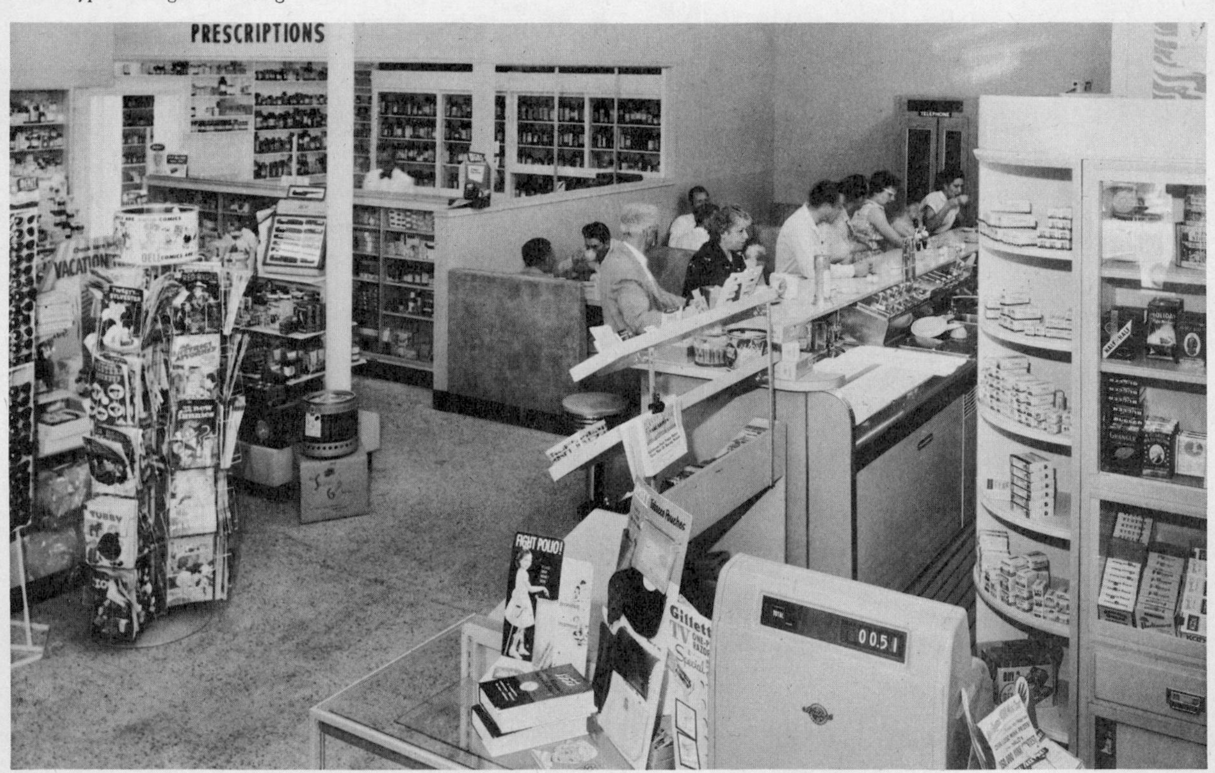

the pharmacist is in a situation where he is capable of either reinforcing or destroying the patient's attitude as developed by the physician.

It is also important whether or not the person comes to the pharmacy with the intention of having a prescription filled or of purchasing some item which does not require a prescription. The dispensing of prescribed medications represents the consummation of the entire professional process which began in the physician's office. The success of drug therapy depends partly upon the faith the patient has in his physician as well as in the medication. When the patient leaves the physician's office and enters the pharmacy, he anticipates that the professional conduct of the pharmacist will be equivalent to that of the physician. It is at this moment that the pharmacist can have a positive or negative effect on the success of the drug therapy. During the dispensing of the prescribed medication, the pharmacist assumes a dominant role and the patient willingly accepts a more passive role.[39] After all, the patient has entered the pharmacy with the knowledge that he is ill and needs help.

On the other hand, when the individual comes to the "drugstore" to buy an item that does not require a prescription, he enters with the attitude of a consumer.[39] He carries purchasing power in his pocket and usually knows what he wants to buy. Even if the pharmacist questions the safety or suitability of the medicament he has chosen, he does not have complete control over the person's final decision. The pharmacist has only persuasive power and the client is not obliged to accept his advice. In addition, the customer occasionally requests the pharmacist for his professional opinion on such commodities as charcoal briquets, garden or panty hose, beer and wine, motor oil, hardware and clothing items and picture frames which are sold in many drugstores. Under these circumstances, the customer equates the pharmacy with any other commercial outlet and forces the pharmacist into a submissive role.[39] This situation is deplorable and incompatible with the education and the role of the pharmacist in society.

The pharmacy-patient consultation offices introduced by Brands into the hospitals of the Public Health Service's Indian Health Service

Figure 2. The waiting room in the Indian Health Medical Center, Public Health Service, Phoenix, showing two private consultation rooms for pharmacist-patient communication

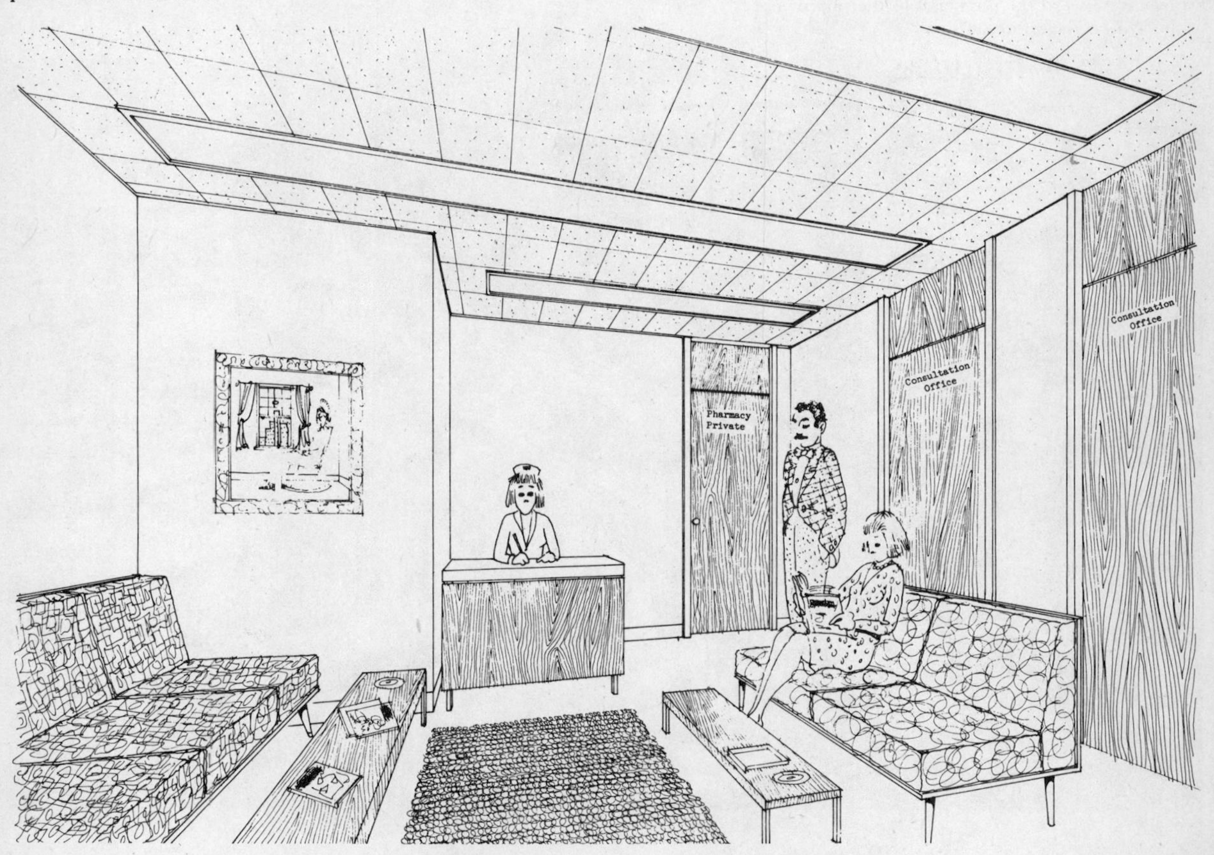

are pioneering efforts.[41] The consultation office is used for the pharmacists to instruct and advise patients in the correct use of their prescription medications. The office provides privacy in a professional setting for the pharmacist and the patient in this important function.

The pharmacy has two consultation offices located adjacent to the pharmacy waiting room. A receptionist is located in the waiting room. Prescriptions are written in the patient's health record. The health record is sent to the pharmacy by pneumatic tube or carried by an aide from the outpatient department. By receiving the patient's health record, the pharmacist has the complete medical history and current diagnosis and treatment prescribed for the patient, and he can serve as a true drug therapy advisor to the patient. With incomplete patient information, it is not possible to serve as a true consultant and advisor to the patient and the physician.

In the privacy of the patient consultation office it is possible to give thorough and complete instructions on the use of prescription medication to the patient without embarrassment to him and to maintain the confidentiality of the prescription, which cannot generally be done over an open counter or through a dispensing window with other people nearby. The pharmacist can even demonstrate the use of the medicine, use models, pictures and drawings for a better understanding by the patient. He can show the patient how full to fill an insulin syringe, how much ointment to use, and what a 1/3 dropperful is. Then he can assure himself that the patient understands, and the patient can ask questions.

One patient consultation office is planned for each 15,000 prescriptions filled annually. This amounts to 60 prescriptions a day for each office. There is one outpatient pharmacist for each 15,000 annual prescriptions or fraction thereof. The pharmacy is connected to the waiting room by a door and pharmacy activities are not visible from the waiting room area. The waiting room area and offices have paneled walls and carpeting. Educational material is in the waiting room with seasonable health subjects stressed.

Brands has also outlined the characteristic

Figure 3. The floor plan of the Indian Medical Center Pharmacy showing the patient waiting area and two consultation offices

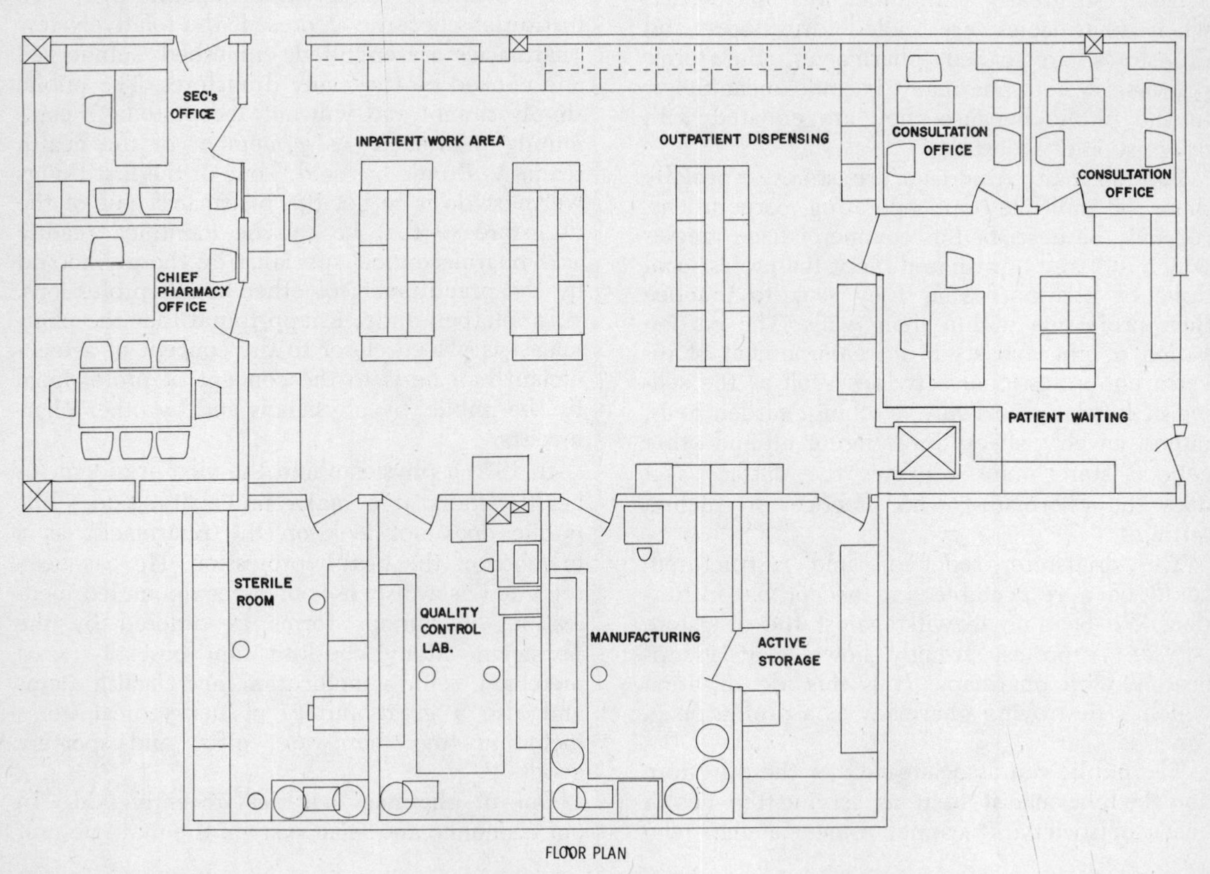

dialogue that should take place between the pharmacist and patient.[42] The pharmacist should instruct the patient:

1. Who the medicine is for
2. What the medicine is to be used for or its general classification
3. The name of the medicine
4. How to use the medicine
5. When to use the medicine
6. How long to use the medicine
7. Maximum amount that may be taken safely in one day
8. The side reactions he might expect
9. What to avoid in activities, such as driving, working machinery, eating, drinking and taking other drugs
10. Special storage and special handling of the medicine

Separation of Pharmacies and Drugstores

The United States has more than 50,000 retail establishments known as drugstores with which are included a few thousand pharmacies. This great heterogeneous mass makes it impossible for the public and the allied professions to clearly discern, to carefully distinguish or to recognize in any way the pharmacist practicing in them as a professional person. Drugstores in America so greatly outnumber pharmacies that when pharmacies are called drugstores and drugstores are called pharmacies, the terms pharmacist and pharmacy become meaningless to the public because they are equated with druggist and drugstore.[43]

Far too many American drugstores, especially those of multiple unit operating corporations, can only be described as commercialized jungles which dull and tarnish and blunt the professional drive of pharmacists as they seek to practice their profession within their walls. The participation of pharmacists in an environment of diverse nonprofessional activities such as the selling of lunches, hardware, clothing, garden tools, radios, jewelry, sheep dung, motor oil and other general store items confuses the public as it does the pharmacist who practices in such a setting.

The drugstore, redefined and restructured, could be a respectable and acceptable institution. We bear no ill will against the drugstore *per se*. We protest strongly, however, its identification with pharmacy. It is this identification which is destroying pharmacy as a profession in America.

The public can associate neither the drugstore nor the pharmacist in it as serving the health needs of society. It cannot esteem a man who works in such an environment; he may sell a health-related product—but he is not accepted as a member of a health profession.

One can find no fault with society's judgment of pharmacists when one reads the studies by the Professors Knapp and their colleagues.[44] As a drug adviser to the physician, pharmacists in their sample failed five out of six questions; as an advisor on self-medication, 83 percent of pharmacists sold patients they believed to be diabetic, products contraindicated in this condition; and several similar actions. The authors state:

> It is painfully and deadly obvious that the pharmacists in our sample utterly failed the tasks presented them—failed to the point of exposing their patients to the unnecessary risk of possible death in the third phase. Statistics are of little use in cases such as this, both because of the overwhelming nature of the incorrect responses and the severity of the consequences of the pharmacists' actions.

The interests, motivations and rewards of the community pharmacist are so greatly diluted and dispersed by all the other activities of his store that he cannot help but fail when tested as a professional practitioner concerned with public health.

We must find some way to separate these two institutions because at present the relatively few pharmacies are engulfed, enmeshed, submerged and choked by the many drugstores. The public simply cannot and will not accept today's community pharmacist as a member of the health team. As Brodie has said,[45] one of the first things we must do is to get the pharmacist out of the drugstore so that he can be identified readily as a pharmaceutical specialist by the public and by the practitioners of other health professions.

In another study, Knapp found that the pharmacist is placed closer to the concept of a technician than he is to the concept of professional by the public, by physicians and by other pharmacists.[44]

In 1970 a physician and the vice president for health affairs at a major university, said, "The public does not look on the pharmacist as a member of the health profession. He has been regarded as a dispenser of precompounded medications in various forms as ordered by the physician. Many consider him basically as a merchant selling medication and health items and also a great variety of nonmedical items including toys, hardware, gifts, and sporting goods."[47]

One of pharmacy's leaders recently said, "In our economic and legal system, the multiple unit

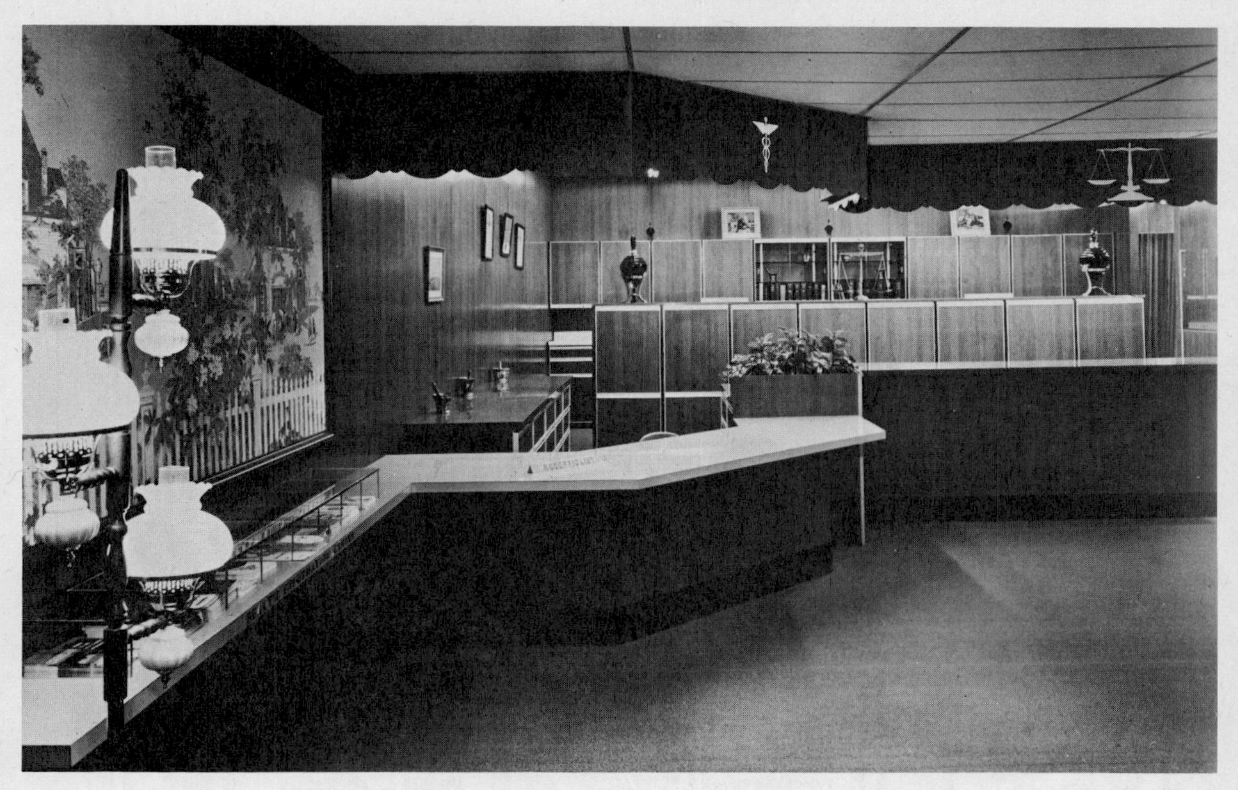

Figure 4. This pharmacy reflects professional dignity; however, the public's image of pharmacy and pharmacists is molded more often by daily newspaper advertisements such as those shown on pages 54 and 55

operating corporation has as much right to own a pharmacy as the individual practitioner."[48] Perhaps it does have the economic and legal right but does it have the moral right to merchandise with such abandon and lack of constraint that it prostitutes and degrades the profession whose name it uses and abuses? Yes, anyone can own a drugstore but not everyone can practice pharmacy.

In his "Essay on Civil Disobedience," David Thoreau employs a sentence which the profession could use in its relationship to many drugstores as they exist today. He said "We can no longer lend our cooperation to an evil system."[49] When pharmacy ceases its cooperation perhaps the system will change. If it continues, then there undoubtedly will develop two types of pharmacists, the clinical pharmacist who practices in a health-care institution and a pharmacist or pharmacy technician who functions in the drugstore emporium. The young men and women being trained in clinical practice will not be content to practice in such a setting.

Discrimination in Selecting Tasks

If pharmacists want to play a role beyond that of a technician, they must select appropriate tasks when dealing with patients. Gone are the days when prescriptions for patients are compounded or prepared in the pharmacy. About 98 percent or more of medications come to the pharmacist in ready-made form. Formerly, the pharmacist compounded and dispensed. Today, he dispenses and consults. Too often, he dispenses in a mechanical, indifferent way, quite oblivious of the patient and his needs. Often, he only dispenses and never talks with the patient.

The public's attitude toward pharmacy is not strong and there is considerable under-utilization of the pharmacist's talents in society. If pharmacists would assume a greater role in drug usage education, society would not only benefit but the public image of pharmacy would improve. It is certainly within the jurisdiction of the pharmacist to teach the patient proper drug usage. Hopefully, if patients are taught more about their medications, they will make fewer errors and become more effective participants in their medical plan of care.

The pharmacist may teach the patient proper drug usage whether he works in a hospital or a community setting. Time and trouble must be spent with patients in learning their drug histories and drug hypersensitivities, in teaching

THE WASHINGTON POST

drug mart

Due to space limitations items marked with THIS SYMBOL are NOT available in D.C. Stores or in the following other stores:

Don't say 'Drug Store', say drug mart

15.88 LADY SCHICK
TOTE & DRY HAIR DRYER
12.44

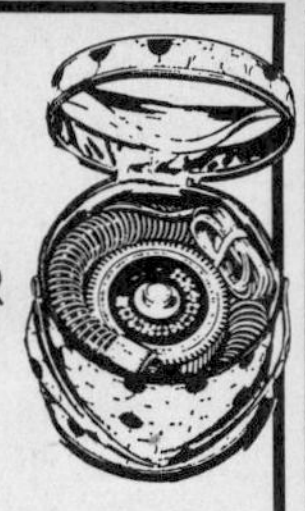

Totes along with you in a colorful vinyl case. New "Floating Bonnet" fits the largest rollers. 4 temperature settings.

18.88 LADY NORELCO
HARD HAT HAIR DRYER
14.88

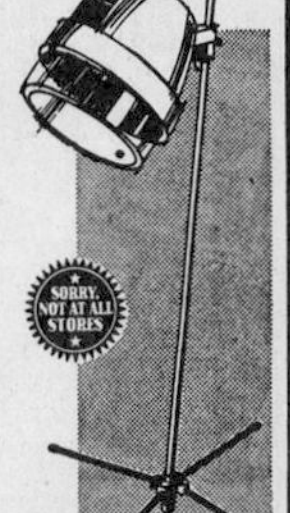

Enjoy professional-results in at-home comfort. Fully adjustable hood and floor stand set to a perfect angle. Fold up floor stand.

Valentine

FRAGRANCES FOR YOUR VALENTINE

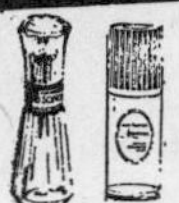
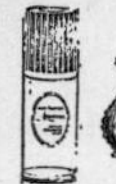
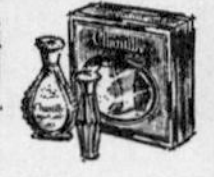
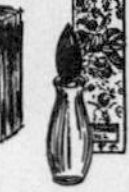

FABERGE MUSIC SPRAY COLOGNE, 2 oz.	3.50
FABERGE MUSIC DUSTING POWDER	2.50
FABERGE SPRAY DUET	5.00
MATCHABELLI SPRAY MIST SPECIAL	2.25
MAX FACTOR SPRAY MIST COLOGNE	1.75
REVLON INTIMATE SPRAY MIST, 2 oz.	2.50
LANVIN ARPEGE SPRAY MIST, 1.3 oz.	3.00
LANVIN MY SIN SPRAY MIST, 1.3 oz.	3.00
CHANTILLY SACHET & PERFUME	3.00
DANA SPRAY COLOGNE	2.00

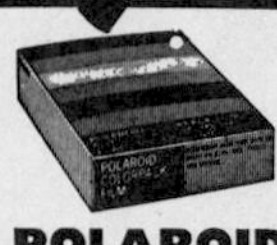

POLAROID
108 COLOR FILM
Reg. 4.18 3.66
88 COLOR FILM
Reg. 3.54 2.88

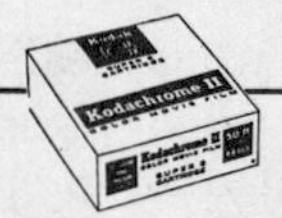

2.58 KODAK KA464
MOVIE FILM
Color movie cartridge for Super 8 cameras. 2.09

1.14 GE
HI-POWER CUBES
77¢
Pk. of 2 for Polaroid Focussed Flash Cameras.

1.38 GE
FLASHCUBES
Pk. of 3 74¢

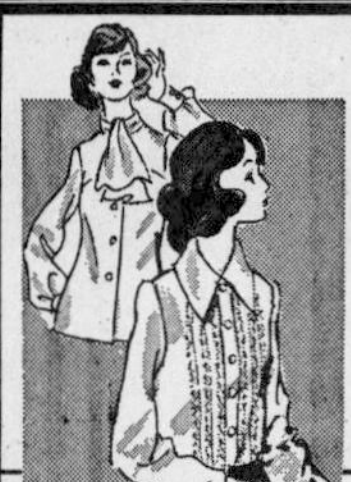

REG. 2.97 TO 3.97
LADIES' NEW SPRING
BLOUSES
2.44 & 2.88
A great collection of the newest styles and fabrics in white and fashion colors. Regular and extra-large sizes.

REG. 2.27 & 2.57
LADIES' NEW SPRING
SHIRTS
Permanent-press fabrics in lovely solid colors and beautiful new prints. Regular and extra-large sizes.
1.77

REG. 3.27 TO 4.97
LADIES'
SLACKS
2.27 to 3.57
Straight and flare leg styles in new Spring fabrics. Solid colors, prints, plaids and stripes. Regular and extra-large sizes.

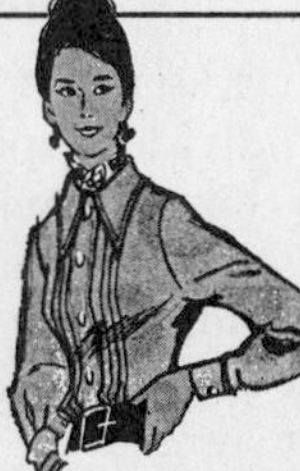

REG. 2.97 TO 5.97
LADIES' NEW SPRING
HANDBAGS
1.97 to 4.17
See all the top new fashion hit sizes, shapes and colors for spring. Pick your favorites to give winter-weary wardrobes new chic.

Soft-wear available at most suburban stores

Photo Special!

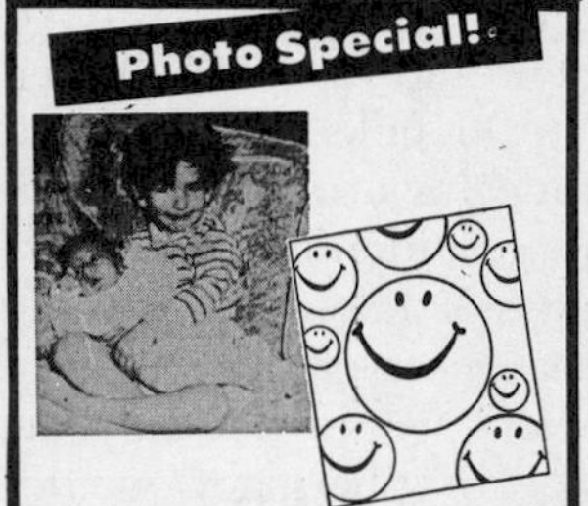

8 KODACOLOR REPRINTS PLUS 8 PHOTO BRAG CARDS
1.99
. . . when your order is accompanied by the guarantee panel from one pack of GE FLASHBULBS or CUBES. Photo Brag Cards come in a choice of colorful, humorous and memorable designs.
Made From Square Kodacolor Neg. Only.

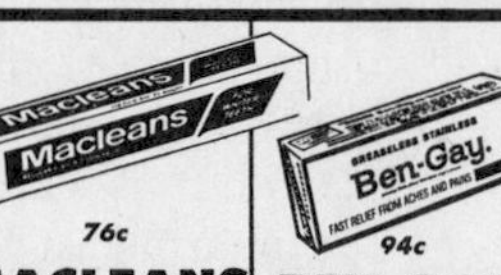

76c
MACLEANS TOOTHPASTE 6¾ oz.
56¢
Spearmint and Freshmint

94c
BEN-GAY GREASELESS OINTMENT 1¼ oz.
64¢

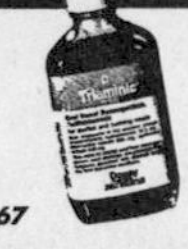

99c
LAVORIS MOUTHWASH 14 oz.
79¢

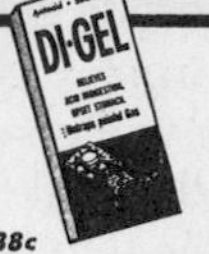

1.67
TRIAMINIC NASAL DECONGESTANT SYRUP 4 oz.
1.18

88c
DI-GEL ANTACID TABLETS 30's
64¢

drug mart

For Emergencies and Your Convenience
DRUG MART
OPEN ALL NIGHT
EVERY NIGHT
24-HOUR PRESCRIPTION SERVICE

MARYLAND:

VIRGINIA:

THE WASHINGTON POST

THERE'S A BIG DIFFERENCE!

drug mart

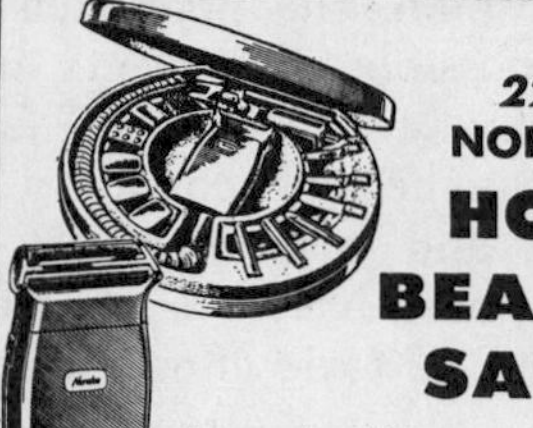

22.44
NORELCO
HOME BEAUTY SALON

A super fast lady's shaver plus eleven grooming attachments. With big, beautiful case.

18.88

AS SEEN ON TV! PROTEL

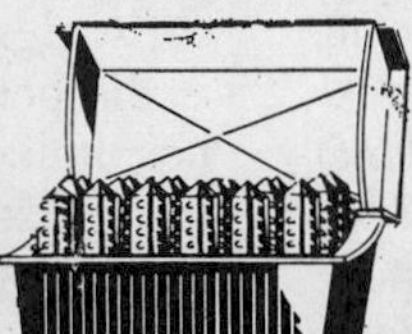

STEAMSET HAIR SETTER

6.99

Fast, non-drying hairsetter with 18 large rollers. Includes facial sauna attachment and carrying case.

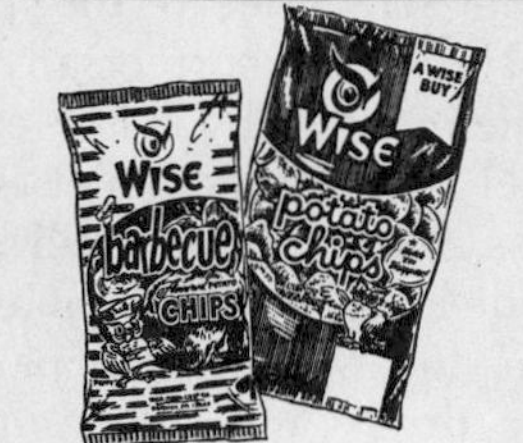

43¢
WISE

- POTATO CHIPS
- BARBECUE CHIPS
- ONION & GARLIC CHIPS

Your Choice

5 oz. **3 for 99¢**

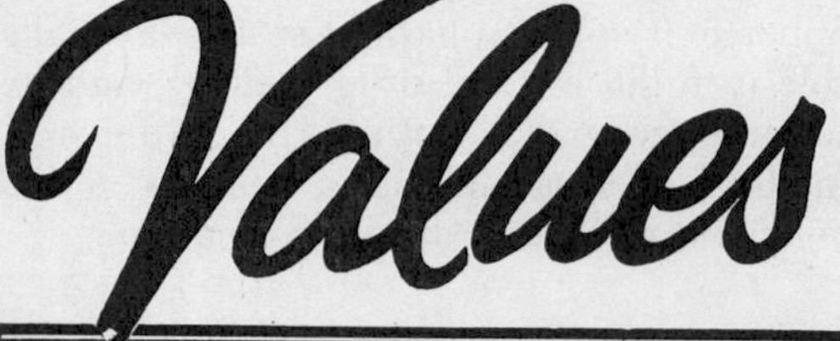

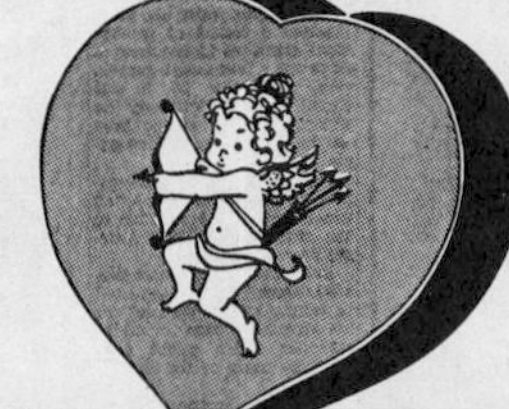

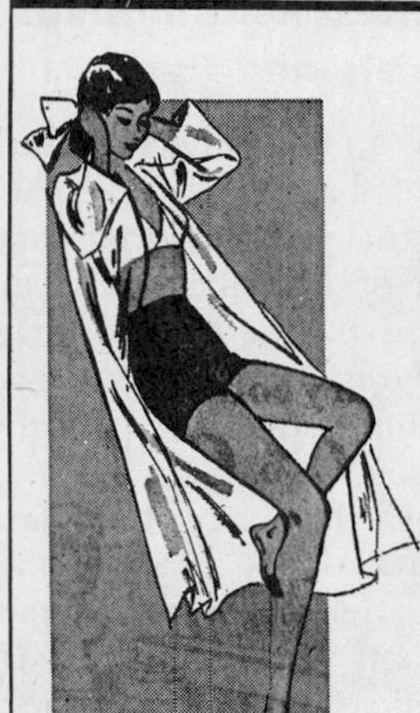

REG. 1.27
MIRACLE FIT
PANTY HOSE

71¢

All nude super-sheer Wonderlon nylon. In Camel, Brown, Beige, Gray and Black. Sizes: Petite/Medium and Medium/Tall.

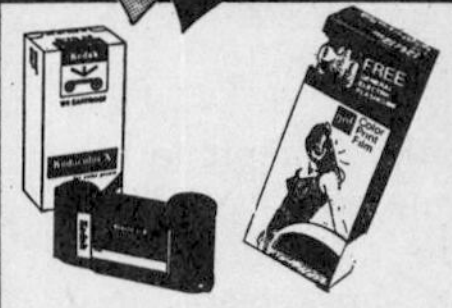

KODAK or GAF
FILM REPLACEMENT PLAN

HERE'S ALL YOU DO:

1 Bring in any of these popular size rolls of GAF Color film, Kodacolor or Kodak Black White film for developing and printing: 126, 135, 120, 127, 620, 616, 116, 828.

2 When you pick up your finished prints we will give you a REPLACEMENT ROLL OF GAF 126-12 FILM PLUS A FREE FLASHCUBE, OR A REPLACEMENT ROLL OF KODAK FILM for each and every roll you had developed and printed. You will receive the same size and type processed, providing at least 50% of the pictures on each roll are printed.

3 The replacement film offer DOES NOT apply to slide or movie film such as Kodachrome, Anscochrome, etc. However, you will receive a substanial discount on the processing of this film.

NEITHER PLAN APPLIES TO WORK SENT DIRECTLY TO KODAK OR GAF.

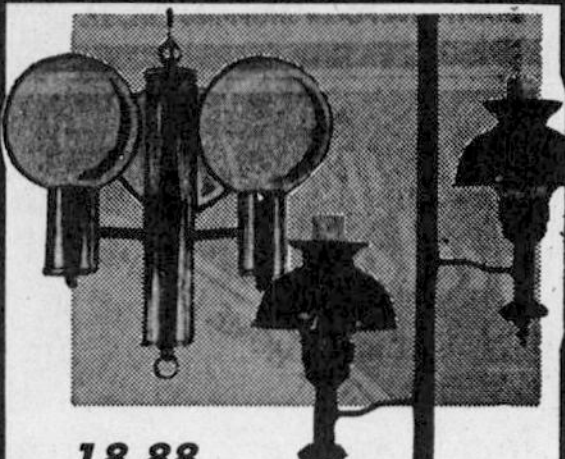

18.88
Lamps

- WET LOOK TOLE POLE LAMP
- CHROME CHAIN LIGHT

Your Choice **15.88**

WET LOOK with two 9" metal shades with frosted glass chimneys. CHAIN LIGHT with three 5" bulbs and chrome hanging chain.

AVAILABLE AT THE FOLLOWING STORES ONLY:

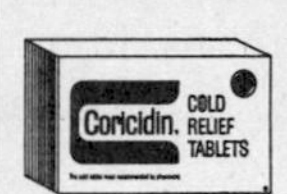

1.17
CORICIDIN
COLD TABLETS
25's **87¢**

4.67
GERITOL
FORTIFIED TONIC TABLETS
100's **3.67**

1.78
PERTUSSIN
8 HOUR COUGH FORMULA
6 oz. **1.18**

1.68
BARNES-HIND WETTING SOLUTION
FOR CONTACT LENSES
2 oz. **1.08**

1.47
BRYLCREEM
MEN'S HAIR GROOM
6½ oz. **99¢**

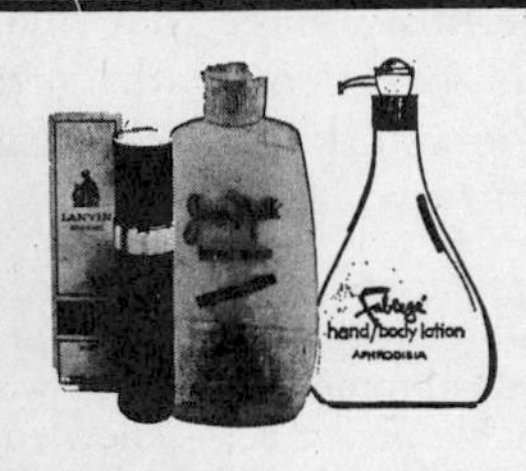

JEAN NATE HAND TONE LOTION, 8 oz. ... **1.50**

FABERGE HAND & BODY LOTION WITH PUMP **1.00**

Just Say **"Charge It"**

OPEN YOUR CHARGE ACCOUNT AT ANY DRUG MART

"USE IT AT ALL OF THEM"

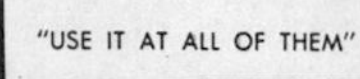

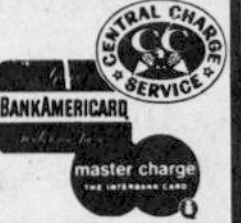

AMERICAN EXPRESS
Money Orders
SOLD HERE

Special prices in this ad effective thru Tues., Feb. 8. Rights reserved to limit quantities.

drug mart

them the importance of their medications, the proper methods of administration, and the early signs of untoward effects. The pharmacist should assist the patient and the physician in adjusting the drug schedule to the patient's pattern of living. He should correct any misunderstandings the patient may have. For example, the patient may feel that if *one* tablet is good, *two* will be twice as good. Society still relies heavily upon self-medication and the pharmacist is in a key position to oversee the patient's use of proprietary drugs and, when necessary, to advise these patients to seek medical help. In the community, the pharmacist should become more involved in health education and accept invitations to speak to various groups. Communication should be designed to inform the general public of the role which pharmacy plays in society in the delivery of comprehensive health care. Public relations are important to every profession—and pharmacy is certainly no exception.

> By playing an active role with the patients rather than his traditionally passive one, he can make contributions to their health. The average patient is psychologically prepared to appreciate any special attention paid to him and he will remember impressions made on him during his stay in the hospital. Any service he receives that is identified with the pharmacist can mold his opinion and attitudes toward pharmacy and the use of drugs. If interest is expressed over what medicines he takes and how he takes them, the patient may realize the importance of having respect for all drugs and may, in time, show more respect toward drugs used in his home environment.[48]

In addition to the traditional aspects of dispensing drug products, the pharmacist is assuming more responsibility in the dispensing of drug information to physicians, nurses, and related health practitioners. Many health practitioners have the false image that pharmacy is little more than the practice of drug distribution and do not understand this increasingly important responsibility:

> Pharmacists are sometimes highly professional and readily available sources of drug information for medical practitioners. It would be good to have reliable and precise knowledge of what their functions actually are in this respect and, better still, what they might more usefully become.[40]

The word "sometimes" in the above statement should irk pharmacists. The pharmacist must become recognized as an authority on drugs. Through the use of medication records, he can provide the physician and dentist with a profile of the patient's drug therapy and medication history. The drug profile is a tool by which he can assist in the rational selection and use of drugs and in the discovery of a drug-related problem. In the hospital, the pharmacist must alert the nurse to possible side effects and the early signs of toxicity due to drugs. The nurse is the person who has the most contact with the hospitalized patient and it follows that she is the person who is most likely to observe any signs of drug toxicity. If toxic effects are recognized soon enough, they can often be counteracted. The opportunity to improve hospital drug education is at every hospital pharmacist's fingertips. All he must do is reach out and grasp this opportunity. The pharmacist has a challenging role to fulfill in total drug therapy, and he must become recognized both by the public and other medical professionals as a reliable and readily available source of drug information.

Factors Which Disturb Relationships Between Pharmacists and Patients

Two prime factors, among others, disturb the relationships between pharmacists and patients: one is concern over the price of drugs and the second is the image of the pharmacist and of pharmacy as projected by the typical drugstore and particularly the large chain drugstores. Each of these factors is interrelated, and one of them has been already discussed.

In many countries, the price that may be charged the public for drugs is established by negotiation between the pharmacists' national professional society and the Ministry of Health representing the public. Once this is done, price is no longer a factor in the patronage of a pharmacy and the caliber of pharmaceutical service assumes paramount importance. With the price the same in all pharmacies, for the same medication, then the scope and breadth of public health service rendered by the pharmacist, his personality, the work of his staff, his interest in the patient and his needs and his humaneness and compassion become the overriding considerations in the patient's choice of a pharmacy from which to obtain his health needs.

The American public has come to equate quality of pharmacy service almost solely with the price of the drug product. Many pharmacists have encouraged this. Others who want to give a more comprehensive public health service are discouraged by competition from offering it because their profit is too closely related to the cost of the drug. In addition, there has been for years—justified or not—a public clamor about the excessive cost of drugs to the public and the high profits of the pharmaceutical industry.

The greatest advantage of these price controlling plans is that the public is represented and, therefore, its interests are protected. At the same time a professional fee and other items of remuneration and reimbursement can be worked into the formula for compensating the pharmacist, based on the level of pharmaceutical service he gives. Perhaps a capitation fee for each person registered with a community pharmacy could be paid in addition to the fee for each prescription, as is done in The Netherlands.[51] Since the government will soon be paying most of the bills for drugs and related professional service, it is inevitable that it, as a representative of society, will exercise some control over them.

A cooperative scheme to adjust the price of drugs to the public makes much more sense than current plans by many health agencies to control the price of drugs by putting a ceiling on the amount they will pay for certain drugs, often ignoring completely the reliability of the source of supply or the quality of the drug product.

PHARMACIST'S RELATIONSHIPS WITH PHYSICIANS

The central core responsibility of the pharmacist in society is the control of prescription legend drugs. He shares this responsibility with physicians; in all state laws, the physician is given equal authority to dispense prescription legend drugs. On the other hand, the sale of nonprescription drugs and medicines is open to any dealer. As Fischelis has noted; "Somewhere along the line someone in authority has either lost faith in registered pharmacists as guardians of the public health with respect to the use of drugs, or pharmacists, as a class, have failed to impress themselves upon the public and the government as sufficiently interested to do the job which they are trained and licensed to carry out.[52]

The physician accepts legal and professional responsibility for the primary care of the patient. Talcott Parsons has observed that the modern physician achieves a depth of intimacy with his patient that is unequaled in our society: The patient is never so naked a creature as when he is with his physician.[53] The sick patient places himself in the hands of his physician who examines him, counsels him, makes a diagnosis of his illness, prescribes medication for him and arranges additional appointments to monitor his progress toward health. Within the context of these acts, the physician himself is a potent therapeutic agent and influences greatly the effectiveness of the medication he prescribes. It has been estimated that 25 to 50 percent of patients who consult general practitioners come to them with neurotic and functional illness.[54] Gowers once said "if every drug in the world were abolished, the physician would still be a useful member of society."[54]

It is the relationship of the patient to his physician and the physician's relationship to his patient that sets the parameters of the relationship of the pharmacist to the physician. This relationship has come to the forefront recently because of the stand taken by the Board of Trustees of the American Pharmaceutical Association relative to the repeal of the antisubstitution laws.[55] In its White Paper the Board has said that the pharmacist should be authorized to be the sole judge of the source of the particular drug product prescribed by the physician for his patient.

In his Remington Address, Francke discusses this question at some length and argues that the physician must remain a partner in the drug selection process and that the pharmacist should not act unilaterally without the physician's knowledge or consent.[56] This argument seems to be reinforced by the significant effect the physician has on the therapeutic action of the drug he selects for his patient and the great dependence the patient places on his physician. Traditionally and historically, community pharmacists in dialogue with physicians have been able to obtain their consent to dispense alternative brands of drug products. In the hospital, pharmacists and physicians coordinate their efforts through the Pharmacy and Therapeutics Committee. Here the physician daily visits his patients and can readily monitor the evidence of physiological and therapeutic effect of the drugs prescribed for his patient. Also the pharmacist is readily at hand and easily identifiable to receive any complaints relative to the ineffectiveness of the drug and he can take appropriate action. Drugs dispensed to outpatients are produced by the same manufacturer as the medication given to inpatients and hence one serves as a control on the quality of the other. The same controlled or controllable situation does not exist in community practice and the physician seldom knows where his patient obtained his medication.

In discussing the pharmacists' relations with the medical profession Fischelis said:[57]

> In the actual everyday routine practice of medicine and pharmacy, physicians and pharmacists reach

a mutual understanding and regard for each other's function and responsibility in the best interest of the patient.

Such understandings are not negotiated in legal terms. They require no policing. They cannot be forced into being by law or regulation. Nor can they be created by intra- or interprofessional codes of conduct or etiquette or resolutions. They happen and exist because dedicated practitioners want both paying and non-paying clients to receive honest, high quality, humane and thoroughly competent medical care.

Levy, a pharmaceutical scientist, in commenting on the White Paper concludes that: "The selection of drug products should be a matter of pharmacists and physicians working in concert, and not independent of one another."[58] Further, he challenges the concepts of ethics and professionalism which gave rise to The White Paper and accuses its authors of distorting science to serve their own political and economic needs.

Commenting editorially on The White Paper, representatives of The American Medical Association after noting that the pharmacist works in a partial vacuum of information about the patient and what the physician is trying to accomplish:[59]

The AMA and its Council on Drugs believe that the antisubstitution laws protect the patient, the pharmacist, and the physician. Accordingly, it is difficult to understand why a prominent branch of organized pharmacy would want the repeal of laws that in no way inhibit the pharmacist from practicing his profession or from having an intimate working relationship with any individual physician concerning the choice of drugs the physician may want to use—laws that allow the physician to maintain control over the medication his patient is receiving, an absolute must if a patient is to receive the full benefit of the physician's training and knowledge—laws that effectively help bridle the unprincipled pharmacist and the drug counterfeiter. Yet, such is the case.

The pharmacist must develop his own status, one which he can earn by being a part of the health team and working cooperatively with its members for the benefit of the patient and of society. He must develop an area of unquestioned competence and then his social psychological role in drug usage in all its aspects will be great. This he has not yet done, but more of the newly developing clinical pharmacists will do it, hopefully not unmindful of all who over the years have practiced as clinical pharmacists under another name.

References

1. Sanders, Irwin T.: "Public Health in the Community," in Howard E. Freeman, Sol Levine and Leo G. Reader, eds., *Handbook of Medical Sociology,* Englewood Cliffs, N. J. Prentice-Hall, Inc., 1963, pp. 369-396.

2. Francke, D. E.: Career Opportunities for Students of Social Studies in Pharmacy, *Am. J. Pharm. Educ. 34*: 567-586 (Nov.) 1970.

3. Modell, W.: To Protect the American Public, *Clin. Pharmacol. Therap. 9*:413-420 (Apr.) 1968.

4. Huntington, Mary Jean: "The Development of a Professional Self-Image," in *The Student-Physician,* edited by Robert K. Merton, George G. Reader and Patricia L. Kendall, Harvard University Press, 1957, pp. 179-187.

5. Levinson, D. J.: Medical Education and the Theory of Adult Socialization, *J. Health Soc. Behavior 8*:253-265 (Dec.) 1967.

6. Menke, Wayne G.: Professional Values in Medical Practice, *New Engl. J. Med. 280*:930-936 (Apr. 24) 1969.

7. Dee, D. A.: News from MSPhA Headquarters, *Minn. Pharm.* (July 30) 1968.

8. Hardy, C. T., Jr.: Group Practice by Medical School Faculty, *J. Med. Educ. 43*:907-911 (Aug.) 1968.

9. Jaco, E. Gartley: "Medicine and Behavioral Science," in *Patients, Physicians and Illness,* Gartley A. Jaco, ed., The Free Press, Glencoe, Illinois, 1958, pp. 1-10.

10. Wilson, Robert N.: "Patient-Practitioner Relationships," in Howard E. Freeman, Sol Levine and Leo G. Reader, eds., *Handbook of Medical Sociology,* Englewood Cliffs, N.J. Prentice-Hall, Inc. 1963, pp. 273-295.

11. Flexner, Abraham, quoted by Samuel W. Bloom in "Some Implications of Studies in the Professionalization of the Physician," in E. Gartley Jaco, ed., *Patients, Physicians and Illness,* The Free Press, Glencoe, Ill., 1958. pp. 313.

12. Mechanic, D.: *Medical Sociology, A Selective View,* Free Press, University of Wisconsin, Madison, 1968, 504 pp.

13. Blaylock, Jerry: The Psychological and Cultural Influences on the Reaction to Pain: A Review of the Literature, *Nurs. Forum, 7*:262-274, 1968.

14. Smith, Lawrence and Kane, Robert: Health Knowledge and Symptom Perception: A Study of a Rural Kentucky County, *Soc. Sci. Med. 4*:557-567 (Dec.) 1970.

15. Apple, D.: *Sociological Studies on Health and Sickness,* McGraw-Hill Book Company, Inc., New York, 1960. pp. 123-133.

16. Nall, Frank C. and Speilberg, Joseph: Social and Cultural Factors in the Responses of Mexican-Americans to Medical Treatment, *J. Health Social Behavior 8*:299-308 (Dec.) 1967.

17. Mumford, E.: *Sociology in Hospital Care,* Harper and Row, New York, 1967, p. 228.

18. Tagliacozzo, D. M. and Ima, K.: Knowledge of Illness as a Predictor of Patient Behavior, *J. Chronic Diseases 22*:765-775, 1970.

19. Hyman, Martin D.: Some Links Between Economic Status and Untreated Illness, *Soc. Sci. Med. 4*:387-399 (Nov.) 1970.

20. Mechanic, D.: The Influence of Mothers on Their Children's Health Attitudes and Behavior, *Pediatrics 33*:444-453 (Mar.) 1964.

21. Davis, M. S.: Variation in Patients' Compliance with Doctors' Orders: Analysis of Consequence Between Survey Responses and Results of Empirical Investigation, *J. Med. Educ. 41*:1037-1048 (Nov.) 1966.

22. Marston, Mary-'Vesta: Compliance with Medical Regimens, A Review of the Literature, *Nursing Res. 19*: 312-323 (July-Aug.) 1970.

23. Schwartz, D. *et al.*: Medication Errors Made by Elderly, Chronically Ill Patients, *Am. J. Public Health 52*:2018-2029 (Dec.) 1962.

24. Francis, V. *et al.*: Gaps in Doctor-Patient Communication, *New Engl. J. Med. 280*:535-540 (Mar. 6) 1969.

25. Overall, John E. *et al.*: Extrinsic Factors Influencing Responses to Psychotherapeutic Drugs, *Arch. Gen. Psychiat. 21*:89-94 (July) 1969.

26. Moulding, Thomas and Sbarbaro: Supervision of Outpatient Drug Therapy with the Medication Monitor, *Ann. Internal Med. 73*:559-564 (Oct.) 1970.

27. Proter, A. M. W.: Drug Defaulting in General Practice, *Brit. Med. J. 1*:218-222 (Jan.) 1969.

28. Bergman, A. B. and Werner, R. J.: Failure of Children to Receive Penicillin by Mouth, *New Engl. J. Med. 268*: 1334-1338 (June 13) 1963.

29. Report No. 148 of the General Practitioner Group: Dosage Schedules in General Practice, *Practitioner 204*:719-723 (May) 1970.

30. Davis, Milton S.: Variations in Patients' Compliance with Doctors' Advice: An Empirical Analysis of Communication, *Am. J. Public Health 58*:274-288 (Feb.) 1968.

31. Luntz, G. and Austin, R.: New Stick Test for P.A.S. in Urine, *Brit. Med. J. 1*:1679-1684 (June 4) 1960.

32. Cooley, Carol H.: *Social Aspects of Illness,* W. B. Saunders Company, Philadelphia, 1951, 305 p.

33. Shapiro, Arthur K.: The Placebo Effect of Treatment, *Drug Therapy 1*:45-54 (Dec.) 1971.

34. Honigfeld, G.: Non-Specific Factors in Treatment, *Diseases Nervous System 25*:225-289 (Apr.) 1964.

35. Rickels, K., Lipman, R. and Raab, E.: Previous Medication, Duration of Illness and Placebo Response, *J. Nervous Mental Diseases 142*:548-554 (June) 1966.

36. Honigfeld, G.: Non-Specific Factors in Treatment I. Review of Placebo Reactions and Placebo Reactors, *Diseases Nervous System 25*:145-156 (Mar.) 1964.

37. Kast, Eric C. and Leosch, John: Influence of the Doctor-Patient Relationship on Drug Action, *Illinois Med. J. 119*:390-393 (June) 1961.

38. Stern, Bernhard J.: "The Specialist and the General Practitioner" in E. Gartley Jaco, ed., *Patients, Physicians and Illness,* The Free Press, Glencoe, Ill. 1958, p. 357.

39. Smečka, Vladimir: A Study of Pharmacy Dispatch Work II, *Acta Fac. Pharm.* (Bratislava) *16*:169-211, 1968.

40. Barber, Bernard: *Drugs and Society,* Russell Sage Foundation, New York, 1967, pp. 39-133.

41. Brands, Allen J.: Pharmacy Patient Consultation Offices, Staff Paper dated May 6, 1969, Department of Health, Education and Welfare, Indian Health Service.

42. Brands, Allen J.: Complete Directions for Prescription Medication, *J. Am. Pharm. Assoc. NS7*:634-635 (Dec.) 1967.

43. Francke, D. E.: Let's Separate Pharmacies and Drugstores, *Am. J. Pharm. 141*:161-170 (Sept.-Oct.) 1969.

44. Knapp, D. A., Wolf, H. H., Knapp, D. E. and Rudy, T. A.: The Pharmacist as a Drug Advisor, *J. Am. Pharm. Assoc. NS9*:502-505 (Oct.) 1969.

45. Brodie, D. C.: "Emerging Patterns of Education and Practice in the Health Professions—Pharmacy," *Proceedings, Pharmacy-Medicine-Nursing Conference on Health Education,* University of Michigan, 1967, pp. 23-25.

46. Knapp, D. A., Knapp, D. E. and Edwards, J. D.: The Pharmacist as Perceived by Physicians, Patrons, and Other Pharmacists, *J. Am. Pharm. Assoc. NS9*:80-84 (Feb.) 1969.

47. Castleton, K. B.: A Medical Educator Looks at Pharmacy Education, mimeographed talk of Vice President for Medical Affairs, University of Utah, 1971.

48. Apple, W. A.: Report to APhA House of Delegates, *APhA Newsletter 7*:3 (May 18) 1968.

49. Thoreau, David: Essay on Civil Disobedience, quoted by Martin Luther King in his lecture "The Quest for Peace and Justice," the Nobel Peace Lecture, December 11, 1964, in *Les Prix Nobel en 1964,* Stockholm, P.A. Norstedt & Sons, 1965.

50. Pfau, J. E. and Sperandio, G. J.: The Hospitalized Patient, Eli Lilly's *Hospital Pharmacy Notes, 5*: (Aug.) 1968.

51. Anon.: Pharmacy in the Common Market, *Pharm. J. 200*:535-541 (May 11) 1968.

52. Fischelis, Robert P.: Things We Can or Cannot Change II. About Regulating Essential Services, *Drug Intelligence Clin. Pharm. 5*:275 (Sept.) 1971.

53. Parsons, Talcott: "Definitions of Health and Illness in the Light of American Values and Social Structure," in E. Gartley Jaco, ed., *Patients, Physicians and Illness,* The Free Press, Glencoe, Ill., 1958, p. 117.

54. Ferguson, R. S.: "The Doctor-Patient Relationship and Function Illness," in E. Gartley Jaco, ed., *Patients, Physicians and Illness,* The Free Press, Glencoe, Ill., 1958, p. 436.

55. Anon.: A White Paper on the Pharmacist's Role in Product Selection, *J. Am. Pharm. Assoc. NS11*:181-199 (Apr.) 1971.

56. Francke, Donald E.: Medicines, Medical Care, Manpower and Mankind, *Am. J. Hosp. Pharm. 28*:410-421 (June) 1971.

57. Fischelis, Robert P.: Things We Can or Cannot Change, I. About Relations With the Medical Profession, *Drug Intelligence Clin. Pharm. 5*:387 (Dec.) 1971.

58. Levy, Gerhard: A Pharmaceutical Scientist's View of the White Paper on the Pharmacist's Role in Drug Selection, *Drug Intelligence Clin. Pharm. 6*:18-20 (Jan.) 1972.

59. Anon.: Drug Substitution—How to Turn Order Into Chaos, *J. Am. Med. Assoc. 217*:817-818 (Aug. 9) 1971.

60. Beecher, Henry K.: Increased Stress and Effectiveness of Placebos and "Active" Drugs, *Science 132*:91-92 (July 8) 1960.

4

The triumvirate of the health team — physician, pharmacist and nurse

by John A. Oliver

Whatever the status of the relationships between pharmacists and other health professionals, its genesis will largely be found in a hospital pharmacist who was a part of the physician's or nurse's first professional experience. Virtually every worker in the health field received preprofessional clinical training in a hospital; that hospital had a pharmacy service and a pharmacist, each of whom made an impression—of one kind or another.

On the average, the relationship of the pharmacist with other health disciplines is passive.[1] (All health professionals will be treated as a generic group in this chapter, but physicians and nurses will be singled out for special emphasis because they play a greater role in the pharmacist's interprofessional relationships.) There are a few—a very, very few—examples of a close professional rapport enjoyed by pharmacists with other members of the health team. The fact there are so very few makes them unique. Even more rare is a situation where there is outright conflict or antagonism, but these are generally based on personal and emotional reasons and not on professional competence. By far the most common is the passive relationship between the pharmacist and his colleagues on the health team, and it is this group who can be influenced toward a more substantial and rewarding professional relationship with the pharmacist, based on mutual respect.

Historical Precedent and Background

It was not always thus. Pharmacy in its origins was a respected specialty, and it maintained this respect for several centuries.[2] Even today, the pharmacist in several European countries enjoys a respect and professional status quite out of proportion to that generally known in the United States. In Denmark this is referred to as the "handicraft tradition," and it is still a significant, integral part of pharmacists' practice, in which they take great pride.[3] Their mode of practice is different, more closely reflecting traditional precepts. The pharmacist has traditionally been acknowledged as a man with unique knowledge and skill. The magical way the pharmacist could take the crude drug of plant, animal or mineral origin, manipulate it with the aid of curiously shaped glass equipment and strange solvents commanded respect and admiration. He could do something no one else could do; moreover, his product had a salutary and beneficial effect on the recipient.

Pharmacists were noted not only for the marvels of compounding, but for breakthroughs in the understanding and comprehension of drugs and their active components. One need only recall Sertürner, Scheele and several others whose scientific ability reflected favorably on pharmacy and pharmacists. The purpose here is not to bask in reflected glories of the past but to document the basis for respectful recognition of the pharmacist by professional colleagues as well as society. These men and traditions of history have their present-day counterparts, but in the main these modern contributions and influence are diluted, if not overshadowed, by a larger population of practicing pharmacists who are not scientifically or professionally motivated and are instead oriented to the commercial adventure. This is true in the United States, and although there are to be found occasional outstanding professional, men like Charles Rice* of the Bellevue Hospital and the *USP,* Martin I. Wilbert of the German Hospital in Philadelphia and the U. S. Public Health Service,[4] H. A. K. Whitney of the University of Michigan and Edward Spease from Western Reserve University,[5,6,7] the mainstream of pharmacy practice in this country has been influenced by other factors. It is interesting to note in passing that there is no emphasis on tradition nor historical contributors in the education of pharmacists in the U. S. This may or may not have a bearing on interprofessional relationships today, but there is reason to believe it has influenced professional attitudes, and this in turn is a factor in the pharmacist's relationship with other health professions.

Current Philosophy of Health Care

Before embarking on an examination of interprofessional relationships among pharmacists and others in the health field, it may be well to examine the current philosophy of health. Within the past decade society has adopted a new set of standards with respect to health.**[8,9,10] A few years ago everyone was entitled to enjoy good health; today everyone has *the right* to enjoy good health. There is a difference in emphasis here, a shift of the burden of responsibility from the individual to the provider. The individual has always been entitled to good health for himself and his family—if he could find a provider and if he could afford the service. When health care was unavailable, he did without or he made use of home remedies and trusted to Providence.

Now society has said that all men have the right to good health, and to assure them of this right society itself will be the provider. (Providence has been omitted. This may be an oversight or a reflection of the tenor of the times; however, it is perhaps the subject for another discussion.) Society will be the provider of health, and all resources will be marshalled and organized to carry out this mandate. These resources will include pharmacists as well as other health professionals and, with this, another factor has been added to the pharmaceutical service equation: the public will.

---

*A German immigrant to the United States with a phenomenal knowledge of languages, Charles Rice began in a menial job at the Bellevue Hospital in New York City, and advanced to the position of Chemist of the Department of Public Charities and Correction of the City of New York and Superintendent of the General Drug Department. He distinguished himself in the profession and in education, becoming Chairman of the Committee of Revision of the United States Pharmacopeia and also a member of the Board of Trustees of Columbia University College of Pharmacy. In many respects, Charles Rice remains a man of mystery until this day. The best information about Rice has been brought together in a biographical article by H. George Wolfe.[11]

**The genesis of these new standards, however, may be found in the Social Security legislation of 1933. The amendments of 1965 (Medicare and Medicaid) accelerated the trend.

It was noted that scientific and professional, as well as commercial motivations influenced pharmacy practice in this country. In the overwhelming majority of cases the commercial influence predominated often to the total exclusion of pharmaceutical science and virtual elimination of professionalism.[12,13] There was, however, no conflict with society because this is what the community wanted and had come to expect. The public wanted a convenient place to serve as a resource for patented nostrums and the occasional prescription medication, as well as advice on personal health problems. It was perfectly natural that such places take on the atmosphere of a commercial purveyor rather than that of a professional service because the pharmacist was regarded as one of the leading businessmen in town and he had to run his establishment as a *business*. So professionalism and science were sacrificed on the altar of commerce and everyone got what he wanted and paid for what he got.

In retrospect, however, that sacrifice probably never took place. A sacrifice is a precipitous event, but the demise of profession and science was more like a slow, wasting process. They atrophied from disuse. The traditional handicrafts of the pharmacist were gradually laid aside as industrial technology grew. Tinctures and extracts need not be percolated any longer because they could be bought from a vendor, as could pills and filled capsules. Tablets were made available and pills became a thing of the past. Industry was even willing to make up simple mixtures, so that gradually the pharmacist had not a single traditional handicraft left. To be sure, the products of the pharmaceutical industry were more elegant and more accurate and of greater purity and the patient was well-served. But where had the magic gone? The skills and the techniques that had inspired wonder and admiration and respect had slipped away so gradually and so quietly their passing was scarcely noticed. Society, however, respected the successful businessman, and relationships with doctors and even the nurses were healthy; more social than professional, but healthy.

The refreshing breeze of social conscience is rearranging priorities for the suppliers of health services and goods. It is no longer an attitude of "you get what you pay for and pay for what you get"; the prevailing doctrine is: "This—is our right and we shall have it." This will apply to professional services as much as, if not more than, goods. It should be clear, then, that it will be possible no longer for the pharmacist to shunt aside professional and scientific precepts in favor of commercial considerations. Society will demand professional competence, and each of the health disciplines will similarly expect competence from other members of the health team. In a sense each profession will be society's agent in evaluating professional competence in the others. The commercial aspects of pharmacy are without value in this concept.[14]

Another ground-swell of potential influence to conjur with is the manner of health delivery. There seems to be little reason to doubt that the solo practice that has characterized the past will give way to group practice and to institutionalized health centers. This concept has been explored by Samuel Martin[15] and Sidney Garfield[16] as well as others,[10] the recurring themes being organization and planning for efficiency and the practice of preventive medicine. Some of the characteristics of this approach to health care will be an increased fund of knowledge, increasing specialization and increasing demands for service. It is axiomatic that in the face of all this there will result an increased cost per professional unit because of the need for highly trained personnel and sophisticated equipment.

There is one other point to consider. It has been said that public health moves forward by a successive redefining of unacceptables.[17] Any number of unacceptables could be listed based on the premise of "health is a right," but one perhaps has special meaning and significance for the pharmacist: any service, or any cost of service, that cannot be justified by a utilization review will not be acceptable to society. This is interpreted to mean that a health service (pharmacy?) whose contribution to health care is not based on sound professional principles will not be tolerated; if the pharmacist does not assume a significant role and make a meaningful contribution to patient care he will not be able to withstand the scrutiny of utilization review by peers in the health professions. In this context, interprofessional relationships may be seen to assume added importance and significance. Thus the imperatives of the Age of Social Conscience, accented by the influences of historical precept, conspire to force an examination and assessment of pharmacy's consanguinity with the other health professions. The focus of this affinity is the patient, and it is this patient and his health status that will provide the means for reconciliation of pharmacy with other health disciplines so that the interrelationship is truly professional. These relationships will be based in the clinical setting where the application of professional expertise has currency. Clinical pharmacy is the application of the principles and sum total knowledge of pharmacy at the clinical level in direct observation of, or involvement with, the patient. Clinical pharmacy, therefore, is the vehicle to bring about more substantial and rewarding interprofessional relationships. It will be further shown that interprofessional relationships are a natural by-product of professional activity, not something to campaign for as an end within itself.

Precursor to Professional Relationships

This chapter opened with a statement to the effect that the hospital pharmacist was responsible for the current state of concord between pharmacists and physicians, nurses and members of the other health professions. This is partly true but it goes much deeper. The fundamental reason for the situation as it is characterized today is the academic training and preceptorship under which the pharmacist begins his professional life. The pharmacist learns his trade in a vacuum. Until recent innovations were introduced, using the clinical setting for the educational preparation of the student, the academic preceptor had little or no clinical experience and used none of it in training. Pharmacy alone among all the health professions prepared its candidates in virtually complete isolation from patients, from the clinical environment and from other health disciplines. Francke quotes some original words and thoughts by L. Wait Rising in this field, and the dismal reception the ideas received from pharmaceutical educators.[18] Even as an intern, the neophyte pharmacist was denied the intellectual and professional stimulation of the clinical setting and other health workers. Small wonder then, that what relationships he has are passive. (It should be noted that pharmacy has never even developed *intra*professional relationships to a very high degree. Except for formal organizations there is little professional exchange or dependence among pharmacists.)

It is in this confused, inconsistent and ambiguous setting one begins the search for a thread of continuity on which to base relationships with colleagues in other health professions. Interdisciplinary relationships are not created or campaigned for; they evolve. The pharmacist must understand that his deeds and solutions to practical problems need to be questioned for their motivation and presuppositions. Solutions based on yesterday's ideas about the mode and purpose of pharmacy have not proven sufficient for today or tomorrow, nor have they enhanced pharmacy's position in the health care scheme. Its relative position in the health care system of the future must be planned with care, not using the old formulas, but infused with new ideas, daring thoughts and a complete understanding of the forces and concepts that will influence the future. The pharmacist will achieve appropriate recognition when his contributions are recognized for their worth. Cato is reported to have said to his friend Sempronius, "'Tis not in mortals to command success; but we'll do more, we'll deserve it." How can pharmacists deserve success? In the first place by assuring health care colleagues of a high degree of professional competence, and secondly, by bringing a body of knowledge into the patient care arena, knowledge to make a contribution to patient care.

Responsibility and Roles

The pharmacist has a unique body of knowledge, and his responsibility is to utilize this knowledge in the arena of patient care. It is this knowledge and this setting that transforms him into a clinical pharmacist. Only here has his contribution currency of equal value to all concerned: the patient, the physician, the nurse and all other supporting health professionals. Knowledge and the communication of knowledge are the clinical pharmacist's responsibility and obligation; he has no other. This is what distinguishes a pharmacist as a professional, as contrasted with skilled technicians. The competent discharge of this responsibility will provide the cement for close interprofessional relationships so necessary to the effective health care team.

There are many roles to assume for the clinical pharmacist in the discharge of his responsibility. He will of course have the role of the professional. He will share his knowledge in the resolution of a problem in therapeutic management. The role of the administrator, or manager, will be a not infrequent pose, as he organizes, plans and directs a system for distributing drugs to patients, safely, efficiently and economically. In the field of technology, the pharmacist will resolve problems of compounding, packaging and storage with his knowledge of pharmacy and pharmaceutics.

In the hospital setting, the pharmacist's roles will, in addition, parallel those of the hospital. The hospital is a center for patient care, and it is also in varying degrees a center for teaching and a center for research. The consummate clinical pharmacist participates in each of these.

Thus the aspiring pharmacist is—or can be—many things. Within these roles there are several functions, and it is these practical aspects within the spectrum of responsibility that focus on the pharmacist and form the basis of respect and recognition.

The Role of the Professional

The role of a professional is of primary interest. "A professional," in the words of William Hubbard, former Dean of the College of Medicine of the University of Michigan, "is a person identified by society to serve on their behalf in an essential role. He must have special knowledge and skill to justify this appointment, and he must be willing to accept personal responsibility for his actions. He must also provide leadership."[19] How does this description reflect the current standard of practice, and how can the pharmacist adapt his practice to fulfill this role? The fundamental responsibility of the pharmacist is to provide knowledge; therefore, to accommodate the professional role he should be providing drug intelligence to other members of the health care team. This is best done on a personal, firsthand basis, and the clinical pharmacist should be spending his time with patients, with physicians and nurses and other pharmacists, consulting, discussing and researching patient care. Or he may be involved in solitary, reflective study to reconcile his knowledge and experience in a problem of therapeutic management. This cannot be done by extrasensory perception from a remote base of operations in the basement pharmacy of a hospital or from a drugstore several blocks from a physician's office. The pharmacist must be where the action is, in the patient care arena with other members of the health team. This is where he belongs. This is also where interdisciplinary relationships begin and flourish.

The Pharmacist Consultant

What is a pharmacist, if he is not, *a priori*, a counselor on drugs and drug use? He has no function, as a professional—or in the professional spectrum—other than an individual who is a reasonable authority on drugs. The role of a consultant in information about drugs is important to the pharmacist because knowledge of drugs is perhaps the last possession he has. Machines can formulate and prepare dosage forms; machines can dispense, record, charge and even reorder without the pharmacist's help. The pharmacist cannot compete with the machine in the function of materials management.

Information about drugs and about the use of drugs must be a part of the pattern of pharmacy service. Medical science and public health disciplines have a sharp appetite for information, and there is a continuing and constant use of information in available forms. The pharmacist can satisfy this demand and is in a position to do so. It can be done by creating an "environment of information," so that "pharmacy" and "information" are thought of in the same context. Be assured if an "information gap" is allowed to develop a vacuum, some other enterprising group will respond to the need, and the pharmacist will be on the outside looking in.*

Again, drug information is part of the pattern of service. The body of practice and the body of knowledge cannot be separated; they must be as one in service to the patient, the physician, nurse and to the institution. Drug information should not be restricted to proscribed channels of communication and procedure if it is to have currency in patient care. Drug information should not be regarded as a special function; it is a part and parcel of the profession of pharmacy, a natural resource, so to speak, of the body and practice of pharmacy. The role as a drug consultant is more enhanced, to paraphrase Emerson, by what is done and how it is done, more than any claim by right of profession or any other reason. This signifies that the role of a drug information consultant must have visual exposure as it resides in the pharmacist who practices in the clinical setting, in preference to relegating it to a central, formal but remote office.

Other Functions in the Professional Role

Information in the clinical setting is not at all restricted to drugs, of course. Of equal, if not primary, importance is information about the patient. It should be recognized in this discussion of relationships between pharmacists and physicians and nurses that drug information *per se* is of little value if it is not relevant to the case at hand. It is imperative, therefore, that the function of the information consultant include knowledge of the patient and disease, and one of the ways to do this is to compose a patient profile.

*To gain the advantage of another perspective in the drug information milieu, the reader should consult an editorial entitled, "The Medical-Legal Aspects of Adverse Drug Reactions," by F. L. Tozer and J. E. Kasik.[20]

A profile is a sketch, an outline; it is also a vivid biography. It gives information needed to be able to make an intelligent assessment of the patient's status or perhaps a decision in the course of therapeutic management. A medication profile provides facts about the patient, physical and physiological, including current diagnoses. It will indicate who the attending physician is and to which teaching service the patient is assigned. It will of course include all drugs ordered for the patient, their dosage and interval of administration, whether on a regular schedule or just one dose, when they were started and when they were stopped. The various diagnostic procedures and clinical laboratory tests should also be included, especially if they have any potential in the resolution of the therapeutic plan for the patient. With such a document the patient begins to come into focus, and is something more than just a statistic in a hospital census. At this point the title "clinical pharmacist" begins to be something more than just a nice sounding phrase, because there is personal, direct involvement with and observation of the patient. This is clinical pharmacy.

Another value of the medication profile, and one which has yet to be fully exploited, is to prepare the pharmacist to play a leading role in therapeutic management. This is not a farfetched dream of the idle mind, but a real possibility, consistent with Dean Hubbard's statement that a professional must provide leadership. Where else shall the pharmacist aspire to provide leadership if it is not in the field of drugs and drug therapy? This outline can be put to another use, and that is to provide logistical control. With all his patient profiles, the pharmacist has the necessary documents to determine the flow of drugs in his area. He can know in the space of minutes just what drugs he will need to carry out his function at any point in time. This is drug control and it is the mainstream of professional practice.

The reality of a medication profile is a virtual impossibility without some form of direct communication with the doctor's original order. This can be done in several ways, and it is unnecessary here to describe these several ways, except to note that the success of such communication is directly proportional to the amount of personal and direct involvement by the pharmacist. The pharmacist who is a familiar sight working with physicians in group practice or on the hospital wards is more likely to become a part of the equation as these professionals resolve their problems with patient care. The pharmacist's counsel will be much more highly regarded than if he is an absentee performer, participating by remote control from his isolated pharmacy. Contrary to the old adage, familiarity breeds confidence. This can make a significant difference in the deliberations of a pharmacy and therapeutics committee, for example.

The Pharmacy and Therapeutics Committee

The pharmacy and therapeutics committee (P & T Committee) is an example of interprofessional relationships in the classical setting. It is also perhaps the ultimate configuration of the fulfillment of the pharmacist's basic responsibility: the contribution and communication of knowledge on drugs and therapeutics. Ideally envisioned, it is a peer committee charged with counseling and recommending rational drug therapy. The pharmacist's role is extremely important and often is the difference between a passive or dynamic group. Although usually associated with hospital practice, the pharmacy and therapeutics committee can function equally well in a physician-pharmacist group practice environment for the benefit of ambulatory patients.

The prescribing of drugs is an act so ancient its origins belong with the beginings of the art and science of medicine. The art, however, may be said to have become the victim of the science, for the armamentarium of the physician has, from an humble collection of selected remedies, proliferated into thousands of therapeutic specialties. Perhaps as recently as 20 years ago, but most certainly at the beginning of the Second World War, the competent physician could retain in his mind and one or two reference books his personal selection of drugs; his "formulary," so to speak. Two decades later, however, there has been a dramatic change in the number and in the dynamism of therapeutic agents. It is within this context that the P & T committee fulfills its mission. One often hears this period—the latter half of the 20th Century—referred to as the Atomic Age, the Electronic Age or the Space Age. Therapeutics have more than kept pace with these other technological and scientific advances, and one could just as well name this the Therapeutic Age. It may be appropriate, therefore, that in this age the pharmacist may realize the ultimate fulfillment in his role as a therapeutic consultant and in his relationships with physicians.

The function of the P & T committee is not the province of this chapter; this has been discussed well and at length in the literature of pharmacy.* It is, however, germane to the discussion to explore the many facets of the role of the pharmacist on this committee. Traditionally the pharmacist serves as the secretary of this committee of the medical staff. As such he has the opportunity to exercise several roles already mentioned, the professional, educational and, in a limited sense, the research role. As secretary he is often the de facto administrator of the committee, organizing the agenda, calling the meeting, reasoning with the members of the committee, recording the minutes and maintaining the files. The importance of this needs no emphasis, and the excellence of this performance is expected and taken for granted. Competence here generates confidence.

The real work of the committee is pursued in the promotion of rational drug therapy. Rational therapy is defined as the best possible therapy, consistent with patient safety, therapeutic efficiency and economy. It is here perhaps that the professional role of the pharmacist, in concert with the roles of education and research, achieves a lasting foundation for interprofessional relationships. For it is with his professional background and knowledge of drug therapy and pharmaceutical sciences the pharmacist accumulates the documentation necessary for the committee to make possible an intelligent and informed evaluation of drugs and therapy. The pharmacist will research the literature to bring current opinions and concepts to the attention of the committee members. He will communicate this documentation objectively and without bias, as befits a health scientist and educator. Thus the pharmacist participates as a peer, and in this context establishes the basis for mutually rewarding interdisciplinary cooperation.

Drugs today have assumed characteristics in a context similar to those that identify the other, infinitely precise surgical and therapeutic tools in the physician's armamentarium. The traditional function of the P & T committee has been to offer counsel on their appropriate use. The authority to command compliance with this counsel or to exercise sanctions against those who do not comply has not been part of the committee's charge. Recent comment and opinion, as well as the developing social philosophy on health care, indicate the role of the P & T committee may assume broader and more authoritative dimensions in the area of drug utilization or drug monitoring. This may manifest itself in a drug audit program and further enlarge the scope and quantity of work of the committee. The role of the pharmacist will not change, but his importance may be reinforced. This growing trend toward review and control of drug use, from prescription order through administration to the patient, will place added emphasis on the relative position of the pharmacist in the health care team.

Historically the pharmacist has been presented with opportunities to develop meaningful relationships with the medical fraternity. From the first formulary of the New York Hospital in 1816, through the endorsement of the pharmacy and therapeutics committee by the American College of Surgeons in 1933, the recommendations of the Joint Committee on Accreditation of Hospitals and including the Conditions for Participation for Title XVIII of the 1965 Amendments to the Social Security Act, there have been opportunities for the pharmacist to enhance his professional position. This has not been exploited, however, and it is interesting to speculate on the reasons and influences that led the pharmacist to emphasize his distributive or logistical function in the administrative echelons rather than professional roles with other health professionals in direct patient care. Theo Van Gogh is reported to have chided his brother Vincent with the observation that "you have all the attributes of greatness in you: the flair for design and the mastery of color and the genius of composition, but so far . . . "[22] One could chide pharmacy similarly: it has the academic preparation and the professional credentials, and opportunity beckons, but so far . . . So far the pharmacist has seen fit to attach himself to merchandising in drugstores, or to the administrative or corporate functions in the hospital, as contrasted with patient care or clinical functions. As a consequence he is often seen by physicians as a retail merchant or a junior member of a hospital's administration, and not at all a part of the patient care team. This may not interfere with the rapport between physicians and pharmacists, but it will not go far toward enhancing interprofessional respect and confidence at the professional, patient care level.

This situation will need to be reversed if the pharmacist wishes to be included in peer groups involved in patient care. The pharmacist professionally, ideologically and clinically must be more closely aligned with the physician as a health professional. This is not to say the phar-

*A recent series of articles appearing in *Drug Intelligence and Clinical Pharmacy* by H. J. Derewicz is recommended as a comprehensive treatment of this important facet of the pharmacist's responsibility.[21]

macist should become a junior physician any more than he is a junior hospital administrator, but it does mean that the thrust of his *professional* activity must be directed toward the patient and the therapeutic management of that patient rather than logistical and administrative consideration for a system, of which the patient is a consumer.

Hospital Roles

Other roles parallel the mission of the hospital. They are not less professional, to be sure; in fact, some may not give these roles separate distinction. It helps, however, to view these from a slightly different perspective, and they should be considered.

The primary role of the hospital is patient care, and that of the pharmacist, therefore, the same. This is the essence of clinical pharmacy discussed earlier as a feature of the professional role. Some activities one may consider under the aegis of the hospital role are I.V. additive programs, preparation of patient doses and even their administration, and 24-hour pharmacy service. The common denominator here is drug-related services for patients that are largely performed by other than pharmacists or pharmacy-supervised personnel. Every general hospital has an I.V. additive program, but with few outstanding exceptions, it is a nursing service program. Is this or is it not a pharmaceutical function in the classical definition of pharmacy? Pharmacists in the majority have avoided making a decision on this issue with the excuse of lack of time and personnel . . . but excuses do not build alliances. The adding of drugs to I.V. fluids is an activity performed daily by hospital personnel; the pharmacist must rethink and reorganize the function so it can be placed under the jurisdiction of the pharmacy department. This is leadership, and this is the way to develop strong interprofessional relationships.

Similarly, the preparation of unusual doses or dosage forms is left to the ward nurse if it cannot be bought on the open market. If an oral solid dosage is to be administered by tube it is generally the nurse who pulverizes the tablet, suspends it in tap water and prepares the dose for administration. It is usually the nurse who has to figure out how to get a 200 mg dose of an oral liquid when it is labeled 150 mg per 5 ml; The nurse reconstitutes PPD tablets and other multiple dose diagnostic drugs for use on the ward, and is generally involved in other *pharmaceutical tasks* so the patient can get the right dose in the right form. Where is the pharmacist? Where is the leadership, where is the professional involvement here? Is it any wonder that pharmacists are not considered in the mainstream of patient care?

The Educational Role

Almost every function performed by a pharmacist in his professional capacity is a potential educational experience for someone. One thing to consider is the training of an intern or resident. What professional who believes strongly and passionately in his goals and objectives does not yearn for the opportunity to pass these on to someone else, to have his disciples? This is what an internship is, a dynamic educational experience and in it the pharmacist is the educator. Intraprofessional as well as interprofessional recognition is in no small way dependent upon the influence the pharmacist has on those who learn from him. It is no accident that the overwhelming majority of recognized leaders in any profession are those who taught well and whose disciples have dignified their teaching. The role of an educator gives an added dimension of dignity to the practitioner and fosters respect from colleagues allied in the programs of health care.

There are several classes and grades of health care personnel who would respond readily to an opportunity to learn more about drugs and how they act. The pharmacist can fulfill this need in the hospital in a variety of ways: in refresher courses for nurses or drug conferences, similar to nursing conferences, on each ward. A drug bulletin is another way to communicate and teach. An educational program may be tailored to fit into the hospital's in-service training program that reaches all personnel. The pharmacist must approach this role with all the dignity and sincerity education commands. It will not do to treat it is a episodic venture; it must be organized and planned to provide a continuing fund of usable information. This is a real service and a necessary service, and it could teach respect for drugs. Respect for drugs brings also respect for those who shoulder the responsibility for drugs and drug use.

Administrative Role

Tradition and custom are precious precepts. Years ago the pharmacist practiced the art of pharmacy with a high degree of skill. The advent of pharmaceutical technology, however, has largely replaced and made these obsolete. The pharmacist responded to this and substituted other manipulative skills, skills that did not justify or dignify his rigorous academic training nor his high professional calling. Even these have now come under attack, and while not universally endorsed, there is a growing acceptance of the belief these manipulative, technical tasks can be assigned to nonprofessional personnel to carry out under the supervision of a pharmacist. It is a question of time before this will be accomplished and what then shall the pharmacist do? If he is to succeed, and if he is to be recognized as a peer in the ranks of health professionals he will marshall his skills as an administrator, or as a manager. One feature of this role will be to design and implement a drug distribution system. Another would be to assure the financial and economic integrity of his pharmacy in the community or of the department or pharmacy in the hospital. This is true of all pharmacists, regardless of the size and scope of their managerial responsibility, including the one-man pharmacy and the so-called "staff" pharmacist.

Management, in its simplest definition, is the art of getting things done through people. The function of a manager is to plan, organize and control the activities for which he has responsibility and authority so that all concerned enjoy success, the consumer and user as well as the producer. In this role the pharmacist will need to reconcile his knowledge, ability and intellectual approach to the current social and professional philosophy. It is beyond the scope of this discussion to go into detail in the several functions of the administrative role, but perhaps it is worth stating again that solutions based on yesterday's ideas and concepts will not be sufficient for the tasks confronting pharmacy today. The clinical pharmacist must make use of the new technology and embrace new concepts of personnel utilization. As Will Durant said, when writing of Francis Bacon: "Of theory and practice, one without the other is useless and perilous; knowledge that does not generate achievement is a pale bloodless thing unworthy of mankind. We strive to learn the form of things, not for the sake of form but by knowing the forms, the laws, we can remake things in the image of our own desires."[23] The pharmacist may interpret this as an invitation to learn the "forms—and laws" of EDP, unit dose technology, mechanical dispensing aids, technicians and more; learn them and use them and remake things in the image of his own desires.

One could continue at length about the roles the pharmacist assumes and how, through the performance of these roles, the pharmacist may develop close rapport and lasting relationships with other members of the health team. There would be too much of a tendency, however, to let this exercise decline into a session of image making through imagination. Pharmacists have been known to do this and, like Narcissus,* they become so enraptured with the image they create they lose sight of the goals and purposes of the profession. *Service* is the nourishment of a profession, not imagery. Recognition, status, respect will come only as a result of dedicated competent service.

Pharmacy is a professional practice that exists as a dichotomy: there is the logistical service that encompasses the distributive function and there is the intelligence service that embodies the heart and brain of the science and art of pharmacy. The latter completely dominates the other in its potential for professional credentials, but the paradox is that the pharmacist is more often judged by the quality of his supply services than by the quality of his intelligence service. It is, however, a situation of the pharmacist's own making, and perhaps one of the first strategic objectives should be to shift the focus of recognition to the intelligence service. Knowledge is the only possession the pharmacist has of lasting value, and his sole responsibility is to communicate, to share and to utilize this in patient care in the clinical setting. Thus an immediate tactical objective is to get into the patient care arena. This arena may be in the hospital ward or in professional intellectual communication with a physician regarding his patient in the community. Clinical pharmacy has application with all patients, whether ambulant or hospitalized, just as interprofessional relationships will be found in the community as well as in the hospital. It is the responsibility of the pharmacist to attain these tactical and strategic objectives, and when this is done the ultimate goal of professional recognition will be within his grasp.

*Narcissus is a character in Greek mythology who became captivated by his own reflection in a pool. He became so enamored with his image he was completely oblivious to opportunities for fulfillment. He withered away and died looking at his reflection in the pool, and where he lay there grew up a slender lovely flower we now call the narcissus.[24]

References

1. Darley, W. and Somers, A. R.: Medicine, Money and Manpower — The Challenge to Professional Education, *New Engl. J. Med. 276*:1414-1423 (June 22) 1967.

2. Suppan, L.: The Monastic Dispensaries of the Middle Ages, *J. Am. Pharm. Assoc. 4*:383-396 (Sept.) 1915.

3. Nuppenau, H.: Hospital Pharmacy in Denmark and Abroad, *J. Mondial Pharm. 8*:33-46 (Jan.-Mar.) 1965.

4. Burkholder, D.: Martin Inventius Wilbert: Hospital Pharmacist, Scientist and Historian, *Am. J. Hosp. Pharm. 25*:330-343 (July) 1968.

5. Anon.: Dedication to Harvey A. K. Whitney, *Am. J. Hosp. Pharm. 15*:4-5 (Jan.) 1958.

6. Lee, C. O.: Edward Spease, A Memorial, *Am. J. Hosp. Pharm. 15*:64-65 (Jan.) 1958.

7. Sonnedecker, G.: Harvey A. K. Whitney and Edward Spease; In Memoriam, *Am. J. Hosp. Pharm. 15*:507-509 (June) 1958.

8. Anon.: National Health Insurance, *Congressional Record 116*:E6317 (July 7) 1970 (Griffiths Health Insurance Bill).

9. Anon.: The Fulton-Broyhill Bill: National Health Insurance Through the Medicredit Tax Incentive Plan, *Congressional Record 116*:H7122 (July 23) 1970.

10. Anon.: The Perloff Committee, *Hospitals 44*:39-42, History of the Committee; The Committee Report, 43-46; Analysis of the Report, 47-52 (Dec. 16) 1970.

11. Wolfe, H. G.: Charles Rice (1841-1901), An Immigrant in Pharmacy, *Am. J. Pharm. Educ. 14*:285-305 (Apr.) 1950.

12. Denzin, N. K. and Mettlin, C. J.: Incomplete Professionalization: The Case of Pharmacy, *Social Forces 46*: 375-381 (Mar.) 1968.

13. Montague, J. B., Jr.: Pharmacy and the Concept of Professionalism, *J. Am. Pharm. Assoc. NS8*:228 (May) 1968.

14. Anon.: Task Force on Prescription Drugs — Background Papers — The Drug Makers and The Drug Distributors, U. S. Dept. HEW, Washington, D.C., Dec. 1968 p. 83-85.

15. Martin, S. P.: Patient Care Yesterday, Today and Tomorrow, *Am. J. Hosp. Pharm. 24*:170-177 (Apr.) 1967.

16. Garfield, S.: The Delivery of Medical Care, *Sci. Am. 222*:15-23 (Apr.) 1970.

17. Vickers, G.: What Sets the Goals of Public Health, *Lancet 1*:599-604 (Mar. 22) 1958.

18. Francke, D. E.: Let's Separate Pharmacies and Drugstores, *Am. J. Pharm. 141*:161-176 (Sept.-Oct.) 1969.

19. Hubbard, W. N., Jr.: "Emerging Patterns of Education and Practice in the Health Professions — Medicine," in Deno, R. A. (ed.): *Proceedings Pharmacy — Medicine — Nursing Conference on Health Education*, University of Michigan Press, Ann Arbor, Mich., 1967, p. 5-9.

20. Tozer, F. L. and Kasik, J. E.: The Medical-Legal Aspects of Adverse Drug Reactions, *Clin. Pharmacol. Therap. 8*:637-646 (Sept.-Oct.) 1967.

21. Derewicz, H. J.: Why a Pharmacy and Therapeutics Committee, *Drug Intelligence 1*:30-32 (Jan.) 1967, *et seq.*

22. Stone, I.: *Lust for Life,* Random House, Inc., New York, NY, 1934.

23. Durant, W.: *The Story of Philosophy,* Simon and Schuster, 1933 (Time, Inc. Ed.), p. 127.

24. Bulfinch, T.: *Bulfinch's Mythology,* Random House, Inc., New York, NY, 1934, p. 84-87.

5

Developing a clinical pharmacy program in the hospital

by William E. Smith and Dennis W. Mackewicz

Within the last five to ten years, pharmaceutical literature and educational meetings have emphasized the responsibilities of the pharmacist to serve the patient. Such terms as clinical pharmacy, clinical pharmacist, clinical clerkship, clinical drug information services and pharmacist participation in the patient care area activities have dominated the literature and thinking of hospital pharmacists. Why the sudden and dynamic thrust for change in providing pharmaceutical services and pharmaceutical education? The authors believe the reasons for change are just as important as the methods to implement change. Therefore, some description of the history, justification for and objectives of clinical pharmacy services will be given at the beginning of this chapter. As the component parts of clinical pharmacy services are presented, the emphasis will be on how to develop, define, implement and manage the new clinical services.

HISTORICAL DEVELOPMENT AND OBJECTIVES OF CLINICAL PHARMACY

No one would dispute the statement that drugs play a significant role in the treatment of most disease states. Also, no one would disagree that drugs are potent and that the drugs of tomorrow will be more potent than those of today. Yet the extensive prescribing of drugs results in patient care problems. Drugs are distributed by a hospital medication system which is so complicated, inefficient and prone to errors that it defies description.

The problem of medication errors was first reported in the literature in 1962 by Barker and McConnell.[1] The study reported one error in every six doses administered. Even though such statistics have been disputed, there is a general agreement that medication errors do exist in modern drug therapy at a significant rate. In 1970, an article by Hynniman and co-workers reported medication error rates of traditional medication systems in four hospitals ranging from 8 to 20 percent.[2]

Appearing in the medical literature in the mid-1960's were epidemiologic studies of adverse drug reactions of patients treated in hospitals. In general, the statistics from these studies showed:

1. Ten to 15 percent of hospital patients experience an adverse drug reaction during hospitalization
2. Hospital stay for patients with a reaction is prolonged an average of nine days when compared to patients with no reaction
3. A direct proportional increase in adverse drug reaction exists with the increase in number of drugs prescribed
4. The majority of reactions (81 percent) are due to pharmacological action of the drug and are, therefore, predictable and preventable[3-5]*

*Refer to Chapter 11 for more extensive information.

Drug distribution in hospitals revolves around the nurse and her supportive personnel. In addition to her nursing duties, she has been charged with the responsibility to maintain an adequate drug inventory on the floor, prepare and administer the medications, prepare drug admixtures for intravenous solutions, return the unused drugs to the pharmacy for credit, maintain narcotic and hypnotic records, and so on. In a recent study, 22 percent of total nursing time was devoted to medication activities.[6] The traditional system of drug distribution results in a tremendous duplication of effort by the nurse and pharmacist, and the nurse practices more pharmacy than does the pharmacist.[7] She interviews the patient on admission for drug allergies, has accepted the major responsibility for initial detection of a potentially undesirable drug reaction and she is supposed "to know about" all of the drugs she administers. Oftentimes, the physician requests drug information from the nurse. In reality, she does not have the time, pharmacological background nor current drug knowledge to perform adequately these responsibilities she has reluctantly assumed.

During the 1960's, pharmacists in hospitals responded aggressively to the problems associated with drug distribution and drug therapy. New services designed, developed and implemented included:

1. Unit dose drug distribution systems
2. Intravenous drug admixture programs
3. Patient medication profiles
4. Drug information centers
5. Pharmacist participation in patient care rounds
6. Practice in patient care areas in pharmacy substations
7. Clinical clerkship teaching programs
8. Drug therapy conferences for physicians and nurses
9. Patient drug monitoring services

The services listed are justified from and based upon the reference point "what is best for the patient." The composite of these services has been called by their advocates "clinical pharmacy services."[8]

In addition to the problems inherent in modern drug therapy, the need for clinical drug information and the inadequacies of traditional hospital medication systems, pharmacists have actively made changes occur for many personal reasons. Pharmacists want to utilize their knowledge and are becoming tired of the mechanical functions of drug dispensing such as typing labels, counting and pouring. They seek acceptance as a professional, as experts on drugs, from physicians, nurses, patients, hospital administrators and other hospital personnel. They are seeking a daily academic challenge. They are fearful of the future, the rapidly changing health care systems, mechanization and what their future might or might not be. Most important, they recognize the drug problems of modern patient care and believe they can help solve those problems and provide better patient care. These reasons coupled with experiences of the past five to ten years are why clinical pharmacy has captured the interest and imagination of many pharmacists and other health professionals. The authors believe clinical pharmacy services should be provided to all patients, inpatient and outpatient. The challenge to pharmacists of the 1970's and 1980's is to provide clinical services to all patients.

Objectives of Clinical Pharmacy Services

A basic objective of clinical pharmacy services is to provide the right drug to the right patient at the right time. To meet this objective two components of pharmacy service are mandatory: (1) drug distribution and (2) clinical drug information. Both components are interrelated and must be provided concurrently for clinical pharmacy services to be beneficial. The problems of manpower utilization, and services at a reasonable cost do not allow for the two components to be separated in the development of clinical pharmacy services in the hospital.

Several goals of the drug distribution element of clinical pharmacy services should be kept in mind when changes are planned and made in the traditional methods of distributing drugs. Some of these are listed below:

1. Minimal medication errors
2. Patient safety
3. Efficient utilization of hospital personnel
4. Drug product control
5. Cost controls

A unit dose system of drug distribution achieves these ends where the traditional methods of drug distribution do not. For these reasons, unit dose is an integral part of the development of clinical pharmacy services.

In order to provide the "right drug" to a particular patient, the use of current clinical drug information is necessary. The pharmacist in clinical practice must work *cooperatively* with the physician in meeting this fundamental purpose of clinical pharmacy. Drug information is provided through the various clinical practice activities of the pharmacist as listed below:

1. Practice in the patient care areas
2. Review, interpret and personalize all prescribed drug orders
3. Patient drug monitoring service
4. Attend and participate in patient care rounds
5. Provide drug therapy conferences for physicians
6. Participation in an organized drug information service

It is through the performance of these clinical activities that the pharmacist plays an active role in patient care by providing clinical drug information.

Figure 1. An abstract representation of pharmacy services in a hospital

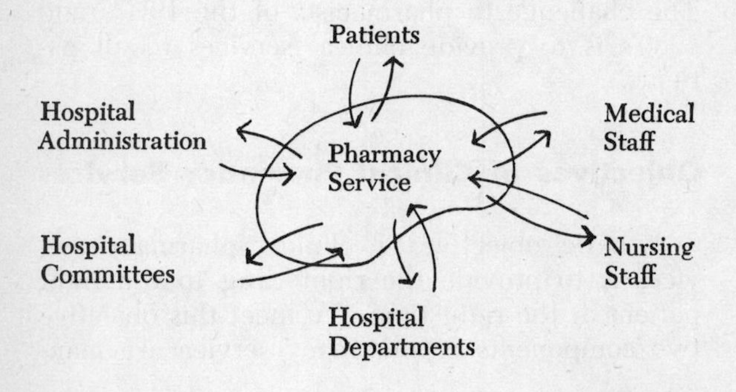

The pharmacy department has been represented abstractly by the region within the closed curve. The interaction between the pharmacy department and other groups within the hospital is indicated by the arrows which also depict the flow of information and materials. Clinical pharmacy services require goals for each group identified. Examples of goals for patients, medical staff and nursing staff are listed below:

Patients

1. To provide safe and effective drug therapy at the lowest possible cost.
2. To provide a safe and efficient drug distribution system for all patients treated.

Medical Staff

1. To provide high quality drug information as needed and when needed.
2. To work cooperatively with the medical staff to provide safe and effective drug therapy for all patients.

Nursing Staff

1. To provide drugs in unit doses accurately and when needed.
2. To provide high quality drug information as needed and when needed.

These goals are reciprocal, that is, the patients, physicians and nurses are users of pharmacy services. Their intent for placing demands on pharmacy for clinical services is in concert with those of the pharmacy department.

If the goals for both the users and providers for pharmacy services are the same, why then is it so difficult to develop and implement a clinical pharmacy service in a hospital? As with any change in patient services, this does not come easily. Pharmacy departments are usually small in size and small in staff. Pharmacists frequently have not adequately defined their service objectives. Many hospital administrators have not been too concerned about hospital medication systems and drug therapy problems, but this is really the fault of pharmacists for not presenting facts about such problems. The most significant difficulty to overcome in order to implement a successful clinical pharmacy service is changing traditional attitudes, philosophies and responsibilities of each component of the drug utilization axis as defined by Brodie and shown in Figure 2.[9]

Figure 2. Drug Utilization Axis

Drug Utilization Axis

Physician - Pharmacist - Nurse - Patient

What are the desired professional relationships and responsibilities among the physician-pharmacist-nurse to provide the safest drug therapy possible? What are effective communications? How can changes in traditional habits and attitudes that need modification for better patient care be implemented? In the sections of this chapter relating to pharmacist-nurse and pharmacist-physician relationships, answers to these questions will be discussed.

HOSPITAL MEDICATION SYSTEM

The hospital medication system has been undergoing critical re-examination on the basis of patient safety and cost in recent years. The hospital medication system beginning with a physician's order for a drug, encompasses a variety of steps involving nursing and pharmacy, ultimately to administer drugs to patients. Traditional medication systems involve the nurse in many more tasks than the pharmacist. Table 1 illustrates the number of steps required of the nurse in the traditional system as compared to the pharmacist.

Table 1. Steps in the Traditional Medication System

Physician	— orders drug
Nursing	— writes orders into medication record
	— writes orders into patient care plan
	— writes orders on medication card
	— writes and/or sends order to pharmacy if not floor stock
Pharmacy	— fills orders (copies of chart, transcribed or ward stock orders)
Nursing	— receives and stores drugs
	— prepares doses at designated time intervals
	— administers doses
	— charts doses at end of nursing shift
	— returns drugs to pharmacy upon discontinuation of order
	— sends credits to pharmacy

The unit dose drug distribution system has been intimately associated with the growth of the pharmacist's clinical practice in the hospital. The unit dose system, however, can stand on its own merit as being safer for the patient[10] and more economical for the hospital as a whole.[11] The patient benefits directly from the unit dose system in several ways: (1) medication errors are fewer, (2) he pays only for the drugs administered to him and (3) prescribed drugs are administered more promptly. The nurse is removed from the drug distribution system except for administering and recording of medications. The pharmacist can safely delegate the majority of the routine and mechanical dispensing duties to a technician.

Probably the first thing one must think about in developing a unit dose system in a hospital is how to approach the hospital administrator. A proposal to design and implement a pilot project for evaluation should be submitted to administration listing the present problems with the existing system and the expected benefits of a unit dose system. Once the go-ahead is given, the first step in planning a unit dose system is to gather as much workload information as possible. The medication record can be studied to determine: (1) the average number of doses per patient day by patient area and (2) the volume of oral solids, oral liquids, injectables and suppositories administered.

From this information an approximate number of doses to be prepared per day can be determined giving an idea of the pharmacy technician's workload. As will be discussed later, the number of unit dose oral solids, liquids, injectables and suppositories which can be purchased as such or need to be packaged is necessary to determine what the packaging and equipment needs will be. In addition, the number of new orders and what time of day they are written can be determined giving some idea of the pharmacist's workload and staffing requirements. To get a more accurate picture, all types of demands to be handled from the unit dose preparation area such as narcotic replacements and I.V. additives should be considered.

If at all possible the amount of nursing time spent in various aspects of the present drug distribution system should be studied. The Commission on Administrative Services to Hospitals (C.A.S.H.) has performed industrial engineering studies and has developed various standard times that can be utilized.[12] For example, the average amount of time necessary to prepare oral medications equals 0.021 hours per dose prepared. The steps in this task include the following:

1. Secure med card for each medicine to be adminstered
2. Arrange cards in room sequence
3. Read name and medication on med card
4. Locate medicine on shelf of medicine cabinet
5. Count medicine to assure 24-hour supply
6. Compare label on medicine container with the label on med card
7. Pour prescribed amount into medicine cup and read the label a second time
8. Wipe rim of bottle, replace cap, read label a third time and replace bottle in medicine cabinet
9. Dispense capsules, tablets and powders. Check each medication against card three times during dispensing procedure
10. Transfer medication dispensed with dropper into medicine cup, add water, milk or juices as prescribed.

The described dose preparation task is removed from the nursing workload and represents the most obvious savings of nursing personnel time upon implementing a unit dose system.

Implementing A Unit Dose System

Implementation of a unit dose system involves the hospital pharmacist in many areas directly affecting the physician and nurse. At the onset, and prerequisite to the more complex changes, a system to provide a chart copy of the physician's order to the pharmacist should first be implemented. Two copies of the physician's order should be considered, one going to the pharmacist and the other to the nurse since the second copy can contribute to saving nursing time. In implementing a new physician order sheet to provide copies, one should avoid having to modify the physician's habits if at all possible, especially in a community hospital.

The design of a unit dose system must be tailor-made to fit each individual hospital's needs. An interdisciplinary approach within the hospital is very important. For example, developing the medication record for the unit dose system is the one area that causes the greatest difficulty and physician input here is essential. The unit dose drug distribution system must be conceptualized and procedures worked out with nursing.

As with any system, a reliable communication and delivery system to handle new drug orders is very important. The location of the unit dose storage and preparation area (centralized or decentralized) will affect these requirements which will include:

- All chart orders - new, discontinue drug orders, etc.
- Admission, transfer and discharge notices
- Non-physician ordered supplies and sundry item requests
- Narcotics replacements
- Missing or dropped unit doses requested
- NPO and surgery orders

Both written and verbal communications may be satisfactory depending upon individual hospital system requirements. Communication demands between pharmacy and nursing are greater as noted above; a timely and accurate current record of the patient's drug therapy is a necessity. Patient location, scheduled surgeries and discontinued orders are necessary to update the patient's current drug therapy record from which to prepare doses. Pneumatic tubes going directly between the dose preparation area and the nursing station (mini-tubes), letter drop chutes and dumbwaiters are some approaches used in routing information and drugs to and from the dose preparation area and each nursing station. Various lateral and vertical communication and delivery systems should be seriously considered when pharmacy and nursing areas are not immediately adjacent to one another. A note pad form (Pharmacy Drug Notice) is used by nursing to record special requests for medication doses and to alert pharmacy as to why some scheduled doses were not administered (Figure 3). A Special Dosage Schedule Drug envelope (Figure 4) is used to issue initial doses of new drugs to nursing. It also serves as a communications notice. Some of nursing communication forms sent to pharmacy are listed below:

Figure 3. Pharmacy Drug Notice. In pad form these are used by nursing service to (1) request drugs and (2) note scheduled drugs not given

PHARMACY DRUG NOTICE

Date __________
Shift— AM PM MN

PATIENT'S NAME __________

ROOM—BED NO. __________

Scheduled Drugs Not Given

- ☐ Refused
- ☐ NPO
- ☐ Discontinued
- ☐ Drug Not Ordered
- ☐ Other (explain): __________
- ☐ Patient Discharged
- ☐ Patient Expired
- ☐ Incorrect Dosage

Drug(s): __________

Drug Request (other than new orders)

- ☐ Missing
- ☐ Dropped
- ☐ Other (explain): __________
- ☐ Stat VERBAL ORDER

Number of Doses Needed to 3:00 P.M.	DRUG	Strength	Route

Noted or Requested by __________

Checked or Prepared by __________

1212/25

Rm. Number____________________

Pt. Name____________________

SPECIAL DOSAGE SCHEDULE
DRUG:

FIRST DOSE = X

AM 1 2 3 4 5 6 7 8 9 10 11 12

PM 1 2 3 4 5 6 7 8 9 10 11 12

GENERIC EQUIVALENT DISPENSED

__________ = __________
Dispensed Ordered

AUTOMATIC STOP ORDER ☐

1.____________________

2.____________________

3.____________________

MISC.:

Figure 4. Drug Envelope. A drug envelope is used to issue initial doses of new drugs to nursing service. The envelope also serves as a communications notice

1. Copies of physician's order sheet
2. Admission/Blank charge slip
3. Transfer/Discharge slip
4. Discharge prescriptions
5. NPO notice
6. Controlled Drug Disposition Record
7. Pharmacy Drug Notice (Figure 3)

The most apparent new piece of equipment in a hospital on a unit dose system is the medication cart (Figure 5). The medication cart usually contains one drawer for each patient with enough drawers for one nursing team. One cart is assigned to a nurse or nursing team responsible for administering drugs to a designated number of patients. The medication cart replaces the nurse's need for a "med room." The medication cart should relieve the nurse of having to return to the nursing station while on her medication rounds. Therefore, the cart should carry an adequate supply of narcotics, syringes and needles and other medical supplies, PRN medications and the medication record.

The medication cart is used by the nurse. She should be consulted on which of the many available designs suits her needs. Height, ease in moving, location of narcotics cabinet, sundry storage areas, trash disposal and light accessories will particularly interest the nurse. Drawer size, drawer dividability, drawers per cassette unit and unit weight will be of interest to the pharmacist as well as the cost. The pharmacist will have to determine from nursing how many patient drawers per cart will be needed in each area.

The next decision is to determine when the patient drawers will be exchanged. At least two sets of patient drawer units are necessary – one set in the medication cart and the other set in the dose preparation area. The frequency of patient drawer exchanges will also affect the way

Figure 5. Medication Cart. The nurse is opening a patient drawer in which all the unit doses for the patient are stored, except those in the narcotics cabinet

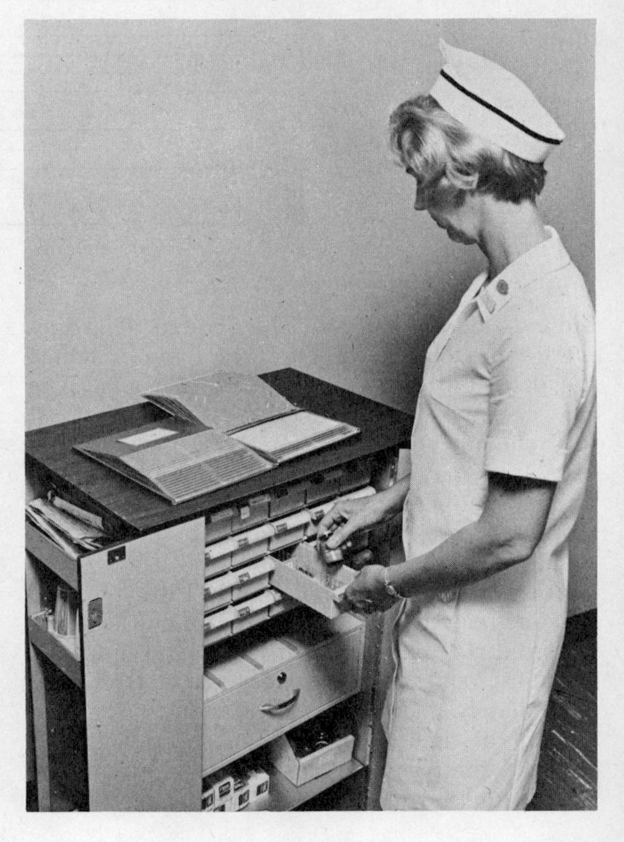

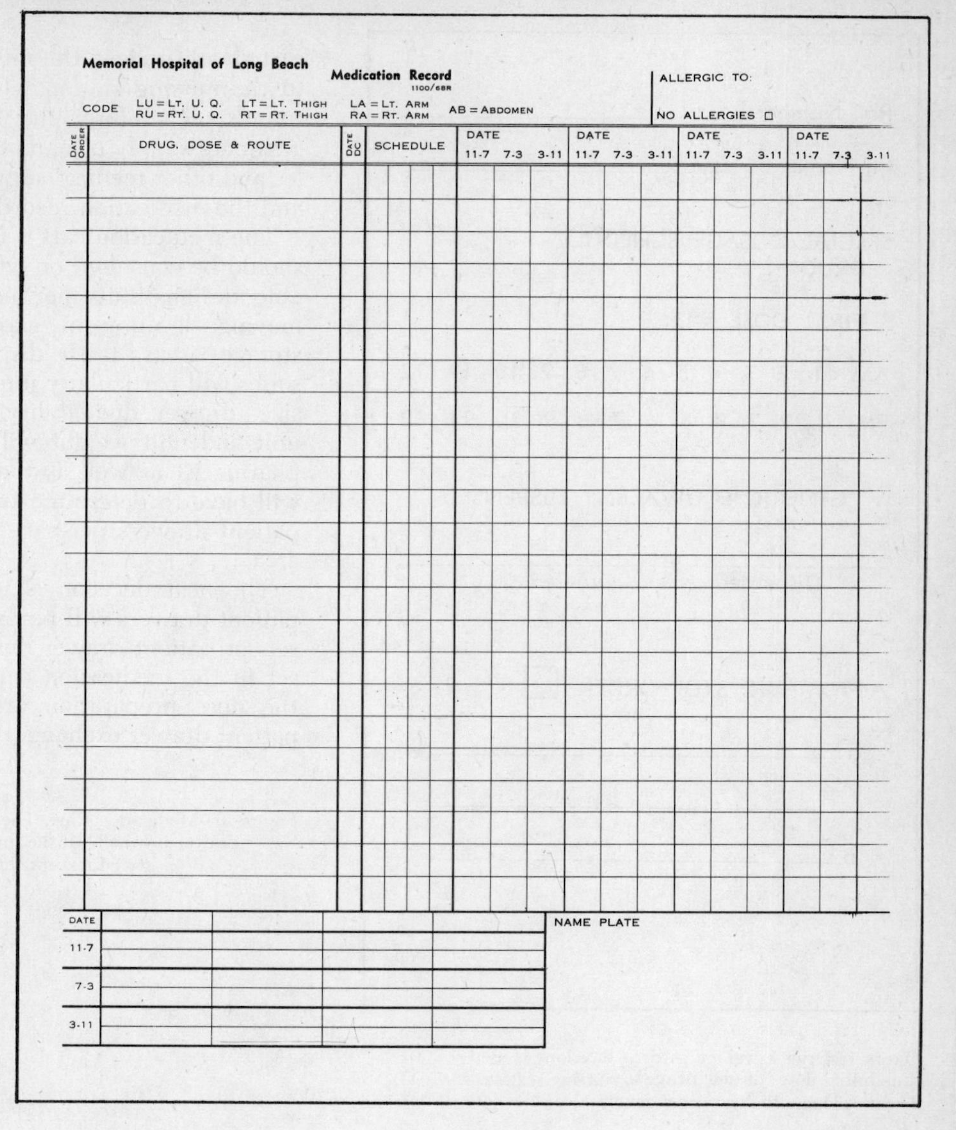

Memorial Hospital of Long Beach
Medication Record
1100/68R

ALLERGIC TO:

NO ALLERGIES ☐

CODE LU = LT. U. Q. LT = LT. THIGH LA = LT. ARM AB = ABDOMEN
RU = RT. U. Q. RT = RT. THIGH RA = RT. ARM

DATE ORDER	DRUG, DOSE & ROUTE	DATE DC	SCHEDULE	DATE			DATE			DATE			DATE		
				11-7	7-3	3-11	11-7	7-3	3-11	11-7	7-3	3-11	11-7	7-3	3-11

DATE				
11-7				
7-3				
3-11				

NAME PLATE

Figure 6. Nurses' Medication Record. Four copies, one posted in the patient's chart each midnight, plus one copy used as a charge document, are below the original sheet

the individual drawer will be divided. The simplest approach is to prepare doses and exchange the patient drawers once every 24 hours. The drawer may simply be divided into two sections: (1) scheduled doses and (2) PRN doses. Scheduled doses may also be put into multiple sections of the patient's drawer indicating particular morning, evening or midnight medication rounds.

The nurse's medication record (Figure 6) and narcotic records will usually remain on the medication cart. The cart can be rolled into the patient's room, doses administered and charted immediately thereafter. Besides increasing the amount of time the nurse can spend with her patients, the charting can always be up to date and should be more accurate.

A pharmacy medication nurse has been used in some institutions in combination with the unit dose system. The concept is based on the theory of task functionalization. The nurse, and in some cases a technician employed by the pharmacy, utilizes the medication cart to administer medications among other tasks. Special exemption from state law may be required to use technicians to administer drugs. The system appears to be a logical step beyond the basic unit dose system. Less interdepartmental procedures are necessary. In practice, the utilization of medication nurses works well for scheduled doses but generally requires a second system to handle PRN doses which do not benefit from the advantages of using the medication cart with all medications for each patient in his drawer.

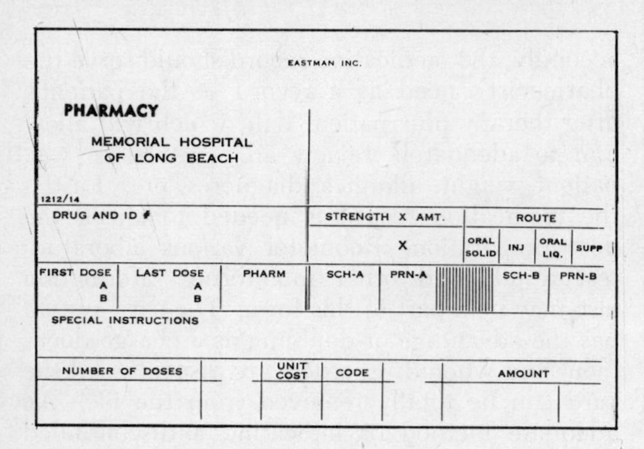

EASTMAN INC.

PHARMACY

MEMORIAL HOSPITAL
OF LONG BEACH

1212/14

DRUG AND ID #		STRENGTH X AMT.	ROUTE			
		X	ORAL SOLID	INJ	ORAL LIQ.	SUPP

FIRST DOSE A B	LAST DOSE A B	PHARM	SCH-A	PRN-A		SCH-B	PRN-B

SPECIAL INSTRUCTIONS

NUMBER OF DOSES	UNIT COST	CODE	AMOUNT

Figure 7. Rolodex Drug Card. One drug order per card is used to fill ongoing unit dose and to charge patient

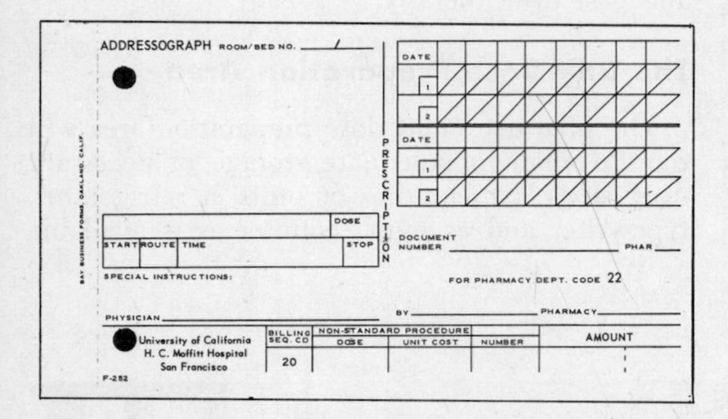

ADDRESSOGRAPH ROOM/BED NO. /

DATE 1 2

DATE 1 2

PRESCRIPTION

DOSE

START ROUTE TIME STOP

DOCUMENT NUMBER PHAR

SPECIAL INSTRUCTIONS:

FOR PHARMACY DEPT. CODE 22

PHYSICIAN BY PHARMACY

University of California
H. C. Moffitt Hospital
San Francisco

BILLING SEQ. CO	NON-STANDARD PROCEDURE			AMOUNT
	DOSE	UNIT COST	NUMBER	
20				

F-282

Figure 8. Drug Card. Another example of a drug card used to fill ongoing unit dose and to charge patient

The medication record used on the cart will have to be designed to meet the demands of the medical staff in order to avoid double charting at the end of each nursing shift. The physician will either agree to forego a current medication record in the patient's chart altogether and use the one on the cart or he will want a "timely" medication record put into each chart. If the latter amounts to a daily update as opposed to one every eight hours, double charting can be avoided by posting a carbon, NCR or machine copy of the medication record each night for the previous 24 hours.

A copy of the medication record also can be used by the pharmacy as a charge document. The medication record works well in charging for all unit doses administered including narcotics. Medications and sundry items not charted on the medication record (as determined by nursing) will still require another charge document. An alternative to utilizing the patient's medication record as a charge document is to generate a charge document card that can be used to prepare the patient's doses each day. When doses are placed in or removed from a patient's drawer, the number is recorded on the card. In either case, the work involved with credits and non-creditable drug returns is eliminated as is the economic loss of discarding returns from the nursing stations.

Recording the number of doses placed in or taken out of the patient's drawer on the drug card, even if by exception, requires additional technician time to prepare doses. It is also a

MEMORIAL HOSPITAL OF LONG BEACH — PHARMACEUTICAL SERVICE RECORD

FIRST DOSE LAST	CD NUMBER	SCH DRUGS	STRENGTH X UNITS PER DOSE	A	B	FIRST DOSE LAST	CD NUMBER	PRN DRUGS	STRENGTH X UNITS PER DOSE	
			ORAL SOLID / INJ. / ORAL LIQ. X	PHARM.				ASPIRIN /ACETAMINOPHEN	ORAL SOLID / SUPP. / ORAL LIQ. X	PHARM.
			ORAL SOLID / INJ. / ORAL LIQ. X	PHARM.					ORAL SOLID / INJ. / ORAL LIQ. X	PHARM.
			ORAL SOLID / INJ. / ORAL LIQ. X	PHARM.				DARVON /TALWIN	ORAL SOLID / INJ. X	PHARM.
			ORAL SOLID / INJ. / ORAL LIQ. X	PHARM.					ORAL SOLID / INJ. / ORAL LIQ. X	PHARM.
			ORAL SOLID / INJ. / ORAL LIQ. X	PHARM.				DRAMAMINE/MAREZINE/COMPAZINE	ORAL SOLID / INJ. / SUPP. X	PHARM.
			ORAL SOLID / INJ. / ORAL LIQ. X	PHARM.					ORAL SOLID / INJ. / ORAL LIQ. X	PHARM.
			ORAL SOLID / INJ. / ORAL LIQ. X	PHARM.				VALIUM /HYDROXYZINE	ORAL SOLID / INJ. / ORAL LIQ. X	PHARM.
			ORAL SOLID / INJ. / ORAL LIQ. X	PHARM.					ORAL SOLID / INJ. / ORAL LIQ. X	PHARM.
			ORAL SOLID / INJ. / ORAL LIQ. X	PHARM.					ORAL SOLID / INJ. / ORAL LIQ. X	PHARM.
			ORAL SOLID / INJ. / ORAL LIQ. X	PHARM.				PENTOBARB/SECOBARB/CHLORAL HYD	ORAL SOLID / INJ. X SCH. PRN	PHARM.

DATE	DIAGNOSIS	DATE	SURGERY - PROCEDURES	DRUG SENSITIVITIES AND ALLERGIES

ROOM	NAME	ID#	WEIGHT	AGE	DOCTOR

MONITOR □

Figure 9. Pharmaceutical Service Record. This part of the form contains a patient's current drug therapy and is filed in a Kardex. It is used by the technicians to fill ongoing unit dose. The inside of the form allows room for monitoring notes

more complicated system from which to calculate the number of doses to be charged, particularly for periodic in-house billings and still requires a special charge system for non-unit dose drugs (*e.g.*, ointments, ophthalmic drops, etc.) and narcotics. In general, using a copy of the medication record is simpler and probably more accurate in charging the patient for what he received, since the nurse now charts immediately after administering a medication. Wasted and dropped medications are not charged to the patient and, therefore, patient charges reflect accurate drug utilization data that can be studied for the whole hospital or a particular patient population.

The pharmacy must maintain a current record of every patient's drug orders (Figure 9). New drug orders which will be on-going may be entered on individual cards and filed by room and bed number or all drug orders for a patient can be recorded on a single sheet. First and foremost, the current medication records should be designed for ease in preparing doses. The form used must be as error free as possible. Secondly, the medication record should serve the pharmacist's need as a record of the patient's drug therapy plus patient data which will allow him to adequately review all new orders, *e.g.*, patient weight, allergies, diagnoses, etc. Lastly, the medication record is needed to check the dose preparation. Room for various laboratory test results and other monitoring information also may be a part of this form. The card system has the advantage of doubling as a charge document and when drug orders are discontinued the card can be totally removed from the file. An adequate method of indicating a discontinued order must be used with the single sheet system but it reduces the chance of misplacing cards and provides a clearer overview of the current and past drug therapy.

The Unit Dose Preparation Area

The pharmacy unit dose preparation area will require room for adequate storage of necessary drug stock, patient drawer units, a refrigerator, typewriter and as much counter as is available

Figure 10. Unit Dose Preparation Area. Unit dose stock stored in bins on six inch shelves. Pharmacist is checking dose preparation against Pharmaceutical Service Record

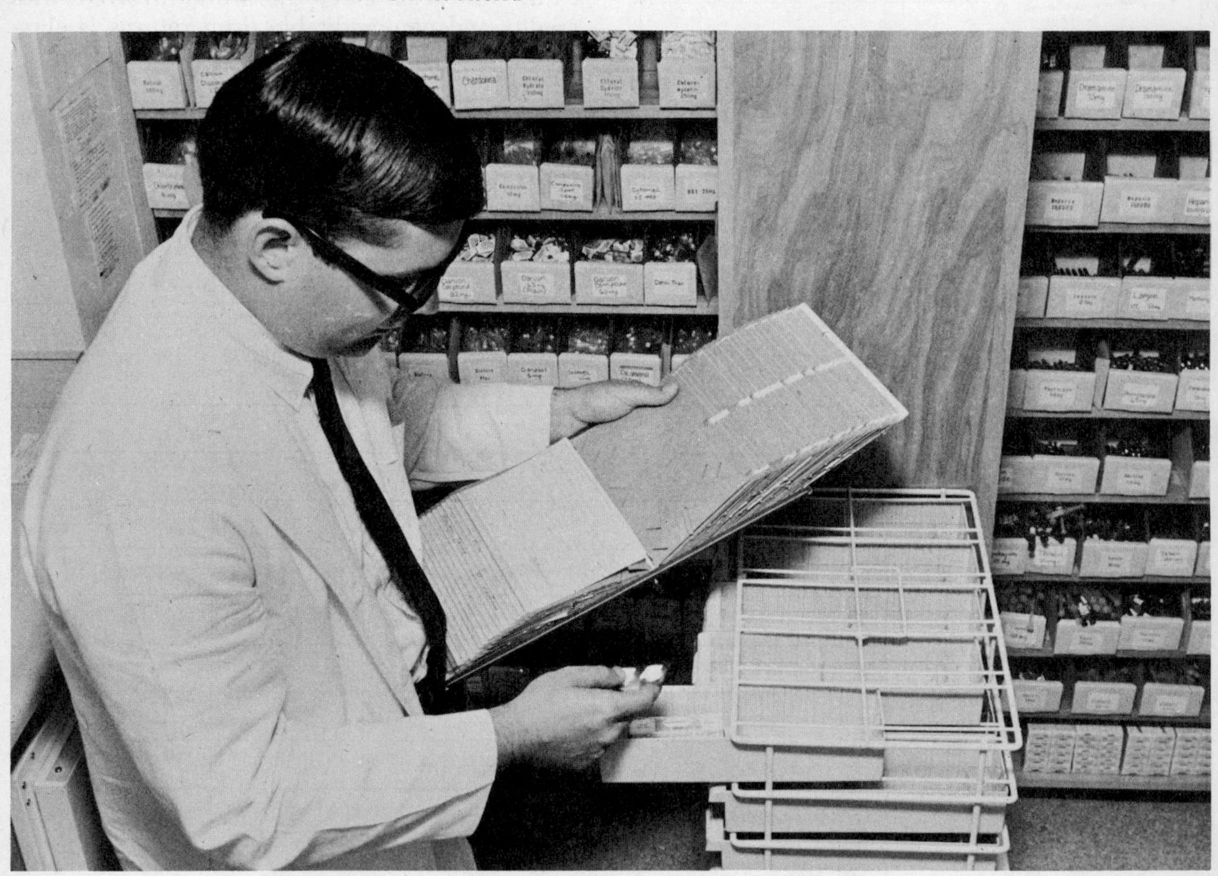

to process the paperwork. Approximately 20 linear feet of shelving (floor to arm's length height) will be necessary to store the unit dose stock. The number of unit dose stock items may vary from 500 to 800. The type of storage bin, box or drawer in which the unit dose stock is kept greatly affects the storage space necessary. See example in Figures 10 and 11.

The dose preparation area usually will require provisions to extemporaneously unit dose package bulk drugs. A clean air flow hood and sink therefore, also can be considered part of the floor space requirements. If the pharmacist's reference books and notes are to be stored and utilized in this area, the room should be designed with an understanding of where the pharmacy technician and where the pharmacist will be working. See Figures 12-15 for examples of floor plans of decentralized satellite pharmacies. The floor space ranges from approximately 160 square feet to 330 square feet.

The hospital's physical facility may dictate from the beginning whether the dose preparation activity should be centralized or decentralized. If this is not the case, there are a number of points to be considered in deciding upon satellite pharmacies or a central unit dose area. The advantages and disadvantages lie either in facilitating the drug distribution system or facilitating the pharmacist's clinical practice. Since the authors have had more experience with a decentralized satellite pharmacy system, the advantages and disadvantages of the decentralized system are enumerated below.

Advantages of a Decentralized Unit Dose System

1. Patients receive initial doses faster
2. There is closer communication between the pharmacist and nurse
3. Nursing is the least involved with drug procurement
4. The narcotic system is streamlined with minimum supplies on cart
5. There is greater pharmacist supervision over technicians
6. Pharmacist can combine clinical activities requiring his presence in a patient care area with supervising the drug distribution system
7. Pharmacists are routinely on patient care areas

Figure 11. Dose Preparation from Rolodex Drug Cards. Cards are on file by room and bed numbers

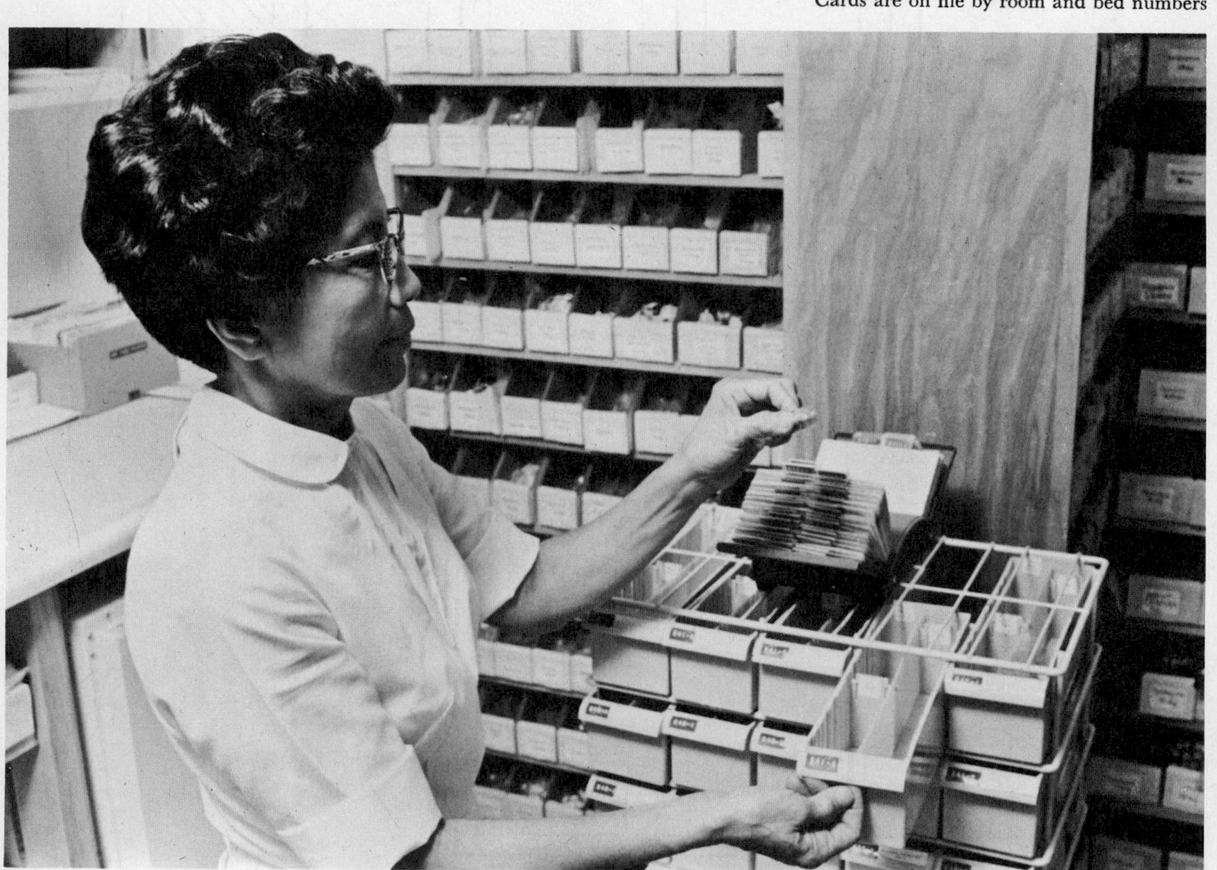

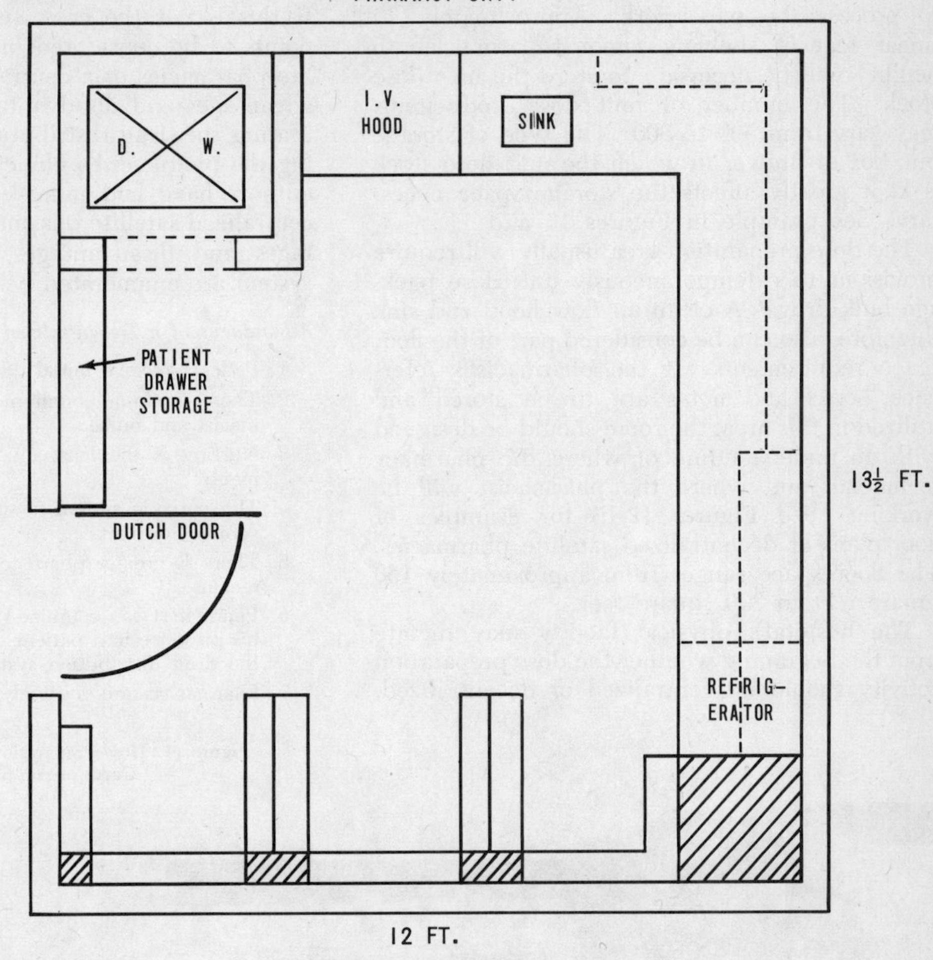

Figure 12. Floor plan of Decentralized Pharmacy Units on 2nd, 3rd, 4th and 5th floors at Memorial Medical Center at Long Beach

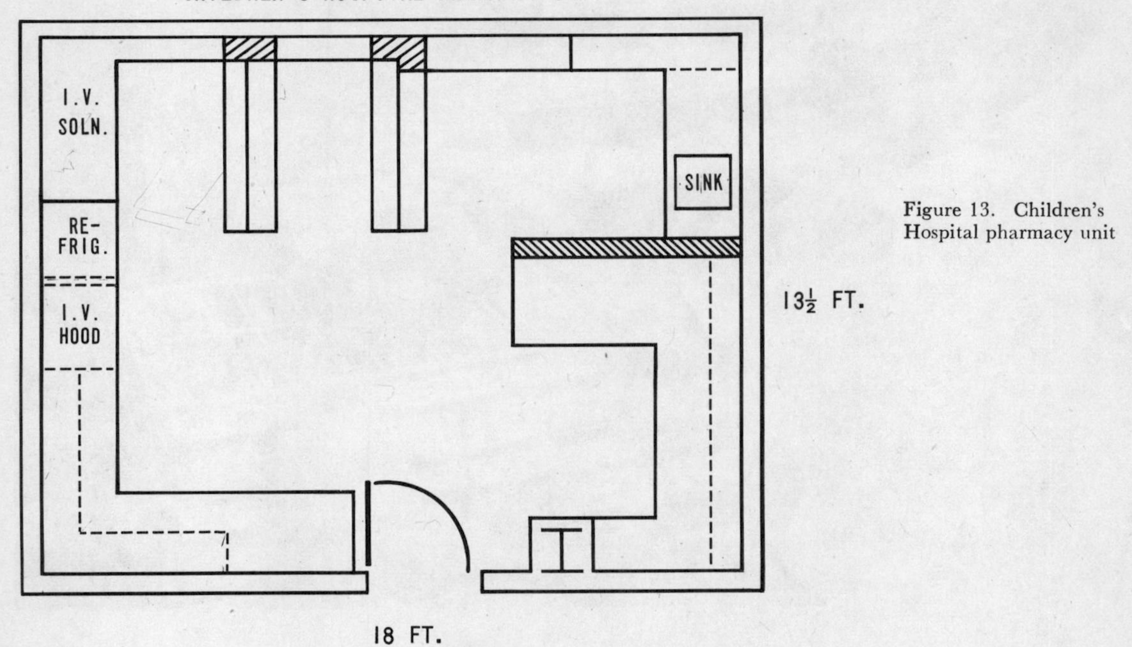

Figure 13. Children's Hospital pharmacy unit

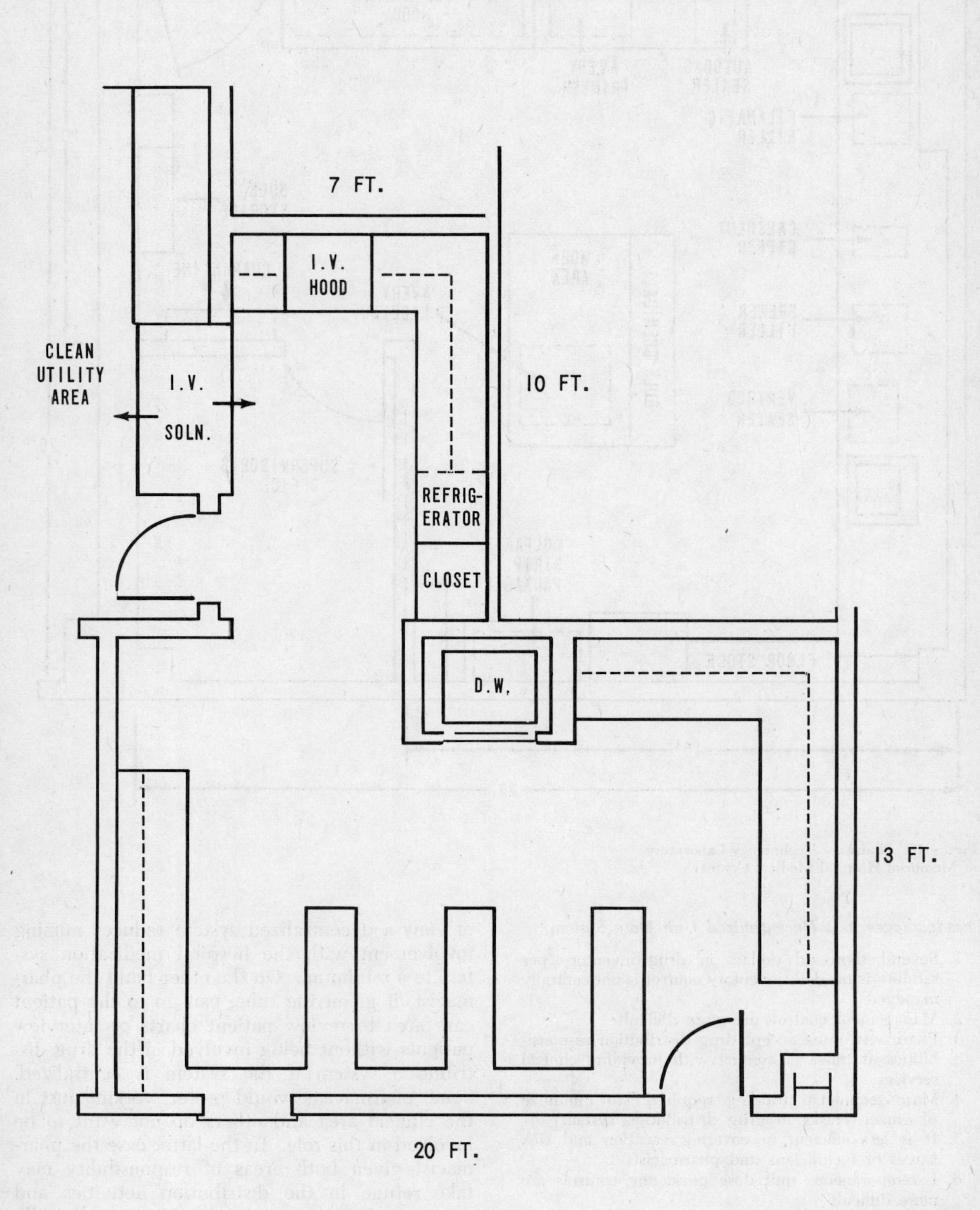

Figure 14. Sixth floor pharmacy unit at Memorial Hospital Medical Center

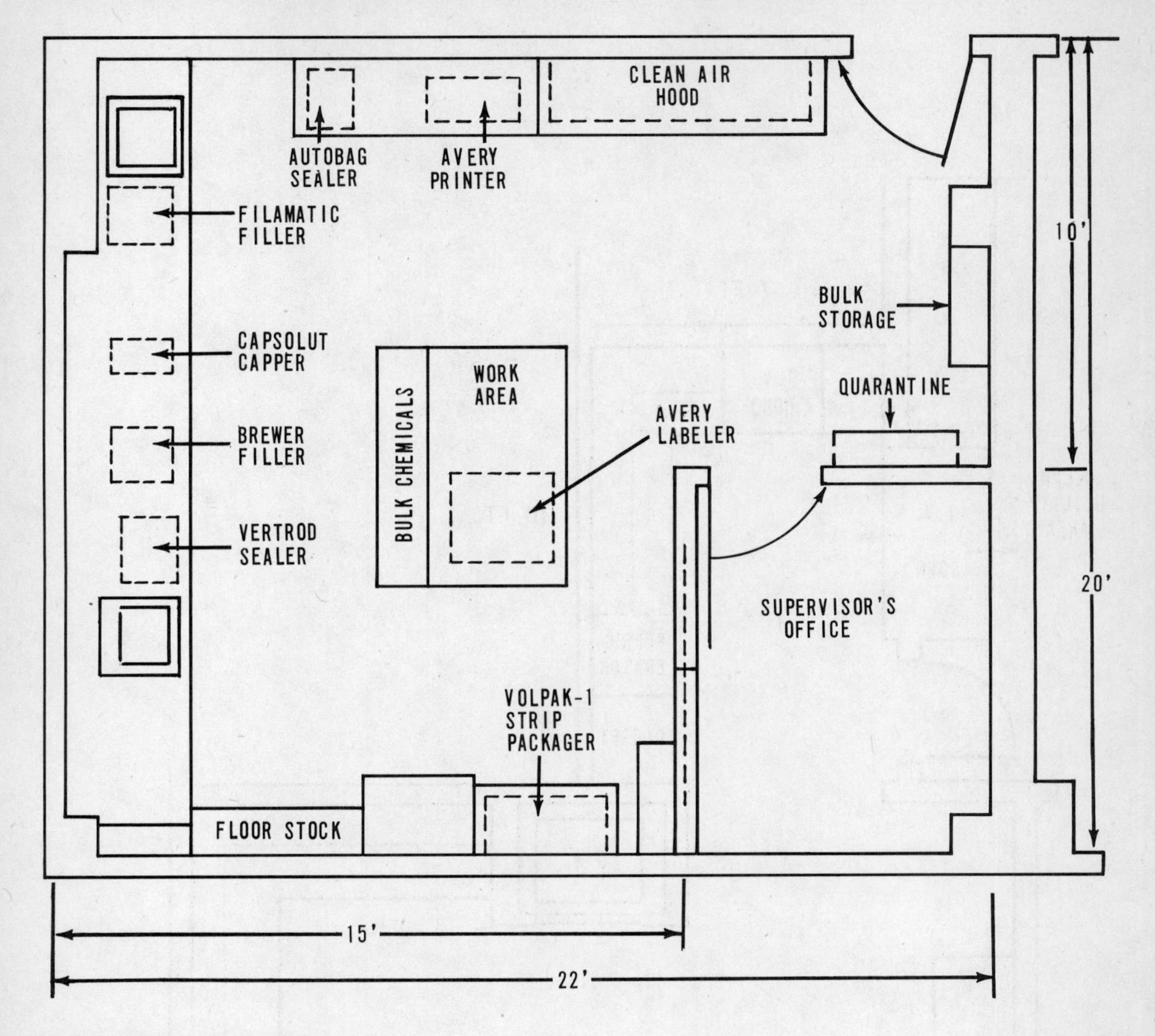

Figure 15. Pharmacy Technology Laboratory at Memorial Hospital Medical Center

Disadvantages to a Decentralized Unit Dose System

1. Several thousand dollars in drug inventory per satellite is needed; inventory control is not centrally managed
2. Management controls are more difficult
3. Pharmacist must accept drug distribution responsibilities at times in conflict with providing clinical services
4. More technician training required (to minimize pharmacist tasks in drug distribution system)
5. It is less efficient in covering vacation and sick leaves of technicians and pharmacists
6. Extemporaneous unit dose packaging controls are more difficult

In general the advantages and disadvantages of the decentralized system conversely apply to a centralized system. From a distribution point of view a decentralized system reduces nursing involvement with the hospital medication system to a minimum. On the other hand the pharmacist, if given the time, can go to the patient care area to review patient charts or interview patients without being involved in the drug distribution system if the system is centralized. Some pharmacists would prefer working just in the clinical area and others do not want to be involved in this role. In the latter case the pharmacist given both areas of responsibility may take refuge in the distribution activities and never manage to get time to become clinically involved, and the opposite can happen. There are also pharmacists who can do both well. A decentralized pharmacy system encourages all pharmacists to be involved in both drug distribution and clinical activities for better or worse!

The number of hours the pharmacy unit dose preparation area will need to be open may be 8, 16 or 24 hours. Pharmacy hours are not particularly affected by the unit dose drug distribution system. The length of time the pharmacy is open should logically depend upon when new orders are written by the physician and the *clinical* activities in which the pharmacist is involved. If the pharmacist is to participate in cardiac resuscitations he cannot be available just part of the time. If the pharmacist is going to interview patients on admission then he must be in the hospital in the evening if this is when patients are admitted. If the pharmacist is to review every new drug order before the patient receives a dose and half of the new orders are written in the afternoon and evening for post-op patients and new admissions, the pharmacist must be available — in this case for a clinical as well as drug distribution activity.

UNIT DOSE PACKAGING AND STORAGE

In many ways, unit dose packaging technology, developing within the hospital pharmacy is reminiscent of past years' emphasis on bulk compounding. As traditional bulk compounding continues to diminish in importance and hospitals implement unit dose systems, unit dose packaging will by and large supplant compounding activities. A growing variety of packaging equipment is becoming available for small and large unit dose packaging needs. A substantial expenditure in equipment may be necessary for large hospitals. There is a concern with quality control and good record keeping, as with bulk compounding. Pharmacy technicians can perform much of the workload with proper supervision. The subsequent section will consider the various aspects in setting up and operating a unit dose packaging laboratory.

Packaging Drugs in Unit Dose

Early in the planning stages of a unit dose drug distribution system, decisions must be made as to what packaging equipment will be required. Before evaluating available equipment on the market, the volume of unit dose packaging required for the institution should be studied. Copies of the medication record, charge requisitions or other such documents can be used to determine, for as long a trial period as possible, the number of each unit dose drug administered. This study can be made first just for a pilot wing or floor on which the unit dose system will begin. The usage rate of each drug can then be evaluated as follows:

1. Is it available commercially in unit dose or must it be packaged?
2. How much should be packaged?
3. How much should be purchased (when available as unit dose)?
4. What volume constitutes grounds for packaging in advance?

From this information the drugs not available commercially in unit dose can be determined. An annual utilization can be calculated. An estimate of annual turnover will determine the annual packaging demands of the institution, *i.e.*, average batch size and total number of batches per year. The evaluation of the unit dose packaging equipment to meet these demands can then follow, considering possible expansion of the hospital. In general, it can be assumed that more and more drug products will become available in unit dose thus decreasing this activity. On the other hand, a large number of moderate to low volume drugs may not be available in unit dose for a long time to come. Oral liquids and injectables probably will never be available in all doses prescribed. The purchase of quality equipment to last some years appears to be a wise investment at present. Figure 15 illustrates a floor plan of a packaging laboratory.

For those products available in unit dose the problem is simple. A study can provide the inventory requirements for inpatient consumption. If unit dose will be dispensed for outpatient prescriptions, past inventory requirements for non-unit dose can be applied to unit dose. Occasionally unit dose drugs procured on bid for inpatient units will be less expensive than non-unit dose in bulk containers.

Two considerations prevail in deciding whether to purchase already available unit dose products as opposed to packaging them: cost and stability. The latter is a matter of real concern and must favor purchasing unit dose whenever available commercially since the shelf-life is then guaranteed by the manufacturer. The other reason, cost, also will lead one to purchasing unit dose whenever available with few exceptions. Suffice it to say, there are so many things for the pharmacist to do, he cannot afford spending his time to do packaging if it can be done by industry. In years back, prestige came from the number of items manufactured by the hospital pharmacy. We are quickly moving beyond that kind of thinking.

PERMANENT PACKAGING RECORD
PHARMACY TECHNOLOGY

MEMORIAL HOSPITAL OF LONG BEACH

DRUG NAME ____________ STRENGTH ____________

UNIT SIZE ____________ DOSAGE FORM ____________

Special Instructions:

LABEL SAMPLE

DATE PACKED	BY	NUMBER PACKED	LOT NO.	MANUFACTURER & LOT NO.	EXP. DATE	DRUG & STRENGTH CHECKED	PACKAGE CHECKED	LABEL CHECKED	LOT & EXP. CHECKED	O.K. FOR USE

Form 1212-14 ATTACH LABEL SAMPLE TO BACK OF PAGE

Figure 16. Permanent packaging record form

What is left then are those drugs not available commercially in unit dose which must be packaged. Two approaches should be planned in packaging drugs: (1) to handle high volume and (2) to handle low volume units. Institutions without a strict formulary are generally faced with a number of products that do not warrant packaging ahead of time and, therefore, some plan needs to be developed to do so on request. This approach will also be of value in packaging new drug products before the inventory status can be determined. Approximately 500 units a year or more probably justifies maintaining an in-house unit dose stock. Another approach would be to package all drugs upon receipt in unit dose, eliminating any dual inventory and delay to unit dose package the drug when it is ordered.

Just as the hospital is allowed to manufacture pharmaceuticals for use within the institution without a manufacturer's license, it can also prepackage on the same basis providing good manufacturing procedures (G.M.P.) are followed. Such procedures are essential for adequate recall capability, inventory controls and management of the unit dose packaging activity. The utilization of pharmacy technicians in packaging drugs likewise dictates thorough record keeping procedures. The Federal Food and Cosmetic Act provides legal authority that could be used by FDA to regulate the repackaging of drugs within hospitals. The FDA's present thinking, however, is that local or state agencies should regulate what is primarily a local operation considering the FDA's limited manpower.[13]

Most hospitals do not have the resources to chemically and physically analyze the hundreds of repackaged unit dose drugs employed in the unit dose system. Some schools of pharmacy and state food and drug agencies may be able to provide some assays of official U.S.P. and N.F. drugs for a modest fee. A sizeable number of repackaged drugs cannot be so tested and thus some guidelines for shelf-life should be decided upon. Obviously, exposure to light, moisture and temperature must be controlled after packaging.

Guidelines for the labeling of unit dose packages are important from the standpoint of the nurse and pharmacy technician who must read these labels on a daily basis. The American Society of Hospital Pharmacists has approved guidelines for single unit packages of drugs directed toward the pharmaceutical manufacturers.[14] Impetus to clarify the legal requirements in labeling single unit packaging has come from those who want to provide unit dose systems to nursing homes and other hospitals. The following information on labels of single unit packages of drugs is recommended:

1. Nonproprietary (generic) and/or proprietary name of the drug

2. Strength of ingredients
3. Institution packaging drug
4. Lot or control number
5. Route of administration, if not oral
6. Expiration date

It should be noted that these recommendations do *not* meet current legal requirements if such units are to be used outside the institution that packaged them such as in a nursing home.

The following sections will deal with each type of dosage form packaged in unit dose.

Oral Solid Unit Dose Packaging. Tablets and capsules represent the highest volume of unit dose packaging to be performed. A number of machines are available ranging in price from $3,000-$10,000. The majority are strip packaging machines that print the label, heat seal and cut or perforate the strip between each unit. Some machines have attachments that automatically feed the tablet or capsule into the machine one at a time. Two disadvantages of some of these attachments are: (1) it may be slower than a manual or semimanual feed and (2) it may require considerably more set up time. The automatic feed attachment generally does not allow the operator to leave the machine, so in the long run the production rate may be slower without saving personnel time.

The capability of the labeling device on these machines is also important in determining how fast a machine can operate in practice. Several options on the same machine may be available. It is worth purchasing the best printing device available since constant attention and adjustment, when necessary, greatly reduce production rates. For example, a chase with individual spring loaded lines is superior to other types that occasionally print one line less distinct than another. In general, little maintenance is required; however, adequate service capabilities by the company should be considered for the area where the machine will be used. In practice, someone in the pharmacy must learn the machine and how to maintain it since the time lag for service is frequently too long.

For extemporaneously packing small batches of oral solids (10 to 100 units), a number of hand operations can be used. The same degree of record keeping should be kept in either case. A small Monarch label machine will save a lot of time usually spent typing labels for each unit packaged and will provide a label for the control sheet. The Maxi-Pak and other larger machines also can be used to package very small batches of 15 or 30 tablets or capsules. Labeling, however, is generally more efficiently done on the Monarch label machine and hand applied as opposed to setting up type on the larger packaging machines.

The following examples of sources of supply for packaging equipment and supplies for oral solids will be helpful for those who wish to obtain additional information.

Packaging Equipment	*Source*
Mark II strip packager and Maxi-Pak strip packager	Becton Dickinson, Inc. Rutherford, New Jersey
SM/V and SM/VI strip packager	Chemical and Pharmaceutical Industry Co. New York, New York
Vol-Pak I strip packager	Crompton Knowles Agawam, Massachusetts
Mercury U-Pak strip packager	G-L Industries, Inc. Westville, New Jersey
Uhlman strip packager	Uhlman Company West Germany
Pharma-Packager	Wrap-Ade Company Clifton, New Jersey
Labeling Equipment	
Mark 60 hand labeling machine	Monarch Marketing Systems Gardena, California
Plastic Bags	
Plastic bags	Assorted Bag Milwaukee, Wisconsin
	Bradley Bag Los Angeles, California

Oral Liquids. Unit dose oral liquids are probably the least efficient dosage form packaged in the hospital. Fortunately, upwards of 80 percent of all oral liquids administered in hospitals may be already available from the pharmaceutical industry. The degree to which a strict hospital formulary is adhered to and the size of the pediatrics department will affect the amount of oral liquids remaining to be unit dose packaged by the pharmacy. A number of machines can be used which can be calibrated to deliver 5, 10, 15, 30, etc. milliliters into amber glass vials. Since a variety of viscous liquids may be encountered for packaging, a machine with a relatively low gear ratio will provide a more consistently accurate delivery of liquid. The vials are then capped with an aluminum closure requiring some sort of crimping device. There are two primary manufacturers of vials, each with a different mouth size and, therefore, requiring a different crimping device.

Since small volumes are involved (5 milliliters or less at times) the quantity on the label should refer to the dose to be delivered which must be determined before packaging each batch of liquids.

After the filling and capping steps are completed a label must be printed and applied. Hospital pharmacies have traditionally made use of labeling machines. The volume of labels necessary for unit dose packaging is enormous in comparison. The investment in a quality machine will be well worthwhile. If the printer can use rubber base ink, the machine will not require disassembly and cleaning at the end of the day, reducing the amount of set-up time required per batch. Another piece of equipment which can quickly pay for itself in man-hours saved is a device to peel off gummed labels from their backing. The operation is still manual to one degree or another but the efficiency of the operator is greatly increased.

Small batches of unit dose oral liquids can be hand poured, capped with a hand crimper and labeled with a typed or Monarch machine label. Regular glass prescription vials with plastic snap-on caps can also be used but often leak if laid on their side or evaporate if stored for any length of time. Small hand devices for delivering a calibrated quantity of liquid are available but are not very accurate, particularly if the liquid is even moderately viscous, and require an excessive time to clean after each batch. Small batches of oral antibiotic suspensions and solutions also must be packaged extemporaneously on demand due to their instability. Preprinted labels can be made in advance for these products. Strength, lot number and expiration date can then be added to the preprinted label as needed.

An example of a permanent packaging record for oral solids and liquids is seen in Figure 16. One form is used for each unit packaged routinely. Besides providing the necessary quality control records it also provides information from which the desired inventory turnover can be based. The turnover is important for both monetary as well as quality control since the shelf-life of such packages is only a conservative estimate.

The following examples of sources of supply for packaging equipment and supplies for oral liquids should prove useful.

Filling Machines	*Source*
Brewer filler; West capper; amber glass vials (Wheaton); caps (West)	Becton Dickinson, Inc. Rutherford, New Jersey
Filimatic filler (DAB6, other models)	National Instrument Baltimore, Maryland
Amber glass vials; caps (Alcoa), Capsulot capper, manual and pneumatic	Owens Illinois Toledo, Ohio
Fill, cap and label machines	Raytron Corp. Toledo, Ohio
Plastic hand pump	Scientific Products (various vendors)
Containers	
Plastic tubes, 1 ml, 2.5 ml, 5.0 ml	Colonial Applicator Vineland, New Jersey
Vertrod heat sealer, model 8H/HTJ	Weber Marking Systems, Inc. Arlington Heights, Illinois
Labeling Equipment	
Super-Etiprint printer; label removers	Avery Monrovia, California
Tick-O-Pres printers; label removers	Monarch Marking Systems Gardena, California
Weber Model 50 printer	Weber Marking Systems, Inc. Arlington Heights, Illinois

Injectables. Although unit dose packaging of injectables is basically a manual operation, it probably represents the greatest improvement per unit in terms of saving time, eliminating drug wastage and providing a safer injectable than the traditional multiple dose vial. The packaging materials are approximately the same as the cost of a syringe and needle which must be used sooner or later. The pharmacy technician prepares the unit dose syringe instead of a nurse. Assembly line techniques are employed in the packaging laboratory ultimately providing the patient with a safer, prelabeled unit for injection.

A number of injectables are available in unit dose syringes of various design and desirability. A decision must be made either to accept what is available from the pharmaceutical industry with all its variety, or package a number of injectables already available in a common syringe unit. Since no company producing empty sterile syringe units is able to provide stability information on various proprietary drugs or even their formulation for the rubber components on which the drug will come in contact, it seems unlikely that the second alternative will be acceptable in the long run. Long-term stability studies of proprietary drugs in single unit syringes may provide an area of interest for schools of pharmacy to study in the future. For such studies to be valid, however, adequate information on the uniformity of rubber components will have to be obtained.

A number of different manual techniques have been developed to fill empty sterile unit dose syringe units in a rapid and efficient manner. No doubt a great many new devices will be developed in the years ahead that will speed up

INJECTABLE PACKAGING RECORD
PHARMACY TECHNOLOGY
MEMORIAL HOSPITAL OF LONG BEACH

DRUG & STRENGTH ____
VOLUME IN UNIT ____
STOCK SOLUTION ____
SPECIAL INSTRUCTIONS:

LABEL SAMPLE

DATE PACKAGED ____ QUANTITY PACKED ____
CONTROL NUMBER ____ PACKED BY ____

UNIT DOSE DATA	PACKAGING DATA
DRUG	DISPOSABLE SYRINGE
MANUFACTURER ____	SIZE ____
LOT NUMBER ____	MANUFACTURER ____
EXP. DATE ____	LOT NUMBER ____
AMOUNT USED ____	
DISPOSABLE UNIT USED	TRANSFER OR DISPOSABLE NEEDLE
SIZE ____	SIZE ____
MANUFACTURER ____	MANUFACTURER ____
LOT NUMBER ____	LOT NUMBER ____
	TIP CAPS
	MANUFACTURER ____
	LOT NUMBER ____

CONTROL DATA

DRUG & STRENGTH CHECKED ____	STERILITY REPORT ATTACHED YES [ ] NO [ ]
MANUFACTURER & LOT NO. CHECKED ____	PYROGEN REPORT ATTACHED YES [ ] NO [ ]
DISPOSABLE UNIT CHECKED ____	
LABEL CHECKED ____	
CONTROL NO. CHECKED ____	DATE RELEASED ____
EXP. DATE CHECKED ____	
PACKAGING DATA CHECKED ____	RELEASED BY ____

Figure 17. Injectable packaging record form

this process. The unit to be used in a particular hospital should be determined by considering the following points and deciding what items have priority for your institution.

1. Speed in filling
2. Largest syringe volume available
3. Storage space required while in inventory and in the patient's drawer – length and width
4. Nursing evaluation
   – Sturdiness
   – Ease of aspirating
   – Ease in adding additional milliliters of drug
   – Needle cover requirements
5. Needle attached or not; options on needle size
6. Plunger detachable
7. Need for auxiliary devices to administer

In all systems, the final product has a needle on the syringe that has not been used in the fill operation and, therefore, remains sharp. The packaging records necessary for adequate controls require more details than with oral dosage forms. Figure 17 is an example of a form used to record the manufacturer's name, the lot number, the disposable syringe size and other packaging information.

The examples of equipment and supplies for injectables and suppositories should prove of value.

Containers	*Source*
Autobag heat seal; plastic bags	Automated Packaging Bedford Heights, Ohio
Sterile glass syringes; sterile rubber tip caps; filling jig	Becton Dickinson Rutherford, New Jersey
Sterile glass cartridge and holder	Ciba Summit, New Jersey
Sterile glass syringe; sterile rubber tip caps; filling jig	Owens Illinois Toledo, Ohio
Sterile glass cartridge and holder; sterile glass syringes and filling device	Sherwood Medical Industries, Inc. St. Louis, Missouri
Tubex syringes and holders	Wyeth Philadelphia, Pennsylvania
Clean Air Hoods	
Clean air hood	Abbott Laboratories North Chicago, Illinois
	Parke-Davis Company Detroit, Michigan
	Becton Dickinson Rutherford, New Jersey

Memorial Hospital of Long Beach Pharmacy Technology Laboratory

EXTEMPORANEOUS PACKAGING LOG

Date Packaged (Control #)	Drug Packaged	Size Or Strength	Mfgr.	Lot Number	Expiration Date	Number Packaged	Packaged By	Check By

Figure 18. Extemporaneous packaging log

Suppositories. Packaging suppositories is a minor part of the packaging workload but is necessary to complete the line of single unit dosage forms. Nursing time can be saved by providing a unit containing the suppository, lubricant and a finger cot since the nurse requires all three for each administration. These can be put into a small plastic bag, heat sealed and labeled.

An additional packaging control form can be utilized in preparing extemporaneous single unit packages. Figure 18 illustrates a form used for drugs not regularly stored as unit dose. Such a log can be used to determine if a particular drug should be packaged routinely for unit dose stock. The quantities packaged are quite small and generally administered shortly after packaging. This type of packaging usually is performed by a number of people in the department as the demand arises. For large institutions with a high extemporaneous packaging volume, more consistent quality and maximum control can be best obtained by assigning one, well-trained pharmacy technician to package the majority of these drugs. Centrally stored, they can be more easily checked for expiration datings and can be more readily procured if ever reordered. Extemporaneous packaging by others then can be done to cover only their immediate needs until more can be packaged by the packaging technician.

Cost of Unit Dose Packaging

As stated earlier, the cost of packaging your own unit dose drugs, all things considered, is frequently more expensive than purchasing what is commercially available. The cost to the institution to package each type of unit is important in determining a reasonable charge to the patient. For example, the cost incurred by the hospital to purchase a drug in unit dose syringes will obviously be more than the drug itself since the cost must cover the syringe. In packaging your own unit dose syringe, the cost of materials and labor as well as drug should be included to obtain the same base price from which to calculate a patient charge.

Batch size, equipment speed and a variety of other factors will affect each institution's packaging costs. Table 2 is an example of data from a study on unit dose packaging costs. There are two time components for each batch: (1) set-up time and (2) production time. Set-up time includes setting up the machine, clean-up and record keeping. Production time includes the time running the machine, bagging or packaging the unit dose, filling, capping, labeling liquids, and so forth.

There is great temptation, when adequate records are not kept, to overpackage since the set-up time is such a large part of a run, particularly for oral solids and liquids. Table 3 gives an example of the packaging workload of a 500-bed hospital without a strict formulary. Unit dose drugs were purchased whenever available. The work of approximately 1.5 FTE's (full-time employees) spent in direct packaging activities was needed to package almost 700,000 units. In addition to this, 150,000 units were packaged extemporaneously requiring approximately one FTE.

Technician staffing requirements for unit dose packaging can be considered along with other non-packaging activities they will be performing to realistically assess their total workload. Filling orders, recording narcotics, preparing intravenous additive and hyperalimentation solutions, manufacturing and bulk prepackaging are possible activities in addition to unit dose packaging. Holiday, vacation and sick leave coverage for technicians also must be included. These activities can amount to as much demand as the unit dose packaging workload.

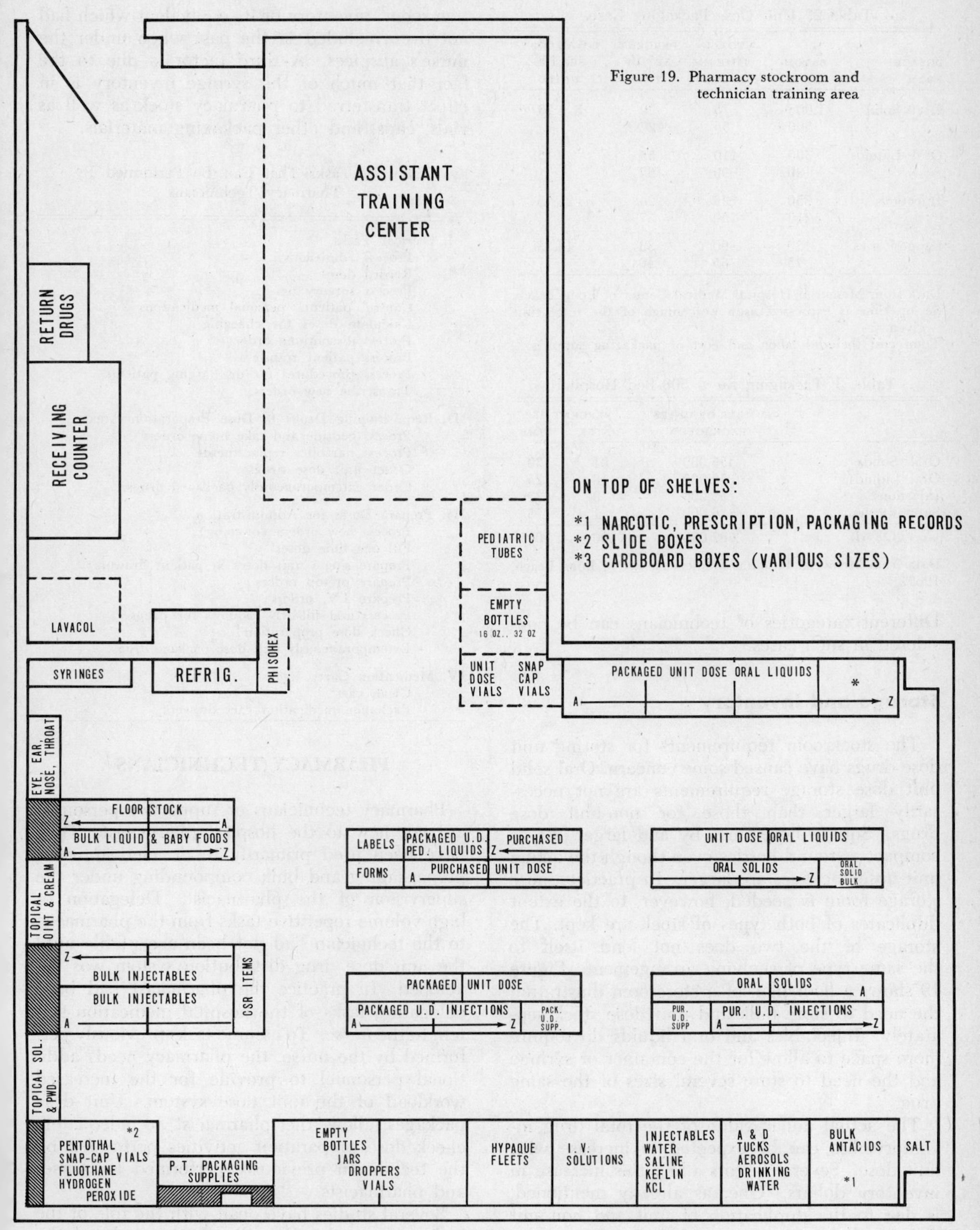

Figure 19. Pharmacy stockroom and technician training area

Table 2. Unit Dose Packaging Costs

DOSAGE FORM	BATCH SIZE	TOTAL TIME IN MINUTES	PERCENT SET-UP TIME	TOTAL COST PER 100 UNITS
Oral Solid	1,000	75	20	$ 1.23
	500	55	27	
Oral Liquids	300	110	55	9.15
	180	90	67	
Injections	350	225	24	21.75
	210	150	37	
Suppositories	130	90	33	14.33
	75	65	40	

Data from Memorial Hospital Medical Center of Long Beach.
Set-up time is expressed as a percentage of the total time given.
Total cost includes labor and cost of packaging supplies.

Table 3. Packaging for a 500-Bed Hospital

	NUMBER OF UNITS PACKAGED	PERCENT OF	
		UNITS	TIME
Oral Solids	556,000	81	38
Oral Liquids	72,000	10	25
Injections	53,000	8	32
Suppositories	6,000	1	5
TOTAL	687,000	100	100

Data from Memorial Hospital Medical Center of Long Beach, 1969.

Different categories of technicians can be considered in such cases.

Storage and Inventory

The stockroom requirements for storing unit dose drugs have caused some concern. Oral solid unit dose storage requirements are not necessarily larger than those for non-unit dose drugs. Square boxes are, by and large, just as compact as round bottles even though the actual unit dose packages are larger. In practice, more storage room *is* needed, however, to the extent duplicates of both types of stock are kept. The storage of the two does not lend itself to the same type of shelving arrangement. Figure 19 shows a floor plan of a storeroom illustrating the need to store bulk and unit dose stock separately. Injectables and oral liquids do require more space to allow for the container or syringe and the need to store several sizes of the same drug.

The actual dollar value of the total drug inventory also can be expected to increase with unit dose. Several factors affect this increase in inventory dollars. One, as already mentioned, is due to the duplication of unit and non-unit dose stock for inpatient and outpatient use. A second factor is due to the inclusion of "medication room" inventory or its equivalent which had not been included in the past when under the nurse's auspices. A third factor is due to the fact that much of the syringe inventory is in effect transferred to pharmacy stock as well as vials, caps, and other packaging materials.

Table 4. Tasks That Can Be Performed By Pharmacy Technicians

I. Clerical Tasks
- Process admissions
- Record doses
- Process surgery list
- Control patients' personal medications
- Calculate doses for charging
- Process discontinue orders
- Process patient transfers
- Process procedures for discharging patients
- Transcribe new orders

II. Requisitioning Drugs to Dose Preparation Area
- Process bedside and take home orders
- Process narcotics replacements
- Order unit dose drugs
- Order extemporaneously packaged drugs

III. Prepare Doses for Administration
- Process new orders (ongoing)
- Fill one time doses
- Prepare single unit doses in patient drawers
- Prepare pre-op orders
- Prepare I.V. orders
- Process and fill RN requests for drugs
- Check dose preparation
- Extemporaneously unit dose package drugs.

IV. Medication Cart
- Clean cart
- Exchange medication cart drawers

PHARMACY TECHNICIANS

Pharmacy technicians or supportive personnel are not new to the hospital pharmacist. They have been used primarily to do clerical work, prepackaging and bulk compounding under the supervision of the pharmacist. Delegation of high volume repetitive tasks from the pharmacist to the technician had not been acceptable until the unit dose drug distribution system was developed. In practice the pharmacist had been delegating tasks of the hospital medication system to the nurse. To assume tasks previously performed by the nurse, the pharmacy needs additional personnel to provide for the increased workload of the unit dose system. Unit dose packages allow the pharmacist to adequately check dose preparation activities performed by the technician previously performed by nurses and pharmacists.

Several studies have dealt with the role of the technician in the drug distribution tasks of the pharmacy.[15,16,17,18] None has explored the tasks involved in a unit dose drug distribution system which includes a number of additional tasks to be performed. Table 4 lists 23 tasks identified from a task analysis of technicians working in a decentralized unit dose drug distribution system.[19] They are grouped into clerical, drug procuring, dose preparation and medication cart tasks. Additional tasks no doubt could be added without too much difficulty. The key to delegating these tasks, however, lies in the training of the technician. Since this burden falls on the institution hiring technicians, this topic will be explored in some depth further on.

A procedural manual, primarily for the technician, delineating each step of each task is most important. This is a difficult chore since constant change and refinement of procedures will probably be ongoing for some time after implementing the first pilot area. Often these procedures are interrelated with nursing so that changes in their procedures affect pharmacy procedures and vice versa. The need for written procedures is more acute in a decentralized service and when technicians are used on two shifts (day and evening). The technician's work schedule may not coincide with a particular pharmacist's so that the technician may work with different pharmacists from day to day. If left to the pharmacist's direction, differing procedures will evolve from each pharmacist. Pharmacy technicians who work in satellite pharmacies, in addition, must understand the interfacing of pharmacy/nursing procedures, must be able to communicate well with nursing and understand how to handle a variety of demands when the pharmacist is not in the satellite pharmacy. In short, the pharmacy technician's job is generally not an easy one and requires as much support in terms of training, morale and remuneration as possible.

The pharmacist must understand the capabilities and limitations of the technicians with whom he works. If he is not personally training the technician, he needs to know how the training progresses and when the technician is qualified to do specific tasks. It is very easy for the pharmacist to be indifferent to the problems and limitations of the technicians. The pharmacist must realize that they are both performing important tasks and that to take the attitude that the pharmacist is superior to the technician will accomplish nothing and in the long run be destructive in working together. The technician is sensitive to derogatory language and references made to imply that they are inferior such as the term "sub-professional" has come to connote.[20]

Technicians must clearly understand their responsibilities and role in relationship to the pharmacists. In setting up a unit dose drug distribution system, the pharmacist is at first more involved with the details of the distribution system than he is later on. If the technician does not understand what the pharmacist's clinical objectives are it will appear that the pharmacist is giving more and more work to the technician who will not understand why.

Table 5 gives an example of a job description for a pharmacy technician. A number of potential applicants can be considered for hiring. Hospital employees already familiar with the institution such as LPN's (LVN's), nursing aides or clerks may also be familiar with some drug terminology, transcribing from physician's orders and so forth. Medical corpsmen have excellent training and experience and in some instances the government may reimburse the hospital for additional training and experience provided after their employment. Immigrants with training as pharmacists, pharmacy technicians or other medical training also may serve as technicians with considerable background and experience, thus reducing the amount of time in training required. High school graduates may do perfectly well provided an adequate training program is carried out. One should consider a pharmacy technician applicant's educational background, aptitude, ability to get along with people and willingness to learn. Technicians without an aptitude for simple mathematics seem to have difficulty in a variety of tasks requiring attention to details.

The turnover of technicians can be expected to be higher than that of the pharmacists. Matching the person with the job and providing a salary commensurate with the demands and responsibilities are not easy. The technician works under a certain amount of pressure to get the dose preparation done on time, he may be interrupted frequently and is expected to be accurate. It has been the experience of the authors that technicians have resigned for many reasons including the pressure of the job, but never from being bored.

One question that must be reviewed is exactly what a pharmacy technician can and cannot do legally. Each state has differing statutes affecting the practice of pharmacy and the dispensing of prescriptions. First to be examined is whether within the context of the inpatient unit dose drug distribution system, the state's pharmacy laws, rules and regulations make a distinction between a prescription and a chart order. When

Table 5. Job Description for a Pharmacy Technician

JOB REQUIREMENTS

I. Education required:
One year of college with chemistry and science courses preferred

II. Experience required:
Hospital background helpful. Knowledge of drugs, biological terminology very helpful. Can be trained on the job. Three to twelve months' training depending upon education and experience

III. Contacts required:
Works with pharmacist. Frequent contact with nurses and other pharmacy personnel. Some contact with physicians and other hospital personnel. Has access to and works with confidential information

GENERAL STATEMENT OF DUTIES

Prepares, issues and records drug doses in unit doses in the patient care area under supervision of the registered pharmacist

SPECIFIC DUTIES

1. Maintains each patient's medication record file of drugs
2. Fills patient medication drawer from medication record with appropriate number of doses for each drug preparation time period. Work checked by pharmacist
3. Orders unit dose drugs, extemporaneously packaged drugs and supplies and maintains inventory control of same
4. Fills one time and other new orders for drugs. Work checked by pharmacist
5. Calculates the number of drug doses administered upon discontinuance of order or every seven days
6. Keeps patient's name and drugs in the medication drawer with correct room and bed number, subject to new admissions, discharges and transfers
7. Keeps patient's medication records, charge documents, I.V. drugs and personal medications properly filed subject to transfers
8. Exchanges medication cassettes, restocks drug cart supplies and empties trash containers
9. Issues supplies, narcotics and other drugs to nursing, upon request, following procedures
10. Maintains pharmacy areas in clean orderly fashion
11. Processes surgery list orders, drug discontinuation orders, bedside and take home orders, pre-op and I.V. orders
12. Responsible for pharmacy area when pharmacist gone
13. Advises pharmacist on scheduled dose returns and other discrepancies related to drug utilization
14. Performs related duties as requested

drugs in units of one or whatever quantity are not issued directly to the patient but rather to a qualified nurse, exemptions may exist from outpatient dispensing procedures allowing technicians to prepare unit doses for the nurse. In addition, (as for example in the State of California) the satellite pharmacy may not be considered different from a medication room under state pharmacy regulations and would, therefore, not be under the jurisdiction of the State Board of Pharmacy. Technically, the existence of satellite pharmacies is a loophole of sorts since technician activities in a centralized, licensed pharmacy area would put these activities under Board jurisdiction. This situation is not necessarily correct or sacrosanct, but the distinction between the inpatient drug order provided to the nurse as opposed to the patient for self-medication is a valid one.

Technician Training

Adequate pharmacy technician training represents an investment which can pay off big dividends by allowing the pharmacist more time to provide clinical services. The investment is considerable since for the time being the availability of applicants having had pharmacy technician experience is unlikely. In the pilot phase of implementing a unit dose system and for sometime thereafter, the pharmacist working with the technician is generally drug distribution-oriented since such a change requires a great deal of time and attention at first. He is generally well motivated to train the technician with regard to details of the distribution system. As time progresses and technicians leave and new ones are hired the pharmacist is less and less motivated to train technicians as his time becomes committed to clinical activities. If the technicians' and pharmacists' work rotation schedules are not the same such training becomes almost impossible. Thus a need for a formalized training program for new technicians becomes essential to maintain the level of clinical services being provided by the pharmacy. In addition, the formalized training results in fewer short-term terminations and in general improves the morale of the technician.

The initial training beginning immediately upon hiring must deal with the rudiments of basic drug distribution procedures. A procedural manual can serve as the basis for explaining the paperwork and dose preparation activities. A combination of verbal explanations and subsequent performing of these tasks will be required, the duration of which will depend upon the number and complexity of the tasks involved as well as the learning capabilities of the technician. Table 6 is an example of a training outline requiring four weeks which ascends from primarily a classroom component to primarily a performance experience component. Four weeks has been a happy medium between fairness to the technician and prudence on the initial training investment for the material covered. The objective of the initial training is to provide the technician with the capability of performing all the tasks listed in Table 4, except for transcribing physicians' orders and checking the dose preparation of another technician.

Table 6. Pharmacy Technician Training Outline

I. ORIENTATION TO THE HOSPITAL AND PATIENT CARE
II. PHARMACY DEPARTMENT ORGANIZATION
III. PHARMACY PROFESSION
  A. History
  B. Patient Care Environment Pharmacy Service
  C. Ethics
IV. PHARMACY LAWS
  A. Legend Drugs
  B. Non-Legend Drugs
  C. Federal Narcotics and Controlled Drugs
  D. State Pharmacy Laws
  E. State Narcotics and Controlled Drug Laws
V. TERMINOLOGY
  A. Pharmacy
    1. Official Compendia
    2. Dosage Forms (Examples: Solution, Ointment, etc.)
    3. Common Terms for Drug Classification (e.g., Antibiotic)
  B. Patient
VI. PHARMACY TECHNICIAN POSITION DESCRIPTION
  A. Dose Preparation Area (Satellite Pharmacy)
  B. Pharmacy Technology (Packaging Area)
VII. DUTIES OF PHARMACY TECHNICIAN
  A. Dose Preparation Area
    1. Prepare under pharmacist supervision, medications for administration by the nurse
    2. Prepare patient charges for medications
    3. Maintain inventory of drugs and supplies
    4. Process discharge and transfer notices
    5. Prepare drug cards for dose preparation
    6. Maintain pharmacy areas in clean and orderly fashion
    7. Perform related duties as requested
  B. Pharmacy Technology
    1. Single unit drug packaging
    2. Prepackaging
    3. Operation of packaging machines
    4. Records and quality control
    5. Special techniques

After the new technician has worked for two or three months and has developed confidence in procedural details, additional training can provide the technician with a better understanding of why things are done as they are, *e.g.*, why some drugs always seem to go into the PRN section of the patient's drawer and others in the scheduled section. Technicians are by and large eager to learn more about the drugs they handle each day. Information on a drug-oriented plane provides for better understanding and performance. Table 7 lists the topics that can be covered in advanced classes. The classifications are not important *per se* but the specific drugs discussed should be the ones most frequently prepared and handled by the technician in the hospital. Emphasis on identifying unit dose drugs, drug use, synonyms, refrigeration requirements, expiration dates and so forth will help the technician understand the whys and wherefores of the procedures and bring home the responsibilities involved with handling potent and dangerous drugs.

The objective of this additional training also can be directed toward adding on additional technician tasks such as transcribing new orders and checking the dose preparation of another technician. Special training also can be provided for intravenous additive activities and even administering medications to patients, topics which are beyond the scope of this chapter. Technician administration of drugs, both technically and legally, is more involved from the pharmacist's point of view. It appears to be a logical step beyond the dose preparation activity for the technician. Further studies are needed, however, to determine whether such an approach provides better patient care. Specialized training in a variety of areas beyond what has been discussed here may open up to the technician in due time.

INTERPROFESSIONAL RELATIONSHIPS

Pharmacist-Nurse Relationship

The nurse is responsible for administering drugs to patients as ordered by the physician. Often the hospital pharmacist has developed an

Table 7. Advanced Topics for Technicians

1. Introduction
   Pretest, drug classifications, nomenclature, synonyms, trade names and generic names, drug manufacturers, outline of course, *American Drug Index*
2. Drug Dosage Forms
   Description of and reasons for tablets, capsules, injections, oral liquids, suppositories, topical preparations, etc.; special dosage forms, *i.e.*, extended release preparations
3. Potency of Drugs
   Weights and measures, avoirdupois, metric, apothecary, units
4. Anti-Infectives - I
   Tetracyclines, Sulfas, Penicillins, etc.
5. Anti-Infectives - II
6. Central Nervous System Drugs - I
   Drugs used for nausea and vomiting, pain, insomnia, nervousness and mental illness
7. Central Nervous System Drugs - II
8. Hormones and Diuretics
9. Electrolytes, Caloric Agents, Vitamins and Minerals
10. Gastrointestinal Drugs
11. Antihistamine, Autonomic and Cardiovascular Drugs
12. Mathematical Calculations
    Weights and measures, solution percentages, dose fractions, dose calculations
13. Inventory Storage and Control
    Storage groups-organizational arrangement, special storage requirements-refrigeration requirements, signs of drug deterioration
14. Pharmaceutical Manipulations - I
    Dilution, reconstitution, unit packaging techniques, sterile technique-clean air hoods
15. Pharmaceutical Manipulations - II
16. Examination
    Identification, practical, written

elaborate set of rules through which the nurse struggles to procure drugs — pharmacy open 8:00 AM to 6:00 PM, requisitions filled three times a week, narcotics replacements at certain hours and so forth. All this makes the pharmacy operation neat and tidy at the expense of not only the nurse but the patient as well. The pharmacy sends multiple dose supplies of drugs to the nursing unit. Patients take drugs in individual doses, so the nurse has to fill the gap. The medication system is but one of too many responsibilities the nurse tries to meet. A classic contemporary description of the nurse preparing to administer a medication to a patient was described as follows: "While taking a group of visitors through one of our (nursing) units a short time ago, I observed one of our team nurses preparing an injectable pain medication while:

1. A secretary informed her that a physician with whom she wanted to talk, was on the phone;
2. An x-ray technician waited to complain about an improperly checked block on a requisition which had resulted in the delay of an important test;
3. Some students strolled up to ask rather dumb questions so they wouldn't have to study;
4. She instructed the dietitian regarding the likes and dislikes of a particular patient who was off the unit and couldn't see the dietitian before lunch;
5. One of her team members reported ill, and the nursing office said, "make do;"
6. She instructed her unit secretary to call the home care coordinator regarding one of the patients; and
7. Came up with a pin for a broken strap or something for a horrified and rather awkward looking visitor."[13]

It does not take very much time on a patient floor to discover that the nurse is expected to do and be all things to too many people. If the nurse looks at you in disbelief when you confront her with this revelation it won't be because she doesn't believe you, it will be because she is wondering where you've been all these years.

In hospitals that have implemented a unit dose drug distribution system the nursing department often is its most enthusiastic supporter. This is not surprising since the pharmacy takes on part of the nurse's previous workload. Table 8 illustrates the shift in tasks from nursing to pharmacy with a unit dose system. This, of course, will vary somewhat from one system to another.

The unit dose system does not encompass providing clinical service *per se*. To emphasize what has already been stated, it is difficult for the pharmacist to provide clinical services, be physically present on the patient floor with nursing and provide nursing with drug information and ignore the drug distribution problems facing a nurse. It would appear incongruous and incomprehensible to the nurse (and to the authors) to attempt it. The pharmacist and nurse must first straighten out the drug distribution system.

Table 8. Nursing and Pharmacy Tasks Before and After Decentralized Unit Dose Drug Distribution System

FUNCTION	BEFORE NURSING	BEFORE PHARMACY	AFTER NURSING	AFTER PHARMACY
1. M.D. prescribes order				
2. Interpret and transcribe order	X		X	X‡
3. Nursing patient care Kardex	X		X	
4. Prepare med card	X†			
5. Prepare med record-charting	X		X	
6. Requisition drugs to patient floor	X†			X‡
7. Prepare doses for administration	X†			X
8. Administer doses	X		X	
9. Chart doses administered	X		X	
10. Clean up med tray	X†			
11. Clean up med cart			X	X‡
12. Check med cards 3 times daily	X†			
13. Pharmaceutical Service Record				X‡
14. Narcotic control records	X	X	X	X
15. Hypnotic records	X†			
16. Credit meds	X†	X		

Note: Some nursing duties pre- and post-unit dose have changed to improve efficiency by changing forms, records and location of performing duty. Example: duties 2, 5, 8, 9, 11 and 14.

Key: X†—nursing tasks eliminated; X‡—new pharmacy tasks

The pharmacist and the nurse must work together if the hospital medication system is to run smoothly getting drugs to patients in a safe and efficient manner. The unit dose drug distribution system is one method for the pharmacy to assume a much greater portion of the total hospital medication system. The efficiency of the dose preparation step is improved and a double check for each dose administered to the patient is provided.

Obviously to make any major changes in the hospital medication system, the cooperation and support of nursing are necessary. A great deal of rethinking is required on the part of nursing if unit dose is instituted. Where does the nurse's role logically begin in the medication system? An honest appraisal from nursing of nursing time saved when the doses are prepared in medication carts by the pharmacy and what benefits to nursing the additional workload and cost in pharmacy will have is essential. Preparing doses is a time honored nursing task and taught in some detail in schools of nursing, which always stress that a nurse never administers doses she has not "poured" or prepared. Since the unit dose package is labeled with drug name and strength, the acceptance of this change in nursing tradition has been universally received with enthusiasm once it was tried.

Specific procedures dealing with the receipt and delivery of new orders and initial doses must be agreed upon. Adequate and timely communications are essential. If the nurse is to deal with pharmacy technicians she must understand who they are and what rules and regulations are imposed on them. Table 9 provides a list of topics which illustrate the variety of details necessary to have worked out prior to initiating a unit dose pilot area.

Table 9. Nursing Procedures Involving Unit Dose Drug Distribution

Cleaning and removing trash from medication cart
Patient drawer divisions for scheduled and PRN doses
Controlled drug distribution system
Time of exchanging patient drawers
Delivery of new orders and initial doses, time schedule
Drug renewal requests
Stat orders
Medication record system
Pre-ops
I.V. additives
Discontinued orders
New admission processing
Patient's own medications on admission
Patient transfers
Patient discharge processing
Discharge prescriptions
Communications with pharmacist
Scheduled doses not given
Drug requests for missing or dropped doses

Once the tentative details have been worked out, the total system should be reexamined to see from an overview of the system whether it will accomplish the objectives originally sought. Will it be a more efficient system and will it provide double checks for new orders and routine ongoing doses? It is very easy for the pharmacist to find himself wondering why he cannot do more and more of the nurses' tasks related to the medication system in the planning stages. Particularly if satellite pharmacies will be located next to the nursing stations, all kinds of possibilities emerge for transferring nursing tasks to the pharmacy such as preparing stop order drug lists, bringing initial doses of new orders to the medication cart and removing discontinued doses from the cart, preparing the nurse medication record and many other tasks. Suffice it to say that tasks should not be transferred from a nursing clerk or the nurse to the *pharmacist* without careful consideration and justification. Too frequently the pharmacist finds himself with insufficient technical help, tied down to mountains of clerical work and as a consequence, is unable to meet the professional opportunities that the patient care environment affords. For example the pharmacist, if immediately available on the patient floor, could interview patients on admission for drug allergies as opposed to doing some of the nurses' paperwork. Looking at the system on paper, the pharmacist is usually concerned about what he will do with all his time, if given a pharmacy technician to prepare all the doses. The clinical services are often *in utero* in the planning stages of the unit dose system. Once on the patient floors, however, the number of clinical services can grow to an incomprehensible degree, demanding more and more pharmacist time.

A pilot wing or floor of the hospital can be used to test nursing/pharmacy procedures among other aspects of the unit dose system. Many orientation meetings with nursing, preferably in small groups, will be necessary to adequately instruct nurses prior to implementing the new system. The proposed system should be explained in detail with a nursing representative. Show what the unit-packaged drugs will look like, what the medication cart will be like and how the drugs will be placed in the cart. Remember, "a picture is worth a thousand words."

Because the pharmacist and nurse are forced into a much closer working relationship with each other with the unit dose system, nurses will ask more questions of the pharmacist about drugs. The nurses' recognition of the pharmacist's *clinical* role beyond this, however, is not as automatic as the pharmacist might assume. The nurse has pretty much decided what the BID, TID and QID schedules should be, when to start the first dose of a new order and what drugs should and should not be given with food. The pharmacist must recognize the limitations in the nurse's ability to handle special dosage schedules but on the other hand he would be remiss in not providing her with information concerning the best administration times for the drugs she will administer. A policy, therefore, must be agreed upon as to whether the pharmacist can dictate special dosage schedules, decide when the first dose will be given and so on, when this would otherwise be left up to the nurse.

Obviously the nurse should expect the pharmacist to explain the rationale of the special instructions he gives her. The pharmacist should take the initiative here and offer inservice discussions for nursing from which a more cooperative attitude will result. There are many areas of interest to the pharmacist that mutually concern the nurse about which the pharmacist can offer continuing educational discussions for nursing. Topics such as how laboratory values relate to particular drug therapy; rationale for dosing time schedules; adverse drug reactions, sources, detection and prevention; absorption, distribution and elimination of drugs, clinical importance and specific drug therapy — provide a better understanding of the pharmacist's capabilities and role on the health care team beyond drug distribution. This level of discussion helps to put the day-to-day drug distribution talk in perspective and gives nurses and pharmacists a better chance to get to know one another. Even 15 minute discussions can go a long way to maintain a good rapport and encourage nurses to help keep the pharmacist aware of drug therapy problems they see in their patients. As the pharmacist continues to expand his clinical role, the nurse will appreciate what the pharmacist has to offer to improve patient care when he advises a physician or interviews a patient.

Pharmacist-Physician Relationship

In traditional pharmacy services the pharmacist-physician relationship is predominately drug-system and drug-product oriented. The basic objective of the physician as a user of traditional pharmacy service and the pharmacist as provider of service is to distribute drugs to patients accurately, efficiently and quickly. The subjects on the agendas of pharmacy and therapeutic committees for the past several years reflect the domination of system problems, such as: hospital formulary system, narcotic controls, emergency drug list, stop order procedures, physician order forms, drug availablity, etc. Drug information as an interprofessional activity has been minimal. Possibly the apparent lack of published studies on the drug information demands by the medical staff in the traditional pharmacy department will illustrate the virtual nonexistent nature of this interprofessional activity.

Whether or not one is discussing traditional or clinical pharmacy services, the basic objective of a safe, accurate and efficient hospital medication system is valid. The physician and patient should not receive anything less from pharmacy services. If the drug distribution component of clinical pharmacy services is not reliable it will be very difficult to gain physician acceptance for the pharmacist's clinical practice. Pharmacists must avoid finding themselves in the following position with the physician, "When you can't even get drugs to patients accurately, should I have confidence in your drug information?"

The physician's drug order is an important initial step to implementing a unit dose system. The interpretation of the physician's order by the pharmacist is the initial bridge to changing the pharmacist's practice from traditional to clinical. In a traditional pharmacy service, what professional judgments does the pharmacist make on physician drug orders? At this level the basic question becomes: "Is the dose prescribed within the usual range recommended by the manufacturer and approved by FDA?" Where is the patient in such a decision? Is the prescribed dose intended as the correct dose for either a 70-pound man, a 240-pound man, a patient with liver disease, kidney disease? Is there a possible drug-drug interaction? How can the pharmacist's interpretation and, therefore, decision be patient-oriented if he does not have access to patient information, total current drug therapy, etc.?[21] If he decides the prescribed dose is inaccurate for a patient, how can he discuss the order with the physician intelligently if he knows little or nothing about the patient? Is not the traditional pharmacy service basically a sophisticated stock room operation? The lack of drug information as an interprofessional activity has resulted from physical isolation and information isolation between the physician and pharmacist. Figure 20 is an attempt to diagram this physical and information isolation of traditional drug information. Of note is that the pharmacist is not included.

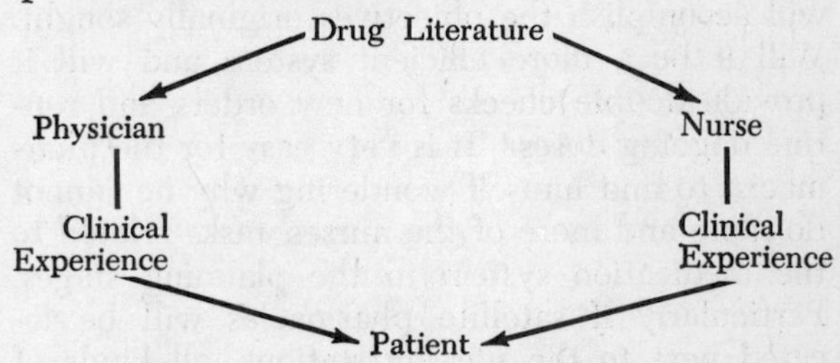

Figure 20. Traditional drug information

Drug therapy as experienced by the patient is predominately a combination of the physician's knowledge of drug literature coupled with clinical experience. Drug literature is composed of education, journal reading, attending seminars and so forth. The result of this traditional drug therapy approach has been for the most part, good therapy. However, a significant adverse drug reaction rate[24] does exist which tends to cause prolonged hospitalization. For additional information on adverse drug reactions, refer to Chapter 11.

A basic component of clinical pharmacy service is drug information. Figure 21 labeled Clinical Drug Information, is an attempt to diagram the interprofessional relationships that result from the pharmacist's clinical practice.

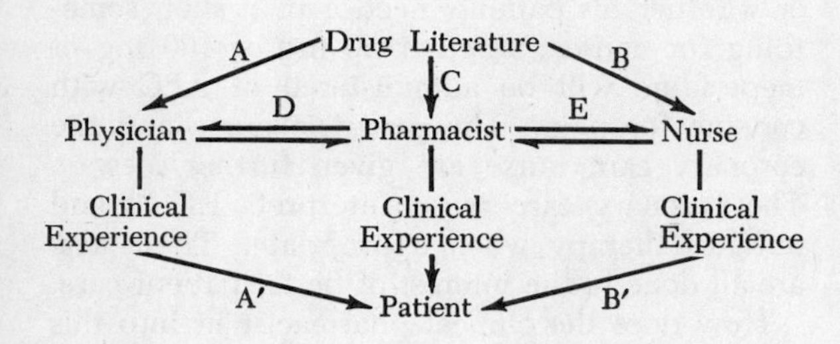

Figure 21. Clinical drug information

Historically, the physician, and to a certain extent the nurse, have acted as their own interpreters in correlating the drug literature with their clinical experience. (Pathways A, A′, B, B′.) This role was satisfactory in the past due to the relative non-sophistication of drug information. Today, the physician and the nurse still rely to a major degree on their clinical experience (Pathways A′, B′) in their respective roles of prescribing and administering. However, the input into the system, Pathways A and B, becomes less desirable as the complexity of drug knowledge, physician specialization and drug utilization increases. Consequently, the pharmacist's input, Pathways C, D, and E, takes on a major character in assuring that the patient receives the best possible drug therapy. The pharmacist has the responsibility both professionally and legally to promote patient safety in the use of drugs.

The opportunity for a pharmacist to provide clinical drug information depends on the creation of an environment for clinical practice. The pharmacist's clinical practice will be discussed later in this chapter.

The ability of the pharmacist to provide clinical drug information depends on his own talents and knowledge plus the cooperation he can develop with physicians and nurses. The pharmacist is recognized as being knowledgeable about drugs so what talents does the pharmacist need, to develop a personally satisfying clinical practice? A successful pharmacist in clinical practice must possess the following:

1. Clinical drug knowledge
2. Commitment to clinical practice
3. Competence in both oral and written communication skills
4. Ability to work cooperatively with people
5. Initially, a high frustration level

Knowledge is essential but knowledge is of no value to patients unless it can be communicated to physicians, nurses and patients. A commitment to clinical practice is essential because no one can ever learn "all" about drugs. A high frustration level is needed because clinical pharmacy is a radical change from traditional practice, and physicians are reluctant to adapt easily to change in pharmacy services. The most important talent requirement is the ability to work with people. No one, especially physicians, will accept a know-it-all, overly aggressive pharmacist.

In Figure 21 line D between physician and pharmacist is most important. A justification for clinical pharmacy service is one of the many problems inherent in modern drug therapy which result from traditional responsibilities as diagrammed. Yet at the same time, physician acceptance of the pharmacist's clinical practice is absolutely necessary. This paradox cannot be ignored and must be approached head on. A physician who is not receptive to clinical pharmacy or who is not well-known by the pharmacist should not be placed in a defensive position about his drug prescribing. No individual likes to be criticized or placed in a defensive position. The normal and predicted response when one is placed in such a posture is saving face, or defending one's decision. When a pharmacist places a physician in such a position, the information the pharmacist provides most likely will not be used nor the desired objective achieved. The ability to approach physicians about their prescribing is an individual matter and will develop with training and effort. A good method for the pharmacist to start out with is to ask questions about the questionable situation to improve his understanding and knowledge. Other guides are:

1. Do not contact the physician over trivia, don't be a pest
2. Contact the physician only when you are concerned about a real problem for the patient
3. Present your information in a factual manner and be capable of documentation using respected medical and pharmacological literature
4. Give your *opinion* only when requested. Never start the discussion with your opinion which places the physician in a defensive posture. This is the quickest and surest road to disaster

A suggested approach to the subject of drug interactions will further illustrate the type and depth of knowledge the pharmacist should have before contacting the physician. A pharmacist should not contact a physician on a drug-drug interaction unless he can:

1. Discuss the interaction on a biochemical, pharmacological, etc. level or in other words know what the requirements for and mechanism of action of the interaction are
2. Discuss the potential for the interaction to occur in the physician's patient
3. Offer alternatives to the present drug therapy regimen

Unless the pharmacist can perform at these three levels, how can he answer the following questions which may be proposed by the physician.

1. What is the proposed drug interaction?
2. What is the potential of this interaction in my patient?
3. What should I do about it?

Unless the pharmacist can answer these predictable questions, the physician should not be contacted.

If the question to the physician on his prescribing is valid, and the physician responds favorably, and the pharmacist "delivers the goods," the patient benefits and both physician and pharmacist are satisfied. The other side of the coin is when the physician is not receptive to the pharmacist's interest in his prescribing. If the physician responds in a curt, defensive, obtuse or negative way which makes the pharmacist want to tell the physician "to go jump," the patient may suffer. The next time the pharmacist should call the physician, he may not call. The patient then loses the opportunity for the combination of the knowledge and clinical experience of the physician and pharmacist. So, line D is extremely important and can only operate if both the physician and pharmacist understand each other's responsibilities, interests, motives, knowledge, etc. The pharmacist must not forget the physician is the person responsible for the patient. The pharmacist should support the physician in what ever way possible, yet at the same time question the physician's prescribing when in the best interest of the patient. If the physician and pharmacist cannot work together, no exchange of clinical drug information takes place.

THE PHARMACIST'S CLINICAL PRACTICE

The delegation of various aspects of medical care for patients by private physicians to interns and nurses is an accepted fact in patient care. The intern, when treating a private physician's patient, may prescribe the majority of treatments and drugs. The intern understands that if he does not know how to handle a given situation he seeks advice from the private physician or resident. Likewise the private physician will utilize consultants whenever he desires additional advice about the treatment of a patient. The physician delegates to the nurse the decision of whether his patients need a pain shot, something for nausea, whether 50 mg or 100 mg of meperidine will be administered or APC with codeine for pain. The pediatric nurse and the coronary care nurse are given further leeway. The coronary care nurse interprets EKG's and initiates therapy when appropriate. These acts are all done in the interest of better patient care.

How does the clinical pharmacist fit into this picture; that is, how much responsibility will he be able to assume for the patient? This section of the chapter will attempt to describe where one can begin a clinical role and approaches that have worked and some that have failed. Suggestions as to what direction pharmacists should pursue in the future will be given.

The pharmacist's clinical practice is composed of many activities. Clinical practice includes those activities in which the pharmacist applies knowledge of the biological and pharmaceutical sciences along with clinical experience to specific questions of drug therapy. Judgment is required of the pharmacist who is now dealing with a particular patient's drug therapy. A clinical practice *requires* that a major portion of the pharmacist's time be devoted to clinical activities. This is true because both experience and keeping current on drug therapy are essential to practice at a high standard of performance.[8]

Activities Performed in Clinical Practice

The activities listed below are performed by pharmacists in clinical practice. The activities have been divided into drug distribution and clinical.

Drug Distribution Activities

1. Supervise pharmacy technician
2. Perform pharmacy technician duties as needed
3. Interpret all physicians' drug orders
4. Check pharmacy technician dose preparations
5. Prepare intravenous drug admixtures

Clinical Activities

6. Question physician drug orders when applicable
7. Suggest laboratory tests, drug therapy changes, etc. to the physician
8. Answer questions asked by the physician

9. Answer questions asked by nurses
10. Participate on the hospital emergency team
11. Attend and participate in patient care rounds
12. Interview patients—admission drug history interviews, drug therapy evaluation, discharge interview
13. Present drug therapy conferences to physicians, nurses and pharmacists
14. Review and monitor drug therapy
15. Ask questions of the Drug Information Service concerning patient drug therapy

Which of the above require judgment, evaluation? How does the pharmacist's judgment affect patient care? What is good patient care, from the standpoint of drug therapy?

The pharmacist's contributions to patient care are interrelated in the following manner as shown in Figure 22.

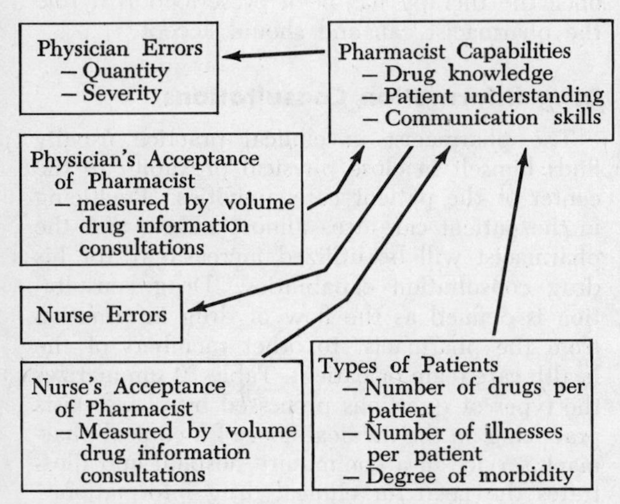

Figure 22. Interrelationship of pharmacist's contributions to patient care

The importance and quantity of the pharmacist's impact on patient care are affected by this complex interrelationship. In practice the limiting factor is the pharmacist's capabilities resulting from lack of experience and lack of a clinically-oriented education. The pharmacist placed in the clinical environment or the environment of the bedside discovers, in effect, a multitude of drug information questions that the busy physician and nurse either do not see or have become conditioned to the point that they seem unimportant, *i.e.*, the level of importance of drug therapy is not that great.

Most pharmacists realize that they are not clinically oriented. Also they need to realize that a review of basic drug information is equally essential in order to contribute to the health care team. Each drug must be reviewed to delineate the specific essential data needed for monitoring patients, *e.g.*, laboratory values, side effects, dose, drug interactions. This essential information should also be listed or understood in order of priorities. The availability of drug information resources is essential to the pharmacist in clinical practice.

Pharmacist Training and Education

The training and education of pharmacists for clinical practice must be directed at two levels: (1) students currently in schools of pharmacy and (2) pharmacists already in practice. It is beyond the scope of this chapter to discuss clinical pharmacy education in depth but some general comments are necessary. Every pharmacy student should receive the best possible and most extensive clinical clerkship teaching program possible. The student upon graduation should have knowledge as to what can happen to patients receiving drugs; how to evaluate critically the drug literature; how to use the medical library effectively; how to communicate in both oral and written form drug information to physicians, pharmacists and nurses; and should have received the most extensive biological science education possible. The student should have been able to witness and participate in an active clinical pharmacy service in the institution used for his clinical clerkship. Some students should receive additional training in management skills so they can be capable of developing and managing a clinical pharmacy service.

What can and should be done to assist pharmacists already in practice to be capable of practicing clinical pharmacy adequately? The individual pharmacist must want to develop his own successful clinical practice. He must be committed and willing to put forth the effort to successfully change his daily practice and provide a new kind of pharmacy service. He should keep in mind that the first pharmacists initiating clinical practice were not specifically educated for such a practice and had to develop their capabilities on their own.

There are several things a pharmacy department staff can do to assist each other in developing themselves for clinical pharmacy services. The department and institution must create the environment and commitment for clinical pharmacy services to grow and mature. An environment for learning and honest evaluation of each pharmacist's strong and weak abilities must be developed. Initial areas for study include: medical terminology; laboratory test values and significance; patient information in the chart; and study of primary disease states — hypertension, diabetes, cardiac, abnormalities; clinical pharmacology of drugs — antibiotics, CNS, electrolytes, etc.

Department conferences can be held with selected subjects given by invited speakers, as well as having pharmacists speak to their colleagues. The staff should be allowed and encouraged to attend medical staff educational conferences. Each pharmacist will have to develop his own self-study program. Reading current journals is a necessity. The pharmacist should first read what the intern, resident and private physician reads. Consult the medical librarian or medical education coordinator to determine most frequently read books and journals. The specialty journals of the clinical area in which the pharmacist practices should be routinely reviewed. Most importantly, the pharmacist must practice in the clinical area daily. He must be willing to work cooperatively with physicians and nurses and display such willingness by his actions. It is best if he can provide precise drug information services on the spot. If he does not know the answer to the question, he should say "I don't know," but get the answer and respond as soon as possible. Follow-through to complete an answer or meet a need is very important. It is the authors' estimate that at least six to 12 months of daily practice in the patient care area is needed before a pharmacist begins to perform adequately in the clinical area. Remembering drug therapy details is easier when study is coupled with monitoring patients' drug therapy. When seen in a patient these details will never be forgotten. A high frustration level and restrained impatience will make the transition from traditional to clinical practice much easier. When the transition is successfully made, the pharmacist must then expand his knowledge beyond that of the physician's.

Some drug therapy areas will be more of a problem to physicians than others. The pharmacist should specialize in specific drug therapy areas where he believes he can have the greatest impact on patient care. Such specialization must be in concert with physician receptivity to such help. The drugs most frequently used in the hospital should be studied in depth. The pharmacist will eventually gain greater experience than the physician with drugs used primarily in the hospital which are the drugs in which he is primarily interested anyway.

Drug allergies, effects of drugs on electrolytes, effect of drugs on blood elements and drug interactions should be studied in some depth. The pharmacist must learn to utilize the patient's chart as: (1) a textbook to help study the patient's clinical progress; (2) a background to give a feeling of confidence; and (3) a working document to review, analyze and suggest as a consultant.[22]

The "clinical" aspect of pharmacy service in its most positive sense is the pharmacist's concern for giving the *best* drug to a *particular* patient, *e.g.*, Mrs. Smith, who has a systemic infection, is allergic to penicillin and has some renal impairment. The pharmacist in clinical practice, after reviewing the diagnosis with the physician, should be capable of accepting the responsibility to recommend the best medication regimen for the patient. This should be done in concert with the physician; however, monitoring the patient once the therapy has been prescribed is a role the pharmacist can and should accept.[22]

Drug Information Consultations

The pharmacist in clinical practice usually finds himself in close physical proximity to the center of the patient care activities. Practicing in the patient care area almost assures that the pharmacist will be utilized increasingly for his drug consultation capabilities. Drug consultation is defined as the flow of drug information from the pharmacist to other members of the health care team or patient. Table 10 summarizes the types of questions processed by pharmacists practicing on the medical floor of a clinical pharmacy service in a community hospital and illustrates the need for clinical drug information.[23] The consultations tallied were collected over a two-month period, May-June 1970.

It can be concluded from this data that the pharmacist was being consulted by physicians, including private physicians. The consultations pertain to important drug categories and relate to many specific patients rather than general information. Many of the consultations take place prior to an actual problem. Most of the information provided by the pharmacist was accepted by the physicians.

Hospital Emergency Team

Success of treatment in an emergency depends on immediate action and availability of supplies and drugs. A valuable service of clinical pharmacy is to have the pharmacist as a member of the hospital emergency team.[24,25] This service should go hand-in-hand with 24-hour clinical pharmacy practice. The pharmacist should participate actively in resuscitation by performing the following:

Table 10. Types of Questions Processed by Pharmacists on the Medical Floor of a Community Hospital

1. The number of questions from physicians to pharmacists was 107; number from pharmacists to physicians was 124.
2. Thirty-six (16 percent) of the questions arose on ward rounds, and 195 (84 percent) arose in other areas, predominately in the pharmacy satellite unit.
3. Consultations by physicians' category was: private physician 75 (32 percent); residents 20 (9 percent); interns 123 (53 percent).
4. Consultations by drug category were (only first six categories listed):
   Antibiotics — 64
   CNS drugs — 36
   Electrolytic, caloric, water balance — 33
   Blood formation and coagulation — 31
   Cardiovascular drugs — 24
   Autonomic drugs — 10
5. Types of consultations were tallied as follows (only top five listed):

TYPE OF CONSULTATION					RECOMMENDATION					
	Patient Specific	Information Provided	Potential Problem	Actual Problem	No Change	Change	New Drug	Discontinue Drug	Accepted	Rejected
Drug of Choice	56	15	7	27	1	4	37	15	37	8
Toxicity (Adverse Rx)	21	6	7	8	–	2	3	9	12	–
Overdose	11	4	5	4	1	5	–	3	7	1
Dose and/or Schedule	80	28	12	22	2	37	5	4	47	3
Comparison 2 or more	11	7	1	–	–	–	1	1	1	–
Other (Specify)	46	19	10	1	–	12	1	–	12	–

6. Physician's acceptance to rejection ratio of the pharmacist's information was 89 to 11 percent.

1. Answer the "Code" page immediately
2. If he is near the emergency cart, move it to the resuscitation scene
3. On arrival, assume responsibility for the preparation of medications for various routes of administration
4. Record medications administered and procedures performed
5. Be a consultant and resource for the physician regarding dosages, compatibilities, timing of doses administered and other drug-related questions
6. Maintain medication inventory on the emergency carts
7. Participate in evaluation and teaching of cardiopulmonary resuscitation

In addition to cardiopulmonary resuscitation emergencies, the pharmacist should have a role to play in the emergency department if a large number of casualties need treatment from a disaster. His responsibilities should be to assist with preparing medications, maintaining an adequate drug supply in the treatment area and participation in cardiopulmonary emergencies if they occur.

Patient Care Rounds

One of the pharmacist's responsibilities in clinical practice should be to attend and participate in patient care rounds. Such an activity will broaden the pharmacist's clinical experience and give him patient contact and exposure. Many decisions about the patient's diagnosis, treatment and prognosis are discussed during rounds. Pharmacist attendance and participation facilitate providing a high quality pharmacy service as he is readily available as a resource person on drug therapy. He will also have a greater understanding of the physician's drug orders when received.[26]

Patient rounds will serve as a learning experience for the pharmacist as he will be exposed to the physician's logic and concern for treating patients. This learning experience will be temporary. Ongoing benefits to the pharmacist from participation in patient rounds are contributions to patient care decisions, particularly if patients are being monitored, and increased rapport with physicians. To maximize participation and contribution, the pharmacist should be familiar with the patient's status and drug therapy prior to the actual patient care rounds. Patient medication profiles which can be carried on patient rounds are of immense value since the number of patients the pharmacist is concerned about may be extensive.

DATE	CHEMISTRY
Temp.	FBS
HEMATOLOGY	BUN
Hgb	Sodium
Hct	Potassium
R.B.C. x 10^6	Chloride
W.B.C. x 10^3	CO_2
Seg. PMN'S	pH
Bands	Calcium
Lymphocytes	Phosphorus
Monocytes	Creatinine
Eosinophils	Uric Acid
Metamyelocytes	SGOT
Myelocytes	SGPT
Progranulocytes	L.D.H.
Blast Cells	Alk P'tase
Platelet Est.	Bilirubin, Conj.
URINALYSIS	Bilirubin, Total
Glucose	Cholesterol
Protein	C.P.K.
W.B.C.	P.B.I.
R.B.C.	T^3
Bacteria	
DATE	
Anticoagulant/Dose	
Prothrombin	
Lee-White	

PATIENT HISTORY; DRUGS AND DISEASES; PROGRESS NOTES

Liver ☐ Bone Mar ☐
Kidney ☐ Drug Interaction ☐ Low Na+ DIET ☐

ANTIBIOTIC SENSITIVITY — DATE:

Ampicillin	Oxacillin
Chloramphenicol	Penicillin G
Colistimethate	Polymyxin B
Erythromycin	Streptomycin
Nitrofurantoin	Tetracycline
Gentamicin	
Kanamycin	
Cephalothin	
Lincomycin	
Methicillin	
Neomycin	

DIAGNOSTIC: X-RAY, BIOPSY, EKG

NARCOTICS, BEDSIDE, SINGLE DOSES AND SUPPLIES

DATE	DATE

NARCOTICS, BEDSIDE, SINGLE DOSES AND SUPPLIES

DATE	DATE

Percodan/Phen-Cod/APC-Cod
MS/Meperidine

Patients Own Drugs ☐ Discharge Rx's ☐ Save PSR ☐

DATE	DIAGNOSIS	DATE	SURGERY - PROCEDURES	DRUG SENSITIVITIES AND ALLERGIES

ROOM	NAME	ID#	WEIGHT	AGE	DOCTOR	MONITOR ☐

Figure 23. Pharmaceutical Service Record. Laboratory and other data can be recorded here. The arrangement should match the order in which the laboratory reports its results

Monitor Drug Therapy

The intent of the patient drug profile is to consolidate the pertinent facts relating to a patient's drug therapy to allow the pharmacist to render a professional judgment regarding the effectiveness and safety of the patient's drug therapy. Patient medication profiles or Pharmaceutical Service Records (Figure 23) are designed usually to record the patient's name, age, diagnosis, drug sensitivities and allergies and to record the patient's history, *i.e.*, past drugs and diseases, physical findings, progress notes and other essential information. The pharmacist must gain the ability to apply drug information to specific patients. He must maintain a questioning attitude in his own mind regarding the appropriateness of every drug ordered initially and its continued use subsequently. The end product of monitoring is an evaluation of each drug order for a particular patient. This is oversimplified to the extent that the individual patient's status must be relevant in a practical sense. The pharmacist should be generating questions in his own mind while monitoring which should be researched and documented (by himself or a drug information service). Every answer should either confirm or recommend change in a particular patient's regimen. The ability to recognize basic drug therapy problems for a given patient is probably more important and difficult for the pharmacist initially than researching the answer to the question and only can be gained by actual experience.

The collection of required information regarding the patient, single drugs, drug-drug interactions and drug-laboratory test interferences cannot be used effectively for the patient's benefit unless the pharmacist understands and can communicate the data to other health professionals. Effective use of the patient drug profile results only from experience, trial and error and aggressiveness on the part of the pharmacist.[22]

Interview Patients

Pharmacists should interview patients upon admission, during their hospitalization and at the time of discharge. A brief review is presented here, but the reader should refer to Chapter 12 for more information on this subject.

Admission. The basic objectives of an admission interview are to obtain a drug history including over-the-counter (O-T-C) drugs prior to admission and to determine if the patient is allergic to any drugs and the background of his allergies.

A specific interview form, (Figure 24) can be used or a narrative report can be written. An approach for interviewing the patient is outlined below.

1. Introduce yourself to the patient
2. Inform the patient of the purpose of interview
3. Inquire how the patient is feeling and whether he is comfortable. If patient is in acute distress, report this to the nurse or physician. Do not conduct an interview
4. Find out reason for hospitalization and symptoms presented by the patient, and whether the symptoms are being relieved during hospitalization
5. Prepare a drug profile of medications, including OTC items, the patient is taking routinely. Learn of reasons for taking the drugs, how much and how long. If patient is a drug abuser, find out how patient is using the drugs, dose, duration and route of administration
6. Ask questions specifically to detect any adverse effects due to prescribed drugs. Questions should not be suggestive, *e.g.*, if patient is on reserpine, do not suggest whether patient has nightmare or stuffy nose. Instead, ask whether patient has problem of sleeping at night, frequent dreams or using excessive amount of nose drops
7. If an adverse drug reaction is suspected, complete the report form immediately

A written report of the interview should be completed and placed either with patient-monitoring records in the pharmacy or in the patient's chart.

Figure 24. Pharmacy interview form

Memorial Hospital of Long Beach — Name Plate
PHARMACY INTERVIEW FORM

Present Illness(es):
Past Illness(es):
Race:
Body Weight:

DRUG HISTORY:

Have you ever taken or been given:

Penicillin ____ X-Ray dyes ____
Sulfonamides ____ Prescription and OTC meds. taken
Novacaine (Procaine) ____ in the past and just preceding
Hypnotics & Narcotics ____ admission. (Meds. brought in)
Corticosteroids ____
Hormones ____
Have you ever received a "shot"? ____
What drugs do you keep in your medicine cabinet at home? ____

DRUG REACTIONS AND ALLERGIES:

Do you avoid taking any drugs? Why?

A. What drug(s) ____
Dose? ____ Route? ____
B. What happened? ____
Did you see a physician? ____
How long after taking the drug did this reaction start? ____
C. Year reaction occurred? ____ Had you taken this drug before? ____
D. Have you been hospitalized before? ____
Cooperation of patient:

During Hospitalization. Interviews of patients may be conducted during the patient's stay in the hospital. The objectives of such interviews may include monitoring patient's drug therapy effectiveness, adverse reactions and drugs affecting a specific laboratory test such as PBI or hemogram. A written record of each interview should be made. If the interview is for a specific project such as PBI test or hemogram study, a copy of the interview may be sent to the pathology department.

Discharge. At the time of discharge, the pharmacist may deliver discharge prescriptions and explain the correct method of self-administration and storage of drugs in the home. Answers to any drug therapy questions of the patient may also be given at this time.[27]

Drug Therapy Conferences

In a community hospital, a well-planned drug therapy conference will be well received by many physicians. A monthly conference one hour in length is suggested. Whenever possible, drug therapy experiences of the institution should be included. The conference should include physician participation both in the planning and the actual conference. Audio-visual aids should be used. Time for question and answers always should be available. In an hour conference, the formal presentation should be no longer than 30-40 minutes in length. It is important to determine what the audience will be concerned about and to present data so they can be used immediately after the conference. Chemistry should be discussed minimally. Topics might include: iron therapy, drug interactions, drug interactions in the G.I. tract, ulcerogenic drugs, heparin therapy.

Drug Information Resources

A clinically-oriented drug information service is discussed in Chapter 8. The intent of briefly discussing a drug information service in this chapter is to emphasize the need for drug information resources to pharmacists in clinical practice. The objective of a drug information service is to provide for the physician, better information pertaining to drug therapy. The pharmacist can bring organization to the vast number of drugs used, present concise unbiased drug information and evaluate the many contradictory articles on product efficacy for the physician. The service will provide the necessary resources pharmacists need to respond adequately to the physician's need for drug information. The pharmacist in clinical practice will also find nurses asking many questions which need answers.

In addition to answering questions, the service should coordinate other pharmacy department drug information programs such as:

1. Drug therapy conferences for physicians
2. Drug therapy conferences for nurses
3. Drug reviews on old and new drugs for the pharmacy and therapeutics committee
4. Drug bulletin for medical and nursing staffs
5. Review new journals for drug related articles
6. Coordinate adverse drug reaction reporting program
7. Pharmacy staff in-service education program

Substantial resources are required to provide such a service and include reference materials, personnel, office equipment and supplies.

The drug information service as a component of clinical pharmacy service lends itself to regionalization. Regionalization is defined as one service center serving several hospitals and surrounding communities with the costs of the service being shared by hospitals and other users. Such approaches to drug information service needs are being studied. Their development in the future is very important.

Management of Clinical Pharmacy Service

Successful implementation of a clinical pharmacy service requires a management approach which will define and implement services, achieve desired results and patient care benefits and, at the same time, keep informed all personnel that are affected by the change in pharmacy services. It is no small task to change a hospital medication system and alter the responsibilities of the physician, pharmacist and nurse in modern drug therapy to achieve working harmony and improved patient care.

Where does one begin? Approaches to implement clinical pharmacy services must be developed for the pharmacy staff, nursing service, hospital administration and medical staff. The pharmacist who wants to implement change must be committed to his objective and knowledgeable about his desired services so he can adequately explain and present his ideas. He must develop an understanding of nursing service systems, problems and needs. He must be able to relate change in terms of better patient care, costs and potential savings to the administrator. He must anticipate and recognize concerns of the medical staff and be able to provide direct explanations to those concerns. For the pharmacy staff, they must want to implement change because no change is easy and they will have to put forth the effort and hard work required to be successful.

The initial place to begin is with the one pharmacist who will direct and be responsible for the change. What is his true motivation? Is it to be respected as a health professional by the physician? Is it to be a pioneer in his profession and thus receive attention and publicity? Is it no longer to "count and pour" medicines? Is it to implement unit dose and clinical pharmacy because these seem to be the things to do? Is it to show up the physician because of his poor drug therapy? Is it no longer to be a second class citizen to the physician? Or, is it to serve the patient and assist in providing the safest and best possible drug therapy? There are other possible motivations, but the only motivation that can withstand all the questions, skepticism, abuse and negative attitudes associated with this type of change in interprofessional relationships is "to serve the patient." This motivation can and will withstand the challenges in the development of clinical pharmacy services in an institution.

This motivation to truly serve the patient must be balanced with knowledge, facts and figures. The development of clinical pharmacy services requires an interdisciplinary effort but it must be understood by pharmacy at the beginning that a pharmacist will be responsible and the catalyst for getting the job done. It requires a full-time effort; sometimes it will seem like a day and night effort. If the chief pharmacist cannot put forth such a commitment, then the job must be delegated. The person to whom the job is delegated must receive the needed support from his superior to implement change.

The first thing for the pharmacist to do is to read and study the literature on unit dose and clinical pharmacy services. Visit by appointment any unit dose system and clinical pharmacy service close by. Identify the basic objectives of each program studied and in particular the responsibilities and interprofessional relationships of each program. Attempt to identify the costs and savings of each program. Attempt to learn the problems of each program. Problems are seldom written in the literature but they do exist in every program.

When the pharmacist completes his homework well, he should attempt to outline a program for his institution. He should keep in mind the concerns of each discipline he must approach as he designs a program for his institution. Some major concerns of each discipline are listed as follows:

A. Hospital Administration
   1. Why unit dose
   2. Why clinical pharmacy
   3. Cost to hospital
   4. Pharmacist or pharmacy hours per patient day
   5. Evaluation of change in services

B. Nursing
   1. Accuracy and quality control of unit dose packaging and dose preparation
   2. Communications
   3. Orientation of personnel
   4. Change in the nurse's responsibilities
   5. Impact on nursing staffing

C. Medical Staff
   1. Change in habits; writing orders, charting record
   2. "Threat" to the physician; pharmacist telling physician how to practice medicine
   3. Increased costs to patients
   4. Why the change to unit dose and clinical pharmacy

D. Pharmacy Staff
   1. Why the changes
   2. Support for change from administration, nursing and medical staff
   3. Training and education

Answers to these areas of concern should be developed and understood by the pharmacist before approaching the different disciplines.

Nursing management should be approached as early as possible to discuss possible methods to improve the hospital medication system and pharmacy services. The pharmacist should be capable of presenting briefly the various new pharmacy service programs, the advantages and disadvantages of each. He should present his ideas on possible changes at his institution. Nursing should be requested to appoint personnel to work out the details of their proposed changes. The interdisciplinary group of nursing and pharmacy should meet frequently to solve mutual problems. Such questions as: central *vs.* decentral pharmacy, flow of communications — nursing to pharmacy and pharmacy to nursing, nurse's responsibilities, pharmacist's clinical practice and so on, need to be discussed. Flow charts and tables to compare old and new systems and services should be developed. Objectives of the new services and a proposed method to test changes should be outlined.

Hospital administration should be kept informed of the discussions with nursing. When ready, both nursing and pharmacy should present their study and proposals to evaluate proposed changes in systems and services. When to consult with the representatives of the medical staff, *e.g.*, pharmacy and therapeutics committee, on proposed changes should be agreed upon by hospital administration, nursing and pharmacy.

Keep in mind that the three greatest concerns of the medical staff are: (1) change in their habits; (2) pharmacist - physician responsibilities; and (3) increased costs to their patients.

This approach should result in an agreed upon method to implement and study the proposed changes. A pilot study in an area of the hospital will most likely be the method of study and is a desirable way to proceed. The pilot study should be at least 30-50 beds and the study period should last long enough to break traditional habits and concepts. The evaluation of the pilot study should be interdisciplinary and relate to the objectives established for the study period. The pharmacist must live with the pilot study "night and day" if necessary. He should participate in the new pharmacy operations and check frequently with individual nurses and physicians as to their attitudes and concerns about the progress of the study. The nursing and pharmacy interdisciplinary group should be the only personnel who can make changes in the study protocol and procedures. The staff participating in the study should not be allowed to make any change they personally believe should be done. The nurses should contact the nurse coordinator and the pharmacy staff the pharmacy coordinator with problems and suggestions.

The pharmacy staff must recognize the need for developing facts and figures and make the necessary extra effort to collect them. If at all possible, a baseline of the existing system should be established. Listed below are examples of data to be collected:

1. Number of doses prepared and administered
2. Number of orders processed, types and time of day
3. Medication error rate
4. Drug information consultations between physician-pharmacist and pharmacist-nurse
5. Nursing time saved
6. Case studies of benefits to specific patients from pharmacist's clinical practice
7. Reduction in drug wastage

The significance of the pilot study in addition to collecting facts and figures and to refining proposed changes is to give actual experience to the new system. Nurses, pharmacists and physicians can experience the benefits of the new services. With good experiences, the expansion of the program will proceed much easier. It is obvious that the pilot study is very important and, therefore, must receive the necessary planning, orientation of personnel, evaluation and reporting of the advantages and disadvantages of the new system and services. The pharmacist must demonstrate his willingness and ability to work with others, solicit and accept the comments of the disciplines and then implement changes as necessary. A bullheaded, all or none attitude will most likely result in an unsuccessful pilot study as measured by no approval to expand.

When approval to expand the pilot study is received, it is important to plan the expansion program to a hospital-wide basis. Equipment and personnel needs, orientation, facilities, supply needs plus a schedule by area for expansion with target dates for each should be outlined. The expansion should be a step-wise procedure. When the hospital is about 50-50, old versus new systems, every effort should be made to reach 100 percent new as soon as possible. In this way the workload trade-offs and final staffing needs will be achieved with the least amount of time spent by personnel providing two services, old and new, at the same time.

Management-Implemented Service

The development of a clinical pharmacy service in an institution probably will be a four- to six-year project. Planning will taxe six months to one year; implementation will be one to two years and refinements will take two to three years. A management approach to manage a service that will and should be continually undergoing change is necessary. A management team will probably have to be established and responsibilities assigned to different supervisors for areas such as training and supervision of pharmacy technicians, drug information services, training and supervision of the pharmacists in clinical practice, educational programs of the department, fiscal responsibility, interdepartmental and interprofessional relationships. The authors have found a "management by objectives" system[28] to be an effective management approach for clinical pharmacy services. Each supervisor and pharmacist determines his objectives for each fiscal year to perform his respective responsibilities. The objectives are reviewed and modified as necessary by the director of pharmacy services. The net result is agreement with department priorities to meet service objectives for the year.

If all the problems associated with developing a clinical pharmacy service were listed, the greatest problem to overcome is the pharmacist himself and his reluctance to initiate change. Descriptions of this problem are listed below:

1. Lack of willingness to work hard to bring about change
2. Questionable commitment to add responsibility to

provide better patient care by improving patient drug therapy
3. Inadequate management skills and abilities of the director of pharmacy services
4. Inadequate training and education for clinical practice

The pharmacist must want clinical pharmacy service and make it happen if the patient is to receive the benefits of the pharmacist's clinical practice!

The time required to perform each of the clinical activities is very difficult to find and at the same time have a cost effective clinical pharmacy service. The utilization of pharmacy technicians enables the pharmacist to assume additional clinical activities without raising the overall cost to the patient.[11] A drug information service program will increase the efficacy of the drug information component of clinical pharmacy services. The work load statistic – doses per patient day – is probably the most convenient tool to measure workload and also revenue. Most unit dose systems charge a dispensing fee per dose so the product of doses times fee will give revenue and at the same time workload. Doses per patient per day differ according to patient types as listed in Table 11 from a study in a community hospital medical center.

Table 11. Variation in Doses per Patient Day on Different Services

SERVICE	NUMBER OF DOSES PER PATIENT DAY
Medicine	10.0
General Surgery	9.76
Psychiatry	8.2
Isolation	7.56
Obstetrics and Gynecology	5.6
Pediatrics	5.1

Data from Memorial Hospital Medical Center, Long Beach, Calif.

Another workload statistic that can be calculated easily is doses prepared per man-hour. This statistic will give an idea as to efficiency and output of a unit dose preparation area. It is calculated as follows:

Number of patient days × doses per patient day ÷ pharmacy man-hours = doses per man-hour

It is possible to develop a profit and loss statement per month per satellite pharmacy area. The basic data for this management tool will consist of:

1. Total revenue
   a. Revenue from fees
   b. Revenue from cost of goods sold
2. Payroll

The director of pharmacy, armed with such statistics and profit and loss data, will be better able to effectively manage a decentralized pharmacy service. Computer applications will facilitate the acquisition of such management data for the drug distribution component of clinical pharmacy services.

How does one manage and supervise the pharmacist's clinical activities? The most effective methods have probably not been developed as yet. Some initial attempts are described below:

1. Drug Information Consultations
   The types and numbers of drug information consultations between the physicians and pharmacists and nurses and pharmacists can be collected. Trends in the types, numbers and so forth can be determined. If there is an increase in the number of consultations it will indicate to some degree the value of clinical pharmacy service. The collection of drug information consultations can be individualized to each pharmacist. This data can be used for improving the pharmacist's clinical practice.
2. Drug Information Service (DIS)
   The tally of activity in the DIS will indicate either an expanding or decreasing service. Also, the types of questions answered will give an indication to the type of services provided.
3. Patient Drug Monitoring
   If the pharmacist is assigned a specific patient population to monitor, periodic reviews either by visual inspection or review of completed profiles can help measure the pharmacist's clinical activities.
4. Drug Information Projects
   The interest of pharmacists in clinical practice will vary. Some will desire to spend time on special drug information projects, some on department educational programs and others on articles for drug bulletins. A continual review of each pharmacist's area(s) of special interest is another method to manage the pharmacist's clinical performance.

More direct and effective ways to supervise the pharmacist's clinical practice activities still need development.

Possibly the most important aspect of management of clinical pharmacy services is for the director of pharmacy services to be responsive to the needs of patients and to the needs of the different disciplines. Proper communications both written and oral are essential. Written reports of the development of clinical pharmacy services should be completed in detail as needed. The development of clinical pharmacy services in an institution is and must be interdisciplinary. The nurse, pharmacist, administrator and physician must be consulted, informed and requested to participate in the monitoring and evaluation of the service if clinical pharmacy services are to be implemented on a hospital-wide basis.

References

1. Barker, K. N. and McConnell, W. E.: How to Detect Medication Errors, *Mod. Hosp. 99*:95,97,98,100,102,106 (July) 1962.

2. Hynniman, C. E., *et al.*: A Comparison of Medication Errors Under the University of Kentucky Unit-Dose System and Traditional Drug Distribution Systems in Four Hospitals, *Am. J. Hosp. Pharm. 27*:803-814 (Oct.) 1970.

3. Seidl, C. G., *et al.*: Studies on the Epidemiology of Adverse Drug Reactions, *Bull. Johns Hopkins Hosp. 119*: 299-315 (Nov.) 1966.

4. Ogilvie, R. I. and Ruedy, J.: Adverse Reactions During Hospitalization, *Can. Med. Assoc. J. 97*:1445-1457(Dec. 9) 1967.

5. Schimmel, E. M.: The Hazards of Hospitalization, *Ann. Internal Med. 60*:100-110 (Jan.) 1964.

6. Drug Distribution Study - II Nursing Involvement in Drug Distribution, Hospital Systems Study Group, University of Saskatchewan, Saskatoon, Saskatchewan, (Jan.) 1968.

7. Henderson, C. K.: The Dispensing Trilemma, *Am. J. Nursing 65*:58-62 (Dec. 1) 1965.

8. Smith, W. E.: Clinical Pharmacy, *Drug Intelligence Clin. Pharm. 3*:322-323 (Nov.) 1969.

9. Brodie, D. C.: Drug Utilization and Drug Utilization Review and Control, Department of Health, Education, and Welfare (Apr.) 1970.

10. Barker, K. N.: The Demonstration and Evaluation of an Experimental Medication System for the U.A.M.C. Hospital, Vols. 1-2, Drug Systems Research, University of Arkansas Medical Center, Little Rock, Arkansas, (July) 1967.

11. Smith, W. E. and Mackewicz, D. W.: An Economic Analysis of the PACE Pharmacy Service, *Am. J. Hosp. Pharm. 27*:123-126 (Feb.) 1970.

12. Commission on Administrative Services to Hospitals, 3345 Wilshire Blvd. #817, Los Angeles, California 90005.

13. Anon.: Proceedings of the First Nation-Wide Seminar on Unit Packaging for Pharmaceuticals, The Packaging Institute and the American Society of Hospital Pharmacists, Washington, D.C. (Mar. 27-28) 1969.

14. Anon.: Guidelines for Single Unit Packages of Drugs, *Am. J. Hosp. Pharm. 28*:110-112 (Feb.) 1971.

15. Sonnedecker, G.: Report of the Task Force on Roles of the Practitioner of Pharmacy and the Subprofessional in Pharmacy, Am. Pharm. Assoc. (May) 1969.

16. Ellison, M.: Meeting Report National Technical Advisory Committee for Pharmacy Allied Health Professions Projects, Division of Vocational Education, University of California, Los Angeles, California (May) 1969.

17. Ellison, M.: Second Meeting National Technical Advisory Committee for Pharmacy Allied Health Professions Projects, Division of Vocational Education, University of California, Los Angeles, California (Sept.) 1969.

18. Anon.: American Society of Hospital Pharmacists Workshop on Subprofessional Personnel in Hospital Pharmacy, *Am. J. Hosp. Pharm. 26*:224-232 (Apr.) 1969.

19. Mackewicz, D. W., Owen, R. L. and Smith, W. E.: Pharmacy Technicians in Unit Dose Drug Distribution, Presented at the 5th Annual Midyear Clinical Meeting of the American Society of Hospital Pharmacists, Anaheim, California (Dec. 7) 1970.

20. Shank, D.: A Technician Expresses His Viewpoint, *Hosp. Pharm. 5*:23-24 (Feb.) 1970.

21. Smith, W. E.: Using the Patient Drug Profile, *Drug Intelligence Clin. Pharm. 4*:73-76 (Mar.) 1970.

22. Zilz, D. A.: The Pharmacist Utilizes the Patient's Chart, *Drug Intelligence Clin. Pharm. 3*:218-223 (Aug.) 1969.

23. Smith, W. E.: Drug Information and Clinical Pharmacy in the United States, *Drug Intelligence Clin. Pharm.* (in Press).

24. Cardiopulmonary Resuscitation Program, Memorial Hospital of Long Beach, California 1970.

25. Edwards, G. A. and Samuels, T.: The Role of the Hospital Pharmacist in Emergency Situations, *Am. J. Hosp. Pharm. 25*:128-133 (Mar.) 1968.

26. Smith, W. E.: The Future Role of the Hospital Pharmacist in the Patient Care Area, *Am. J. Hosp. Pharm. 24*: 288-231 (Apr.) 1967.

27. Owyang, E., Miller, R. A. and Brodie, D. C.: The Pharmacist's New Role in Institutional Patient Care, *Am. J. Hosp. Pharm. 25*:624-630 (Nov.) 1968.

28. Smith, W. E.: Clinical Pharmacy Services - Management by Objectives, Presented at Annual Meeting American Society of Hospital Pharmacists, San Francisco, Calif., 1971.

6

Recent advances in drug distribution systems and their economic feasibility

by William W. Tester

Clinical pharmacy is a constellation of ideas and functions which are logical extensions of investigations and innovations in drug distribution systems. Within pharmacy, the 1950's, "the manufacturing years," and the 1960's, "the drug distribution decade," witnessed extensive research and development into nearly every aspect of drug distribution systems: safety,[1] legal liabilities,[2] cost,[3] professional responsibilities,[4-7] and technological innovations.[8-12] This chapter will discuss the factors which influenced these investigations into hospital drug distribution systems with an historical review of pertinent literature. However, its main emphasis will be on the basic functions of drug distribution systems while outlining the elements of the "new" distribution and control systems. Further, a methodology of economic analysis for these systems within the health care delivery system will be presented. Throughout, the "perspective of clinical pharmacy" is that of an idea come of age from within the tradition of pharmacy practice.

Since 1950, numerous professional and societal factors have influenced the study of hospital drug distribution systems. The significance of these events and ideas has been variously interpreted,[13-16] but any historical reconstruction into the reasons for the reevaluation of hospital drug distribution systems must include some discussion of the following factors.

The Philosophy of Service

While the shift from community to institutional practice was evolving during the two decades under consideration, a generation of pharmacy practitioners was rediscovering the service aspects of pharmacy. The same philosophy which had contributed to the founding of the

American Society of Hospital Pharmacists in the preceding decade, was urgently extended to the profession as a whole.

> The strategic position which hospital pharmacy holds in the relationship between pharmacy and all the future practitioners of medicine is one of the major determining factors to the future survival of pharmacy as a profession.[17]

The basic philosophic awareness was that pharmacy was not simply an entrepreneurship but rather a profession whose basic attributes were:

1. A relatively specific, socially necessary function upon which the regular performance of the practitioner depends for his livelihood and social status;
2. A special technique, competence in which is demanded, resting upon;
3. A body of knowledge embracing generalized principles, the mastery of which requires theoretic study;
4. A traditional and generally accepted ethic subordinating its adherents' immediate private interests to the most effective performance of the function; and
5. A formal association fostering the ethic and improvement of performance.[18]

Within this conceptual framework, the pharmacist's purpose for existence, regardless of his place of practice, was:

> to provide pharmaceutical services as an integral part of the total patient care concept in the interest, safety, and welfare of the public health.[19]

While this philosophy of service engendered searches for the "role of the pharmacist,"[20-23] it brought to the fore the patient orientation inherent within the profession and spurred demands for higher professional educational standards to meet society's health needs. It seemed a natural outgrowth of these beliefs that the drug distribution system should be investigated, as it encompassed all the elements this philosophy of service highlighted: the patient, the professional pharmacist and the health care centered environment, the hospital.

Staffing and Personnel Patterns

A severe shortage of nurses and pharmacists is often cited as a motivating reason for investigation into hospital drug distribution systems.[24] It was deemed essential that the most efficient use of professional talent be effected by the delineation of specific role responsibilities into administering and dispensing functions,[25] and it was believed that the medication distribution systems within hospitals consumed valuable nursing and pharmacy time on nonprofessional tasks.[26] Earliest studies focused on the possibility of adjusting the medication distribution system to release significant nursing time for patient care[27] although only recently have the methodology and economic implications of this approach been documented.[28]

The concern for maximum utilization of trained personnel foreshadowed a decade-long discussion of the functions of the pharmacist within the drug distribution system,[29-31] the use of pharmacy technicians[32-34] and the relationship among medicine, nursing and pharmacy.[35-36]

Hospital Influences

The increasing use of hospitals as community health centers focused more public attention upon hospitals and their operation. The safety of the institutional drug distribution system was emphasized by the concern for the "medication error rate," definitions of which abounded.[1,37-39] Its importance is suggested by the fact that error rate was the first major evaluation standard, before nursing-time-saved or cost, upon which new drug distribution systems were judged. The extension of the philosophy of service to the hospital established the main criterion for the success of drug distribution systems: the welfare of the patient.

TECHNOLOGICAL INNOVATIONS

Unitized and disposable packaging and the application of new storage media (*i.e.*, glass, aerosols, plastics, etc.) for pharmaceuticals were technological advances which revolutionized pharmacy practice. Although parenteral technology advanced markedly, the development of oral unit packages has been inhibited due to difficulty in determining the configuration of the ultimate package. The packaging methodology for oral solids extended its vocabulary of packaging into pharmacy practice. The term "unit dose" was used, officially defined, redefined and extended commercially into numerous shapes, sizes and types.[40-44] The variety of packaging types created systems and multi-systems while leaving certain medications in traditional packaging. The lack of packaging standardization handicapped installation of the newer drug distribution systems in many hospitals.[45] Methods of packaging the many medication forms into single unit packages are reflected in the plethora of articles in the literature of the past 15 years.

Simultaneously, for the institutional practitioner, the technology of communication of both information and materials burst upon the scene transforming the mobile drug wagon into a "medication cart" and the inventory stock book into a computer printout.[46-47] The application of automated techniques to the dispensing function within the hospital was discussed and debated.[48-50] In the initial stages, the automation of the drug distribution system was being prophesied before it was completely understood. Prototype automated systems designed on the enthusiasm of the potential of the hardware rather than on the actual communication and materials management needs of the institution, faded into history. By the 1970's the hospital pharmacist had developed considerable acquaintance with computer applications. The extension of computer science to hospital pharmacy included, at least on a demonstration basis, inventory control, the patient medication record, formulary preparation and drug information.[51-55] By the late 1960's, the community practitioner was becoming involved in the challenges of these packaging and communication changes.

Other factors which affected the investigation into drug distribution systems included:

1. Increased application of multidisciplinary research teams to resolve health care problems;
2. Governmental programs, particularly Medicare and Medicaid;
3. Increased concern over medication losses from nursing stations within hospitals;
4. Pharmacists' increased interest in engaging in research activity; and
5. Extension of pharmacy service to nursing homes and extended care facilities.

The state-of-the-art in hospital drug distribution research can be followed through reference to the numerous bibliographies compiled on the subject.[13,56-58]

System Concepts

Drug distribution systems can be examined methodically through the "system point of view." This conceptual framework borrows from cybernetics the idea of a "system being anything that consists of parts connected together."[59] The focus is the dynamic interaction of the whole organism with the flow, the connections and the interrelationships assuming maximum study importance.

> What one specifies as a system is entirely arbitrary, for no matter how it is done, no system exists in complete independence. It can be abstracted from reality and treated as if it had independence, but the independence is something the observer ascribes—it is not an inherent part of the system. . . . and systems do not function aimlessly. . . . The purpose relates it to, encompasses it in, a larger system. . . . This circuitously brings us back to the major proposition that the natural world is either made up of, or can be conceptualized as if it were made up of systems; and human knowledge of the natural world is possible only because it is capable of being studied as sets of relatively autonomous systems.[60]

Usually drug distribution is defined simply as "the physical transfer of drugs from their storage area in the hospital to the patient's bedside."[39] The definition is expanded when system is added to refer to an organization forming a network especially for distribution and/or accomplishment of specified purposes. The "system point of view" emphasizes that drug distribution is part of a large system, for example, the health care delivery system; and simultaneously composed of sub-systems such as the communication cycle. Most systems are composed of a number of complex activities, often called operations, performed by a large number of individuals. The first look at the hospital drug distribution system will be through an abbreviated list of the individuals involved in the drug distribution system and their respective functions.

I. Physician
   A. Drug specification as part of pharmacy and therapeutics committee.
   B. Ordering a particular medication for a specific patient.

II. Pharmacist and Pharmacy Personnel
   A. Select the vendor of the medication.
   B. Order the medication from the vendor.
   C. Receive, inspect, inventory and store the medication.
   D. Receive, interpret and fill drug orders, requisitions or requests from the nursing stations.
   E. Transport the medication to the nursing unit.

III. Nursing Personnel
   A. Initiate and/or direct the request for medication to the pharmacy.
   B. Receive, inspect and store medication at the nursing unit.
   C. Prepare medication for administration to the patient.
   D. Administer the medication to the patient.
   E. Record the administration of the medication.
   F. Observe the effects of the medication upon the patient.
   G. Evaluate the effects of the medication.
   H. If necessary, act upon this evaluation.

IV. Business Office Personnel
   A. Process the orders for medication and send them to the vendor.
   B. Charge the patient for medications administered.[61-63]

Obviously, even the simplest drug distribution system involves the efforts of many individuals to accomplish the distribution of medications from vendor to patient's bedside.

The first three functions outlined for pharmacy encompass concerns of drug purchasing, inventory control and drug storage and are all significant sub-systems of any drug distribution system. However, the last two operations are the core of any drug distribution system design and operation since here a vital interaction occurs among pharmacist, physician, nurse and patient. Sometimes referred to as the "medication cycle," it is this aspect of the drug distribution system which is most usually included in the term drug distribution system.[64] Figure 1 is a general flow chart of the drug distribution system highlighting the functions of the various health professionals involved.[64]

Although no two drug distribution systems function alike, three classifications have been defined and traditionally used:

1. Complete Floor Stock System
   A system whereby all but dangerous or rarely used medications are stocked at the nursing station in stock containers.
2. Individual Prescription Order System
   A system whereby virtually all medications are dispensed from the pharmacy upon receipt of a prescription or drug order for an individual patient.
3. Combination of Individual Prescription Order and Floor Stock System
   Systems which combine some of the features of Classes 1 and 2, with the intention of eliminating the disadvantages of both. The drug distribution systems of most American hospitals fall within this third classification.[65,66]

Within each class of drug distribution system, phases can be defined and the most common

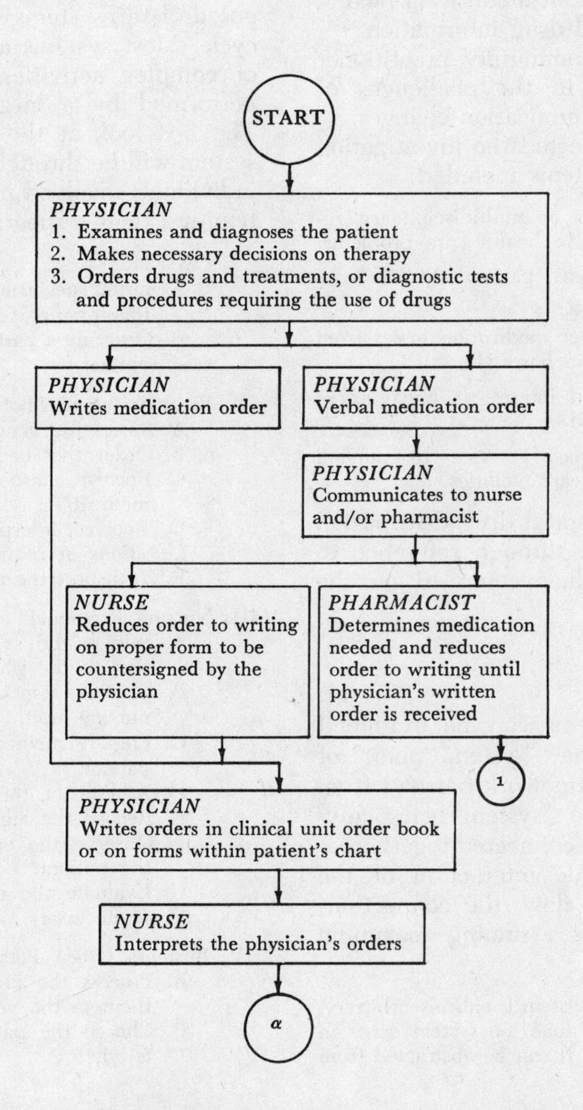

Figure 1. General flow chart of the hospital Drug Distribution System

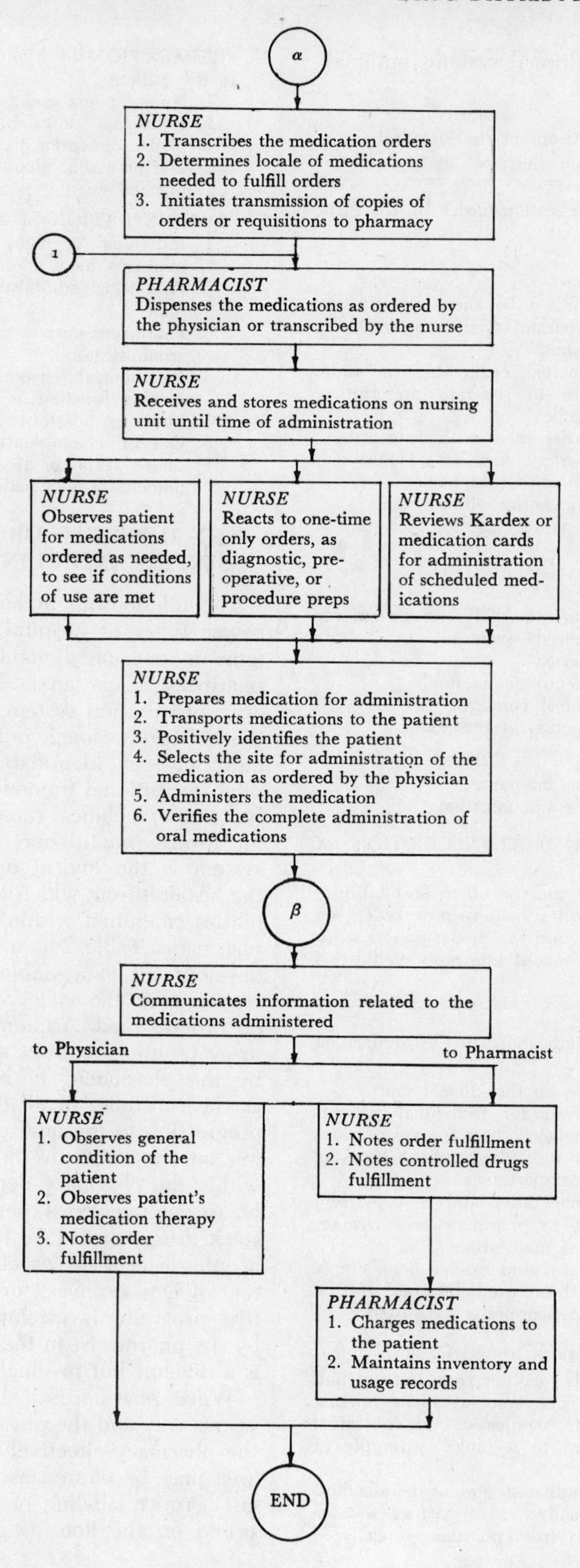

Figure 1. Flow chart, continued

variations from the traditional systems outlined (Table 1).

Table 1. Phases and Variations of the Hospital Drug Distribution System

A. INITIATION of the Medication Order by the Physician
  1. Written orders
    A. Documentation
      1. Physician's order sheet
        a. Separate order form for drug orders
        b. Doctor's order sheet in addition to separate prescription blank
        c. Order sheet with drug orders, therapy, diet, etc., inclusive
      2. Clinical unit order book
        a. For entire clinical unit
        b. Separate page for each patient
    B. Transmission
      1. Human courier
      2. Copy
        a. Carbon, NCR (no carbon required) paper
        b. Xerox
        c. Electronic facsimile
      3. Mechanical conveyor
      4. Combination of the above
  2. Verbal orders
    A. Telephone or intercom
    B. Face-to-face communication

B. INTERPRETATION AND TRANSCRIPTION of the Medication Order
  1. Nurse, pharmacist and/or other hospital professional or nonprofessional records orders on medication cards and/or medication Kardex
  2. Nurse and/or pharmacist interprets medication orders
  3. Copy of original order replaces transcribed copy

C. PROCUREMENT of Medications to Fill Medication order
  1. All stock drugs are on the clinical unit
  2. Some drugs ordered for individual patients from central pharmacy, others from floor stock
  3. Drugs ordered for individual patient are kept in some type of compartment
  4. Requisition, original order and/or copy sent from nursing unit to pharmacy or pharmacy satellite to procure medications
  5. Controlled drugs are used from a floor supply with records of those used returned to the pharmacy when the supply is exhausted

D. DELIVERY of Medications to the Clinical Unit
  1. Pharmacy responds to order from nursing unit with medications delivered at times ranging from just prior to medication administration time for a patient to a multiday supply of medications
  2. Nurse and/or pharmacist and/or paramedical personnel individually, or as part of a team secure medications from pharmacy area

E. PREPARATION of Medications for Administration to the Patient
  1. Nurse "pours and passes" at nursing unit
  2. Individual doses prepared by nurse and/or pharmacist prior to administration, at nursing unit or within pharmacy area. Pharmacy technicians, nursing paramedicals assist

F. ADMINISTRATION of Medications to the Patient
  1. Individual or team of nursing personnel administers medications to the patient
  2. Pharmacist administers medications to the patient
  3. Pharmacist-nurse teams function as medication administrators
  4. Paramedical personnel from pharmacy and/or nursing function or assist in above capacities
  5. Physician administers drugs to the patient
  6. One or a combination of the above note patient's response to medication and note fulfillment of medication administration

THE HOSPITAL DRUG DISTRIBUTION SYSTEM AND CLINICAL PHARMACY

The relationship of clinical pharmacy to the newer types of hospital drug distribution systems is one of dynamic integration. Clinical pharmacy is not an addendum to the hospital drug distribution system but an integral operation of professional practice. The pharmacist must have an identifiable role within the hospital institutional framework from which he can function in a clinical capacity and create a model for future practitioners. The drug distribution system is the logical operating system within the hospital from which to program the responsibilities contained within the practice of clinical pharmacy. Table 2 is a list of priorities in the development of a viable clinical pharmacy operation and the staff preparation which must be programmed. Attainment of a clinical pharmacy program requires an educational overview by the pharmacist of his role in the hospital as the controller of all drugs in use. A rational progression to the final goal is started by building on the strengths of the present operation within the pharmacy department. Simultaneously, areas of weakness, perhaps the status of ward stock drugs, should be brought up to standards of pharmaceutical excellence before the addition of new services, for example, an I.V. additive program, is attempted. This involvement by the pharmacist in the basic pharmacy service is a difficult but invaluable self-educative effort.

When pharmaceutical talents are maximized in this way and the physical environment within the pharmacy effectively organized, the nursing area may be offered assistance by the pharmacist. Proper labeling of drugs, control of drugs stored on the floor (*e.g.*, expiration dates, re-

Table 2. Clinical Pharmacy As Part of the Hospital Drug Distribution System

Development of the Program
1. Improve basic practice within pharmacy area
2. Improve basic practice of pharmacy on nursing unit
3. Improve drug distribution system:
Automatic replacement
Controlled drugs
Drug reconstitution
4. Twenty-four hour service
5. Use of technicians
6. EDP program
7. Drug information center
8. Unit dose packaging
9. Unit dose dispensing: I.V. additive program
10. Clinical pharmacy as an extension of service
Staff Preparation
1. Assignment of pharmacists to specific areas in hospital
2. Orientation of pharmacy to nursing unit activity
3. Facilities tour
4. Review pharmacy problems in area
5. Nursing rounds
6. Patient assignment and follow up
7. Orientation of physician activities on nursing unit
8. Pharmacist attending "doctors' rounds"
9. Orientation to medical records
Physician and how he uses medical records
Nurse and how she uses medical records
10. Diagnostic procedures and conclusions
11. Orientation to disease
12. Involvement and review of drugs in use
Drug-drug interactions, drug-laboratory test interference, drug-food incompatibilities

frigeration), placement of conversion charts and establishment of an emergency system of drugs, are only a few examples of ways the pharmacist can assist the nursing staff. Automatic replacement programs, systematic accounting for controlled drugs and pharmacy preparation of penicillins and similar drugs, are services which are in basic demand by the nurse. By providing these services the pharmacist will achieve a deeper insight into the daily activities and problems in the patient care area. These fundamental programs give the pharmacist a clearer perception of the broader problems of drug control and establish communication and rapport with other health professionals within the institution.

Advancement into certain activities, for example, the installation of electronic data processing (EDP) systems, obviously depends on the external support available to the pharmacist. The last set of operations, to be attempted when the initial priorities have been met to the best of individual talents and available resources, is an outgrowth of the pharmacist's knowledge and experience. From a management standpoint, this may seem like a painful way to achieve change, but to realize a meaningful program in clinical pharmacy, based on the drug distribution system, this empirical methodology is the procedure which offers the opportunity for lasting and significant extensions of service.

Unit Dose Terminology

In any examination of newer types of drug distribution systems a clear distinction must be maintained between unit dose drug distribution *systems* and unit dose *packages*. The terminology of unit dose packaging has been defined by the American Society of Hospital Pharmacists.

> A single unit package is one which contains one discrete pharmaceutical dosage form, i.e., one tablet, one capsule, one 2 ml quantity of a liquid, etc. A single unit package becomes a unit dose package when the physician happens to order that particular amount for a particular patient. In either case the package should be labeled and patient-ready so that the contents can be administered *directly from the package.*[41]

The general advantages of using a single unit package within any type of drug distribution system are as follows:

1. Positive identification of each dose to the point of administration;
2. Identity reduces possibility of medication errors;
3. Drug form is ready for administration, resulting in saving of nursing time;
4. Minimizes drug waste in that doses not administered can be returned to pharmacy stock;
5. Alleviates waste of having to discard partially used injectable vials;
6. Package eliminates possibility of contamination;
7. Less chance of deterioration of medications; and
8. Facilitates inventory control.

Within a ward stock system all of the advantages stated above *can* be realized. However, the *pharmacist* has little or no control over drug identification, contamination, errors, deterioration, loss and so forth after fulfilling the nurse's requisition as these responsibilities are deferred to the nurse. Although quantities dispensed are completely and properly labeled, the pharmacist has little opportunity to continuously monitor the drug products or to offer his professional knowledge and judgment. The individual prescription system can also realize all the advantages cited and in addition, when drugs are returned for credit they can be easily accounted for and these drugs should be free from contamination. However, drug control is again abdicated by the pharmacist. When single unit packages are incorporated into the combination of ward stock and individual prescription system, all the advantages and disadvantages cited for each of the systems individually will be present. Within automated drug storage and dispensing devices the use of single unit packages eliminates prepackaging errors that are occasionally encountered and enhances the stocking and storage of medications. There are other uses of single unit packages which do not fall into any specific drug distribution system: emergency kits and cardiac carts, narcotic dispensing and medications for self-administration.

Incorporating single unit packages into existing methods of drug distribution will not create a *unit dose* drug distribution *system*. The main characteristic of such a system has been stated to be the receipt of the physician's medication order prior to the administration of the drug to the patient. The significance of this function is that it gives the pharmacist the responsibility and opportunity for directing the entire drug cycle. The pharmacist's receipt of the medication order is more than a clerical operation. It must be tied to systematic controls over the pharmaceutical entity, *e.g.*, drug administration, automatic replacement and stop orders, and a command over the information flow to physician, nurse and patient. Only when these controls are built into the drug distribution process can complete pharmacy service be offered and a unit dose drug distribution system function.

Of still further confusion has been the application of the terms "centralized" and "decentralized" to unit dose drug distribution systems. Because of the many different hospital applications and service components of unit dose drug distribution systems these terms have been used to mean: the location of the pharmacist,[7,67,68] the type of medication delivery system,[69] the site of medication order interpretation and transcription,[70] the site of medication preparation[71-73] and the system of medication administration.[74] Consequently, they now convey little information and, when used to categorize unit dose drug distribution systems, generate confusion. For example, a "decentralized" unit dose drug distribution system within a 600-bed hospital may be so called because it has satellite pharmacies or substations throughout the hospital. However, this type of installation often "centralizes" drug storage by the severe reduction or elimination of ward stock medications. Conversely, "centralized" systems often call for a "roving" pharmacist thus drastically redistributing his professional availability to many areas of the patient care environment. And finally, a "decentralized" system in a large hospital when installed in a smaller institution seems to function as a "centralized" operation. In short, while the terms have served their historical purpose they are no longer sufficiently descriptive to explain the operations of unit dose drug distribution systems.

The philosophy underlying unit dose drug distribution systems is to create an efficient, error-free and professionally directed system of drug distribution which promotes rational drug therapy, maximizes the cost effectiveness of materials handling and enhances professional decision-making roles. Rational drug therapy, the right drug for the right patient in the right amount at the right time, involves decision making at many levels. The safety and efficacy of the drug for the clinical problem, the advantages or disadvantages of alternative forms of therapy, the most appropriate dosage form, the length and intensity of treatment, the possible side effects, adverse reactions and drug interactions, are all encompassed by this concept.[75]

Communications and materials management are the twin subsystems of the newer drug distribution systems. This means that in a viable unit dose drug distribution system the pharmacist must control all drugs in use and be available and accessible to the physician, nurse and patient. All communications must be programmed through and via the pharmacist. At the point of maximum pharmacy control it is assumed that the pharmacist is responsible for control and preparation of all medications. It is this role of the pharmacist as the controller of information and materials which is the basic characteristic of the newer drug distribution systems. However, the means by which the pharmacist accomplishes this, the technology he uses to meet this goal and/or where he locates his activities within the hospital can vary because of numerous factors impinging on the design of any particular installation of a drug distribution system (Table 3).

Within communication transfers of unit dose drug distribution systems there are two types of information processes, *i.e.*, continuous and interrupted communication which result from scheduled and nonscheduled medication orders. Generally, the greater the increase of scheduled medication orders, hence continuous communications, the more effective the drug distribution system will be. From both an engineering and pharmacy viewpoint, the more that procedures

Table 3. Factors Which Affect Design and Implementation of Unit Dose Drug Distribution Systems

Availability of drugs in single unit packages
Size of hospital
Location of pharmacy
Space available
Initial costs
Acceptance by hospital administration, physicians and nurses
Availability of personnel
Restricted hours of pharmacy service
Nursing shortage
Doctor's order form
Concepts of practice by pharmacist

are pre-set, scheduled and systematized, the more successful the system will be in meeting its goals. Professional time consignments reflect the dichotomy between these two types of communications which are invariably linked to materials management. Scheduled medication activity might represent 70 percent of activity measured by volume of medications dispensed, number of medication orders handled, and so forth, while taking only 30 percent of a pharmacist's time. The remaining 30 percent of volume activity is for nonscheduled medications reflecting the communication process initiated by the patient and his condition, and consuming perhaps 70 percent of the pharmacist's professional contribution. Since this type of nonscheduled activity reflects direct patient needs, and involves an "interruption" of the normal channels of both materials management and the communication process, the pharmacist will often find himself contributing the major part of his time in this area. Conceptually, if there are few nonscheduled activities and information-transfer situations are continuous, a "centralization" of activity tends to occur because the communication from patient-to-physician-to-nurse-to-pharmacist is systematized.

Any classification schema which attempts to describe unit dose drug distribution systems must explicitly state the nature of the communications and materials management affected by that system for both scheduled and nonscheduled elements. Table 4 lists an initial attempt to categorize the functions of the unit dose drug distribution system which encompass both communications and materials management.

Communications and Materials Management: Subsystems

Receipt of the physician's medication order prior to the administration of a drug to a patient is of basic concern to the pharmacist. The significance of this operation can be appreciated

Table 4. Communications and Materials Management Subsystems of Unit Dose Drug Distribution Systems: Categorization by Functioning Personnel

FUNCTIONS	PERSONNEL					
	M.D.	R.N.	R.Ph.	Tech.	Other	None
Patient drug history taken by:						
Order interpretation from:						
Original						
Copy						
carbon						
NCR-carbonless						
Xerox						
mechanical						
other						
Order transcription by:						
Kardex prepared by:						
Med-cards prepared by:						
Patient profile prepared by:						
Review of patient's drug therapy						
drug-drug interactions						
drug vs. lab test						
drug vs. diet						
drug vs. allergies						
adverse drug reactions						
Medication prepackaging:						
I.V. preparation (including additives):						
Preparation of injections:						
Medications prepared:						
All						
All except narcotics						
All except narcotics and barbiturates						
Other						
Medications checked:						
Medications delivered to nurse by:						
Medications administered to patient by:						

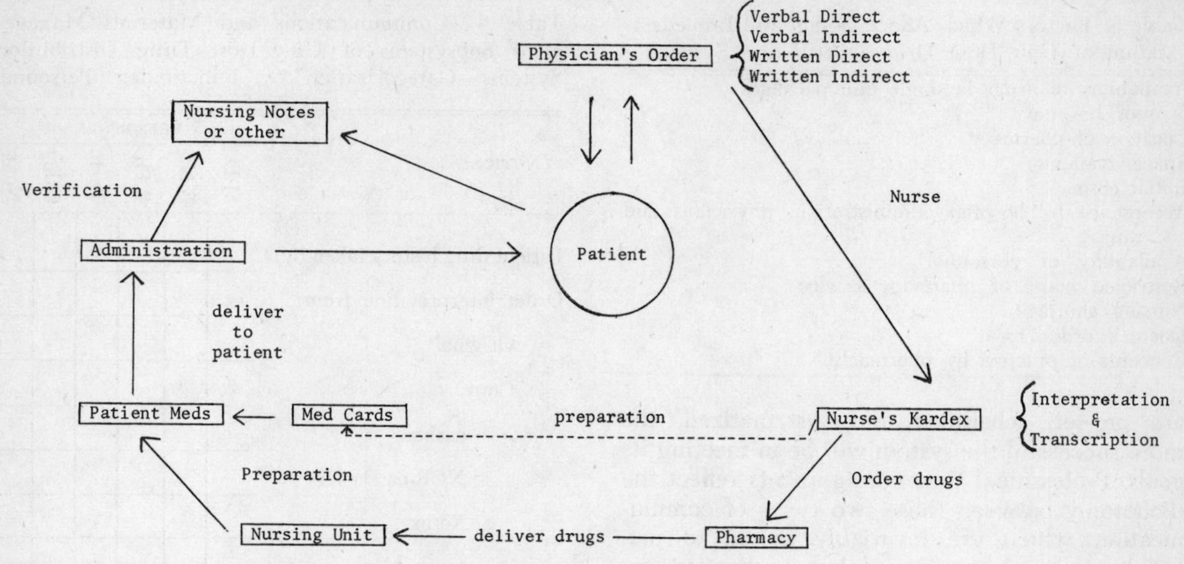

Figure 2. Conventional drug cycle

through a thorough understanding of medication orders as a means of communication within the hospital. The distinction between professional judgments and mechanical transmissions within this communication process must be understood. One route of progress of the medication order within the drug distribution cycle is shown in Figure 2.

THE PHYSICIAN

Following his examination and diagnosis the physician makes his decisions on the therapy needed for a particular patient. Among the choices and determinations he must make are those of the drug, the dosage form, the dose, the duration of therapy and inclusion of special instructions when necessary. While some suggestions have been offered that would transfer these decisions to the pharmacist, presently these decisions are usually made by the physician. Each decision made is monitored by the person to whom it is directed which serves as a control on those decisions.

The physician's orders are communicated in writing or verbally to the nurse or pharmacist or both for their interpretation and transcription. The physician's orders are written on various types of forms in different hospitals. Each has advantages and disadvantages which can lead to a decrease or increase of the possibility of error in the fulfillment of the orders and of extraneous communication between the personnel involved. *Direct medication orders* specify the medication and other information necessary for the complete fulfillment of the orders. Personnel receiving the orders do not have to make the decision concerning the medication needed, since it is stated explicitly. Direct medication orders may be given verbally when necessary or written by the physician. Verbal medication orders are given by the physician in emergency situations, when the patient's chart or order form is not immediately available, and when the physician is not in the area and telephones in an order. *Indirect medication orders* are usually a by-product of other orders. They are either written or verbal and are often initiated when certain laboratory and diagnostic procedures are called for, *e.g.*, in the preparation of the patient for a series of x-rays. The problems of indirect orders are numerous in that the medication needed is determined by someone other than the physician when the procedure or treatment is not standardized.

The communication of written orders to the pharmacist is frequently the responsibility of nursing personnel, but may be initiated directly by the physician. The type of document used by the physician to write his orders for medications may be one of the following.

1. Clinical Unit Order Book
2. Physician's Order Sheet plus a separate Prescription Blank
3. A Physician's Order Sheet, including all orders (*i.e.*, drugs, therapy, lab tests, etc.)
4. Physician's Order Sheet with a Separate Area for Drug Orders Only
5. Separate Medication Order Sheet for Drug Orders Only

The document received by the pharmacist will be either a physical copy of the physician's orders, an individual prescription written by the physician in addition to the orders written in the chart or order book or a transcription of the orders to a requisition by nursing personnel or by the pharmacist on the nursing unit.

Examples of the types of copies of the physician's original orders that are used are those made by carbon paper, NCR (no carbon required) paper, Xerox copy or electronic facsimile machines. Copies may be of the entire order form each time a new series of orders is written or of only that part of the form containing the new orders.

THE NURSE

Upon receipt of the physician's order the nurse traditionally interprets it and makes a professional judgment on its acceptability. At this time a judgment must be made about the nature of the drug, the desired effect, the average dose, the mathematical preparation of the dose, the toxic symptoms, the method of preparation and administration and the antidote. In addition, the patient's allergies, sensitivities, physical condition and ability to accept the medication in the dosage form and by the route ordered must be known. Within unit dose drug distribution systems most of these decisions are made the responsibility of the pharmacist. However, the nurse must still be educated to these facts if she retains medication administration responsibilities.

Transcription

Probably the most common system in use today is that in which a nurse or even more commonly a lay person such as a ward clerk, transcribes the physician's order onto another document and sends it to the pharmacy. The documents usually used for transcription are a medication Kardex and medication cards. On the Kardex, nonscheduled and scheduled medications are recorded in designated sections, with the conditions of use for nonscheduled orders and the hours of administration for the scheduled orders included.

Medication cards, when used, are the nurse's guide for preparation and administration of the ordered medications. A separate card is prepared for each drug. The fact that a precise record of the patient's total medication therapy, allergies and sensitivities is not listed when medication cards are used alone is a major disadvantage.

Procurement

After nursing personnel have interpreted and transcribed the physician's orders, they must decide where to obtain the medications. To do so without causing undue delay, they must be knowledgeable of the methods of drug distribution in use at that particular hospital.

THE PHARMACIST

Upon receipt of the orders from the nursing unit the pharmacist dispenses enough of the medication ordered for a single dose up to a three- or four-day supply. In many, if not a great majority of hospitals, pharmaceutical service is not available 24 hours a day. When this is the case, the fulfillment of medication orders written during the off-hours must be by a different means than is found during the day. Some of the methods in use when pharmacy service is not available include: the use of the evening and night nursing supervisor to provide a limited type of service; the placing of a night drug supply cabinet on each nursing unit or in the nursing office; the use of a physician to enter the pharmacy; the use of a pharmacist on-call; and the use of purchased service from the local community pharmacy. In most instances, a combination of methods is used.

It is essential that certain drugs always be available for instant use in the case of emergencies. This is done by placing an emergency box on each nursing unit. The box should be kept in an easily accessible place known to all ward personnel, and should be ready for use at all times. The medications to be prepared for administration are determined by observing the patient for his need for a drug ordered, by the nurse's reaction to a new one-time-only medication order, and by the review of the Kardex or medication cards for the hours of administration of the scheduled medications.

Depending on the physical state of the drug, one of two actions is taken at the time of preparation. Either the dose ordered can be taken directly out of the stock container and placed in a medication cup or special device necessary for administration, as a syringe, or the stored form of the drug must be physically altered, as reconstituted or diluted. If the latter is necessary, the quantity needed to administer the ordered dose must be calculated. In conventional drug distribution systems, these functions are often performed by nursing personnel. In unit dose drug distribution systems these functions are controlled by the pharmacist and performed by a pharmacist or pharmacy technician under the pharmacist's supervision.

Once prepared, the medications are transported to the individual patient's bedside, where traditionally the nurse checks the bed tag or the patient's wrist identification band, and asks the patient his name. The nurse may check the patient for physical conditions relative to the medication, and then administers the medication to the patient.

Order Fulfillment

Communications initiated by the nurse and directed to the physician and pharmacist include her verification of administration of the drugs ordered and her subsequent observation of the patient and her fulfillment of the various records required by the hospital. In some hospitals, every dose of every drug is recorded in a designated place, usually the "medication record," as being given, which is a very time-consuming procedure. In other hospitals only the more potent drugs are recorded, or those not administered as scheduled are recorded and it is simply assumed that all of the drugs ordered have been administered as long as the physician's order is still in effect.

Fulfillment may be noted on a special form in the patient's chart each time the drug is administered or only once with fulfillment recorded for several days on the same line. The use of only a single entry with multiple fulfillment takes less time and space, and generates a concise record of medications administered (Figure 3A). Fulfillment may also be recorded on the same form as the physician's orders with enough

MEDICATION CHART

NAME OF DRUG OR I.V. FLUID STRENGTH AND FORM	DOSAGE	ROUTE GIVEN				DATE			DATE			DATE			DO NOT WRITE IN THIS COLUMN
		ORAL	I.M.	I.V.	MISC.	7-3	3-11	11-7	7-3	3-11	11-7	7-3	3-11	11-7	
MEDICATION NURSE 7-3															
MEDICATION NURSE 3-11															
MEDICATION NURSE 11-7															TOTAL

MEDICATION CHART
AFTER 3 CONSECUTIVE DAYS AND UPON DISCHARGE:
1. DETACH PHARMACY COPY OF CHART.
2. IMPRINT MISCELLANEOUS TAB CARD FORM WITH PATIENT'S IDENTIFICATION PLATE.
3. SEND BOTH TO PHARMACY TOGETHER.

THE UNIVERSITY OF TEXAS MEDICAL BRANCH HOSPITALS
GALVESTON, TEXAS
FORM NO. 2594 (CHART COPY)

Figure 3a. Medication chart, copy for chart

fulfillment columns adjacent to the space for each order to record several days administrations. Using the physician's order form to note fulfillment relieves the nurse from the job of rewriting the medication orders on a special form. If there is only room enough on the form to "X" fulfillment, it could be difficult to determine at which hours medications were given, withheld or refused, unless a supplementary record is kept.

The pharmacist's use of the fulfillment record as a document for charging the patient eliminates the need for the giving of credits to the patient and their subsequent extra transcriptions (Figure 3B). The success of this type of charging is dependent on the prompt transmission of the pharmacy fulfillment copy to keep the patient's charges current.

Several local laws and most hospitals require that each individual dose of a narcotic and many of the medications subject to the Drug Abuse Prevention and Control Act as well as spirits be accounted for on a separate record by the nurse. This record is then maintained by the pharmacist after its completion to maintain a perpetual inventory and for proof of use of the drugs involved. The completion of such forms and the other procedures that are related to the control of these types of drugs takes more nursing time than any other group of medications.

This brief review has indicated some of the variance in procedures for communicating and

MEDICATION CHART

NAME OF DRUG OR I.V. FLUID STRENGTH AND FORM	DOSAGE	ROUTE GIVEN				DATE			DATE			DATE			PRICE OF DRUGS
		ORAL	I.M.	I.V.	MISC.	7-3	3-11	11-7	7-3	3-11	11-7	7-3	3-11	11-7	
MEDICATION NURSE 7-3															
MEDICATION NURSE 3-11															
MEDICATION NURSE 11-7															TOTAL

PHARMACY: **MEDICATION CHART**

1. ENTER PRICE FOR EACH DRUG OR FLUID.
2. ADD COLUMN AND ENTER FIGURE IN TOTAL BLOCK.
3. ENTER DATES GIVEN ON PATIENT'S TAB CARD FORM AND IMPRINT WITH ITEM CARD AND TOTAL PRICE.
4. SEND TAB CARD TO DATA PROCESSING - SEND MEDICATION CHART AND TAB CARD SLIP TO INS. OFFICE.

THE UNIVERSITY OF TEXAS MEDICAL BRANCH HOSPITALS
GALVESTON, TEXAS

FORM NO. 2594 (PHARMACY COPY)

Figure 3b. Medication chart, copy for pharmacy

processing the medication order. Examination must be directed also to means used to transmit the documented information relative to the medication order and the actual medications.

Transmission of Documentation and Materials

Whatever type of documentation is used for written drug orders, a number of methods may be utilized to transmit the drug order or requisition to the pharmacy. Human couriers of varying training may physically carry the order to the pharmacy. Nurses, nurse's aides, ward clerks and hospital volunteers may perform this task also. Professional or nonprofessional pharmacy personnel can also function in this capacity.

In addition or in place of human couriers, various mechanical conveyor devices may be used for transmission of orders. Dumbwaiters in certain institutions are used to transport documents as well as materials. Elevators will often be used in combination with other methods. Pneumatic tube systems and trayveyors are other fairly common means. Electronic facsimile equipment which includes units functioning as transmitting devices on the nursing unit and receiving units in the pharmacy are also in operation. Presently less common, but certainly of future application, is the use of computer software, terminals, cathode ray tube consuls and so forth, to transmit information traditionally placed on the medication order.

Verbal orders reach the pharmacy through face-to-face communication, telephone and intercom devices. Automatic voice-activated recording devices may be available to provide playback capabilities for verbal orders.

The methods used by the pharmacy to send the medication to the nursing unit also fall within the major categories of human and mechanical conveyors. Nonprofessional or professional pharmacy or hospital staff might use some type of medication cart to deliver medications to the nursing area. Again, dumbwaiters, elevators, pneumatic tubes or trayveyors may be used in this task. Automatic delivery stations which are programmed for a particular destination within the hospital and follow a radio beam or buried floor strips on a specified route are newer types of material transmission equipment.

ECONOMIC FEASIBILITY OF UNIT DOSE DRUG DISTRIBUTION SYSTEMS

Implementation and analysis of unit dose drug distribution systems have been achieved predominantly by trial and error methods. Historically, the study methodology evolved from an "investigator," a multidisciplinary research team, within a "laboratory," the on-going patient care environment of a hospital. The research design comprised an analysis of the conventional drug distribution system during a base period, followed by a "demonstration" of a new, previously developed system during an experimental phase. While data during both periods were similarly collected and analyzed, the success of the "experiment" was determined not only by the comparative results but also by the ability of the new system to survive in the hospital. Each system that has been developed has been formed from the mold of the hospital in which it was developed. Facilities, manpower, budget, communications technology and individual initiative all played important roles in developing a workable drug distribution system. It has often been impossible with such a methodological procedure to achieve environmental stability and control of variables or to replicate data collection and analysis in a different institution.

Unit dose cost factors which have been studied include packaging costs, pharmacy labor costs, nursing labor costs, inventory cost, and pilferage and wastage costs.[74,76-84] These factors are obvious components of any cost structure for a drug distribution system and are documented with varying exactness in the hospital pharmacy literature. Presently, while data may be collected and analyzed on isolated cost factors in an institution, there has been little documentation offered for a complete cost analysis methodology which might be used in measuring all costs associated with a unit dose drug distribution system in any type of hospital environment.

The discussion which follows is the first publication of a complete cost structure analysis of unit dose drug distribution systems. Developed at the University of Iowa, the model has been tested at other hospitals and modifications noted. While the following presentation should be considered simply preliminary documentation prior to more complete publication, the conceptual framework outlined for the cost analysis structure and the mathematical computations are of immediate interest to all concerned with the economic feasibility of unit dose drug distribution systems.

Model Theory

An academic dimension must be added to the method of calculating costs associated with hospital pharmacy unit dose drug distribution systems. One such academic dimension is the use of model theory. A model refers to

> . . . an abstraction of the actual system for which we wish to predict performance. A model is useful when it accurately duplicates the behavior of the real world system.[85]

The rationale is to devise a model which will contain the fixed and variable elements to be considered in an economic analysis of drug distribution systems. The modeling tool is valuable because it focuses on the component parts of a system and allows critical evaluation of each factor. Any developed model must be capable of being manipulated to predict the costs associated with a variety of unit dose drug distribution systems. The simplicity of any working model should make it possible for the practicing hospital pharmacist to insert certain variable values in the model and predict the costs for a particular unit dose drug distribution system. However, pharmacists must be prepared to familiarize themselves with basic concepts from statistics, systems analysis and operations research.

To assist in the evaluation of expected costs of operating a unit dose drug distribution system the primary step is an investigation of the components of the system. Actual costs of a unit dose drug distribution system must be audited where expenses are incurred. These costs are then allocated to cost centers where direct cost data are analyzed on a per dose basis whenever possible. Variable indirect costs are also related to this independent variable. All costs are considered in terms of the short run or annual accounting period. While a detailed time work study methodology is not explained in each cost center for data collection, due to space limitations, the concepts imply a strict data collection procedure.

Five cost centers applicable to unit dose drug distribution systems are:

1. Packaging
2. Inventory
3. Pharmacy service
4. Medication administration
5. Raw drug costs

Packaging Costs

Expenses generated by the *packaging* operation are categorized by the type of medication involved. The cost factors are identical for all types: oral solids, oral liquids, injectables and miscellaneous. These factors include direct labor, indirect labor, containers, capital equipment and supplies.

Labor and equipment are considered fixed, while the other cost factors vary directly with production level. Although labor is measured separately for each type of medication in terms of time required per dose, the short run labor commitment is best determined in view of total packaging requirements since operators can be alternately assigned to any of the types. Equipment needs depend upon the level of production for each type of medication since, in general, they are not interchangeable among the three types of packages. Container and supply costs vary directly with the number of medications packaged and are different for each type of package.

Inventory Costs

The *inventory* and supply operation of any drug distribution system is characterized by various factors such as physical plant design, available floor space and individual ward area operation which are independent of the distribution system itself. Consequently, many expenses of the inventory operation are not unique to a unit dose system. Warehousing costs such as floor space maintenance, insurance and internal handling cannot be measured and generalized for any unit dose program. Similarly, inventory transfer costs within the hospital are determined, in part, by the particular central supply service arrangement.

The storage space and capital costs of drug inventory in the pharmacy and on the ward area are directly influenced by the unit dose operation. Again, these expenses will depend to some degree upon specific design of the pharmacy system. Storage space is measured in cubic feet of volume and includes shelves, cabinets and refrigerators which contain medications. The volume required for medication storage is measured on several ward areas and then averaged in order to eliminate potential bias resulting from the physical arrangement of a single ward area.

The capital investment in medication inventory is measured by a detailed audit of the pharmacy and ward area supplies. If a prescribed inventory level is maintained, the date of this audit is not critical.

The costs associated with inventory floor space and investment are indirect and fixed in nature. The values of these factors are related to the operational capacity of the pharmacy and the number of items maintained in ward stock. Once the capacity and ward stock are determined these costs will remain constant in the short run.

Pharmacy Service

The *service* cost center includes all expenses that are incurred by the pharmacy operation. The factors which account for these costs are labor, equipment, supplies and fixtures.

Equipment and fixture expenses do not vary. These costs are prescribed by the type of communication system used, mode of delivery, inventory and physical layout. Straight line depreciation accounting is used to assign the appropriate fixed costs to the short run term.

The staffing requirements of a unit dose system depend upon the design "capacity" of the operation for either a main pharmacy or satellite pharmacies. Capacity is estimated in terms of total minutes of pharmacy service required per patient day for the particular drug distribution system. It is derived from average daily census and number of doses dispensed (prepackaged and extemporaneous) of each type of medication. Therefore, labor costs are fixed according to the capacity as determined by patient population and number of doses dispensed.

The various individual activities performed by pharmacy personnel account for constant proportions of the total, non-idle time prescribed by the work load. As the number of doses dispensed and patient census decrease, more idle time occurs, but the time required for each productive activity remains the same percentage of non-idle time.

A work measurement study conducted for the unit dose drug distribution system at the University of Iowa defined individual activities within the drug distribution cycle and then measured them by continuous observation. Average daily time requirements of groups of activities are shown in Table 5. By correlating the daily allocation of time to each group of activities with the number of doses dispensed and patient census of each day, a model may be formulated for capacity prediction. The number of minutes required each day is given by:

$$y = -107.9 + 10.85X_1 + 0.751X_2 + 0.423X_3 + 0.404X_4 + 0.700X_5 + 0.59X_6 + 1.606X_7 + 4.870X_8$$

where:

X_1 = average daily and previous day's census
X_2 = total doses/day
X_3 = total prepackaged oral solid doses/day
X_4 = total prepackaged oral liquid doses/day
X_5 = total prepackaged injectable doses/day
X_6 = total extemporaneous oral solid doses/day
X_7 = total extemporaneous oral liquid doses/day
X_8 = total extemporaneous injectable doses/day

Table 5. Average Daily Time Requirements of Activities within A Unit Dose Drug Distribution System

ACTIVITY		PERCENT OF NON-IDLE TIME
Medication Preparation		31.0
Oral solids	11.8	
Oral liquids	4.7	
Injectables	10.4	
I.V.'s	3.1	
Miscellaneous	1.0	
Internal transportation		3.7
Checking order preparations		6.3
Medication delivery		12.1
Communication		9.3
Patient record keeping		13.1
Labeling and recording		9.2
Inventory		6.2
Drug research and consulting		5.6
Housekeeping		3.5
		100.0

Why is it necessary to establish the "capacity" of a pharmacy installation? Once the capacity of the pharmacy operation is established, then the average cost per unit of medication is based upon the fixed costs of labor and equipment as established at capacity. Therefore, if patient census and number of doses dispensed drop below capacity, pharmacy activities may be shifted to consultation, drug information or idle time. Average costs will increase since fewer doses are dispensed but fixed costs will continue at a capacity level. Supply costs are variable but relatively low compared to fixed expenses.

Medication Administration

The activities involved in conventional drug distribution from the point of delivery to the ward to administration of the medication to the patient are performed usually by nursing personnel. These activities include preparation, inventory control and ordering, medication and treatment order processing, and medication administration. The expenses relative to these activities are essentially variable labor costs.

Unit dose drug distribution systems assign the preparation responsibility to the pharmacy operation rather than to nursing. Therefore, nursing labor costs for this activity are eliminated. The times required for inventory control, Kardex preparation, medication preparation, medication administrating and charting fulfillment are measured by time study analysis. The data generated by this analysis are then used to estimate the time per day and time per dose required for each activity. The observed time data are converted to per patient day and per dose estimates by relating elapsed time to frequency of occurrence.

Raw Drug Costs

Raw drug cost is a direct variable cost which is related to pharmacy acquisition price, losses resulting from missed charges, pilferage, contamination and waste. Several proponents of the unit dose system have suggested a cost savings could be realized due to the improved efficiency and control afforded by single unit packaging. Since medications need not be removed from the packages until the exact time of administration, unused and unopened packages may be returned to pharmacy for future use. Waste expense may also be reduced since one or several single unit packages may furnish the exact quantity of medication ordered, whereas multiple dose containers frequently result in unused waste. Furthermore, the unit dose system may promote additional drug control and thus reduces the revenue loss due to pilferage and missed charges.

A measurement and quantification of each of these costs would necessitate a lengthy, tedious study of each. Alternately, the combined cost can be determined by dividing average per diem drug costs per patient by the average number of doses administered per patient per day.

The total direct material cost per dose of drugs is determined by dividing the dollar value of drug material used during a given time period by the number of doses administered during the same period. The dollar value represents total acquisition costs to the pharmacy of all drug items administered, wasted or lost. Defined in this manner, raw drug costs consists of individual but related expense factors which may be conveniently quantified as a single value.

Other Costs

All other costs of the unit dose drug distribution system are considered to be either impractical to measure or nearly identical in both a unit dose and a traditional drug distribution system. Indirect pharmacy expenses such as salaries for purchasing and clerical functions, and the director and his staff are similar in each system. A central material operation is necessary regardless of the characteristics of the drug distribution system. With the exception of the drug inventory system, variations in the central material costs are primarily influenced by local conditions. Since these costs are not influenced by the type of drug distribution system, it is assumed they are extraneous to an evaluation of the unit dose drug distribution system and are therefore not included.

The Economic Model

The total cost (tc) generated at each cost center is represented by the sum of fixed (f) and variable (v) expenses allocated to that activity. For Cost Center X,

$$tc_x = fc_x + vc_x \quad \text{(Equation 1)}$$

Since these cost values are evaluated at a specified volume of activity, Equation 1 can be restated to indicate the dosage or census level (N).

$$tc_x(N) = fc_x + vc(N)_x \quad \text{(Equation 2)}$$

The variable cost portion of the total cost equation is not a predetermined value but rather a function V of the volume N.

$$tc_x(N) = fc_x + V(N)_x \quad \text{(Equation 3)}$$

It must also be kept in mind that each of the right hand members of Equation 3 are sums of individual cost factors. The summation of costs in each behavior category may be indicated in the total cost function. Symbolically,

$$tc_x(N) = (\sum_{\alpha} fc)_x + (\sum_{\beta} V(N))_x \quad \text{(Equation 4)}$$

where $\sum_{\alpha}$ and $\sum_{\beta}$ equal the number of fixed and variable costs, respectively, evaluated in cost center X.

The following list of symbols will be established for use throughout the formulation of the economic model.

TC	total cost of entire unit dose drug distribution system
tc	total cost of a cost center
fc	fixed cost of a cost center
V(N)	variable cost function of a cost center
P	packaging cost center
RD	raw drug cost center
INV	inventory cost center
MA	medication administration cost center
SER	pharmacy service cost center
N	annual volume of activity in number of doses dispensed
T	processing time
s	oral solid medications
l	oral liquid medications
i	injectable medications
m	miscellaneous medications
(N_s)	annual volume of oral solid doses dispensed
N_{sli}	annual volume of oral solid doses plus annual volume of oral liquid doses plus annual volume of injectables doses
DL	direct labor cost factor
IL	indirect labor cost factor
E	equipment cost factor
C	container cost factor
F	fixture cost factor
S	supplies cost factor
ARC	average raw drug cost factor
CC	capital cost factor
IC	inventory control and ordering cost factor
OP	order form processing cost factor
A	medication administration cost factor
PR	medication preparation cost factor
CF	charting fulfillment cost factor

The costs incurred by the Packaging Cost Center (P) include the fixed and variable costs for each of the three types of medications: oral solids (s), oral liquids (1) and injectables (i).

$$tc_P(N) = [\sum fc]_P + [\sum V(N)]_P \quad \text{(Equation 6)}$$

Using the form of Equation 4, fixed costs are:

$$fc_P(N) = \sum DL_P + \sum IL_P + \sum E_P \quad \text{(Equation 7)}$$

where DL is direct labor, IL is indirect labor, and E is equipment. Expanding to include the three medication types,

$$fc_P(N) = DL_s + IL_s + E_s + DL_l + IL_l + E_l + DL_i + IL_i + E_i \quad \text{(Equation 8)}$$

Equation 7 now includes the nine fixed cost factors which were evaluated in the packaging cost center.

Annual equipment costs can be taken directly from the several depreciation expenses of the three packaging processes, as measured in the unit dose system at the University of Iowa.

$$E_P = E_s + E_l + E_i = \$480.33 + \$113.33 + \$350.00 = \$943.66 \quad \text{(Equation 9)}$$

Fixed labor costs, both indirect and direct, are also summed for the oral solid, oral liquid and injectable operations. Within each of the three types, the cost factors become more manageable if the direct and indirect terms are combined. This is possible since both direct and indirect labor were measured in minutes per dose and evaluated at the same labor rate.

$$DL_P + IL_P = \sum (DL_P + IL_P) = (DL + IL)_{Ps} + (DL + IL)_{Pl} + (DL + IL)_{Pi} \quad \text{(Equation 10)}$$

At this point, it is important to note the characteristics of the terms in Equation 10. Labor cost, the combination of direct and indirect factors, is directly proportional to the time required to process one unit, a dose of medication. Since labor expenditures are to be considered fixed in this analysis, the overall packaging labor cost is determined by the total number of doses to be packaged in the short run. However, the processing time per dose and the total number of doses to be packaged are different for each type of medication. Short run packaging time, the product of these two parameters, will also be of unique value for each of the three medication forms. It is necessary, therefore, to establish three separate labor time requirements for packaging costs. Each short run time requirement reflects the processing time and annual usage rate of a particular type of medication and is, consequently, independent of the other two types.

Packaging labor costs for oral solid medications is given by

$$(DL + IL)_{Ps} = \$/hr \times (N_s \times T_s) \quad \text{(Equation 11a)}$$

where N_s is the volume of oral solid doses and T_s is the processing time, direct plus indirect, per dose of oral solids stated in hours. The labor cost of oral liquids and injectables can also be expressed in this form.

$$(DL + IL)_{Pl} = \$/hr \times (N_l \times T_l) \quad \text{(Equation 11b)}$$

$$(DL + IL)_{Pi} = \$/hr \times (N_i \times T_i) \quad \text{(Equation 11c)}$$

The annual labor time required to package N_x medications is given by the term $(N_x \times T_x)$ in the three equations above. Although the labor cost has been formulated individually for the three types of medications, the labor times from each equation could be combined to yield one short run packaging labor time for the system as a whole.

$$\text{Total Packaging Time} = (N_s \times T_s) + (N_l \times T_l) + (N_i \times T_i) \quad \text{(Equation 12)}$$

This combination is feasible because operators can be interchanged among the three packaging processes. That is, the labor time required to package N_s doses of oral solids given by Equation 11a is independent of the other two processes. Since an operator can perform any and all functions of the three packaging activities, the total labor time can be given by the sum of the three independently determined labor times.

It will be assumed that the minimum unit of labor which can be supplied to the packaging process is one full-time operator employed throughout the short run. Therefore, the anticipated number of man hours required for the short run must be rounded upward to the next highest increment of the labor unit. An operator working eight hours per day, 250 days per year represents a labor unit resource of 2000 hours. The number of packaging operators required at the anticipated volume of activity can be found by dividing the 2000 hour unit into the total packaging labor hours expressed on the right side of Equation 12. That is,

$$\text{Number of Packaging operators} = \frac{(N_s \times T_s) + (N_l \times T_l) + (N_i \times T_i)}{2000} \quad \text{(Equation 13)}$$

Time values measured in the Iowa system are:

$$T_s = .00167 \text{ hrs/dose} \qquad T_l = .0115 \text{ hrs/dose} \qquad T_i = .0335 \text{ hrs/dose}$$

If the number of operators given by Equation 13 is a fraction, it is then necessary to round up to the next highest integral value.

Packaging labor cost can then be ascertained by assigning the appropriate labor rate to total labor time represented by the integral number of operators.

$$\Sigma\,(DL_P + IL_P) = \text{Number of Operators} \times 2000 \text{ hrs/operator} \times \$/\text{hr} \quad \text{(Equation 14)}$$

This labor cost is fixed at the anticipated level of activity during the short run period. Once programmed at this level, fixed labor cost will not fluctuate with variations in activity.

Variable packaging costs, those represented by the right hand member of Equation 6, include the container (C_P) and supply (S_P) costs for each medication type. When expanded these variable cost factors resemble the terms in Equations 7 and 8.

$$\begin{aligned}\Sigma V(N)_P &= \Sigma C_P(N) + \Sigma S_P(N)\\ &= C_{Ps}(N_s) + C_{Pl}(N_l) + C_{Pi}(N_i)\\ &\quad + S_{Ps}(N_s) + S_{Pl}(N_l) + S_{Pi}(N_i)\end{aligned} \quad \text{(Equation 15)}$$

The value of each cost factor in Equation 15 is determined by the packaging cost per unit (C_{Px} or S_{Px}) and the volume of activity given by the number of doses dispensed (N_x). Both container cost and supply cost for each type of medication vary with the volume of doses dispensed of that particular type. Therefore, the variable costs of the three medication forms may be shown individually by adding container and supply costs and evaluating at the respective dosage volumes. Mathematically this is accomplished by factoring the three volume terms.

$$\begin{aligned}V(N_s)_P &= [C_{Ps} + S_{Ps}]\ (N_s)\\ &\quad\ \text{(Container + Supply)}\\ &= [\$.00065 + \$.00033]\ (N_s)\end{aligned} \quad \text{(Equation 16a)}$$

$$\begin{aligned}V(N_l)_P &= [C_{Pl} + S_{Pl}]\ (N_l)\\ &\quad\ \text{(Container + Supply)}\\ &= [\$.03800 + \$.00196]\ (N_l)\end{aligned} \quad \text{(Equation 16b)}$$

$$\begin{aligned}V(N_i)_P &= [C_{Pi} + S_{Pi}]\ (N_i)\\ &\quad\ \text{(Container + Supply)}\\ &= [\$.10350 + \$.01695]\ (N_i)\end{aligned} \quad \text{(Equation 16c)}$$

Stated in these three equations, it is obvious that the variable packaging cost of each type of medication is an independent function, void of influence from either of the other types. Combining the terms within brackets and summing the three functions, variable packaging cost is

$$\Sigma V(N)_P = [\$.00098(N_s)] + [\$.03996(N_l)] + [\$.12045(N_i)] \quad \text{(Equation 17)}$$

The total cost function of the packaging cost center is composed of the fixed costs given in Equations 9 and 14 and the variable costs from Equation 17.

$$\begin{aligned}tc_P(N_{all}) = {} & [\$943.66] + [\text{No. operators} \times 2000 \text{ hrs/operator} \times \$/\text{hr}] + [\$.0098(N_s)\\ & + .03996(N_l) + \$.12045(N_i)]\end{aligned} \quad \text{(Equation 18)}$$

The expenses allocated to the second cost center, *Raw Drug Cost,* are expressed by a single cost factor. This factor is a direct, average cost which varies with the total volume of all doses dispensed (N_{all}). In equation form,

$$tc_{RD}(N_{all}) = V_{RD}(N_{all}) = ARC_{RD}(N_{all}) \quad \text{(Equation 19)}$$

The average raw drug cost (ARC) of all types of medications dispensed by the Iowa unit dose operation was evaluated at \$.20/dose.

$$tc_{RD}(N_{all}) = \$.20(N_{all}) \quad \text{(Equation 20)}$$

The *Inventory Cost Center* of the unit dose system is a fixed indirect factor, capital cost (CC). Based on the dollar value of inventory, the expense remains constant in the short run. A percentage of the total dollar value of inventory will be used to calculate the investment cost of inventory. Based on current investment interest rates, 8 percent will be used here to compute the inventory cost center.

$$tc_{INV} = fc_{INV} = CC_{INV} \quad \text{(Equation 21)}$$

Inserting the cost values tc_{INV} = 8 percent of \$6986 (pharmacy inventory) = \$558.88.

Allocated to the *Medication Administration Cost Center* are the various direct nursing labor costs resulting from medication related activities. Three cost factors, inventory control and ordering (IC), order processing (OP) and administration (A), account for these nursing expenses. A fourth cost factor, preparation (PR), has no value in this model since there are virtually no preparation activities for the nurse in a unit dose system. Each of these costs vary directly with the volume of medication activity in terms of total number of doses dispensed.

$$tc_{MA}(N_{s11}) = V_{MA}(N_{s11}) = IC_{MA}(N_{s11}) + OP_{MA}(N_{s11}) = A_{MA}(N_{s11}) + PR_{MA}(N_{s11}) \quad \text{(Equation 22)}$$

Using the cost per dose values of these variables as measured in the unit dose operation, the function of this cost center becomes

$$tc_{MA}(N_{s11}) = \$.0094\ (N_{s11}) + \$.0105\ (N_{s11}) + \$.0673\ (N_{s11}) \quad \text{(Equation 23)}$$

The cost per dose values were calculated using a nursing wage rate of \$3.77/hr, and these activity times:

IC = .150 minutes/dose, OP = .167 minutes/dose, A = 1.072 minutes/dose.

The final cost center to be described by this economic model is *Pharmacy Service*. Fixed direct labor costs, equipment costs, fixture costs, plus a variable indirect supply expense, are cost factors employed to identify expenditures assigned to this center. Supply charges increase or decrease as the level of activity in the pharmacy changes. The logical measure of variability of this factor is again, total doses dispensed.

Labor cost is fixed by the number and kind of personnel employed in the pharmacy. The service features provided by the pharmacy operation, the hours of service offered per day, and the volume of activity to be maintained determine these staffing requirements.

Three fixed cost factors and one variable cost factor are specified in the formulation of pharmacy service costs.

$$tc_{SER}(N_{s11}) = fc_{SER} + V_{SER}(N_{s11}) = DL_{SER} + E_{SER} + F_{SER} + S_{SER}\ (N_{s11}) \quad \text{(Equation 24)}$$

Substituting unit dose cost values measured at the University of Iowa into this function,

$$tc_{SER}(N_{s11}) = \$97{,}284 + \$1998 + \$749 + \$.0081\ (N_{s11}) \quad \text{(Equation 25)}$$

All of the cost factors have now been evaluated and formulated into five cost functions. Each function describes one of the cost centers and together comprise a model of the entire cost structure of a unit dose drug distribution system. Thus the total cost of the system could be equated to a summation of the five individual cost center functions.

$$TC = tc_P(N_{s11}) = tc_{RD}(N_{s11}) + tc_{INV} + tc_{MA}(N_{s11}) + tc_{SER}\ (N_{s11})$$

Inserting the values obtained in measurement of the University of Iowa unit dose system the structure becomes

$$\begin{aligned} TC = {} & \$943.66 + \#\text{ of Operators x 2000 hrs x \$/hr} \\ & + \$.00098\ (N_s) + \$.03996\ (N_1) + \$.12045\ (N_1) \\ & + \$.20\ (N_{s11}) \\ & + 8\%\text{ of }\$6{,}986 = \$557 \\ & + \$.0094\ (N_{s11}) + \$.0105\ (N_{s11}) + \$.0673\ (N_{s11}) \\ & + \$97{,}284 + \$1998 + \$.0081\ (N_{s11}) \end{aligned} \quad \text{(Equation 26)}$$

SUMMARY AND CONCLUSIONS

The design and implementation of a hospital unit dose drug distribution system is a challenge to any pharmacist's professional knowledge and to his ability to establish effective working relationships within an institution. Whether a recent graduate or a seasoned practitioner, the pharmacist developing a unit dose drug distribution system must accept responsibility for his self-education to a considerable extent. Since the drug distribution system extends to the most basic level of patient care throughout the hospital, communication with members of the health care team is of paramount importance at all planning stages. This need for a viable relationship with one's colleagues in terms of program development, operation and evaluation cannot be overstressed. While any institutional committee developing a new drug distribution system must represent members of the institution's administration, it is equally important to include actual staff representatives and to maintain close contact with those individuals who will be most affected by the day-to-day activities of the new drug distribution system.

It is conceded that fiscal information about conventional drug distribution systems is too often inadequate. However, the pharmacist must assume the task of compiling financial data about the operations of his department in its present state, that is, base line data, before revisions are instituted. Minimally, the approach to implementing a unit dose drug distribution system should entail a pilot program, that is, the extension of the new concept of service to a limited patient census along with data collection and allowing time for evaluation and program modification before installing the new drug distribution system as a complete service component.

While the literature of the health professions continues to discuss the impact of computer science on the delivery of health care, it can be asserted that for the average size hospital most of these predictions are still several years away. However, it is not too soon for the pharmacist to prepare for the advent of the computer by the analysis and standardization of procedures and operations within his department. When the pharmacist has an organized drug distribution system in operation at a fully professional level, then the transition to automated information and materials handling systems is relatively painless and less complicated.

While the general consensus of many pharmacists and hospital administrators is that unit dose drug distribution systems are costly and expensive, this is contradicted by the many pilot studies and on-line service applications of these systems in both large and small hospitals. Without denying that direct pharmacy costs will usually increase under unit dose drug distribution systems, a total economic analysis reveals that the revenues saved by such factors as nursing time released from medication activities, reduction of medication inventory and reduction of medication wastage, loss and pilferage, combine to balance out the economic situation most favorably. This is aside from the non-economic assets inherent within the design of unit dose drug distribution systems: increased patient safety, better medication control and improved utilization of professional talents.

Hospital pharmacy has advanced markedly in the last two decades. And yet, the best years are yet to come, when a new generation of pharmacists fulfill the still unmet health needs of our society.

References

1. Tester, W.: *A Study of Patient Care Involving A Unit Dose System,* Final Report, University of Iowa, College of Pharmacy, Iowa City, Iowa, January, 1967.
2. Anon.: *Selected References on Medication Error and Law,* U.S. Dept. HEW, PHS, Health Services and Mental Health Administration, Health Facilities Planning and Construction Service, Office of Consultation on Hospital Functions, Rockville, Md. 20852.
3. Hepler, C. D.: A Study of Direct Labor Costs in Hospital Pharmacy Systems Using the Model Concept, *Am. J. Hosp. Pharm. 23*:645-661 (Dec.) 1966.
4. Owyang, E., Miller, R. A. and Brodie, D. C.: The Pharmacist's New Role in Institutional Patient Care, *Am. J. Hosp. Pharm. 25*:624-630 (Nov.) 1968.
5. Levine, M. E.: The Pharmacist in the Clinical Setting: A Nurse's Viewpoint, *Am. J. Hosp. Pharm. 25*:168-171 (Apr.) 1968.
6. Burkholder, D. F.: The Future Role of the Hospital Pharmacist in Drug Information Services, *Am. J. Hosp. Pharm. 24*:216-219 (Apr.) 1967.
7. Greth, P. A., Tester, W. W. and Black, H. J.: Drug Information Services and Utilization in a Decentralized Pharmacy Substation, *Am. J. Hosp. Pharm. 22*:558-563 (Oct.) 1965.
8. Advertisement: Brewer Pharmacal Engineering Corporation, "Our Brewer System Installation Increases Hospital Revenue — Saves Nurses' Time, Helps Control Cost of Patient Care," *Mod. Hosp. 103*:174-175 (Aug.) 1964.
9. Slavin, M.: Design of An Automated Medication Subsystem, *Am. J. Hosp. Pharm. 24*:254-261 (May) 1967.
10. Samuels, T. M. and Guthrie, D. L.: Unit Dose Packaging—A New Machine for Strip Packaging Tablets and Capsules, *Am. J. Hosp. Pharm. 23*:5-11 (Jan.) 1966.
11. Bourn, I. F., Flack, H. L. and Browneller, E. R.: The Feasibility of a Hospital Pharmacy to Prepare Disposal-Unit Injectable Medication for the Nursing Units (Abstract of paper presented to 4th Pan-American Congress of Pharmacy and Biochemistry), *Am. J. Hosp. Pharm. 15*:68 (Jan.) 1958.
12. Seibert, S. *et al.*: Utilization of Computer Equipment and Techniques in Prescription Processing at Los Angeles County General Hospital, *Drug Intelligence 1*:342-350 (Nov.) 1967.
13. Stauffer, I. E.: A Review of Drug Distribution Systems in Hospitals, presented at a Symposium on Drug Distribution Systems, Hospital Pharmacy Institute, Faculty of Pharmacy, University of Toronto, Toronto, Ontario, April 30, 1966.
14. Bowles, G. C.: Better Drug Distribution Is Goal of Research Studies, *Mod. Hosp. 102*:134 (Apr.) 1964
15. Brown, R. E.: Some Forces That Will Affect the Hospital and Hospital Pharmacy, *Hosp. Management 89*: 92-98 (Apr.) 1960.
16. Smythe, H. A.: Basic Considerations in a Study of Unit Dose Dispensing, *Hosp. Pharmacist 16*:181 (July-Aug.) 1963.
17. Francke, D. E. *et al.*: *Mirror to Hospital Pharmacy,* American Society of Hospital Pharmacists, Washington, D.C., 1964, p. 37
18. Sonnedecker, G.: To Be or Not to Be—Professional, *Am. J. Pharm. 133*:243-254 (July) 1961.
19. Francke, D. E. *et al.*: *op. cit.*, p. 36.
20. Smith, W. E.: Role of a Pharmacist in Improving Rational Drug Therapy as Part of the Patient Care Team, *Drug Intelligence 1*:244-249 (Aug.) 1967.
21. Godwin, H. N.: Developing a Clinical Role for the Hospital Pharmacist, *Drug Intelligence 2*:152-157 (June) 1968.
22. Brown, R. E.: The Changing Hospital and the Changing Role of the Hospital Pharmacist, *Am. J. Hosp. Pharm. 24*:178-187 (Apr.) 1967.
23. Kenna, F. R.: The Future Role of the Hospital Pharmacist in Departmental Administration and Management, *Am. J. Hosp. Pharm. 24*:239-241 (Apr.) 1967.
24. Bowles, G. C.: Extending Pharmacist's Duties Helps Alleviate Nurse Shortage, *Mod. Hosp. 108*:106 (Jan.) 1967.
25. Henderson, C. K.: The Dispensing Trilemma, *Am. J. Nursing 65*:58-62 (Dec.) 1965.
26. Aydelotte, M. K. and Hudson, W. R.: *An Investigation of the Relation Between Nursing Activity and Patient Welfare,* University of Iowa, Iowa City, Iowa 1960.
27. Daggett, J. E.: *The Establishment and Preliminary Evaluation of a Decentralized Drug Distribution System, Incorporating the Unit Dose Concept,* (Unpublished Master's Thesis, University of Iowa, College of Pharmacy) 1962.
28. Black, H. J. and Upham, R. T.: *The Impact of Unit Dose Pharmacy Service on the Time Involvement of Registered Nurses with Medication Activities,* Health Care Demonstration Series, No. 1, University of Iowa Press, Iowa City, Iowa 1971.
29. Bowles, G. C.: Debate Over Dispensing Systems Stirs Review of Pharmacist's Role, *Mod. Hosp. 101*:120 (July) 1963.
30. Blumberg, M. S.: What's Ahead for the Hospital Pharmacy?, *Mod. Hosp. 99*:14 (July) 1962.
31. Bartscht, K. G., Estrella, M. A. and Rothenbuhler, E. F.: Pharmacy Staffing Methodology—A Management Tool, *Am. J. Hosp. Pharm. 22*:564-569 (Oct.) 1965.
32. Sister M. Gonzales: Couriers Speed Pharmacy Service, *Hosp. Pharmacist 9*:212-214, 216 (July-Aug.) 1956. Also, *Hosp. Progr. 36*:88, 90, 94, 96 (July) 1955.
33. Francke, D. E. (editorial): Hospital Pharmacy Technicians, *Drug Intelligence 2*:259 (Oct.) 1968.
34. Oddis, J. A.: Facing up to Hospital Pharmacy Manpower Needs, *Am. J. Hosp. Pharm. 24*:300-305 (June) 1967.
35. Merton, R. K.: Status Orientations in Nursing, *Am. J. Nursing 62*:70-73 (Oct.) 1962.
36. Willig, S.: Drugs—Dispensing, Administering, *Am. J. Nursing 64*:126-131 (June) 1964.
37. Barker, K. N., Kimbrough, W. W. and Heller, W. M.: *A Study of Medication Errors in a Hospital,* University of Arkansas, Fayetteville, Ark., Nov., 1966.
38. Francke, D. E. (editorial): The Interdisciplinary Nature of Medication Errors, *Drug Intelligence 1*:341 (Nov.) 1967.
39. McConnell, W. E., Barker, K. N. and Garrity, L. F.: Centralized Unit Dose Dispensing: Report of a Study, *Am. J. Hosp. Pharm. 18*:530-541 (Sept.) 1961.
40. Anon.: Guidelines For Single Unit Packages of Drugs, *Am. J. Hosp. Pharm. 24*:79-80 (Feb.) 1967.
41. Anon.: Guidelines For Single Unit Packages of Drugs, *Am. J. Hosp. Pharm. 28*:110-112 (Feb.) 1971.
42. McLeod, D. C.: Single Unit Packages of Drugs Available Today I: Oral Medications, *Am. J. Hosp. Pharm. 24*: 502-509 (Sept.) 1967.

43. McLeod, D. C.: Single Unit Packages of Drugs Available Today II: Injections in Prefilled Disposable Syringes, *Am. J. Hosp. Pharm. 24*:696-703 (Dec.) 1967.

44. McLeod, D. C.: Current Status of Single Unit Packaging of Medications, *Am. J. Hosp. Pharm. 27*:742-749 (Sept.) 1970.

45. Tester, W. W.: Unit Dose Packaging, (Film) Audio Visual Unit, University of Iowa, Iowa City, Iowa, 1968.

46. Nuckolls, H. B.: Individual Medication Boxes, *Nursing Outlook 16*:57 (Sept.) 1968.

47. Wirth, B. P.: A Computerized System for Restricted Drug Control and Inventory, *Am. J. Hosp. Pharm. 24*: 556-560 (Oct.) 1967.

48. Slavin, M.: *Hospital Pharmacy and Automation*, Santa Monica System Development Corporation, Santa Monica, California, 1963.

49. Tober, T. W.: Applications of Data Processing to Hospital Pharmacy, *Am. J. Hosp. Pharm. 21*:105-111 (Mar.) 1964.

50. Herner and Company: *The Use of Computers in Hospitals*, Dept. HEW, PHS, Health Service and Mental Health Administration, National Center for Health Services Research and Development, Contract No. PH 110-223, Nov. 1970.

51. Title, I and Richardson, C. A.: Preparation of an Inventory Deck and a Drug Locator List by Electronic Data Processing, *Am. J. Hosp. Pharm. 24*:26-27 (Jan.) 1967.

52. Ashour, S.: A Computerized Hospital Information System, Proceedings of the 19th Annual Institute Conference and Convention, American Institute of Industrial Engineers, May, 1968.

53. Flack, H. L., Downs, G. E. and Lanning, L. E.: Electronic Data Processing and the Hospital Formulary, *Am. J. Hosp. Pharm. 24*:4-17 (Jan.) 1967.

54. Frankenfeld, F. M., Black, H. J. and Dick, R. W.: Automated Formulary Printing from a Computerized Drug Information File, *Am. J. Hosp. Pharm. 28*:155-161 (Mar.) 1971.

55. Greth, P. A.: Data Processing Application to Drug Information Services, *Hosp. Pharm. 1*:26-30 (June) 1966.

56. U.S. Dept. HEW, PHS, Health Services and Mental Health Administration, Health Facilities Planning and Construction Service, Office of Consultation on Hospital Functions: (1) Selected References on Drug Distribution Systems; (2) Selected References on Unit Dose Dispensing; (3) Selected References on Automation in Hospital Pharmacy, 5600 Fishers Lane, Rockville, Maryland.

57. Hill, W. T., Jr.: Systems of Drug Distribution and Control, Selected Bibliography, Distributed by Philips Roxane Laboratories, Inc., Columbus, Ohio, 1968.

58. Annual Administrative Reviews: Pharmacy, *Hospitals*, Annotated bibliographies appear annually in the April 1st issue.

59. Beer, S.: *Cybernetics and Management*, John Wiley and Sons, Inc. New York, 1959, p.9.

60. O'Donahue, J. D.: Developing a Conceptual Framework for Planning, *Hosp. Admin. (USA) 14*:35-54 (Fall) 1969.

61. Latiolais, C. J.: What Can Be Done to Improve Drug Distribution, *Hospitals 39*:105-110 (Nov. 16) 1965.

62. Barker, K. N.: Trends in Drug Distribution Systems in Hospitals, *Am. J. Hosp. Pharm. 19*:595-602 (Dec.) 1962.

63. Nickel, R. O.: A Study of a Unit Dose Drug Distribution System in a Chronic Disease Hospital (Unpublished Master's Thesis, University of Iowa, College of Pharmacy) June, 1969.

64. Bernstein, E. L.: Variables and Restrictions of the Hospital Medication Cycle (Unpublished Master's Thesis, University of Iowa, College of Pharmacy) Aug., 1967.

65. Heard, J. S.: Considerations in Inpatient Dispensing, *Am. J. Hosp. Pharm. 15*:388-393 (May) 1958.

66. Anon.: Statement on Hospital Drug Distribution Systems, *Am. J. Hosp. Pharm. 21*:535-536 (Nov.) 1964.

67. Barker, K. N.: *The Demonstration and Evaluation of an Experimental Medication System for the U.A.M.C. Hospital*, Vols. 1,2 Drug Systems Research, University of Arkansas Medical Center, Little Rock, Arkansas, July, 1967.

68. Durant, W. J., Hamill, H. T. and Zilz, D. A.: A Unique Decentralized Unit Dose Project, *Am. J. Hosp. Pharm. 24*:113-119 (Mar.) 1967.

69. Smith, W. E. and Mackewicz, D. W.: An Economic Analysis of the PACE Pharmacy Service, *Am. J. Hosp. Pharm. 27*:123-126 (Feb.) 1970.

70. Sister M. Naomi Holysko and Ravin, R. L.: A Pharmacy Centralized Intravenous Additive Service, *Am. J. Hosp. Pharm. 22*:266-271 (May) 1965.

71. Walsh, H. C., Thomason, M. R. and Davis, N. M.: Effective Decentralized Unit Dose Dispensing on a One-Shift Basis, *Am. J. Hosp. Pharm. 25*:249-255 (May) 1968.

72. Bohl, J. C. *et al.*: A Trinity of Units—Patient, Pharmacist and Doses; Part One, The Medication System, *Am. J. Hosp. Pharm. 26*:316-323 (June) 1969.

73. Harrison, W. L. and McConnell, W. E.: A Study of Centralized Interpretation and Distribution of Physicians' Orders, *Am. J. Hosp. Pharm. 25*:634-640 (Nov.) 1968.

74. Beste, D. F., Jr.: An Integrated Pharmacist-Nurse Approach to the Unit Dose Concept, *Am. J. Hosp. Pharm. 25*: 396-407 (Aug.) 1968.

75. Anon.: *Task Force on Prescription Drugs, Final Report*, U.S. Dept. HEW, pub. 333-366, Supt. of Documents, U.S. Govt. Printing Office, Feb. 7, 1969, p. 21.

76. Blumberg, M. S.: Packaging of Hospital Medications, *Am. J. Hosp. Pharm. 19*:270-273 (June) 1962.

77. Schwartau, N. and Sturdavant, M.: A System of Packaging and Dispensing Drugs in Single Doses, *Am. J. Hosp. Pharm. 18*:542-559 (Sept.) 1961.

78. Kurtz, A. R. and Smith, J. L.: Three Dimensional Drug Losses, *Hosp. Topics 39*:53-58, 60-61 (Apr.) 1961.

79. Naylor, M. J. V. and Tester, W. W.: Analyzing and Predicting Hospital Pharmacy Costs Using Stepwise Regression, *Am. J. Hosp. Pharm. 28*:162-171 (Mar.) 1971.

80. Barker, K. N.: The Effects of an Experimental Medication System on Medication Errors and Costs; Part Two, The Cost Study, *Am. J. Hosp. Pharm. 26*:388-397 (July) 1969.

81. Petrick, R. J. and Kleinmann, K.: An Evaluation of a Drug Distribution System Using the Physician's Order, *Am. J. Hosp. Pharm. 22*:512-515 (Sept.) 1965.

82. Slater, W. E. and Hripko, J. R.: The Unit Dose System in a Private Hospital, Part Two: Evaluation, *Am. J. Hosp. Pharm. 25*:641-648 (Nov.) 1968.

83. Winship, H. W. and Mc Evilla, J. D.: The Determination of Pharmacy Department Dispensing Costs in Selected Hospitals, presented at the Annual Meeting of the American Pharmaceutical Association, Miami Beach, Florida, May 6, 1968.

84. Upham, R. T.: An Evaluation of Nursing Time and Labor Costs Resulting from the Implementation of a Unit Dose Drug Distribution System, (Master's Thesis, University of Iowa, College of Business Administration) 1969.

85. Buffa, E. S.: *Models for Production and Operations Management*, John Wiley and Sons, Inc., New York, 1963.

7

Developing a parenteral admixture service

by Robert L. Ravin

The utilization of sterile fluids for maintaining and replacing fluids as well as a method for providing a vehicle for the administration of medications is rapidly increasing. Drug products are increasingly being added to both sterile solutions administered intravenously and to irrigating solutions used in bladder irrigation, peritoneal dialysis and in the treatment of burns.

William E. Morris, formerly Professional Services Manager for Baxter Laboratories, estimated that nationally, more than 75,000,000 units of parenteral fluids were administered in 1969. Out of 25,000,000 patients admitted to hospitals during this period, almost 15,000,000 would have surgery during their hospitalization. These figures represent an average of four plus units of fluids used on each surgical patient. He noted also that the severely dehydrated patient may receive as many as eight to ten liters of parenteral solutions during the first 24 hours of hospitalization.[1] It has also been estimated that 25,000,000 intravenous prescriptions contain one or more additives.[2]

Today, the trend in hospitals is toward actively involving the pharmacy department in the safe and efficient preparation of admixtures of both intravenous and irrigating solutions to which drug products are admixed. Support of this concept is recognized in the *Standards for Accreditation of Hospitals* of the Joint Commission on Accreditation of Hospitals. Standard III, Scope of Pharmacy Service, became effective April, 1971, and states:

The scope of the pharmaceutical service shall be consistent with the medication needs of the patient and shall include a program for the control and accountability of drug products throughout the hospital.

Interpretation:
Within this framework, the director of pharmaceutical service should be responsible for at least the following:

Manufacturing pharmaceuticals, when this is done in the hospital, including the admixture of parenteral products, when feasible.[3]

In discussing the injectable route of administration, Goodman and Gilman have noted that:

The injection of medicinals has at times certain distinct advantages over oral administration. . . . Absorption is usually more rapid and more predictable than when a drug is given by mouth. The effective dose can therefore be more accurately selected. In emergency therapy, parenteral administration is particularly serviceable. If a patient is unconscious, uncooperative, or unable to retain anything given by mouth, parenteral therapy may become a necessity . . . . Strict asepsis must be maintained in order to avoid infection.[4]

A wide range of pharmaceuticals is administered by the intravenous route, including electrolytes, blood derivatives, carbohydrates, proteins, vitamins and anti-infective agents. One of the primary reasons for the pharmacist's involvement in sterile solution additive services is to utilize the pharmacist's knowledge and experience in drug compounding to assure that such sterile admixtures will be: (1) therapeutically active and stable during the preparation and administration period; (2) free of bacteria and particulate matter; and (3) correctly and legibly labeled as to contents, date and time of compounding, storage requirements, expiration time, etc. The pharmacist should also assure availability at the time needed.[5]

Published guidelines relative to the utilization of intravenous fluids and intravenous medicinal therapy are available from the major manufacturers of such pharmaceutical products.[6,7,8] It is not the purpose of this chapter to discuss in detail the clinical application of intravenous and irrigation therapy, but rather to orient the student and assist the pharmacy practitioner in assuming the pharmaceutical responsibilities associated with properly providing a support service such as a "parenteral admixture service." These responsibilities include the following:

1. Assisting the hospital's pharmacy and therapeutics committee in developing appropriate policies and procedures for the preparation and administration of intravenous admixtures, as well as stock solutions and blood.
2. Assisting in designing and equipping an area for preparation of I.V. admixtures, including an area for aseptic preparation. This includes floor-plan design, selection of specific laminar-flow hoods and selection of storage shelving and carts.
3. Training those who will prepare the admixtures to properly use the laminar flow hoods, to utilize reference sources regarding reported incompatibilities and to label properly the admixtures.
4. Maintaining accurate and current compatibility and stability data for convenient use by those who will prepare the admixtures.
5. Reconstituting and properly labeling stable, frequently administered lyophilized additives.

Another objective of this chapter is to orient the student and pharmaceutical practitioner to intravenous administration systems and associated apparatus.

Continuous Drip versus Intermittent Therapy

Basically, drug additives are administered via continuous slow intravenous drip over a several hour period or by intermittent intravenous administration over a period of minutes, rather than hours.

In continuous slow intravenous drip, the drug product is added to a large volume (usually 500 to 1,000 ml) solution and is administered over a 4- to 24-hour period. This method is suitable for drug products that are compatible together, are stable at the resultant pH and are not especially irritating at the site of injection.

In contrast, in intermittent intravenous administration the drug product is administered in a small volume (2 to 50 ml) of solution over a period of several minutes, rather than hours. Intermittent I.V. therapy is used to avoid anticipated or potential stability or compatibility problems, to reduce the potential of thrombophlebitis due to a very irritating drug product by minimizing the length of time the solution is in contact with the vein and to promote better diffusion of antibiotics into tissues because of the greater concentration gradient. Intermittent intravenous therapy techniques require more personnel time because the drug product may have to be prepared and injected as often as every four hours around the clock.

Intermittent intravenous therapy is accomplished in three ways:

(1) The pharmacy sends "mini-bottles" (usually 50 ml) containing the drug product to the patient care area. The preparation and labeling procedure is very similar to preparing large volume I.V. admixtures. The "mini-bottle" is then piggy-backed to the large volume primary bottle already hanging by inserting the needle from the mini-bottle administration set into an injection

site of the administration set of the primary bottle.

(2) The pharmacy sends the drug product, either reconstituted or not reconstituted, and the nurse injects it into a special volumetric I.V. administration set, *e.g.*, Soluset, Volu-Trole or Buretrol, which is used in place of the routine administration set. This is somewhat similar to "mini-bottle" therapy in that the nurse fills this set with 25 to 50 ml of solution from the primary bottle, injects the drug into this volume, and then administers the 25 to 50 ml. However, the set is not labeled as to drug contents while the additive is being administered.

(3) The pharmacy sends the drug product, either reconstituted or not reconstituted, and the nurse injects it directly via an injection site on the I.V. administration set tubing. This is commonly referred to as an "I.V. push."

Intermittent therapy is used primarily for the administration of antibiotics, for several reasons. Some antibiotics (*e.g.*, ampicillin and erythromycin) are unstable and lose a significant amount of potency when left standing over the period of time normally taken to infuse fluids by slow, continuous drip. Other antibiotics are incompatible in solution with other additives (*e.g.*, buffered penicillin G potassium with vitamin B complex and ascorbic acid). Still other antibiotics are irritating to the vein. Some physicians believe that slow continuous drip, wherein the drug is in constant contact with the vein, is more toxic and has a greater potential to cause thrombophlebitis than does the intermittent therapy approach. Another reason for the intermittent intravenous administration of antibiotics is the belief by some physicians that the higher concentration of antibiotics in the blood following their more rapid administration *might* produce better diffusion into tissues because of the greater concentration gradient.

Intermittent therapy, however, is not recommended for all antibiotics. For example, potassium penicillin G, which contains 1.7 mEq of potassium per million units, is more likely to produce a dangerous elevation of serum potassium after rapid injection of large doses than after continuous slow infusion, particularly in patients with renal insufficiency. Colistimethate and kanamycin can cause muscular paralysis which is more easily detected before complete paralysis occurs if slow continuous infusion is used.

In commenting on the relative advantages and disadvantages of the intermittant intravenous administration of antibiotics, *Medical Letter* has stated that, "In most cases, either method of administration will be clinically effective, and the available evidence does not show that either is generally more reliable or safe." It also notes that, "Continuous intravenous administration does not require frequent manipulation of the intravenous apparatus; in contrast, intermittent therapy requires more attention. The antibiotic must be injected as often as every four hours around the clock. In many hospitals, intravenous injections of drugs must be given by physicians; continuous infusion of antibiotics can therefore ease the burdens of the house staff."[9]

The usefulness of intermittent therapy is not restricted to antibiotics. For example, in the intensive care unit where patient needs may change rapidly, intermittent therapy provides a method of meeting changing electrolyte and steroid requirements without constantly changing the primary solution. Table 1 shows the results of a literature survey conducted in March, 1970 by Charles Osborn, R.Ph., of the St. Joseph Mercy Hospital staff, regarding the desirability of administering certain drug products by "direct push", which constitutes one method of intermittent therapy. It should be noted many manufacturers recommend if drugs not further diluted are administered via injection sites in the I.V. tubing, that such be done very slowly.

Intravenous Administration Systems

At present, the vast majority of intravenous solutions are packaged in glass bottles, although the major parenteral solution manufacturers are presently evaluating the use of plastic bottles and bags. Plastic is less expensive to ship due to lighter weight and is potentially less dangerous to the patient should a hanging bottle fall. The plastic containers are presently being evaluated for solution-container interactions, stability, freedom from particulate matter, etc.

Many of the following comments regarding the various intravenous fluid administration systems are based upon a presentation by Flynn Warren, Jr. of the School of Pharmacy of the University of Georgia, in February, 1970. At the time, he noted that his comments were based upon "information obtained from complaining nurses and physicians, information supplied from the various manufacturers and information presented in published professional and scientific journals."[10]

All current intravenous fluid systems utilizing glass bottles operate by gravity flow with room

Table 1. Results of Literature Review Pertaining to "Direct I.V. Pushes"

I.V. ADDITIVE	LITERATURE FINDINGS: RECOMMENDED DIRECT I.V. PUSH	CAUTION	INFORMATION SOURCE
Aminophylline	No	Should be well diluted.	Hospital Formulary Product Literature
Ampicillin	Qualified Yes	Very slow rate (100 mg/min.) Rapid administration—convulsions	Product Literature
Aqua Mephyton	Qualified Yes	5-10 mg/min	Product Literature Hospital Formulary
Benadryl	Yes		Product Literature
Calcium Gluconate	Qualified Yes	10% solution very slowly (5-20 ml)	Hospital Pharmacy
Chloromycetin	Qualified Yes	10% solution (1 g/10 ml) over 1 minute intervals	Hospital Formulary
Deslanoside (Cedilanid-D)	Qualified Yes	In 4 ml portions	Product Literature
Digitoxin	Yes		Product Literature
Digoxin	Yes		Product Literature
Erythromycin	No	Dilute 100-250 ml Infuse 20-60 min.	Product Literature
Gantrisin	Qualified Yes	Slowly—no rate in literature	Product Literature
Heparin	Yes		Product Literature
Histamine Acid PO_4	No	Must be diluted	Product Literature
Insulin			
Isuprel	No	Well diluted	Product Literature
Keflin	Qualified Yes	1 g/10 ml in 3-5 minutes	Product Literature
Levophed	No	Well diluted	Product Literature
Lincomycin	No	600 mg/250 ml Infused slowly	Product Literature Hospital Formulary
Mannitol	Qualified Yes		Product Literature
Metaraminol (Aramine)	No	Dilute for drip. Emerg: 5-500 mg direct for severe shock	Hospital Formulary
M.V.I.	No	Must be well diluted	Product Literature
Penicillin G	No		Hospital Pharmacy
Potassium Chloride	No	Slowly 30 mEq/L./hr.	Hospital Formulary
Prostaphlin	Qualified Yes	Administer over 10 min. after special dilute	Product Literature
Serum Albumin	Qualified Yes	Slow administration	Product Literature
Sodium Bicarbonate	Qualified Yes	Infused very slowly	Product Literature Hospital Formulary
Sodium Iodide	No		Product Literature
Solu B & C	Qualified Yes		Product Literature
Solu B Forte	Qualified Yes	Infused very slowly Check for thiamine sensitivity	Product Literature
Solu Cortef	Qualified Yes	100-500 mg over 30 seconds	Product Literature
Staphcillin	No	1 g/6 hr. in 50 ml	Product Literature
Sulfadiazine	Qualified Yes	Dilute 50 mg/ml (5%)	Hospital Formulary
Tetracycline	No	Should be diluted Infusion 20 mg/min.	Product Literature Hospital Formulary
Xylocaine	No		Product Literature

Recommendations: Direct IV pushes be limited to physician administration, except possibly heparin and Benadryl.

air replacing the lost volume of fluid administered. Abbott, Baxter, Cutter and McGaw all package their intravenous solutions under vacuum, which must be returned to atmospheric pressure with room air prior to fluid administration. The presence of the inrush (whoosh) of air and the resulting bubbles supposedly indicate that the bottle has been sterilized and that sterility has been maintained during shipping and storage to the immediate point of use. This latter point is open to question since it has been reported that a vacuum can be maintained even if there is a hairline crack in the bottle, yet mold will grow.

The major difference between the various manufacturers of intravenous fluid systems utilizing glass bottles is the presence or absence of an airway in the bottle. As already mentioned, all intravenous fluids flow by gravity and the fluid that empties from the bottle must be replaced by air from the surrounding atmosphere. The Baxter and McGaw systems utilize a plastic airway tube that extends from the rubber stopper above the level of the fluid when the bottle is hanging for administration. This airway means that the air that comes into the bottle does not pass through the fluid and this reduces the danger of oxidation of the drugs in the fluid. There is also a disadvantage to this system, however. The airway does not contain any mechanism for filtering the air admitted to the bottle. Contamination in the room air or due to poor technique in removing the latex diaphragm when attaching the administration set theoretically can be introduced into the bottle while it is running. Both companies counter this idea with the fact that any contaminants which might gain entrance to the bottle will layer on top of the solution and remain there throughout the period of fluid therapy. Since there is always some amount of fluid in the bottle and the administration set that is not administered, these contaminants will remain in the bottle and not be administered to the patient—unless someone shakes the bottle or hooks up a secondary solution.

The Abbott and Cutter systems both utilize a filtered airway on the administration set for the admission of air to the bottle. This filter has the capability of filtering some microorganisms from the air before the air enters the fluid. While the air can probably increase the susceptibility of easily oxidized drugs to damaging oxidation, it does have at least one advantage. If during the period of administration the needle should adhere to the side of the vein and stop the flow of the fluid, the bubbles will not rise through the fluid. This may be the nurse's first clue that something is wrong with the infusion.

The proper attachment of the set to the bottle of various systems is a fairly simple process. However, strict aseptic technique must be followed and the FDA (Food and Drug Administration) and CDC (Center for Disease Control), in a joint communique in March 1971, stated: "Hospitals are also being advised to change IV apparatus at least every 24 hours. The CDC studies have demonstrated that any brand of IV apparatus is more likely to cause infection if left in place longer."[11]

With the Baxter and McGaw systems, the latex diaphragm is removed breaking the vacuum and allowing room air into the bottle. Care must be taken not to touch the rim of the air vent tube to avoid touch contamination. The spike of the set is then inserted into the proper hole in the rubber closure. If the spike is inserted into the airway hole by mistake, the airway will be pushed out of place and the system rendered unusable.

The set is attached to the Abbott and Cutter systems by plunging the plastic spike on the administration set through the indicated puncture site on the rubber closure. The room air that is admitted into this system enters the bottle through an air filter on the administration set, thereby lessening potential contamination.

Once the fluid has been started, the flow rate of the fluid must be adjusted to determine the length of time over which the fluid will be administered. The exact flow rate that is determined is a function of the drops per milliliter delivered by the administration set. Most of the standard sets will deliver either 10 or 15 drops per milliliter and will convey this information on the package. Since pediatric patients normally receive relatively small volumes of fluid over long periods of time, all pediatric administration sets deliver 60 drops per milliliter of fluid.

Each administration set consists of several parts: an airway for admitting air into the bottle (in the Baxter/McGaw systems this is not an integral part of the set); a drip chamber for counting the drops to determine the flow rate and also to act as a reservoir to insure continuous flow; a length of tubing of sufficient length to reach from the hanging bottle to the patient's arm; a flow control meter; an injection site for adding medications to the bottle of fluid (again in the McGaw and Baxter systems this is not an integral part of the administration set); an

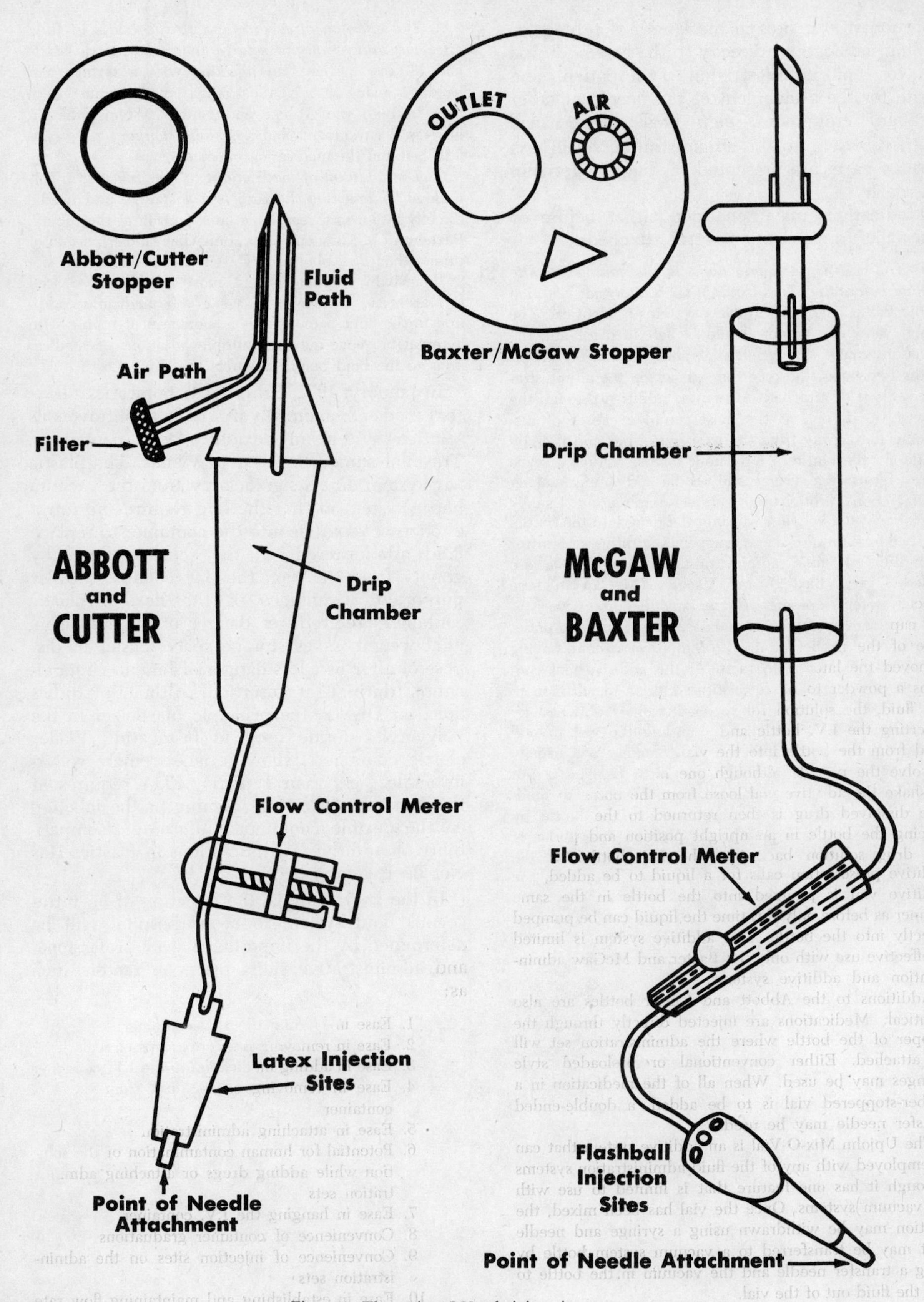

Figure 1. The various I.V. administration systems

injection site or sites in the length of tubing for adding medications directly to the flowing liquid and for rapid administration to the patient; and a site for the attachment of the needle or other auxiliary equipment, *e.g.*, final filters, small scalp vein sets, to the administration set. These various parts are presented in diagram form in Figure 1.

Medications may be added either before or after the administration set is attached:

1. *The addition of medications to the complete bottle of fluid before the administration set is attached.* Addition to the Baxter glass and McGaw systems is identical. The rubber latex diaphragm should be left in place and the injections made through the diaphragm into the larger of the two holes, the hole through which the administration set will be attached. Attempted addition through the airway site is one of the most common causes of displacing the airway from the rubber stopper and thereby rendering the bottle of fluid unfit for use. Drugs may be added by using a syringe and needle and simply making an injection through the rubber diaphragm. Usually the force of the vacuum will pull the drug into the bottle. Both companies also market a special additive system for their type of fluid administration system. These are called Incert (Baxter) and Vacojet (McGaw). These special systems operate by removing the protective rubber cap from the additive and inserting it into the outlet hole of the rubber stopper, preferably without having removed the latex diaphragm. If the additive vial contains a powder to be reconstituted prior to addition to the fluid, the solution for reconstitution is obtained by inverting the I.V. bottle and pumping the vial to pull fluid from the bottle into the vial. Shaking will usually dissolve the powder although one must be careful not to shake the additive vial loose from the bottle of fluid. The dissolved drug is then returned to the bottle by placing the bottle in an upright position and pumping the drug solution back into the I.V. bottle. If the additive prescription calls for a liquid to be added, the additive vial is plugged into the bottle in the same manner as before only this time the liquid can be pumped directly into the bottle. This additive system is limited to effective use with only the Baxter and McGaw administration and additive systems.

Additions to the Abbott and Cutter bottles are also identical. Medications are injected directly through the stopper of the bottle where the administration set will be attached. Either conventional or preloaded style syringes may be used. When all of the medication in a rubber-stoppered vial is to be added, a double-ended transfer needle may be used.

The Upjohn Mix-O-Vial is an additive system that can be employed with any of the fluid administration systems although it has one feature that is limited to use with the vacuum systems. Once the vial has been mixed, the solution may be withdrawn using a syringe and needle or it may be transferred to a vacuum system bottle by using a transfer needle and the vacuum in the bottle to pull the fluid out of the vial.

2. *The addition of medications to the bottle of fluid after attachment of the set.* In the Baxter glass bottle and McGaw systems, an injection with a syringe and needle is made through the triangle on the rubber stopper. In both the Abbott and Cutter systems, the air filter is first removed and a syringe, *without needle*, is attached and the medication injected.

3. *The addition of medications to the fluid path.* This is done by injecting the drug via a syringe and needle directly into a soft, resealable latex portion of the tubing. Baxter and McGaw employ a somewhat fancier portion of tubing than do Abbott and Cutter. Baxter calls their site a "Flashball" site. Some sets, most notably those used in anesthesia, come with a "y-site" for medication addition to the fluid path. This is a short arm of tubing with a resealable covering for multiple additions of medications to the fluid before it enters the vein.

In January, 1971, Travenol Laboratories (Baxter) made commercially available an intravenous solution system in flexible plastic containers. Travenol named this system Viaflex. The plastic bag system differs significantly from the vacuum bottle system in that the bag requires no introduction of room air into the container to replace fluid administered; as the solution flows by gravity from the bag, the bag collapses. Other purported advantages of the flexible plastic container are: reduces danger of air embolism, light weight, saves storage space, easier to dispose of after use, less danger of human contamination during set insertion. Although studies done on DEMP, the principle plasticizer in the polyvinyl chloride used in fabricating Viaflex plastic containers, show it is extremely water-insoluble (less than 1 ppm), FDA requires at this time the following warning in the labeling on the flexible containers "*Warning*: Compatibility of Additives with Solutions in Plastics Has Not Been Established."

In the final analysis, the selection of an intravenous fluid system for your hospital will be determined by the importance your professional and administrative staffs place on factors such as:

1. Ease in holding the I.V. container
2. Ease in removing protective caps or seals
3. Ease in adding medication to the I.V. container
4. Ease in removing excess fluid from the I.V. container
5. Ease in attaching administration sets
6. Potential for human contamination of the solution while adding drugs or attaching administration sets
7. Ease in hanging the I.V. container
8. Convenience of container graduations
9. Convenience of injection sites on the administration sets
10. Ease in establishing and maintaining flow rate

11. Availability of specific administration sets to meet special needs (or desires)
12. Cost of the system
13. Delivery
14. Service

FORECASTING THE SERVICE POTENTIAL

Once the hospital pharmacist agrees to assume the responsibility for the admixture of parenteral products, the question that immediately arises is, "What do we need in staffing, equipment and facilities to implement a parenteral admixture program?" Unfortunately, there does not appear to be a simple mathematical formula wherein one can answer this question by merely inserting into an equation information pertaining to patient census, number of surgical procedures, and so forth.

The first step is to estimate the number of solutions containing drug additives that are administered daily. This should include both the addition of drugs to large volume intravenous solutions for continuous slow drip, and the intermittent rapid drip administration of drugs by piggy-backing small-volume bottles, using volumetric sets or injecting into sites on the I.V. tubing. Both continuous drip and intermittent administration may require reconstituting (of lyophilized parenterals), repackaging (into large-volume bottles, volumetric sets or syringes) and labeling services.

Rather than attempting to survey all patient charts, you might consider sampling a specific percentage of all charts every day, at all nursing stations, using a random-sampling technique for a period of three to six weeks. When using this technique:

1. Decide upon a specific percentage of charts that conveniently can be reviewed daily (*e.g.,* 20 percent).
2. Write all the bed numbers for each nursing unit on separate pieces of paper.
3. Put the numbers for each individual nursing unit in a large container.
4. Shake the container well, and withdraw the number of slips that constitutes the percentage of charts to be checked.
5. Repeat for each nursing unit.
6. Repeat this random-sampling technique daily at each nursing station for the three-to-six week period.
7. Record the results of chart surveys on a form such as shown in Figure 2.
8. Estimate potential workload:
   a. Determine the sample factor by dividing the total number of beds by the number of charts surveyed. (In the example below, this is 50 beds divided by 10 charts, or a sample factor of 5.)
   b. Multiply the total number of preparations charted by the sample factor to estimate potential workload. (The form indicates a workload of 50 preparations by continuous slow drip and 55 by intermittent therapy.)
9. The longer the survey period, the better your workload forecast will be.

Figure 2. Form for I.V. admixture survey

I.V. ADMIXTURE SURVEY FORM

Day (Wed.) Date (7/29/70) Sample (20) %

Nursing Station	Total Beds	Number of Beds Surveyed	Patient Charts Surveyed	Number of Preparations by Continuous, Slow Drip	Number of Preparations by Intermittent Therapy
4 North	20	4	402-1	0	0
			411	2	4
			417-2	3	0
			419-1	0	0
4 South	30	6	428	3	4
			432-2	0	0
			433-1	0	0
			437-1	0	0
			437-2	2	3
			439	0	0
TOTALS	50	10	10	10	11

Estimating Personnel Needs

Once the projected workload is determined, staffing must be forecast.

The estimated number of personnel and the skills needed to provide a centralized intravenous additive service depend on such factors as the number of units of I.V. solutions to be prepared daily, the functions to be included in the service (*e.g.*, delivery), the efficiency of the work flow, the division (and delegation) of specific functions and the method of preparing doses for intermittent therapy compared to preparing doses to be administered by continuous slow drip.

Two studies, however, can serve as a guide in estimating the time required for preparing doses to be administered by continuous slow drip; information regarding time requirements for preparing doses for administration through volumetric sets or by injections into sites on the tubing of administration sets is apparently lacking at this time. Godwin found that an average of 7.8 minutes was required per admixture, of which 2.7 minutes (35 percent) were devoted by pharmacists and 5.1 minutes (65 percent) by auxiliary personnel.[12] The auxiliary time included prepackaging, reconstitution, obtaining supplies, delivering completed admixtures to the nursing stations, cleaning up and pricing completed orders. Petruconis and Newman determined that it took an average of 9.2 minutes per admixture to perform approximately the same functions.[13] Differences, of course, will occur because of the factors previously noted. Personal experience gained by providing I.V. additive service to one or more nursing units on a trial basis will give you a valuable indication as to whether these guidelines are applicable in your hospital.

Therefore, it seems reasonably safe to predict staffing requirements of between 7.8 and 9.2 minutes (*e.g.*, 8.5 minutes) per intravenous admixture. Moreover, approximately 65 percent of this time may be delegated to trained auxiliary personnel such as technicians. Experience at St. Joseph Mercy Hospital, Ann Arbor, Michigan, shows that approximately 80 percent of the admixtures are prepared between 8 a.m. and 5 p.m., 10 percent between 5 p.m. and midnight, and 10 percent between midnight and 8 a.m.

What can be done if the pharmacy department cannot provide an admixture service 24 hours daily? Some such pharmacies provide nurses with printed instructions for reconstitution and mixing procedures to be followed when the pharmacist is not present to prepare the admixture himself.

Developing a Compatibility-Stability Information File

Until rather recently, it has been very difficult for the pharmaceutical practitioner to obtain information regarding the potential compatibility and/or stability of intravenous admixtures. Several charts have been developed by hospital pharmacists regarding visual signs of incompatibility, *e.g.*, precipitates, turbidity, color changes. Then, in 1969, Eugene A. Parker, a former hospital pharmacist who is now Director of Parenteral Products for Abbott Laboratories, began to edit a column in the *American Journal of Hospital Pharmacy* entitled "Compatibility Digest".[14-20]

The information regarding specific drug

Table 2. Stability of Penicillin G Potassium (1,000,000 units/L.) with Various Additives in Dextrose 5% (25°C.)

ADDITIVE	CONCENTRATION/L	ADMIXTURE pH	ACTIVITY (UNITS/ML) AFTER MIXING 0 HRS.	6 HRS.	24 HRS.
Aminophyllin (Searle)	500 mg	8.7	940	730	525
Aramine Bitartrate	100 mg	4.35	850	790	350
Bejectal w/C	10 ml	3.9	920	580	127
Benadryl HCl	50 mg	6.5	870	860	870
Compazine Edisylate	10 mg	6.45	870	890	888
Gantrisin Ethanolamine	4 g	7.4	900	870	868
Heparin Sodium (Abbott)	20,000 units	6.65	920	900	965
Nembutal Sodium	500 mg	9.0	920	760	535
Sodium Bicarbonate (Abbott)	3.75 g	8.1	900	930	663
Sodium Iodide (Abbott)	1 g	6.8	860	870	904

products (additives) presented in this column includes a product definition; the therapeutic and non-therapeutic ingredients; physical constants (molecular weight of the salt, solubility in water, pKa, product pH range); storage stability of the dry form and/or reconstituted solution; special techniques for reconstitution if applicable; and discussions of visual and chemical compatibility.

Table 2, a reproducton of a table appearing in the September, 1969, Compatibility Digest pertaining to potassium penicillin G injection (buffered), is typical of the helpful information presented. From information such as this, the pharmacist can evaluate objectively many of the admixtures frequently prescribed.*

In developing a compatibility-stability information file, we found that the use of 8x5 cards that can be stored in a Kardex-type book provides both ease in handling and a convenient means of revising information.

As shown in Figures 3 and 4, one side of the card lists general compatibility-stability information and the other side shows the resultant pH's of admixtures prepared in our department.

*Refer to Chapter 21 for further discussion and a compilation of incompatibilities.

Figure 3. Compatibility-stability information file card

pH Stability Range: pH 6.7-7.0 for 24 hours in 5% D/W & Sodium Chloride Injection

INCOMPATIBILITIES	REASONS	SOURCE
Aminophyllin, Na bicarbonate and neut	basic admixture: penicillin inactivated	'Compatibility Digest' *Am. J. Hosp. Pharm.* Sept. 1969 pages 543-544
B complex and C, Tetracycline HCL	acidic admixture: penicillin inactivated	"

GENERAL INFORMATION	REASONS	SOURCE

PENICILLIN G POTASSIUM BUFFERED (E. R. SQUIBB)

Figure 4. Sample card showing resultant pH's of admixtures

PENICILLIN G POTASSIUM BUFFERED (E. R. SQUIBB)

pH Determinations:

DATE	VEHICLE	VOLUME	ADDITIVE(S)	MFG.	AMOUNT	TIME	PH
	5% D/W	1000 ml.	K + Penicillin G Buffered	Squibb	5M u.	10 min.	8.5
			Aminophyllin	Searle	500 mg.		
	5% D/W	1000 ml.	K + Penicillin G Buffered	Squibb	5M u.	22 hr.	7.8
			Aminophyllin	Searle	500 mg.		
	5% D/W	1000 ml.	K + Penicillin G Buffered	Squibb	5M u.	10 min.	4.25
			Solu B & C	Upjohn	5 ml.		
	5% D/W	1000 ml.	K + Penicillin G Buffered	Squibb	5M u.	22 hr.	5.3
			Solu B & C	Upjohn	5 ml.		

Rather than duplicating this information and making it available at all nursing stations, which presents revision problems, we have a hospital policy that states: "Prior to the addition of second and subsequent drugs to an intravenous solution already flowing, a pharmacist shall be consulted regarding drug compatibility."

Recommended Equipment and Facilities

One of the primary objectives of an intravenous admixture program is to create a "clean air" environment that will minimize the potential for contaminating admixtures with airborne particles such as dirt, lint, exhalations and microscopic debris sloughed off by human bodies—all of which can carry bacteria. This is most easily accomplished through the use of a laminar flow work area incorporating a HEPA (high efficiency particulate air) filter. These work areas are available in both counter-top and floor models of varying linear dimensions, usually from three to eight feet. Prefiltered air delivered under pressure passes in a uniform manner through the HEPA filter which filters out 99.97 percent of all particles 0.3 microns or larger, which includes airborne bacteria. The uniform outward flow of "clean air" prevents "dirty" room air from entering the protected area.

The expenditure for this equipment varies from $650 to $2,000. The specific model to purchase, of course, will depend primarily upon the work flow system to be adopted. Some sources of supply include:

(1) Abbott Laboratories
Hospital Product Division
North Chicago, Illinois 60064
(2) Air Control, Inc.
125 Noble Street
Norristown, Penn. 19401
(3) Pure Aire
15544 Cabrito Road
Van Nuys, California
(4) Becton-Dickinson
Rutherford, New Jersey 07070
(5) Market Forge, Inc.
Everett, Massachusetts 02149
(6) Travenol Laboratories, Inc.
Morton Grove, Ilinois 60053

Many pharmacists also utilize their clean air environment to provide services related to intravenous admixtures, such as reconstituting lyophilized intramuscular injectables and intravenous anesthetics, preparing of admixtures for peritoneal dialysis, extemporaneously compounding small volume injections, packaging sterile unit dose parenterals and preparing admixtures for IPPB treatments.

Equipment for reconstituting lyophilized injectables is helpful and quite inexpensive, usually costing less than $50 for complete sets of syringes, control handles (*e.g.*, Luer-Lok), two-way valves, and rubber tubing. Sources of supply include:

(1) Becton-Dickinson
Rutherford, New Jersey 07070
Re: B.-D. Yale Luer-Lok Syringes
B.-D. Automatic Double Valve No. 3094
Medical Grade Rubber Tubing
(2) American Hospital Supply Corp.
McGaw Park, Illinois 60085
Re: Tomac Three-Way Stopcock,
Sterile No. 17108-010

A small refrigerator is also desirable for the storage of reconstituted lyophilized additives and "opened" multiple dose vials to promote stability and sterility. Small refrigerators, between 1.0 and 2.0 cubic feet, are available from many sources for less than $100.00.

A candling unit, incorporating a high intensity light, can be helpful in detecting particulate matter in solutions, physical incompatibilities and hairline cracks in containers. High intensity light microscope illuminators can be used at a cost of less than $50.00 and are available through many scientific instrument supply houses.

A pH meter will be of value for determining whether the resultant pH of an admixture containing two or more drug additives is within the known stability range of each ingredient. Meters accurate to tenths are available from scientific instrument supply houses for as little as $225.00.

Prefabricated work counters, shelf storage units, supply carts, typewriters, etc., must also be considered and are available through many suppliers. The hospital's purchasing agent can be of great assistance here.

From personal experience, we have found it to be very uncomfortable without cooling mechanisms if the laminar flow stations are confined to a small room where the heat generated by them cannot be dissipated over a sufficiently large area. The decision as to whether to further cool the air and the specific method for accomplishment should be made by a consulting engineer specializing in air handling. The cost-to-benefit relationship of adding an electrostatic precipitating device to the air conditioner to prolong the life of the laminar flow HEPA filters also should be determined by the consulting engineer.

It is not necessary, of course, to use a separate physical facility in addition to using laminar flow clean air centers for the purpose of controlling the level of air-borne contamination; the clean air centers are themselves adequate. There is, however, a distinct safety factor in locating the admixture service in an area where the respective individuals are not subjected to to the traffic and noise associated with other department functions. We have found that movable partitions, such as those used for constructing offices, are quite satisfactory for constructing a separate facility. These partitions cost between $15.00 and $30.00 per linear foot installed and are available through most lumber supply dealers and many office suppliers. The following manufacturers of movable partitions can supply you with the names of distributors in your geographical areas:

(1) Royalmetal Corporation
One Park Avenue
New York, New York 10016
(2) Brewster Corporation
Old Lyme, Connecticut
(3) Brunswick Corporation
Contract Furniture Division
Kalamazoo, Michigan
(4) Workwall Division
L. A. Darling Co.
Bronson, Michigan

The area to be used, whether a separate room or not, should be designed to provide for the proper flow of materials during processing and to permit convenient accessibility to supplier. Again, consulting industrial engineers can be very helpful in reviewing your initial plans and suggesting alternatives.

DEVELOPING INTRAVENOUS THERAPY POLICIES

According to the Joint Commission on Accreditation of Hospitals, "Written policies and procedures that pertain to the intrahospital drug distribution system . . . [and] that govern the safe administration of drugs shall be developed by the medical staff in cooperation with the pharmacist and representatives of the disciplines, as necessary."[3]

The pharmacy director and the other members of the hospital's pharmacy and therapeutics committee should develop and recommend policies pertaining to the prescribing, preparation, and administration of intravenous medications, such as:

1. What procedures are to be used for the I.V. order:
   a. What method will be used to transmit the physician's order to the pharmacy? It is desirable for the pharmacist to receive the prescriber's original order or a direct copy.
   b. When are verbal orders by the physician acceptable, if ever?
   c. How frequently shall orders for intravenous therapy be reevaluated? How frequently shall orders for I.V. therapy be rewritten, if to be continued?
2. Who shall be responsible for preparing routine (non-emergency) intravenous solutions to which drugs are added:
   a. Days?
   b. Afternoons (evenings)?
   c. Nights?
   What provisions will be made for the 24-hour availability of the use of a laminar flow "clean air center"? What arrangements will be made for the proper training of pharmacy and nursing personnel in the use of the laminar flow hood?
3. Who shall be responsible for preparing emergency intravenous solutions to which drugs are added?
4. How will intermittent intravenous therapy be prepared and administered:
   a. By piggy-backing small-volume bottles (*e.g.*, 50 to 100 ml)?
   b. By use of volumetric sets?
   c. By direct injection into the injection site of the I.V. set?
   (If (b) or (c), who will reconstitute, if necessary, the lyophilized additives, and who will package and label the syringes containing the additives?)
5. How will compatibility information be made available to those responsible for preparing intravenous admixtures?
6. Who may perform venipunctures:
   a. Physicians only?
   b. Any registered nurse?
   c. Nurses who have demonstrated competence?
   d. Nurses who have completed the hospital's in-service program pertaining to intravenous therapy?
7. What are the recommended sites for venipuncture and the respective needle lengths and gauges?[21]
8. If nurses are authorized by the medical staff to administer intravenous solutions:
   a. What, if any, doses of drugs must be started initially by a physician, but can be continued by the nurse? *e.g.*, metaraminol (Aramine), levarterenol (Levophed), lidocaine (Xylocaine), oxytocin (Pitocin), papaverine. What exceptions will be made? (*e.g.*, I.C.U., C.C.U., E. R., Delivery, Recovery).
   b. What special policies, if any, will apply to newborn nursery and pediatrics?
   c. What intravenous doses must always be administered by a physician? *e.g.*, antineoplastic agents, BSP, PSP, histamine, isoxsuprine (Vasodilan).
9. If a physician fails to prescribe the flow rate:
   a. What is the recommended rate, if any, for intermittent therapy? (*e.g.*, 25 to 50 drops/minute).
10. Who may administer blood and blood derivatives, and what, if any, special precautions shall be taken? (*e.g.*, check by a physician or a second nurse).
11. What procedure shall be followed if infiltration occurs?

12. If an adverse reaction occurs during I.V. administration to a patient, what procedures should be followed for:
    a. Allergic reaction?
    b. Shock?
    c. Cardiac arrest?

PARENTERAL HYPERALIMENTATION

The history of the healing arts has witnessed many ways to introduce medicaments into or onto the afflicted body. Although parenteral injection of drugs is one of the more recent of the routine routes of administration, interest in it dates back to the time of Sir Christopher Wren who intravenously injected medication into dogs in the mid-seventeenth century, some 40 years after Harvey discovered the circulation of blood. The historical antecedents of the state of today's art make interesting reading, particularly in the search for efficacious parenteral alimentation. Almost 100 years ago milk was given by intravenous injection successfully in man, and before that, Claude Bernard had injected a variety of nutrients in animals, including sugar and egg white as well as milk.[23] The need for an intravenous solution high in calories and small in volume has been recognized for a long time, but the fulfillment of the need is of fairly recent vintage.

The seriously ill surgical patient requires two to three times the caloric intake of a healthy person. Nutritional intake should be balanced according to the body's needs for carbohydrate, protein, fat, water, salts and vitamins. This is a relatively new concept since the prevailing practice in the nineteenth century, the work and theories of Bernard and Hodder notwithstanding, was to severely restrict dietary intake in the presence of serious or wasting disease. Malgaigne's account of observations on wounded soldiers following Napoleon's first defeat in 1814 provides an interesting case in point. Soldiers of the French army were treated according to the standard of practice of the day, including dietary deprivation. Russian soldiers, on the other hand, received the same quality of medical treatment but were allowed to eat all they wanted. Wound mortality among the French troops was four times that of the Russian army but the significance of these observations had little effect and fifty years later Florence Nightingale was decrying the "abysmal habit of starving those who need nutrition most and are least able to receive it."[24] Tradition and habit are hard to change.

The clinical indications for parenteral hyperalimentation include:

1. *Patients who cannot eat.* Esophogeal carcinoma, gastric carcinoma, obstructing peptic ulcer, paralytic ileus, etc.
2. *Patients who should not eat.* Traumatic or inflammatory enterocutaneous fistulas, regional enteritis, granulomatous colitis, pancreatitis, laryngeal incompetence, etc.
3. *Patients who cannot eat enough.* Multiple injuries (especially long bone fractures), major full thickness burns, ulcerative colitis, short bowel syndrome, malabsorption syndrome, etc.
4. *Patients who will not eat enough.* Postoperative geriatric patients, anorexia nervosa, etc.
5. *Infants who have congenital anomalies or chronic diarrhea.*

A recent advance in nutritional therapy is parenteral hyperalimentation which has been well documented in the current literature.[22-33] (Refer to Chapter 13, page 244 for a brief discussion on hyperalimentation in infants and children.)

As recently as 1966 it was believed that parenteral hyperalimentation without fat was not possible because of the high caloric value of fat (9 calories per gram *vs* 4 calories per gram of carbohydrate), the small volume necessary, and the fact that fat has no osmotic effect.[25] In 1895 Laube injected camphor oil into cardiac patients to provide a source of calories, and it was rumored that the Germans used camphorated oil intravenously during World War I.[26] The Japanese, notably Yamakawa and his associates, were the first to emulsify oils (castor oil) for intravenous use in the 1920's,[27] and Holt and others used fat emulsions as a source of calories in extremely emaciated children.[28] During the Second World War a Task Force on Intravenous Alimentation was formed under the aegis of the Surgeon General of the Army. Meng and coworkers[29] studied parenteral alimentation in dogs injecting carbohydrate, fat, protein, minerals and vitamins for as long as ten weeks at a time. One dog, on a diet minus the fat, lost 14 percent of his weight, developed lesions, became apathetic and emaciated. This perhaps reinforced the theory of the essentiality of fat, and much of the work in clinical nutrition focused on this aspect. Not until the 1950's was an emulsified oil available or marketed suitable for routine I.V. use. Success was short-lived, however, for it was soon found that long-term use of this form of parenteral hyperalimentation resulted in a delayed "fat-overloading syndrome," characterized by fever, hemorrhage, abdominal discomfort, anemia, jaundice and several other symptoms. Wherefore, the search in America began anew, although parenteral alimentation solutions con-

Table 3. Concentration of Protein Hydrolysates, Amino Acids and Various Salts per 100 ml of Commercially Available Products

AMIGEN 5% WITH DEXTROSE 5% (BAXTER)		AMINOSOL 5% (ABBOTT)		HYPROTIGEN 10% (MCGAW)		CUTTER PROTEIN HYDROLYSATE (C.P.H.)	
Dextrose (Hydrous)	5 g			Casein Hydrolysate	10 g	Casein Hydrolysate	5 g
Casein Hydrolysate	5 g						
Sodium Bisulfite	0.05 g						
		Modified Fibrin Hydrolysate	5 g				
		KCl	0.5 g				
				K-Bisulfite	60 mg		
K-Metabisulfite	0.056 g	K-Metabisulfite	0.06 g				
Leucine	410 mg	1-Leucine	636 mg	1-Leucine	820 mg	Leucine	415 mg
Valine	310 mg	1-Valine	163 mg	1-Valine	600 mg	Valine	300 mg
Lysine	310 mg	1-Lysine	400 mg	1-Lysine	700 mg	Lysine	350 mg
Isoleucine	260 mg	1-Isoleucine	218 mg	1-Isoleucine	500 mg	Isoleucine	240 mg
Phenylalanine	200 mg	1-Phenylalanine	100 mg	1-Phenylalanine	400 mg	Phenylalanine	230 mg
						Arginine	150 mg
Threonine	190 mg	1-Threonine	232 mg	1-Threonine	380 mg	Threonine	180 mg
Methionine	130 mg	1-Methionine	100 mg	1-Methione	320 mg	Methionine	220 mg
				dl-Methionine	130 mg		
						Histidine	120 mg
Histidine	130 mg	1-Histidine	116 mg	1-Tryptophan	80 mg	Tryptophan	50 mg
Tryptophan	35 mg	1-Tryptophan	50 mg	dl-Tryptophan	32 mg		
Na (80 mg/100 ml)	3.5 mEq	Na (23 mg/100 ml)	1.0 mEq	Na	5.0 mEq	Na	3.9 mEq
K (75 mg/100 ml)	7.9 mEq	K (66 mg/100 ml)	1.7 mEq	K	3.6 mEq	K	1.8 mEq
Ca	0.5 mEq			Ca	1.0 mEq		
Mg	0.2 mEq			Mg	0.4 mEq		
Cl	2.0 mEq			Cl	3.6 mEq		
PO_4	3.0 mEq			PO_4	5.0 mEq		
		1-Arginine	290 mg				
		1-Tyrosine	110 mg				
		1-Glutamic Acid	30 mg				
		1-Aspartic Acid	30 mg				
		1-Cysteine HCl	30 mg				
		Glycine	208 mg				

taining fat have been used successfully in Europe for some years.

Solutions containing 5 percent protein hydrolysate and 5 percent dextrose in water have been available for years; however, they lack the ability to increase lean tissue mass. A minimum of 120 to 150 nonprotein calories must be given with each gram of parenteral nitrogen to supply the energy necessary for protein synthesis. When protein hydrolysate is infused without sufficient nonprotein calories, the amino acids in the hydrolysate are deaminated and oxidized to supply energy.[42] Although a number of other carbohydrates have been used including fructose, invert sugar and sorbitol, hypertonic glucose in the presence of adequate insulin is today the least expensive and practical caloric source.[34]

A healthy adult male who requires about 2800 calories and 100 g of protein per day would need approximately 2 liters of 5 percent protein hydrolysate in 5 percent dextrose in water and over 10 liters of 5 percent dextrose and water to supply the necessary calories and protein found in his normal diet. This amount of fluid could not be given safely without danger of fluid overload and pulmonary edema.[48]

Dudrick, *et al.* have shown that the infusion of 3.5 percent protein hydrolysate in 19.5 percent dextrose in water with added electrolytes and multivitamins can be tolerated by patients for over a month under certain circumstances. Infusion of such a high concentration of dextrose as this, however, into the peripheral veins would be impossible because of its irritating and necrosing properties. Successful hyperalimentation techniques are based primarily on the subclavian venipuncture technique developed by the Frenchman Aubaniac in 1942 and used by him

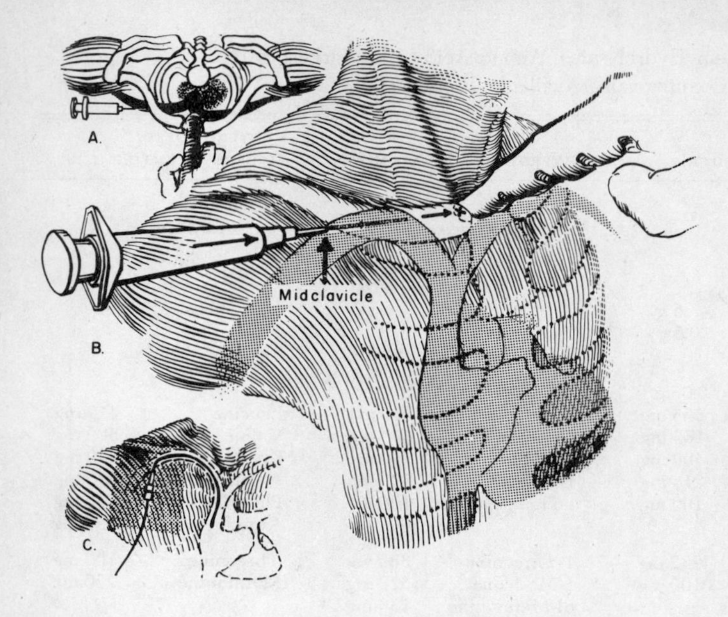

Figure 5. Technique of percutaneous infraclavicular subclavian catheterization. The needle, inserted under the mid-clavicle and aimed in three dimensions at the top of the posterior aspect of the sternal manubrium (indicated by the fingertip in the suprasternal notch), lies in a plane parallel with the frontal plane of the patient and will enter the anterior wall of the subclavian vein[34]

during the Italian campaign to treat soldiers in shock.[43] Despite the early development and numerous reports of this technique in the literature, it was slow to be investigated by Americans until the work of Dudrick and his co-workers.[44-47] Other large veins which permit rapid dilution, such as the superior vena cava, are also used. For example, infants weighing less than 10 kg do not have a sufficiently well-developed subclavian vein, so the catheter is inserted through the external or internal jugular vein and threaded into the superior vena cava.

Composition of Solutions

The ideal solution for intravenous hyperalimentation should contain the same balance of nutrients as provided by a well-balanced oral diet. The composition of a number of commercially available hyperalimentation solutions is shown in Table 3. For use, these solutions are mixed with concentrated dextrose solutions so that the resulting volume of 1100 ml contains 5.25 g of nitrogen, 212 g of glucose, 7 mEq of Na, 13 mEq of K, and approximately 1000 calories.[34]

To date, protein hydrolysates from enzymatic hydrolysis of casein or acid hydrolysis of fibrin have been the major sources of intravenous nitrogen. These solutions provide about two-thirds of the available nitrogen as amino acids and one-third as dipeptides and tripeptides. When infused with sufficient calories, minerals and vitamins, the hydrolysates supply the substrates needed for synthesis of protein.

Minerals and vitamins are added to the base solution prior to use (Table 4).[34] For the aver-

Table 4. Composition of Daily Intravenous Nutrient Ration in the Average Adult

Water	2,500-3,500 ml	Vitamin A	5,000-10,000 U.S.P. units
Protein hydrolysates (amino acids	100-140 g	Vitamin D	500-1,000 U.S.P. units
Nitrogen	12-20 g	Vitamin E	2.5-5.0 I.U.
Carbohydrate (dextrose)	525-750 g	Vitamin C	250-500 mg
Calories	2,500-3,500 Kcal	Thiamine	25-50 mg
Sodium	125-150 mEq	Riboflavin	5-10 mg
Potassium	75-100 mEq	Pyridoxine	7.5-15 mg
Magnesium	4-8 mEq	Niacin	50-100 mg
		Pantothenic acid	12.5-25 mg

age adult, 50 mEq of NaCl and 40 mEq of KCl are added to each bottle of solution. To at least one bottle daily is added 10 ml of a multivitamin mixture, containing fat-soluble and water-soluble vitamins. Magnesium (4 to 8 mEq) as the sulfate salt is also added daily. Vitamin B_{12}, folic acid, and vitamin K are given intramuscularly or added to the intravenous solution if desired. Calcium (gluconate) and phosphorus (potassium acid phosphate) are added as indicated by blood chemical studies.[34]

Table 5. Composition of 100 ml Essential Amino Acid Solution

ESSENTIAL AMINO ACIDS	MINIMUM DAILY REQUIREMENTS (G)
L-isoleucine	0.70
L-leucine	1.10
L-lysine	0.80
L-methionine	1.10
L-phenylalanine	1.10
L-threonine	0.50
L-tryptophane	0.25
L-valine	0.80
Total	6.35 g/100 ml

The use of solutions of essential amino acids, rather than protein hydrolysates, in uremic patients has resulted in utilization of retained endogenous urea nitrogen with prompt return of the BUN toward normal. The composition of an essential amino acid solution is shown in Table 5.

Preparation of Solutions

This brief account of a problem in therapeutic management has significance for the clinical pharmacist, and hence its inclusion in this chapter. Flack and co-workers[37,38] have discussed this in capable fashion, as have others in the recent literature of pharmacy.[39,40] Pharmacists early in the research studies recognized the combining of solutions and electrolytes and vitamins was in truth a sophisticated prescription, requiring the utmost skill in the essentials of pharmacy, compounding accuracy and careful handling in storage. There are several pharmaceutical problems present in the compounding of parenteral hyperalimentation solutions, and they require resolution by a pharmacist.

There are three methods of preparing nutritional feedings, the 'dry' method, the 'wet' method, both using a commercial form of the protein hydrolysate,[37] and a third method that consists of a solution of synthetic essential amino acids and a solution of 50 percent dextrose. This latter, a two-flask combination package is still in the developmental stage. Each of these methods requires aseptic technic in compounding, and with the dry method, sterilization using membrane filtration.

A comparison of the single unit and the bulk compounding methods is shown in Table 6.

The Hospital of the University of Pennsylvania (HUP), where much of the pharmaceutical intelligence in this new area of service originated, uses the 'dry' method of preparing intravenous nutrients. The dry method differs from the wet method in that anhydrous dextrose is mixed with the hydrolysate solution and is sterilized by membrane filtration. Most other hospitals use

Table 6. Quantity, Caloric Content and Nitrogen Content of Single Unit and Bulk Compounding Methods[38]

	QUANTITY	CALORIC CONTENT	NITROGEN CONTENT
1. single unit method modified fibrin hydrolysate 5%-dextrose 5% injection	750 ml	140 cal	5.25 g
dextrose injection 50%	350 ml	700 cal	0.0
	1,100 ml	840 cal	5.25 g
2. bulk compounding method modified fibrin hydrolysate 5%-dextrose 5% injection	865	173 cal	6.0 g
dextrose anhydrous	185 g	740 cal	0.0
	1,000 ml	913 cal	6.0 g

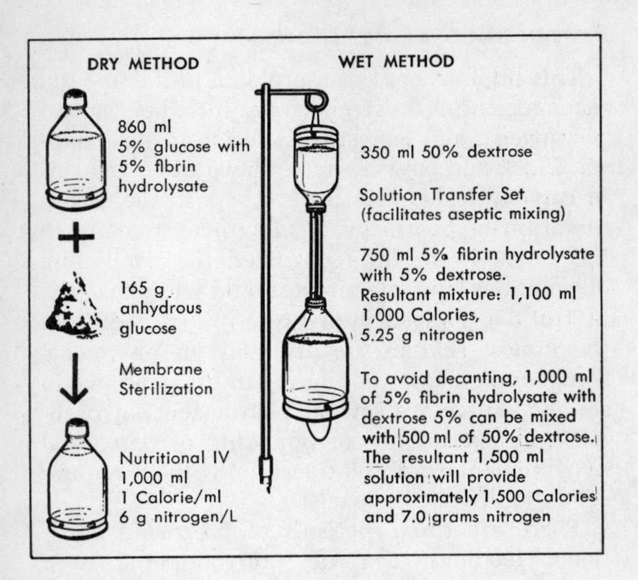

Figure 6. Comparison of the "dry" method and the "wet" method of preparing parenteral hyperalimentation solutions

the wet method, wherein the appropriate volumes of protein hydrolysate and 50 percent dextrose in water are combined to provide the desired nitrogen content and calories. Strict aseptic technic must be followed in all steps of both methods, preferably working in a laminar flow hood. The resultant solution in the 'wet' method does not require further sterilization. The combination two-flask kit is a variation of the wet method except, instead of using a protein hydrolysate solution, a solution of synthetic amino acids is provided for combination with sterile dextrose solution for injection. Most hospitals use fibrin hydrolysate (Aminosol, Abbott) or casein hydrolysate (CPH, Cutter; Amigen, Baxter; Hyprotigen, McGaw) for the source of nitrogen.

Precautions

As mentioned earlier, the parenteral hyperalimentation solution consists of multiple components. Several precautions are necessary to assure a quality product with each prescription. The sterile integrity of the product is of primary concern, and for two reasons. Most hospitals use the 'wet' method of preparation, and this requires multiple handling, decanting, measuring and combining of solutions; these procedures in turn provide multiple opportunities to introduce contaminants. This can be minimized by using a laminar air flow hood and maintaining scrupulous aseptic technic. The second reason is that the combination of dextrose and protein hydrolysate solution provides an excellent medium for bacterial and fungal growth. With appropriate care, however, sterility can be maintained. Bacterial contamination should be monitored by culturing a sample of the solution in thioglycolate broth; fungal contamination is monitored using Sabouraud's broth. The efficiency of the laminar air flow hood should be monitored on a regular basis.

Another precaution deals with the delicate balance of the solution. All authorities with experience in extemporaneous and bulk preparation of hyperosmolar nutrient solutions stress the need for following the correct order of mixing,[37,40] and even using ingredients of the same manufacturer and same lot or batch number when a successful formula has been prepared. The basic solution may be prepared in advance but should be stored under refrigeration and given a 30-day dating. The dating may be renewed if the solution presents no color changes or other obvious signs of deterioration. A color change may indicate a Maillard reaction, similar to the carmelization of glucose, but caused by a chemical reaction between the amino group on the amino acid and the hydroxyl group on the glucose. It is for this reason that refrigeration is recommended, because heat tends to influence the Maillard reaction. Some pharmacists use a darkening of the solution as an indicator of the terminal point of storage.[48] Heat sterilization is, of course, contraindicated because of the high glucose content.

Electrolyte and vitamin additives are included according to the individual needs of the patient as determined by laboratory tests, and are introduced only at the time of dispensing. A 24-to 48-hour dating is placed on the prescription after additives have been included. Drugs, such as steroids, antibiotics, hypotensives and others should be administered separately and should not be combined with the nutrient solution. It may be considered good practice not to add any drug to a parenteral hyperalimentation solution that is not a component of the nutrient formula for that patient.

Technique of Administration

The administration of the hyperalimentation solution presents its own set of precautions. The solution is hypertonic and hyperosmolar exerting 1800 - 2200 milliosmoles per liter pressure and, until the technique of the subclavian vein catheterization was perfected, it was too irritating and inflammatory using the usual routes of parenteral administration. Peripheral veins are not used in the administration of hypertonic nutrients because of insufficient blood flow to provide the necessary dilution and protect the intima of the vessel.[31,33]

The potential for infection from indwelling catheters is well documented. For example, twenty-two of thirty-three patients receiving parenteral hyperalimentation solutions for severe gastrointestinal function developed fungal septicemia during the course of therapy.[49] The relationship between the development of septicemia and the duration of parenteral alimentation and prolonged intravenous catheterization is shown in Table 7.

Recent studies indicate that antibiotic ointments containing polymyxin, bacitracin and neomycin applied to the catheter site progressively inhibit bacterial flora but at the same time increase the number of fungal colonies and thus the risk of fungal sepsis.

Meticulous care of the indwelling central venous catheter is essential for safe long-term parenteral feeding. The current practice is to prepare a sterile field at the site of insertion, to suture the catheter in place after placement, to apply an antibiotic ointment around the catheter site and then to cover the entire area with a sterile dressing. Meticulous and routine catheter care is thereafter necessary to prevent infection. Every two or three days the intravenous tubing is changed and the dressing over the puncture site is removed and the site again redressed. Patients are carefully watched for sudden elevation of temperature since pyrexia is presumptive evidence for sepsis and its appearance may necessitate removal of the indwelling catheter.

For maximum metabolic effect the solution is infused at a constant rate twenty-four hours a day at an average rate of about 2 ml per minute which assures dilution of the hyperosmolar solution.[37] Administration of the fluid at a more rapid rate may result in dehydration caused by osmotic diuresis produced by the concentrated glucose solutions. Glucose overload is combatted by maintaining urine glucose at 3+ or less (2 percent glucosuria). As the normal pancreas responds to the large glucose stimulus by increasing insulin output, the amount of glucose given can be gradually increased. When the pancreas is incapable of an adequate response, as in diabetes mellitus, crystalline insulin is added to the nutrient solutions or given in evenly divided doses subcutaneously. The use of supplementary insulin has enhanced glucose utilization and positive nitrogen balance in the elderly, in those with pancreatic dysfunction, and in critically ill and nutritionally depleted patients in whom early achievement of positive nitrogen balance is essential to survival. Use of 5 to 25 units of regular insulin in each liter of hyperalimentation solution may be required.[34] The dynamic changes in glucose and insulin must be carefully monitored to insure patient safety. Sudden cessation of high concentration of glucose may result in hypoglycemia due to a rebound phenomena resulting from a delay in endogenous insulin production.

Table 7. Relation of Septicemia to Duration of Parenteral Hyperalimentation and Venous Catheterization in 47 Patients

DURATION OF HYPER-ALIMENTATION (DAYS)	TOTAL PATIENTS	PATIENTS WITH SEPTICEMIA	PERCENTAGE WITH SEPTICEMIA
1-5	13	1	7.7
6-10	11	3	27.2
11-20	14	4	28.6
> 20	9	5	55.5
Interval from Last Catheter Change to Septicemia (Days)			
1-5	11	1	9.1
6-10	19	5	26.3
11-20	12	4	33.3
> 20	5	3	60.0

Guidelines for Intravenous Nutrition of Critically Ill Patients

Guidelines for safe administration of hyperalimentation solutions include daily body weight, daily fluid balance, urine specific gravity and fractional determinations of sugar and acetone every 6 hours, serum electrolytes 3 days weekly, and blood urea nitrogen, blood sugar, and other indicated studies weekly. Periodic determinations of calcium, phosphorous, serum protein, prothrombin time, and complete blood count are advisable.[34] A proposed set of Guidelines for the intravenous nutrition of pediatric patients has been discussed by physicians at the Departments of Pediatrics and Surgery, Columbia Presbyterian

Medical Center in New York.[49,51] The following excerpt is pertinent to this discussion:

> In our opinion the successful application of the technique of parenteral alimentation requires the development of a team approach to the patient. A close working relationship between the pediatrician, the pediatric surgeon, and the nurse is the primary requirement of such a team. Another essential member of the team is the pharmacist who mixes the fluids. A responsive laboratory service is also essential for serial monitoring of relevant plasma, blood, and urine constituents, as well as for screening of the fluid for possible microbial contamination and for culture and sensitivity tests in patients with suspected sepsis. In addition, a research group should be a part of the team in order that the many questions concerning the technique can be studied in a systematic way.
>
> It is the authors' strong opinion that hospitals which are unable to provide such a team should not use this technique; rather, patients requiring parenteral nutrition should be referred to a center where such a team is functioning and where all ancillary facilities are available on a 24-hour a day basis. Otherwise the complications of the technique, which are being reported in dramatically increasing numbers, will outweigh the benefits.
>
> One final aspect of intravenous alimentation concerns the fact that the technique is a life-support system and as such is subject to all the practical and ethical considerations applicable to other life support systems. In most centers where the technique has been used for a reasonable period of time, patients (usually those with a very short bowel) have been encountered who are unable to survive without intravenous alimentation, even after as long as 18 months. Unfortunately, the technique has not been used sufficiently to warrant establishing definite guidelines that would avoid such problems. At present each center employing the technique of intravenous alimentation would probably benefit from establishing a patient selection committee composed of members who are knowledgable about the technique of intravenous alimentation and experienced in caring for patients with the underlying disease state requiring its use.[49]

Usually, 40 mEq of KCl is required for each liter of hypertonic glucose solution to maintain normal serum levels and to provide the 3.5 : 1 potassium to nitrogen ratio necessary for protein synthesis. Patients with extensive burns, enterocutaneous fistulas or other causes of unusual potassium loss may require even more.[34]

Sodium requirements require 50 mEq of sodium as sodium chloride or as $\frac{2}{3}$ sodium chloride and $\frac{1}{3}$ sodium bicarbonate per liter.[34]

Clinical Pharmacy Considerations

It is imperative that the pharmacist maintain a close liaison with the physician and the nurse when involved with a patient requiring hyperalimentation. The medical status of such patients is critical and their condition dynamic, so that modest or even precipitate changes in therapy may be needed. As the patient responds to attempts at metabolic correction the indicators being monitored may indicate the need to make a change. The pharmacist is well-served if he keeps himself advised and up-dated on the status of the patient. He may thus anticipate a change in the physician's orders and prepare to expedite the change, or he may help provide essential intelligence to help the physician reach a decision. It might be noted that this format of service is consistent with the accepted standard of practice in clinical pharmacy.

It is reasonable to assume that parenteral hyperalimentation will become an even more routine method of therapeutic management. If the history of health care is any indicator it is also reasonable to expect changes to make the procedure more efficient and safer in terms of stable solutions. Some pharmacists will possibly contribute to this expected advancement, but in the meantime thousands of patients and hundreds of doctors and nurses will have to depend on the expertise and pharmaceutical know-how of pharmacists in hospitals of all types and sizes to prepare and dispense parenteral nutrients. Every pharmacist should be knowledgeable and capable of providing this service.

References

1. Morris, W. E.: The Objectives of Parenteral Therapy, paper presented at the Intravenous Admixture Seminar, Ohio State University Hospitals, Columbus, Ohio, unpublished (Nov.) 1969.
2. Anon.: *I.V. Additives — Steps to Safety,* Abbott Laboratories, North Chicago, (Feb.) 1970, p. 1.
3. "Standards for Accreditation of Hospitals plus Interpretations"—Pharmaceutical Service.
4. Goodman, L. S. and Gilman, A.: *The Pharmacological Basis of Therapeutics,* ed. 4, The Macmillan Co., New York, N.Y., 1970, p. 7.
5. Anon.: *I.V. Additives — Steps to Safety,* op. cit., p. 2.
6. Anon.: *Fluid and Electrolytes,* 97-0738/R14-100, Abbott Laboratories, North Chicago, Illinois (Dec.) 1969.
7. Snively, W. D. and Westerman, R. L. (editors): *Guide to Fluid Therapy,* E104-37, Baxter Laboratories, Morton Grove, Illinois (Oct.) 1969.
8. Anon.: *Parenteral Solutions Handbook, A Guide to Optimal Utilization,* 12-6J-NK, Cutter Laboratories, Berkley, California.
9. Anon.: Continuous versus Intermittent Intravenous Antibiotics, *Med. Letter Drugs Therap. 10*:57-58 (July 26) 1968.
10. Warren, F., Jr.: A Review of Intravenous Fluid Administration Systems, paper presented at I.V. Additive Seminar, University of Georgia, Athens, Ga., unpublished (Feb.) 1970.
11. Anon.: Special Supplement to Vol. 20, No. 9, *Morbidity and Mortality Report,* Public Health Service.
12. Godwin, H. N.: Developing a Parenteral Admixture Service in a Teaching Hospital, (Master's Thesis) Ohio State University, College of Pharmacy, Columbus, Ohio, 1966, p. 33-34.
13. Petruconis, S. and Newman, M.: I.V.'s and Additives—Testing an Experience, unpublished, USPHS Hospital, San Francisco, 1969.
14. Parker, E. A.: Compatibility Digest, *Am. J. Hosp. Pharm. 26*:412-413 (July) 1969.
15. Ibid.: *26*:543-544 (Sept.) 1969.
16. Ibid.: *26*:653-655 (Nov.) 1969.
17. Ibid.: *27*:67-69 (Jan.) 1970.
18. Ibid.: *27*:327-329 (Apr.) 1970.
19. Ibid.: *27*:492-493 (June) 1970.
20. Ibid.: *27*:672-673 (Aug.) 1970.
21. Anon.: *Parenteral Administration,* Abbott Laboratories, North Chicago, Illinois, pp. 9 and 11.
22. Dudrick, S. J., *et al.*: Long-Term Total Parenteral Nutrition with Growth, Development, and Positive Nitrogen Balance, *Surgery 64*:134-142 (July) 1968.
23. Dudrick, S. J.: Rational Intravenous Therapy, *Am. J. Hosp. Pharm. 28*:82-91 (Feb.) 1971.
24. Elman, R.: *Surgical Care,* Appleton Century Crofts, New York, N.Y. 1951.
25. Jones, R. J.: Present Knowledge of Fat Emulsions, *Nutritional Rev. 24*:225-228 (June) 1966.
26. Mueller, J. F. and Canham, J. E.: Prefaces to a Symposium on Fat Emulsions, *Am. J. Clin. Nutr. 16*:1-4 (Jan.) 1965.
27. Elman, R.: *Parenteral Alimentation in Surgery,* Hoeber, New York, N. Y. 1947.
28. Watkin, D. M. and Steinfeld, J. K.: Nutrient and Energy Metabolism with Fat Administered Intravenously, *Am. J. Clin. Nutr. 16*:182-219 (Jan.) 1965.
29. Meng, H. C. and Early, F.: Study of Complete Parenteral Alimentation in Dogs, *J. Lab. Clin. Med. 34*:1121-1131 (Oct.) 1949.
30. Rhode, C. M., Parkins, W. M. and Vars, H. M.: Nitrogen Balance in Dogs with Continuously Infused 50 Percent Glucose and Protein Preparations, *Am. J. Physiol. 159*:415-425 (Dec.) 1949.
31. Wilmore, D. W. and Dudrick, S. J.: Growth and Development of an Infant Receiving all Nutrients Exclusively by Vein, *J. Am. Med. Assoc. 203*:140-144 (Mar. 4) 1968.
32. Dudrick, S. J., Wilmore, D. W., Vars, H. M. and Rhoads, J. E.: Can Intravenous Feeding as the Sole Means of Nutrition Support Growth in the Child and Restore Weight Loss in an Adult?, *Trans. S. Surg. Assoc. 80*:307, 1969.
33. Taylor, F. K.: Parenteral Nutrition by Subclavian Catheter, *Hosp. Physician 10*:53-56 (Nov.) 1970.
34. Dudrick, S. J., Long, J. M., Steiger, E. and Rhoads, J. E.: Intravenous Hyperalimentation. *Med. Clinics N. Am. 54*:577-589 (May) 1970.
35. Das, J. B., Filler, R. M., Rubin, V. G. and Eraklis, A. J.: Intravenous Dextrose-Amino Acid Feeding: The Metabolic Response in the Surgical Neonate. *J. Ped. Surg. 5*: 127-135 (Apr.) 1970.
36. Rea, W. J., Wyrick, W. J., McClelland, R. N. and Webb, W. R.: Intravenous Hyperosmolar Alimentation, *Arch. Surg. 100*:393-398 (Apr.) 1970.
37. Flack, H. L., Gans, J. A., Dudrick, S. J. and Serlick, S. E.: Current Status of Parenteral Hyperalimentation, *Am. J. Hosp. Pharm. 28*:326-335 (May) 1971.
38. Serlick, S. E., Dudrick, S. J. and Flack, H. L.: Nutritional Intravenous Feeding, *Bull. Parenteral Drug Assoc. 23*: 166-173 (July-Aug.) 1969.
39. Sauve, Sr. F.: The Pharmacist and a Nutritional Intravenous Therapy Program, *Am. J. Hosp. Pharm. 28*: 106-109 (Feb.) 1971.
40. Klotz, R., Sherman, J. O. and Egan, T.: Preparation of Hyperalimentation Solutions for the Pediatric Patient, *Am. J. Hosp. Pharm. 28*:102-105 (Feb.) 1971.
41. Wilmore, D. W. and Dudrick, S. J.: In-Line Filter for Intravenous Solutions, *Arch. Surg. 99*:462-3 (Oct.) 1969.
42. Sherman, J. O., Egan, T. and Macalad, F. V.: Parenteral Hyperalimentation, *Surg. Clin. N. Am. 51*:37-47 (Feb.) 1971.
43. Aubaniac, R.: Une Nouvelle Voie d'Injection ou de Ponction Veineuse: La Voie Sous-Claviculair, *Sem. Hosp. Paris 28*:3445-3447 (Nov. 18) 1952.
44. Defalque, R. J.: Subclavian Venipuncture: A Review, *Anesthesia Analgesia Current Res. 47*:677-682 (Nov.-Dec.) 1968.
45. Ashbaugh, D.: Subclavian-Vein Infusion, *Lancet 1*:1138-1139 (Nov. 30) 1963.
46. Davidson, J. T., Ben-Hur, N. and Nathan, H.: Subclavian Venipuncture, *Lancet 1*:1139-1140 (Nov. 30) 1963.
47. Keéri-Szātó, M.: The Subclavian Vein, a Constant and Convenient Intravenous Site, *Arch. Surg. 72*:179-181 (Feb.) 1956.
48. Klotz, R., Sherman, J. O. and Egan, T.: Preparation of Hyperalimentation Solutions for the Pediatric Patient, *Am. J. Hosp. Pharm. 28*:102-105 (Feb.) 1971.
49. Winters, Robert: Guidelines for Intravenous Nutrition of Critically Ill Patients, *Proceedings, Symposium on Total Parenteral Nutrition,* Council on Foods and Nutrition, Am. Med. Assoc., Chicago, 1972.
50. Curry, C. R. and Quie, P. G.: Fungal Septicemia in Patients Receiving Parenteral Hyperalimentation, *New Engl. J. Med. 285*:1221-1225 (Nov. 25) 1971.
51. Heird, W. C. *et al.*: Medical Progress — Intravenous Alimentation in Pediatric Patients, *J. Pediatrics 80*:3:351-372 (Mar.) 1972.

8

Building a clinically-oriented drug information service

by Joseph L. Hirschman

The pharmacist as a provider of drug information, in the generic sense, is nothing new. It is probably safe to say that pharmacists have been dispensing information as well as drugs as part of their responsibilities since the beginnings of the profession. Traditionally, this information has been usually confined to the physical or chemical properties, dosages, sources, formulations and the like. What is new, however, is the development of the concept of the pharmacist as a provider of clinically useful drug information that can be applied to the therapeutic management of patients. The evolution of this concept resulted in the formation of organized, centralized drug information services. The formation of these information centers was indeed evolutionary in the Darwinian sense of the word, that is, it was a result of natural selection. Just as the efficient delivery of health care to increasing patient populations has led to the centralization of these services, the dissemination of drug information by pharmacists has had to be organized in a similar manner. In this fashion, the greatest possible utility of information centers is achieved. Prevailing logistical requirements resulted in the elimination of less efficient methods of drug information dissemination from the environment.

Evolution of Drug Information Specialization

The origin of this species culminated in 1962 with the establishment of the Drug Information Center at the University of Kentucky. This center has served as the prototype of the modern drug information service.[1] Naturally, the species continues to be refined, but for practical purposes the concept as implemented in 1962 remains substantially unchanged.

There are many factors which played major roles in determining the present state of pharmacy practice in the area of drug information. Paramount among these are the biomedical information explosion, the existence of specialization in the health professions, the continuing development of new drug entities and pharmacologic and therapeutic principles, and the increasing clinical involvement of pharmacists. These are the basic parameters of the health care environment that have led to the development of pharmacist-operated drug information services and thus they require some explanation.

The information explosion is the predominant factor in the growth of drug information services and underlies all of the other prodding influences. The biomedical literature is growing exponentially. This is forcing specialization and drug information is no small part of it. The first national scientific societies in the modern tradition were founded in the late 17th century. These societies established the first scientific periodicals, and scientists found themselves beginning to write scientific papers instead of the books, which heretofore had been their only outlet. By 1963, there was a world list of 50,000 scientific periodicals that had been founded of which 30,000 were still being published. These journals had published a world total of about six million scientific papers and were increasing at a rate of at least half a million a year.[2] At least 10 percent of these are biomedical in nature. As an illustration of this phenomenon, the library of the University of California, San Francisco lists 9,500 periodical titles of which 6,000 are currently active.[3]

Obviously, no individual can presume to be competent in all areas of medical practice with the existence of such imponderable amounts of published knowledge. Simple logic dictates that one must specialize in a given limited area if one is to be effective. As a consequence we have an era of specialization. Pharmacy is not exempt from this and a "drug information specialist" is evolving at present.

As a fallout to the knowledge explosion, new pharmacologic and therapeutic principles are being established with new drugs developed to take advantage of these principles. Although the introduction of new drugs is declining over what it was ten years ago, it is still quite substantial. In fact, what seems to be the current trend is that more laboratory and clinical studies with drugs are being carried out today than ever before. The literature is expanding in areas, such as drug interactions, which were not fully understood when the drugs were originally introduced. So, in reality, information on drugs is growing as rapidly as ever, if not more so.[4] Drug investigations are taking more of a scientific rather than a purely clinical viewpoint, that is, in terms of understanding why things work, not just the observing of the effects. Interpreting this data, communicating it and applying it is becoming the realm of the drug information pharmacist.

For the pharmacist to function as an interface between the biomedical literature and the clinician and his patient, he must assume a posture of clinical involvement. This, too, is part of the evolutionary pattern. Like all health professions today, the pharmacist is seeking a role proper for himself within the framework of a collaborative approach to the patient's problem. In seeking to define his role or establish his identity in modern health care delivery, the pharmacist has entered the clinical area and by his aggressiveness has been able to contribute to the rational use of drugs. This clinical involvement was on an informal, casual basis in the beginning, but the success of such relationships has naturally led to the establishment of organized, formal mechanisms for providing this contribution. The result, of course, is the consultative-type drug information center.

Definition and Philosophy of Drug Information Service

The term "drug information" is fast becoming a cliché. But what is drug information really? Drug information as used in "drug information center," "drug information service" or "drug information specialist" should not be construed as being the basic factual information that can be gleaned from the literature. On the contrary, it should imply the ability to communicate to the practitioner the clinically relevant information that can be used to facilitate the practice of rational therapeutics. However, one should not be deceived by this seemingly simple definition. The complexity of the drug literature creates enormous problems for the pharmacist in filling this need. The problems and some of the solutions for providing drug information services are essentially those of how to best communicate existing information.

I have characterized the activities of a drug information service as being primarily communicative in nature. The scope of these communication activities is essentially divided into two broad categories, *i.e.*, the collection and dissemination of drug information. The net result of both activities should be improved patient care through more rational drug therapy as influenced by the efforts of the drug information service.

When contemplating the establishment of an information service, one must give first priority to adopting basic principles and a philosophy for the operation. Decisions have to be made as to whether the emphasis will be clinical or nonclinical, whether the service will be one of consultation or data collection, who is to provide the service and who is to receive the service.

The question of whether to be a clinical or a nonclinical service is hardly subject to debate anymore. One cannot expect to provide a meaningful service if he does not understand the problems of the patient, of the physician and of the nurse. In addition, drug information *per se* is not nearly as useful as information that is tempered by clinical judgment. Without clinical training and involvement a drug information pharmacist can not possibly be empathetic with the problems of the patient or those responsible for his care, nor can he make any valid clinical judgments. The only real measure of the success of a drug information service is its utilization. Experience has shown that without a clinically oriented service, utilization dwindles to a point where the continuing existence of the service cannot be justified.

Scope of Services

Establishment of a consultative service is really not an optional choice, if one adopts a clinical orientation. Provision of a consultative operation is really a corollary to clinical service. Of course, the word consultant can have many definitions. For our purposes, a consultant is one who is able to be selective and discriminating and who uses critical judgment in assessing the information available, but, above all, is able to interpret this information, place it into clinical perspective and communicate it effectively. Alternatively, placing the emphasis on the transmission of superficial factual information will fill no immediate gaps in the delivery of health care and as a consequence will not be a viable service. Viewing things logically, the pharmacist is the most obvious professional who should provide drug information services of a clinical, consultative bent. For a pharmacist to do this he has to become more patient-conscious and suppress his traditional drug product preoccupation. In addition, the drug information pharmacist cannot be encumbered with other responsibilities simultaneously with his drug information activities. There is no way that information and consultation can be a piecemeal operation; it requires full attention to be successful.

Because a few drug information pharmacists with continuing experience in this area perform more competently than those who rotate only infrequently through the service, this does not mean that a service cannot involve the entire pharmacy staff. The logistics of a rotational position can be worked out. Nevertheless, this does require appropriate training and interest. There is no reason why such pharmacists could not provide an adequate service on a periodic basis. In any event, specialization is the name-of-the-game and should be the aim. With either alternative, it cannot be overemphasized that when someone is assigned to the drug information division, he should not have other encumbering responsibilities.

In the current scheme of health care delivery, the physician is the central figure. As a consequence, most drug information services orient the operation toward the needs of the physician. Few, if any, however, limit their service exclusively to physicians. Generally, most services are available to all health professionals. Occasionally service will be provided to lay people as well. There are also some information operations that limit the use of their facilities to patient-care area pharmacists, but these usually evolve to the point where they are providing information directly to clinicians as well.

Virtually all drug information centers are located in medical institutions and are supported financially by the administration of these institutions. As a consequence, quite often the services are limited to the staff of that hospital. However, a number of centers are available to the health professional community at large as a public service. The extent of a center's service area is an operating parameter that must be determined at the outset.

Providing drug information to lay people can have some legal implications and liabilities that probably are best avoided at present. Generally, it is more prudent to refer a layman to his pharmacist or physician for advice and information. Occasionally, one can make exceptions for laymen who are involved in professional or voluntary aspects of health care services or to attorneys with medical-legal problems.

Patient-Specific Consultations

The range of services that can be provided by an information operation is only limited by the imagination of the individuals who are involved. There are an enormous number of useful functions that can be provided that fall into the areas of dissemination and gathering of drug information. They range from patient-specific consultations to teaching. The "bread and butter" service and that which will determine the ultimate place of the center and its effect on patient care, is the patient-specific consultation. Providing this service well will indeed result in the pharmacist being known as a drug consultant. Preparing this type of consultation requires a knowledge of the patient's history and the understanding of it. These consultations may range from dosage instruction to suggesting or outlining a course of drug therapy for the patient's particular problem. A drug information pharmacist should only be limited in this area by one parameter: where the problem is sufficiently complex that it requires a physical examination of the patient. At this point, the consultation becomes the prerogative of the physician. However, one should not use this as an excuse to avoid complex problems as in the end it is the ability to solve the difficult and out-of-ordinary problems that will have the most substantial impact on health care.

Drug-Oriented Information

In most drug information centers, the second most common service will consist of providing non-patient, drug- and product-oriented information. Frequently these requests are generated as a result of previous patient problems or anticipated patient problems. Many questions in this category are of a relatively trivial nature, *e.g.*, identification of foreign drug products, dosage forms, product availability and so on. Nevertheless, they can range the full spectrum from the trivial to the very complex. It is important not to minimize the value of the information to the inquirer. The information is almost always important to that individual no matter how trivial the question may seem. If one is to provide drug information, he must be prepared to contend with the routine as well as the sophisticated.

Information for Poisonings

A rather large and demanding service function is poison control. If poison control activities are to be engaged in, they should be embraced wholeheartedly or not at all. There is no practical way that a poison control service can be provided on a limited or selective basis. The difficulty most drug information pharmacists encounter is a result of many users of the service who consider drug information and poison control synonymous. Experience indicates that a good drug information service also makes an excellent poison control center. In view of the difficulty of avoiding this responsibility, it is wise to consider preparing for and accepting it prior to implementation of the operation.

Investigational Drug Information

Involvement in investigational drug control may be an area that an information service might wish to pursue. Such things as preparational assistance for IND applications, maintaining records of use on investigational drugs, reviewing the literature in preparation for writing protocols and communicating investigational usages of drugs to physicians are activities engaged in by some centers. The minimum in this area that should be met is providing advice on the investigational uses of drugs and maintaining sufficient records of investigational drug usage within the parent institution. These records should contain, of course, the drug's and the investigator's names. Extensive participation in investigational drug programs may drain off energy from more directly patient-oriented activities.

P & T Committee Functions

Participation in pharmacy and therapeutics (P & T) committee functions should be a high priority of any information service. This is the most important non-patient specific activity of a drug information center. In the organization and establishment of a new service, efforts should be made to have the director of the service appointed to the P & T committee. In addition, it should be the responsibility of the center to provide drug reports for evaluation by the committee. These reports should serve as a basis for the committee's deliberations and decisions. If the drug information service reports prove to be reliable, the influence upon drug usage in that hospital will be profound. A center's work for the P & T committee may be one of the most effective ways in which a pharmacist exerts an influence on the use of drugs. This assumes that the formulary system is in effect and enforced, which should be a goal of every hospital pharmacy. The committee's drug reports should be prepared by analyzing critically the therapeutic merits of the drugs on the basis of objective evidence. Included in these reports should be definite recommendations to the committee for action on the particular drugs in question. Such things as whether the drug should be admitted or deleted from the formulary, whether the drug should be placed in a restricted category or whether the drug should be re-evaluated when further evidence is obtained should be spelled out. Since most P & T committees, without the services of a drug information pharmacist, function on a rather subjective level, usually basing decisions upon the collective, limited personal experience of the committee members, the influence of objective reports prepared by drug information centers can have a dramatic impact on the makeup of a hospital's formulary.

Publication of Newsletters

The majority of information centers participate in the publication of a newsletter. Some centers play an active, primary role in this endeavor while others perform more of an advisory function. In many cases the drug information service has taken over the publication and distribution of existing hospital pharmacy bulletins. It seems appropriate that an information service should be responsible for a pharmacy newsletter describing drug usage and reporting on other drug-related bits of knowledge. If this function is undertaken, there should be a predetermined set of goals. There is not much point in grinding out a newsletter every month that is a bunch of abstracts from other easily available sources. Such a newsletter will be essentially a pile of scratch paper. If, however, relevant information is gathered together in one package, such as a survey of the literature on drug interactions, then the publication becomes quite useful. Also, it is a practicable vehicle within one's own institution to highlight aspects of drug usage that may need amplification or changing because of newly available information or because of traditional drug usage patterns. A newsletter is also an ideal mechanism for disseminating P & T committee actions to the staff at large. In any event, this function should not be undertaken by a drug information service unless one can spend the time to do the job necessary for providing a quality publication without compromising the more directly patient related activities. Publication of a newsletter always must be considered a subordinate function.

Literature Searches

Literature searches and bibliographic services are activities that may be engaged in by information centers. However, where adequate medical library facilities are available to the professional staff, provision of these services is probably not warranted. The expertise required is not within the exclusive domain of a pharmacist and, in fact, these functions are probably better performed by a trained librarian. Furthermore, every health professional should be able to perform these functions for himself or engage the assistance of a librarian for them. In most cases, it would be a waste of time for a pharmacist to provide these services at the expense of more patient-directed endeavors. In circumstances where a medical library facility is not readily available, but where a drug information service has the resources necessary for literature searches or bibliographic compilations, then these services may be provided. But these functions are clearly of low priority and should not be engaged in unless there is adequate time available. In no case should these services be the primary responsibility of the drug information center. These activities do not, in themselves, justify the existence of a center or the talents of a drug information pharmacist.

Teaching Functions

Almost every drug information center will be, at one time or another, engaged in teaching. Those services associated with schools of pharmacy will be involved with the undergraduate education of pharmacy students. Those associated with medical centers, in many cases, will be responsible for the training of pharmacy residents and virtually all information services, regardless of their location will be involved in the continuing education of their own staff pharmacists. In most cases, the teaching function is on a preceptor basis. This essentially consists of an orientation followed by continuing on-the-job training, that is, learning by experience. The burden placed upon the staff of the center in the preceptor-type situation is usually not excessive and can even be useful in providing additional manpower for the service. However, those centers associated with schools of pharmacy must have additional teaching staff, beyond what is required for drug information service, to train undergraduate students. It should be noted also that students have considerably less experience and as a result they do not contribute to the service aspect as much as a resident or a staff pharmacist might. Regardless of the burden placed upon the service, teaching responsibilities should not be avoided. The training of pharmacists in the area of drug information is a vital necessity to the continuing growth of pharmacy practice.

Other Services

Any number of activities performed by traditional hospital pharmacy services may be considered to be within the domain of the drug information center depending upon one's point of view. Information services that are relatively inactive in terms of patient-specific consultations may be used as "garbage cans" for activities that the dispensing pharmacy service does not wish to be bothered with but which might "justify" the continuing operation of an information center. With the possible exceptions of controlling pharmaceutical detailing activities and performing patient monitoring within the hospital, any additional functions, other than those that have already been described above, probably are not appropriate for a well conceived and adequately utilized drug information center. The logistics involved in regulating detailing are not within the scope of this chapter. Because of the time-consuming activities that may be involved with this function, it should probably be left for others. The drug information center, though, is always indirectly involved in detailing. In fact, it should serve to counterbalance the detailing activities of the manufacturers' representatives.

The selective monitoring of patients' drug therapy is within the purview of the drug information pharmacist where no ward-based clinical pharmacy staff exists. This requires participation in such activities as patient rounds with physicians, drug history taking, and so on. Obviously, access to the patient's chart is also needed. All of these tasks should be directed toward uncovering therapeutic misadventures and hopefully preventing their adverse effects. In other words, this is taking the initiative and soliciting business rather than waiting passively for it. Of course, this cannot be done by a drug information pharmacist routinely on every patient, but it can be performed selectively on certain patients where experience has shown that difficulties are most likely to be encountered. Where a clinical pharmacy staff is functioning, this activity should be left to their expertise. In this situation, the drug information pharmacist and a clinical pharmacist can work in unison with each other.

Facilities

The pharmacist who provides the various informational services described must have adequate facilities. Just as a drug information pharmacist should not have any other responsibilities, such as dispensing, simultaneously with his drug information activities, he should not have to share physical facilities in areas where these other activities are being performed. He should be provided with a location that is physically isolated from the rest of the pharmacy department. The ideal location for a center is within the confines of the institution's medical library. The reasons for this are obvious; that is where the information can be found. Thus, the main criterion for determining location is accessibility to the information, that is to say, accessibility to the pharmaceutical and medical literature. The accessibility of the center to users of the service is relatively unimportant since the vast majority of them will request information over the telephone rather than by their physical presence. Consequently, locating a drug information center in a heavy traffic area of the hospital is of little importance.

Space required for a center's activities is really determined by whether or not the facilities of a medical library are readily available. If they are, then a service can operate with a very minimum amount of space. Ample space for several desks, three or four file cabinets and a couple of bookshelves is all that is necessary. On the other hand, if access to a medical library is not available, then considerably more space will be required. The number of textbooks and reference books is pretty much the same for any service, but without library facilities the storage area needed for journal collections and reprint files becomes the main determinant of space requirements. If extensive journal collections and reprint files are maintained then several hundred square feet as a minimum will be required. However, if microfilming is used, space can be reduced substantially.

In addition to desks, file cabinets and bookshelves, a typewriter and telephone are obvious necessities. Less obvious equipment that should be part of an information center is a telephone answering device that will give and take a message. These devices are available either from the Bell System or from other private sources. They are very useful when no one is available to answer the phone, such as after hours or when the drug information pharmacist is on rounds or gathering information outside of the center. A small blackboard and a bulletin board are also handy items to have.

Personnel Requirements

We have determined what drug information is, what the scope of drug information is, what services a drug information center may provide and the physical facilities required for a drug information center, but we have not discussed any specifics in regard to the people who actually provide the service. The individuals who provide drug information may be called drug information specialists, clinical pharmacists or clinical drug communications specialists. The title is unimportant, but their experience and training is paramount. The training and experience of a drug information service pharmacist must be clinically based. There is no way that a drug information service in the context of what has been discussed so far can be provided without a clinical orientation. The user population for any information service is going to be primarily clinicians and to communicate with these people effectively you must be speaking their language. This cannot be done without having the clinician's frame of reference, *i.e.*, the patient. While it is true that many pharmacy schools are restructuring their curriculum to provide a more clinically relevant undergraduate education, it is still a necessity for a pharmacist to gain his clinical experience by on-the-job activities. Becoming involved with the medical team on ward rounds, attending various speciality conferences and grand rounds, taking patient's drug histories and providing informal drug information consultations during this training phase is prerequisite to full-time service in a drug information center. The length of this "clinical internship" is dependent upon the intensity of the exposure and the aggressiveness of the individual in becoming involved in the patient-care area. Thus, the duration of this period cannot be set arbitrarily, but a reasonable end point could be one where the pharmacist feels that he has confidence in his ability to communicate on an equal level with other clinicians.

In addition to clinical experience, which does not stop when one becomes a full-time "drug information specialist" but must be continually supplemented by participation in medical rounds, conferences and the like, one must be proficient in literature retrieval, analysis and evaluation. Also, one must be able to comprehend the full range of the biomedical literature. Demonstrated ability at all levels of communication, written and verbal, is also a prerequisite for a drug information pharmacist.

The necessity to obtain clinical experience before assuming the responsibilities of drug information should not be considered as a discouragement or as an obstacle. Also, it does not imply that one needs clinical training as a pharmacy student. A pharmacist who has kept reasonably abreast with his profession and therapeutic innovations and developments is required to have only the desire and ambition to become clinically oriented. It is safe to say that virtually all pharmacists who consider themselves clinical types achieve this through their own postgraduate efforts rather than through any formal training. This is very likely going to be the situation in most instances for some time to come.

The assignment of additional pharmacists to a center should be based upon the utilization rate and the teaching burden imposed upon the service. Nonprofessional personnel required for the service functions of a center are usually limited to the employment of one capable clerk-typist. Ordinarily, this is adequate for all but the busiest services. This individual should have a familiarity with medical and pharmacological terminology, in addition to the normal clerical and secretarial skills. Some services may get along with a half-time individual, but the majority will require one full-time individual for this position. This person should be responsible for maintaining the library, filing, maintenance of reprint and other files, updating index and abstract services and other nonprofessional clerical functions.

In addition to physical and staff requirements, the problem of anticipating the relative workload in certain aspects of drug information, *e.g.*, adverse reactions and dosages, is frequently considered. There has been published at least one survey of the information needs of health professionals in the hospital, particularly nurses and physicians.[5] Such studies are done in anticipation of establishing a drug information center in an effort to allow for organization of reference materials to meet the anticipated needs. It is questionable whether it needs to be given serious consideration. Generally this type of survey is an exercise in futility. There is absolutely no doubt that the need for information exists, but the question of how to fill the need is quite another story. It cannot be readily determined by superficial surveys. If an individual is not aware of the information he needs, no amount of interviewing or questionnaire forms will bring this out. Unquestionably a large amount of information is needed by nurses and physicians that is fairly unsophisticated and can be found in most existing reference sources, but this is by no means the real problem. The real problem is promoting the rational usage of drugs, the absence of which is usually the result of ignorance. The real job of a drug information service is to identify those areas where knowledge is lacking and to pursue them vigorously to provide the information that is really essential in patient care. What people think they want and what they really need are quite often two different things.

Operational Procedures

Naturally, as with any other organized service function there has to be a defined hierarchy with delineated responsibilities. Most information centers have a pharmacist who is responsible for the administration and formulation of policy. In most cases, the administrative functions are relatively routine and do not require a great deal of time, but because the organized information aspect of pharmacy practice is still in the development phase, the formulation of policies and methods of operation are extremely important responsibilities. Those responsible for this should have a great deal of clinical and drug information experience. Acceptance of drug information services by the other health professions is still by no means an assured occurrence, thus all policy decisions must be contemplated with thoroughness before implementation. The basic guideline that should be used for justifying policy decisions is to consider what effect it might have on promoting the rational usage of drugs. Considerations as to pleasing the users are important but they should not take precedence over what is ultimately good for the patient. In other words, service should not be provided solely on the basis of the desires of the user.

Hours of Service

After deciding on general policies and the service areas that are to be embraced by the drug information service, the routine operating procedures must be delineated. The most basic operating parameter that must be established is the hours of operation. If the responsibility of poison control is assumed then this decision is made for you. Providing poison control services demands a 24-hour operation. It does not mean that somebody has to be physically present within the confines of the center 24 hours a day and, in fact, few if any services do this. What is usually done in a 24-hour service is to have one of two shifts a day (*i.e.*, 16 hours) covered by drug information pharmacists with the remaining 8 hours, usually the night shift and holidays, covered by an on-call clinical pharmacist who is always within the institution but may be assigned to another area of the pharmacy department. This is the only time you can compromise the basic principle that a drug information pharmacist should not be encumbered by other responsibilities. The demands on a night time pharmacist in the hospital are usually not of such magnitude that he cannot handle both his primary responsibilities and any poison control or drug information problems that may arise during this period of the day. Variations will occur in demands depending upon the institution's size.

If poison control is not to be included as a service then the hours should be based on anticipated or realized utilization and available resources for personnel. The experiences at the 553-bed, University of California Hospital, San Francisco, has been that the operating hours of 8 a.m. to 11 p.m., Monday through Friday and 2 p.m. to 11 p.m. on weekends and holidays with on-call clinical pharmacists coverage at other times, have been feasible to meet the utilization demands placed on the service. The staff required for this is two full-time pharmacists, one half-time pharmacist and one full-time clerk typist. Periods of peak utilization at U.C.S.F. are late mornings and early evenings and this pattern would probably hold true for most large teaching hospitals.

Records

Drug information practice is not devoid of paper work. Just as the dispensing pharmacist has his prescriptions and other records, a drug information specialist must maintain records of his activities as well. The most basic record is the daily log book (Figure 1). The log book serves as a record for utilization, the patterns of utilization, the type of professional utilizing the service and similar data. This record is a statistical profile of the overall use of the service. It can be relatively simple as is the one utilized by the Drug Information Analysis Service (DIAS) at U.C.S.F. or it can be as elaborate as one wants to make it. It depends upon how much information on utilization patterns is required.

The DIAS utilizes a simple laboratory log book with prenumbered pages. The information noted for each drug information request is the date, the time, the professional classification of the caller, *e.g.*, M.D., Pharm. D., the source of the call, *e.g.*, County Hospital, a brief, two or three-word statement as to the nature of the request and the pharmacist's initials. This simple record-keeping chore, admirably fulfills the need for a utilization profile. Needless to say, the record keeping does not stop with the log book. A permanent record of consultations or requests is kept by most drug information centers. Here again, there are a var-

112

Date	Time	Caller	Source	Question	Pharm
11/20	7:00 PM	Layman	SF	PCP? Procaine HCl?	JR
11/21/70	2:00 PM	PharmD	9th	dosing - IM vs PO digoxin	LKD
11/21/70	2:50 PM	Pharm.	E. Bay-Oakland	GI effects of Vit. C	LKD
11/21/70	5:30 PM	Pharm Stdt.	St Francis Hosp.	IV incompatibility	LKD
11/21/70	7:30 PM	RN	ICU	reconstitution of drug	LKD
11/21/70	9:30 PM	MD	SFGH	pKa of drug (tx of poisoning)	LKD
11/22/70	1:30 PM	PharmD	10th fl.	drug interaction-significance	LKD
11/22/70	1:40 PM	RN (student)	UCSF	use of drug	LKD
11/22/70	2:40 PM	RN	UCSF	poisoning - Atarax + $FeSO_4$	LKD
11/22/70	4:50 PM	PharmD	9th fl.	efficacy (steroids for mood elev.)	LKD
11/22/70	6:00 PM	Nurs. Stdt.	UCSF	drug use & effects	LKD
11/22/70	9/15	MD	[illegible]	[illegible] toxicity (Kidney)	[illegible]
11/22/70	9:15	MD	10th Flr	Kanamycin Dosing with Peritoneal Dialysis	DA
11/23	8:45 AM	PharmD	UC	Adverse React.	ETH
11/23	8:45	PharmD	UC	Use + adverse effect	ETH
11/23	9:00	MD	UCER	Ingestion - Thorazine	ETH
11/23	10 am	MD	UCER	Ingestion	ETH
11/23	9:30	PharmD	El Cerrito	Availability	ETH
11/23	9:30	PharmD	Palo Alto	Ingredients	ETH
11/23	10:07	[illegible]	SF	Drug Abuse	ETH
11/23	10:25	MD	U.C	Drug I.D.	ETH
11/23	11:25	RN	UC	Sterility + Indication	ETH
11/23	11:30	PharmD	Oakland	Drug I.D.	ETH
11/23	12:45	PharmD	SF	Analysis of drug	ETH
11/23	12:30	MD	UC	Use of drug	ETH
11/23	1:58	PharmD	Stanford	Dose in Uremia	ETH
11/23	2:00 PM	PharmD	Oakland	Toxicity	DA

(Margin notes: Saturday; Sunday; Monday)

Figure 1. Page from daily log book

UNIVERSITY OF CALIFORNIA HOSPITALS – DRUG INFORMATION ANALYSIS SERVICE

REQUESTED BY: ______ DATE: ______

ADDRESS: ______ TELEPHONE: ______

PATIENT HISTORY:

REQUEST:

RESPONSE:

REFERENCES:

______, Pharm.D.

DIAS-I

Figure 2. DIAS report form

Figure 3. DIAS business card

UNIVERSITY OF CALIFORNIA, SAN FRANCISCO
SAN FRANCISCO, CALIF. 94122

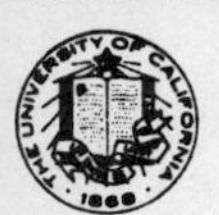

DRUG INFORMATION ANALYSIS SERVICE

HOURS: 8 A.M.–11 P.M.
MONDAY–FRIDAY
(415) 666-4346

24 HOUR EMERGENCY SERVICE
(415) 666-2155

iety of forms but the experience of the DIAS with a number of variations has shown that the simpler the better. The form currently used (Figure 2) by the DIAS contains information on the individual requesting the information, the patient's history, the request, the response and the reference used. Forms that are too severely structured inhibit the consultative aspect of the service. If one is to be a consultant, he should feel free to communicate any information in his own style with a free hand. So basically, all that is really needed is a blank piece of paper with a minimum of preprinted data. The latter should serve the purpose only of providing for the efficient storing of the information for future reference. The DIAS form, incidently, is printed on a heavy-gauged paper so it files easier. The space in the upper right hand corner is used as a subject heading for indexing these records. They are filed under the nonproprietary name of the drug involved or the disease state as primary classification headings and then they are cross-indexed under the circumstance that prompted the request. For example, if a request were for the proper dosage of kanamycin in a patient with renal failure, the consult would be filed under the generic name of the drug involved, *i.e.*, kanamycin, and cross-indexed under uremia. If more than one drug is involved in a response, the primary heading is usually the disease state involved, with cross-indexing under each of the drugs.

Work Priorities

I have established the personnel requirements, hours of operation and the records necessary for use. When the first request for information arrives, what do we do with it? The first thing that has to be done with every request for information is to assign a priority to it. The most appropriate way to establish priority is to determine the acuteness of the situation. Obviously, patient-oriented problems take precedence over hypothetical or purely informational problems. Of course, poisonings take precedence over everything. With experience, one can mentally assess the amount of time that will be required to fulfill a consulting responsibility and establish its priority relative to the current workload. In this way the caller can be given a reasonable estimate of the time when he will receive his reply. One other factor that enters into priority as well, is when a center is servicing the professional community outside its own institution. In this situation, priority will usually be given to staff members of the parent institution.

Management of Requests

After establishing priority for the question, the next step is to classify the request. This is necessary for efficient handling. The classification will dictate the approach to gathering the information necessary to base a consultation on. Following initial classification, the request is further refined to enable a search. The entire procedure consists of mentally classifying the question in a broad sense, *e.g.*, adverse reaction, and then refining it to specific terms such as a drug causing a specific unwanted effect, interference of lab tests and so on. With experience, this whole procedure can be done mentally, but Pearson and Salter at the University of Michigan have worked out a formalized set of aids to classifying the nature of drug information requests.[6]

Besides classifying and refining the requests to aid the search, it is very important to insure that all of the pertinent information is received from the caller. Not infrequently, a physician will request a single, isolated bit of information, *e.g.*, the half-life or pKa of a drug, in the hope of solving a much larger problem which depends on that one piece of information. In other words, he thinks that he has the key to the puzzle. On careful questioning it frequently turns out that his isolated piece of information may not solve the problem and in fact may even complicate things by misleading the caller. So as a consequence, a drug information pharmacist must question every caller for a complete background, the reasons why the question has been asked and for all pertinent information on the patient involved. In a sense the drug information pharmacist asks more questions than he answers. The classic example of this sort of situation is the problem of adverse reactions. The usual circumstance is similar to the following: somebody calls and asks whether or not a certain drug is known to produce a maculopapular rash. If this question is taken at face value you may find out the drug does, but you may not note that the patient is taking three or four other drugs that could be at fault and because of circumstantial evidence may indeed be responsible. Even a very simple question, such as dosage, requires knowledge of the patient; such things as kidney function, liver function, weight and the disease state may require substantial modifications of the dose. Responding with the usual empirical dose as an answer may be quite wrong. Examples of this sort are endless. It cannot be over-emphasized that to be effective in drug information one has to obtain all the pertinent information of the circumstances surrounding the request. This is one of the reasons why clinical experience is so important for drug information pharmacists. With a clinical orientation, the gathering of the appropriate patient parameters for a specific request comes naturally.

Dissemination of Information

Assuming that the consultation has been completed, the problem arises as to how best to communicate this information. Simply providing a photocopy of published information is inadequate even if it fulfills the need of the inquirer. You do not need a pharmacist to perform this function and as a consequence it cannot be justified as a professional service. The best approach is to give oral replies whenever possible. Since the pharmacist-operated drug information center is a consultative service rather than one of simple information retrieval, it is better to discuss the problem with the individual with whom you are consulting. In this way, clarification can be made of ambiguous points and understanding is guaranteed. These things may not be resolved on a written report. Of course, the oral consultation can and in many cases should be supplemented by a written report. The latter situation should prevail when a written report is requested or when the information pharmacist believes that the information is sufficiently complex to warrant a written document for reference purposes.

Every request requires documentation. This does not mean that every statement that is made must have a reference index number attached to it followed by a literature citation. On the contrary, documentation can take the form of personal knowledge and experience or it can be based on interpretation and extrapolation of existing data. Of course, it can be based upon literature citations as well, but it should not be restricted to the latter. In fact, if one is truly providing a consulting service, it becomes apparent that a consultation of merit depends on documentation of fact and the personal experiences of the consultant. The essence of clinical orientation is really the experience gained in achieving this perspective. When one speaks with the authority of experience, he is often more effective than if he essentially says the same thing without the confidence that experience provides. The personal knowledge and experience of a drug information pharmacist should play a major role in the formulation of drug information consults.

Frequently information that is available in the literature is contradictory, equivocal or scanty on a particular subject. When faced with these situations a drug information pharmacist should be able to analyze and interpret the data to arrive at the best possible solutions based upon his training and his experience. This is also a legitimate source of documentation, but it should be labeled as interpretation or speculation so there are no misunderstandings. Fortunately, however, the majority of the situations have a reasonable parallel in the literature and it is comforting to be able to answer a problem unequivocally based on a wealth of published data. Obviously, when this approach is available it is the most reasonable to take. Unless one's personal experience is overwhelmingly contradictory to what is in the literature it is probably, at this stage in the game anyway, better to suppress one's limited experience and accept the judgment of many investigators. This assumes that one has already made a judgment as to the validity of the published material.

The actual preparation of written reports should not be a time-consuming project. When utilization of the service becomes significant, the information pharmacist will not have the time to write definitive, exhaustive reports on every request. Whenever written reports are indicated they should be preceded by a thorough oral reply to the user. The oral reply should not be terminated until the information pharmacist feels that the caller has a firm grasp of the consultation subject matter. Then the written report can be a summary document which presumes that the recipient will have a thorough background and thus the report does not require the inclusion of a lot of background discussion. For example, if one is asked to evaluate the efficacy of a certain drug, the written report should not go into exhaustive detail on the pharmacology of the drug. Any gaps in the caller's knowledge in this area should have been cleared up orally. The reply should be simply a discussion of the virtues or lack of them compared to equivalent drugs for the same use.

Evaluation of Services

Every drug information center must have procedures whereby the effectiveness of the service can be evaluated on a continuing basis. Monitoring and assessing the effectiveness of a service are not only necessary to increase the quality of the service rendered but also to justify its continuing existence to the department responsible for financing its activities. In general, the utilization rate is the most important measurement of effectiveness. Ordinarily, it is safe to assume that if utilization begins to drop off or never really gets off the ground, the quality and utility of the information being provided are not sufficient. There are, however, other parameters that should also be measured. Such things as the response time to requests for information, the types of information being requested and, most importtantly, the effect of the service on patient care. Also, one may wish to solicit evaluations from the health professionals who utilize the service. The latter procedure may be done by following-up on requests and by asking the recipient to respond as to whether the answer was sufficient or not sufficient. In addition, any other comments on the service may be requested. This procedure is used by the Michigan Drug Information Network[7] and others may also find it useful.

Utilization rate, time spent in responding, types of requests asked, the area served and the type of professional utilizing the service all can be measured by the maintenance of a log book or form. However, measuring the direct effect of the service on patient care is quite another problem. There are several alternatives available to determine this parameter of effectiveness, although none of them is fully reliable. The easiest procedure is to follow-up the patient-specific consultations at some later date by procuring the patient's chart and determining the effect of the drug information consultation on that patient's course. Determine whether or not the information provided was utilized in the patient's care and, if used, whether or not it was effective or solved the particular problem at hand. It is also valuable to determine what the patient's course was when the information provided was not utilized and to make some speculations as to what might have happened if the consultation was accepted. In this manner, one can get a fair view of the overall effectiveness relative to patient drug therapy. The deficiency of this procedure is that not all requests for information are patient-specific or if they are they may not all be within one's own institution. Getting follow-ups on patients in other institutions has logistical problems that usually preclude follow-up by the drug information pharmacist himself. However, in this situation one can request follow-ups from the individual using the drug information service.

The other method of measuring the contribution of an information service to patient care is to establish a review committee composed of, for example, an internist, a clinical pharmacologist and a clinical pharmacist, or any other qualified individuals, to evaluate the written reports provided by the service for their accuracy and validity. This advisory panel can be quite useful in providing constructive criticism and advice in addition to evaluating the service rendered. The major drawback to this procedure is that the written reports which are or should be a summary of the consultation may not always tell the full story. In fact, the consultation may have been quite adequate when communicated orally, but appears weak in the written form. In any event, if utilization rate continues to increase, particularly from health professionals within the local institution, it can be assumed that the service is effective. However, this is not an excuse to adopt a complacent attitude. An information center must be a dynamic operation.

Publicizing the Center

In addition to providing all the services associated with a drug information center, there should be an effort to promote its utilization. Promoting the use of the center really can be considered part of an overall scheme encouraging the rational use of drugs. A big obstacle to rational drug therapy is ignorance. Encouraging health professionals to develop the habit of utilizing a drug information service will go a long way in replacing ignorance with knowledge. There are many ways of publicizing a center. The pharmacist can discuss its use at medical intern and resident orientation programs, at speciality conferences, at pharmacy and therapeutic committee meetings, through a bulletin or newsletter and through various memos. Also, the distribution of business cards (Figure 3) to the appropriate individuals can help increase utilization of a drug information service.

Sources of Information

We have been discussing information services without mentioning where the information comes from. Eventually, of course, the information can be said to come from the drug information pharmacist communicating it. This is a primary source of information in many instances. The use of personal experience and knowledge as a source of documentation was previously discussed. Experience is also a source of information. For the same reasons that experience is a good source of documentation, it is also a good source of information. Observations made over the course of the last few years at the DIAS indicate that it is one of the better sources of information. The next best thing to one's own experience are the experiences of one's colleagues. Sharing clinical experiences among colleagues can be a successful teaching exercise as well as an excellent source of information. Since most of us tend to specialize our interests in one or several areas of drug usage, *e.g.*, antibiotics and antihypertensives, the limits of experience as a source of information are relatively narrow. Nevertheless, where experience does exist, it should be a primary source.

Periodical Literature and Books

When experience is inadequate there are a number of alternative sources of information that can be exploited. The periodical biomedical literature in association with medical records is the foundation of most drug information services. Whenever possible the current literature should be utilized as a source of information. Reference and textbooks, although quite useful in many situations, should play a secondary role to the literature as sources of information. When dealing with patient-specific problems, it is best to have the most up-to-date information for evaluation and application to the problem at hand. Books have a built in factor of obsolescence because of the time involved in preparation, publication and distribution. Of course, for factual data of a nature that would not change, *e.g.*, chemical and physical properties, reference books can be a primary source. Books are also a good jumping off point into the literature. It is well to know what is considered to be the relevant knowledge of a subject up to a certain point in time *i.e.*, the publication date of the book. Following this up with the current literature will determine whether or not the newer information adds anything to what can be found in the reference book.

Card Systems, Patients' Records and Consultants

Additional sources that are often maintained by centers include card filing systems. These may consist of 4 x 7 inch cards with drug monograph-like information consistent with or approximating that of a package insert. They may contain a specialized area of information such as drug interactions which may be extracted and compiled from the literature and put on the cards for easy retrieval. Medical records of patients can also be useful sources of information. By analyzing the effects of drugs in patients with similar problems one can frequently make some judgments and extrapolate the data to other patients. Another source of information is the use of consultants. However, since drug information pharmacists are themselves consultants, it is generally a good rule to avoid the use of other specialists. Just as you would expect them to call you for drug information you should refer individuals with problems outside your area to the appropriate consultant rather than performing the function of the middle man. If a consultant is required for the problem it is probably out of the domain of a drug information center. Of course, there are situations where reliance on a consultant may be indicated. This situation might occur when most of the problem is resolved, but a few pieces of information necessary to complete the consultation are missing. The use of consultants with personal experience in the particular area may provide the information when it cannot be found in the literature.

Information Retrieval

The most important technical activity of a drug information pharmacist is the retrieval of information. This will be a determining factor in the response time to requests for information and also a determinant of the validity of the information in the sense that the retrieval and search must be thorough. Combining thoroughness with speed is the primary goal when selecting index and abstracting services for a drug information service.

Among the most useful manual retrieval systems available are the *Paul de Haen Drug Card Systems*, the *FDA Clinical Experience Abstracts*, various National Library of Medicine publications such as *Index Medicus, International Pharmaceutical Abstracts* and Excerpta Medica abstract and title publications. In addition to manual retrieval systems, there are a number of automated literature search systems including the *Iowa Drug Information Service, MEDLARS* and *Excerpta Medica Drug Information Systems.*

Manual Retrieval Systems

The selection of a literature retrieval system, either manual or automated, is based on several criteria. They include the acceptable period of lag time between publication of the original article and the appearance of its citation in the retrieval system, the total number and scope of journals indexed by the retrieval system, whether an abstract or just a citation is required, and the ease and speed with which a search can be done with the system. Unless a center has the facilities of a large medical library available, the number and scope of the journals, within certain minimal limits, indexed and abstracted by a retrieval system is not a primary factor in selection. It does little good to invest in a system that indexes 5,000 journals if you have only 100 or so available. The probable minimum necessary is the 100 English language journals indexed by the *NLM Abridged Index Medicus.* Although 100 quality journals may provide 80 or 90 percent of the information that one is most likely to need, it should still be considered the bare minimum requirement. If a service is to provide information of a sort that is not always easily found, it should have a retrieval system that supplements and expands upon what is covered by the *Abridged Index Medicus.* This requirement assumes that the original journals or their reprints are readily available.

At the other end of the spectrum, in terms of depth of coverage, is the *Index Medicus* itself. This is a monthly bibliographic listing of references to current articles from approximately 2300 of the world's biomedical journals. Some of the Excerpta Medica publications, such as *Adverse Reaction Titles,* approach or exceed this number of journals also. These publications, of course, represent exhaustive index services and, again, are only useful if the journals cited are available, in as much as these services do not provide abstracts.

Although the *Index Medicus* and similar indexing services that provide only a literature citation are all-inclusive in terms of the number of journals covered, they are relatively cumbersome to use. The lack of an abstract usually means that the cited article almost always has to be retrieved and perused before accepting or rejecting it as a potential source of information. As a consequence, these services should not be used by a drug information center as primary retrieval systems. They are, however, necessary for the performance of thorough searches of the literature.

The primary system should be one that can be used rapidly, that has a short lag time from appearance of the original article to the citation and covers a relatively broad scope of journals. Of the manual systems available, only the *Paul de Haen Drug Card Systems* fulfills all these criteria. Although de Haen has several card index services, the most useful to a drug information center is the *Drugs in Use System.* At U.C.S.F. we have found that this system works quite well. It should be pointed out, however, that unless the original journals or reprints are available this system has limited utility. Although they are in a tabulated abstract form, it must be emphasized that a pharmacist should never make judgments based on abstracts alone. This principle is not limited to the de Haen System, but to all abstract services. *Drugs in Use* reviews about 500 journals, both domestic and foreign, providing about 7,000 abstracts per year. These abstracts are printed on 4 x 7 inch cards which contain such information as: number of patients involved in the study, type of study, dosages used, routes of administration, descriptions of the subjects, *e.g.*, sex, age and the disease state, purpose of the study, adverse reactions, laboratory values and the author's comments and conclusions. This information is displayed in a manner that is logical and uniform with regard to the facts contained in the original study. This makes it very easy to quickly retrieve a pertinent study because of the manner in which the information is visually displayed. This allows for correlation of patients and their disease states to articles that may provide information useful in solving their therapeutic problems.

Other abstract-index systems available that may be useful are the *International Pharmaceutical Abstracts (IPA), Excerpta Medica: Pharmacology and Toxicology* and some of the other Excerpta Medica speciality abstracts, and the *FDA Clinical Experience Abstracts.* All of these services are deficient in one area or another in meeting the criteria outlined as being necessary for an effective index and retrieval system. The major drawback of all of these publications is the narrative form of their abstracts. The narrative format makes it necessary to read the abstract, usually in its entirety, to make a determination as to whether the original article is relevant to the problem at hand. This makes them somewhat slower at retrieval than the *Drugs in Use System.* They also have a relatively longer lag time between appearance of the original article and the abstract. However, this problem is being solved by *IPA* and the FDA abstracts. Both the *de Haen Drugs in Use* and the *FDA Clinical Experience Abstracts,* because they are provided on index cards, can be retrieved for a particular drug much more rapidly than can a monthly collection of abstracts published in a magazine form. *IPA* and the Excerpta Medica abstracts are of the latter type and for the most recent issues it requires perusing the individual monthly issues to gather the appropriate citations. They do provide semiannual or annual cumulative indexes which reduce the search time for the slightly older literature.

IPA does have some advantages over the others for information published on pharmacokinetic and biopharmaceutical data which is not easily found in de Haen, in Excerpta Medica or in the FDA abstracts. It is more pharmaceutically oriented and in this respect serves as a valuable secondary source to one of the more clinically directed literature indexes such as de Haen.

Automated Retrieval Systems

In addition to the manual retrieval systems described above, there are several automated systems available. For practical everyday application in a drug information center there are only two proprietary systems generally available and only one of these, the *Iowa Drug Information System,* is within reach of the average center. The other is the *Excerpta Medica Drug Literature Index* which is quite an extensive computer-based index system, but it is extremely expensive. The MEDLARS system is an operation of NLM (National Library of Medicine) and is also a computerized service, but it is not one to which a center can avail itself on an instantaneous or regular basis. Some services may wish to use MEDLARS from time to time, but for most practical purposes, it is not of much value to a service-oriented drug information center. If, on occasion, comprehensive literature searches on particular subjects are required, then MEDLARS may be useful.

The Excerpta Medica drug information system sounds like the ultimate in index and literature retrieval systems, but because of the price, it is impractical at present. However, a description of the system is warranted in hopes that it will become economically feasible in the future. The drug literature index section of the system covers the total world output of biomedical journals. It gives rapid access to any article, concerning any drug, published anywhere in the world. All articles on drugs from 3,000 biomedical journals are included in the data base. The information recorded on computer tape includes the full title of the article in English, the names of the authors, their affiliation, the title of the journal and its volume, page and date. Also included in the indexing are the generic names of the drugs, their trade names, as well as such medical indexing terms as clinical indications, contraindications, clinical effects and pharmacologic effects. In addition, adverse reactions that are noted are also included on the tape. Retrieval can be approached through the generic names index, or a new product index. Thus, access to the system is available through a number of routes and appears to be quite comprehensive in this respect. The system should be extremely fast in retrieving citations but, as with the other systems, it is only useful when the original journals are available to the user.

The more available system is the Drug Literature Microfilm File of the Iowa Drug Information Service, College of Pharmacy, University of Iowa. This system goes one step beyond the citation and abstract format characteristics of the other available alternatives since it provides the user with a copy of the entire article cited. Thus, it is particularly useful for information centers isolated from traditional medical library facilities. Approximately 200 English language medical and pharmaceutical journals are covered by this service and all articles from these periodicals which discuss the clinical use of drugs are microfilmed in total. The microfilm provided to the user is a handy 7" x 3" microfiche which contains an average of nine sequentially numbered articles. Indexing information is stored in a computer and also printed out on index cards which are used for manual retrieval by each user. The indexing schema is simple, with manual retrieval done alphabetically either by generic name of the drug discussed in an article or the clinical classification discussed, which includes diseases, operations, tests and adverse reactions to chemical substances. Approximately 2,800 generic entities are documented and the clinical index contains 1,500 terms from the International Classification of Diseases, Adapted Index. Secondary index terms which appear on every index card include: title, author, microfilm number of the complete article, source, and descriptors, which are brief pharmaceutical key words used to describe the contents of the article or define its structure.

Although this system does require the purchase or lease of a microfilm reader or reader/printer, it does conserve storage space of information. Retrieval by each user, who receives monthly updates of new articles and matching index cards, is completely manual and no computer equipment is needed. Computer searches of the entire data base which is retroactive to January, 1966 and includes as of 1970 approximately 15,000 articles are run by the Iowa Drug Information Service on demand. However, computer searches are not practical for problems of an immediate nature.

The journal coverage is not as extensive as in the de Haen system, nor data as research-oriented. However, the indexing schema is considerably simplified and access to the complete article may be a compensating advantage, depending on the environment of the information center.

Specialized Manual Retrieval Systems

Up to now, we have discussed retrieval systems for the general biomedical literature. There are a number of specialized index citation and abstract services available. The *NLM Toxicity Bibliography, Clin-Alert, Unlisted Drugs* and *Excerpta Medica Adverse Reactions Titles* are useful publications to have available in a drug information center. The *Toxicity Bibliography* appears quarterly and covers the adverse and toxic effects of drugs and chemicals reported in the 2300 journals used by *Index Medicus.* This is a useful index for background information on toxicological problems. It is not of much use in the acute situations but there are circumstances where a thorough search of the literature in this area is indicated. Chronic exposure to insecticides, for example, may be a patient problem where the *Toxicity Bibliography* may serve as a retrieval instrument for information pertinent to that patient's problem.

Clin-Alert is a collection of abstracts of articles published in other journals reporting adverse reactions and side effects of drugs. It is issued about every two weeks and is most useful as a continuing review of adverse reactions for the pharmacist rather than as a primary source for information. This is because there is little indication as to how thorough the coverage of the literature is and it is poorly indexed. On the other hand, the *Adverse Reactions Titles* covers about 3,000 biomedical journals published throughout the world. It is an exhaustive index of adverse reactions. However, it provides only journal citations, not abstracts, so one must have the original journal for this system to be useful in any manner. If the journals are available, *Adverse Reaction Titles* is the last word in attempting to document the occurrence of a particular reaction.

Unlisted Drugs is a monthly publication that deals with new drugs, investigational drugs and foreign drugs. It identifies and describes, on a current basis, all those newly reported drug compounds and products which as yet are not listed by name, manufacturer and composition in a basic set of common drug reference compendia. It is most useful to the drug information pharmacist in identifying foreign drugs and investigational drugs for interested people. It provides a basic profile of the drug such as other names, chemistry and usage as well as the original literature citation.

In this discussion, the various retrieval systems available have been analyzed. No attempts have been made to evaluate other reference sources such as textbooks and reference manuals. A suggested reference list of these sources can be found on page 175. Since the current literature and access to it are the primary problems of most drug information centers, the retrieval systems are far more important considerations than are reference books.

Organization and Storage of Information

Every center must maintain informational files in addition to reference books and the selected retrieval systems. There must be an organized method established for storing reprints, tear sheets, photostatic copies, etc. This material should be stored and organized in such a fashion that easy retrieval is provided for. There are a number of methods for doing this and the best one is really dependent upon the needs of the service. A service located in a large medical library will be unlikely to require a large file of reprints. On the other hand, a center located away from a library will be very dependent upon reprints and will need a more sophisticated system.

A prototype system for filing medical literature has been described by Fuller.[8] This system is based on the method developed originally by Maxwell Wintrobe. It is a unified method for filing medical literature that can be adapted and individually tailored to meet the needs of varying disciplines and interests. The system is based on a numbered index that is developed by the user and can be expanded and modified. Reprints are filed in manila folders marked with the same index number.

An adaptation of the Wintrobe method for a drug information service has been developed by Dr. Philip Hansten who was formerly the Director of the Alta Bates Community Hospital Drug Information Service in Berkeley, California. His system involves using a consecutive numbering system combined with the *American Hospital Formulary Service (AHFS)* drug classification numbering system. An index is maintained under the AHFS classification. For example, a reprint of an article concerning tetracycline would be indexed on the page headed 8:12.24 in the index. On this index page a number is stamped with a prescription numbering machine with the same number stamped on the reprint itself. The reprint is then filed numerically in a binder, file drawer or some similar manner. Thus, if reprints are needed for tetracycline all one simply does is to look up the appropriate section in the index binder and get the numbers of the articles cited. These then can be retrieved from the file drawer by their numerical order. No manila folders are required and processing of a large number of incoming reprints is relatively simple under this system.

The U.C.S.F.-DIAS method of filing reprints is also based on the Wintrobe method. A large reprint file is not necessary for this service so a numerical listing of all reprints on file is also unnecessary. What is needed is a general classification system that maintains order between the location of the reprints and the index. Instead of using the AHFS numerical drug code, a broad therapeutic group classification designed by Paul de Haen is utilized. Although this does not break it down to the individual drug, it does provide a sufficiently structured classification for the maintenance of a small file. An index binder is maintained with a sheet for each therapeutic group classification, for example broad-spectrum antibiotics, on which articles fitting into this classification are indexed. The article is then coded with the same therapeutic group number and filed in a filing folder corresponding to that group number. Retrieval requires going through the entire folder for that therapeutic group for one particular article, but since the total number of articles is small it is not a problem. If a large number of reprints are filed, then a system similar to the Hansten method is more appropriate. The foregoing are examples of filing systems which are presented to illustrate alternatives. These are adequate for the particular centers that utilize them, but they may not be sufficient in all situations. Every service should take the time to design a filing system to meet its individual needs.

Information can be stored on microfilm and microfiche or computer tapes. For an individual center to do this on its own probably is not worth the expenditure in terms of what can be gained from such procedures. Undoubtedly, in the future, to save space and to ease retrieval, more mechanized approaches to filing and retrieving information will be utilized. The technology is available at present and it is only a question of time until the demand will justify the expenditure. It should be emphasized that one should not expect a computer based information system to replace or infringe upon the responsibilities of a drug information pharmacist. Computers will be very useful tools to a drug information service, but they will never be able to make judgments or interpretations of the literature. Individuals responsible for providing a consultative drug information service will always be an interface between the clinician and the machine. Someone has to be available to interpret the information, to analyze the information and to apply the information that comes out of a machine. In addition, a machine is limited in the number of questions that it can ask a user. There are many patient parameters that must be considered when applying a piece of drug information. This can be provided in a computer program, but it will be relatively inflexible and will always require a human being that is capable of judgment.

Evaluating Information

Evaluation of the literature is an extremely important task and represents a basic skill for the drug information pharmacist. As has been noted there is no lack of information available. In fact, the amount of information available can be overwhelming. Unfortunately the information published is not of uniform quality and a lot of poor material and duplication of effort are apparent in the literature. Drug information specialists must be able to recognize the good, pertinent work. A lot of the literature is just plain irrelevant and inaccurate. There are a number of basic factors that should be considered when evaluating the literature. These factors will determine whether an article reflects the true picture of the clinical effectiveness and deficiencies of a drug. These include the clinical investigator, the place of the study, the test patients used, the techniques of the study and the interpretation of the results.

THE CLINICAL INVESTIGATOR

There are essentially four broad types of clinical investigators. There is the *clinical pharmacologist* who probably is the best qualified by training to observe and interpret drug actions accurately and to recognize pharmacological or toxic effects more readily. Unfortunately, there are not too many of these scientists around. Many investigators are the *special interest type, e.g.*, the physician who is an authority on the liver and is not primarily interested in drugs or their interactions unless they excite his interest by virtue of some unique property. Many combined studies are done by this type of investigator or by groups of them. There are many *specialists* such as surgeons, internists and so on who conduct studies. They usually do not have the knowledge and training of the clinical pharmacologist, but they do have a broad clinical knowledge in their particular speciality. This type of investigator is the most prevalent and is responsible for the vast majority of clinical drug studies. The last type of investigator is the *general physician.* These people are usually poor investigators because they do not have any of the attributes of the other three types except that they generally know their patients better.

Study Location and Patients Tested

Location of the study is of prime importance. Most investigations are best done in the controlled atmosphere of a hospital, especially a university teaching hospital where records, facilities and staff are better. There are, however, situations where these studies should not be carried out in such a controlled environment. For example, anti-anxiety drugs are probably better studied on outpatients to measure their true effects under the ordinary stresses of everyday living, whereas cardiac drugs can be assessed by quantitative monitoring devices and thus are better studied in the hospital setting. Studies emanating from private office patients usually are poor quality because of the lack of proper controls and generally their validity should be discounted. Obviously the test patients used must be appropriate and representative of the problem being studied if the results are to be extrapolated. For example, the results of studying a hypertensive drug on relatively sick hospitalized patients may not be extrapolatable to ambulatory outpatient hypertensives.

Study Techniques

Among the most critical factors that must be looked for when evaluating studies are the techniques used. They must be analyzed and interpreted carefully. There are very few situations in which the double-blind technique does not apply. An exception to the use of rigid controls is when quantitative measurements are used as a criteria for results of the study. This never applies in efficacy studies, but only for such things as measurement of blood levels, metabolic pathways and so on. The rotation of a placebo with active agents in some standard pattern is almost always necessary to secure proper perspective in any clinical drug study. The use of a placebo establishes a base line of activity. One may read studies where the authors explain that placebos were not used because the drug is known to be effective. This is not a valid argument. Additional information on this subject may be found in Chapter 25.

Interpretation of Results

Interpretation of the results of any study must be based on critical analysis. There are many considerations. Toxicity, for example, should be carefully evaluated against the relative merits of the drug. If the agent represents an essential advance where no satisfactory agent is presently available, as in cancer chemotherapeutics, the toxicity becomes a relatively lesser factor. Conversely to this principle, a new congener of existing drugs, such as phenothiazine, with exaggerated toxicity would offer no advantage and in fact would be considered a less efficacious agent. Side effects or adverse reactions observed with an agent may be the precursor of toxicity, especially in studies with new drugs. One should also look at how long a drug has been in use and its relative efficacy to alternative agents. All of these things must be considered when interpreting the results of a study.

Expediting the Evaluation

There are a few rules of thumb for a fast evaluation of a literature reference that can be used. These rules are particularly useful when looking at an abstract in an attempt to make a determination of whether or not to retrieve the original. The number of patients used can be a fair indication of the scope of the study and whether or not it is likely to be valid. Clinical trials for evaluating the efficacy of a new or old drug should involve relatively large numbers of patients. For determining the efficacy of a drug, 12 patients are usually not sufficient and a study often can be rejected on this basis alone. On the other hand, adverse reaction reports are valid even when based on a few patients, if the observers have carefully established a causal relationship. The number of patients used really depends upon what one is looking for. Another good rule of thumb is to look at a study to see whether or not side effects and adverse reactions are observed. If an author is purporting to evaluate the efficacy of an agent and cites that no side effects or adverse reactions were observed, you can automatically reject the study as being invalid. This is an indication that the investigators were not very observant. Any drug that has therapeutic effects also has side effects. Since they were not observant in this area one cannot have faith in their ability to observe the desired effects of the drugs.

As mentioned, controls such as the double-blind technique are usually imperative. In scanning abstracts, noting the use of controls can be a guide as to whether the original article is worth retrieving. A less objective method for quick evaluation of the literature is to note the name of the journal in which the work is published, who the investigators were and where the work was done. Although no journal, even of the highest quality, consistently publishes entirely valid material, one can nevertheless get an indication of the quality of the work. Articles published in the *New England Journal of Medicine*, for example, are much more likely to be valid then those published in a proprietary throwaway journal which is essentially used as a vehicle for advertising. As for the authors, we have already discussed the types of investigators and this can be a clue to the validity of a study. University hospital-affiliated clinical pharmacologists are much more likely to produce quality work than an internist located in a small town doing work sponsored by a drug manufacturer. Of course, some of the work done by proprietary interests and some of the work done away from university hospitals are quite good, as is some of the work published in lesser journals or those with a reputation for not consistently publishing good work. However, as a general rule of thumb, these things can be used to make the process of literature evaluation and retrieval a faster procedure.

Suggested References

A fairly inclusive list of suggested references is given on page 175. There are a number of references that carry an asterisk. These are the references that should be considered essential to every drug information center. A number of these are useful in one specific area such as adverse reactions while others are of a general type such as some of the pharmacology references. What can be said, however, is that a number of years of experience using these references in a drug information service has proved their utility time and again. The preferential list with the asterisk represents a sizeable and continuing investment as revisions are published. If this basic investment cannot be met, then the establishment of a drug information service probably should not be considered. Without the tools to do the job, it is better not to attempt it. These sources do not replace, but supplement the periodical literature and the retrieval systems necessary to enter the literature. It should be noted that some of the listed titles do not deal directly with drug information but with the medical sciences in general. Since one's clinical experience is usually not all-encompassing, it must be supplemented with such reference material. This is necessary if clinically relevant information is to be dispensed. There must be a thorough understanding of each patient's pathology before an appropriate drug information consultation can be synthesized.

The facilities and resources necessary to provide a first-class consultative drug information service will probably confine the existence of such operations to the larger medical center type institutions. However, there is no compelling reason why these larger institutions could not function as a central information center for a regional network of satellite information services. The latter could screen requests for information based upon the local resources and the sophistication of the problem. This would obviate the necessity to duplicate efforts in the same areas and provide for more efficient use of manpower and facilities. This concept of a regional network is already operable in some areas and is under study by others. It appears that this is the most logical approach to the dissemination of drug information for the promotion of rational therapeutics.

Professional Organizations for Drug Information

Most of the existing pharmaceutical associations and societies are promoting the concept of the drug information pharmacist and drug information service. There are two organizations, however, which are involved in this area of practice to a much greater extent. They are the American Society of Hospital Pharmacists and the Drug Information Association.

The American Society of Hospital Pharmacists (ASHP)

The ASHP through its publications, meetings and committees has done much over the years to promote the acceptance of the concept and practice. Much of the published material on drug information services and the pharmacists' involvement in them has appeared in the *American Journal of Hospital Pharmacy*, published by the Society.

The Drug Information Association (DIA)[13]

The Drug Information Association is a newer association founded in 1965. The DIA is an independent society designed to further modern technology of communication of medical, pharmaceutical and allied fields. It is: (1) a medium for free expression of ideas of individuals from all professional, industrial, governmental and related groups concerned with drug information; (2) a medium for mutual instruction in the technology of drug information processing in all its ramifications—collecting, selecting, abstracting, indexing, coding, vocabulary building, terminology standardizing, computerizing data storage and retrieval, tabulating, correlating, computing, evaluating, writing, editing, reporting and publishing; and (3) a medium for a reciprocal interchange of know-how about drug information handling.

Examples of Drug Information Consultations

Regardless of the location of a drug information service, the type of information that should be provided is represented by the following examples of drug information consultations from the files of the DIAS at U.C.S.F. These are typical of a consultative type drug information service. Some of these problems undoubtedly could not have been handled by a satellite service, but they certainly could be referred to the main center for disposition. However, any drug information specialist should be able to produce this type of work with the appropriate resources available. All of these examples have previously appeared in volume 4 of *Drug Intelligence and Clinical Pharmacy*.[9,10,11,12]

Request Number 1

Patient History:

The admitting diagnosis is cerebrovascular disease with fleeting blindness. As part of the work-up, an aortogram was done on August 7, 1969. The contrast medium used was Conray. The patient has been taking alpha-methyldopa 250 mg once a day, chlorothiazide 250 mg once a day and reserpine 0.1 mg once a day. The admitting blood pressure was 220/120, which dropped to 140/90 at 12 noon during the aortogram.

Request:

Could this drop in blood pressure be attributed to any of the drugs used?

Background:

This request is illustrative of several aspects of our operation. First of all, a problem very similar to this one had occurred about eight months previously and the write-up was in our file. Our file of "old" consults frequently proves to be a valuable source of information as it was in this case.

Secondly, we offered advice on the therapy of the reaction even though it was not specifically requested. Nothing is lost by doing this, and often enough we are able to provide information that proves useful in treating the patient.

Essentially, this request was answered with information obtained from our previous experience with this problem. The initial case, however, was solved by searching the current literature with the assistance of the de Haen system.

An interesting aspect of this problem is that in each case the medical team responsible for the patient's care had never encountered this reaction before, even though both patients were on the same service, *i.e.*, vascular surgery. Also, the diagnosis and work-up of these two patients were not unusual. The facts lead us to believe that this reaction may occur more often than realized but is usually not attributed to the contrast media.

Response:

Transient drops in blood pressures have been observed following intravenous injections of contrast media. Maluf and McCoy[1] reported a consistent fall in peripheral arterial pressure immediately after the injection of contrast media during aortography. Amundsen *et al.*[2] stated that the blood pressure dropped during aortography which they attributed to a peripheral vasodilatation effect of the contrast medium. Greitz[3] reported no local pressure changes in the carotid artery during the injection of the contrast media into that artery. He did note, however, a decrease in the heart rate and a lowering of the blood pressure after the injection of the contrast media, but not following the administration of normal saline. The literature is replete with data showing that Conray, Renografin and Hypaque cause first an increase in blood pressure due to the high pressure injection, but secondly cause a transient lowering of blood pressure due to a peripheral vasodilatation effect of the contrast media. According to the patient's history she has been on reserpine for some time. Since the depletion of catechols by reserpine is at maximal limits in 24 hours and since daily doses accumulate, it is safe to assume that there is a fair degree of catechol depletion in this patient, although depletion may not be total. Hence any assault which would tend to lower the blood pressure in this patient would not be counteracted by a homeostatic sympathetic response. It is reasonable to think that these contrast media would contribute to the morbidity, and even mortality, for slowing or momentary stopping of the heart and fall in blood pressure are not always well tolerated by the patient, particularly one with embarrassed cardiovascular or cerebrovascular reserve.[4] In summary, the prolonged fall in blood pressure is due to the peripheral vasodilatation action of the media and it is aggravated by the reserpinized state of this patient. The contrast media mentioned above, *i.e.*, Conray, Renografin and Hypaque, are rapidly excreted by glomerular filtration and should be eliminated from the body in a short time. In the meantime, blood pressure should be maintained or supported by a *direct* acting sympathomimetic amine such as levarterenol. If catechol depletion is not total, the use of an indirect sympathomimetic in adequate doses may be satisfactory, *e.g.*, metaraminol.

References:

1. Maluf, N. S. R. and McCoy, C. B.: Translumbar Aortography as a Diagnostic Procedure in Urology, *Am. J. Roentgenol. 73*:533-573 (Apr.) 1955.
2. Amundsen, A., Amundsen, P. and Muller, V.: Blood Pressure and Heart Rate During Angiocardiography, Abdominal Aortography, and Arteriography of the Lower Extremities, *Acta Radiol. 45*:452-458, 1956.
3. Greitz, T.: A Radiologic Study of the Brain Circulation by Rapid Serial Angiography of the Carotid Artery, *Acta Radiol. Suppl. 140,* 1956.
4. Pen-tze Fin, Joseph, *et al.*: Blood Pressure Changes During Retrograde Brachial Angiography, *Radiology 83*:640-646 (Oct.) 1964.
5. Chase, N. and Kricheff, Irvin: The Comparison of the Complication Rates of Meglumine Iothalamate and Sodium Diatrizoate in Cerebral Angiography, *Am. J. Roentgenol. 95*:852-856 (Dec.) 1965.
6. Tindall, George, *et al.*: Effect of 50 Percent Sodium Diatrizoate (Hypaque) on Blood Flow in the Internal Carotid Artery of Man, *Am. Heart J. 69*:215-219 (Feb.) 1965.
7. Pen-tze Fin, Joseph, *et al.*: Comparative Blood Pressure Changes in Angiography with Meglumine Iothalamate 60% (60% Conray) and 50% Sodium Diatrizoate (50% Hypaque), *Radiology 85*:1033-1035 (Dec.) 1965.

Request Number 2

Patient History:

The patient is a 35-year-old white woman with severe psoriasis. She is currently taking methotrexate 20 mg twice a week and prednisone 25 mg every day to control pustular lesions that would be life-threatening without the drugs. Reducing the prednisone to 5 mg a day or the methotrexate to 2.5 mg a week, results in an exacerbation of the lesions. The psoriasis is well controlled by these drugs, but the patient suffers a great deal of vomiting. The vomiting has been treated symptomatically with prochlorperazine 20 mg orally but was ineffective for this purpose. Her physicians would like to try folinic acid (Leucovorin) in an attempt to reduce the vomiting without reducing the dosage of methotrexate. The patient is slightly cushingoid, but her white count is fairly good.

Request:

Is the proposed treatment with folinic acid rational? If it is not, what do you suggest be done?

Background:

There is a great temptation to respond to a request like this "off the top of your head." Our first inclination was to just point out that the drugs are directly antagonistic and thus the combination would not work. However, we try to resist such temptations. There is always the possibility that there is something that we are not aware of. Even though the possibility that we would find anything to change our initial appraisal seemed remote, we pursued it by doing a thorough literature search. We approached the literature search from two points. First, digging out all the information we could on folinic acid. We felt that there was likely to be a lot less material available on this drug, and thus a less strenuous effort would be needed to search it. Although this presumption was correct we did not find any information other than confirmation of what we already knew. So next we searched the literature for methotrexate. We did not find anything startling but we did come across various means of reducing methotrexate toxicity which were helpful in formulating our response. A curious thing occurred when we presented our answer to the resident who had called us initially. His chief of service had mentioned to him that he had seen animal studies confirming one of our speculations, *i.e.*, methotrexate has a greater affinity for skin tissues than do the folates. We asked for the references, but he could not recall where he had seen them, and we were unable to locate them. We followed this patient's progress for several months. Attempts to reduce the methotrexate doses and the vomiting were unsuccessful. Alternative therapy with thiamiprine (Guaneran), an investigational purine analog, was begun. Along with this change in therapy, strong psychological enforcement was given to the patient so that she would not vomit with the new medication. She did fairly well on this therapy with an appreciable decrease in the number of episodes of nausea and vomiting. Folinic acid was never tried.

Response:

At first look, this approach appears to be irrational. Folinic acid is a direct antagonist to methotrexate and as such is an antidote for methotrexate toxicity. It will reverse methotrexate's therapeutic effects as well as its toxic effects. However, there may be factors that might allow one to use these drugs in combination to the benefit of the patient. It is possible that folic acid and its congeners may not have as high a tissue concentration in the skin as they do in other organ systems. There is also the possibility that methotrexate may get to the tissues, *i.e.*, skin, sooner than the folates. These are, at the moment, just speculations. There are no clinical or human studies available describing the use of a combination of methotrexate and folinic acid in dermatological diseases. Other factors that should be considered in this patient are her nutritional state and the folate content of her diet. It would be beneficial to insure that she has a relatively folate–free diet and advise her not to take vitamin preparations as they may contain folic acid. Lowering of the folate intake, if not already done, may allow some lowering of the methotrexate dose. Nutrition is important as malnourished patients are more susceptible to methotrexate toxicity. Since we are unable to find any evidence, either human or animal, for tissue concentration variances between folinic acid and methotrexate, it appears that folinic acid will not be of value in this patient. Indeed, it is quite likely that folinic acid would aggravate this patient's psoriasis.

References:

1. Spiro, J. M. and Dennis, D. J.: Treatment of Psoriasis with Minute Divided Oral Doses of Methotrexate, *Arch. Dermatol. 99*:459-464 (Apr.) 1969.
2. Fry, L. and McMinn, R. M. H.: Topical Methotrexate in Psoriasis, *Arch. Dermatol. 96*:483-488 (Nov.) 1967.
3. McDonald, C. J.: High Dose Methotrexate and Leucovorin in Refractory Mycosis Fungoides and Psoriasis, *Clin. Res. 17*:276 (Apr.) 1969.
4. Ryan, T. J. and Baker, H.: Systemic Corticosteroids and Folic Acid Antagonists in the Treatment of Generalized Pustular Psoriasis, *Brit. J. Dermatol. 81*:134-145 (Feb.) 1969.

Request Number 3

Patient History:

Our patient is a 61-year-old man who has had extensive small bowel resections, with a result that he has relatively little small bowel left. Most of his electrolytes are normal at present, but his serum calcium is low (8.6). We suspect a magnesium deficiency as well, but so far we have not been able to confirm this. We are treating his calcium deficit with calcium gluconogalactogluconate syrup 20 ml orally four times a day.

Request:

Would orally administered magnesium salts be effective in treating hypomagnesemia in this patient?

Background:

At face value this request could have been simply answered "yes." However, there were more implications to this problem than the request itself would indicate. When the surgical intern, with the problem, called us we had to question him on the patient to get the background found above. It was not volunteered. If we had not done this, we would not have known about the equivocal nature of the diagnosis for hypomagnesemia in this patient or of the fact that he was receiving calcium supplementation. At the time we received the request, we were not aware of the potential effects of calcium on magnesium absorption. Just because of situations like this we always make an effort to find out all medications a patient is taking. Although our response may seem a little long-winded, we felt we should clarify the principles of determining magnesium deficiencies. The intern seemed to us to be somewhat unsure of himself on the subject. Also, we were surprised that magnesium salts could be used in the presence of diarrhea, especially milk of magnesia since it can be a laxative. The long explanation was partly to convince ourselves, as well as the intern, of their efficacy in this situation. We find that by anticipating other problems related to the primary one, as we did in this case, quite frequently results in our consultation having a more positive impact on the caller.

Response:

A negative magnesium balance can co-exist with a normal serum magnesium concentration. Since the vascular space represents only a fractional portion of the body involved in magnesium homeostasis the determination of serum magnesium does not always give a true indication of the total body magnesium stored. If the clinical situation is suggestive of magnesium depletion, and serum values are normal as they are in this patient, then the erythrocyte content and 24-hour urinary excretion of magnesium should be measured. When the magnesium content of the erythrocytes or the urinary excretion is normal, magnesium deficiency is very unlikely.[1,2]

The presence of magnesium depletion in this patient would not be too surprising. Magnesium deficiencies have been well documented following extensive small bowel resections.[3,4] Other factors that may contribute to magnesium depletion include prolonged nasal-gastric suction without repletion of lost magnesium, prolonged diarrhea and steatorrhea, the last being an important cause of magnesium soaps formed by reactions in the gut between magnesium and the fatty contents of the stool. This phenomenon was illustrated in a patient with extensive resection of the distal small intestine whose dietary fat intake was excessive.[1,2]

Another factor that may contribute to excessive fecal loss of magnesium is vigorous calcium supplementation administered orally, *e.g.*, calcium gluconogalactogluconate syrup. It has been shown in animal studies that magnesium absorption from the intestine varies inversely with calcium intake, possibly because of competition for a common transport system.[1,2]

Magnesium administration is specifically indicated when symptoms of magnesium depletion develop and when the depletion is documented by measurements of serum or tissue concentrations. Oral replacement therapy with magnesium salts can be successful. Furthermore, the anticipation of diarrhea or a worsening of a malabsorption syndrome should not be a deterrent to the oral administration of magnesium. Patients can often tolerate magnesium salts, which will restore a positive magnesium balance without causing diarrhea.[1,2] In fact, there is a reported case[3] of magnesium deficiency secondary to small bowel resection where 60 mEq of magnesium hydroxide (20 ml milk of magnesia) was given daily in the presence of diarrhea. This patient had a restoration of the normal magnesium balance in one week on this regimen, with a corresponding abatement of the diarrhea. Thus, to answer the initial question, orally administered magnesium supplementation can be effective in hypomagnesemia.

References:

1. Wacker, W. E. C. and Parisi, A. F.: Magnesium Metabolism, *New Engl. J. Med. 278*:712-717 (Mar. 28) 1968; *ibid.*, 772-776 (Apr. 4) 1968.
2. Ibid.
3. Fletcher, R. F. *et al.*: Magnesium Deficiency Following Massive Intestinal Resection, *Lancet 1*:522-525 (Mar. 5) 1960.
4. Opie, L. H., Hunt, B. G. and Finlay, J. M.: Massive Small Bowel Resection with Malabsorption and Negative Magnesium Balance, *Gastroenterology 47*:415-420 (Oct.) 1964.

Request Number 4

Patient History:

The patient is a 62-year-old woman weighing 52 kilograms. She has a history of headaches over the past 35 years following an attack of acute glaucoma, retinal detachment and loss of an eye. In the past four years, she has taken eight [aspirin] tablets, with a cup of coffee, each morning upon arising. If this does not work she takes three or four Excedrin or two Empirin Compound with Codeine 30 mg. She entered the hospital with a large antral ulcer and a long-standing iron deficiency anemia. She is now taking ferrous sulfate 300 mg three times a day, thyroid 300 mg daily (has had a partial thyroidectomy), diazepam 5 mg prn and hydrochlorothiazide 50 mg daily.

Request:

Can aspirin cause a large ulcer in the antrum of the stomach?

Background:

This request was prompted by a raging controversy on one of our surgery services. The chief resident was insistent that aspirin does not cause frank ulceration; gastrointestinal bleeding perhaps, but never ulceration. At opposite ends were the assistant resident and intern who argued that aspirin could very possibly have been the cause of this woman's ulcer. Complicating the management of this patient was the possibility that this ulcer was malignant. Radiology consults were equivocal, but leaned toward the possibility of a carcinoma. Cytology had been ordered but had not been done at the time our service was consulted. The chief resident was positive that she had a carcinoma, based upon the radiology consults and his belief that aspirin could not have induced an ulcer. We were brought into the case as a sort of a referee to settle the debate on whether or not aspirin is indeed ulcerogenic. The importance of establishing an unequivocal diagnosis is apparent when one considers the fact that she could be spared surgery if the ulcer were proved benign.

After we completed our consult, cytology came back negative, but it was felt that an exploratory operation was necessary because of the adverse radiological findings. At laparotomy an inactive ulcer was found that appeared to be benign on gross inspection. Also, the ulcer was in the antrum, but it was only 4-5 mm in diameter, not "large" as the radiologist described it. Pathology later confirmed the benign nature of the ulcer.

Response:

Ever since the gastroscopic observations of Douthwaite and Lintott[1] in 1938 it has been known that aspirin can cause gastrointestinal bleeding, even hemorrhaging, especially if taken on an empty stomach. Experimental animals given aspirin on an empty stomach (in some cases intravenously) have developed hemorrhages and severe ulcerations. In numerous studies in humans, ingestion of aspirin has resulted in detection of blood in the stool (when before there was none), and often in aspirated gastric contents.

Various reports indicate that particles of aspirin often lodge in mucosal folds in the antrum and other areas. Gastroscopic examination following ingestion of the tablets shows them lying in the mucosal folds in small pools of fresh blood.

Muir and Cossar[2] did studies of aspirin effects in patients about to undergo gastrectomy. In one series 20 patients received commercial aspirin tablets about two hours before surgery; two uncrushed 5 grain tablets were taken on an empty stomach. Twelve of 20 patients showed macroscopic evidence of irritation in the form of an acute gastritis; in three cases this was severe. Multiple erosions visible to the naked eye were observed in five cases, and in all cases the lesions were most marked in the antrum along the greater curvature.

In the three severe cases the aspirin was present in large particles, and the mucus production was low. Erosions were larger in these patients, and obviously produced by the firmly adherent particles.

In one case half an aspirin tablet was found deeply enbedded in a mucosal fold in the antrum. When the firmly attached particle was removed, a lesion "showing the features of an acute peptic ulcer rather than a simple erosion" was seen. The lesion was the shape of the aspirin fragment, punched-out in appearance, and clearly visible on inspection.

Because this patient had no previous history of ulcer diseases, had had no corticosteroids or other drugs predisposing to ulcer formation and had taken aspirin for so long and recently in such high single doses, if carcinoma is ruled out this ulcer can be blamed on the salicylate in our opinion. It is quite likely that the very high doses taken on an empty stomach, along with the stress factor accompanying the large doses of thyroid extract, have brought a long-standing gastritis to a full-blown ulcer in the last few months.

In patients with a documented pre-existing peptic ulcer, massive hemorrhaging and re-activation of the ulcer have followed the ingestion of even small amounts of aspirin. In one especially striking case a patient with an 11-year history of duodenal ulcer had had only three recurrences of his ulcer symptoms, one of which resulted in massive bleeding. Each of these three flare-ups had been immediately preceded by the only occasions on which he had taken aspirin.[3]

One controlled study of emergency admissions showed that 54 of 166 patients admitted for gastrointestinal hemorrhage had taken salicylates within six hours before the incident. In 21 cases aspirin "was the major factor in precipitating the hemorrhage, beyond any reasonable doubt." Some were known ulcer patients, in whom ulcers were re-activated, and some had had previous gastrointestinal disease.[4]

Therefore, even if this patient had had previous ulcer disease the aspirin could be blamed for the worsening of the condition or for its recurrence. The anemia is undoubtedly due to chronic aspirin ingestion; this has been well documented.

Although the patient has taken iron for three to four months the anemia is still present; blood loss may be exceeding regeneration, and the iron is probably adding to the irritation. This patient is a candidate for parenteral iron until her gastrointestinal tract is in better shape.

References:

1. Douthwaite, H. and Lintott, A.: Gastroscopic Observation of the Effect of Aspirin and Certain Other Substances on the Stomach, *Lancet 2*:1222 (Nov. 26) 1938.

2. Muir, A. and Cossen, I.: Aspirin and Ulcer, *Brit. Med. J. 2*:7 (July 2) 1955.

3. Alvarez, D. and Summerskill, J.: Gastrointestinal Hemorrhages and Salicylates, *Lancet 2*:92 (Nov. 1) 1958.

4. Scott, J. *et al.*: Studies of Gastrointestinal Bleeding Caused by Corticosteroids, Salicylates, and Other Analgesics, *Quart. J. Med. 30*:167 (Apr.) 1961.

5. Weiss, A. *et al.*: Aspirin and Gastric Bleeding, *Am. J. Med. 31*:266 (Aug.) 1961.

6. Vickers, F. and Stanley, L.: Gastroduodenoscopic Observations, Four Case Reports, *Gastroenterology 44*:419 (Apr.) 1963.

Request Number 5

Patient History:

The patient is a 10-kg girl, with bilateral Wilms's tumors. At present she is essentially anephric, probably secondary to obstruction, as well as being septic. There are no immediate plans to hemodialyze this patient. However, we will attempt to relieve the obstruction.

Request:

We would like to treat the sepsis with kanamycin and ampicillin. What should be the dosage and the regimen for these drugs in this patient?

Background:

In the early days of our service, we felt a little overwhelmed by a question of this sort. It is critical that we answer these accurately and we were acutely aware of this responsibility. The overwhelmed feeling arose because we simply did not have the necessary data at hand. The pharmacology books usually did not have the information necessary for us to respond to these questions adequately. We were fortunate, however, to find the necessary information in the current literature for most of the commonly used antibiotics. Now, whenever we come across an article dealing with the dosing of agents in the presence of renal impairment, we photocopy it and keep it on file for future reference. Thus, in the present case, we simply referred to some articles on file. There are two parameters, however, that we must know in these patients before calculating the dose and the dosing interval. These are the serum creatinine or the creatinine clearance and the patient's weight. Liver function also may be important with particular drugs, *e.g.*, chloramphenicol. With this information, we can usually answer the request promptly.

Response:

In this patient a single loading dose of 7 mg/kg, *i.e.*, 70 mg, kanamycin, will give adequate circulating levels of kanamycin for the entire treatment period and need not be repeated. If dialysis is eventually decided upon, a 7 mg/kg dose after every other hemodialysis should be adequate for this patient. About 50 percent of the administered dose of kanamycin will be removed in a 6-8 hour run of hemodialysis.[1]

As for the ampicillin, extrapolating from adult anephric patient data, where one-fourth the daily dose suffices, a dose of 400 mg I.V. in a single daily dose should be adequate for this patient. Clinical studies have shown that using standard ampicillin dosing regimens in the presence of renal failure results in a nine-fold increase in the incidence of complications. Ampicillin blood levels of 2-3 mcg/ml are adequate for therapeutic results. Using the above regimen should achieve these levels without any difficulty.[2]

References:

1. Culter, R. E. and Orme, B. M.: Correlation of Serum Creatinine Concentration and Kanamycin Half-Life, *J. Am. Med. Assoc.* *209*:539 (July) 1969.

2. Lee, H. A. and Hill, L. F.: The Use of Ampicillin in Renal Disease, *Brit. J. Clin. Pract.* *22*:354 (Aug.) 1968.

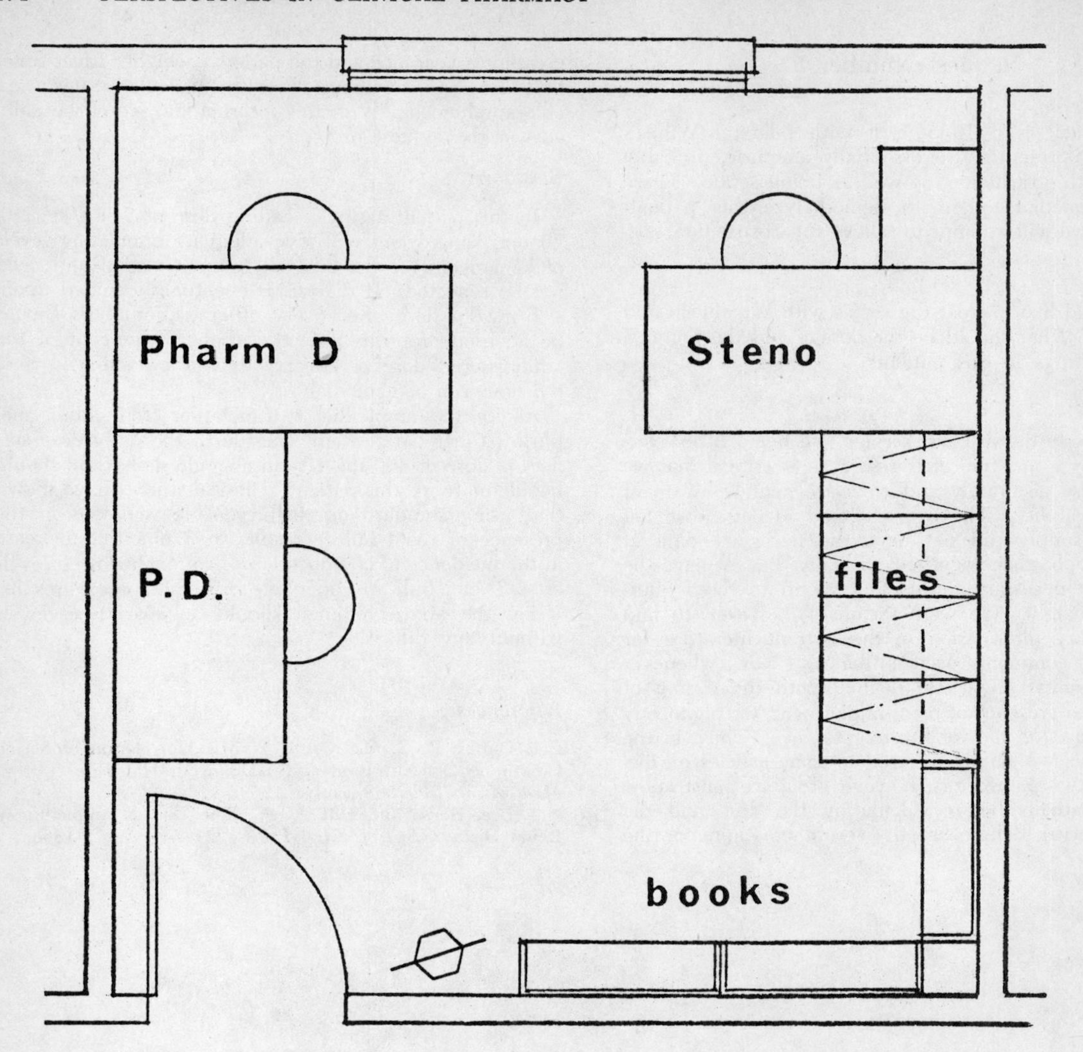

Figure 4. Prototype of a drug information service calling for 169 sq. ft.

References

1. Burkholder, D.: Some Experiences in the Establishment and Operation of a Drug Information Center, *Am. J. Hosp. Pharm. 20*:506-513, (Oct.) 1963.
2. Price, D. J. de S.: *Little Science, Big Science,* Columbia University Press, New York, N. Y. 1963, 119 pp.
3. *The Library: Serials Title List, Health Sciences Collection,* University of California, San Francisco, California, (Oct.) 1970, 240 pp.
4. de Haen, P.: *New Products Parade,* 1969, 16th edition, Paul de Haen, Inc. New York, N. Y. (Jan.) 1970, page 1.
5. Benson, S. and Kabat, H.: Drug Information Needs in the Hospital Environment, *Am. J. Hosp. Pharm. 24*:263-267 (May) 1967.
6. Pearson, R. and Salter, F.: *Drug Information Center Job Aids,* University of Michigan Hospital Pharmacy Service and University of Michigan College of Pharmacy Drug Information Network. Philips Roxane Laboratories, Inc., Columbus, Ohio, 1969, 20 pp.
7. Pearson, R.: Evaluation of the Effectiveness of a Hospital Center, *Drug Information Bull. 4*:45-49 (Jan.-June) 1970.
8. Fuller, E.: A System for Filing Medical Literature: Based on a Method Developed by Dr. Maxwell M. Wintrobe, *Ann. Internal Med. 69*:684 (Mar.) 1968.
9. Hirschman, J. L. and Maudlin, R. K.: The DIAS Rounds, *Drug Intelligence Clin. Pharm. 4*:45-48 (Feb.) 1970.
10. *Ibid. 4*:64-66 (Mar.) 1970.
11. *Ibid. 4*:307-310 (Nov.) 1970.
12. *Ibid. 4*:45-48 (Feb.) 1970.
13. Martin, E.: The DIA Idea, *Am. J. Hosp. Pharm. 23*: 50-54 (Feb.) 1966.

Additional References

1. Reilly, M. J.: *Drug Information—A Literature Review of Needs, Resources and Services,* National Center for Health Services Research and Development, Dept. of HEW, Rockville, Maryland, (Sept.) 1971.
2. Anon.: *Proceedings of the Institute of Drug Literature Evaluation,* American Society of Hospital Pharmacists, Rockville, Maryland, (Sept.) 1971.

Drug Information Service Reference Sources

Adverse Reactions

1. *Adverse Reaction Titles,* monthly. Excerpta Medica Foundation, N. Y., N. Y.

*2. *Clin-Alert,* published p.r.n., Science Editors, Louisville, Ky.

*3. Moser, R. (ed.): *Diseases of Medical Progress: A Study of Iatrogenic Disease,* 3rd edition, Charles C Thomas, Springfield, Ill., 1969, 925 pp.

*4. Meyler, L. and Herxheimer, A. (ed.): *Side Effects of Drugs: A Survey of Unwanted Effects of Drugs Reported 1965-1967,* Volume VI, The Williams and Wilkins Company, Baltimore, Md., and Excerpta Medica Foundation, Amsterdam, The Netherlands, 1968, 561 pp. (previous volumes cover periods from 1955-1965).

Biopharmaceutics

1. Wagner, J. G.: *Biopharmaceutics and Relevant Pharmacokinetics,* Drug Intelligence Publications, Hamilton, Ill., 1971, 375 pp.

2. Ritschel, W. A.: *Applied Biopharmaceutics I and II,* College of Pharmacy, University of Cincinnati, Cincinnati, Ohio 45221.

Chemistry

*1. *The Merck Index,* 8th edition, Merck and Company, Rahway, N. J., 1968, 1713 pp.

2. Wilson, C., Gisvold, O. and Doerge, R. F. (ed.): *Textbook of Organic Medicinal and Pharmaceutical Chemistry,* 6th edition, J. B. Lippincott, Philadelphia, Pa., 1971, 1053 pp.

3. Harper, H.: *Review of Physiological Chemistry,* 12th edition, Lange Medical Publications, Los Altos, Cal., 1969, 569 pp.

Clinical Pathology

*1. Goodale, R. and Widmann, F.: *Clinical Interpretation of Laboratory Tests,* 6th edition, F. A. Davis, Philadelphia, Pa., 1969, 568 pp.

2. Levinson, S. and MacFate, R.: *Clinical Laboratory Diagnosis,* 7th edition, Lea and Febiger, Philadelphia, Pa., 1969, 1323 pp.

Dentistry

1. *Accepted Dental Therapeutics, 1969/1970,* 33rd edition, Council on Dental Therapeutics, American Dental Association, Chicago, Ill., 1968, 317 pp.

Dermatology

*1. Sauer, G.: *Manual of Skin Disease,* 2nd edition, J. B. Lippincott, Philadelphia, Pa., 1966, 284 pp.

2. Criep, L. H.: Clinical Immunology, 2nd edition, Grune and Stratton, New York, 1969, 962 pp.

Drug Identification

*1. *Facts and Comparisons,* monthly, Facts and Comparisons, Inc., St. Louis, Mo.

*2. *Pharmacological and Chemical Synonyms,* 4th edition, Excerpta Medica Foundation, N. Y., N. Y. 1967, 349 pp.

*Considered essential for all drug information centers

3. Gupta, R. and Kofoed, J.: *Identification Guide for Tablets and Capsules,* Canada Law Book Company, Toronto, Canada, 1967.
*4. *Physicians' Desk Reference to Pharmaceutical Specialities and Biologicals,* 26th edition, Medical Economics, Inc. Oradell, N.J., 1972, 1508 pp.
*5. Wilson, C. and Jones, T. (ed.): *American Drug Index,* 1972, J. B. Lippincott, Philadelphia, Pa., 1972, 699 pp.

Drug Interactions

1. Hartshorn, E. A.: *Handbook of Drug Interactions,* D. E. Francke, Publisher, Cincinnati, Ohio, 1970, 88 pp.
2. Hansten, P. D.: *Drug Interactions,* Lea and Febiger, Philadelphia, Pa., 1971, 437 pp.

Drug Monographs

*1. *American Hospital Formulary Service,* volumes 1 and 2, supplemented 4 to 6 times annually, American Society of Hospital Pharmacists, Washington, D. C., 1972.
*2. Todd, R. G. (ed.): *Martindale's Extra Pharmacopoeia,* 25th edition, The Pharmaceutical Press, London, England, 1967, 1804 pp.
3. *AMA Drug Evaluations,* American Medical Association, Chicago, Ill., 1971, 984 pp.

Endocrinology

1. Williams, R. (ed.): *Textbook of Endocrinology,* 4th edition, W. B. Saunders, Philadelphia, Pa., 1968, 1258 pp.

Intravenous Therapeutics

1. *Parenteral Solutions Handbook: A Guide to Optimal Utilization,* Cutter Laboratories, Berkeley, Cal., 1965, 44 pp.
2. Francke, D. E. (ed.): *Handbook of I.V. Additive Reviews,* 1970, D. E. Francke, Publisher, Cincinnati, Ohio, 1970, 48 pp.
3. Francke, D. E. (ed.): *Handbook of I.V. Additive Reviews,* 1971, D. E. Francke, Publisher, Cincinnati, Ohio, 1971, 58 pp.
4. Plumer, A. L.: *Principles and Practice of Intravenous Therapy,* Little, Brown and Co., Boston, Mass., 1970, 262 pp.

Liver Disease

1. Sherlock, S.: *Diseases of the Liver and Biliary System,* 4th edition, F. A. Davis, Philadelphia, Pa., 1968, 809 pp.

Medicine

1. Beeson, P. B. and McDermott, W. (ed.): *Cecil-Loeb Textbook of Medicine,* 13th edition, W. B. Saunders, Philadelphia, Pa., 1967, 1923 pp.
*2. Brainerd, H., *et al.*: *Current Diagnosis and Treatment,* Lange Medical Publications, Los Altos, Cal., 1970, 884 pp.
3. Rosenfeld, M. G. (ed.): *Manual of Medical Therapeutics,* 20th edition, Little, Brown and Co., Boston, Mass., 1971, 476 pp.
4. Grupp, M., *et al.*: *Physician's Handbook,* 16th edition, Lange Medical Publications, Los Altos, Cal., 1970, 660 pp.
5. Chatton, M., *et al.* (ed.): *Handbook of Medical Treatment,* 12th edition, Lange Medical Publications, Los Altos, Cal., 1970, 789 pp.
6. Wintrobe, M., *et al.* (ed.): *Harrison's Principles of Internal Medicine,* 6th edition, McGraw-Hill, New York, N. Y., 1970. 2016 pp.

Microbiology

*1. Jawetz, E., *et al.*: *Review of Medical Microbiology,* 9th edition, Lange Medical Publications, Los Altos, Cal., 1970, 484 pp.
2. Davis, B., *et al.*: *Microbiology,* Hoeber, New York, N. Y., 1967, 1464 pp.

Miscellaneous

*1. Chatton, M. and Sanazaro, P. (ed.): *Current Medical References,* 6th edition, Lange Medical Publications, Los Altos, Cal., 1970, 673 pp.
*2. *Stedman's Medical Dictionary,* 21st edition, Williams and Wilkins, Baltimore, Md., 1966, 1836 pp.
3. Diem, K. (ed.): *Documenta Geigy-Scientific Tables,* 7th edition, Geigy Pharmaceuticals, Ardsley, N. Y., 1970, 809 pp.

Neurology

1. Merritt, H.: *A Textbook of Neurology,* 4th edition, Lea and Febiger, Philadelphia, Pa., 1967, 844 pp.

Obstetrics and Gynecology

1. Benson, R.: *Handbook of Obstetrics and Gynecology,* 4th edition, Lange Medical Publications, Los Altos, Cal., 1971, 774 pp.

Ophthalmology

1. Newell, F.: *Ophthalmology-Principles and Concepts,* 2nd edition, C. V. Mosby, St. Louis, Mo., 1969, 527 pp.

O-T-C Drugs

*1. Griffenhagen, G.: *Handbook of Non-Prescription Drugs,* American Pharmaceutical Association, Washington, D. C., 1971, 202 pp.

Parasitology

*1. Markell, E. and Voge, M.: *Medical Parasitology,* 2nd edition, W. B. Saunders, Philadelphia, Pa., 1965, 317 pp.
2. Faust, E. and Russell, P.: *Craig and Faust's Clinical Parasitology,* 7th edition, Lea and Febiger, Philadelphia, Pa., 1964, 1099 pp.

Pathology

1. Robbins, S.: *Pathology,* 3rd edition, W. B. Saunders, Philadelphia, Pa., 1967, 1434 pp.

---
* Considered essential for all drug information centers

Pediatrics

*1. Silver, H., *et al.*: *Handbook of Pediatrics,* 9th edition, Lange Medical Publications, Los Altos, Cal., 1971, 713 pp.
2. Kempe, C., *et al.*: *Current Pediatric Diagnosis and Treatment,* Lange Medical Publications, Los Altos, Cal., 1970, 883 pp.
*3. Shirkey, H. (ed.): *Pediatric Therapy,* 3rd edition, C. V. Mosby, St. Louis, Mo., 1968, 1294 pp.
4. Nelson, W. (ed.): *Textbook of Pediatrics,* 9th edition, W. B. Saunders, Philadelphia, Pa., 1969, 1589 pp.
5. Winkelstein, J. (ed.): *The Harriet Lane Handbook—A Manual for Pediatric House Officers,* 5th edition, Year Book Medical Publishers, Chicago, Ill., 1969, 264 pp.

Pharmacology

*1. Goodman, L. and Gilman, A. (ed.): *The Pharmacological Basis of Therapeutics,* 4th edition, Macmillan, New York, N. Y., 1970, 1794 pp.
*2. Goldstein, A., *et al.*: *Principles of Drug Action, The Basis of Pharmacology,* Hoeber, New York, N. Y., 1968, 884 pp.
3. Ban, T.: *Psychopharmacology,* Williams and Wilkins, Baltimore, Md., 1969, 485 pp.
*4. Havener, W.: *Ocular Pharmacology,* 2nd edition, C. V. Mosby, St. Louis, Mo., 1970, 556 pp.
*5. Meyers, F., *et al.*: *Review of Medical Pharmacology,* 2nd edition, Lange Medical Publications, Los Altos, Cal., 1970, 663 pp.
*6. Gravenstein, J. (ed.): Pharmacology for the Preoperative Visit, *Intern. Anesth. Clinics* Volume 6, No. 1, (Spring) 1968.
*7. Beckman, H.: *Dilemmas in Drug Therapy,* W. B. Saunders, Philadelphia, Pa., 1967, 404 pp.
*8. *Pharmacology for Physicians,* monthly, W. B. Saunders, Philadelphia, Pa.

Pharmacy

*1. Osol, A., *et al.* (ed.): *The United States Dispensatory and Physicians' Pharmacology,* 26th edition, J. B. Lippincott, Philadelphia, Pa., 1967, 1277 pp.
*2. Martin, E., *et al.* (ed.): *Remington's Pharmaceutical Sciences,* 14th edition, Mack, Easton, Pa., 1970, 2074 pp.
3. *The Pharmacopeia of the United States of America,* 18th revision, The United States Pharmacopeial Convention, Washington, D. C., 1970, 1115 pp.
4. *The National Formulary,* 13th edition, American Pharmaceutical Association, Washington, D. C., 1970, 1012 pp.

Physiology

1. Ganong, W.: *Review of Medical Physiology,* 4th edition, Lange Medical Publications, Los Altos, Cal., 1969, 628 pp.

Surgery

1. Wilson, J. (ed.): *Handbook of Surgery,* 4th edition, Lange Medical Publications, Los Altos, Cal., 1969, 781 pp.
2. Condon, R. and Nyhus, L. (ed.): *Manual of Surgical Therapeutics,* Little, Brown, and Company, Boston, Mass., 1969, 379 pp.

Therapeutics

*1. Conn, H. (ed.): *Current Therapy-1971* W. B. Saunders, Philadelphia, Pa., 836 pp.
*2. Thomas, P.: *Guide to Steroid Therapy,* J. B. Lippincott, Philadelphia, Pa., 1968, 223 pp.
3. Modell, W. (ed.): *Drugs of Choice 1972-1973,* C. V. Mosby, St. Louis, Mo., 1972, 924 pp.
*4. *The Medical Letter of Drugs and Therapeutics,* Volumes 1-current, fortnightly, Drug and Therapeutic Information, New York, N. Y.

Toxicology

1. Williams, R.: *Detoxification Mechanisms,* 2nd edition, John Wiley and Sons, New York, N. Y., 1959, 796 pp.
*2. Gleason, M., *et al.*: *Clinical Toxicology of Commercial Products,* 3rd edition, Williams and Wilkins, Baltimore, Md., 1969, 1411 pp.
*3. Dreisbach, R.: *Handbook of Poisoning,* 6th edition, Lange Medical Publications, Los Altos, Cal., 1969, 477 pp.
4. Poison Cards, National Clearinghouse for Poison Control Centers, Washington, D. C.
5. Deichmann, W. and Gerarde, H.: *Toxicology of Drugs and Chemicals,* Academic Press, New York, N. Y., 1969, 805 pp.
6. Arena, J.: *Poisoning,* 2nd edition, Charles C. Thomas, Springfield, Ill., 1970, 715 pp.

Urology

1. Smith, D.: *General Urology,* 6th edition, Lange Medical Publications, Los Altos, Cal., 1969, 409 pp.

9

Drug interactions and their therapeutic implications

by Edward A. Hartshorn

Definitions and Philosophy

One part of the pharmacist's drug knowledge which draws from all areas of both the theoretical and clinical components of pharmacy is that of drug interactions. The term "interactions" is used advisably, and preferred over "therapeutic incompatibilities." The connotation of the word "incompatible" is that the two drugs cannot be used together when, in fact, many drugs which "interact" are used concomitantly with no serious sequelae and indeed may be deliberately used together for a specific beneficial effect.

The term drug interaction has been defined as the phenomenon which occurs when the action of one drug is modified by the prior or concurrent administration of another (or the same) drug.[1] This is a fairly restrictive definition, describing a drug-drug interaction. Practical use of the term has enlarged the scope so that the drug interaction literature considers the alteration of net effect of one substance (be it drug, chemical, food stuff, physiological substance or environmental agent) by another substance. Furthermore, alteration of laboratory test results by ingested drugs is popularly considered in the drug interaction literature when, in fact, this may involve anything from an increase or decrease of an endogenous substance to a simple production of an interfering color. The literature on drug interactions includes alterations in drug effect on living animals and humans as well as isolated organs, tissues and even subcellular components. This chapter, however, will be concerned primarily with clinically important interactions as reported in the literature and the mechanism of their interaction. Animal or *in vitro* data will be considered only as they relate to the establishment of a mechanism of action. There will be no effort to list or review all reported interactions. Likewise, there will be no attempt to give a complete bibliography; only a representative reference will be included.*

As indicated in the definition, *concurrent* administration of two drugs is not necessary for an interaction to occur. Consider, for example, the prolonged effect of the monoamine oxidase inhibitors, the irreversible cholinesterase inhibitors or reserpine, each of which may have residual effects for some time after the drug is discontinued. In some instances, chronic administration of one drug (*e.g.*, meprobamate, glutethimide) may alter its own metabolism and hence its effectiveness. In other cases, a drug may have a different effect upon another substance depending on whether the drug is given acutely or chronically.[2]

Drug interactions may occur as a result of one or more of about a dozen different mechanisms such as: a direct effect of one compound upon another, by modification of intestinal absorption, by affecting the transport of a drug or substance across cell membranes, by altering the distribution of a drug in the various body compartments, by modification of a drug's action at its receptor site, by altering the binding of a drug to inactive binding sites, by acceleration or retardation of the metabolism of a drug, by affecting the rate of excretion or by modification of the sensitivity of the receptor site. Such mechanisms have been termed "pharmacodynamic" actions.[3] "Pharmacologic" actions would include the apparent enhancement or antagonism of a drug's effect via the second drug acting on the same or a related physiologic system and producing either a similar or an opposite pharmacologic effect. Still other reported interactions defy a simplified method of categorization. In essence, a drug interaction may occur when a substance either alters the ability of a drug to reach its receptor site in its usual manner and concentration, or alters the body's response to the drug.

* For a thorough discussion of drug interactions and an extensive bibliography, see: Hartshorn, E. A.: *Handbook of Drug Interactions,* D. E. Francke, Publisher, Hamilton Press, Hamilton, Illinois 62341.

Perspective

This chapter will consider clinical examples of drug interactions according to the proposed mechanism of action. One must, however, put the subject into perspective. First of all, an adverse effect from an interaction does not occur in each patient who receives two particular drugs and, in fact, occasionally the interaction is beneficial. Unfortunately, we have no idea how often an interaction may occur when two drugs are given. Second, the clinical importance of the interaction varies tremendously. There are only a few drugs whose effect can be objectively monitored; with many drugs, alteration of the effects may or may not be important or may not even be noticed. Finally, there are a host of factors which affect drug action, and hence affect drug interaction. Pharmaceutically this would include, for example, dose, dosage form, method of administration, time of administration (*e.g.*, before or after meals) and the various biopharmaceutical implications. Physically, factors such as diet, habits and even the psychological milieu may alter the response of a patient to a drug and hence to a drug interaction. Physiological factors (such as age, sex, weight and *p*H of the urine), genetic variances (particularly where there may be deficiency of certain enzyme systems) and pathological conditions all have the propensity to alter the effects of a drug and the results of a drug interaction. To make the situation even more complex, it is a rare patient who is receiving only two drugs. Polypharmacy is *not* dead.

MECHANISMS OF DRUG INTERACTIONS

Alteration of Absorption from the Gastrointestinal Tract

A number of factors may alter the rate of passage of food and other substances through the GI tract and thus may affect drug action. Variation between individuals, the type of food eaten (*e.g.*, fats, very cold) and even psychological factors may alter emptying time of the stomach and intestinal motility. Any substance which alters one of these factors or alters the *p*H of the GI tract has the potential for altering the effect of a drug. However, there are only a few examples of drug interactions via this mechanism which have been clinically important enough to be recognized in the medical literature.

Much is made of the effect of *p*H on the absorption of weak acids and bases. Apparently the body has a great capacity to return the contents of the GI tract to the physiological *p*H; while this theory may make sense, there are very few reports of clinically important altered drug effects via this mechanism. Absorption of levodopa may be enhanced if administered concurrently with an antacid.[4] Penicillin G potassium, a weak acid, should be most readily absorbed from an acid stomach; however, the drug is acid-labile and recommendations are for its administration at least 45 minutes before meals when the degree of stomach acidity is at its lowest ebb.

Diminished absorption of the tetracyclines by chelation by di- and tri-valent cations, and particularly aluminum, is a well-known interaction.[5] Yet the physician often uses magnesium, calcium or aluminum-containing antacids or milk to decrease the incidence of GI upset; the patients do get better. It would seem that rational therapeutics dictates that such a combination should not be used. However, the interaction is apparently of importance only if the decreased antibiotic blood level falls below the minimal inhibitory concentration needed for the organism causing the infection. Data seem to indicate that therapeutic doses of aluminum hydroxide gel cause a marked decrease in tetracycline blood levels but that commonly used doses of magnesium trisilicate, magnesium hydroxide or milk may not cause significant changes in antibiotic blood levels.[6,7]

Certain drug combinations are used for their interactions. Ganglionic blocking agents (*e.g.*, pentolinium), which are only partially absorbed from the GI tract, decrease peristaltic activity and cause constipation. This delays the excretion of the unabsorbed drug, permits more of the drug to be absorbed and results in an increased and unpredictable hypotension.[8] To prevent this, peristaltic stimulants, such as bethanechol or neostigmine, are sometimes administered. On the other hand, certain laxatives might be considered improper therapy if the increased rate of propulsion of substances through the GI tract prevents absorption of a drug. As with the *p*H problem above, there is little if any information which indicates this to be a problem of clinical importance. Perhaps this information is so well known that problems which arise do not warrant a published report.

Other Sites for Absorption

Drugs which affect the circulation to the site of absorption may likewise affect a drug's absorption. While we generally think of absorption from the GI tract, drugs administered intramuscularly or subcutaneously must also be absorbed for systemic effect. One of the most commonly used drug interactions as far as altering the absorption of a drug is the use of epinephrine with a local anesthetic. By its vasoconstrictor effect, epinephrine decreases bleeding, slows the rate of absorption of the local anesthetic, prolongs its local effect and decreases the potential for systemic toxicity.

Passage of drugs across cell membranes is necessary for absorption, excretion and, frequently, action. Such passage may be a passive phenomenom for many drugs, but there are substances which require specialized transport systems such as active transport or facilitated diffusion. Carrier systems which exhibit selectivity, saturability and, in some instances, a requirement for energy, may be involved. One drug may alter the effect of another drug by blocking, competing for or poisoning an essential enzyme system. Such reactions have been known to pharmacologists and biochemists for years and are not generally thought of as a drug interaction, yet the mechanism of action and the end result certainly fit the definition as described earlier. The ability of p-aminohippuric acid (PAH) or probenecid to alter the excretion of penicillin is probably the classical example.

Modification of Drug Action at the Receptor Site

In the distribution of a drug, some portion must go to a receptor site where it interacts and causes biochemical changes ultimately resulting in the effect of the drug. A number of drugs apparently increase the sensitivity of the receptor site to certain neurohormones in some vague way, other drugs act by blocking the receptor site to make it unavailable to the neurohormone and still other substances alter the enzyme systems which either synthesize or destroy the neurohormone at the receptor site. Certain of these effects have been considered the pharmacological action of the drug; others have been reported in recent literature as drug interactions.

The antihyperlipemic drugs clofibrate and dextrothyroxine reportedly enhance the effect of certain oral anticoagulants by increasing the sensitivity of the receptor substance.[9] This enhancement of anticoagulant effect apparently appears in a sizeable percentage of patients taking both drugs.

Atropine, phentolamine and propranolol are

classical drugs whose primary action is simply blocking the cholinergic, alpha-adrenergic or beta-adrenergic receptor sites, respectively. Certain drug interactions as, for example, potentiation of the hypoglycemia of insulin therapy by propranolol, are explainable in pharmacologic terms. Propranolol probably interferes with the body's compensating response to hypoglycemia.[10]

The cholinesterase inhibitors produce their effect by preventing or delaying the destruction of acetylcholine. The potentiation of succinylcholine in patients exposed to organo-phosphate insecticides or eye drops is the result of an inhibition of the enzyme normally responsible for the metabolism of the succinylcholine.[11]

Some drugs may block another drug from a receptor and yet have a weak effect in themselves. Such agents are called partial agonists and may be represented by nalorphine.

Alteration of Binding of a Drug

Once drugs are in the circulatory system, they are transported via the plasma to sites of action, excretion and metabolism. Drug action depends upon the absorption of the drug by an active receptor; the drug on the receptor is in equilibrium with the drug in the plasma. Hence, the response to a drug is determined in part by the concentration of unbound drug in the plasma which, in turn, is dependent upon a number of factors, not the least of which is the amount of "bound" drug.

The "bound" drug, as intimated above, is inactive. Binding may be to plasma proteins, to connective tissue, to fat, in transcellular areas or even within cells. These many areas of the body serve as reservoirs, since the pharmacologically inactive stored drug is in equilibrium with the free drug in the plasma and is released as the drug is metabolized, accumulated in other tissues or excreted. Binding of drugs may be useful in that it prolongs the action of a drug and prevents steep peaks and valleys in blood levels. But binding may also result in subtherapeutic levels of active drug. The degree of binding varies considerably with the various drugs; phenylbutazone is found primarily in the bound state while alcohol is hardly bound at all.

One drug may affect the concentration of another at the receptor site by displacing the second drug from inactive binding sites. This action not only increases the amount of free drug available for action at the receptor site, but also for metabolism and excretion. Hence, displacing a drug from its inactive binding site may result in a shortened biological half-life. This must be distinguished from a shortened biological half-life caused by increased rate of metabolism via enzyme induction.

A number of reported interactions appear to relate to the binding of certain acidic drugs to a specific site on the albumin molecule (Table 1).

Table 1. Drugs Bound to the Same Albumin Site

(Bilirubin)
Bishydroxycoumarin
Ethyl biscoumacetate
Methotrexate
Penicillin
Phenylbutazone
Salicylic acid
Sulfinpyrazone
Sulfonamides
Tolbutamide
Trichloroacetic acid (metabolite of chloral hydrate)

The protein has a limited carrying capacity and there may be competition between the drugs for the binding site. Several suggestions of relative affinity of drugs for this binding site have been proposed; however, there is no evidence that these proposed arrangements have clinical validity.

Possibly the most significant drug interaction involving displacement of one drug from its binding sites by another is the enhancement of the anticoagulant effect of warfarin and other coumarin congeners by phenylbutazone.[12] It should, however, be noted that phenylbutazone may also stimulate the microsomal enzyme systems which metabolize the coumarin in anticoagulants. Chronic use of phenylbutazone may decrease the effectiveness of the anticoagulant and order of administration of drug may be important.[13]

A case history suggested that chloral hydrate decreased the effectiveness of bishydroxycoumarin (Dicumarol) by stimulating the microsomal enzymes.[14] More recent data generated by a carefully controlled study by Sellers and Koch-Weser indicate that a metabolite of chloral hydrate, trichloroacetic acid, is strongly bound to the same albumin site as warfarin. Patients receiving warfarin showed an excessive hypoprothrombinemia after a dose of chloral hydrate.[15]

Bilirubin is an endogenous substance bound to this albumin binding site. It is normally metabolized by glucuronyl transferase found in the microsomal fraction of liver cells. Premature infants, whose limited amount of albumin is quickly saturated with bilirubin, may have a deficiency in this enzyme.[16] Displacement of bilirubin from the albumin binding site by drugs such as sulfonamides or salicylates may result in hyperbilirubinemia and kernicterus in these babies.[17,18]

Drugs may be bound or concentrated in other tissues. A reported interaction deals with the displacement of highly bound pamaquine by quinacrine. Plasma concentration of the pamaquine is increased five- to tenfold.[19]

Norepinephrine is stored in granules and different pools at adrenergic nerve endings and is metabolized, in part, by the enzyme monoamine oxidase. Tyramine, found in a number of foods, and certain sympathomimetic amines commonly incorporated into non-prescription preparations, cause norepinephrine to be released from these storage sites resulting in symptoms of hypertension in patients receiving monoamine oxidase inhibitors.[20,21] On the other hand, reserpine depletes norepinephrine from these binding sites and produces a hypotensive effect partially via this mechanism.[22]

Alteration of Metabolism of a Drug

Enzyme systems involved in drug metabolism are found throughout the body. Some are very specific; others appear to catalyze rather general reactions. One function of such enzyme systems is to change lipid-soluble active compounds into less toxic, more polar substances which are less likely to be reabsorbed in the kidney tubules (although occasionally a more active or more toxic substance is produced). The enzyme systems most commonly considered in the literature on drug interaction are those found in what is called the microsomal portion of the liver cell. The same enzyme systems are found to a lesser extent in heart, lung and kidney cells. These enzyme systems may be influenced by a number of factors such as age, temperature, pathological status and, most important to this discussion, by various drugs. Table 2 lists some drugs and endogenous substances metabolized by hepatic microsomal enzymes.

Table 2. Drugs Metabolized by Microsomal Enzymes

Anticoagulants (oral)
Barbiturates (some)
(Bilirubin)
Diphenylhydantoin
Glutethimide
Griseofulvin
Hydrocortisone
Meprobamate
Testosterone
Tolbutamide

It has been demonstrated both in animal experiments and *in vitro* studies that certain drugs are capable of increasing the amount of enzyme substance, termed "enzyme induction" (Table 3).

Table 3. Drugs Shown to Stimulate Hepatic Microsomal Enzymes in Man

Barbiturates (some)
Chlordane
Diphenylhydantoin
DDT
Ethanol
Glutethimide
Griseofulvin
Meprobamate
Phenylbutazone

There are considerable differences between species. Conney has listed 200 drugs and other substances which have been shown to induce enzyme activity in animals.[13] The list of importance to humans is considerably smaller. Furthermore, there is no indication that all drugs stimulate the same enzyme systems or to the same degree. Phenobarbital is considered to be a wide spectrum enzyme stimulant; 3-methylcholanthrene appears to stimulate only a few systems.[13] Chronic administration of an enzyme inducer can reduce the pharmacological activity of another drug and sometimes itself by stimulating its metabolic inactivation. Two points must be considered. Certain drugs may be metabolized to active or more active congeners. The enhanced toxicity in animals of cyclophosphamide by halogenated insecticides illustrates this point.[23] Also, while concurrent administration of two drugs may result in decreased activity or difficulty in attaining a controlled effect by one of the agents, when the enzyme inducer is discontinued, the drug whose metabolism was affected may then produce toxic effects as the metabolizing enzymes return to their normal level of activity.

Probably the best known interaction involving enzyme induction is that of phenobarbital and warfarin. Case histories as well as studies which demonstrate altered anticoagulant blood levels or prothrombin times have been published.[24,25,26] How many of the barbiturates are enzyme inducers is not known; phenobarbital and hexobarbital have been used most frequently; secobarbital and amobarbital recently have been shown to have enzyme-inducing properties in man.[27] Warfarin and bishydroxycoumarin have been the anticoagulants most frequently named. There are few clinical reports relating altered metabolism of phenindione by drug-induced enzyme induction. Other sedatives, particularly glutethimide and ethchlorvynol, have likewise been reported to stimulate the metabolism of the orally administered anticoagulants.[28] Griseofulvin, haloperidol and meprobamate may also stimulate the microsomal enzymes which metabolize the oral anticoagulants. With griseofulvin, at least, the effect is dose related and not all patients respond with altered metabolism.[24,29] Interactions with oral anticoagulants are frequently reported because their action can be fairly accurately monitored objectively by the prothrombin time test.

Alcohol and phenobarbital, when administered to a pregnant woman, apparently can cross the placental barrier and stimulate the activity of the enzyme glucuronyl transferase in the fetus. This action has been used clinically to reduce serum bilirubin levels in infants.[30,31] Chronic use of alcoholic beverages has been shown to reduce the half-life of tolbutamide nearly 50 percent as compared to control patients.[32] Phenobarbital has been shown to stimulate the enzyme systems which metabolize other barbiturates, hydrocortisone, digitoxin, griseofulvin and others. Additional substances which reportedly stimulate enzymes are the chlorinated insecticides, chlordane and DDT, but not the organic phosphate insecticides (which have an inhibiting effect on the enzymes).[13,23,33,34]

A number of other drugs have their metabolism stimulated by enzyme inducers; the significance of many of these interactions is questionable. For example, the blood level and half-life of diphenylhydantoin is decreased by concurrent administration of phenobarbital; however, this combination of drugs is used effectively in the treatment of grand mal epilepsy.

Just as certain drugs may stimulate microsomal enzymes, other drugs can inhibit these same enzymes. Inhibition of the metabolizing enzymes will, of course, result in delayed metabolism, hence prolonged or increased activity of the drug (Table 4).

Table 4. Drugs Shown to Inhibit Microsomal Enzymes in Man

Allopurinol
Bishydroxycoumarin
Disulfiram
Isoniazid
MAO Inhibitors
Methylphenidate

Several case histories appear in the literature indicating drug intoxication due to enzyme inhibition. Several patients receiving bishydroxycoumarin and methylphenidate had a hypoprothrombinemic response attributed to reduced metabolism of the anticoagulant. Toxicity to diphenylhydantoin has been reported in epileptics who were later given bishydroxycoumarin, isoniazid or chloramphenicol.[35,36,37] Chloramphenicol and bishydroxycoumarin may also inhibit the metabolism of tolbutamide.

The monoamine oxidase inhibitors are a deceptive group of drugs involved in many interactions because of a dual enzyme inhibiting phenomenon. As indicated by their name, they inhibit the enzyme, monoamine oxidase, which is found at adrenergic nerve endings, and whose function is to destroy norepinephrine. A number of drugs are monoamine compounds; thus a drug which inhibits monoamine oxidase has the potential for enhancing the effect of levarterenol (norepinephrine) on drugs and other substances which either mimic norepinephrine or cause its release. Numerous articles have reported hypertensive crisis and even death in patients on MAO inhibitors who were given sympathomimetics,[38] had taken non-prescription cold medications containing sympathomimetics,[21] or had ingested foods high in tryramine content, the tyramine displacing norepinephrine from inactive binding sites at the adrenergic nerve ending.[20] Because of their microsomal enzyme inhibiting activity, the list of drugs which the MAO inhibits *could* potentiate is quite long.

Other drugs may inhibit specific enzymes. Mercaptopurine is normally metabolized by the enzyme xanthine oxidase which is inhibited by allopurinol. When the drugs are used concomitantly the dose of mercaptopurine should be reduced to 25 to 33 percent of the usual therapeutic dose.[39]

Alteration of Excretion

The kidney is the most important excretory organ for the body. Excretion of drugs in the urine involves several processes including passive glomerular filtration, active tubular secretion and passive tubular diffusion. In the proximal and distal tubules, the un-ionized forms of weak acids and bases undergo reabsorption or excretion by passive diffusion. The direction is potentially bidirectional, the direction of the diffusion depending upon the concentrations of the drug and the *p*H on the two sides of the tubular cells. The same acid-base phenomenon affecting passage of drugs across cell walls in absorption from the gastrointestinal tract applies in the excretion of drugs in the kidneys. Weak acids with a *p*Ka of 3.0 to 7.5 (Table5) and weak bases with a *p*Ka of 7.5 to 10.5 (Table 6) seem to have the greatest changes in lipid solubility at physiological *p*H range.

Table 5. Weak Acids with pKa of 3.0 - 7.5

Barbiturates	Phenylbutazone
Coumarins	Salicylic acid
Nalidixic acid	Sulfonamides
Nitrofurantoin	

Table 6. Weak Bases with pKa of 7.5 - 10.5

Amitriptyline	Morphine
Amphetamine	Procaine
Chloroquine	Quinacrine
Ephedrine	Quinidine
Imipramine	Quinine
Levorphanol	Theophylline
Mecamylamine	Tolazoline
Meperidine	

Application of the Henderson-Hasselbach equation shows graphically this phenomenon.

$$\frac{[H+]\,[A-]}{[HA]} = K$$

Enzyme systems generally function to convert non-polar compounds into more water-soluble, polar (or ionized) substances. Such substances, after being filtered into the tubular urine at the Bowman capsule, are less likely to cross tubular cell membranes and be reabsorbed into the blood stream. Because the lipid solubility of the above-named weak acids and bases can be altered several fold by physiologically possible *pH* changes, change in the *p*H of the urine can result in markedly altered excretion rates of such products.

Clinical examples of interactions affecting the patient because of altered excretion of compounds are difficult to find. However, the effect may be the insidious cause of unexplainable reactions. For example, individual variability may explain the discrepancy between Koch-Weser's and Udall's report on warfarin-quinidine interaction (or non-interaction).[40,41] However, neither investigator considered the *p*H of the urine of the patient. Work by Gerhardt and co-workers[42] indicated that changes of urinary *p*H can markedly alter the effectiveness of quinidine, changing the quinidine excretion from 115 mg/L at urinary *p*H 6.0 to 13 mg/L at *p*H 7.5 with concomitant changes in EKG findings.

The effectiveness of certain antibiotics is somewhat *p*H-dependent. For example, the aminoglycoside antibiotics, neomycin, kanamycin and streptomycin, are reportedly more active in an alkaline urine than an acid urine.[43]

Certain drugs may be excreted via the same enzyme system. Aminosalicylic acid (PAS) is said to prolong the blood level of isoniazid (INH) by competing with INH for sites on the enzyme involved in excretion.[44] PAH apparently acts in a similar fashion with penicillin while probenecid may act by inhibiting the enzyme system (there are other theories for the action of probenecid).

Just as drugs which alter urinary *p*H can affect the action of other drugs, so likewise can drugs which alter excretion of ions. Most common is the hypokalemia induced primarily by thiazide diuretics, but also other diuretic agents. Increased digitalis toxicity is one outcome of hypokalemia;[45] increased potency of skeletal muscle relaxants is not well documented.[46]

PHARMACOLOGICAL EFFECTS AND INTERACTIONS

Two drugs may have similar or opposite pharmacological effects and, hence, if administered concurrently, may produce additive or antagonistic results. Most health practitioners are familiar with the primary pharmacological action of a drug or at least its main use. The secondary pharmacological effects, which are often obscure or ignored, are the ones which seem to have produced some clinically important adverse results.

Alcohol, of course, is a CNS depressant. When ingested by a patient taking other CNS depressant drugs, the expected result is an additive depression.[47]

The phenothiazine tranquilizers have a number of secondary pharmacological actions. Their alpha-adrenergic blocking action results in warnings in the literature that epinephrine should not be used to combat phenothiazine-induced hypotension because of "epinephrine-reversal."[48] Less well known is the anticholinergic effect of the phenothiazines which, when combined with other anticholinergic drugs, including the antihistamines, has resulted in loss of teeth and adynamic ileus.[49,50]

Quinidine and quinine have a mild hypoprothrombinemic effect which apparently seldom causes any problems. Four case histories appear in the literature indicating that this effect of quinidine may be additive with that of the oral anticoagulants.[40,51] Not all patients receiving this combination of drugs[41] (*e.g.*, quinidine and warfarin) seem to exhibit the additive effect, and since quinidine is a weak base whose excretion rate is markedly affected by urine *p*H, this interaction might have a third component.

Quinidine also has a myoneural blocking effect, and one or two cases of "recurarization" have been reported in patients receiving quinidine shortly after an operation in which ether or a skeletal muscle relaxant was used.[52,53,54] More commonly reported, however, is apnea following administration, usually intraperitoneally, of an aminoglycoside antibiotic (*e.g.*, streptomycin, neomycin, kanamycin) during or immediately after an operative procedure in which ether or a skeletal muscle relaxant was used.[55,56,57]

Neostigmine, the cholinesterase inhibitor, is recommended as an antagonist for the curare-type (non-depolarizing) relaxants but may potentiate the succinylcholine-type (depolarizing).[58] Patients may have contact with cholinesterase inhibitors without the physician being aware of this fact; for example, the patient may be using eye drops such as echothiophate or may be exposed to polyphosphate insecticides such as parathion.[59,60]

A number of hypotensive agents act by displacing or replacing norepinephrine at adrenergic nerve endings. This effect of guanethidine, particularly, may be reversed by a number of agents such as amphetamine-type adrenergics, other CNS stimulants such as methylphenidate or diethylpropion, monoamine oxidase inhibitors and the pharmacologically related tricyclic antidepressants.[61]

Miscellaneous Interactions

A number of interactions defy simple classification. The antagonistic effect of the bacteriostatic antibiotics (*e.g.*, chloramphenicol, tetracyclines) to penicillin has been reported.[62,63] The bacteriostatic antibiotic modifies certain characteristics of the bacterial population making them less susceptible to the action of penicillin. Only in rare instances has this been of clinical importance for, if the organism is susceptible to the bacteriostatic agent, a clinical cure will occur.

Many drugs interfere with laboratory test results. They may do it by forming a substance which enters into the reaction, by providing a metabolite which is chemically similar to the substance being measured or by producing a masking color. This subject is considered in Chapter 23 and the reader also may refer to one of the review articles in the literature.[64,65]

Nonproprietary and Trade Names of Drugs:

Allopurinol	Zyloprim
Amitriptyline	Elavil
Bethanechol	Urecholine
Bishydroxycoumarin	Dicumarol
Chloroquine	Aralen (withdrawn from market)
Clofibrate	Atromid-S
Cyclophosphamide	Cytoxan
Diethylpropion	Tenuate, Tepanil
Dextrothyroxine	Choloxin
Disulfiram	Antabuse
Echothiophate	Phospholine
Ethchlorvynol	Placidyl
Ethyl Biscoumacetate	Tromexan (withdrawn from market)
Glutethimide	Doriden
Haloperidol	Haldol
Hexobarbital	Sombucaps, Sombulex
Imipramine	Tofranil
Levarterenol	Levophed
Levodopa	Dopar, Larodopa
Levorphanol	Levo-Dromoran
Mecamylamine	Inversine
Mercaptopurine	Purinethol
Methylphenidate	Ritalin
Nalidixic Acid	NegGram
Neostigmine	Prostigmin
Norepinephrine	Levophed
Pentolinium	Ansolysen
Phentolamine	Regitine
Phenylbutazone	Butazolidin
Probenecid	Benemid
Propranolol	Inderal
Quinacrine	Atabrine
Sulfinpyrazone	Anturane
Tolazoline	Priscoline
Tolbutamide	Orinase
Warfarin	Coumadin, Panwarfin

Conclusion

What should the clinical pharmacist do if he notes that a patient is receiving two drugs which may interact? This is a matter of personal judgment. The pharmacist should contact the prescriber if the pharmacist believes the prescriber is unaware of the potential problem. It is important that the pharmacist refer to original clinical reports in commenting on the possibility of adverse effects due to an interaction. Furthermore, the pharmacist should be prepared to offer alternative suggestions for the prescribed drug and, perhaps, a professional evaluation on the possible incidence and clinical importance of the interaction as well as an evaluation of the published reports.

Drug interactions is a complex subject of unknown clinical importance. A myriad of factors may be responsible for the lack or incidence of interactions and their severity. Drug interactions is an area requiring professional competence in reading, interpreting and evaluating the literature of drug therapy and disseminating information of clinical relevance.

References

1. Hartshorn, E. A.: Drug Interactions. General Considerations, *Drug Intelligence* *2*:4-7, (Jan.) 1968.

2. Douglas, J. F. *et al.*: Studies on the Metabolism of Meprobamate, *Proc. Soc. Exptl. Biol. Med.* *112*:436-438 (Feb.) 1963.

3. Hartshorn, E. A.: Drug Interactions—2. How Drugs Interact, *Drug Intelligence* *2*:58-65 (Mar.) 1968.

4. Bianchine, J. *et al.*: L-Dopa Absorption and Metabolism by the Human Stomach, Johns Hopkins University, Baltimore, Md. From paper presented at the New York Academy of Sciences Conference on Drug Metabolism in Man, June 29 - July 1, 1970.

5. Kunin, C. M. and Finland, M.: Clinical Pharmacology of the Tetracycline Antibiotics, *Clin. Pharmacol. Therap.* *2*:51-69 (Jan.-Feb.) 1961.

6. Michel, J. C. *et al.*: Effect of Food and Antacids on Blood Levels of Aureomycin and Terramycin, *J. Lab. Clin. Med.* *36*:632-634, 1950.

7. Harcourt, R. S. and Hamburger, M.: The Effect of Magnesium Sulfate in Lowering Tetracycline Blood Levels, *J. Lab. Clin. Med.* *50*:464-468 (Sept.) 1957.

8. Goodman, L. S. and Gilman, A.: *The Pharmacological Basis of Therapeutics*, ed. 4, The Macmillan Co., New York, N. Y., 1970, p. 597.

9. Solomon, H. M. and Schrogie, J. J.: Change in Receptor Site Affinity—A Proposed Explanation for the Potentiating Effect of D-Thyroxine on the Anticoagulant Response to Warfarin, *Clin. Pharmacol. Therap.* *8*:797-799 (Nov.-Dec.) 1967.

10. Kotler, M. M. *et al.*: Hypoglycemia Precipitated By Propranolol, *Lancet* *2*:1389-1390 (Dec. 24) 1966.

11. Muray McGavi, D. D. M.: Depressed Levels of Serum-Pseudocholinesterase with Ecothiophate-Iodine Eye Drops, *Lancet* *2*:272-3 (Aug. 7) 1965.

12. Aggeler, P. M. *et al.*: Potentiation of Anticoagulant Effect of Warfarin by Phenylbutazone, *New Engl. J. Med.* *276*:496-501 (Mar. 2) 1967.

13. Conney, A. H.: Pharmacological Implications of Microsomal Enzyme Induction, *Pharmacol. Rev.* *19*:317-366 (Sept.) 1967.

14. Cucinell, S. A. *et al.*: The Effect of Chloral Hydrate on Bishydroxycoumarin Metabolism—A Fatal Outcome, *J. Am. Med. Assoc.* *197*:366-368 (Aug. 1) 1966.

15. Sellers, E. M. and Koch-Weser, J.: Potentiation of Warfarin-Induced Hypoprothrombinemia by Chloral Hydrate, *New Engl. J. Med.* *283*:827-831 (Oct. 15) 1970.

16. Done, A. K.: Developmental Pharmacology, *Clin. Pharmacol. Therap.* *5*:432-479 (July-Aug.) 1964.

17. Odell, G. B.: The Dissociation of Bilirubin from Albumin and Its Clinical Implications, *J. Pediat.* *55*:268-279 (Sept.) 1959.

18. Silverman, W. A.: *et al.*: A Difference in Mortality Rate and Incidence of Kernicterus Among Premature Infants Allotted to Two Prophylactic Antibacterial Regimens, *Pediatrics* *18*:614-625 (Sept.) 1956.

19. Zubrod, C. G. *et al.*: Studies on the Chemotherapy of Human Malarias; VIII. The Physiological Disposition of Pamaquine, *J. Clin. Invest.* *27*:114-120 (May) 1948.

20. Asatoor, A. M., Levi, A. J. and Milne, M. D.: Tranylcypromine and Cheese, *Lancet* *2*:733-734 (Oct. 5) 1963.

21. Cuthbert, M. F., Greenberg, M. P., and Morley, S. W.: Cough and Cold Remedies—A Potential Danger to Patients on Monoamine Oxidase Inhibitors, *Brit. Med. J.* *1*:404-406 (Feb. 15) 1969.

22. Goodman and Gilman, op. cit., p. 425.

23. Dixon, R. L.: Effect of Chlordan Pretreatment on the Metabolism and Lethality of Cyclophosphamide, *J. Pharm. Sci.* *57*:1351-1353 (Aug.) 1968.

24. Cucinell, S. A. *et al.*: Drug Interactions in Man, *Clin. Pharmacol. Therap. 6*:420-429 (July-Aug.) 1965.

25. Orrenius, S. *et al.*: Phenobarbital-Induced Synthesis of the Microsomal Drug-Metabolizing Enzymes System and Its Relationship to the Proliferation of Endoplasmic Membranes, *J. Cell. Biol. 25*:627-639 (June) 1965.

26. MacDonald, M. G. *et al.*: The Effects of Phenobarbital, Chloral Betaine and Glutethimide Administration on Warfarin Plasma Levels and Hypoprothrombinemic Responses In Man, *Clin. Pharmacol. Therap. 10*:80-84 (Jan.-Feb.) 1969.

27. Robinson, D. S. and Sylwester, D.: Interaction of Commonly Prescribed Drugs and Warfarin, *Ann. Internal. Med. 72*:853-856 (June) 1970.

28. Catalano, P. M. and Cullen, S. I.: Warfarin Antagonism by Griseofulvin (Abstract), *Clin. Res. 14*:266 (Apr.) 1966.

29. Cullen, S. I. and Catalano, P. M.: Griseofulvin-Warfarin Antagonism, *J. Am. Med. Assoc. 199*:582-583 (Feb.) 1967.

30. Yaffe, S. J. *et al.*: Enhancement of Glucuronide-Conjugating Capacity in a Hyperbilirubinemic Infant Due to Apparent Enzyme Induction by Phenobarbital, *New Engl. J. Med. 275*:1461-1466 (Dec. 29) 1966.

31. Lieber, C. S. and DeCarli, L. M.: Ethanol Oxidation by Hepatic Microsomes—Adaptive Increase after Ethanol Feeding, *Science 162*:917-918 (Nov. 22) 1968.

32. Kater, R. M. H. *et al.*: Increased Rate of Tolbutamide Metabolism in Alcoholic Patients, *J. Am. Med. Assoc. 207*: 363-365 (Jan. 13) 1969.

33. Bledsoe, T. *et al.*: An Effect of o,p'-DDD on the Extra-Adrenal Metabolism of Cortisol in Man, *J. Clin. Endocrinol. Metab. 24*:1303-1311 (Dec.) 1964.

34. Southren, A. L. *et al.*: Remission in Cushing's Syndrome with o,p'-DDD, *J. Clin. Endocrinol. Metab. 26*:268-278 (Mar.) 1966.

35. Christensen, L. K. and Skovsted, L.: Inhibition of Drug Metabolism by Chloramphenicol, *Lancet 2*:1397-1399 (Dec. 27) 1969.

36. Hansen, J. M. *et al.*: Dicumarol-Induced Diphenylhydantoin Intoxication, *Lancet 2*:265-266 (July 30) 1966.

37. Kristensen, M. and Hansen, J. M.: Potentiation of the Tolbutamide Effect by Dicumarol, *Diabetes 16*:211-214 (Apr.) 1967.

38. Elis, J. *et al.*: Modification by Monoamine Oxidase Inhibitors of the Effect of Some Sympathomimetics on Blood Pressure, *Brit. Med. J. 2*:75-78 (Apr. 8) 1967.

39. Reilly, M. J. *et al.*, eds.: American Hospital Formulary Service (AHFS), Am. Soc. Hosp. Pharm., Washington, D.C., (Mar.) 1967, p. 92:00 (Allopurinol).

40. Koch-Weser, J.: Quinidine-Induced Hypoprothrombinemic Hemorrhage in Patients on Chronic Warfarin Therapy, *Ann. Internal Med. 68*:511-517 (Mar.) 1968.

41. Udall, J. A., Quinidine and Hypoprothrombinemia, *Ann. Internal Med. 69*:403-404 (Aug.) 1968.

42. Gerhardt, R. E. *et al.*: Quinidine Excretion in Aciduria and Alkaluria, *Ann. Internal Med. 71*:927-933 (Nov.) 1969.

43. Anon.: Effect of *p*H of the Urine on Antimicrobial Therapy of Urinary Tract Infections, *Med. Letter Drugs Therap. 9*:47-48 (June 16) 1967.

44. Reilly: AHFS, op. cit. (May) 1963, p. 8:16 (Aminosalicylic Acid).

45. Lown, B. *et al.*: Paroxysmal Atrial Tachycardia with Block, *Circulation 21*:129-143 (Jan.) 1960.

46. Foster, P.: Potassium Depletion and the Central Action of Curare, *Brit. J. Anaesthesia 28*:488 (Nov.) 1956.

47. Chelton, L. G. and Whisnant, C. L.: The Combination of Alcohol and Drug Intoxication, *Southern Med. J. 59*: 393 (Apr.) 1966.

48. Reilly: AHFS, op. cit., (Mar.) 1970, p. 28:16.08 (The Phenothiazines).

49. Warnes, H., Lehmann, H. E. and Ban, T. A.: Adynamic Ileus During Psychoactive Medication—A Report of Three Fatal and Five Severe Cases, *Can. Med. Assoc. J. 96*:1112-1113 (Apr. 15) 1967.

50. Winer, J. A. and Bahn, S.: Loss of Teeth with Antidepressent Drug Therapy, *Arch. Gen. Psychiat. 16*:239-240 (Feb.) 1967.

51. Gazzaniga, A. B. and Stewart, D. R.: Possible Quinidine-Induced Hemorrhage in a Patient on Warfarin Sodium, *New Engl. J. Med. 280*:711 (Mar. 27) 1969.

52. Miller, R. D., Way, W. L. and Katzung, B. G.: The Potentiation of Neuromuscular Blocking Agents by Quinidine, *Anesthesiology 28*:1036-1041 (Nov.-Dec.) 1967.

53. Schmidt, J. L. *et al.*: The Effect of Quinidine on the Action of Muscle Relaxants, *J. Am. Med. Assoc. 183*:669-673 (Feb. 23) 1963.

54. Cuthbert, M. F.: The Effect of Quinidine and Procainamide on the Neuromuscular Blocking Action of Suxamethonium, *Brit. J. Anaesthesia 38*:775-9 (Oct.) 1966.

55. Belam, O. H.: Anaesthesia and Therapeutic Drugs, *Postgrad. Med. J. 42*:374-377 (June) 1966.

56. Bell, R. W. and Jenicek, J. A.: Respiratory Failure Following Intramural Bowel Injection of Neomycin—Report of a Case, *Med. Ann. D.C. 35*:603-604 (Nov.) 1966.

57. Blake-Knox, P. E. A.: Neuromuscular Block with Streptomycin, *Brit. Med. J. 1*:1319 (May 6) 1961.

58. Goodman, L. S. and Gilman, A.: op. cit. p. 613.

59. Anon.: Adverse Effects of Topical Antiglaucoma Drugs, *Med. Letter Drugs Therap. 9*:92 (Nov. 17) 1967.

60. Reilly: AHFS, op. cit., (Mar.) 1967, p. 52:20 (Echothiophate).

61. Gulati, O. D. *et al.*: Antagonism of Adrenergic Neuron Blockade in Hypertensive Subjects, *Clin. Pharmacol. Therap. 7*:510-514 (July-Aug.) 1966.

62. Lepper, M. H. and Dowling, H. F.: Treatment of Pneumococcic Meningitis with Penicillin Compared with Penicillin Plus Aureomycin, *Arch. Internal Med. 88*:489-494 (Oct.) 1951.

63. Wallace, J. F. *et al.*: Studies on the Pathogenesis of Meningitis; VI. Antagonism Between Penicillin and Chloramphenicol in Experimental Pneumococcal Meningitis, *J. Lab. Clin. Med. 70*:408-418 (Sept.) 1967.

64. Cross, F. C., Canada, A. T., Jr. and Davis, N. M.: The Effect of Certain Drugs on the Results of Some Common Laboratory Diagnostic Procedures, *Am. J. Hosp. Pharm. 23*: 234-239 (May) 1966.

65. Elking, Sr. M. P. and Kabat, H. F.: Drug-Induced Modifications of Laboratory Test Values, *Am. J. Hosp. Pharm. 25*:485-519 (Sept.) 1968.

Additional References

1. Bernstein, D.: Drugs Known to Interact with Coumarin-Type Anticoagulants, *Drug Intelligence Clin. Pharm. 5*:276-278 (Sept.) 1971.

2. Hansten, P.: *Drug Interactions,* Lea & Febiger, Philadelphia, Pa., 1971.

3. Hartshorn, E. A.: Central Nervous System Drugs—Anesthetics, *Drug Intelligence Clin. Pharm. 5*:202-206 (July) 1971.

4. Hartshorn, E. A.: CNS Drugs—Analgesics and Antipyretics, *Drug Intelligence Clin. Pharm. 5*:356-360 (Nov.) 1971.

5. Hartshorn, E. A.: Drug Interactions—Analgesics, Salicylates, *Drug Intelligence Clin. Pharm. 5*:388-392 (Dec.) 1971.

6. Hartshorn, E. A.: Drug Interactions—Pyrazolone Derivatives, *Drug Intelligence Clin. Pharm. 6*:6-10 (Jan.) 1972.

7. Hartshorn, E. A.: Drug Interactions—Miscellaneous Analgesics, *Drug Intelligence Clin. Pharm. 6*:50-54 (Feb.) 1972.

8. Inglott, A. S.: Significance of Drug Interactions, *Drug Intelligence Clin. Pharm. 6*:11-13 (Jan.) 1972.

9. Ku, L. L. J. H., Ward, C. O. and Durgin, Sr. J. M.: A Clinical Study of Drug Interaction and Anticoagulant Therapy, *Drug Intelligence Clin. Pharm. 4*:300-306 (Nov.) 1970.

10. Anon.: Drug Interactions—I. American Society of Hospital Pharmacists, Bethesda, Md., 1971.

10

Drug therapy and diet

by Paul G. Pierpaoli

A previous chapter on clinically significant drug interactions and their therapeutic implications has dealt with mechanisms of drug interactions and the limitations inherent in interpreting and disseminating such information in a clinical setting. To date, most reports of drug interaction phenomena have been largely limited to the effects of one drug being modified by another drug or the effects of drug-induced changes in clinical laboratory values. Interactions of drugs and dietary components, on the other hand, have been primarily directed toward reports of drug-induced malabsorption phenomena or drug effects on nutritional status. Studies on the effects of food upon drug absorption and drug response have been only sporadically cited in the literature.

Changing dietary patterns, the advent of food processing technology, unintentional or intentional alterations in the quality of the food chain, and the resultant impact on nutritional status and disease are now considered major elements in health care maintenance. Relationships between drugs and diet is a subject fraught with much speculation and uncertainty with minor exceptions. Foods are known to contain a variety of pharmacologically active substances, some of which are capable of producing severe toxicity and even death. The reader is directed to Sapeika's text for a more detailed and comprehensive treatment of this subject.[1] Pharmacologically active substances present in foods can be categorized and topically exemplified in the following manner:

1. *Foods of Plant and Animal Origin.* In this class one can cite the presence of 5-hydroxytryptamine in pineapples and bananas,[2,3] 3,4-dihydroxyphenylalanine (DOPA) in broad beans,[4] oxalates in spinach, rhubarb and celery, and various metals such as selenium, potassium, calcium, magnesium and sodium in grains and other foods. Also the presence of tyramine in various cheeses and chicken livers as well as fatty acids and lipids in meats has been noted.
2. *Foods of Marine Origin.* Neurotoxins have been found in species of poisonous fish and paralytic toxins in polluted shellfish. Pesticide and heavy metal residues also have been detected in several species of edible fish.
3. *Food Additives and Contaminants.* Increasing quantities of intended food additives such as preservatives, antioxidants, sequestrants, surface-active agents, stabilizers and thickeners, bleaching and maturing agents, buffers, acidulants, food colors, nonnutritive and special dietary sweetners, flavors, and so forth are used in food processing technology to enhance the taste, structure or storage life of food.[5] Examples of naturally occurring contaminants are the potent mycotoxins and bacterial toxins which result from fungal or bacterial contamination of foods. Man-made contaminants include antibiotics, pesticides, radionuclides, metals, and processing degradation products.
4. *Water, Soft Drinks and Alcoholic Beverages.* These dietary constituents may contain various metals, xanthines, histamines, alcohol and congeners.

The Nature of Drug-Food Interactions

There are two major areas of concern with regard to drug effects and food: (1) some drugs are capable of impairing the absorption and utilization of nutrients and (2) certain foods or patterns of dietary consumption may alter drug absorption and response. There are numerous examples of the first phenomenon, which in some instances may result in markedly altered nutritional states. With the exception of anti-infective agents, most of those drugs implicated in the impairment of absorption and utilization of nutrients are used for long-term treatment and hence are more prone to induce malabsorption syndromes.

The absorption characteristics of drugs and foods are strikingly dissimilar. The absorption of most drugs is governed to a large extent by (1) relative lipid solubility (the more lipid-soluble the greater the extent of absorption), (2) rate of dissociation (characterized by pKa), (3) pH of the medium, (4) particle size or molecular size, and (5) physical form (crystal state, etc.). Transport across gastric or intestinal mucosa is mostly by passive non-ionic diffusion rather than active transport. (Exceptions are digitalis glycosides and pyrimidine compounds which are believed to be actively transported.) Weak acids (those with a pKa less than 2) are as a rule absorbed in the stomach, while weak bases (those with a pKa less than 8) are usually absorbed in the upper intestine.[6] Digestive enzymes or competitive inhibition are not thought to be factors in drug absorption.

The absorption of food, unlike the absorption of drugs, is largely dependent on gastrointestinal secretions, pH and enzyme activity. Transport mechanisms are not limited to passive diffusion, and lipid solubility is only of significance in lipid absorption.[7]

Various dietary constituents also have been shown to alter clinical laboratory test values. Bananas, pineapples, coffee, chocolate, tea and vanilla may alter results of vanilmandelic acid, catecholamine and 5-hydroxyindole acetic acid determinations, while carrots may interfere with serum bilirubin determinations. Dietary restriction of these substances for at least twenty-four hours prior to the respective test is therefore advisable.

Effects of Drugs on Nutrient and Electrolyte Absorption and Utilization

There are numerous citations of drug-induced impairment of nutrient and electrolyte absorption and utilization in man. They can be classified accordingly:

1. *Drugs Affecting Gastric and/or Intestinal Motility.* Mineral oil has been shown to decrease the absorption of carotenes, vitamins A, D, E, and K.[8] Chronic use of certain cathartics such as podophyllin, jalop and colocynth may cause calcium and potassium loss, and steatorrhea,[9] while oxyphenisatin, bisacodyl and phenolphthalein are capable of inhibiting intestinal uptake of glucose.[6] It also has been suggested that chronic and excessive antacid use can lead to thiamine deficiency, presumably because of alkaline destruction of thiamine within the bowel lumen.[8] Orally administered calcium carbonate and mannitol have been implicated in causing steatorrhea by possible intraluminal fat binding[10] and direct injury to absorptive mucosal cells.[11] In addition, certain ganglionic blocking agents and anticholinergic substances may be capable of inhibiting the absorption of some nutrients by their action on the autonomic system of the gastrointestinal tract.[12] Examples of such drugs are methantheline, propantheline and mecamylamine.

2. *Hypocholesterolemic Agents.* In light of current dietary trends in patients with coronary heart disease, the hypocholesterolemic agents are being used with increasing frequency. Neomycin, clofibrate and cholestyramine resin, while being relatively effective hypocholesterolemic agents, have been associated with a variety of malabsorption phenomena including vitamin B_{12}, d-xylose, carotene, medium chain triglyceride, electrolyte, iron and sugar absorption.[8,9]
3. *Surfactants.* Stool softening agents are capable of affecting fat dispersion and permeability of the lipoprotein membrane of mucosal cells with resultant changes in the absorption of a number of nutritional factors.[6]
4. *Anti-Infective Agents.* Cycloserine, para-aminosalicylic acid, neomycin, erythromycin, sulfonamides, broad spectrum antibiotics such as the tetracyclines, penicillins, isoniazid, chloramphenicol and others have been implicated in decreased folic acid utilization, vitamin B_{12} malabsorption, decreased bacterial synthesis of vitamin K, impaired absorption of calcium and magnesium, pyridoxine inactivation and impaired amino acid transfer in protein synthesis.[8,13]
5. *Cytotoxic Drugs.* Methotrexate, aminopterin and other folic acid antagonists are inhibitors of folic acid, interfere with vitamin B_{12} and d-xylose absorption and are responsible for nonspecific changes in the jejunal mucosa.[13,14] Colchicine, a specific therapeutic tool in the management of acute episodes of gout, is also associated with vitamin B_{12}, carotene, fat, lactose and electrolyte and d-xylose malabsorption.[15,16]
6. *Anticonvulsant Drugs.* Diphenylhydantoin, primidone and phenobarbital have been specifically indicted for their role in the impairment and utilization of folic acid, vitamin B_{12} and d-xylose.[17]
7. *Alcohol.* The effects of alcohol on nutritional status are well-known with malabsorption of folic acid, vitamin B_{12} and increased excretion of magnesium.[9,18] Transient hypomagnesemia has been observed in alcoholic patients undergoing convulsive seizures during acute withdrawal phases.
8. *Diuretics.* Most diuretics with the exception of triamterene and spironolactone are capable of precipitating dangerous episodes of hypokalemia through excessive renal clearance of potassium. Some diuretics such as the thiazides also have been reported to be diabetogenic.[19]
9. *Oral Contraceptives.* Some oral contraceptives have been implicated in impaired folic acid absorption and utilization.[20-22]

In addition to these broad groupings of drugs there are recent citations of chlorpromazine-induced hypercholesterolemia.[23] This may well be a serious problem since this agent and other phenothiazine drugs are used quite widely in the management of psychiatric patients over long periods of time.

Drug Effects on Taste and Appetite

Recently there have been reports of decreased taste acuity and unpleasant or altered taste sensation associated with griseofulvin, D-penicillamine, clofibrate, lincomycin, oxyphedrin and some tranquilizers.[24] It should be noted that these reports are not associated exclusively with concomitant ingestion of foods, but appear to be systemically mediated. Exact mechanisms explaining these effects remain obscure at this time.

Any unpleasant tasting drugs, on the other hand, such as chloral hydrate, paraldehyde, vitamin B complex, uncoated penicillin preparations as well as suspensions, and a host of other drugs may precipitate transient states of altered taste sensation or aftertastes when foods are administered concomitantly or shortly after ingestion of such drugs. The long-term use of many of the psychotropic agents such as the phenothiazines, benzodiazepines and tricyclic antidepressants also has been associated with substantial weight gain in some patients. Such effects appear to be secondary to altered mental status and resultant appetite improvement.

Effects of Food Upon Drug Absorption and Response

There have been relatively few citations devoted to this phenomenon exclusive of the classic monoamine oxidase inhibition and tyramine-containing food interaction, selected studies on food impaired antibiotic absorption, and alcohol-drug interactions. Four possible means in which drug-food interaction phenomena might theoretically occur include:

1. The effect of food upon drug absorption.
2. Dietary constituents may alter drug metabolism (*i.e.*, through enzyme induction or inhibition, etc.).
3. Foods may possibly alter the rate of excretion of certain drugs (*i.e.*, excessive acidification or alkalinization of urine).
4. Pharmacologically active substances present in foods may alter the response of a concomitantly administered drug (*i.e.*, monoamine oxidase inhibitors and tyramine-containing foods with resultant increases in pressor responses).

From a practical therapeutic view point, the bulk of such interactions (at least those of clinical significance) probably relate to impaired drug absorption. The exact mechanisms of food effects on absorption of drugs are poorly understood and do not appear to be uniform in nature. The presence of food in the gastrointestinal tract may precipitate changes in pH, osmolality, motility and secretion. Such effects are largely functions of the composition of the meal. In turn, they may have an effect on ionization, stability, solubility, intestinal transit time, stomach emptying time, and drug absorption.[6] Insoluble complex formation between drugs and food constituents also has been demonstrated.[25] The absorption of lincomycin has been shown to be reduced when administered with sodium or calcium cyclamate sweetened beverages. The exact mechanism has not been completely elucidated, but it is postulated that the cyclamate may form a complex with lincomycin which is not absorbed.

Antibiotic and Sulfonamide Drugs

Perhaps the antibiotic and sulfonamide drugs have received more attention than any other group of therapeutic agents with regard to impairment of absorption by foods. Food has been shown to reduce the efficiency of absorption of tetracycline, demethylchlortetracycline, chlortetracylcline and methacycline. Penicillin G, penicillin V, nafcillin, oxacillin, ampicillin, erythromycin base, erythromycin propionate, erythromycin stearate, triacetyloleandomycin and lincomycin absorption also have been reportedly delayed by concomitant administration with food.[26-32] It should be noted, however, that none of these reports alludes to clinical failures and that by and large they represent delays in absorption rather than a diminution of effect. This same effect has been observed with the sulfonamide drugs. There is conclusive evidence that absorption is delayed but not reduced by concomitant administration of food.[33] The concomitant administration of tetracyclines and dairy products containing large amounts of calcium presumably could result in complex formations with calcium caseinate present in such foods and result in impaired absorption of the antibiotic.[34] To date, however, no clinical failures have been reported despite the widespread dissemination of this interaction report. Recent *in vitro* studies which compare the relative calcium binding capacity of tetracycline derivatives show that demethylchlortetracycline is 74.5 percent bound, chlortetracycline 52.7 percent, tetracycline and methacycline 39.5 percent, oxytetracycline 36 percent and doxycycline 19-22 percent.[35] Perhaps more significant in this regard, is a recent report of impaired tetracycline absorption through concomitant administration with iron salts. This report clearly established declines in plasma levels of the tetracyclines from 10-50 percent.[36]

Griseofulvin levels have been found to be markedly increased after ingestion of a high fat content meal.[37] This could be a significant problem in patients receiving anticoagulant therapy, as there have been several case reports of decreased prothrombin time when griseofulvin and warfarin were administered concurrently.[38]

Tetrachloroethylene is often used to treat hookworm, a problem prevalent in many Puerto Rican communities. Patients should be cautioned against excessive fat intake when taking this anthelmintic in order to avoid systemic absorption and possible central nervous system toxicity.

Drug Administration and Food Ingestion

Inasmuch as there are many drugs whose absorption may be apparently delayed or impaired by concomitant administration of foods, there are a number of drugs which are intrinsically irritating to gastric mucosa and should therefore be taken immediately before, with or immediately after meals or with food or milk. This list is quite extensive but the more popular drugs are indomethacin, diphenylhydantoin, phenylbutazone, nitrofurantoin, steroids, metronidazole, iron salts, aminophylline, potassium supplements, reserpine and many others. The following drugs should be taken on an empty stomach, preferably one hour before meals or three hours after meals: ampicillin, cloxacillin, erythromycin base, lincomycin, penicillin G potassium, pentaerythritol tetranitrate and penicillamine.

Drugs are often mixed with various juices and beverages in an attempt to mask their unpleasant taste or assist in oral administration in patients having difficulty swallowing oral solid dosage forms. This is very often the case in pediatric or geriatric patient populations. The practice of extemporaneously mixing drugs with various juices and beverages may precipitate problems with regard to acid labile substances whose absorption might be impaired in the stomach through decreased gastric pH or *in vitro* inactivation in acidic media. Most beverages and juices as seen in Tables 1 and 2 are quite acidic. Whole milk, by contrast, has an approximate pH range of 6.4 - 6.8. In light of the relative acidity of most beverages other than milk, acid labile antibiotics such as ampicillin, erythromycin base, and penicillin G potassium should not be mixed and allowed to stand for any length of time in the beverages represented

Table 1. pH Range of Selected Commercially Canned Juices and Other Beverages[68]

CANNED JUICES	APPROXIMATE pH RANGE
Cherry	3.4 - 3.6
Cider	2.9 - 3.3
Cranberry	2.5 - 2.7
Currant	3.0
Grapefruit	2.9 - 3.4
Grape	3.5 - 4.5
Lemon	2.2 - 2.6
Lime	2.2 - 2,4
Pineapple	3.4 - 3.7
Prune	3.7 - 4.3
Tomato	3.9 - 4.4
OTHER BEVERAGES	
Milk (cow's)	6.4 - 6.8
Milk (evaporated)	5.9 - 6.3
Beers	4.0 - 5.0
Wines	2.3 - 3.8

Table 2. Approximate pH of Carbonated Beverages[69]

BEVERAGE	pH
Club soda	4.7
Cream soda	3.9
Cherry soda	3.0
Cola	2.4
Ginger ale (pale dry)	2.7
Grape	3.0
Grapefruit	3.0
Lemon	2.9
Lemon-lime	3.1
Orange	3.2
Quinine	2.5
Raspberry	3.1
Root beer	4.0
Sarsaparilla	4.0

in the tables. Concomitant ingestion of large volumes of such beverages (*i.e.*, in excess of 8 fluid ounces) with any acid labile substances also should be avoided whenever possible.

Dietary Constituents and Drug Metabolism

There are numerous literature citations of apparent enzyme induction as well as enzyme inhibition caused by drugs and their resultant impact on rates of drug metabolism; however, reports of diet-induced changes in human drug metabolism have been limited to food contaminants. Pesticide residues such as DDT (chlorophenothane), lindane (gamma benzene hexachloride), aldrin and dieldrin can be found in all levels of the food chain in varying concentrations. These residual concentrations are a function of such factors as the nature of the pest control treatment used in seed preparation, spraying and sprinkling, weathering, climate and soil conditions. Untreated plants may also absorb pesticides from the soil. Organo-chlorine insecticides are stored for prolonged periods in the body fat and livers of man and animals after having been absorbed from contaminated food. Such accumulations to date, however, have been considerably below the minimum toxic dose of such substances. Although acute toxicity from such accumulation has not been observed in man thus far, residuals of certain pesticides (*e.g.*, DDT, aldrin and dieldrin) have been shown in a number of studies to induce microsomal enzymes.[39,40] On the other hand, a recent study by Davies indicated that DDT levels in patients taking phenobarbital and diphenylhydantoin were significantly lower than in those patients not taking these drugs.[41] Since both of these drugs are known to be microsomal enzyme inducers, it has been suggested that this may be the mechanism by which these drugs act to reduce tissue storage of DDT.

Whether such findings are of therapeutic significance is still a matter of considerable speculation. It is becoming readily apparent, however, that advances in food processing technology will continue to add a variety of chemical congeners to the food chain of man. This is a matter which demands a great deal of attention in light of the potential long-term effects of such food consumption on drug metabolism.

Alcohol has been shown to stimulate a microsomal enzyme system responsible for the metabolism of the oral hypoglycemic agent, tolbutamide. Resultant twofold reductions in the half-life of this drug have been observed in chronic alcoholic patients. This may well explain the relatively high failure rate in treating diabetics in this population.[42] It should be noted that this observation to date has been limited to tolbutamide.

Alteration Urinary Excretion

Changes in urinary pH have been shown to markedly influence the activity of some drugs by altering their respective rates of excretion. Such alterations in rates of excretion are functions of pH influence on the ionization of weak acids and weak bases. A drug in its nondissociated form, for example, will more readily diffuse from the urine back into the blood. The action of acidic drugs will be prolonged in an acid urine because there is a larger proportion of the drug in its nondissociated form in an acid urine than in an alkaline urine where it would exist primarily as an ionized salt. The opposite phenomenon will occur for a basic drug such as amphetamine or quinidine.

Although it is generally thought that extreme shifts in urinary pH (*i.e.*, well below 5 and above 8) are difficult to achieve through changes in dietary patterns alone, increased urinary acidification or alkalinization has been observed with concomitant ingestion of acid—or alkaline—ash diets and urinary acidifying or alkalinizing drugs (*i.e.*, ammonium chloride and carbonic anhydrase inhibitors, respectively). That extreme shifts in urinary pH can have important clinical significance is illustrated by a recently cited case of quinidine intoxication which was caused by ingestion of antacids and an alkaline-ash diet during maintenance therapy with quinidine.[43] This patient consumed eight tablets daily of a proprietary antacid preparation containing 200 mg of magnesium hydroxide, 200 mg of dried aluminum hydroxide gel and 20 mg of simethicone. In addition, he consumed one quart daily of fresh orange-grapefruit juice (in a 1:1 ratio). It should be noted that the fruit juice mixture would be equal to ingestion of about 50 mEq of bicarbonate ion daily. This combination of antacid therapy and excessive alkaline-ash diet intake was capable of producing a consistent alkaluria and a resultant decrease in quinidine excretion culminating in a serious abnormal sinus rhythm requiring hospitalization of the patient.

Tables 3 and 4 represent examples of potentially acid or acid-ash foods and basic or alkaline-ash foods.[44] This should be considered in obtaining drug histories from patients receiving acidic or alkaline drugs whose excretion might be altered by shifts in urinary pH and in whom drug toxicity is suspect. Patients receiving quinidine preparations should also be cautioned against taking drugs or foods which might render the urine alkaline. It should be noted that strict vegetarian diets or excessive and chronic alkaline-ash foods would more than likely produce an alkaline urine.

Table 3. Potentially Acid or Acid-Ash Foods[44]

MEAT	VEGETABLE
Meat, fish, fowl, shellfish Eggs Cheese (all types) Peanut butter	Corn and lentils
FAT	FRUIT
Bacon Nuts: Brazil, filberts, peanuts, walnuts	Cranberries, plums, prunes
BREAD	DESSERT
Breads (all types), crackers Macaroni, spaghetti, noodles	Cakes and cookies, plain

Table 4. Potentially Basic or Alkaline-Ash Foods[44]

Milk, cream and Buttermilk

Nuts
Almonds, chestnuts, coconut

Vegetable
All types (except corn and lentils)

Fruit
All types (except cranberries, prunes, plums)

PHARMACOLOGICALLY ACTIVE SUBSTANCES PRESENT IN FOODS

Tyramine-Containing Foods and MAO Inhibitors

Pharmacologically active substances present in some foods have been shown to alter the response of a concomitantly administered drug. This type of interaction has been observed with the concomitant administration of monoamine oxidase inhibitors (*e.g.*, pargyline, phenelzine, nialamide, tranylcypromine and isocarboxazid) and the ingestion of foods containing large amounts of tyramine and other biologically active amines. Several deaths were initially reported from this interaction as a result of exaggerated pressor responses and subsequent hypertensive crisis with intracranial bleeding. Severe attacks have followed the ingestion of as little as one ounce of cheddar cheese. The hypertensive syndrome observed in this drug/food interaction has been described as being clinically similar to that seen in pheochromocytoma. Headache usually heralds the onset of the syndrome, with fever frequently accompanying the hypertensive episode. Most of the attacks have occurred between a half-hour and two hours after patients have eaten the cheese. Monoamine oxidase inhibition appears to modify and intensify the effects of endogenous biogenic amines as well as the precursors of biogenic amines (*i.e.,* DOPA and 5-hydroxytryptophan). Evidence accumulated thus far, also indicates that the indirectly acting sympathomimetic amines such as amphetamine and tyramine are more potentiated than the direct acting amines such as norepinephrine and epinephrine. Amphetamine and tyramine have been shown to act peripherally, primarily by releasing the stores of catecholamines in nerve endings. With monoamine oxidase inhibition, the levels of catecholamines are raised significantly, thereby producing profound potentiation of effects such as pressor actions.[45]

Tyramine-containing foods (notably cheeses) and beverages (specifically Chianti wine) have been the major offenders in this interaction, although DOPA (3,4-dihyroxyphenylalanine) containing substances also have been implicated. The initial warnings resulting from the early cases of hypertensive crisis which were reported in the literature, prompted a number of investigations into the tyramine content of various foods and beverages. These studies clearly indicated that the tyramine content of various cheeses and beverages varied considerably.[46-48] It has been clearly established that the major tyramine-containing foods are certain cheeses (*i.e.,* Stilton, New York State Cheddar, Gruyere and Ermentaler varieties especially), chicken livers, pickled herring and Chianti wine. Broad beans, which also have been implicated in this interaction phenomenon, have been shown to contain significant quantities of DOPA.[46] Table 5 represents a tabulation of the tyramine content of various foods and beverages. It is imperative that patients receiving MAO inhibitors be appropriately counseled to avoid those foods which contain unusually high amounts of tyramine.

Table 5. Tyramine Content of Various Foods[46]

FOOD	MCG/G OR MCG/ML
Cheeses	
Camembert	86
Stilton	466
Brie	180
Ermantaler	225
N. Y. State Cheddar	1,416
Gruyere	516
Processed American	50
Cream	N.D.*
Cottage	N.D.
Yeast	N.D.
Yogurt	N.D.
Beer	
Brand A	1.8
Brand B	2.3
Brand C	4.4
Wine	
Sherry	3.6
Sauterne	0.4
Riesling	0.6
Chianti	25.4
Port	N.D.

*N.D. = not detected

Other Foods

Licorice, when ingested in excessive amounts, has caused hypokalemic myopathy and myoglobinuria.[49] This is thought to be due to an active principle, the 18-beta isomer of glycyrrhetinic acid, which has mineralocorticoid, antidiuretic and anti-inflammatory activity. This compound's structure is steroidal in nature and possesses structural features related to the desoxycorticosterone as well as the glucocorticoid series. In addition to hypokalemia, excessive licorice ingestion has been associated with salt and water retention, hypertension, paresthesias, and alkalosis.[50] Although this substance is only found in the root of the *Glycyrrhiza* species, the natural extract of this plant is still used in some candy manufacturing as a licorice flavor. It should be noted, however, that most American candy manufacturers now use a synthetic licorice flavor in the processing of various candies. On the other hand, many imported varieties of licorice candies (especially those from Italy, France, Switzerland and Holland) contain the natural extract. Chronic excessive consumption of such imported licorice candies may be contraindicated in patients with chronic cardiovascular disease who are maintained on non-potassium sparing diuretics or who are on a salt-free diet.

Monosodium L-Glutamate

The widely used food additive monosodium L-glutamate has definitely been implicated as the causative agent in the "Chinese restaurant syndrome" in certain predisposed individuals.[51] This syndrome is characterized by headaches, burning sensations of the extremities, facial pressure, and chest pain which may mimic the pain of angina. The pharmacological effects appear to be dose related. However, there is a considerable variation in oral threshold doses among individuals.[52] One postulated mechanism of action for this phenomenon is a transient hyponatremia. Chinese and Cantonese cuisine are known to contain large quantities of monosodium L-glutamate, especially the very popular Won Ton soup which has been shown to contain excessive amounts. Perhaps caution should be urged in patients consuming significant quantities of such foods when on long-term diuretic therapy.

Goiterogenic Foods

Brussel sprouts, cabbage, cauliflower, kale, turnips and rutabaga long have been known to possess goiterogenic activity as a result of their thio-oxazolidine content.[53] Under normal circumstances, however, there is usually enough iodine in the normal diet to counteract any such effect.

Potassium Replacement in Diuretic Therapy

Potassium depletion is an ever present problem especially with patients on thiazide therapy. This is particularly true in long-term therapy for patients with hepatic cirrhosis or congestive heart failure. Although potassium supplementation has gained much popularity over the past two or three years, dietary potassium supplementation is also desirable and perhaps more acceptable to some patients. In these patients, high potassium and low sodium containing foods such as dried apricots, peaches, dates and figs, raisins, bananas and prunes are advisable.[54] Orange juice has become popular in this regard, but it should be noted that there are only approximately 6 mEq of potassium in a four ounce portion of fresh juice. Tomato juice has been recommended for potassium supplementation, but a recent report indicates that sodium concentrations in various samples of tomato juice range from 12 to 35 mEq of sodium per 100 ml, despite their relatively high potassium content. It has been suggested that large amounts of tomato juice be withheld from patients with a history of heart failure in light of the unreliable sodium content.[55] Other foods containing relatively high amounts of potassium but concomitantly high sodium content are ham, bacon, sardines, scallops, bran flakes, milk and ketchup. Table 6 represents a list of dietary components which are relatively rich in potassium. Note that breads and cereals, with the exception of bran, are extremely low in potassium.

It should be noted that considerable quantities of sodium and potassium can be contributed unknowingly in many drugs. Some antacids, for instance contain appreciable amounts of sodium and intravenous penicillin G preparations contain considerable quantities of potassium. Comprehensive lists of such values are now available and are of assistance to the pharmacist.[56]

Table 6. Potassium-Rich Foods (300 - 600 mg per serving)

MEAT, FISH, POULTRY	FRUIT	FRUIT JUICES	VEGETABLES
AVERAGE SERVING 3 OUNCES (COOKED)	AVERAGE SERVING AS STATED	AVERAGE SERVING 1 CUP	AVERAGE SERVING 1 CUP OR AS STATED
All fresh fish	*Dried apricots, 12 med. halves	Prune juice	*Yam, 1 medium
Veal	*Dried peaches, uncooked, 1/2 c.	Low sodium tomato juice	*Squash, winter
Chicken (Light meat only)	Banana, 1 medium	Orange juice	Lentils, dry, 1/3 c.
Beef liver	Prunes, 7 large	Orange-grapefruit	Broccoli
Beef	Cantaloupe, 1/2	Tangerine juice	White potato, 1 med.
Pork	Figs, dry, 4 large	Pineapple juice	Sweet potato, 1 med.
	Dates, 6 to 7		Brussels sprouts, 8
	Watermelon, 1/2 slice 3/4″ x 10″		Cauliflower

All breads and cereals (except bran) have a low potassium content.
High potassium but high sodium foods include ham, bacon, sardines, scallops, bran flakes, milk, ketchup, tomato juice.
*Over 600 mg of potassium per average serving.

Table 7. Sodium Content of Some Commonly Used Foods

FOODS	GRAMS PER SERVING	APPROX. MG OF SODIUM PER SERVING
Bread and Cereal Products		
Bread, French	40	200
Bread, raisin, plain or toasted	23	80
Bread, white or whole wheat, plain or toasted	23	120
Crackers, saltines, salted top	25	300
Crackers, graham, honey	50	250
Doughnut, cake type	30	160
Doughnut, yeast	30	70
Pancake, plain	45	200
Waffle, plain	75	360
Most ready to serve breakfast cereals	30	300
Puffed rice, puffed wheat, shredded wheat	15	1
Most cereals including rice, macaroni, cooked, unsalted	140	10
Most cakes with icing	100	375
Most pies, 9"	160	425
Dairy Products		
Milk, whole	240	120
Milk, evaporated	120	120
Milk, skim	24	150
Buttermilk, commercial	240	310
Cheese, cheddar	30	180
Cheese, cottage, creamed	70	140
Cheese, process	30	350
Cream, half and half	60	30
Ice cream, vanilla	70	70
Sherbet, orange	100	20
Yogurt	120	65
Butter or margarine, salted	14	140
Butter or margarine, unsalted	14	1-2
Egg	50	70
Fruits		
Apple, fresh	100	1
Applesauce, canned sweetened	100	2
Apricots, fresh or canned	100	1
Banana	100	1
Cantaloupe	100	12
Grapefruit, pink or white	100	1
Orange	100	1
Peaches, fresh or canned	100	1-2
Pears, fresh or canned	100	2
Pineapple, fresh or canned	100	1-2
Prunes, cooked	100	4
Strawberries	100	1
Watermelon	100	1
Meat, Chicken, Fish		
Bacon, crisp	25	400
Hash, canned corned beef	100	600
Frankfurter, cooked	50	550
Most plain beef, veal, pork, lamb, cooked unsalted	30	25
Beef liver, cooked without salt or salted fat	90	120
Potted meat	90	440
Ham, cooked	30	350
TV Dinners: meat or fish, potato, vegetable	350	1100
Bologna	30	400
Chicken, boneless, cooked, unsalted	85	80
Crab meat, fresh, boiled	100	400
Oysters, fresh	100	75
Salmon, canned	60	300
Sardines, canned in oil	50	260
Shrimp, fresh, cooked	100	150
Tuna, canned in oil	100	800
Vegetables		
Asparagus, cooked, unsalted	100	1
Asparagus, canned	100	300
Beans, dry, most varieties, unsalted	100	5-20
Beans, canned, most varieties	100	300
Beets, cooked, unsalted	100	60
Carrots, raw or cooked, unsalted	100	30
Celery, raw	50	60
Celery, cooked, unsalted	100	90
Eggplant, cooked, unsalted	100	1
Lettuce, plain	50	10
Olives, green	15	350
Peas, English, fresh, cooked, unsalted	100	1
Peas, English, canned	100	275
Peas, English, frozen, cooked unsalted	100	110
Pickles	100	1200
Potato, plain, baked or boiled	100	10
Potato, mashed, creamed	100	325
Potato chips	20	250
Sauerkraut, canned	100	750
Sweet potato, canned in syrup	100	75
Sweet potato, fresh, baked	100	12
Tomato, raw	100	5
Tomato catsup	35	300
Tomato juice, canned	100	200
Tomato paste, canned	100	40
Tomato puree, canned	100	400
Miscellaneous		
Table salt	1 tsp.	2300
Baking powder	1 tsp.	400
Baking soda	1 tsp.	1200
Mustard, prepared, brown	5	65
Tabasco sauce	2	6
Bouillon cube, beef	4	400
Gelatin dessert, flavored	85	80
Mints, chocolate covered	30	60
Fudge, chocolate with nuts	30	60

Sodium Restriction and Diet

Many patients with chronic congestive heart failure and other cardiovascular diseases may be placed on low sodium diets. A comprehensive list of the relative sodium content of commonly used foods is represented in Table 7. It is also interesting to note that recent studies have confirmed speculation that a relatively high carbohydrate intake has an inhibitory effect on sodium excretion. This, in turn, may have an impact on diet, the use of diuretics and the treatment of heart failure, cyclical edema, obesity, diabetes and hypertension. Presently this is still under clinical investigation.[57]

Leafy Vegetables and Anticoagulant Therapy

A number of interesting reports on leafy vegetable consumption (*i.e.*, spinach, kale, etc.) and altered prothrombin time have implications for the patient stabilized on an anticoagulant regimen.[58] In fact, any excessive dietary consumption of foods rich in vitamin K is capable of producing this phenomenon.

Alcoholic Beverages and Drugs

Alcohol has been shown to potentiate or markedly affect the response to antihistamines, barbiturates, benzodiazepine compounds, chlorpromazine, tranylcypromine, tricyclic antidepressants and other substances affecting the central nervous system. For a detailed review of such interactions the reader is directed to Polascek's extensive annotated bibliography.[59] It should be noted that absorption rates of various alcoholic beverages can vary widely and should be taken into consideration when assessing such potential interactions with alcohol. Wines possess a relatively high buffer capacity and are hence absorbed less rapidly than distilled liquors. This results in the absence of high alcohol levels seen after ingestion of distilled liquors on an empty stomach.[60] Blood levels of alcohol have been shown to be markedly reduced by the intravenous infusion of fructose. This lowering of alcohol levels by fructose may occur because the dissociation of the alcohol dehydrogenase-NADH complex (nicotinamide adenine nucleotide) is apparently accelerated by intermediary metabolites of fructose.[61] This finding may have some practical value in the treatment of critically acute alcoholic patients.

UNUSUAL REACTIONS TO FOODS

Food Allergenicity

Allergic reactions to various foods are not infrequent phenomena. Some individuals react abnormally under certain conditions to specific foodstuffs that do not affect the vast majority of people. For example, there is the well recognized sensitivity of certain individuals to strawberries, shellfish, milk, or eggs. Common manifestations of such sensitivities include abdominal symptoms and skin rashes, although almost any type of reaction can be evoked in certain food-sensitive individuals. Individuals have shown hypersensitivity to drugs present in food, for example, as in the case of cow's milk containing penicillin. It is also possible that attacks of migraine may be produced in susceptible individuals by tyramine and other amines present in certain foods such as cheese, fish, beans, milk, dairy products, chocolate and alcoholic beverages.[62] The smell of fish has been shown to induce violent allergic attacks in asthmatic children. Allergies to the smell of other foods such as garlic, onions, coffee, cooked peas, beans and lentils have been documented.[63,64] Certain artificial food colors are known to have caused urticaria in children who have eaten colored candies. Severe asthma has been reported from tartrazine and other dyes commonly used to color various drug preparations.[65] Food allergenicity should aways be ruled out as an etiologic factor in suspected allergic drug reactions.

Common Foods Harmful in Certain Individuals

Many seemingly innocuous foods may cause disturbances in certain individuals having basic disorders that may be aggravated or precipitated by an offending food substance. Some examples are:

1. *Celiac disease or gluten-induced enteropathy.* In susceptible persons, gluten (a protein found in wheat and rye flour) is capable of producing a serious malabsorption phenomenon secondary to enteropathy. A gluten-free diet in conjunction with certain supplements is indicated in this situation.
2. *Hepatic cirrhosis with liver failure.* Proteins and any nitrogenous substances should be withheld in order to avoid hepatic encephalopathy.
3. *Favism*—a hemolytic disorder induced by the ingestion of fava beans or by contact with the pollen of the plant. Red blood cells in these patients are deficient in glucose-6-phosphate

dehydrogenase, an enzyme system which plays a vital role in the metabolism of glucose and is necessary for the continued integrity of the cell. It should be noted that these deficient cells are also sensitive to a number of drugs (primaquin, sulfonamides and vitamin K analogs).

4. *Phenylketonuria* is an example of an inborn metabolic error of amino acid metabolism in which mental deficiency will occur unless a diet sufficiently low in phenylalanine content is started early.
5. *Galactosemia* is a rare inborn error of metabolism in which the red blood cells are deficient in galactose-1-phosphate-uridyl-transferase. The body is unable to convert dietary galactose to glucose, resulting in vomiting, jaundice, failure of growth, cirrhosis and lenticular cataracts in later life.

Vitamin Toxicity

Vitamins are a group of substances which are not wholly innocuous. Vitamins A and D as well as niacin have all been implicated in various forms of toxicity. Acute vitamin A toxicity has been observed in infants and children. A single dose (300,000 units) in infants, for example, has produced bulging fontanelles from increased intracranial pressure, vomiting and other symptoms. Chronic toxicity has resulted from the daily ingestion of moderately high doses of the vitamin over long periods of time. Impairment of skeletal development, hepatomegaly, splenomegaly and anemia may also occur. This has been observed especially in the food faddist population.[66]

Idiopathic hypercalcemia in children has occurred from chronic ingestion of an alkaline-ash diet combined with vitamin D and cow's milk. (Cow's milk contains five times as much calcium and phosphorus as breast milk.) An idiopathic factor and hypersensitivity to the vitamin also appear to be involved. Potent vitamin D preparations have caused loss of appetite, emaciation, diarrhea, and metastatic calcification in children.

Niacin when taken in large amounts may produce pharmacological and harmful effects. Food poisoning has occurred from the eating of adulterated meat to which niacin was added to prevent darkening of the meat. Large doses of niacin consumed over long periods of time have also been shown to produce hyperglycemia, jaundice, and gastrointestinal symptoms including peptic ulcer. Accordingly, large doses should be avoided in diabetic patients.[67]

Conclusion

Although it is apparent that relationships between diet and drug therapy are not as common place or as frequent as drug-drug interactions, the pharmacist should be constantly aware of their potential contribution to therapeutic failures and adverse effects in the clinical setting. A constant vigil of the clinical literature as well as a balanced perspective of judgment will indeed facilitate the appropriate application of drug-food relationships in therapeutics.

References

1. Sapeika, N.: *Food Pharmacology,* Charles C Thomas Publishing Co., Springfield, Ill., 1969.
2. Foy, J. M. and Parrott, J. R.: 5-Hydroxytryptamine in Pineapples, *J. Pharm. Pharmacol. 13*:382-383, 1961.
3. Woolkes, T. P. *et al.*: Serotonin, Norepinephrine and Related Compounds in Bananas, *Science 127*:648-650 (Feb. 12) 1958.
4. Hodge, J. V. *et al.*: Monoamine Oxidase Inhibitors, Broad Beans and Hypertension, *Lancet 1*:1108 (May 16) 1964.
5. Potter, N. N.: *Food Science,* Avi Publishing Co., Inc., Westport, Conn., 1968, p. 597-600.
6. Krondl, A.: Present Understanding of the Interaction of Drugs and Food Drug Absorption, *Can. Med. Assoc. J. 103*:360-364, 1970.
7. Code, C. F.: *Handbook of Physiology,* section 6. Alimentary Canal, Intestinal Absorption, Williams and Willkins Co., Baltimore, Md., Vol. 3, 1968.
8. Christakis, G. and Miridjanian, A.: Diets, Drugs, and Their Relationships, *J. Am. Dietetic Assoc. 52*:22 (Jan.) 1958.
9. Faloon, W. W.: Drug Production of Intestinal Malabsorption, *N. Y. State J. Med. 70*:2189-2192 (Sept.) 1970.
10. Dobbins, W. O.: Drug-Induced Steatorrhea, *Gastroenterology 54*:1193 (June) 1968.
11. Nasrallah, S. M., Coburn, W. M., Jr. and Iber, F. L.: The Effect of Hypertonic Mannitol on the Intestine of Man, *Johns Hopkins Med. J. 123*:134-137, 1968.
12. Fordtran, J. S. *et al.*: Ionic Constituents and Osmolality of Gastric and Small Intestine Fluids After Eating, *Am. J. Digestive Diseases 11*:503, 1966.
13. Waxman, S. *et al.*: Drugs, Toxins and Dietary Amino Acids Affecting Vitamin B_{12} or Folic Acid Absorption, *Am. J. Med. 48*:600 (May) 1970.

14. Trier, J. S.: Morphologic Alterations Induced by Methotrexate in the Mucosa of Human Proximal Intestine, *Gastroenterology 43*:407, 1962.
15. Rice, T. R. *et al.*: Intestinal Malabsorption Induced by Oral Colchicine, *Am. J. Med. Sci. 259*:32 (Jan.) 1970.
16. Webb, D. I. *et al.*: Mechanisms of B_{12} Malabsorption in Patients Treated with Colchicine, *New Engl. J. Med. 279*:845, 1968.
17. Reynolds, E. H. *et al.*: Reversible Absorptive Defects in Anticonvulsant Megaloblastic Anemia, *J. Clin. Pathol. 18*: 593, 1965.
18. Heaton, F. W. and Pyroh, L. N.: Hypomagnesemia in Chronic Alcoholism, *Lancet 2*:802-805 (Oct.) 1957.
19. Anon.: Drug-Induced Diabetes, *Lancet 2*:328, 1965.
20. Shejania, A. M. *et al.*: Oral Contraceptives and Serum Folate Levels, *Lancet 1*:1376, 1968.
21. Streiff, R. R.: Malabsorption of Polyglutamic Acid Folic Acid Secondary to Oral Contraceptives, *J. Clin. Res. 17*:345, 1969.
22. Streiff, R. R.: Megaloblastic Anemia Due to Folyl-Conjugase Inhibitions by Oral Contraceptive Agents, *J. Am. Med. Assoc.* (in press).
23. Clark, M. *et al.*: The Effect of Chlorpromazine on Serum Cholesterol in Chronic Schizophrenic Patients, *Clin. Pharmacol. Therap. 11*:883-890 (Nov.-Dec.) 1970.
24. Fagan, L.: Griseofulvin and Dysgeusia: Implications? (letters), *Ann. Internal Med. 74*:795-796 (May) 1971.
25. Wagner, J. G.: Aspects of Pharmacokinetics and Biopharmaceutics in Relation to Drug Activity, Proceedings of a Symposium "Determinants of Drug Activity," Philadelphia College of Pharmacy and Sciences, Nov. 14, 1968, p. 3-18.
26. Kirby, W. M., Roberts, C. E. and Burdick, R. E.: "Comparison of Two New Tetracyclines with Tetracycline and Demethylchlortetracycline," in Finland, M. and Savage, G. M., eds.: *Antimicrobial Agents and Chemotherapy*, American Society for Microbiology, Detroit, Mich., 1961, p. 286-292.
27. Heatley, N. G.: Comparative Serum Concentration and Excretion Experiments with Benzyl Penicillin (G) and Phenoxymethyl Penicillin (V) on a Single Subject, *Antibiotic Medicine Clinical Therapy 2*:33, 1956.
28. Klein, J. O. and Finland, M.: Nafcillin. Antibacterial Action *in Vitro* and Absorption and Excretion in Normal Young Men, *Am. J. Med. Sci. 246*:10-26 (July) 1963.
29. Klein, J. O. and Finland, M.: Ampicillin. Activity *in Vitro* and Absorption and Excretion in Normal Young Men, *Am. J. Med. Sci. 245*:544-555 (May) 1963.
30. Klein, J. O. *et al.*: Laboratory Studies on Oxacillin: I. *in Vitro* Activity Against Staphylococci and Some Other Bacterial Pathogens; II. Absorption and Urinary Excretion in Normal Young Men, *Am. J. Med. Sci. 245*:399, 1963.
31. Hirsch, H. H. and Finland, M.: Effect of Food on the Absorption of Erythromycin Propionate, Erythromycin Stearate and Triacetyloleandomycin, *Am. J. Med. Sci. 237*:693, 1959.
32. McCall, C. E. *et al.*: Lincomycin: Activity *in Vitro* and Absorption and Excretion in Normal Young Men, *Am. J. Med. Sci. 254*:144, 1967.
33. MacDonald, V. A. *et al.*: Effect of Food on Absorption of Sulfonamides in Man, *Chemotherapia 12*:282-285, 1967.
34. Kunin, C. M. and Finland, M.: Clinical Pharmacology of the Tetracycline Antibiotics, *Clin. Pharmacol. Therap. 2*: 51 (Jan.-Feb.) 1961.
35. Seneca, H.: *Biological Basis of Chemotherapy of Infections and Infestations,* F. D. Davis Co., Philadelphia, Pa., 1971.
36. Neuvonen, P. J. *et al.*: Interference of Iron with the Absorption of Tetracyclines in Man, *Brit. Med. J. 4*:532 (Nov. 28) 1970.
37. Crounse, R. G.: Effective Use of Griseofulvin, *Arch. Dermatol. 87*:176 (Feb.) 1963.
38. Cullen, S. I. and Catalano, P. M.: Griseofulvin-Warfarin Antagonism, *J. Am. Med. Assoc. 199*:582, 1967.
39. Conney, A. H.: Pharmacological Implications of Microsomal Enzyme Induction, *Pharmacol. Rev. 19*:317-366, 1967.
40. Juchare, M. R. *et al.*: Stimulation of Hepatic Microsomal Drug-Metabolizing Enzyme Systems in Primates by DDT, *Gastroenterology 51*:213-218, 1966.
41. Davies, J. E. *et al.*: Effect of Anticonvulsant Drugs on Dicophane (DDT) Residues in Man, *Lancet 2*:7, 1969.
42. Kater, R. *et al.*: Increased Rate of Tolbutamide Metabolism in Alcoholic Patients, *J. Am. Med. Assoc. 207*:363-365 (Jan. 13) 1969.
43. Zinn, M.: Quinidine Intoxication from Alkali Ingestion, *Texas Med. 66*:64-66 (Dec.) 1970.
44. *Mayo Clinic Diet Manual,* ed. 3, W. B. Saunders Co., Philadelphia, Pa. 1961, p. 137.
45. Goodman, L. S. and Gilman, A. eds.: *The Pharmacological Basis of Therapeutics,* ed. 4, The Macmillan Company, New York, 1970, p. 183-184.
46. Horwitz, D. *et al.*: Monoamine Oxidase Inhibitors, Tyramine and Cheese, *J. Am. Med. Assoc. 188*:90-92 (June 29) 1964.
47. Blackwell, B. *et al.*: Tyramine in Cheese Related to Hypertensive Crises After Monoamine Oxidase Inhibition, *Lancet 1*:938-940 (May) 1965.
48. Sjoquist, F.: Psychotropic Drugs Interaction Between Monoamine Oxidase Inhibitors and Other Substances, *Proc. Roy. Soc. Med. 58*:967-977, 1965.
49. Gross, E. G.: *et al.*: Hypokalemic Myopathy with Myoglobinuria Associated with Licorice Ingestion, *New Engl. J. Med. 274*:602, 1966.
50. Meyler, L.: *Side Effects of Drugs,* Excerpta Medica Foundation, New York, Vol. 5, 1966.
51. Schaumburg, H. H. and Byck, R.: *New. Engl. J. Med. 279*:105, 1968.
52. Schaumburg, H. H. *et al.*: Monosodium L-Glutamate: Its Pharmacology and Role in the Chinese Restaurant Syndrome, *Science 163*:826 (Feb.) 1965.
53. Lamy, P. P. and Blake, D.: Therapeutic Incompatabilities, *J. Am. Pharm. Assoc. NS10*:72-77 (Feb.) 1970.
54. Anon.: Potassium Formulations and Therapy, *Med. Letter Drugs Therap. 11*:77-79 (Sept. 9) 1969.
55. Pipe-Wolferstan, M. W.: Dangers of Tomato Juice, *New Engl. J. Med. 284*:1105, 1971.
56. Anon.: *Potassium Content of Selected Medicinals* and *Sodium Content of Selected Medicinals*, prepared by Michigan Regional Drug Information Network, University of Michigan Hospital Pharmacy, College of Pharmacy, Ann Arbor, Michigan.
57. Weinsier, R. L.: Fasting—A Review with Emphasis on the Electrolytes, *Am. J. Med. 50*:233-240 (Feb.) 1971.
58. Leafy Vegetables in Diet Alter Prothrombin Time in Patients Taking Anticoagulant Drugs (medical news), *J. Am. Med. Assoc. 187*:27, 1964.
59. Polascek, E.: *Interactions of Alcohol and Other Drugs —An Annotated Bibliography*, The Addiction Research Foundation, Ontario, 1970.
60. Newman, H. and Abramson, M.: Absorption of Various Alcoholic Beverages, *Science 143*:43-44 (July 10) 1962.
61. Lowenstein, L. M. *et al.*: Effect of Fructose on Alcohol Concentrations in the Blood in Man, *J. Am. Med. Assoc. 213*:1889-1901 (Sept. 14) 1970.
62. Harrington, E.: Preliminary Report on Tyramine Headache, *Brit. Med. J. 1*:550, 1967.
63. Aas, K.: Studies of Hypersensitivity to Fish. A Clinical Study, *Intern. Arch. Allergy 29*:346, 1966.
64. Urback, E. and Gottlieb, P. M.: *Allergy,* William Heinemann Publishers, London, 1946.
65. Sapeika, N.: *op. cit.*, p. 5.
66. Bergen, S. S. *et al.*: Hypervitaminosis A, *Am. J. Clin. Nutrition 16*:265, 1965.
67. Molnar, G. D. *et al.*: The Effect of Nicotinic Acid in Diabetes Mellitus, *Metabolism 13*:181, 1964.
68. Anon.: *Bacteriological Analytical Manual,* Food and Drug Administration, U.S. Dept. HEW, Aug., 1966.
69. Gardner, W. H.: *Food Acidulants,* Allied Chemical Corporation, New York, N. Y., 1966.

11

Drug surveillance for patient safety

by Andrew T. Canada, Jr.

It has long been recognized that one of the basic functions of a pharmacist is that of drug control. In hospital practice this aspect has been looked upon in terms of inventory control, packaging and manufacturing control, narcotic control and various dispensing controls. Most control systems have been designed to assure that the pharmacist would dispense the correct drug ordered by the physician to the correct patient and in the correct dosage form. Until recently, however, few efforts had been made to expand this concept of drug control to the actual utilization of drugs in the most rational way based on current therapeutics. The pharmacist by virtue of his control of drug distribution, especially in institutions, is in a unique position to monitor and subsequently to influence drug utilization in his institution.

The Philosophy of Drug Use

"That drugs are two edged swords" is a fact well recognized among those knowledgeable in drug misuse. Each time a drug is prescribed and then administered to a patient, the patient automatically assumes a degree of risk that the drug may actually produce a harmful effect rather than a beneficial one. Studies by Cluff and Sidel demonstrated that if a patient was receiving a drug, each time another drug was added to a therapeutic regimen the chances of the patient developing a harmful effect to the combination more than doubled.[1-3] The greatest problem in therapeutics now facing those whose basic activity is drug control is that of reducing drug usage to an absolute minimum consistent with optimal therapeutics. Physicians and pharmacists of today are products of a drug-oriented society. There is a tendency of the majority of prescribing and dispensing practitioners to think in terms of what drug should be prescribed and dispensed rather than whether a drug should be prescribed at all. Recent statements by medical authorities have pointed out that 70 percent of medications are prescribed needlessly. Other estimates have suggested that in 1968 over 80 percent of the chloramphenicol prescribed was for uses inconsistent with company brochure recommendations and recognized medical uses for this highly effective but dangerous antibiotic.[4] The economic and patient safety implications of the preceding figures are staggering.

Drugs have, since 1940, become the answer for many conditions which, prior to the advent of chemotherapy, were self-limiting and required a minimum of clinical intervention. The most common example of this is anxiety. The anxieties of motherhood, menopause, college examinations and puberty are now labeled disease states requiring intervention through chemical means.[5] Recent trends in therapeutics have been to continue to expand the indications for drugs in general and more specifically, the minor tranquilizers. Each time a new condition falls before the onslaught of chemotherapy the practitioners of medicine and pharmacy become just a little more drug-oriented. It is the feeling of many authorities in the area of drug abuse that this concept of a drug for each condition, no matter what, has contributed substantially to the creation of our drug-oriented society. The young people of today are aware of the fact that one out of every five of their elders finds it impossible to sleep without a chemical sleeping aid coursing through his veins. They see their parents taking legally prescribed tranquilizers for minor anxieties. Medicine cabinets are filled to overflowing with depressants and antidepressants, sedatives and stimulants, pain killers and cold killers. It is inevitable that with adult society so oriented toward drugs, the young of today would go the same road. Many of the barbiturates and amphetamines first abused by a young person come from his parents' medicine cabinet and before that, from a legal prescription emanating from a physician and dispensed by a pharmacist. One of the most effective ways a pharmacist can reduce the chances a drug may be misused is to prevent its use in the hospital or community where he practices if the drug does not represent a significant advance in drug therapy. This is best accomplished through the mechanism of the hospital pharmacy and therapeutics (P&T) committee or the formulary board of the state or community, when the latter exists.[6]

Restrictions on Drug Use

The Kefauver-Harris drug amendments of 1962 required proof of drug effectiveness before a drug could be marketed for human consumption. It is, therefore, a safe assumption that any new drug is effective for the uses claimed by the manufacturer. The value of each new drug may be judged on the criterion of *relative* efficacy and that being equal, *relative* safety as compared with other available drugs used to produce the same therapeutic results. Once it has been decided that a new drug released to the market represents a significant enough advance in drug therapy to be admitted to the "formulary," the reduction of known side effects to a minimum consistent with proper therapy is a logical goal. This reduction of side effects to an absolute minimum may be accomplished by any of the following P & T committee-approved regulations:

(1) Restriction of drug use to specific physicians in the community or hospital.

Example: Succinylcholine restricted to anesthesiologists or levodopa restricted to board-certified neurologists.

(2) Requirement that certain laboratory procedures have to be performed routinely for specific drugs.

Example: Serum blood lithium levels weekly for maintenance patients taking lithium carbonate and complete blood counts on patients taking carbamazepine.

(3) Limitation on ambulatory dispensing.

Example: Prohibit the dispensing to ambulatory patients of chloramphenicol or limit the quantity of sedative-hypnotic which could be dispensed at any one time.

Each of the preceding examples of regulations which could emanate from the P & T committee should go far in reducing potential adverse effects to a minimum. Needless to say, the dissemination of information on such regulations to the medical staff before their enforcement is absolutely necessary in order to reduce friction to an absolute minimum. Such dissemination is best done by a specific mailing to each medical staff member with a detailed explanation as to why such action was taken. In the event such regulations become official, a mechanism should exist to enable a physician, at his own risk and with the informed consent of the patient, to deviate from the stated P & T recommendations for rational drug use. Most institutions with such a policy of restricted use allow a physician to break out of the system utilizing a nonformulary route. Most frequently this is accomplished by the completion of a form (Figure 1). This completion of this form would probably remove the hospital from any liability accruing from a physician's not following hospital recommendations. Such deviations from hospital recommendations may require the prior approval of a particular medical staff member, medical staff committee or department head.

The Need for Surveillance

Despite all the efforts to prevent both the misuse of drugs and their adverse effects, some drug misadventures will inevitably occur. It is necessary that such occurrences be detected as soon as they happen. Surveillance is necessary to be able to: (1) detect when a drug is not being used according to recommendations; (2) detect adverse reactions which may be avoided in the future if correct remedial measures are taken; and (3) detect adverse reactions and interactions to drugs so unusual as not to have been discovered in the clinical testing which took place prior to marketing. A drug surveillance system is necessary in order to be able to monitor the quality of drug therapy within a hospital. This is the most important function of a surveillance program. The second most important aspect is to convey to appropriate private and governmental agencies the information so derived.[7]

Occurrence of Adverse Drug Reactions

There are varying statistics on the occurrence of adverse drug reactions in a hospital as shown in Table 1. The incidence of reactions discovered ranges from 0.4 percent to 24 percent with some suggestions of even higher percentages. It must be kept in mind that each of the studies citing figures used different interpretations of what they considered to be an adverse drug reaction. Each investigator used a definition suitable for his own purposes. These purposes can be broken down on three bases: (1) investigators who were interested solely in statistics, (2) authors interested in reporting reactions through the normal reporting programs in the FDA and AMA and (3) authors interested in adverse drug reactions because of their relevance to patient care in their own institutions. The first report which brought the study of adverse drug reactions to the forefront of contemporary medical thinking was the work done in 1964 at Johns Hopkins Hospital.[11] In this study patients on a medical ward were surveyed on a daily basis for the occurrence of an adverse drug reaction. The criteria used in the Hopkins program for what constituted an adverse drug reaction was *any* effect produced by a drug and not desired by the attending physician. This work showed that 14 percent of the patients surveyed had experienced an adverse effect to a drug. The study at Johns Hopkins and later data by Jick *et al.* relied heavily on nursing personnel to detect these reactions.[12] The work at Johns Hopkins set off a flurry of investigations, some attempting to substantiate and some attempting to refute the high percentage. It is important to remember that the 14 percent figure resulted from patients on the medical service. The percentage when projected to the entire hospital would be much lower because patients on the medical service receive many more drugs and are therefore more likely to have adverse drug reactions than most other patients.[9] Most people involved in adverse drug reaction programs become so concerned with statistics and incidence data that they forget about the patient suffering from the reaction. Many programs studying adverse drug reactions report drowsiness to antihistamines, nausea with nitrofurantoin and sedation with narcotics as adverse drug reactions.

A few things are known about the incidence of adverse drug reactions, some of which are obvious, some are not.[3]

Table 1. The Varying Incidences of Adverse Drug Reactions

GROUP	TYPE PATIENT	TOTAL PATIENTS WITH REACTION	PATIENTS STUDIED	PERCENTAGE REACTIONS*
1. Erslev and Smith (1966)[8]	All	—	—	0.7
2. Erslev and Smith (1966)[8]	All	37	1,504	2.4
3. Seidl, L. *et al.* (1966)[2]	Medical	184	122	14.3
4. Ridenberg (1968)[9]	All	351	86,100	0.41
5. Schimmel[10]	Medical	119	990	12.0
6. Ogilvie[11]	Medical	177	731	24.0

*Not recorded as percentage of patients but a percentage of ordered drugs.

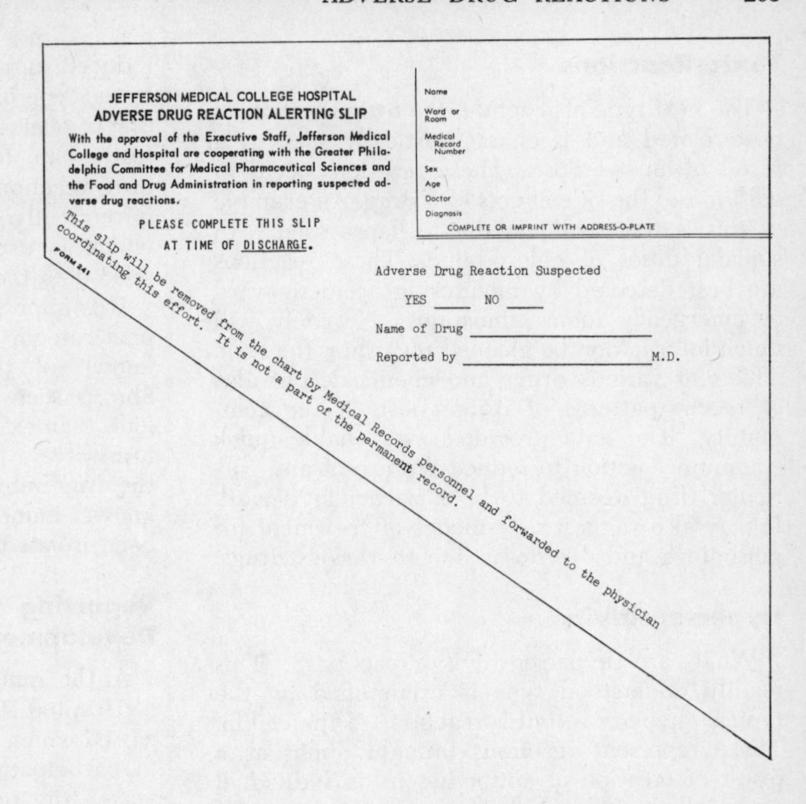

JEFFERSON MEDICAL COLLEGE HOSPITAL
ADVERSE DRUG REACTION ALERTING SLIP

With the approval of the Executive Staff, Jefferson Medical College and Hospital are cooperating with the Greater Philadelphia Committee for Medical Pharmaceutical Sciences and the Food and Drug Administration in reporting suspected adverse drug reactions.

PLEASE COMPLETE THIS SLIP AT TIME OF DISCHARGE.

Name
Ward or Room
Medical Record Number
Sex
Age
Doctor
Diagnosis
COMPLETE OR IMPRINT WITH ADDRESS-O-PLATE

Adverse Drug Reaction Suspected
YES ____ NO ____
Name of Drug ____________
Reported by ____________ M.D.

This slip will be removed from the chart by Medical Records personnel and forwarded to the physician coordinating this effort. It is not a part of the permanent record.

FORM 241

Figure 1. Adverse drug reactions alerting slip

(1) The more medications a patient receives the greater the chance of his having an adverse drug reaction. This is a synergistic phenomenon: a person receiving two drugs has better than twice the chance of having a reaction than has a person receiving one drug. In one study of patients having adverse drug reactions, the average number of drugs received during the period of hospitalization was 14, in another study, 11 drugs. This complicates the problem of identifying specific drugs responsible for adverse reactions.

(2) A patient admitted to a hospital for treatment of an adverse drug reaction is a likely candidate for additional reactions to other drugs.

(3) Certain kinds of diseases appear to be more commonly associated with adverse drug reactions than others.

(4) Age and race do not influence the overall incidence of adverse drug reactions. This is not to say that race will not influence the reactions seen with certain drugs such as the primaquine sensitivity reaction seen in the Negro.

(5) Men have more allergic reactions to penicillin than women.

(6) Adverse drug reactions constitute an important reason for the admission of individuals to a hospital.

(7) The group of drugs which most often cause reactions are the antimicrobials.

VARIOUS TYPES OF ADVERSE DRUG REACTIONS

Generally, adverse drug reactions may be divided into four specific types: (1) side effects, (2) toxic reactions, (3) hypersensitivity reactions and (4) a category which, for lack of a better term, will be called idiosyncratic.[13]

Side Effects

Side effects of drugs are a dose-related phenomenon and are related also to the blood level of the drug. They can be expected to occur with relative frequency in any individual receiving a particular drug. In other words, all patients taking a drug will exhibit the characteristic side effects of the drug if a high enough dose is given. Dryness of the mouth produced by tincture of belladonna is an example of this. This is not to suggest that at any particular dose all patients will exhibit the same side effect. Another example of this category is the bone marrow depression seen with the administration of antineoplastic agents. This is the category of adverse drug reactions we probably know the most about because of the high and predictable frequency of occurrence. However, it is necessary that surveillance be maintained for this type of reaction for the following two reasons: (1) these reactions frequently can be avoided through an intensive educational program of physicians and (2) there needs to be developed some means to predict which patients will exhibit which dose-related side effect at which level.

Toxic Reactions

The next type of reaction, the toxic reaction, is dose-related and is characteristically seen as a result of an overdose. These reactions occur *in addition* to the side effects of a drug. An example of this is the cardiovascular collapse seen with suicidal doses of chloroquine. These reactions are best detected by monitoring accident ward or emergency room admissions. Not only will much information be gleaned regarding the toxic effects of various drugs and chemicals but also of recent patterns of drug abuse in the community. The data provided may enable quick community action to reduce the use of any particular drug deemed to be a particular hazard. It may also suggest new modes of treatment for poisonings and overdoses due to various drugs.

Hypersensitivity

What are hypersensitivity reactions? This readily understood type is exemplified by the typical hypersensitivity reaction to penicillin. These represent reactions brought about as a result of creation of antibodies in an individual against a particular drug. Occurrence of such reactions requires prior exposure to or long-term administration of a drug (there must be time for antibodies to develop). These reactions may be exhibited in many different ways, all characterized by the presence of an antibody against the drug. There may be simple reactions such as puffiness around the eyes, rhinitis or pruritus; more severe reactions such as hives or rashes; or very severe reactions such as hemolytic anemia or cardiovascular collapse. The complete range of severity is covered in this type of reaction. A patient's history of being allergy-prone, such as the presence of asthma, indicates that there is a good possibility also of a future occurrence of drug allergy. McHale and Canada found that approximately 20 percent of the patients admitted to a 700-bed hospital stated a history of a drug hypersensitivity.[14]

Idiosyncratic Reactions

The last category of adverse drug reactions, the idiosyncratic type, is probably of greatest significance. These are usually severe, unpredictable and frequently difficult to diagnose. They range the spectrum of pathological states and include: oral contraceptive-induced pigmentation of the skin; procainamide-induced lupus erythematosus; long-acting sulfa-induced, Stevens-Johnson syndrome; methoxyflurane-induced high output renal damage; and chloramphenicol-induced agranulocytosis. This is the area, due to the type of reaction involved, in which health practitioners find their training and experience inadequate to the demands. The most difficult drug reaction to recognize is one which occurs infrequently and mimics a pathological state which is usually caused by other factors unrelated to the drug therapy.

It is impossible to put many drug reactions in one category or another because so little is known of their mechanisms. Retroperitoneal fibrosis seen in some patients taking methysergide is an example of this type. It is thought not to involve a primary hypersensitivity reaction to the drug but a secondary stimulation of some unknown immune reaction. No antibodies have been isolated.

Reporting Program—Developments and Problems

At the annual meeting of the American Society of Hospital Pharmacists in 1955 a resolution was passed which expressed the interest of the Society in participating in the establishment of an adverse drug reporting program by the Food and Drug Administration. The FDA began its program with a pilot study using five hospitals to report adverse drug reactions.[15] The procedure for reporting in those institutions was as follows:

(1) Suspected adverse reactions were noted on a form by the nurse or physician.

(2) The form was then sent to the medical record librarian who supplied patient information.

(3) It was then sent to the pharmacy where information on the drug source, form and strength was supplied.

(4) The report was then reviewed by the pharmacy and therapeutics committee.

The one-year pilot program was extended to four years evolving into the formal monitoring program in 1960 involving about 200 hospitals which also provided data for the growing system. However, the "early warning" premise so highly regarded as the rationale for the FDA to become deeply involved in adverse drug reactions, has never been completely successful. This is partially due to a lack of a coordinated effort within the FDA to create a workable system and partially to the general disinterest of hospitals in creating effective surveillance programs. The FDA in 1967, in adopting a new philosophy, dropped all but 80 teaching institutions from this program.[16] Indications from the FDA in late 1970 suggested it was becoming interested primarily in supporting intensive surveillance programs, either directed to monitoring carefully all drug therapy on a certain number of patients or all patients receiving a particular drug for collective adverse effects or for a specific one. Although the FDA system involves contractual arrangements with institutions reporting to it, it accepts and likes to receive reports from physicians, pharmacists and hospitals outside of its system.

The Food and Drug Administration publishes two monthly listings of adverse drug reactions on index cards. One reports those significant reactions accepted by the FDA Center for Drug Information. This listing is then fed back to the contractual institutions in the FDA system. The other listing is also on easy-to-file 3"x5" cards and reports on those adverse reactions listed in a significant portion of the medical literature of the world.

Until recently, the American Medical Association accepted reports from sources not reporting to the FDA. Starting with the Registry on Blood Dyscrasias in 1957, and expanding this concept to the Registry on Adverse Reactions in 1963,[17] the program was discontinued last year. Private practitioners and hospitals not in the FDA program reported adverse reactions to the AMA. The major pharmaceutical manufacturers are also recipients of reports from private practitioners of medicine and pharmacy. Not only do they encourage such reports but some of the companies also provide follow-up medical consultations on request to further elucidate on the reactions.

SURVEILLANCE SYSTEMS

Various systems and combinations of systems may be utilized to maintain varying degrees of surveillance on drug usage within the institutional setting. These vary drastically both in their relative effectiveness and cost. The pharmacy and therapeutics committee should be the recipient of any information and subsequent recommendations derived.

The Scuttlebutt System. It is common for a therapeutic misadventure or serious adverse drug reaction to be the subject of discussion by health professionals in the institution where it has occurred. A pharmacist may be made aware of these in a routine nursing station review or at a clinical conference where the reaction is discussed. This method, which may be quite effective in smaller institutions, requires a high degree of communication and rapport between the pharmacist and other health professionals. Obviously the pharmacist should utilize the information gained to try to avoid such an occurrence in the future, if possible. Any remedial steps taken must be as a result of some action by the P & T committee.

Automatic Chart Pulling. The cooperation of the medical records department is essential for this system to be effective. With this system the pharmacist requests the charts possibly denoting drug-produced adverse reactions as having occurred. This would be done with the aid of certain diagnoses. The following is a partial list of such diagnoses.

1. All patient deaths
2. Agranulocytosis, aplastic anemia, leukopenia, thrombocytopenia
3. Stevens-Johnson syndrome, erythema multiformae
4. Renal failure
5. Hepatitis
6. Anaphylactoid reaction
7. Toxic psychosis
8. Any diagnosis containing a drug name
9. Any rash
10. Hemolytic anemia
11. Gastrointestinal bleeding

The pharmacist should review every chart pulled by the medical records department for the possibility of a drug having produced the disease state found in the diagnosis. Frequently it will be found that although the diagnosis review had no relationship to a drug, other valuable information may be found in the chart.

The Voluntary Reporting Sheet. In this case a physician, when noting a reaction, completes an adverse drug reaction reporting sheet and sends it to the P & T committee or the individual assigned the function of collecting the reports by the committee. This system, used commonly in the late 1950's and early 1960's, suffered from extreme under-reporting of adverse occurrences, as have all voluntary systems. Any system which relies on an individual physician to report adverse reactions seen in his patients will experience the same problem of underreporting.[8] This underreporting is due to a combination of factors such as fear of medico-legal aspects, in making it known that such a reaction occurred. However, it has been stated by a number of attorneys, that should a patient seek malpractice damage against a physician, his earlier admission, through such a report, that an adverse drug reaction had indeed occurred would make him less liable than if he had tried to hide the fact.

The Notification Card. This system can utilize both physicians and nurses. The physician or nurse noticing or observing a possible adverse reaction to a drug completes a card stating the patient's name, room number, reaction observed and the suspected drug. This card, which should be located on each nursing unit, is then sent to the individual in the institution responsible for the monitoring of drug usage. That individual then, upon receipt of the card, goes to the patient unit and reviews the chart and interviews the professionals involved in the case. The reaction, if determined to be reportable, is then submitted to the pharmacy and therapeutics committee along with any recommendation for action.

The Completed Chart Check-Off. This is a system that requires each physician completing the chart of a patient to check an alerting slip (Figure 1) for the presence or absence of an adverse reaction to a drug having occurred to his patient. The physician has only to check yes or no regarding the occurrence of a reaction. This tag is completed for every patient discharge, and the chart is not considered complete by the medical records department until this slip is completed. All slips with a positive response are then pulled by medical records and the charts of those patients having a positive response are reviewed retrospectively by the individual responsible for the reporting of adverse drug reactions in the institution. This method of surveillance is four times more effective than the voluntary reporting systems just described.

Chart Scanning. Again this is a retrospective survey which involves scanning the chart of every patient discharged. The patient diagnosis, summary sheet, progress notes and consultation sheets are reviewed for any mention of drug-induced adverse reactions by a specially trained technician. These charts are screened for validity of the suspected reaction by a pharmacist and reported. This is five times more effective than the check-off slip previously described and 20 times more effective than any voluntary system. Charts may be scanned on the basis of patient service, for a particular drug given or for the presence of a particular reaction. One technician can review the charts of approximately 40 to 60 hospital discharges per day. In addition to looking for a physician's mention of any adverse drug reaction, he can also pull keyed diagnoses as described in "automatic chart pulling." In addition, this technician can be trained to pull charts in which the result of a laboratory test indicates a possible adverse drug reaction. As an example, the technician could be instructed to pull all charts where the white blood cell count had dropped below 3000 per square millimeter, indicating a leukopenia. The pharmacist would then investigate whether or not the leukopenia was or was not drug-related.

Individual Drug Studies. This system entails the intensive study of a certain drug or certain disease from a drug-related cause. These may be either retrospective, *i.e.,* looking at the records of patients already seen previously or prospective, reviewing patients while they are still in the hospital or still taking the drug. The type of study, especially the prospective one involving a specific drug, is one especially adapted to a pharmacist's contribution. An example of this would be as follows: A new drug is placed on the market with a claim of minimal but dose-related nephrotoxicity. Presuming a wide enough use of this drug, the pharmacist would initiate his own study to clarify any doubts. Each new order coming to the pharmacy for the drug in question would be noted. A pharmacist would then go to the unit involved and record pertinent patient information: age, sex, weight, working diagnoses, history of renal function and renal function tests as of that date (hopefully blood urea, nitrogen *and* creatinine). Those patients selected could be reviewed daily by the pharmacist for any change in renal function denoting decreased kidney function. It would be of special importance to monitor carefully any patient with initial impaired kidney function or patients with a history of renal disease or impairment. If given normal doses of a nephrotoxic drug, these patients would be among the first to show early damage as their renal reserve is significantly lower than patients without such a history. Positive findings indicating the possibility of such nephrotoxicity problems should first be presented to the kidney specialty group of the institution and then to the pharmacy and therapeutics committee for its review and action. This action could range from deletion of the drug from the formulary to requiring daily renal function tests on each patient receiving the drug.

Intensive Surveillance Programs. These programs usually entail the daily review by specially trained surveillance nurses of all the patients on a particular medical unit. These nurses review the daily progress notes and interview attending staff members as to reactions which may have occurred in the preceding 24 hours. These programs, characterized by the work of Jick *et al.* at the Lemuel Shattuck Hospital in Boston and Cluff *et al.* at Johns Hopkins and the University of Florida, are the most sophisticated surveillance programs in existence. They are also the most expensive.

The retrospective programs involving the review of a patient's chart after discharge suffer because of the lack of a great amount of data necessary to confirm the presence of an adverse drug effect. A prospective study or one detecting a reaction as it occurs would provide for the necessary laboratory tests performed as part of the study. As an example, if a drug is suspected to cause liver damage each of the following tests would be valuable to assess the cause and effect as well as degree of the reaction: serum glutamic-oxaloacetic acid transaminase (SGOT), lactic dehydrogenase (LDH), glutamic pyruvic transaminase (SGPT), alkaline phosphatase (also the isoenzyme to differentiate from bone alkaline phosphatase) and bilirubin, both direct and indirect fractions.

In addition, a prospective program may be able to reduce the severity of a reaction in a particular patient if detected early in its course. A recommendation for drug discontinuance would be the obvious result if such an impending reaction were discovered.

Food and Drug Guidelines for the Reporting of Adverse Drug Reactions

To provide further assistance in the reporting of adverse reactions to drugs, the following summaries of types of reactions and mechanisms of particular importance within selected medical specialities have been included.

Obstetrical Service. There are certain conditions that are of special significance regarding possible adverse effects of drugs as they pertain to patients on the obstetrical service. Since most drugs cross the placental barrier, this effect on the embryo and fetus is a matter of primary concern; and the collection of information regarding these effects is most important. The FDA is desirous of careful reporting of all medications, including over-the-counter preparations taken by the mother in cases of (1) congenital defects, (2) unexplained jaundice in the newborn, (3) unexplained hematologic problems, (4) severe respiratory depression or hypotension in the newborn or (5) other conditions possibly related to medications taken by the mother. We are becoming increasingly aware of the teratogenic effects of certain drugs as well as some of the problems related to the newborn's inability to detoxify certain others. The FDA also would like reports on adverse effects of drugs as they relate to the mother including oxytoxics, perineal sprays, drugs for suppression of lactation and others.

Gynecological Service. All those which are pertinent on the medical and surgical services are included, as well as those associated with diagnostic procedures such as hysterosalpinogography and those associated with use of various douche solutions and with mechanical devices used as contraceptives or abortives, as well as with medications used as contraceptives and abortives.

Surgical Service. Included are all those which are pertinent on the medical services; those associated with diagnostic procedures such as cholecystography, G.I. studies, pyelography, arteriography, radioactive uptake studies and others; those associated with dressings, tapes, sprays, antiseptics, topical medications and others; and those associated with mechanical devices such as orthopedic plates, nails, screws, or the use of newer devices employing Laser beams, high frequency sound, and so forth.

Psychiatric Service. More psychopharmacologic drugs are prescribed by physicians in general practice, internal medicine, surgery and other non-psychiatric specialties both in hospital and office practice, than are prescribed in psychiatric hospitals. Hence, adverse reactions to psychopharmacologic drugs must be sought as diligently in a general hospital as in a psychiatric hospital. All adverse reactions to all psychopharmacologic drugs should be reported. These may be serious reactions as hematologic and hepatotoxic, or may be the less serious and more common reactions such as extrapyramidal reactions and skin reactions. The FDA is also interested in reports of overdosages of these drugs whether prescribed in the hospital, taken by accident, or taken with suicidal intent.

Anesthesiology Service and Dental Service. To be reported are all local anesthetic reactions of the central, allergic or psychogenic type, including reactions related to the vasoconstrictors as well as the reactions to topical anesthetics; all general anesthetic reactions to include respiratory cardiovascular, neurological and miscellaneous effects (*e.g.*, liver and renal effects); all reactions to anesthetic premedication, *i.e.*, effects related to atropine, meperidine, morphine and barbiturates; reactions to analgesics, *i.e.*, salicylates, coal tar derivatives, synthetic non-narcotic and narcotic analgesics; all reactions to the sedatives and hypnotics; all reactions to the antibiotics; and all reactions to the antiseptics and germicides. Include those used for topical application to infectious processes, root canal sterilization and bleaching, as well as those used for cold sterilization.

All local and systemic reactions to hemostatics and astringents should be reported. These are to include hemostatics, blood coagulants (*e.g.*, gelatin sponge), astringents and styptics such as tannic acid and zinc chloride and iron preparations (*e.g.*, Monsel's solution). Also included should be all adverse effects caused by the fluoride compounds; all adverse effects produced by dentifrices and mouthwashes; all injuries resulting from materials and devices used in restorative and prosthetic dentistry (*e.g.*, allergic dermatitis from denture base materials); all reactions from self-medication, *e.g.*, "aspirin burns," home denture-relining kits; all reactions resulting in oral manifestations through medication not prescribed by the dentist, such as Dilantin-hyperplasia and black-hairy tongue; and all reactions to miscellaneous preparations used in the practice of dentistry such as antisialogogues, enzyme preparations, plasminogen activators and steroids.

Medical Service. Examples of significant adverse reactions to drugs which should be reported in internal medicine are as follows: drugs suspected of inducing hematologic reactions; allergic reactions; hepatotoxic reactions; neurologic reactions; cardio-respiratory reactions; alterations in renal functions; and drugs suspected of inducing alterations of metabolic, endocrinological, electrolytic and gastrointestinal functions.

Examples of reactions that need not be reported are: (1) isolated febrile episodes that are very brief in duration and (2) temporary episodes of nausea, vomiting, diarrhea and so forth. Very severe episodes of vomiting or diarrhea should be reported.

Pediatric Service. Examples of significant adverse reactions to drugs which should be reported in pediatrics are as follows.

Drugs inducing hematologic reactions: chloramphenicol-induced aplastic anemia, sulfa-induced hemolytic anemia, thiazide-induced thrombocytopenia, methemoglobinemias and others.

Drugs inducing reactions related to immunological medications: anticonvulsant-induced lupus erythematosus; phenacetin-induced non-thrombocytopenic purpura, sulfa-induced Stevens-Johnson syndrome, allergic dermatitis, anaphylaxia and others.

Drugs administered to the mother during pregnancy, including congenital reactions in the infant: iodide-induced goiter, hormone-induced masculinization, vitamin K-induced hemolytic anemia, thalidomide and metabolite-induced teratogenicity and others.

Drugs interfering with growth: steroid-induced dwarfism, tetracycline-induced hypoplasia of bone and teeth and others.

Drugs inducing neurological reactions: streptomycin-induced 8th nerve damage, tetracycline-induced bulging fontanel syndrome, chloramphenicol-induced optic neuritis (in children with cystic fibrosis) and others.

Drugs inducing renal reactions: Tridione-induced nephrosis, tetracycline-induced Fanconi-like syndrome and others.

Drugs inducing metabolic, endocrinological, electrolytic and gastrointestinal reactions similar to those occurring in internal medicine.

Dermatological Service. Adverse effects to be noted and reported are: (1) contact dermatoses of an allergic or chemical nature and (2) systemic reactions through skin absorption of dermatological drugs and cosmetics (*e.g.*, toxicity to the heavy metal preparations).

The Potential Role of a Pharmacist

A pharmacist's role in the establishment of an adverse drug reaction reporting program in his institution is limited *only* by his interest. It is conceivable that a pharmacist could be responsible for the complete adverse drug reaction reporting program in an institutional setting and thereby contribute to the improvement of patient care to a significant degree. The existence of a surveillance program to monitor the quality of drug therapy and a mechanism to report adverse drug reactions are now recommendations for hospital accreditation by the Joint Commission on Accreditation (JCAH).

What methodology should be followed in establishing such a surveillance system?[18]

(1) The administration of the hospital should be informed of the need to establish such a system and likewise, the attorney of the hospital should receive prior notice. Each should have the opportunity for any positive input into the implementation of the system.

(2) Prior to presentation of the plan to the pharmacy and therapeutics committee as a whole, the following individuals should be contacted with respect to the various proposed systems.

(a) The chairman of the pharmacy and therapeutics committee.

(b) The director of the nursing department.

(c) The director of the medical records department.

(3) The pharmacy and therapeutics committee should be the means for formal implementation of the system. The committee members should be provided with as much background information on the various possible surveillance systems prior to the meetings where the program will be discussed. It would be valuable to have the hospital attorney present for a part of one of the meetings to clarify any medico-legal questions which may arise.

(4) The most workable system for any given hospital would be a combination of the first five surveillance systems described earlier. The first system, not being formal, would not need to be approved by the committee.

(5) The systems chosen should be implemented only after wide dissemination of the aims and objectives of the program, preferably in the form of a group presentation and less desirably, by written communication to all people involved.

After implementation of the program, individual patient cases of which the clinical pharmacist is notified and all charts selected under this program would then be reviewed by him for reportability of the reactions. Many reactions thought to occur and attributed to a particular drug will be found to be due to an entirely different drug when the chart is reviewed. A clinical pharmacist could easily fulfill this role since he, if he does a nominal amount of reading, is frequently more aware of which drugs cause what reactions than the patient's attending staff physicians and nurses. The reactions so recorded should then be presented to the pharmacy and therapeutics committee for review. At this time, difficult cases in which the pharmacist needs the assistance of medical practitioners may be discussed. Both professions could learn from this exchange of information.

Detection and reporting are not enough, however. The principal direction of his activity will be toward prevention of adverse reactions.[19] The pharmacist will investigate circumstances surrounding the occurrence of a specific reaction of a patient so as to prepare a better report and also to determine what factors contributed to the reaction. For example, was the patient who had a primaquine-type reaction to nitrofurantoin Negroid? Among this race and certain other ethnic groups there is a high incidence of glucose-6-phosphate dehydrogenase deficiency, and pretesting for this deficiency might have averted the reaction. Did the patient who had a reaction to kanamycin also have renal impairment which would have predisposed him to a high susceptibility to reaction? What is the incidence of a given adverse reaction in relationship to the total utilization of the drug in the hospital? That is, what is the epidemiology of the reaction: If frequent reactions to a given drug are occurring, what is the pattern of usage? That is, in what disease conditions and age groups, in the presence of what laboratory findings and with what other drugs is it being used? Evaluation of these aspects may be facilitated in the near future as more and more patient medical records are computerized.

At the time of the case review by the P & T committee remedial measures could be suggested which would reduce the chances of such a reaction occurring again, if it could have been avoided. This could result in any one of the following actions:

(1) Deletion of the drug from the formulary
(2) Limit drug use
   (a) To specific cases
   (b) To specific diagnoses
   (c) To set duration of therapy
   (d) To a maximum allowable dose
(3) Prepare a series of recommendations for safe use to be included in the formulary.
(4) Mount an educational campaign utilizing special mailings, the physician's bulletin published by the pharmacy or clinical conferences to encourage correct and rational use of the drug under surveillance.
(5) Implementation of a special drug study as outlined in surveillance system, "individual drug studies."

Monthly feedback reporting of the reactions and difficulties detected by the various systems implemented is essential to maintain continuing interest in the programs on the part of medical, dental and nursing practitioners. Such communication is important if adverse drug reactions are to be avoided or more rapidly recognized and treated in the future. The institutional pharmacist should serve as the individual to disseminate this information. He should utilize the bulletin which he publishes for the physicians, dentists and nurses of his staff to list all reactions reported from his institution in the month prior to publication. He can also include in the bulletin abstracts of articles appearing in the literature concerning new reactions to drugs currently being used in his hospital. It is of little value to use such a bulletin to tell physicians what they already know, for example, that thiazide diuretics precipitate gout or that tetracycline causes tooth staining in infants. Most physicians, however, are probably not aware that the incidence of chloramphenicol aplastic anemia is now estimated at 1:10,000 exposures which is 70 times higher than originally estimated, or that sulfisoxazole may precipitate an acute attack of hypoglycemia in an individual on oral antidiabetic therapy. The pharmacist could, in addition, send to physicians in his hospital, abstracts, reprints or articles about adverse drug reactions he knows will be of particular interest to them either because of their wide use of the particular drug about which the article is written or because the reaction is one that they might be called in as a consultant. An example of this would be an article dealing with the nephrotoxicity of cephaloridine. Copies of this article could be sent to the infectious disease group of the hospital and specialists in renal diseases on the hospital staff.

What else could a pharmacist do? When a physician calls the pharmacy to inquire whether a drug produces a particular type of reaction (if the pharmacist is doing the things previously mentioned, physicians will call), the pharmacist could inquire why the physician asked the question. If it is because one of his patients is exhibiting such a reaction, the pharmacist could review the patient's complete problem with the physician. He could then perform a search of the literature documenting other such cases and send copies of the information to the physician. When a question is directed to a pharmacist about a drug or drug therapy in a particular case, the pharmacist should attempt to encourage the use of the least toxic of drugs in a particular therapeutic class. This, of course, should be that drug which is least toxic and still able to achieve the therapeutic goal desired. As an example of this, rather than suggesting a tricyclic antidepressant for someone with neurotic depression and anxiety, recommend trial of a minor tranquilizer before turning to the tricyclic.

In some institutions where it is the practice for the clinical pharmacist to make patient rounds, he can even discover reactions as they occur, and by immediate discontinuation of the offending drug, prevent possible severe patient injury. He could also suggest a drug less likely to produce a reaction in a specific instance. For example, for an individual in congestive heart failure who requires a high blood sulfa level for fungal infection, triple sulfas would be preferred rather than sulfadiazine alone. The reason for this is that a great amount of fluid must be forced in individuals on oral sulfadiazine therapy in order to avoid sulfa crystal-induced renal damage. Naturally, any further addition of fluid to the patient which will in turn increase the circulatory burden of the heart must be avoided. Since the forcing of fluids is not as relatively important with triple sulfas as with sulfadiazine, triple sulfas would be the recommended drug under these circumstances. He could suggest in a patient with congestive heart failure and a history of alcoholic cirrhosis that digoxin be prescribed rather than digitoxin as the latter must be metabolized through the liver prior to excretion while the former is excreted unchanged via the kidney.

It has been estimated by some that *one out of every five* patients admitted to a hospital can be expected to have an adverse drug reaction. It is the responsibility of a pharmacist, through his obligation to the patient in all aspects of drug surveillance, to hold these drug reactions to a minimum by various programs. If drugs are misused and adverse drug reactions occur despite his endeavors to prevent them, it is also his obligation to provide this information to others so that they may, hopefully, be avoided in the future.

References

1. Cluff, L. E., Thornton, G. F. and Seidl, L. G.: Studies on the Epidemiology of Adverse Drug Reactions. I. Methods of Surveillance, *J. Am. Med. Assoc. 188*:976-983 (June 15) 1964.

2. Seidl, L. G., Thornton, G. F., Smith, J. W. and Cluff, L. E.: Studies on the Epidemiology of Adverse Drug Reactions. III. Reactions in Patients on a General Medical Service, *Bull. Johns Hopkins Hosp. 119*:299-315 (Nov.) 1966.

3. Smith, J. W., Seidl, L. G. and Cluff, L. E.: Studies on the Epidemiology of Adverse Drug Reactions. V. Clinical Factors Influencing Susceptibility, *Ann. Internal Med. 65*: 629-640 (Oct.) 1966.

4. Obrien, W. M.: *The Sun,* Baltimore, p. K1-K2 (May 11) 1969.

5. Lennard, H. L., Epstein, L. J., Bernstein, A. and Ransom, D. C.: Hazards Implicit in Prescribing Psychoactive Drugs, *Science 169*:438-441 (July 31) 1970.

6. Pellegrino, E. D.: The Role of the Hospital Pharmacist in Rational Therapeutics, *Hospitals 37*:102-108 (Feb. 16) 1963.

7. Carr, E. A., Jr. (editorial): Adverse Reactions to Drugs — Should We Have Formal Programs for Reporting Them? *Clin. Pharmacol. Therap. 5*:141-144 (Mar.-Apr.) 1964.

8. Smith, J. E. and Erslev, A. J.: Toward More Effective Drug Reaction Reporting, *Hosp. Pract. 6*:78-83 (Jan.) 1967.

9. Anon.: Registry of Adverse Drug Reactions, *J. Am. Med. Assoc. 203*:31-34 (Jan. 1) 1968.

10. Schimmel, E. M.: The Hazards of Hospitalization, *Ann. Internal Med. 60*:100-110 (Jan.) 1964.

11. Ogilvie, R. I. and Ruedy, J.: Adverse Reactions During Hospitalization, *Can. Med. Assoc. J. 97*:1445-1457 (Dec. 9) 1967.

12. Jick, H. J.: Drug Surveillance Program, *Med. Sci. 18*:41-46 (July) 1967.

13. Canada, A. T., Jr.: Adverse Drug Reactions—Some Problems of Definition, Interpretation and Reporting, *Drug Intelligence 1*:372-377 (Dec.) 1967.

14. McHale, M. K. and Canada, A. T., Jr.: The Use of a Pharmacist in Obtaining Medication Histories, *Drug Intelligence 3*:115-119 (Apr.) 1969.

15. Esch, A. F.: Food and Drug Administration Drug Experience Reporting System, *J. Chem. Doc. 9*:66-70 (May) 1969.

16. Ruskin, A.: Drug Experience Reporting, *FDA Papers 1*:13-16 (Apr.) 1967.

17. Anon.: Registry on Adverse Reactions, *J. Am. Med. Assoc. 188*:374 (Apr. 27) 1964.

18. Hotaling, W. H.: Adverse Drug Reactions, *Hosp. Formulary Management 1*:38-41 (Sept.) 1966.

19. Canada, A. T., Jr.: Adverse Drug Reaction Reporting —A Practical Program, *Am. J. Hosp. Pharm. 26*:18-23 (Jan.) 1969.

Additional References

1. Gardner, P. and Watson, L. J.: Adverse Drug Reactions—A Pharmacist-Based Monitoring System, *Clin. Pharmacol. Therap. II*:802-807 (Nov.-Dec.) 1970.

2. Hutchinson, R. A.: Adverse Drug Reactions—A Review, *Hosp. Topics 48*:69-76 (Sept.) 1970.

3. Parks, J. S.: Drug Surveillance—A Practical Contribution, *Can. J. Hosp. Pharm. 23*:147-151 (July-Aug.) 1970.

4. Wade, O. L.: Pattern of Drug-Induced Disease in the Community, *Brit. Med. Bull. 26*:240-244 (Sept.) 1970.

5. Zilz, D. A.: Drug Surveillance, *Hospitals 45*:89-92 (Apr. 16) 1971.

12

Interviewing and advising the patient

by Tim R. Covington

Basic to effective patient interviewing and advising is the ability to communicate. Communication is defined as a giving and/or receiving of information, signals or messages by talk, gestures, writing or other means. Communication therefore, may be through verbal or nonverbal processes. Effective communication depends largely upon the pharmacist's ability to communicate verbally with the patient and interpret nonverbal responses.

As the clinical role for the pharmacist continues to evolve, it is becoming more essential that the pharmacist communicate directly with the patient. Areas of practice where the pharmacist may communicate directly with the institutionalized patient or ambulatory outpatient include (1) acquisition of medication history, (2) discussions of current therapy and (3) counseling regarding proper home use of prescribed medications or devices. In addition, the pharmacist may find it necessary to interact verbally with hospital inpatients as he monitors drug utilization or participates in structured adverse drug reaction detection and prevention programs.

The importance of effective communication between health professionals and patients is dramatically revealed in the following nursing service incident (accident) report:

Mr. Smith, on April 14, 1966, was given some liquid pHisoHex soap so he could take a shower before going to surgery. Instead of taking a shower with pHisoHex he drank it. Because he didn't go to surgery on April 14, Mr. Smith was again given some liquid pHisoHex soap so he could take a shower. Instead, he drank it again. Another person with Mr. Smith this morning heard me tell him to take a shower with the soap. This morning the patient complained to the doctor that the medicine made him vomit.[1]

In addition, the pharmacy and medical literature is replete with articles demonstrating patient inadequacy in consuming prescribed medication.[2-5] One study revealed that 77 (42.8 percent) of 180 outpatients misused at least one of their medications in some manner.[5] Eight of these patients misused medication to the extent that it posed a serious threat to their health. In another study one patient revealed he did not take his diphenylhydantoin and phenobarbital until he "got bad" while another patient said he took a friend's digitalis for his lower back pain.[6] Obviously the health care team and particularly the pharmacist is not effectively communicating pertinent data to the patient regarding proper drug usage.

The pharmacist must have a basic understanding of methods that will guarantee an appropriate clinical approach to the patient. There is presently little information available concerning patient-pharmacist communicative processes. This chapter enumerates certain communicative methods and points out how they may be utilized by the pharmacist to maximize patient care relative to drug therapy.

PREPARATION FOR INTERVIEW

Before any attempt is made to interview or counsel patients, the pharmacist must familiarize himself with the environment in which he will be working and the professional personnel with whom he will be interacting. All other health professionals involved with a specific patient's care, particularly the physician and nurse, must be aware of the pharmacist's role and responsibility on the patient care unit or in the community pharmacy if a situation conducive to maximum patient care is to exist. The pharmacist, in addition to communicating his role and responsibility and how it may benefit the patient, must develop and express a genuine interest in the responsibilities of other health professionals. Once each professional group thoroughly understands the role of the other and how it contributes to the patient's welfare, a spirit of mutual respect and cooperation is assured.

In preparing to interview and/or counsel hospitalized patients or ambulatory outpatients, it behooves the pharmacist to familiarize himself with the patient's present medical status. This task is more difficult to achieve in community pharmacy because it depends on the patient's knowledge of his pathological condition or the willingness of the patient and physician to cooperate with the pharmacist in providing pertinent information. The pharmacist in the institutional environment generally has access to all patient records and encounters little difficulty in acquiring medical and demographic data that will facilitate the communicative process.

Past experiences in acquiring medication histories of inpatients indicate that the interview by the pharmacist should be performed after the attending physician has examined the patient and made appropriate notes in the chart. The interview by the pharmacist should occur as soon after the initial physician examination as possible so that the medication history may become a working document as an integral part of the patient chart. A quick survey of the nurses' Kardex or patient chart prior to the interview will provide basic medical and demographic data regarding the patient that will facilitate the interviewing process. Information useful in preparing for the interview includes patient age, sex, race, social history, chief complaint on admission, previous and current medical history, physical exam findings, medication history (if physician acquired), laboratory test results, current drug therapy and diagnosis (Table 1). Information regarding these topics should give the pharmacist considerable insight into a patient's psychological and pathological condition, and the clinical approach to the patient may be adjusted accordingly.

It is also helpful to talk with other health professionals on the patient care unit who are involved with a particular patient's care, such as the nurse or physician, as they are generally well aware of a patient's communicative abilities and willingness to cooperate. In certain instances there will be a note in the chart as to whether a patient is or is not cooperative or a reliable historian, but this practice is the exception rather than the rule. As patients will frequently be off the patient care unit for surgery, diagnostic tests, treatments and so forth, professional personnel who are well aware of day-to-day routine activities can be of great assistance to the pharmacist in that they are generally aware of how long patients will be absent. This allows the pharmacist to utilize his time for other activities while waiting for a patient to return. Once the pharmacist has acquired the necessary preliminary data he must then begin to consider his clinical approach to the patient and what interviewing techniques he will utilize.

Table 1. Data Useful in Preparing for the Interview

1. Age
2. Sex
3. Race
4. Social History
5. Chief Complaint on Admission
6. Previous & Current Medical History
7. Physical Exam Findings
8. Medication History (If Physician Acquired)
9. Laboratory Test Results
10. Current Drug Therapy
11. Diagnosis

Pharmacist-Patient Relationship

The professional relationship between the pharmacist and the patient is becoming more visibly recognizable as essential to the maximal well-being of the patient. Interviewing and counseling are the media for the development of this professional relationship, hence the techniques for effective verbal interaction cannot be ignored. For the pharmacist to be an effective communicator with the patient he must be aware of certain communicative techniques and appreciate certain psychological and emotional factors which might influence patient behavior and attitudes.

There are several fundamental communicative techniques that have their primary application in the interview of institutionalized patients during the acquisition of medication histories. The pharmacist should recognize that with certain alterations, most methods employed in the more formal institutional environment have an application in community pharmacy. The degree of success in acquiring a comprehensive medication history in any practice environment is limited only by the initiative of the pharmacist and his expertise in applying certain communicative principles to various clinical situations.

PATIENT BEHAVIORAL AND ATTITUDINAL FACTORS AFFECTING THE INTERVIEW

The pharmacist must first understand factors that might influence the patient's behavior and attitude. Some patients adapt readily to their dependence on the health care team. A few patients find this very difficult and have a tendency to be noncooperative or even antagonistic when approached for an interview. Familiarity with various personality structures can be of significant help in communicating with patients.

Prior Relationship

The patient's *past experience* with and exposure to pharmacists may affect his attitudinal response and willingness to cooperate in providing a thorough medication history. The psychoanalytical phenomenon known as transference indicates how the patient perceives individuals and how he behaves toward them. Transference is the process whereby feelings of love, hate, trust and distrust attached to certain individuals in the past are unconsciously projected onto important individuals in the present. If the prior relationship was a good one the transference is positive; if the patient's feelings are those of hostility and fear, the transference is negative. If the patient perceives the pharmacist as the unseen individual who fills prescriptions and charges too much for them, the response toward the pharmacist may be negative. On the other hand, if the patient had a history of frequent interaction with a pharmacist who was genuinely concerned with the patient's general health, the response should be favorable. Negative transference can generally be countered if the pharmacist will meet the patient's hostility with quiet understanding rather than counterhostility.

Sociological Factors

Basic *sociological factors* relating to the patient's experiences with important persons in his childhood can affect the patient's willingness to interact with the pharmacist. A history of unreliable, rejecting or neglectful parents or family may seriously interfere with the patient's capacity to have confidence in even the most dedicated health professional.[7] Often patients have an unfilled need for approval of their action. Such patients may actually omit or distort facts about drug therapy to gain the pharmacist's approval. For example, an individual on phenothiazine therapy might not want the pharmacist to know he took a tranquilizer prior to admission as this reflects on his mental state. This distorts the reliability of the interview and reveals the importance of reviewing the family and social history beforehand so that appropriate adjustments in approach and evaluation may be made.

Fears

Some patients have major *fears* about the nature of their illness, drug therapy and hospital procedures. Fear may be expressed verbally by direct statements, asking questions, demanding attention or being critical. A few physiological manifestations of fear that the pharmacist should be aware of include pallor, restlessness, sweating, muscular tension, stomach upset, diarrhea and headaches. An example of a verbal expression of fear would be a patient who was coughing and expectorating, asking the pharmacist if the drugs he was receiving were for the treatment of tuberculosis. If a patient relays his fears to the pharmacist, these fears must be considered in evaluating the accuracy of the history obtained. Patients who do not know their diagnosis often tend to be fatalistic and assume the drugs they are receiving are for treatment of more exotic disorders than the disease from which they actually suffer.

Social, Cultural, Educational and Economic Factors

Social, cultural, educational and economic factors significantly affect the interview. Patients from lower socioeconomic strata are less likely to exercise inhibition of aggressive behavior and are more often unwilling to conform to the role of the "good" patient.[8] These patients have relatively less education and often have difficulty in understanding and communicating regarding certain segments of a medication history. For example, the pharmacist may have to define words such as allergy, adverse reaction or antacid in very elementary or colloquial terms. Patients from lower socioeconomic levels are sometimes unaware of the good intentions of health professionals when questions are asked and may tend to be noncooperative. In these instances it may be necessary for the pharmacist to portray a "good guy" image so that the two-way communicative process may begin. The strict professional approach is not indicated in all interviews and a smile, good humor and levity may provide the key to effective interaction in a few clinical situations. Individuals from the middle and upper social, cultural, educational and economic levels tend to be more inquisitive of the pharmacist and he must guard against being interviewed rather than conducting the interview. Patients of middle and upper class society are generally more reliable historians than those from the lower class.[6] Although patients of middle and upper class society are more reliable and cooperative, the need to effectively interview the patient from lower class society is just as great and should be considered a challenge to the interviewer's ingenuity.

Technical Problems

There are a multitude of special technical problems of the interview due to psychological, psychiatric or organic disorders that manifest themselves in patient behavior and attitude, and these will be discussed later in the chapter.

SPECIFIC INTERVIEWING TECHNIQUES

Clinical Approach to the Patient

In developing an appropriate *clinical approach to the patient,* the pharmacist must establish certain modes of behavior. Perhaps the single most essential ingredient of an effective interviewer is the ability to *empathize* with the patient. If, in this age of social awareness and humanism, one can see all mankind as individuals with ideals and values who face conflicts and disappointments, who experience joys and fulfillment and who live in a world of qualities and meanings that individual can be said to have empathy for his fellow man.[9] If the pharmacist has the ability to project himself into the patient's situation and effectively conceptualize the patient's feelings or ideas without becoming distressed, the patient can generally sense this and will respond to questions in a much more effective manner. The greater the pharmacist's "empathy quotient" the greater will be his overall degree of success in obtaining information from patients. One must guard against becoming visibly sympathetic or overly friendly with the patient, however. If the pharmacist becomes overly sympathetic or friendly, he may destroy the professional relationship and the patient may exploit the interviewer's sympathy, thus endangering the validity of the interview.

Professional attitude is an essential component of an effective interviewer and includes attention to such things as dress, hygiene, grooming, language and behavior. The pharmacist should always approach the patient in the appropriate professional attire and appear neat, clean and well-groomed. Such activities as joking in the halls or wards, horseplay, laughter, gum-chewing, smoking and other out-of-the-hospital social behavior are taboo in the clinical environment. Such activities are truly unprofessional and likely to be misinterpreted by the patients. Basic to professional conduct is respect for the patient no matter how deviant his behavior or bizarre his pathological condition. Under no circumstances should the patient be the butt of jokes or ridicule in "bull sessions" among professionals. The pharmacist has a professional responsibility to respect the confidentiality of information gathered or read in the patient's chart and should discuss patients only with appropriate members of the health care team. The pharmacist must be alert to the presence of patients or families when conducting corridor conversations with other professionals. In certain obvious instances statements overheard might be very deleterious to the patient or the family.

Nonverbal Considerations

There are a number of nonverbal behavioral traits of patients that, if recognized, may enhance the effectiveness of the interview. These nonverbal behavioral traits may produce significant insight into a patient's personality, anxieties and apprehensions. Nonverbal communication involves a wide spectrum of behavior which may occur coincidentally with spoken communication, but may reflect more clearly the emotional state of the patient and includes the following components: (1) pitch and tone of voice, (2) sequential phrasing of statements, (3) facial expression, (4) posture of the body and (5) motor movements of the extremities, particularly the hands.[10] To truly assess patient response to questions it is important to recognize not only how the patient answers questions but also how he appears when he answers questions.

The interviewer should be *observant* upon entering the patient's room and throughout the interview so that nonverbal behavioral traits may be recognized. In addition, it is wise to note the general physical appearance of the patient.[11] Needle puncture marks of the limbs would make one think in terms of diabetes or drug addiction and the interviewer should determine the explanation for these marks. In observing the patient's head the pharmacist should be aware of overt symptoms of deficiency diseases such as pallor of lips and skin due to iron deficiency or cheilosis (riboflavin deficiency). The pharmacist should also be aware of visible facial manifestations of hepatic disease, carbon monoxide poisoning, acute alcoholism, phenolic poisoning, complications of corticosteroid therapy, psychotic depression, catatonic schizophrenic stupor and so forth. In addition the pharmacist may wish to note abnormal physiology of the eye such as pupil size, icteric sclera or other deviations from normal that may have a pathological basis.

The Interview

The pharmacist, prior to any dialogue with the patient, should develop a *systematic approach* to the interview. He should have a general idea of the questions to be asked and their sequence. The Medication History Data Sheet (Figure 1) reveals a logical sequence of questions that might be utilized in obtaining a comprehensive medication history. Simple, easily understood phrases are preferred and complex medical or pharmacological terminology is to be avoided.

The first verbal step in interviewing the patient is for the pharmacist to *introduce himself and describe his role.* A logical approach would be to say, "I am John Doe, the pharmacist for this section of the hospital, and I need to ask you a few routine questions about your medication." It is neither necessary nor appropriate for the pharmacist to ask the patient's permission to be interviewed. After having introduced himself, the pharmacist may inquire as to whether it is a convenient time for the patient to be seen. The pharmacist should not feel awkward or insecure in assuming the professional role of obtaining the medication history. Most patients accept him as a member of the professional staff and readily cooperate. The pharmacist has a significant service to render and should proceed with the patient's ultimate welfare in mind.

A very important portion of the interview is *putting the patient at ease.* If a pharmacist has the ability to assess a patient's level of intelligence and translate patient colloquialisms he can structure his conversation using the patient's vocabulary, thus facilitating the interviewing process greatly. The ability to translate patient colloquialisms is often a great challenge as vocabularies are affected by patient sex, socioeconomic level, ethnic and cultural background and geographic origin.[12] The importance of using the patient's vernacular is revealed in the following report.

> Dr. Thomas Orr, at the University of Kansas, insisted that a history on a youngster with acute appendicitis must be incomplete because there was no mention of vomiting. The discussion prompted the surgical resident to return to the parents to inquire further. His questions included the following: 'Did he vomit? Did he throw up or have an emesis? Was he sick at his stomach?' All to no avail, with continuing negative answers. Finally he asked, 'Did he puke?' — to which the father replied, 'Oh, hell yes, he puked all over the place.'[13]

In addition to speaking the patient's "lingo" in putting the patient at ease, the pharmacist must *appear interested, unhurried, tactful and considerate.* As most patients are preoccupied

Figure 1. Medication History Data Sheet

Patient Name ____________ Age ______ Sex ______ Race ______

Case History Number ____________ Diagnosis ____________

Date (and Hour) of Admission ____________ Date (and Hour) of History ____________

Person Acquiring History ____________

1. Name of drugs you were taking prior to admission (legend) ____________
2. Description of drugs (legend) you were taking prior to admission (only if don't know name) ____________
3. Why were you taking these drugs? ____________
4. What drugs have you stopped taking? ____________ Why? ______
5. Did you ever miss a dose at home? ____________

   Frequency? ____________
6. Have you ever taken someone else's prescription medication? ____________

   Why? ____________
7. Did you bring any prescription medications to the hospital with you? ____________

   Which one(s)? ____________
8. Medicines (OTC) you take at home:
   a. Laxatives
   b. Vitamins
   c. Aspirin
   d. Cold medicines
   e. Cough syrup
   f. Pain medicine
   g. Antacids
   h. Topical preparations
   i. Antidiarrheals
   j. Drugs to stay awake
   k. Drugs for insomnia
   l. Drugs for nerves
   m. Drugs for fluid retention
9. Known allergies to drugs ____________
10. Known allergies to food ____________
11. Known allergies to pets ____________
12. Any other members of the family with allergies (relationship and allergy) ____________
13. Do you consume alcoholic beverages (amount)? ____________
14. Do you consume large amounts of tea, coffee or soft drinks (amount)? ____________
15. Have you ever taken drugs that made you "feel bad?" (specify) ____________
16. Have you noticed adverse effects (include side effects) that are due to drugs you have received while hospitalized? ____________

with their immediate distress or pathological condition, the pharmacist must immediately let the individual know that he is concerned. A question regarding drug therapy such as, "Do you think the drugs you are receiving are making you feel better?" is appropriate in that it reveals your concern for the patient and the answer can serve as an entrée into the interview. Careless, random conversation by the pharmacist is to be avoided. Considerable thought must be given to everything asked or told the patient. It is not the pharmacist's responsibility to answer direct questions relative to the patient's condition. This responsibility lies solely with the physician and questions concerning the patient's case should be referred to the attending physician. Also, the pharmacist should not issue irrational statements such as, "I'm sure you will be all right in a few days." Uninformed declarations such as this may only serve to delude or confuse the patient about his actual status.

A truly effective interviewer must be a good *listener*. The patient should feel that he is the sole concern of the interviewer for the duration of the interview, and an attentive attitude which conveys the readiness to listen can create this atmosphere.[14] Listening, rather than talking, will provide the climate in which the patient can communicate. The interviewer should not be too silent, but should avoid an excess of verbiage that might stifle the patient's efforts to respond completely to questions.

To be a good listener the interviewer must devote his attention to the patient, but should not stare hypnotically at the patient as he answers questions. This degree of attentiveness by the interviewer is to be avoided as it tends to make the patient restless and uncomfortable. Brief periods of note taking will allow a break in eye contact, and sketchy notes for later interpretation and transcription generally suffice. Prolonged periods of writing are to be avoided as these make the patient feel that the interviewer's full attention is not directed toward him.

The pharmacist should *maintain control of the interview* at all times. It is the interviewer's responsibility to keep the conversation relevant. Although the pharmacist should encourage the patient to talk, the interview must not become a patient discourse into minutia. Conversely, the pharmacist should not spend too much time and effort in extracting inconsequential information.

Patient *spontaneity* should be encouraged. If the interviewer begins with a burst of short questions the patient may respond by waiting silently for the next question rather than elaborating on particular points. Question and answer sessions are not nearly as productive as the interviews in which the patient is encouraged to speak freely. It is generally easier to guide a talkative person into productive channels than to extract pertinent information from a reticent person.

If a patient insists on asking questions of the pharmacist, the interview may be turned back to the patient by answering his question with a question such as, "Why do you ask?" If this response does not divert the conversation and the interviewer feels he should not comment then the question should be referred to the attending physician. Many times direct eye contact, a firm facial expression and a statement such as, "You were saying — about a particular subject," will guide the interview back into a relevant vein.

The interview should be as *private and free from interruption* as possible. Many patients have qualms about discussing their drug therapy among other patients, friends or relatives. If friends or relatives are in the patient's room, the pharmacist may wish to ask them to step out of the area for a few minutes or delay the interview. In some cases certain family members will insist on remaining at the bedside. In these cases, continue the interview as planned if the patient has no objections. Many patients do not wish others to know they are taking such drugs as analgesics, hormones, tranquilizers or sedatives. The stigma of habituation, addiction, aging or mental defects that is synonymous with certain drugs dictates that the patient be allowed privacy in discussing drug therapy if he so wishes. If the patient is in an open ward or semi-private room, it is a good practice to draw the bed curtain prior to the interview as this conveys a psychological privacy to the patient and puts the interview on a more formal basis.[15]

The *phrasing of questions* is a very important technique of effective interviewing. Questions may be phrased in four basic ways: neutral, simple-direct, leading and loaded. In selecting the phraseology of the question the interviewer should (1) make sure the patient has no difficulty understanding what is being asked, (2) in no way prejudice the patient's response and (3) induce the patient to speak freely.[16] To meet these requirements the following are essential.

1. Questions should be brief and simple. Whenever it is necessary to explain a question the interviewer should stop and think through exactly what it is he wants to find out.
2. The interviewer should use language that is understandable to the patient. This will require taking into account the patient's level of education and his background.

3. Only one question should be asked at a time. To string several questions together or to ask about more than one item leaves the patient uncertain as to what he should answer.
4. In exploring any issue the inquiry should always start with non-directive questions, reserving more direct questions to clarify ambiguities or verify facts. Questions which can be answered with a simple "yes" or "no" should be used sparingly; otherwise the patient may fall into a pattern of waiting silently for the next question.
5. One should use the patient's own terms until there is mutual agreement as to what the term means. Vague terms such as "water pill," "blood builder," "nerve medicine," "pain pill," "heart medicine" and so forth need to be clarified by the interviewer as the patient is often confused about his drug therapy regimen.[16]

The neutral question does not suggest any particular response from a patient and is seldom used in obtaining a medication history. The simple-direct question is used most often. The simple-direct question, if not overly specific and staccato, can yield the most information. The leading question tempts the patient to give a particular answer. These questions are biased and should be used only when it is impossible to obtain information by other means. Loaded questions are very heavily biased and are used primarily in psychological testing to study patient reaction. They have no place in the acquisition of a medication history.

In *bringing the interview to a close,* it is good practice to give the patient an opportunity to mention anything else he may have on his mind that pertains to drug therapy. Also, if the interviewer is not clear about a particular point it may be helpful to recapitulate briefly. Occasionally this post-interview discussion will result in some new piece of pertinent information. The interviewer should be alert to patient fatigue or discomfort, and, if necessary, the interview postponed for a short time. When the interview is completed, the patient should be politely thanked for his cooperation.

Special Problems of the Interview

There are many special problems that may be encountered during the interview and these usually stem from the patient's own problems, be they psychological or organic. Clinical experience helps resolve many of the technical difficulties of the interview, but a consideration of common problems that may occur in an interview can prevent embarrassing inadequacies on the part of the interviewer.

Occasionally patients will ask the interviewer certain *personal questions* or respond in a challenging or aggressive manner to questions of them which are considered personal. The interviewer should respond with a brief, honest statement and assure the patient that the only concern is for the patient and his welfare. Rarely, patients, notably hysterics, manics and a few psychotics, may make seductive or even sexual advances toward the interviewer, and such behavior must be met in a firm professional manner, avoiding involvement in any type of personal exchange.[17]

Silences by the patient in response to questions may complicate the interview and are attributable to a number of factors. Brief silences of 20 or 30 seconds generally reflect a patient's attempt to recall a fact. The proper behavior by the interviewer is simply to wait expectantly and indicate by facial expression or verbally that he wishes the patient to continue. Prolonged or repeated silence is often due to faulty technique on the part of the interviewer. If patients are offended by tactless remarks or note a lack of genuine concern by the interviewer, they may become silent or offer minimal verbal response. Prolonged silence may also be due to manifestations of organic brain disease, depression or psychosis and the pharmacist should delay the interview in these cases pending a consult with the attending physician.

Crying may result if certain questions remind the patient of something very distressing or tragic that has occurred in his past relative to drug therapy. For example, a friend or relation may have sustained an anaphylactic reaction to penicillin or met with a tragic accident while under the influence of drugs. Many individuals are very fearful of drugs and their potentially harmful effects and will reveal this fact during the interview. Crying, however, is a valuable clinical sign as it reveals the importance of the topic under discussion to the patient. The interviewer should allow the patient to cry and let the patient know that he understands by a sympathetic nod or a kindly remark such as, "I understand how you feel."[18] The patient is usually able to resume the interview, feeling relieved and gratified that the interviewer understands.

Various degrees of patient *hostility* may be encountered during the interview. Different situations which may provoke patient anger include: (1) the inconsiderate or angry interviewer; (2) the patient who is already angry; (3) the aggressive, pseudoindependent patient; (4) the demanding, dependent patient; or (5) the paranoid patient.[18]

In dealing with hostile patients the situation

is often helped if the pharmacist will remain passive and reassure the patient that the interview is necessary to maximize health care. If, after a long period of passive understanding and explanation, the patient cannot be calmed, it is best to delay further questioning and try to determine the etiology of the patient's behavior from other professional personnel who have contact with the patient. A patient may apologize for his previous behavior upon the interviewer's return, and the patient should be reassured that his behavior was understood and accepted as part of the stress of illness. If the interviewer erred in his approach to the patient and set off the patient's hostility, he must restructure his clinical approach accordingly. If the second attempt at interviewing the patient proves futile, the pharmacist should then attempt to contact relatives or close friends for the information he desires.

Patients who are *seriously ill* generally cannot give a complete medication history due to weakness, pain, disorganization, confusion or many other manifestations of their pathological condition. The interviewer should, therefore, give priority to those aspects of the interview that are most relevant to the patient's immediate well being. The pharmacist should delay the interview if the patient is suffering severe discomfort or having difficulty in understanding or communicating. The seriously ill patient generally appreciates attentiveness to his comfort and this approach coupled with other interviewing methods should ultimately result in an adequate medication history.

Patients with *organic brain disease* present a real challenge to the interviewer. In delerium the inability to communicate effectively is usually due to a reversible disorder of cerebral metabolism secondary to an inadequate metabolic supply of oxygen or glucose, an electrolyte imbalance or a blocking of the metabolic pathways by endogenous or exogenous toxic substances; in dementia the defect results from the irreversible destruction of brain substance which may develop gradually, as in cerebral atherosclerosis, or abruptly, as in head trauma.[19] These individuals exhibit various degrees of reduced attention and awareness, defects in recall and recent memory and reduced ability to think abstractly. The interviewer must be aware of the patient's mental deficit and be able to evaluate the reliability of the history obtained. Reversible delerium requires a brief delay of the interview, but once the patient's metabolic processes begin to normalize an accurate history is generally obtainable. In more serious brain disorders where the patient appears incapable of giving a reliable history, a relative or friend may be utilized.

The psychotic or depressed patient often elicits behavior that the pharmacist is not trained to cope with. Crude techniques that may be utilized by the pharmacist in an effort to gather pertinent information regarding drug therapy may actually do the patient great harm. It is always best to consult with the attending physician prior to an interview with patients diagnosed as mentally ill. The physician may or may not permit the pharmacist to talk with the patient. If he approves the interview, he may be able to forewarn the pharmacist about patient inhibitions and behavior and assist the pharmacist in developing the appropriate clinical approach to the patient. If the patient is very hostile, aggressive or uncooperative, the physician may offer to perform the medication history and assist in its evaluation. If a medication history is unobtainable then an interview with a relative or close friend is indicated.

Patients who have sustained *cerebral injury*, such as a cerebrovascular accident, may be aphasic, although totally aware and able to comprehend the spoken word. These patients may be interviewed if a system of gestures for yes or no can be developed. Interviews of this type are considerably more difficult and time consuming but are necessary.

There are many other special problems of the interview that are beyond the scope of this chapter. Clinical experience can do much toward producing effective interaction with uncooperative patients. In instances where the interviewer feels he does not have the experience to continue the interview to a productive end point, the interview should be abbreviated. Alternatives available are to (1) re-analyze the patient chart and revise interviewing techniques, (2) consult the attending physician as to how communication obstacles may be overcome, (3) allow the physician to acquire the medication history or (4) interview family member(s) or friends who are familiar with the patient's medication habits.

Interviewing Family or Friends

It is generally best to attempt to interview the patient before turning to others for information. Although a patient may have limited ability to communicate, his responses represent his own feelings as only he can describe them. Patient attitudes about drug therapy are best revealed by the patient himself. Also, patients who sustained subtle or even overt adverse drug reactions may not have related these to a relative or friend

Table 2. Comparison of Physician vs. Pharmacist Acquired Medication History*

	PHYSICIAN-ACQUIRED INFORMATION	PHARMACIST-ACQUIRED INFORMATION
1. Number of legend drugs (based on prescription orders) taken immediately prior to admission	21	129
2. Number of times question 1 was asked by physician as evidenced by information contained in the chart	12	—
3. Number of patients with a history of missing doses at home	0	15
4. Number of patients with a history of taking someone else's medication	0	5
5. Number of patients who brought prescription medication to the hospital	0	5
6. Number of OTC drugs consumed during past year by patients sampled	0	153
7. Prior history of allergies:		
Number of patients with allergies to drugs	2	12
Number of patients with allergies to food	2	8
Number of patients with allergies to pets	1	2
Miscellaneous allergies (ragweed)	0	1
Number of individuals whose immediate family had history of allergies	0	7
8. Number of patients with a history of moderate to heavy drinking (one case of beer or one fifth of hard liquor or more per week)	4	8

*Sample size, 40 patients

and may have even passed them off as a part of the pathological condition for which they were being treated.

If an interview with a family member or close friend is indicated, the patient – when possible – should be informed or asked for his consent. Generally a patient is pleased that the pharmacist will speak to relatives or friends who are concerned with the patient's care.

In interviewing relatives or friends the meeting should be as private as possible. Many interviewing methods used with the patient may also be applied when interviewing visitors. The interview of family members or friends is generally not as thorough as the interview of the patient. Visitors, although not aware of many patient medication habits, may be of great assistance in determining what medications the patient was consuming prior to admission as they may be able to enter the patient's home and obtain prescription vials and other items that provide much absolute data. Also, family members or friends generally will talk more openly regarding topics about which the patient may have guilt feelings or inhibitions such as misuse or abuse of drugs or consumption of alcoholic beverages. The results of the patient interview and visitor interview should be compared and evaluated for discrepancies. If inconsistencies occur it may be desirable to re-direct the original question to the patient. If a harmonious answer cannot be obtained for a question of potentially great clinical significance (*e.g.*, allergy to penicillin) it may be necessary to review previous medical records. As uniformity of response is not always obtainable, the interviewer must then assess the reliability of the individuals providing the data.

Summary

The material presented in the first portion of the chapter is intended to be used as a guide in conducting patient interviews. It is impossible to prepare guidelines applicable to every interview or personality structure. One must bear in mind that the most effective interviews are flexible in format and content so as to be adaptable to individual situations. The material set forth in the previous paragraphs should assist the pharmacist in the basic structuring of the interview.

THE MEDICATION HISTORY

Need

Various communicative techniques have been discussed that can be applied in the acquisition of a medication history, but the importance of the medication history has not been fully revealed (Figure 2). Due to demands on physician time, the physician acquired medication history is often not as thorough as it might be. One study revealed that in a retrospective analysis of 270 patient charts, 42 (16 percent) of the patients were apparently not asked if they had drug allergies, or if they were asked, their responses were not recorded.[20] Of the 228 patients who were asked, 45 (20 percent) had histories of drug allergies. Questions concerning allergies should always be asked and documented lest the patient sustain an unnecessary, expensive and potentially life-threatening allergic reaction.

In another study the pharmacist's expertise in acquiring a comprehensive medication history was evaluated and compared to physician-acquired data recorded in the patient chart.[6] Results indicate the pharmacist has considerable ability in the area of medication history acquisition (Table 2). Many of the questions asked

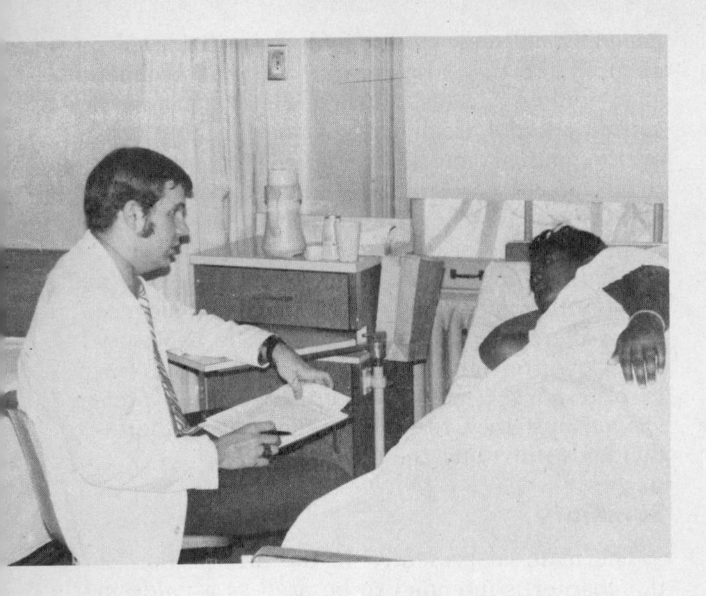

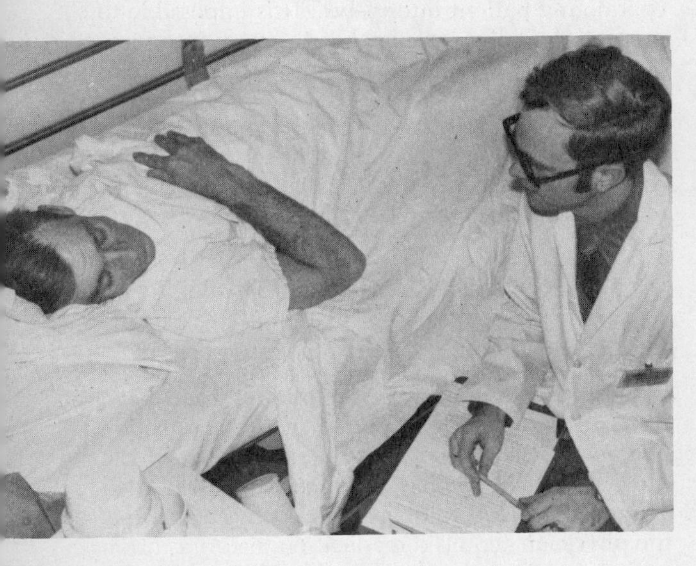

Figure 2. Clinical pharmacists acquiring medication histories from hospitalized patients

were not routine questions in a physician-acquired medication history, but are, nevertheless, essential in maximizing patient safety. Of particular interest in this study was the fact that no physician documented his results of inquiries into proprietary (OTC) drug use. Results obtained by the pharmacist reveal that the average hospitalized patient consumed 3.8 different patent remedies during the previous year. Many of these drugs were flagrantly abused, laxatives being the most abused proprietary. A woman with severe asthmatic episodes was admitted to the hospital five times before it was discovered that her symptoms were brought on by the ingestion of aspirin-containing drugs.[21] As we continue to recognize the potential of over-the-counter remedies as sources of drug-drug interactions, adverse drug reactions and iatrogenic disorders, it is imperative that inquiries be made into patient usage of these products.

Some reasons expressed by patients with a history of unreliability in taking prescribed medication are: "Sometimes I forget," "When I run out I usually get a refill in a day or two," "I stop taking them when I start feeling better" and "I can't afford the medicine." Many patients are too casual about taking drugs. Some individuals take their drugs in excess while others omit doses. It is reliably estimated that only two-thirds of 6000 tuberculosis patients on drug therapy and under the care of the Tuberculosis Control Section of the Philadelphia Department of Health take their medication.[22] Reports of patients from lower socioeconomic levels *selling* their drugs or leaving them on buses are not uncommon.

Medication histories may often reveal patients who have taken someone else's medication in the hope that they will achieve relief from their symptoms. Five patients revealed the following reasons for taking another person's legend drugs: (1) digitalis for lower back pain; (2) pink pain pills for headache; (3) green water pills for fluid; (4) diet pills for energy; and (5) amitriptyline HCl 10 mg to "Make me feel better."[6]

Many patients see more than one physician and it is not uncommon for one physician to prescribe the same drug another physician had previously prescribed. In one instance a patient had two separate prescriptions for pentaerythritol tetranitrate 20 mg tablets. She continued to take both, although they were identical in appearance, because the prescription numbers and directions were different. Situations such as these are not always preventable, but they can be detected and terminated by the pharmacist obtaining a comprehensive medication history.

Table 3. Pharmacist-Detected Adverse Drug Reactions Occurring Prior to Admission*

	DRUG**	ADVERSE EFFECT
1	Furosemide	Ototoxicity (tinnitis and partial deafness)
2	Glutethimide	Nausea and vomiting
3	Chlorpromazine	Extreme drowsiness
4	Theophylline with ephedrine and phenobarbital	Nervousness; vomiting
5	Hydrochlorothiazide	Dizziness
6	A sulfonamide***	Severe rash
7	Aminophylline	Nausea
8	Propoxyphene with APC	Nausea
9	Furosemide	Dizziness; headache
10	Aspirin	Upper gastrointestinal distress
11	Unknown anorexic agent (white tablet)	Extreme nervousness

*All patients reported a dosage schedule within normal limits
**All drugs administered orally
***Exact generic name unknown

The medication history may also reveal overt adverse drug reactions that have occurred to the ambulatory outpatient. Detection of these adverse effects can greatly benefit the patient if the pharmacist will advise the patient regarding proper drug usage and/or consult with the patient's physician regarding an alternative drug regimen. Table 3 reveals adverse drug reactions sustained by hospitalized patients prior to admission as revealed through a pharmacist-obtained medication history.[6]

Finally, the pharmacist should inquire into the patient's drinking habits. Alcohol ingestion and concurrent drug therapy may be the source of some problems for the patient. Guidelines as to what degree of alcohol consumption constitutes a "light," "moderate" or "heavy drinker" should be set, as arbitrary assignment of these terms is of little use.

Cost-Benefit Analysis

Cost and professional time required for patient interviews are factors that cannot be ignored. One hospital study revealed the average time required per interview was 35 minutes.[23] The interview consisted of the following components: (1) nine minutes in personal interview, (2) 14 minutes for telephone follow-up to community pharmacies to see what legend drugs the patient had received the six months prior to the interview as indicated on the patient drug profile and (3) 12 minutes for pre-interview and post-interview write-up. Further analysis revealed that the cost of the medication history per patient per patient day in this study was $0.34. Another study of lesser magnitude revealed an average interviewing time of 4.15 minutes per patient, but this figure does not include follow-up.[24] Benefit of the pharmacist-acquired medication history clearly outweighs cost considerations, and experience in performing this function should lead to innovations that can further decrease cost.

Information sought and obtainable in a medication history may be varied. Guidelines have been established, however, and may be applied in both community and institutional pharmacy.[6,24,25] Evidence such as that presented in this chapter points out the critical need for a health professional who has the time, technique and expertise to procure a comprehensive medication history. This information should become a part of the patient's permanent hospital or community pharmacy record and can serve as a most useful document in promoting rational drug therapy and improving patient care. It is interesting to note that many reasons for the misuse and abuse of drugs, as revealed through the medication history, are due to inadequate counseling regarding their proper use. Most of this responsibility must be accepted by the pharmacist as he is the logical and best qualified health professional to perform this function.

COMPUTERIZED HISTORIES — FOR THE FUTURE

A new approach to the acquisition of important patient data is the utilization of the computer. History taking consumes a large amount of time, and in light of today's rising cost and questionable quality of health care, new methods must be explored to improve patient care. Better methods of collecting and recording detailed clinical information from patients are needed. Several medical questionnaire systems that utilize the speed, efficiency and reliability of the computer have been established and these computer-based automated medical histories (AMH) are being utilized in a few institutions throughout the country.[26-30]

Techniques

One system for collecting the medical histories begins with dialogue between a patient and a computer through a teletypewriter terminal. A paramedical staff member verbally collects and enters basic patient demographic data into the system through the terminal and then instructs the patient in the use of the terminal. The terminal prints out multiple choice questions and the patient chooses the number which designates the appropriate response. Subsequent questions depend on the patient's answers. More sophisticated systems utilize a cathode-ray screen system where questions and choices of answers are flashed upon a screen and the patient's response recorded by depressing the appropriate key, button or similar indicator. A branching logic technique is used to vary succeeding questions in accord with prior answers. The computer may be programmed to go on to the next general question, ask more detailed questions on the same subject or give additional information. A relatively concise, thorough summary can be generated for use by appropriate members of the health care team.

Experience with Computer-Acquired Medical Histories

How do patients and physicians react to this method of acquiring medical histories, and how accurate and complete is the computer-acquired information when compared with physician-acquired histories? In a study performed at Massachusetts General Hospital patient and physician attitudes to the AMH were evaluated.[29]

Patient attitudes toward the AMH were generally favorable. Patients were seldom bored, were satisfied with the choices of answers available, felt the questions were related to their medical problems and thought they were able to give a complete and accurate history. It is not known at this time whether favorable patient attitudes to AMH are due to true acceptance of the technique, the "novel effect" or apprehension to speaking freely about this depersonalized technique. A hint at true patient feelings toward the AMH was revealed in generally mixed responses about the possibility of being interviewed by the computer again and lack of preference of the computer over the physician as an interviewer.

Physician attitudes toward the AMH were not as favorable as those of patients. Physicians perceived little or no measurable difference in their rapport with patients or in their efficiency during their interview with patients that previously received the AMH.

The *accuracy and completeness* of the automated medical history versus the physician-acquired verbal history is extremely difficult to quantitate. The advantage of the dialogue technique is its complete flexibility which allows the interviewer to probe deeply into certain areas and utilize psychological and communicative techniques that assure accuracy of information. Also, although a physician or other interviewer may record fewer facts than those recorded in automated histories, one may be certain that the data collected are considerably more than that which he records. On the other hand, the dialogue consumes a phenomenal amount of a health professional's time. Also, a great amount of variability of interviewing technique and interpretation of patient responses occurs with the dialogue technique, whereas there is greater consistency of response in automated testing. No conclusive objective data comparing the traditional history with the automated history revealing changes in the degree of patient care are presently available, therefore, judgment on the virtues of the automated medical history must await further evaluation.[31]

Automated History and Impact on Evolving Clinical Pharmacy Roles

It may seem paradoxical that the automation of newly elucidated roles for pharmacy requiring verbal interaction with patients by the pharmacist is slowly evolving. The pharmacist should not be discouraged by potential applications of the computer. The contents of this chapter should clearly reveal that the pharmacist is needed *now* to perform certain vital functions such as the acquisition of a comprehensive medication history. As for what the future holds, we can only speculate.

There are many groups of patients whose pathology prohibits the acquisition of an accurate automated history (*e.g.*, psychiatric patients, patients with CNS disorders, patients with impaired brain function, acutely ill patients and so forth). In addition, the pediatric patient, patients without a reading knowledge of English and patients with subnormal intelligence pose a considerable problem. Highly sophisticated computers are required and although their purchase is generally not feasible for private physicians, small hospitals and the community pharmacy, computer capability is available through a shared time arrangement utilizing a teletypewriter and telephone linked to the central facility. The basic question of cost (time and money) versus the benefit (improved patient care) of the automated medical history has not been absolutely demonstrated.

Summary

The technology of data processing in dozens of other fields has been revolutionized by the computer in the last two or three decades but few of these changes have made their way into the medical and paramedical field as they inevitably must. If the computer can serve certain health needs of society more efficiently than certain health practitioners then the function logically belongs to the computer.

There is a great need, however, for the pharmacist of today to project himself more vigorously into the patient care area and contribute his expertise to improved patient care through verbal interaction with patients and the health care team. The pharmacist must not be intimidated into submission or apathy by the computer. The day that the computer may acquire a complete medical history, diagnose, prescribe and advise a significant percentage of patients is a possibility but, realistically speaking, it is many years in the future.

There will *always* be a need for health professionals who have the time, technique and expertise to *evaluate* computer generated data and render *judgmental decisions* that will serve to improve patient care. The key to success in today's changing world is the ability to be flexible in thinking and adaptable to change. With appropriate training, attitude and initiatives the pharmacist can secure his place on the health care team, regardless of technological advances.

ADVISING THE PATIENT

Need

It has been said that if more physicians would reach for their history form instead of their prescription pad, many suicides by drug overdosage could be prevented.[32] If the physician does not have the time to acquire a thorough history regarding the patient's tendency toward drug abuse he certainly cannot be expected to thoroughly advise patients regarding proper use of all drugs. The burden then is upon the pharmacist, where indeed it should be, to educate and advise the public they serve in drug therapy related matters.

Society has a great concern for the acutely ill, hospitalized patient and hospital treatment is generally thorough and up-to-the-minute. Great efforts are often made to see that the inpatient receives the right drug in the right dose at the right time by the right route. However, patients upon discharge from the hospital and ambulatory outpatients are often neglected in being counseled about proper home use of drug products as evidenced by information obtained via the medication history and documented previously. The need for proper counseling of patients about medication therapy can be learned from the following example.

A patient's mother did not know the importance of uninterrupted medication to control her son's epileptic seizures. She had not given the child any medication for approximately two weeks; yet, she did not associate this with an admitted increase in the frequency of his seizures.[25]

Obviously this mother had not been told how to properly utilize her son's medication to most effectively treat his pathological condition.

Communicative Techniques

Certain communicative techniques should be remembered when advising patients. To reiterate previous suggestions in interviewing, the pharmacist must be genuinely empathetic and maintain a professional attitude. Counseling is best performed in a private or semiprivate area. The pharmacist should then introduce himself and describe his role, appearing interested, unhurried, tactful and considerate at all times. Numerous other communicative techniques used in the interview could and should be modified to apply to the counseling process.

Patient Drug Profile

A very useful document allowing a detailed analysis of drug usage that should be maintained if one is to achieve near optimum efficiency in advising patients is the patient drug profile. This document, if appropriately designed and monitored, may provide information that can protect the patient against such things as potential drug-drug interactions, drug-food interactions and receiving duplicate prescriptions. It can also serve to alert the pharmacist to a patient's allergies, drug misuse and conscious abuse. Recognition of these factors can allow the pharmacist to advise the patient or consult with the physician, depending on which action is more appropriate. The pharmacist would certainly not wish to unduly alarm patients with the possibility of every potential drug-drug interaction, for example, but information of potential clinical significance should be referred to the attending physician for appropriate action. A pharmacist skilled in interviewing may subtly gather pertinent facts regarding symptomatology of suspected drug-drug interactions, drug-food interactions or adverse drug reactions and relay this information to the physician or counsel the patient accordingly. In addition, the pharmacist may be able to determine reasons for drug misuse or abuse and correct the situation through proper counseling.

Topics for Counseling

The pharmacist should make the patient aware of the following points at discharge or upon dispensing a prescription.[33-34]

1. *Who the medication is for.* When several prescriptions are dispensed at one time for different family members potential confusion should be recognized and clarified by the pharmacist. The patient should also be told that the medicine is for the individual whose name appears on the label and is never to be used to treat similar symptoms in other individuals.
2. *What the medication is to be used for.* The patient should be told what the medicine is to be used for in general layman's terms (*e.g.*, heart, blood pressure, infection) so he may differentiate more easily the differences between drugs with the same or similar directions. For drugs used in treating acute or terminal illnesses the pharmacist may not wish to relate the specific use of the drug to the patient, as the patient may not be aware of his diagnosis.
3. *The name of the medication.* Labeling a prescription with the name of the drug is becoming a common practice. This policy has been recommended by the American Medical Association's Council on Drugs. This practice allows positive identification of the drug in many poisoning cases.
4. *How to use the medication.* The pharmacist should explain in detail the proper administration of medication to ensure the proper therapeutic response. Aerosol inhalation therapy, rectal and vaginal suppositories, ophthalmic and otic preparations, pediatric liquids, douches, enemas and injectables all require knowledge of certain techniques by the self-medicating public to assure maximum effect of the active ingredient.
5. *When to use the medication.* The pharmacist should make the patient aware of appropriate time intervals between administering doses as the time of administration can affect absorption and blood levels appreciably. Definition of label instructions such as before meals, after meals, every six hours or four times daily should be related verbally to the patient. *As directed* is an inappropriate form of instruction and should be clarified by calling the prescribing physician to determine exact instructions. These instructions should then be placed on the label and explained.
6. *How long to use the medication.* The patient should be instructed to follow the full course of treatment unless the physician tells the patient otherwise. This is particularly important in the use of antibiotics and other antimicrobials.
7. *Maximum daily dose.* The pharmacist should emphasize that the dose recommended on the label should not be exceeded unless the physician has indicated otherwise. This should be emphasized, especially for drugs with a high abuse potential or drugs to be taken "as needed." The patient should be made aware of potential adverse or side effects that may occur if dosage recommendations are exceeded.
8. *Side effects.* Patients should be made aware of side effects that occur with a relatively high frequency at normal dose ranges so they will not become unduly alarmed and can take necessary precautions. Patients should not be terrorized, however, and drugs such as chloramphenicol which produce very

severe, but rare, adverse effects should be dispensed with no comment about its potential ill effects.

9. *What to avoid.* The patient should be made aware of the interaction potential of certain drugs with foods, alcohol and other drugs (legend and over-the-counter).
10. *Storage.* Special storage requirements of certain drugs should be pointed out to the patient. Reasons for precautions regarding the storage of medicines that must be refrigerated, protected from sunlight or moisture or maintained in a "near sterile" state (ophthalmics) should be revealed. The pharmacist should also point out the importance of keeping all medications out of the reach of children.
11. *Miscellaneous auxiliary instructions.* A multitude of specific instructions peculiar to a few single dosage forms are indicated. It is the pharmacist's professional responsibility to render appropriate statements regarding proper use or precautions as he is the only health professional with a comprehensive knowledge and appreciation of information needed by the patient to maximize efficiency of self-medication.

Oral instructions should not take the place of written instructions as many patients cannot always remember who said to do what, and when they were supposed to do it. For information that cannot be placed on the label due to space limitations supplementary sheets are indicated (Figure 3).[34] These data sheets allow for much more information than can be typed on the label, reinforce oral instructions and provide the name and phone number of the pharmacist should the patient become confused about a particular point. The entire efforts of the health team become futile if the patient fails to take his medication correctly while at home. The Supplemental Data Sheet can do much toward decreasing confusion and increasing the reliability of the self-medicating public.

Summary

If the pharamcist is to become a more effective practitioner, he must develop certain communicative skills that will allow greater dialogue with the patient. Pertinent verbal and nonverbal exchanges between pharmacist and patient can result in the collection of a comprehensive medication history and the provision of counsel that may greatly enhance the patient's well-being through proper utilization of drugs. As clinical roles that require direct pharmacist-patient contact continue to evolve, it is hoped that pharmacists will take necessary initiatives to seize this professional practice opportunity. Increased clinical experience in obtaining medication histories and advising patients will hasten the evolution of the pharmacist's appropriate professional identity and greatly benefit patient care.

Figure 3. Supplemental Data Sheet

Prescription No.______ Patient's Name__________

Drug ____________________

M.D. ____________________

Special Directions ________________

Precautions __________________

Possible Side Effects ______________

Storage ____________________

Dosage Instructions _______________

(Date Filled) (Pharmacist)

(Address)

(Phone)

References

1. Zinner, N. R.: Clean Inside and Out (correspondence), *New Engl. J. Med. 281*:853 (Oct. 9) 1969.
2. Anon.: Keep on Taking the Tablets (editorial), *Lancet 2*:195-196 (July 25) 1970.
3. Roth, H. P., *et al*: Measuring Intake of a Prescribed Medication, *Clin. Pharmacol. Therap. 11*:228-237 (Mar.-Apr.) 1970.
4. Moulding, T., Onstad, G. D. and Sbarbaro, J. A.: Supervision of Outpatient Drug Therapy with the Medication Monitor, *Ann. Internal Med. 73*:559-564 (Oct.) 1970.
5. Latiolais, C.J. and Berry, C. C.: Misuse of Prescription Medications by Outpatients, *Drug Intelligence Clin. Pharm. 3*:270-277 (Oct.) 1969.
6. Covington, T. R. and Whitney, H. A. K.: Patient-Pharmacist Communication Techniques, *Drug Intelligence Clin. Pharm.*, to be published.
7. Morgan, W. L., Jr. and Engel, G. L.: *The Clinical Approach to the Patient,* W. B. Saunders Co., Philadelphia, Pennsylvania, 1969, p. 4.
8. Hinkle, L. E., Jr. and Wolff, H. G.: The Nature of Man's Adaptation to His Total Environment and the Relation of This to Illness, *Arch. Internal Med. 99*:442-460 (Mar.) 1957.
9. King, L. S.: Humanism and the Medical Past, *J. Am. Med. Assoc. 213*:580-584 (July 27) 1970.
10. Kabat, H. F.: *Clinical Pharmacy Handbook,* Lea and Febiger, Philadelphia, Pennsylvania, 1969, p. 9.
11. Holden, M. and Sletten, I.: The Patient as an Information Source, *Clin. Toxicol. 3*:195-203 (June) 1970.
12. Millward, C. M.: Familiar English for Foreign Doctors (Editorial), *New Engl. J. Med. 283*:430-431 (Aug. 20) 1970.
13. Riederer, R. E.: Native Language Barriers, *New Engl. J. Med. 283*:768 (Oct. 1) 1970.
14. Bernstein, L. and Dana, R. H.: *Interviewing and the Health Professions,* Appleton-Century-Crofts, New York, 1970, p. 30.
15. *Ibid.*, p. 32.
16. Morgan, W. L. and Engel, G. L., *op. cit.*, p. 46.
17. *Ibid.*, p. 64.
18. *Ibid.*, p. 66.
19. *Ibid.*, p. 73.
20. Yim, M. K.: Drug Hypersensitivities of Hospitalized Patients (Master's thesis), Philadelphia College of Pharmacy, Philadelphia, Pennsylvania, May 1967.
21. Archambault, G. F.: Autotherapy and Prescription Drugs, *Am. J. Hosp. Pharm. 24*:510-515 (Sept.) 1967.
22. Boucot, K. R.: Déja Vue (editorial) *Arch. Environ. Health 20*:449 (Apr.) 1970.
23. Zilz, D. A. and Angaran, D.: Medication History—Development, Evaluation and Cost, Presented at the American Pharmaceutical Association Annual Meeting, Washington, D. C., Apr. 1970.
24. McHale, M. K. and Canada, A. T.: The Use of a Pharmacist in obtaining Medication Histories, *Drug Intelligence 3*:115-119 (Apr.) 1969.
25. Lesshafft, C. T.: An Exploration of the Pharmacist's Role in Outpatient Clinics, *J. Am. Pharm. Assoc. NS10*:205-209 (Apr.) 1970.
26. Slack, W. V., *et al.*: A Computer-Based Medical History System, *New Engl. J. Med. 274*:194-198 (Jan. 27) 1966.
27. Collen, M. F., *et al.*: Automated Multiphasic Screening and Diagnosis, *Am. J. Public Health 54*:741-750 (May) 1964.
28. McCormick, J. B. and Kopp, J. B.: Automated Multiphasic Health Testing — Manpower Considerations, *Hospitals 45*:71-72 (Mar. 1) 1971.
29. Grossman, J. H., *et al.*: Evaluation of Computer-Acquired Patient Histories, *J. Am. Med. Assoc. 215*:1286-1291 (Feb. 22) 1971.
30. Collen, M. F. *et al.*: Reliability of a Self-Administered Medical Questionnaire, *Arch. Internal Med. 123*:664-681 (June) 1969.
31. Simborg, D. W., Rikli, A. E. and Hall, P.: Experimentation in Medical History-Taking, *J. Am. Med. Assoc.* 210: 1443-1445 (Nov. 24) 1969.
32. Anon.: Many Suicides Traced to Careless Prescribing of Drugs, *J. Am. Med. Assoc. 211*:1778 (Mar. 16) 1970.
33. Brands, A. J.: Complete Directions for Prescription Medication, *J. Am. Pharm. Assoc. NS7*:634-635 (Dec.) 1967.
34. Vreugdenhil, P. P.: Patient, Pharmacist, Physician, Prescription, *Can. Pharm. J. 9*:18-21 (Jan.) 1970.

Additional Readings

Browne, K. and Freeling, P.: *The Doctor-Patient Relationship,* E. & S. Livingston, Ltd., London, 1967.

Burton, G.: *Personal, Impersonal and Interpersonal Relations,* Soringer Publishing Co., Inc., New York, 1970.

Froelich, R. E. and Bishop, F. M.: *Medical Interviewing—A Programmed Manual,* C. V. Mosby Co., St. Louis, Mo., 1969.

Ley, P. and Spelman, M. S.: *Communicating with the Patient,* W. H. Green, Inc., St. Louis, Mo., 1967.

Lamm, H. and Willeford, G.: Teach Your Pharmacists to be Silent—Or Careful, *Med. Econ. 46*:188 (Apr. 28) 1969.

Smith, D. L.: Pharmaceutical Communications in the Clinical Environment, *Can. J. Hosp. Pharm. 23*:191-197 (Sept.-Oct.) 1970.

Stevenson, I.: *Medical History Taking,* P. B. Hoeber, New York, 1960.

Wilson, R. S. and Kabat, H. F.: Pharmacist Initiated Patient Drug Histories, *Am. J. Hosp. Pharm. 28*:49-53 (Jan.) 1971.

13

The clinical pediatric specialist

by John J. Piecoro, Jr. and Gregory M. Chudzik

One may possibly think that a discussion of pediatric pharmacy practice is too narrow in scope to find a rightful place in a book on clinical pharmacy. However, there are numerous indicators supporting the thesis that specialization in pharmacy practice will be commonplace in the 1970's, and many pharmacists are choosing the area of clinical practice. Within this field there is and will undoubtedly be further specialization – super specialization if you will. Pediatric pharmacy practice is only one example of such refinement in professional specialization. It would appear to be an attractive selection, since it is an area which encompasses all types of clinical practice, *i.e.*, medicine, surgery, neurology, hematology, etc. Yet it is distinguishable from all other areas because its patient population is unique. The pediatric pharmacy practitioner is therefore a specialist, dealing with children and their special problems, and a generalist, dealing with a wide range of problems and services.

One can see then, that there are compelling reasons for the propagation of the pediatric pharmacy practitioner. Some of these are: (1) the accelerating trend toward specialization in the health professions; (2) the unmanageable scope of knowledge necessary to discuss clinical pharmacy in general terms that apply to all clinical services and patient populations; and (3) the unique nature of the pediatric patient.

There must be a rational approach to attaining competence in the pediatric service. Psychological adjustment, academic preparation, technical competence, development of judgment in practice situations and the ability to create and maintain service objectives all must be attained, and they must flow together until the "complete" pediatric practitioner is ready to assume his professional duties. The approach to attainment of these goals may best be accomplished through segmental study, integration of clinical and academic training along with development of service competence. This training may best be provided through some sort of residency in pediatric pharmacy. This field can be a rewarding one, though not one for all pharmacists, just as clinical practice itself does not appeal to everyone. The pharmacist must make a psychological adjustment to his intimate involvement in any clinical practice situation. In pediatrics, however, the pharmacist's identification with the patient, his special needs and his special place in the lives of his family require a particular kind of adjustment. Nowhere can patient empathy be more complete, more motivating to the achievement of excellence in professional services. Getting to understand the pediatric patient is at once natural, even compelling, but it is also difficult. Perhaps the best method to appreciate the significance of the pediatric patient is to attach a special meaning to each letter in the word PEDIATRIC.

Person
Enchanting
Dependent
Inquisitive
Attentive
Terrified
Recuperative
Individual
Child

PERSON

P The pediatric patient is a person with problems. These problems may range from a minor ailment to something very serious or death dealing. The average pediatric floor may be likened to one large intensive care unit, since children are usually not hospitalized until they are seriously ill. Elective admissions whether for routine work-up or for elective surgery are the exception rather than the rule.

ENCHANTING

E The pediatric patient is enchanting, charming: a heart-winner. His initial shyness and apprehension on being hospitalized appeal to the sensitivity of the pediatric staff. You cannot help loving these sick little ones, you admire their courage and optimism which has not been dampened by "maturity" and you sympathize with their helplessness.

DEPENDENT

D The pediatric patient is dependent upon the health care team for the routine physical care formerly provided by his mother or family; for that unique blend of health care designed not only to restore his health but also renew his potential for the future; and for care designed to educate the child so that he might leave the hospital with better habits of hygiene and a better social outlook if possible.

INQUISITIVE

I The child wonders at all the new sights, the new places, the people, equipment and other children. He asks questions and peers around corners and into closets. He is also *imaginative* and becomes anxious about all his problems, but mostly concerning the unknown environment and what else is going to happen to him in terms of painful treatments.

ATTENTIVE

A The child's attention span may be short but it is intense. It can be shifted from his bodily discomfort to something pleasant. Fresh pleasant stimuli should be provided or he will soon shift his attention back to his physical condition. He must not be allowed to feel he is alone in his difficulties. One advantage of hospitalization (if there can be an advantage) is that he sees others who have problems not too different from his own.

TERRIFIED

T The pediatric patient may be terrified or *trusting* in his reactions toward the "people in white," but worst of all he may be a *tragedy* to the clinical pharmacist. Consider the little two-year-old boy who drinks gasoline from a coke bottle and dies within a few hours because his lungs are destroyed due to aspiration. Or reflect on the beautiful young girl with the devoted adoptive parents who led a normal health life until two weeks ago and now lies dying of acute leukemia. Or think about the married couple who have been trying to have children for many years and finally succeed, but the baby has a multiplicity of congenital defects and is destined for a life of pain and sorrow if he is destined for any life at all.

RECUPERATIVE

R Although he lacks the reserve forces which the adult has to act as a defense mechanism against illness, his body and metabolism are adjusted for growth and regeneration. This allows him to recuperate much faster than an adult or to handle some disease states with a much lower incidence of adverse effects and serious complications (*e.g.*, heart surgery, mumps and infection).

INDIVIDUAL

I Each child is an individual and should never be considered a typical boy or girl; that is, one unit of a group who are all alike. Each child is genetically different from all other children and his capacities and talents are uniquely his own. It is not possible for all children to respond equally to a given therapeutic regimen or to a given dose of medication. The dose and therapy must be tailored to suit the child.

CHILD

C A child is not a miniature adult. His body differs in quality as well as in size from that of an adult. These differences make pediatrics a separate discipline in which modern scientific knowledge in many branches of health care specialties is applied to the total care of the child.

Preparation for Pediatric Practice

Now that a feeling for pediatrics has been developed, how does one get involved in pediatric patient care? In addition to clinical orientation, one must gain a working knowledge of the pediatric area. Reading a textbook of pediatrics from cover to cover is not the best way to accomplish this. The pharmacist must be selective in his reading so that he will understand why children differ from adults in their responses. To assist the pharmacist in selecting topics on which to focus, the following reading list is recommended:

- Drug Dosage for Children[1,2]
- Techniques and Problems in Drug Administration to Children[3]
- Normal Lab Values for Children[4]
- How to Recognize a Sick Child[5,6]
- Fluid and Electrolyte Balance in Children[7]
- Common Accidents and Poisoning — Treatment and Prevention[8,9,10]
- Management of Acute Infections
  - Specifically: Respiratory Infection[11]
  - Meningitis[12]
  - Urinary Infection[13]
  - Septicemia[14]
- Immunization Materials and Their Use[15]
- Jaundice of the Newborn[16]
- Placental Transfer of Drugs[17]
- Drugs Which Appear in Breast Milk[18]
- Anorexia and Enuresis[19]
- Dealing with Families of Chronically Handicapped[20]
- Adverse Reactions to Drugs — Their Relation to Growth and Development[21]
- Pain, Fever, Cough[22]
- Rheumatic Fever [23,24]
- Acute Nephritis and Glomerulonephritis[25]
- Anemia and Related Blood Disorders[26]
- Leukemia and General Patterns of Neoplasms in Infants and Children[27,28]
- Concepts of Inborn Errors of Metabolism[29]
- Concept of Cytogenic Disorders[30]
- Incubation Periods of Infectious Diseases[31]
- Seasonal Factors in Allergic Disorders[32]
- Continuity Symptoms of Allergic Diseases[32]
- Congestive Heart Failure[33]
- Premature Care[34]
- Treatment of Respiratory Distress[35]

In addition to the references provided, there are a number of textbooks of pediatrics in which most of the above topics are covered, as well as the specialty texts which deal with individual topics. The advances in child care have been rapid in recent years, therefore, one must keep abreast of the current trends by judicious use of selected periodicals. A list of selected books and current pediatric literature is included on a following page.

Drug Dosage for Children

Pharmacists, as a rule, pride themselves in their knowledge of average dosage of commonly used drugs, but generally this is only in terms of "average adult dose." This dose is often used as a base for calculating pediatric doses using one of the common rules which we all learned in pharmacy school. Among these rules are:

Bastedo	Hamburger
Brunton	Holt
Clark (two rules)	Ide
Cowling	Martinet
Dilling	Nolsecourt
Fried	Starkenstein
Gaubius	Young
Griffith	

It has been pointed out that "the great number of these rules attests to the fact that they fail to serve their intended purpose. Despite the custom, there is no more reason to use fractions of adult doses for children than to use multiples of known infant doses for adults."[36] These rules are rapidly falling out of use since they have been shown to be scientifically unsound. Clark's weight rule, used for patients 2 years old or over, still maintains some popularity. Scaling down adult doses to children's doses does not take into account the various stages of metabolic development children go through.

$$\frac{\text{wt in lb}}{150} \times \text{adult dose} = \text{child dose}$$

(Clark's Weight Rule)

A more recent method for determining children's dosages is based on body surface area. This method is more acceptable than the "rules" listed above. There exists a fairly direct relationship between the body surface and many physiologic functions including heat production, extracellular fluid volume, plasma volume, cardiac output, glomerular filtration rate, organ size, oxygen consumption, nitrogen requirement, caloric requirement and water and electrolyte requirements. It may also serve as an unusual although not infallible index of metabolic activity. A number of studies have shown that the optimal dose of a variety of drugs is consistently proportional to body surface area. Since the measurement of surface area depends on the dimensions and shapes of objects, the direct measurement of body surface area is impractical. A number of methods to determine body surface area have been developed. One of the most popular is the West Nomogram (Figure 1) which uses correlation of height and weight to determine surface area. In addition, it contains an area which allows rapid determination of surface area by weight alone. This latter method has been shown to have a standard deviation of only eight percent, a relatively insignificant value as far as drug dosage is concerned.[37]

Two major methods which employ body surface area in determining drug dosage for a child are:

A. $\frac{\text{Surface Area of Child}}{\text{Surface Area of Adult}} \times$ Dose for Adult = Child's Dose

B. Surface area of Child (in M^2) × Dose per M^2 = Child's Dose

Method A above still produces the child's dose as a fraction of the adult dose, whereas Method B finally frees the child's dose by using a base other than the adult dose. In fact, the adult dose can accurately be determined using Method B. Tables for pediatric dosage expressed in dose per M^2 as well as dose per kg may be found in the 1971 *Pediatric Dosage Handbook*.[2]

Body surface area may also be estimated by two quick methods. One of these is the "Sitting Height Formula" developed by Snively, *et al.*[38]

Sitting Height Formula:

A. Under 6 Months of Age:
Sitting Height of Child × 0.00017 = Surface area in M^2

B. 6 Months to 14½ years of Age:
Sitting Height of Child × 0.00019 = Surface area in M^2

Sitting Height = $(\text{Crown-Rump Length in cm})^2$

The other method is an empirical formula based on weight which was derived by Costeff.[39]

Costeff's Formula:

$$\frac{4W + 7}{W + 90} = \text{Surface Area}$$

W = Weight in Kg

Just as the weight and age rules had their limitations, drug dosage determined by body surface area is not perfect. We must remember:

(1) No dose, however reached, is better than the skill of the prescribing physician.
(2) Any dose is useful only as a tentative initial dose to be modified in accordance with the patient's tolerance, requirements and clinical progress.
(3) For newborn and premature infants no rule suffices. Doses must be individualized.
(4) No dosage rule protects against drug idiosyncrasy or allergy (which are drug dependent not dose dependent).
(5) With certain types of drugs, doses must be individualized (*e.g.*, morphine, pentobarbital, atropine and scopolamine).[40]

In newborn and premature infants, the prescriber's skill and experience is the ultimate reference for drug dosage. Beargie has developed a dosage table for infants in their first weeks of life (Table 1).[41]

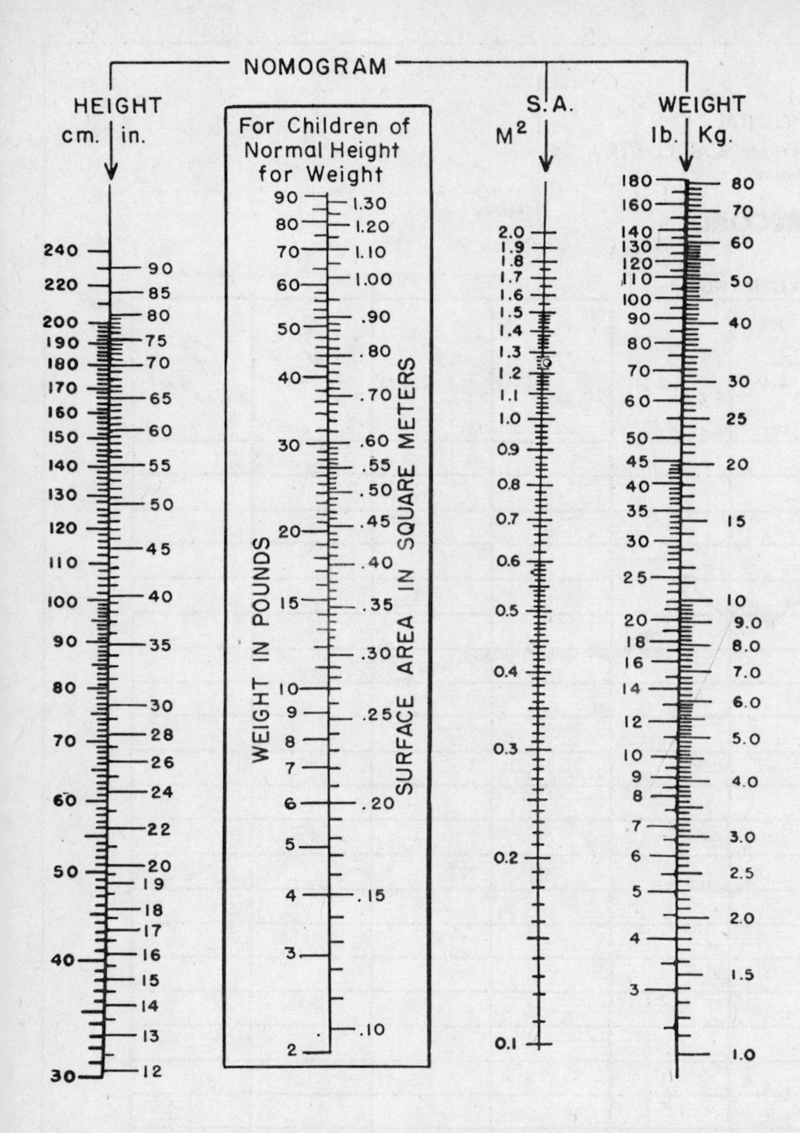

Figure 1. West nomogram (for estimation of surface areas). The surface area is indicated where a straight line connecting the height and weight intersects the surface area (S.A.) column or, if the patient is roughly of average size, from the weight alone (enclosed area). (Nomogram modified from data of E. Boyd by C. D. West; from Shirkey, H. C. and Barba, W. P.: Drug therapy. In Nelson, W. E., editor: Textbook of pediatrics, ed. 8, Philadelphia, 1964, W. B. Saunders Co.)

A more complete discussion of posology may be found in any pediatric text.

Therapeutic Orphans

The drug laws of 1962 were essentially a result of the thalidomide catastrophe and led to the introduction of the term "therapeutic orphans" into the practice of pediatrics.[42] By legal definition, drugs introduced since 1962 must be safe and efficacious, but only a small number of these have been studied in the pediatric age group. Thus, "many of the drugs released since 1962 carry an 'orphaning' clause, *e.g.*, 'Not to be used in children' – 'is not recommended for use in infants and young children, since few studies have been carried out in this age group' – 'clinical studies have been insufficient to establish any recommendations for use in infants and children . . . 'should not be given to children' . . ."[43] This unfortunate set of circumstances causes the age group originally responsible for passage of these laws to be denied the use of many new medications.

It is true that some of the drugs released since 1962 are not acceptable for pediatric use, but it seems unfair that those which may be of some

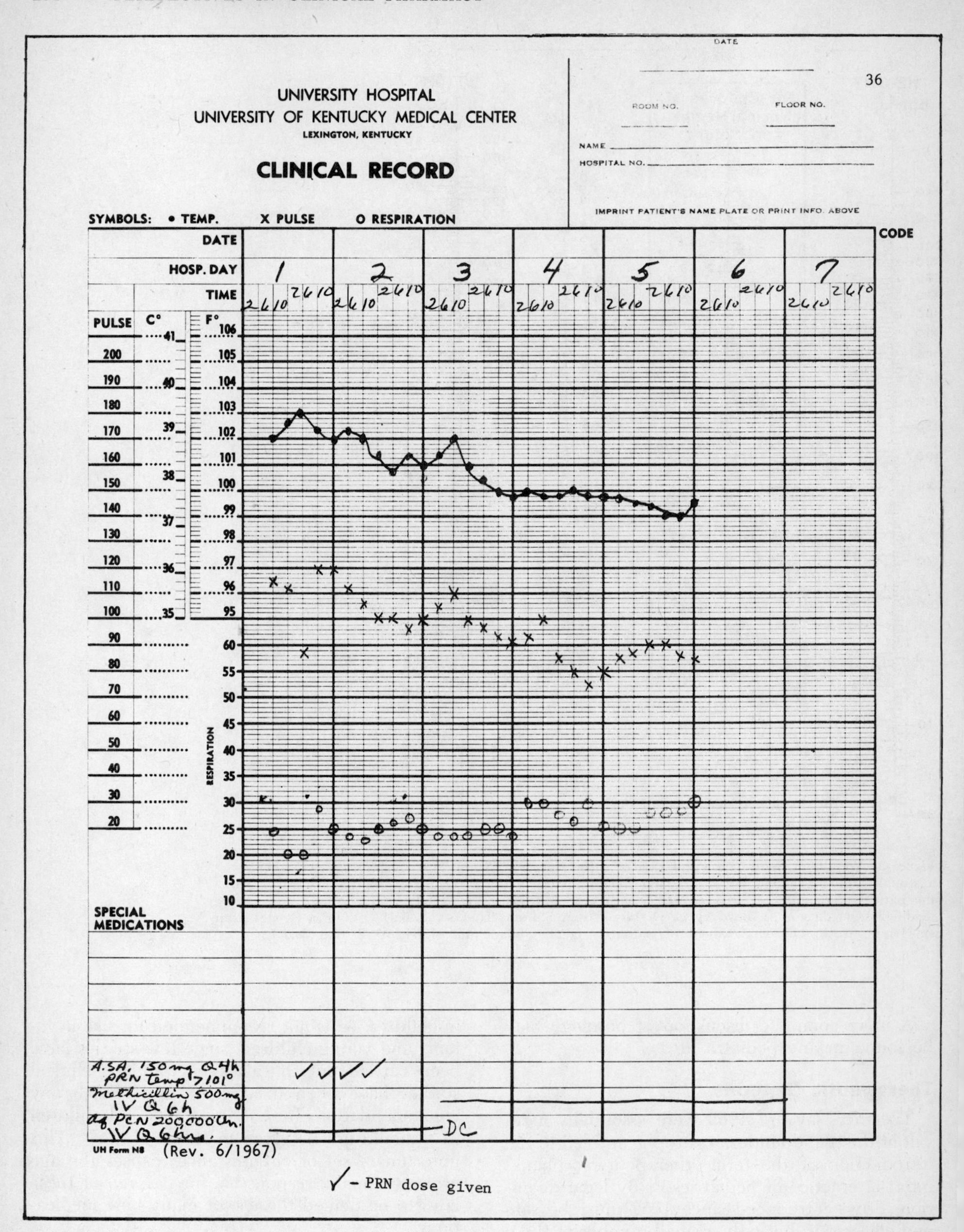
DATE

36

UNIVERSITY HOSPITAL
UNIVERSITY OF KENTUCKY MEDICAL CENTER
LEXINGTON, KENTUCKY

CLINICAL RECORD

ROOM NO. FLOOR NO.
NAME
HOSPITAL NO.

IMPRINT PATIENT'S NAME PLATE OR PRINT INFO. ABOVE

SYMBOLS: • TEMP. X PULSE O RESPIRATION

DATE								CODE
HOSP. DAY	1	2	3	4	5	6	7	
TIME	2 6 10 2 6 10	2 6 10 2 6 10	2 6 10 2 6 10	2 6 10 2 6 10	2 6 10 2 6 10	2 6 10 2 6 10	2 6 10 2 6 10	

PULSE: 200, 190, 180, 170, 160, 150, 140, 130, 120, 110, 100, 90, 80, 70, 60, 50, 40, 30, 20

C°: 41, 40, 39, 38, 37, 36, 35

F°: 106, 105, 104, 103, 102, 101, 100, 99, 98, 97, 96, 95

RESPIRATION: 60, 55, 50, 45, 40, 35, 30, 25, 20, 15, 10

SPECIAL MEDICATIONS

A.S.A. 150 mg Q 4 h PRN temp > 101° ✓ ✓ ✓ ✓
Methicillin 500 mg IV Q 6 h
Aq PCN 200,000 U. IV Q 6 hrs. — DC

UH Form N8 (Rev. 6/1967)

✓ - PRN dose given

Figure 2. Clinical record

potential use are legally denied to the pediatrician. An example of just such a situation is the use of diazepam injection in the treatment of status epilepticus. This drug is the drug of choice for this condition in adults in many medical centers. However, the current package insert states: "The safety and efficacy of injectable Valium (diazepam) in children under age 12 have not been established."[44] Anyone who has ever witnessed a patient in status epilepticus is well aware of the feeling of helplessness one experiences during the episode. The patient is in a constant state of seizure, with everyone around him struggling to prevent his injuring himself, *i.e.*, swallowing tongue, bruising his head, arms, legs and torso. Any one or all of several drugs may be administered by injection in this situation. The most preferred route of administration would be intravenous, if one can be started, but intramuscular is suitable for some cases. The drugs used may be diazepam, phenobarbital, paraldehyde and possibly diphenylhydantoin. With the last three drugs mentioned, control of the seizures may not be achieved until nearly 30 minutes have elapsed. Diazepam injection, however, will control most attacks within a few minutes. Is there any doubt as to the usual choice, especially since its efficacy and safety in adults are well documented in the literature?

To remove these "orphaning" clauses, physicians, pharmacologists, pharmacists and all those involved in child health care should assume greater responsibility in promoting clinical assessment of drugs in infants and children.

Adverse Reactions to Drugs

The common adverse effects of drugs, which are seen so often in adults, are also shared by infants and children. We must remember, however, that children, for many reasons, provide a unique opportunity for "pediatric" adverse reactions. Evidence is accumulating that there are differences in drug-host interactions at all stages of growth and development, not only in the fetus and newborn, but in the older infant and toddler and from the preschool child to the adolescent. A thorough knowledge of both drug action and the metabolic capacity of the organism at a specific stage of its development is essential, even where the dose alone is concerned. Thus, a given dose of chloramphenicol while toxic to the newborn, may be insufficient for therapeutic effectiveness in the same infant just a few weeks later.[45]

Drug metabolism is thought to be a developmental process similar to behavior, physical growth, bone maturation and other processes that change with age. To achieve comparable therapeutic effects in subjects of different ages and sizes, one must know the concentration and distribution of the drug in the body fluids and tissues. These are determined by the relation of intra- and extracellular fluid compartments known to change with age. In the process of maturation, specific tissues have their own rates of development, so that sensitivity to any agent is a function of the state of maturation of that particular target tissue.[46] Also the permeability of the vascular system to specific molecules alters with maturation. These factors lead to marked differences in the rate of elimination, biologic half-life and coefficient of distribution of drugs in different age groups. The growing child is in a continuous state of change with respect to these pharmacologic responses and sensitivities. Seven specific age periods of differential drug response can be demonstrated:[46-48]

1. The first trimester of pregnancy—that critical period of organogenesis when the hazard of teratologic effects is so very high. The toxic effect of a drug is more acute with the more rapid rate of growth and development.[49] A list of maternally ingested drugs which have been known to cause abortions or congenital anomalies is illustrated (Table 2).

2. The last trimester of pregnancy—when abnormal organ growth or severely altered fetal metabolic activity may accompany the ingestion of noxious agents by the mother (Table 3).

3. The immediate prepartum period—another crucial period for the physiology and biochemistry of the infant when drugs which may cross the placental barrier may produce CNS depression, hemolytic anemia, hyperbilirubinemia and possible neonatal death (Table 4).

4. The neonatal period—when the baby is undergoing changes in enzyme competence, as well as the change from anaerobic to aerobic existence. The immature organ systems, notably kidneys and liver, are inadequate with respect to detoxification and excretion of drugs.

5. During lactation—when the young infant is subject to the effects of the drugs which may be transmitted via the mother's milk. We may see untoward pharmacologic effects and be at a loss to explain them until we realize the vast number of drugs which may be transmitted via the mother's milk (Table 5).

6. Early childhood—that period from infancy to three years of age when it is known that certain drugs may be metabolized faster than in adults. Also, the target organs of drug toxicity may be characteristically different in children. As an example, phenobarbital may produce excitement; prochlorperazine may cause dystonia in children; and tetracycline may cause increased intracranial pressure.

7. Adolescence—the period of rapid growth. Changes would be expected to be a pharmacologic milestone since changes in drug sensitivities are linked to these body changes. Little specific knowledge is available for this period.

Table 1. Dosages of Drugs for an Infant in First Weeks of Life

ANTIBIOTICS

Potassium Penicillin G
50,000 units/Kg/24 hrs. IM or IV - q 12 hrs.

Kanamycin Sulfate
15 mg/Kg/24 hrs IM - q 12 hrs.

Methicillin
100-200 mg/Kg/24 hrs. IM or IV

Oxacillin
100-200 mg/Kg/24 hrs. IM or PO

Polymyxin B
1.5 mg/Kg/24 hrs. IM or IV - q 6 hrs.

ANTICONVULSANTS

Dilantin
5-8 mg/Kg/24 hrs. PO, IM, IV - as needed

Phenobarbital
5-8 mg/kg/24 hrs. PO, IM - as needed

Paraldehyde
0.15 ml/Kg/dose IM or rectal
Repeat as needed q 4-6 hrs.

Calcium-Gluconate
(10%) 100 mg to 1.0 g may be diluted and given IV slowly until heart rate decreases

Diazepam
300-800 mcg/Kg/24 hrs. PO, IM, IV - as needed.

Atropine Sulfate
20 mcg/Kg/dose SC

BUFFER:

$NaHCO_3$ (7.5%)
1 to 2 ml/Kg may be given slowly IV. For continuous IV, drip at 75 ml total fluid/Kg/24 hrs.
pH 7.35 to 7.25 - 5 ml $NaHCO_3$/100 ml fluid
pH 7.25 to 7.15 - 10 ml $NaHCO_3$/100 ml fluid
pH 7.15 or less - 15 ml $NaHCO_3$/100 ml fluid

DIGOXIN
40 mcg/Kg total oral digitalizing dose
30 mcg/Kg total IM or IV digitalizing dose

Maintenance = 1/4 total digitalizing dose/day - q 12 hrs.

DIURETICS

Sodium Meralluride
3 Kg and under 0.1 ml IM

Ethacrynic Acid
500 mcg/Kg/dose IV or IM

HYPOGLYCEMIA

Glucose
50% 1 ml/Kg/dose push IV slowly

Glucagon
300 mcg/Kg/dose IV or IM (not to exceed 1 mg)

Epinephrine
1:1000 0.03 ml/Kg/dose IV or IM (not to exceed 1 mg)

Susphrine
1:200 0.01 ml/Kg/dose may be given q 6 hrs. subcutaneously

ACTH
4 units/Kg/24 hrs. IM - q 12 hrs.

MYASTHENIA GRAVIS TEST (unexplained weakness in newborn)

Edrophonium Chloride
200 mcg/Kg single dose IM or SC (keep atropine handy).

NARCOTIC ANTAGONIST

Nalorphine HCl
100 mcg/Kg/dose IM or IV (limit initial dose to 200 mcg).

PHYTONADIONE
0.5 to 1.0 mg IV, IM

—STIMULANT

Caffeine & Sodium Benzoate
8 mg/Kg/dose SC or IM

From Beargie, R. A., Director of Nurseries, University of Kentucky Medical Center, Lexington.

Table 2. Drugs Which May Affect Fetus in the First Trimester

DRUG	ADVERSE EFFECT	REFERENCE
Amethopterin	Cleft palate	50-54
Aminopterin	Cleft palate	50-54
Androgens	Masculinization; labial fusion and clitoral enlargement	54-57
Busulfan	Cleft palate	50-54
Chlorpropamide	Prolonged neonatal hypoglycemia	52, 58
Cholinesterase inhibitors	Transient muscular weakness	57
Cortisone	Cleft palate	54, 59
Cyclophos-phamide	Severe stunting, fetal death, extremity defects	50-54
Estrogens	Masculinization; labial fusion and clitoral enlargement	55, 56, 60
Hexamethonium bromide	Neonatal ileus and death	61
LSD	Chromosomal damage, stunted off-spring	62
Nicotine and smoking	Small babies	50, 59
Oral progestogens	Masculinization; labial fusion and clitoral enlargement	55-57, 60
Phenmetrazine	Skeletal and visceral anomalies	50, 54, 59
Streptomycin	8th nerve damage; micromelia; hearing loss; multiple skeletal anomalies	50, 52, 63
Thalidomide	Phocomelia; hearing defect	50, 51, 53, 55, 64
Tolbutamide	Congenital anomalies	55, 65
Vitamin A	Congenital anomalies; cleft palate; eye damage; syndactyly	54, 66, 67
Vitamin D	Excessive blood calcium; mental retardation	68
Warfarin Sodium	Fetal death; hemorrhage	50,63

Adapted partly from Takata, A.: Adverse Effects of Drugs on the Fetus, *Hosp. Formulary Management 4*:25-29 (June) 1969.

Yet another factor which differentiates pediatric patients is the number of disease entities which are exclusive to pediatrics. These disease factors may alter the usual drug effects and their metabolic pathways. Examples of this phenomenon are: (1) hypersensitivity of children with

Table 3. Drugs Which May Affect Fetus During the Third Trimester

DRUG	ADVERSE EFFECT	REFERENCE
Androgens	Masculinization; labial fusion and clitoris enlargement	54-57
Chlorpropamide	Prolonged neonatal hypoglycemia	52, 58
Cholinesterase inhibitors	Transient muscular weakness	57
Estrogens	Masculinizaton; labial fusion and clitoris enlargement	55, 56, 60
Hexamethonium bromide	Neonatal ileus and death	61
Methimazole	Goiter and mental retardation	50
Nicotine and smoking	Small babies	50, 59
Oral progestogens	Masculinization; labial fusion and clitoris enlargement	55-57, 60
Potassium iodide	Goiter and mental retardation	50, 56, 69
Propylthiouracil	Goiter and mental retardation	50, 70
Radioactive iodine	Congenital hypothyroidism	57
Streptomycin	8th nerve damage; micromelia, hearing loss, multiple skeletal anomalies	50, 52, 63
Tetracyclines	Inhibition of bone growth; discoloration of teeth; micromelia; syndactyly	55, 56, 71
Thiazides	Thrombocytopenia; neonatal death	56, 72
Tolbutamide	Congenital anomalies	55, 65
Vitamin A	Congenital anomalies; cleft palate; eye damage, syndactyly	54, 66, 67
Vitamin D	Excessive blood calcium; mental retardation	68
Warfarin sodium	Fetal death; hemorrhage	50, 63

Adapted partly from Takata, A.: Adverse Effects of Drugs on the Fetus, *Hosp. Formulary Management 4*:25-29 (June) 1969.

Table 4. Drugs Which May Affect Fetus at or Near Term

DRUG	ADVERSE EFFECT	REFERENCE
Chloramphenicol	"Gray syndrome" and death	50, 51, 56, 71, 73
Chlorpropamide	Prolonged neonatal hypoglycemia	52, 58
Cholinesterase inhibitors	Transient muscular weakness	57
Heroin	Respiratory depression; neonatal death	50, 51
Hexamethonium bromide	Neonatal ileus; death	61
Mepivacaine	Fetal bradycardia; neonatal depression	57, 74
Morphine	Respiratory depression; neonatal death	50, 51
Nitrofurantoin	Hemolysis	50, 51, 63
Novobiocin	Hyperbilirubinemia	50, 51, 63
Streptomycin	8th nerve damage; hearing loss	50, 52, 63
Sulfonamides (long-acting)	Hyperbilirubinemia	50, 63, 71, 75, 76
Tetracyclines	Discoloration of teeth	55, 56, 71
Vitamin K analogues	Hyperbilirubinemia	55, 56, 59, 77
Warfarin sodium	Fetal death; hemorrhage	50, 63

Adapted in part from Takata, A.: Adverse Effects of Drugs on the Fetus, *Hosp. Formulary Management 4*:25-29 (June) 1969.

Down's syndrome to atropine and (2) the metabolic deficiency diseases such as phenylketonuria which may alter the effects of epinephrine or ephedrine.

As previously stated there are differences in metabolic capacity at various stages of growth and development. This leads to differences in drug metabolism and biologic half-life of drugs in infants and children. Biological half-life has been defined as the time required for one-half the amount of drug absorbed to be eliminated, whether by excretion, metabolic decomposition or other natural processes following the establishment of equilibrium. This is important for maintaining effective blood levels and for prevention of drug toxicity due to accumulation. Knowledge of the biological half-life of a drug allows one to alter the dosage schedule for maximum therapeutic effect. The biological half-life is not an absolute value for any given drug, but may have variations due to the following reasons:[80]

1. Dosage size effects
2. Variations in urinary excretion
3. Inter-subject variations
4. Effect of age
5. Effect of other drugs
6. Protein binding of drugs
7. Disease

Table 6 provides an excellent comparison of biological half-lives of antibiotics and sulfonamides in newborn, premature and full term infants in comparison to older children and adults.[80]

PHARMACIST'S PRECLINICAL SERVICE OBJECTIVES

It is most important to realize that establishment of a clinical practice in the patient area neither can be obtained nor contemplated until the pharmacy department is providing strong and progressive pharmaceutical services which may be characterized as follows:

1. One of the major functions of a progressive pharmacy is to provide round-the-clock continuous pharmaceutical service. This demonstrates a concern for good patient care, and complete commitment on the part of the pharmacy. It makes the pharmacist a full-time mem-

Table 5. List of Which Drugs May Be Transmitted Via the Mother's Milk[18,78,79]

Acetaminophen	Lead
Alcohol	Magnesium
Aloin	Mercurous chloride, mild
Allergens	Mercury
Cottonseed	Phosphate
Eggs	Potassium
Flax	Sodium
Peanuts	Sulfur
Wheat	Methadone
Ambenonium chloride	Methdilazine
Aminophylline	Methimazole
Aminosalicylic acid and salts	Methocarbamol
Amobarbital	Methohexital
Amphetamine sulfate	Morphine
Aspirin	Neomycin sulfate
Atropine	Niacin
Bishydroxycoumarin	Nicotine
Bromides	Nitrofurantoins (?)
Brompheniramine	Novobiocin
Caffeine	Pantothenic acid
Calomel	Papaverine
Chloral hydrate	Penicillin
Chloramphenicol	Benzyl-
Chloroform	Phenacetin
Chlorpromazine	Phenaglycodol
Cortisone	Phenobarbital
Cyclophosphamide	Phenylbutazone
Cyclopropane	Phenytoin
Cycloserine	Propylthiouracil
Danthron	Pseudoephedrine
DDT	Pyrimethamine
Dextroamphetamine sulfate	Quinidine
Dextropropoxyphene	Quinine
hydrochloride	Reserpine
Diphenhydramine	Rhubarb (?)
hydrochloride	Riboflavin
Diphenylhydantoin	Salicylates
Ephedrine	Scopolamine
Ergot	Secobarbital
Erythromycin	Sodium chloride
Estrogens	Sodium salicylate
Ether	Streptomycin
Ethinamate	Sulfonamides
Ethyl biscoumacetate	Sulfamethoxazole (?)
Folic acid	Sulfadimethoxine
Heroin	Tetracyclines
Hexachlorobenzene	Thiamine
Hydroxyzine	Thiazides
Imipramine hydrochloride	Thiopental
Iodides	Thiouracil
Iopanoic acid	Thyroid (?)
Isoniazid	Tolbutamide
Levopropoxyphene	Trifluoperazine
Mandelic acid	Vitamins
Mephenoxalone	A
Metals, salts, minerals, etc.	B_1
Arsenic	B_{12}
Calcium	C
Chloride	D
Copper	E
Iodide	K

ber of the health care team. The presence of a pharmacist every hour of the day allows the department to provide another important service, direct interpretation of every physician's order. Close scrutiny of every order enables the pharmacist to follow patients and intercept potential problems. In small hospitals continuous pharmacy service can be provided by having a pharmacist on call.

2. Other functions which should be provided are reconstitution of all drugs and unit dose drug distribution. Moreover, the preparation of intravenous additives is another very useful function.

3. Access to a functioning drug information center or service is a necessity for clinical practice, since pharmacists in their traditional setting are often called upon to provide drug information. The "visibility" of the pharmacist is directly proportional to the number and complexity of drug information inquiries. As one might expect, these complex questions may require an extensive literature search. It is in these instances that the aid of a drug information center and possibly a drug information specialist may prove invaluable.

Initiating Clinical Pediatric Service

If a pharmacist feels he is ready to participate in the pediatric clinical area, and provide quality service capable of meeting the drug needs of the pediatric patient, a service that would be comprehensive, intensive and continuing and to the pharmacist a challenging professional practice, how might he begin? A successful approach which the authors have used is a rather direct route. Arrange a meeting with the chairman of the pediatrics department and discuss with him the services you feel competent to render and enthusiastic about developing. Show your sincere desire to help improve patient care and express your willingness to cooperate. Remember this team has existed for a long time without direct pharmacist involvement. It is best therefore to integrate your program into their established patterns to gain acceptance without abruptly disrupting the traditional approach to pediatric patient care. A smooth transition requires a good knowledge of what, when, why, how and who of the ongoing system. This knowledge may be gained by "shadowing" a resident or intern in pediatrics for several weeks, simply following him around, being as helpful as you can and as unobtrusive as possible. Table 7 depicts a rather typical weekly schedule for a pediatric house officer and makes it evident that there are many "standard" meetings or conferences which he attends each week. As one starts attending these meetings and learns the pattern, he might begin to plan his functions so that they can be carried out at the most opportune time.

Before discussing the functions, duties and responsibilities of the clinical pharmacist, it is necessary to consider one personal attribute absolutely essential for active participation in any patient care area, that is: *empathy*.

Table 6. Biological Half-Lives in Newborn, Premature and Full-Term Infants in Comparison to Older Children and Adults (Adapted partly from Sereni, F. and Principi, N.)

DRUG	SUBJECT	AGE	HALF-LIFE OF DRUG [HRS]
Chloramphenicol succinate	Premature Infant	1 day	15-22
	Premature Infant	12-23 days	8-15
	Children	5 years	4.0
	Adult	——	3.5-5.0
Streptomycin	Premature Infant	1.3 days	7.0
	Adult	——	2.2-3.2
Kanamycin	Premature Infant	<48 hours	18
	Premature Infant	5-22 days	6
	Adult	——	2-4
Tetracycline-1-methylene lysine	Newborn Infant	1-2 days	16.2
	Infants	3-7 months	9.8
	Children	5-11 years	6.8
Ampicillin	Premature Infant	3-6 days	3.6
	Premature Infant	21-39 days	1.9
	Term Infant	<24 hours	3.4
	Term Infant	4-5 days	2.2
	Adult	——	0.75-2.0
Methicillin	Premature Infant	4-5 days	3.3
	Premature Infant	4-7 days	2.4
	Premature Infant	13-15 days	2.0
	Premature Infant	17-33 days	1.4
	Premature Infant	26-30 days	1.4
	Term Infant	<24 hours	3.3
	Term Infant	4-5 days	1.3
	Term Infant	8-30 days	0.9
	Adult	——	0.5
Oxacillin	Premature Infants	8-15 days	1.6
	Premature Infants	20-21 days	1.2
	Term Infant	1-6 days	1.5
	Children	1 year	1.1
	Adults		0.7
Neomycin	Premature Infants	4-10 days	5.4
	Premature Infants	13-21 days	3.7
Colistimethate	Premature Infants	4 days	2.6
	Premature Infants	12-51 days	2.3
	Term Infants	1 day	9.0
	Term Infants	3-4 days	2.6
	Adult	——	1.5-2
Cephaloridine	Term Infant	1 day	5.4
	Term Infant	4 days	3.7
	Term Infant	10-14 days	2.1
	Term Infant	2-4 months	1.1
Oleandomycin	Term Infant	2-4 days	3.2
	Term Infant	10-15 days	3.0
	Adult	——	4.0
Sulfonamide 2-Sulfanilamido-3-methoxypyrazine (Sulfamethoxypyrazine)	Term Infants	1-10 days	280.0
	Term Infants	11-30 days	136.8
	Term Infants	2 months	67.8
	Children	1-4 years	44.2
	Adults	——	71.1

From Ritschel, W. A.: Biological Half-Lives of Drugs, *Drug Intelligence Clin. Pharm. 4*:338 (Dec.) 1970.

Table 7. Scheduled Activities of House Staff

	MONDAY	TUESDAY	WEDNESDAY	THURSDAY	FRIDAY	SATURDAY	SUNDAY
7:00				HSR			
	HSR	HSR	HSR		HSR		
8:00				GR			
		AdC	X-RC		AdC	HSR	HSR
9:00							
		KR					
10:00							
11:00	AR	AR	AR	AR	AR		
12:00		RS					
			MRDC				
1:00							
2:00							
3:00					CC		
4:00	PMC	NC	PMC	MER			
5:00	HSCOR	HSCOR	HSCOR	HSCOR	HSCOR		
6:00							

HSR – House Staff Rounds
AR – Attending Rounds
AdC – Admitting Conference
GR – Grand Rounds
HSCOR – House Staff Check Out Rounds
RS – Residents Seminar
X-RC – X-Ray Conference
PMC – Patient Management Conference
NC – Neurology Conference
CC – Chest Conference
KR – Kardex Rounds
MER – Metabolic Endocrine Rounds
MRDC – Mental Retardation Disposition Conference

E EMOTION – The patient is a human being not a disease state or a cold statistic. The clinical pharmacist should get to know him as a person; get a "feel" for him (*i.e.*, "The vegetable in 36" is actually John Doe, a 14-year-old swimming phenomenon involved in a tragic automobile accident).

M MATURITY – Have the maturity to recognize that the patient has problems and may not be his true self. He may not be right, but you do not have to prove it to him.

P PATIENCE – Continue to adapt your procedures and methods to best suit the individual patient. Are you not dependent on him?

A ATTENTION – The patient is not interrupting your work, he came to you with his problems. He rates the most courteous and attentive treatment you can provide him.

T THERAPY – The patient deserves the highest quality care at the most reasonable price and at the proper time.

H HOPE – As an individual becomes ill, he may become despondent. Your concern, your help, your interest in him can provide him with the hope he needs to make it.

Y YOURSELF – Give of yourself as the patient is the heart and soul, the lifeblood of your work, and you must give all you can to treat him as you would want to be treated.

FUNCTIONS, DUTIES AND RESPONSIBILITIES

The major functions, duties and responsibilities of a pediatric clinical pharmacist are much the same as those envisioned for any other clinical pharmacist and may be categorized as in Table 8.

Rounds

House Staff Rounds. House staff rounds are generally conducted twice daily—once early in the morning when the house officers report for

Table 8. Functions, Duties and Responsibilities of a Pediatric Clinical Pharmacist

1. Rounds
   - A. House staff
     - 1. Morning
     - 2. Check out
   - B. Attending
   - C. Nursing report
   - D. Kardex
2. Conferences
   - A. Admitting
   - B. Patient management
   - C. Clinical pathological
   - D. Residents' seminar
   - E. Grand rounds
   - F. Other conferences
3. Service Committees
   - A. Patient care task force
   - B. Planning
   - C. Action
4. Instructional Services
   - A. Inservice education for nurses and students
   - B. Lecturing to pediatric medical clerks
5. Pharmaceutical Services
   - A. Prescription Services
     - 1. Interpreting orders
     - 2. Monitoring Therapy
     - 3. Providing Unit Doses
       - a. high risk nursery
       - b. extemporaneous compounding
     - 4. Parenteral fluids
     - 5. Stop orders
   - B. Cardio-respiratory resuscitation team
   - C. Information source
     - 1. Drug
     - 2. Poison treatment
   - D. Adverse drug reaction reporting program
   - E. Investigational drug program
   - F. Admission interview
     - 1. Drug history
     - 2. Drug identification
   - G. Patient or parent consultations
     - 1. Education
     - 2. Evaluation
     - 3. Adverse drug reaction screen
   - H. Discharge summary
     - 1. Education
     - 2. Review of therapeutic regimen
6. Supplies and equipment responsibilities
   - A. Presence
   - B. Maintenance
   - C. Correct usage
   - D. Safety
   - E. Promote efficient and economical usage
7. Clinical Research and Investigation
   - A. Liaison between clinicians and basic scientists
8. Education — Pharmacy
   - A. B.S. student
   - B. Pharm.D. student
9. Future Functions
   - A. Drug administration responsibilities
   - B. Coordination of services
   - C. Drug prescribing

duty, and again late in the afternoon when those who are to remain on duty for the night receive information concerning each and every patient who will be in their care. During the *morning rounds* each patient is visited by the team responsible for his care, and new patients are "presented" to the team by the member responsible for admission. However, those patients whose hospital stay exceeds one day and who have previously been "presented" to the team are visited, and any further diagnostic information concerning them or any change in their condition is discussed. *Check-out rounds* are usually quite brief and consist of the team's visiting each patient and briefly bringing the "cover" physician up to date on the condition and therapy of each patient.

Both of these situations provide the pharmacist with a first hand opportunity to follow the patient from admission through discharge. He will observe the patient prior to, during and after therapy. Situations and questions involving drugs and drug therapy occur quite often, allowing the pharmacist to gradually make the transition from a passive observing role to an active participating role. What better way is there to learn of the effects of drugs in patients than by direct observation of the patient daily?

Attending Rounds. These rounds are held daily or several times weekly and consist of the house staff along with the attending physician who is ultimately responsible for the care of the patient. Patients are "presented" by the house staff to the attending physician who, in turn, discusses the disease in relation to the patient and then critiques the treatment rendered by the house staff. These encounters are an invaluable learning process for the pharmacist and allow him the opportunity to actively participate in the discussions concerning drug therapy.

Nursing Report. At eight-hour intervals the nursing staff changes. Prior to the actual changeover the outgoing staff reports to the incoming staff on the condition of each patient. Drug therapy, treatments, problems, special precautions, special tests and parameters to follow are reviewed for each patient. The pharmacist's attendance and participation are welcomed. Oftentimes, important facts about the patients may be revealed that otherwise would not be found elsewhere.

Kardex Rounds. Members of the health team meet at weekly or biweekly sessions to discuss the patients in that particular patient care area. The charge nurse usually leads the discussion by asking each member to comment about the patients. The intern or resident physician discusses the diagnosis, treatment and prognosis; the pharmacist discusses drug therapy; the dietitian, the social worker, the recreational therapist and the chaplain or anyone else present may comment on his speciality as it applies to each patient.

Conferences

Admitting Conference. The frequency of these conferences will vary with different services or institutions; generally they are held daily or twice weekly. Attendance at these conferences is open to the attending staff, the house staff, the pharmacist, the social worker, the nurse and others. The chief resident conducts the proceedings. New patients are "presented" and discussed by the group. During the latter part of the conference, important announcements and comments are conveyed to the group. We have used this time to reveal important facts about drugs and to report on the deliberations and recommendations of the Pharmacy and Therapeutics Committee. It is an excellent opportunity to "detail" new drugs in a short concise manner.

Patient Management Conference. At weekly intervals one or several cases of a particular disease or condition are presented to a group consisting of attending staff, house staff, medical students (if they are on board), nurses, pharmacists and others. Following the student's, intern's or resident's presentation of the cases, one of the attending physicians expounds on the particular disease or condition. He will cover diagnosis, pathophysiology, treatment and prognosis. The session is completed with an open discussion. The pharmacist may be asked to participate as the discussant on drug therapy.

Clinical Pathological Conference. Several days prior to this monthly conference on diagnosis, a protocol of the case to be discussed is circulated to the team. The protocol contains information about the case: how the patient presented, initial findings, subsequent findings, laboratory tests performed, x-ray or special reports, etc.; however, some important facts are left out or are sketchy. Thus, many different disease states or conditions may fit the case. The discussant is not informed of the diagnosis beforehand and his job is to put the pieces of the puzzle together, continually ruling out alternative decisions so as to arrive at a conclusive diagnosis. Drugs are quite capable of causing diseases and pathological conditions and one might perceive that the pharmacist's knowledge of pharmacology may be utilized at a conference such as this.

Residents' Seminar. House staff members take turns at weekly intervals presenting timely topics to this group. Drugs and drug therapy may enter into the discussion at one point or another or may be the focus of the seminar. These sessions are held at noon during lunch and offer the pharmacist another opportunity to participate and to build rapport.

Grand Rounds. These sessions are much the same as patient management conferences; however, they are open to the entire community of pediatricians in private practice. Frequently, nationally and internationally prominent experts are invited to be the discussants. On occasion, the pharmacist may, in conjunction with a physician, make presentations to this group on timely topics, *e.g.*, hyperalimentation, practical aspects of pediatric drug therapy and poison control.

Other Conferences. There are a number of other conferences of a special nature that are held at varying intervals. They are open conferences and we need not discuss them other than to list some as follows: allergy, cardiology, clinical genetics, mental retardation disposition, pulmonary, radiology, renal, etc.

Service Committees

Patient Care Task Force. A group such as this would consist of the individuals responsible for the smooth operation of the patient care area. For instance, one such unit with which the authors have had experience is a Pediatric Task Force made up of an assistant administrator, an attending physician, a pediatric surgeon, the chief pediatric resident, the assistant director of nursing for pediatrics and the clinical pediatric pharmacist. Meeting monthly or more often as conditions may dictate, this group: (1) establishes appropriate goals for patient care and clinical teaching; (2) evaluates the patient care program on the pediatric unit and identifies problems which need resolution; (3) formulates recommendations for needed changes in policies, procedures, staffing and other matters relevant for patient care and clinical teaching; and (4) when appropriate implement changes in the patient care program through proper administrative channels. Since the clinical pediatric pharmacist may be responsible for drugs, supplies and equipment for the pediatric patient care area; he is an integral part of the Task Force.

Planning and Action Committees. Special planning and action committees may be appointed to look into a procedure or area and then devise a plan of action to improve the situation. The active concerned pharmacist will find himself on such committees. An example would be "The Intensive Care Unit Planning Committee."

Instructional Services

Inservice Education for Nurses and Students. The pharmacist, with his broad and intensive knowledge of drugs, drug actions, interactions and side effects as well as available dosage forms, may be an invaluable aid for inservice education for nurses. This information may be disseminated through formalized lectures, seminars and informal discussions. New drugs and recent concepts of therapy may be topics of discussion. Information on changes in procedure, equipment or supplies may best be handled by the pharmacist through the inservice education program for nurses.

Lecturing to Pediatric Medical Clerks. In the case of a teaching institution, the pharmacist may be of value as an instructor for the pediatric medical clerks. He may certainly discuss the determination of pediatric dosage in detail, assessing the precision and accuracy of the various "rules" and formulas. Other important topics include classes of drug therapy (*e.g.*, specific, supportive, empiric, therapeutic trial, placebo); dosage forms and their respective intricacies as applied to children; conditions that alter drug therapy; and the use of pertinent medical and pharmacy references (*e.g.*, the *American Hospital Formulary Service*).

Pharmaceutical Services

The traditional role of any pharmacist is built around prescription services. However, now the pharmacist is going to provide not only the traditional service but relatively new clinically-oriented services which are designed to provide better, safer and more economical pharmaceutical care.

Interpreting Orders. Perhaps the most important initial step in providing these newer services is direct interpretation of physicians' orders. This may be accomplished by altering the chart copy so that a physician writing orders for his patient creates a direct copy of that order to be seen and interpreted by the pharmacist rather than his receiving a ward clerk's or nurse's transcription of the order. Direct interpretation of orders allows the pharmacist to screen the order in the form it was written and thereby gives him the opportunity to correct any error before it gets to the patient.

Monitoring Therapy. As the pharmacist interprets and acts on the physician's order he can also monitor each patient's therapy by maintaining an accurate and up-to-date patient profile. This very important tool of the clinical pharmacist is even more important in the pediatric area, since the use of drugs in children is so much more critical. He screens for accurate and suitable doses, drug-drug interactions, drug modifications of laboratory tests, drug efficacy specific for each patient and adverse drug effects. This function also permits an additional check on the drug distribution system. Many methods have been devised for preparing and maintaining a patient profile; one example is shown as the "Clinical Record" (Figure 2). This type of a record offers special advantages since it becomes a permanent part of the patient's chart and is always ready for use by physicans, nurses, pharmacists and other members of the team. Additionally, maintaining the drug profile on the Clinical Record permits easier monitoring of response to therapy (efficacious or deleterious) since some of the vital signs (temperature, pulse and respiration) are also charted there on a daily basis.

Provide Unit Doses to High Risk Nursery. Mention has been made of the importance of unit dose drug distribution and the critical need for precision in determining pediatric doses. Precision in medication preparation becomes more important as the volume of the dose diminishes. Combining these factors most certainly increases the safety and quality of pediatric pharmaceutical care, since the pharmacist may provide the exact dose every time and decrease the possibility of errors which may occur within a traditional system. Errors in drawing up medications for infants in high risk areas such as nurseries, where it is difficult to achieve concentration and precision, may have severe sequelae. A good unit dose drug distribution system, backed by a versatile drug packaging department, can prevent these errors.

At the present time there is no suitable oral liquid unit dose package for use in infants and children under three years of age. The commonly available package for liquid unit doses is not convenient for administering medication to infants. It is made for pouring, and that is difficult with a small child. A nurse receiving liquids packaged in this manner will undoubtedly draw the medication into a syringe without a needle and inject it into the child's mouth. This is an expensive procedure and hazardous in that it creates a potential for a particularly dangerous misadventure by having available an oral medication in a syringe. We have found the use of collapsible plastic tubes suitable for administering medications to young children.* These tubes, available in 1 ml, 2.5 ml and 5 ml sizes, resemble ophthalmic ointment tubes and have an extended tip which permits placing the medication well into the mouth. They are open at the back and can easily be filled by automatic pipetting equipment and then heat sealed. However, we must remember that the stability of liquid medications in plastics is uncertain, and long-term storage in this package is not recommended. Drug manufacturers and the packaging industry are currently investigating suitable economical pediatric liquid packages. One device pending release resembles a syringe but cannot be used for injection.

Extemporaneous Compounding. Because of their relatively infrequent use in pediatrics, or their "orphaning" clause, many important drugs are not commercially available in pediatric dosage forms. This lack of commercially available dosage forms considerably reduces the medication armamentarium of the pediatrician. But when he deems it absolutely necessary to use a drug which falls into this category he turns to the pharmacist for assistance. The pharmacist will usually answer the request with one of two stock replies: either, "This drug is not commercially available in a suitable dosage form, but we will try to make one up for you"; or, "I cannot supply this drug for you since it is not available in a suitable form and the literature does not recommend it for use in children."

The latter extends further the "therapeutic orphan" concept,[43] whereas the former leads the pharmacist into producing an extemporaneous formulation of the drug product. Such formulations must have good short-term stability, provide availability of the drug for absorption and have good general pharmaceutical elegance. The establishment of a list of proven formulas for extemporaneous formulations of pediatric dosage forms would greatly increase the caliber of patient care by: (1) providing pediatric dosage forms when they are not commercially available; (2) establishing formulas which are known to be reliable; and (3) providing a more consistent dosage form which does not change with each pharmacist receiving an order for the drug.

Parenteral Fluids. There is no doubt that intravenous additives can be more safely prepared by the pharmacist than by others who are currently preparing them since he is specially trained to recognize drug interactions, incompatibilities and possible therapeutic problems. He is also better prepared for the actual process of mixing the solutions under conditions utilizing aseptic technique, proper labeling, storage, handling and so forth. Since all intravenous solutions are "legend" drugs and the pharmacist is charged with the responsibility of providing the best pharmaceutical care, it is only common sense that he oversee and direct a well-controlled intravenous admixture program.

Patients undergoing peritoneal dialysis require a stock solution consisting of electrolytes, heparin and an antibiotic to be added to each liter of dialysate fluid. Stock solutions such as this require a good deal of manipulation, should be prepared under aseptic conditions and need a fairly complicated label which includes all additives, expiration hour and date, and directions for use.

Total intravenous hyperalimentation is a special technique which has recently progressed beyond the experimental stage. This technique when properly used is capable of supporting normal growth and development and is now being used widely for a variety of gastrointestinal conditions in which oral feedings are hazardous, inadequate or impossible. Conditions for which this treatment has been used include chronic

*Plastic tubes are available from Colonial Applicator Co., Vineland, New Jersey.

Table 9. Contents of "Pediatric INF"*

1. 5% Amigen	700 ml
K	13 mEq
Na	24.5 mEq
Ca	3.5 mEq (70 mg)
Mg	1.4 mEq (17 mg)
Cl	14 mEq
PO_4	21 mEq (217 mg phosphorus)
2. Dextrose 50%	300 ml
3. KCL	4 mEq
4. Calcium gluconate 10%	12.2 ml (110 mg Ca)
5. Magnesium sulfate 50%	2.25 ml (113 mg Mg)
6. Phytonadione	2 mg
7. Vitamin B-12	50 mcg
8. Folic acid	3 mg
9. MVI	2 ml
10. *Total electrolyte content*:	
K	17 mEq/liter
Na	25 mEq/liter
Ca	180 mg/liter
Mg	130 mg/liter
Cl	18 mEq/liter
PO_4	217 mg/liter

*Intravenous Nutrient Formula
Amigen — Available from Baxter Laboratories, Morton Grove, Ill. 60053
MVI — Available from USV Pharmaceutical Corp., Tuckahoe, N.Y. 10707

intestinal obstruction due to adhesions or peritoneal sepsis, bowel fistulae, inadequate intestinal length, chronic non-remitting severe diarrhea, extensive body burns, abdominal tumors treated by surgery, irradiation and chemotherapy, prematurity, ruptured omphalocele, gastroschisis, anorexia nervosa and atresia of the small bowel.[81-88]

The infusion consists basically of glucose for calories and protein hydrolysate as a source of nitrogen as well as electrolytes, vitamins and trace elements all of which must be tailored for the growth and development of each individual patient. Several different formulas used in the preparation of hyperalimentation solutions and the techniques for their administration have been described in the articles cited previously. As an example, a formula designed for pediatric use is shown in Table 9.*

Stop Orders. Any drug may harm a patient if it is given in sufficient doses for a sufficient length of time. This is especially true in the area of pediatric therapy. For this reason the Joint Commission on Accreditation of Hospitals first required some controls or stop order systems in March 1956 to serve as a protection for the safety and welfare of the patient against indiscriminate, indefinite prescribing of an open-ended type.[89] In most institutions the nursing staff has assumed the responsibility of maintaining stop order controls, but we feel this should be a duty and responsibility of the clinical pharmacist. The maintenance of a good patient profile system can enable the pharmacist to initiate a system whereby he notifies the prescribing physician 24 to 48 hours before a medication order is to expire.

Cardio-Respiratory Resuscitation Team. A pharmacist directly involved in a patient care area must be able to respond and function as a member of the cardio-respiratory resuscitation team. The pharmacist must maintain all equipment and supplies in a state of readiness, be responsible for the preparation and labeling of all medications and record all doses and times of administration as well as responses to these drugs. Finally, he must complete an accurate report of the emergency, including identification of the patient, procedures, medications and professionals involved, and the outcome of the resuscitative efforts. Efficiency and accuracy are essential in a stressful situation such as this and therefore the pharmacist involved must be an experienced individual who can remain calm and collected.

*Refer to Chapter 7 for additional information on total intravenous hyperalimentation.

Information Sources

Drug Information. The pharmacist's background of education and experience includes a special knowledge of drugs, drug products, adverse reactions, precautions, bioavailability, half-lives and other pertinent data including current advances in therapeutics. As he appears in the patient care area the clinical pharmacist will begin to use knowledge as a source of information to physicians and nurses, as well as to medical, nursing and pharmacy students. Initially his participation may be fairly passive, awaiting individual questions, but as he gains experience and the confidence of his associates he will be an active participant in therapeutic deliberations and eventually anticipate inquiries by spontaneously interjecting his comments. Some examples of extemporaneously rendered therapeutic information of interest to pediatric pharmacists are presented below:

1. Chloramphenicol palmitate, although rarely used in pediatrics, is an ester which must be split in the gastrointestinal tract before the active drug can be absorbed. Children with cystic fibrosis, who may require treatment with chloramphenicol for other conditions, are usually incapable of splitting the ester, thus the drug may not be absorbed. This problem has been overcome by oral administration of a freshly prepared solution of chloramphenicol sodium succinate.
2. A few children have shown a gastric intolerance to commercially available penicillin suspensions and syrups. This problem is characterized by a rapid vomiting of any administered preparation. Oral administration of freshly prepared unflavored solutions of intravenous penicillin preparations has successfully overcome this problem.

Combining the skill of the individual pharmacist with a functioning drug information center provides the ideal drug information source — the ideal dissemination system for promoting drug intelligence.

Poison Treatment Information. The number of accidental ingestions of drugs and household products by children is quite alarming, often creating situations which call for quick action based on accurate information. Here again, the pharmacist should be prepared by his education and training to provide valuable information about the ingested product. Firstly, he is familiar with hundreds of drugs and drug products which he may readily identify by sight or by the use of various identification guides. Secondly, he should be thoroughly familiar with such references as *Clinical Toxicology of Commercial Products* and others in which he may obtain descriptive and quantitative information about contents and relative toxicity, as well as the specific or general treatment information.[90] Thirdly, he should have established a working relationship with the local Poison Control Center so that he may obtain back up support and more extensive treatment information. With time and experience the pharmacist will become measurably proficient at acquiring important clinical information and may be able to aid in making critical judgments as to the treatment of the poisoning.

Adverse Drug Reaction Reporting Program. A certain number of adverse drug reactions is bound to occur no matter how well the drug therapy is controlled; these may be idiosyncratic or unforeseeable. On the other hand, the knowledge gained through an adverse experience may lead to recognition of the probable cause and elimination of the chance of its recurring. This knowledge can only be gained by observation and documentation of all adverse reactions. The pharmacist who makes daily rounds with the physicians, consults with the nurses, maintains a good drug profile and reads the patients' charts daily is in the best position to recognize, observe, document, report and file the adverse reactions.

Investigational Drug Program. Traditionally the role of a pharmacist in investigational drug studies has been one of controlling, preparing and distributing the medication for the principal investigator. The clinical pharmacist may very well increase his commitment to include not only these traditional roles, but also the coordination of studies, participation measuring parameters and occasional involvement as a principal investigator. Occasionally, a single course of treatment of an investigational drug may be required for an unusual case. The pharmacist may then be called upon to determine the availability of the drug, and arrange for the procurement and use of the quantity necessary for that case. Perhaps this role can best be illustrated by describing an actual case in which pharmacists were involved.

J. K. is an infant boy who at the age of two weeks underwent a nearly total bowel resection which left him with almost no absorptive surface in his gastrointestinal tract. Prior to the development of parenteral hyperalimentation solutions this condition was incompatible with life. The pharmacy department prepared these solutions using commercially available protein hydrolysates. After several months of therapy the child developed a rash and splenomegaly which disappeared promptly upon withdrawal of the solutions, and reappeared upon challenge with the solutions. Several different protein hydrolysates were tried, with the same results. Skin tests using all the hyperalimentation solutions, as well as the individual protein hydrolysates, gave a positive reaction, versus negative controls.

By this time it had become apparent that the solutions were responsible for the child's hypersensitivity reactions; however, this child could not survive without some sort of hyperalimentation. Consultations between the physicians and pharmacists concerning the availability of some other type of nitrogen source stimulated an extensive search by the pharmacists who finally located FreAmine*—at that time a relatively unknown investigational product prepared from crystalline amino acids rather than modified protein. A supply was procured and new formulations of hyperalimentation solutions were prepared. These new formulations were successfully used in the child for well over a year and no incidences of hypersensitivity were noted.

The clinical pharmacist has responded similarly in other diseases which required experimental or very rare drugs such as Yomesan, an antihelminthic used in a stubborn case of tapeworm acquired in Turkey, and Pentamidine, which was successful in treating several cases of pneumocystis carnii pneumonia.

Admission Interview. Upon admission, the parents should be interviewed as a means of establishing some rapport among the pharmacist, the parents and the patient. It is essential that the pharmacist introduce himself as the man who will be involved in insuring quality pharmaceutical service to the child. He must radiate assurance, confidence and professional ability to promote cooperation and faith in him.

Drug History. The pharmacist should, in his admission interview, obtain a complete drug history, including both prescribed drugs and O-T-C medications. Several methods proposed for eliciting all the necessary information are described in Chapter 12. A number of specific questions may be utilized to stimulate the essential answers. However, the most successful method is that which the interviewer feels comfortable with and achieves the desired results. The authors currently use a medication history outline designed by Dunphy and Hart (Table 10).[91] Initially the form was used as a guide during the interview, but experience has shown that committing the questions to memory and tailoring the interview to the patient is much more successful. Results of this interview are summarized and placed in the history and progress section of the patient's chart. The value of the pharmacist's drug history may be seen in the following examples:

1. A known hemophiliac was admitted to the hospital with a "spontaneous" bleeding episode, coincidental with an upper respiratory infection. While interviewing the

*FreAmine—available from McGaw Laboratories, Glendale, California 91201.

mother, the pharmacist found that she had been giving the child aspirin for his fever, a fact she had not reported to the physician interviewers.

2. A hypertensive patient was admitted for evaluation of a recent increase in blood pressure. During the pharmacist's interview it was noted that the patient had been receiving pseudoephedrine for nasal congestion.

Drug Identification. As part of a drug history any medications brought to the hospital by the patient are identified and recorded. The drugs are retained by the pharmacy until discharge. A Patient's Personal Medications form (Figure 3) is placed in the patient's chart opposite the discharge prescription form. At discharge the physician checks this form and writes new directions or new prescriptions. Unidentifiable drugs should not be returned to the patient. Drug identification in the pediatric area may be facilitated by placing samples of the most commonly used liquid preparations in small clear glass bottles, to be made available for the patients and parents to examine and point out the characteristics (color, odor, etc.) which match the medication they had at home. This system is especially useful when the patient did not bring his medications to the hospital with him.

Patient or Parent Consultations. Daily rounds by the clinical pharmacist should include a personal visit to patients or parents or both to discuss and to educate them on proper use of their drugs, to evaluate the therapy by following the significant parameters, to learn about any problems the patients may be having with the drug or dosage form so that alternatives might be suggested to the physician and to observe patients daily for possible adverse reactions.

Discharge Summary. Upon the patient's discharge, the clinical pharmacist once again should interview him or his parents and check the instructions received from the physician concerning the therapeutic regimen to be followed at home. The clinical pharmacist should inform and instruct the patient or his parents on the proper methods of self administration, cautions, side effects, proper storage and handling and so on of drugs. The interview should be adequately documented. A résumé stating the medications taken and their effectiveness and the occurrence or lack of adverse reactions should be placed in the patient's chart.

FIGURE 3
Patient's Personal Medications

The following medications were brought in by patient ____________________ and have been stored in the PCS room. In order to save expense to this patient and avoid any duplication or interaction with discharge medications please indicate which may be returned to the patient and any changes in instructions.

____________________R.Ph.

The following medications should be returned to patient ____________________ with the following changes in instructions.

____________________M.D.
Discharging Physician

Table 10. Medication History Outline

I. Present Medications
- A. Medications brought to hospital by patient.
  Identify them.
  How long has patient been taking each?
  Does he take them according to directions?
  Does the patient know why he is taking each?
- B. Other medications which patient is taking presently for this illness or an unrelated condition.
  Ask the same four questions as above.

II. Past Medications

Try to determine any medications that have been taken for past illnesses.
Identify them.
How long did he take these? How long ago did he stop taking them?
What directions were followed?
For what reason was each medication taken?

III. Allergies and Adverse Reactions
- A. Has the patient any known allergies?
- B. Has the patient had any of the typical allergic reactions—skin rash, itching, nausea, vomiting, etc.
- C. Has the patient had an adverse drug reaction—was a drug ever discontinued because of intolerance?

IV. Review of Drug Categories

This often uncovers other prescription products that had been forgotten but emphasis should also be placed on O-T-C products.

sleep	iron preps
pain	hormones or birth control pills if appropriate
nerves	constipation, diarrhea, bowels
eye preps	heart burn or indigestion
ear preps	nausea and vomiting
headache	kidney pills
colds	liver pills
hayfever or allergies	fluid pills
nasal preps	any skin preparations
cough	anything else
vitamins	

V. Financial

Who pays for medications?
Has patient not obtained medications at any time because of financial difficulty?

VI. Instructions

Has patient been properly instructed on the use of his medications with regard to proper dosages, potential interactions, side effects, signs of toxicity or adverse reactions?

Supplies and Equipment Responsibilities

In some institutions the clinical pharmacist may have responsibility for supplies and equipment in his particular patient care area. It is a widely accepted practice that the pharmacy department be responsible for central supply functions, but the responsibility for equipment is usually fragmented among several departments. Since no single department has complete control over the equipment a state of confusion may exist when equipment is needed, damaged or obsolete. Centralizing the responsibility for supplies, equipment and drugs under one individual, namely, the clinical pharmacist, with technician support, provides a more efficient system. The clinical pharmacist, through his technicians, will be responsible for the presence, maintenance, correct use, safety and operation of all supplies and equipment in his area; he must also be concerned with the efficient and economical use of this equipment. The pharmacy technician is responsible for the routine daily activities associated with the presence, distribution, charging, recording and minor repair of supplies and equipment. The pharmacist assumes ultimate responsibility for the appropriate use and safety of equipment. As the use of electrical devices increases, the possibility of electrical hazards rises, and the increasing concern over these hazards should interest the pharmacist so that he has all equipment screened for possible dangers. The following examples illustrate the need for involvement by the clinical pharmacist:

While participating in a number of resuscitation efforts the pharmacist noted an alarming rate of failure of the laryngoscope. A number of these important instruments continually failed to light, to the extent that pharmacists carried an "extra" with them. Investigation into the procedure for preparation of the "emergency trays" (Tables 11 and 12) showed that each instrument was inspected and operative prior to processing. Processing consisted of ethylene oxide sterilization which, it turned out, destroyed the batteries of the larynogoscope. Noting this, the pharmacist initiated a change in procedure, whereby the laryngoscope handle was affixed to the tray immediately after sterilization.

Still another role for the pharmacist is to express his knowledge in the choice of equipment to be purchased for use in pediatric patients. As an example, breathing bags* may be very dangerous instruments if used overzealously in a tiny infant. To prevent this possibility some bags are equipped with a safety valve which releases when a certain pressure is reached. The knowledgable pharmacist can advise on the purchase of the breathing bag with the valve, and by doing so may possibly avert an iatrogenic pneumothorax.

Table 11. Infant Resuscitation Tray (Sterile)

Item	Size
1. Infant Laryngoscope Handle	
2. Laryngoscope Blade Miller 0	
3. Laryngoscope Blade Miller 1	
4. Oral Airway 00	
5. Oral Airway 000	
6. Cole Endotracheal Tube with Adapter	8 Fr
7. Cole Endotracheal Tube with 4 mm. Adapter	10 Fr
8. Cole Endotracheal Tube with 4 mm. Adapter	12 Fr
9. Newborn Suction Tube with Regulator	
10. Endotracheal Adapter	15mm
11. Premature Feeding Tube	

NOTE: *This is a limited supply item.* Each item is to be checked by nursing personnel and must be complete before returning to PCS before replacement.

Nursing Personnel ____________ Returned

PCS Personnel ____________ Checked

Table 12. Emergency Kit (Pediatric Supplement)

Item	Quantity
Oral Airway, Size 000	1
Oral Airway, Size 0	1
Oral Airway, Size 1	1
Oral Airway, Size 2	1
Small Laryngoscope Handle	1
Laryngoscope Blade, Wis-Hipple #1½	1
Laryngoscope Blade, Premature	1
Endotracheal tube, Cole tapered	
Size 10 fr.	1
Size 12 fr.	1
Size 14 fr.	1
Endotracheal tube, Murphy, uncuffed	
Size 12 fr., 10 cm.	1
Size 14 fr., 12 cm.	1
Size 16 fr., 12 cm.	1
Size 20 fr., 15 cm.	1
Size 24 fr., 20 cm.	1
Size 26 fr., 20 cm.	1
Size 28 fr., 30 cm.	1

1st check ____________
2nd check ____________

Clinical Research and Investigation

There is a great need for clinical research and investigation in the pediatric area, and the pharmacist may definitely be an important contributor. However, to do so he must have established a strong rapport with the practicing pediatricians and have gained expertise in his field. While achieving this plateau the clinical pharmacist, due to his unique blend of basic science education and clinical training and experience, may become the ideal liaison between the clinician and the basic scientist. An example follows:

One of the current methods of treating neonatal hyperbilirubinemia is the use of phototherapy. Successful as this therapy has been, it is not without hazard; therefore, more beneficial, less hazardous methods are still being sought. The clinical pharmacist was aware of some preliminary investigations, currently being conducted by pharmaceutical scientists, directed at drugs which might enhance the effects of other drugs using phototherapy

*HOPE—Hand Operated Pediatric Emergency Resuscitator, Ohio Medical Products, Madison, Wisc. 53701

as a means of measuring relative activities. His recognition of the therapeutic possibilities of these drugs in conjunction with phototherapy prompted him to introduce the scientist to the pediatrician resulting in a joint grant proposal and a clinical study.

Table 13. Clinical Orientation Clerkship

I. Conferences

A. *Teaching Seminars* - There will be a teaching seminar each Tuesday morning from 9:30 - 11:30 a.m. These seminars will cover various aspects of therapeutics.

B. *Grand Rounds* - All students will attend grand rounds each week.

C. *Admitting Conference* - All students will hold two one-hour admitting conferences with their instructor or resident each week. Each student must be prepared to present a brief summary of any new patients to whom he is assigned and to report on any change in the condition of any of his other patients. During these conferences the student will be expected to provide his instructor or resident with any of the following information about his patients:

1. Why they are in the hospital.
2. Their medication history.
3. Their working diagnosis.
4. Any concomitant disease states.
5. The medications which they are on and why they are on them.
6. The mechanism of action of the drugs being used (where this information is known).
7. The side effects which might be expected to be seen with the use of these drugs.
8. Whether or not the patient exhibits any side effects or adverse reactions due to drugs.
9. Whether or not the patient is exhibiting any efficacious effects due to his drug therapy (*i.e.*, are the drugs doing what they are supposed to be doing?)

D. *Patient Presentations* - Each student will make one patient presentation per week. The student will be informed by his instructor or resident as to which patient he is to present. The discussions should be primarily concerned with the following:

1. The patient's presenting complaints.
2. The working diagnosis.
3. The final diagnosis.
4. Any concomitant disease states which the patient may have had.
5. Drug history.
6. Drugs taken while in the hospital and why. (This portion of the discussion should include mechanisms of drug action where known.)
7. Any effects which the drugs may have had on the disease state(s).
8. Any side effects exhibited.
9. Any adverse drug reactions or interactions.
10. Discharge medications (where applicable).
11. Condition upon discharge (where applicable).
12. Information from the current literature concerning the treatment of the disease state or the drugs discussed.

On the same day that the patient presentation is made a formal write up of the case should be turned into the instructor. Each write up should be accompanied by a bibliography containing a minimum of two articles (reviews on the therapy of the disease state or concerning the use of a particular drug) from the recent literature.

E. *Literature Conference* - Once a week the students will meet to discuss articles of interest from the current literature. Each student will be assigned a specific journal from which he will prepare an abstract to be presented to the rest of the group. The students will be divided into two groups and each group will present abstracts on alternating weeks.

II. Responsibilities

A. You will maintain medication profiles on all patients designated by your instructor.

B. You will take a medication history on all patients to whom you are assigned.

C. You will identify drugs brought into the hospital by patients.

D. You will be responsible for making sure that all patients to whom you are assigned are instructed in the use of their discharge medications.

E. Each morning that you are assigned to the floor you will attend rounds. You should be alert for any information pertaining to possible drug side effects or adverse reactions.

F. You will be responsible for providing any information pertaining to drugs or drug therapy which is requested by physicians on the floor. (You may enlist the help of your instructor or the Drug Information Center Staff in assisting you to acquire this information).

Education in Pharmacy

B.S. Student. The education of pharmacy students should include a clinical orientation course which provides the student the opportunity to: (1) study the clinical application of drugs; (2) study diseases and their treatment with drugs; and (3) interact with other health professionals.

Pediatrics is an ideal area for clinical education of pharmacy students since it provides a diverse range of drugs, diseases and conditions which require medical and surgical attention. Thus, in the pediatric area the student will be exposed to medicine, surgery, neurology, ophthalmology, orthopedics, urology, hematology/oncology, as well as such areas as newborn nursery, high risk nursery, intensive care unit, possibly a care-by-parent unit and pediatric outpatient clinics. Other areas in the hospital usually offer less diversification. Limited student rotation to appropriate adult areas would provide a broader scope of experience. A list of conferences and responsibilities of an undergraduate student involved in a clinical orientation clerkship is shown in Table 13. A typical schedule for students assigned to the pediatric area is shown in Table 14.

Pharm.D. Student. The Pharm.D. degree has been instituted with the basic purpose of de-

APPENDIX

Table 14. Clerkship Schedule Fall, Pediatrics

Instructor:
Resident:

	MONDAY	TUESDAY	WEDNESDAY	THURSDAY	FRIDAY	SATURDAY
7 – 8	1 3 5	2 4 6	1 3 5	1 2 3 4 5 6	1 3 5	
8 – 9	1 3 5	2 4 6	1 3 5	1 2 3 4 5 6 (Pediatric Department Teaching Conference)	1 3 5	2 4 6
9 – 10	1 3 5 1 2 3 4 5 6 (Admitting Conference)	2 4 6 123 ↑ 456	1 3 5 1 2 3 4 5 6 (Admitting Conference)	1 2 3 4 5 6 (Patient Presentation)	1 3 5 1 2 3 4 5 6 (Admitting Conference)	2 4 6
10 – 11	1 2 3 4 5 6 (Admitting Conference)	TEACHING 123 SEMINAR 456	1 2 3 4 5 6 (Admitting Conference)	1 2 3 4 5 6	1 2 3 4 5 6 (Admitting Conference)	2 4 6
11 – 12		123 ↓ 456	1 2 3 4 5 6		1 2 3 4 5 6	
12 – 1						
1 – 2		1 2 3 4 5 6			1 2 3 4 5 6	
2 – 3	1 2 3 4 5 6	1 2 3 4 5 6 (Patient Presentation)	1 2 3 4 5 6	1 2 3 4 5 6 (Literature Conference)	1 2 3 4 5 6	
3 – 4	1 2 3 4 5 6 (Patient Presentation)	1 2 3 4 5 6 (Patient Presentation)	1 2 3 4 5 6 (Patient Presentation)	1 2 3 4 5 6		
4 – 5	1 2 3 4 5 6 (Pediatric Department Teaching Conference)		1 2 3 4 5 6 (Pediatric Department Teaching Conference)	2 4 6		
5 – 6						

Admitting Conference
Patient Presentation
Pediatric Department Teaching Conference
Literature Conference

Students: 1. ____
2. ____
3. ____
4. ____
5. ____
6. ____

veloping a stronger professional program and upgrading the quality of pharmacy. Much of the value of the Pharm.D. program served in pediatrics will result from the personalized supervision of the student by the instructor in the clinical setting. A professional spirit and a sense of competence will be developed through the interaction and counsel between student and practitioner-educator, between student and pediatricians and between the student and the patients.

Future Functions

Just as there has been great conjecture on the future role of the pharmacist in general, emerging specialties within pharmacy such as the pediatric practitioner still speculate on the functional specifics of their emerging specialty. Among the functions currently being discussed and evaluated as part of the future role of the clinical pharmacist are: (1) coordination of patient services; (2) total responsibility for drug administration; and (3) an increasing sophistication of input into product selection, utilization and evaluation. The future role of the pharmacist in the clinical areas certainly hinges on his development and level of sophistication as well as his acceptance by other members of the health team.

Conclusion

It seems especially appropriate to conclude this chapter with an excerpt from Appley which has profoundly influenced the authors' thinking, and is provided with the hope that others may be similarly moved.[92]

> . . . if you want to measure your own effectiveness as a supervisor, as a front-line person, as a person who is so important out there, . . . If you want to know how effective you are, then just take a piece of paper and a pencil and write this down. What has happened in the last 12 months that you made happen that would not have happened had you not been on the job? . . . did you just leave things to chance? Are you just flying by the seat of your pants and letting each day take care of itself or are you really having an impact upon the environment within which you are a leader?

Pediatrics References

General Textbooks

*Barnett, H. L.: *Pediatrics,* ed. 14, Appleton, Century and Crofts, N. Y. 10016, 1968.

Cooke, R. E.: *The Biological Basis of Pediatric Practice,* 2 vol., McGraw-Hill, N. Y. 10036, 1968.

Gellis, S. S. and Kagan, B. M.: *Current Pediatric Therapy,* ed. 4, W. B. Saunders Co., Philadelphia 19105, 1970.

*Nelson, W. E., *et al.*: *Textbook of Pediatrics,* ed. 9, W. B. Saunders Co., Philadelphia 19105, 1969.

*Shirkey, H. C.: *Pediatric Therapy,* ed. 3, The C. V. Mosby Co., St. Louis 63103, 1968.

Other References

*American Academy of Pediatrics: *Report of the Committee on Infectious Diseases,* ed. 16, Am. Academy of Pediatrics, Evanston, Ill. 60204, 1970.

Brennemann: *Practice of Pediatrics,* loose leaf, Harper & Row, N. Y. 10016.

Caffey, J.: *Pediatric X-Ray Diagnosis,* ed. 5, Yearbook Medical Publishers, Inc., Chicago 60601, 1967.

*Dreisbach, R. H.: *Handbook of Poisoning: Diagnosis and Treatment,* ed. 6, Lange Medical Publications, Los Altos, Calif. 94022, 1969.

Dawes, G. S.: *Foetal and Neonatal Physiology,* Yearbook Medical Publishers, Inc., Chicago 60601, 1968.

Ford, F. R.: *Diseases of the Nervous System: In Infancy, Childhood and Adolescence,* ed. 5, Charles C Thomas, Springfield, Ill. 62703, 1966.

Gesell, A. and Amatruda, C. S.: *Developmental Diagnosis,* ed. 2, Harper & Row, N. Y. 10016, 1947.

*Gleason, M. N., *et al.*: *Clinical Toxicology of Commercial Products,* ed. 3, The Williams & Wilkins Co., Baltimore 21202, 1969.

Green, M., and Richmond, J. B.: *Pediatric Diagnosis,* ed. 2, W. B. Saunders Co., Philadelphia 19105, 1962.

Harper, P. A.: *Preventive Pediatrics: Child Health and Development,* Appleton-Century Crofts, N. Y. 10016, 1962.

Hughes, J. G.: *Synopsis of Pediatrics,* ed. 2, The C. V. Mosby Co., St. Louis 63103, 1967.

Ilg, F. L. and Ames, L. B.: *The Gesell Institute's Child Behavior,* Harper & Row, N. Y. 10016.

Kanner, L.: *Child Psychiatry,* ed. 3, Charles C Thomas, Springfield, Ill. 62703, 1960.

Keith, *J. D., *et al.*: *Heart Disease in Infancy and Childhood,* ed. 2, The MacMillan Co., N. Y. 10022, 1967.

Krugman, S. and Ward, R.: *Infectious Diseases of Children,* rev. ed., The C. V. Mosby Co., St. Louis 63103, 1968.

Nadas, A. S.: *Pediatric Cardiology,* ed. 2, W. B. Saunders Co., Philadelphia 19105, 1963.

Potter, E. L.: *Pathology of Fetus and Infant,* ed. 2, Yearbook Medical Publishers, Inc., Chicago 60601, 1961.

Shaffer, A. J.: *Diseases of the Newborn,* ed. 2, W. B. Saunders Co., Philadelphia 19105, 1965.

*Shirkey, H. C.: *Pediatric Dosage Handbook,* The American Pharmaceutical Association, Washington, D. C. 20037, 1971.

Silver, H. K., *et al.*: *Handbook of Pediatrics,* ed. 8, Lange Medical Publications, Los Altos, Calif. 94022, 1969.

Silverman, W. A.: *Dunham's Premature Infants,* ed. 3, Harper & Row, N. Y. 10016, 1961.

Smith, C. H.: *Blood Diseases of Infancy and Childhood,* ed. 2, The C. V. Mosby Co., St. Louis 63103, 1967.

Smith, C. A.: *Physiology of the Newborn Infant,* ed. 3, Charles C Thomas, Springfield, Ill. 62703, 1959.

Speer, F.: *The Allergic Child,* Harper & Row, N. Y. 10016, 1963.

Spock, B.: *Baby & Child Care,* Pocket Books, Inc., N. Y. 10018, 1970.

Top, F. H.: *Communicable and Infectious Diseases,* ed. 6, The C. V. Mosby Co., St. Louis 63103, 1968.

U. S. Department of Health, Education, and Welfare: *Infant Care,* U. S. Government Printing Office, Washington, D. C. 20025, 1962.

U. S. Department of Health, Education, and Welfare: *Your Child from 1 to 6,* U. S. Government Printing Office, Washington, D. C. 20025, 1962.

*Varga, C.: *Handbook of Pediatric Medical Emergencies,* ed. 4, The C. V. Mosby Co., St. Louis 63103, 1968.

Watson, E. H. and Lowery, G. H.: *Growth and Development of Children,* ed. 5, Yearbook Medical Publishers, Inc., Chicago 60601, 1967.

Wilkins, L.: *Diagnosis and Treatment of Endocrine Disorders in Childhood and Adolescence,* ed. 3, Charles C Thomas, Springfield, Ill. 62703, 1965.

*Winkelstein, J. A. and Swick, H. M.: *The Harriet Lane Handbook,* Yearbook Medical Publishers, Inc., Chicago 60601, 1969.

*Essential for a good personal pediatric library.

Current Literature

Pediatrics, American Academy of Pediatrics, Inc., P. O. Box 1034, Evanston, Ill. 60204.

Journal of Pediatrics, The C. V. Mosby Co., 3207 Washington Blvd., St. Louis 63103.

American Journal of Diseases of Children, American Medical Association, 535 N. Dearborn St., Chicago, Ill. 60610.

Pediatric Clinics of North America, W. B. Saunders Co., West Washington Square, Philadelphia 19105.

Advances in Pediatrics, Yearbook Medical Publishers, Inc., 35 E. Wacker Dr., Chicago 60601.

Archives of Disease of Childhood, British Medical Journal, 1172 Commonwealth Ave., Boston 02134.

Acta Pediatrics, Almqvist and Wiksell, Stockholm, Sweden.

Clinical Pediatrics, J. B. Lippincott Co., East Washington Square, Philadelphia, Pa. 19105.

Pharmapediology News, American Society of Hospital Pharmacists, Washington, D. C. 20014.

References

1. Shirkey, H. C., ed.: *Pediatric Therapy*, ed. 3, C. V. Mosby Co., St. Louis, 1968, pp. 35-47.
2. Shirkey, H. C.: *Pediatric Dosage Handbook*, American Pharmaceutical Association, Washington, D. C. 1971.
3. Shirkey, H. C.: "Dosage Administration — With Special Emphasis on Techniques and Problems Related to Infants and Children," in Shirkey, H. C., ed., *Pediatric Therapy, op. cit.*, pp. 14-29.
4. Nelson, W. E., Vaughan, V. C., III and McKay, R. J., eds.: *Textbook of Pediatrics*, ed. 9, W. B. Saunders Co., Philadelphia, 1969, pp. 1533-1538.
5. *Infant Care*, U.S. Dept. of H.E.W.: U. S. Govt. Printing Office, 1962, pp. 74-75.
6. *Your Child from 1 to 6*, U.S. Dept. of H.E.W.: U.S. Govt. Printing Office, 1962, p. 77.
7. West, C. D.: "Parenteral Fluid Therapy," in Shirkey, H. C., ed., *Pediatric Therapy, op.cit.*, pp. 252-265.
8. Dreisbach, R. H.: *Handbook of Poisoning*, ed. 6, Lange Medical Publications, Los Altos, Calif., 1969.
9. Gleason, M. N., *et al.*: *Clinical Toxicology of Commercial Products*, ed. 3, The Williams & Wilkins Co., Baltimore, 1969.
10. Coleman, A. B. and Alpert, J. J., eds.: Poisoning in Children, *Pediat. Clin. N. Am. 17*:471-758 (Aug.) 1970.
11. American Academy of Pediatrics: "Respiratory Infections," in *Report of the Committee on Infectious Diseases*, ed. 16, Am. Acad. Pediat., Evanston, Ill., 1970, pp. 111-122.
12. Bradford, W. L.: "Purulent Meningitis," in Nelson, W. E., *op.cit.*, pp. 571-577.
13. Rubin, M. I.: "Infections of the Urinary Tract," in Nelson, W. E., *op.cit.*, pp. 1119-1124.
14. Hodes, H. L. and Carver, D.: "Infectious Diseases," in Barnett, H. L. and Einhorn, A. H., eds.: *Pediatrics*, ed. 14, Appleton-Century-Crofts, New York, 1968, pp. 574-584.
15. American Academy of Pediatrics: *op.cit.* "Immunization Procedures - General Considerations," pp. 1-20.
16. Schaffer, A. J., Markowitz, M. and Finberg, L.: *Diseases of the Newborn*, ed. 2, W. B. Saunders Co., Philadelphia, 1965, pp. 613-616.
17 Takata, A.: Adverse Effects of Drugs on the Fetus, *Hosp. Formulary Management 4*:25-29 (June) 1969.
18. Knowles, J. A.: Excretion of Drugs in Milk—A Review, *J. Pediat. 66*:1068-1082 (June) 1965.
19. Langford, W. S.: "Abnormalities of Psychological Growth and Development," in Barnett, H. L., *op.cit.*, pp. 266-274.
20. Covert, C.: "Counseling Parents," in Covert, C., ed., *Mental Retardation*, American Medical Association, Chicago, 1965, pp. 58-66.
21. Shirkey, H. C.: "Adverse Reactions to Drugs — Their Relation to Growth and Development," in Shirkey, H. C., ed., *Pediatric Therapy, op.cit.*, pp. 151-174.
22. Shirkey, H. C.: "Pain, Fever, Cough," in Shirkey, H. C., ed., *Pediatric Therapy, op.cit.*, pp. 290-315.
23. Wannamaker, L. W.: "Rheumatic Fever," in Nelson, W. E., *op.cit.*, pp. 533-542.
24. Stollerman, G. H.: "Connective Tissue Diseases," in Barnett, H. L., *op.cit.*, pp. 549-562.
25. Rubin, M. I. and Rahill, W. J.: "Disturbances of the Kidney," in Nelson, W. E., *op. cit.*, pp. 1124-1149.
26. Schulman, I.: "The Blood and Blood-Forming Organs," in Barnett, H. L., *op.cit.*, pp. 1121-1210.
27. Pearson, H. A.: "Disorders of the Leukocytes," in Nelson, W. E., *op.cit.*, pp. 1071-1078.
28. Arey, J. B.: "Neoplasms and Neoplastic-Like Lesions," in Nelson, W. E., *op.cit.*, pp. 1438-1477.
29. Auerbach, V. H., DiGeorge, A. M., Crocker, A. C., and Chisolm, J. J., Jr.: "Inborn Errors of Metabolism," in Nelson, W. E., *op. cit.*, pp. 413-470.
30. Warkany, J., Fraser, F. C. and Wright, S. W.: "Prenatal Disturbances," in Nelson, W. E., *op.cit.*, pp. 318-346.
31. American Academy of Pediatrics: *op. cit.*
32. Vaughan, V. C., III: "Allergic Disorders," in Nelson, W. E., *op.cit.*, pp. 488-510.
33. Kaplan, S.: "Congestive Heart Failure," in Nelson, W. E., *op.cit.*, pp. 1031-1034.
34. Schaffer,, A. J.: *op. cit.*, pp. 949-954.
35. Varga, C., ed.: *Handbook of Pediatric Medical Emergencies*, ed. 4, C. V. Mosby Co., St. Louis, 1968, pp. 149-182.
36. Shirkey, H. C.: Drug Dosage for Infants and Children, *J. Am. Med. Assoc. 193*:443-446 (Aug. 9) 1965.
37. Butler, A. M. and Richie, R. H.: Simplification and Improvement in Estimating Drug Dosage and Fluid and Dietary Allowances for Patients of Varying Sizes, *New Engl. J. Med. 262*:903-908 (May 5) 1960.
38. Snively, W. D., Jr., Montenegro, J. L. B. and Dick, R. G.: Quick Method for Estimating Body Surface Area, *J. Am. Med. Assoc. 197*:208-209 (July 18) 1966.
39. Costeff, H.: A Simple Empirical Formula for Calculating Approximate Surface Area in Children, *Arch. Disease Childhood, 41*:681, 1966.
40. Varga, C.: *op. cit.*, pp. 623-626.
41. Beargie, R. A.: Director of Nurseries, Univ. of Ky. Medical Center, Personal Communication.
42. Shirkey, H. C.: Conference of Professional and Scientific Societies, Chicago, June 27-28, 1963.
43. Shirkey, H. C. (editorial comment): Therapeutic Orphans, *J. Pediat. 72*:119-120 (Jan.) 1968.
44. Roche Laboratories: Valium Injection Package Insert, Roche Labs., Div. of Hoffmann-LaRoche Inc., Nutley, N. J., August, 1970.
45. Shirkey, H. C.: "Adverse Reactions to Drugs - Their Relation to Growth and Development," in Shirkey, H. C., ed., *Pediatric Therapy, op.cit.*, p. 152.
46. Lowe, C. U.: Pediatric Pharmacology, *J. Clin. Pharmacol. J. New Drugs 8*:31-40 (Jan.-Feb.) 1968.
47. Buchanan, R. A. and Weiss, C. V.: Applications of Pediatric Pharmacology, *J. Clin. Pharmacol. J. New Drugs 8*:212-216 (July-Aug.) 1968.
48. Yaffe, S. J.: Fetal and Neonatal Toxicity of Drugs, *Can. Med. Assoc. J. 98*:301-306 (Feb. 10) 1968.
49. Sutherland, J. M. and Light, I. J.: The Effect of Drugs upon the Developing Fetus, *Pediat. Clin. N. Am. 12*: 781-806 (Aug.) 1965.
50. Stuart, D. M.: Teratogenicity and Teratogenic Drugs, *PharmIndex 8*:4-8 (Aug.) 1966.
51. Apgar, V.: Drugs in Pregnancy, *J. Am. Med. Assoc. 190*:840-841 (Nov. 30) 1964.
52. Beckman, H.: "Drugs in the Developing Fetus," in Beckman, H., ed., *Dilemmas in Drug Therapy*, W. B. Saunders Co., Philadelphia, 1967, pp. 140-144.

53. Moser, R. H.: "Miscellaneous Diseases," in Moser, R. H., ed., *Diseases of Medical Progress,* ed. 2, Charles C Thomas, Springfield, Ill., 1964, pp. 250-252.

54. Grumbach, M. M. and Ducharne, J. R.: The Effects of Androgens on Fetal Sexual Development, *Fertility Sterility 11*:157-180 (Mar.-Apr.) 1960.

55. Cohlan, S. Q.: Fetal and Neonatal Hazards from Drugs Administered During Pregnancy, *N. Y. State J. Med. 64*:493-499 (Feb. 15) 1964.

56. Shirkey, H. C.: The Innocent Child, *J. Am. Med. Assoc. 196*:418-421 (May 2) 1966.

57. Adamsons, K., Jr. and Joelsson, I.: The Effects of Pharmacologic Agents Upon the Fetus and Newborn, *Am. J. Obstet. Gynecol. 96*:437-460 (Oct. 1) 1966.

58. Zucker, P. and Simon, G.: Prolonged Symptomatic Neonatal Hypoglycemia Associated with Maternal Chlorpropamide Therapy, *Pediatrics 42*:824-825 (Nov.) 1968.

59. Warkany, J. and Shirkey, H. C.: "Drugs and Teratology," in Shirkey, H. C., ed., *Pediatric Therapy, op.cit.,* pp. 148-174.

60. Wilkins, L.: Masculinization of Female Fetus Due to Use of Orally Given Progestins, *J. Am. Med. Assoc. 172*: 1028-1032 (Mar. 5) 1960.

61. Goldstein, A., Aronson, L. and Kalman, L.: "Chemical Teratogenesis," in *Principles of Drug Action, The Basis of Pharmacology,* Harper & Row, New York, 1968, pp. 711-734.

62. Smart, R. G. and Bateman, K.: The Chromosomal and Teratogenic Effects of Lysergic Acid Diethylamide, *Can. Med. Assoc. J. 99*:805-810 (Oct. 26) 1968.

63. Done, A. K.: Perinatal Pharmacology, A Research Grant Supported Study, Department of Pediatrics, University of Utah, 1965.

64. Mellin, G. W. and Katzenstein, M.: The Saga of Thalidomide, Neuropathy to Embryopathy with Case Reports of Congenital Anomalies, *New Engl. J. Med. 267*: 1184-1193 (Dec. 6) 1962.

65. Larsson, Y. and Sterky, G.: Possible Teratogenic Effect of Tolbutamide in a Pregnant Prediabetic, *Lancet 2*: 1424-1426 (Dec. 31) 1960.

66. Cohlan, S. Q.: Excessive Intake of Vitamin A as a Cause of Congenital Anomalies in the Rat, *Science 117*: 535-536 (May 15) 1953.

67. Cohlan, S. Q.: Congenital Anomalies in the Rat Produced by Excessive Intake of Vitamin A During Pregnancy, *Pediatrics 13*:556-567 (June) 1954.

68. Lenz, W.: Malformations Caused by Drugs in Pregnancy, *Am. J. Diseases Children 112*:99-106 (Aug.) 1966.

69. Galina, M. P., Avnet, M. L. and Einhorn, A.: Iodides During Pregnancy: An Apparent Cause of Neonatal Death, *New Engl. J. Med. 267*:1124-1127 (Nov. 29) 1962.

70. Aaron, H. H., Schneierson, S. J. and Siegel, E.: Goiter in Newborn Infant Due to Mother's Ingestion of Propylthiouracil, *J. Am. Med. Assoc. 159*:848-850 (Oct. 29) 1955.

71. Weinstein, L. and Dalton, A. C.: Host Determinants of Response to Antimicrobial Agents, *New Engl. J. Med. 279*:467-473 (Aug. 29) 1968.

72. Rodriguez, S. U., Leikin, S. L. and Hiller, M. C.: Neonatal Thrombocytopenia Associated with Ante-Partum Administration of Thiazide Drugs, *New Engl. J. Med. 270*:881-884 (Apr. 23) 1964.

73. Sutherland, J. M.: Fatal Cardiovascular Collapse of Infants Receiving Large Amounts of Chloramphenicol, *Am. J. Diseases Children 97*:761-767 (June) 1959.

74. Gordon, H. R.: Fetal Bradycardia After Paracervical Block, *New Engl. J. Med. 279*:910-914 (Oct. 24) 1968.

75. Weinstein, L. and Dalton, C.: Host Determinants of Response to Antimicrobial Agents, *New Engl. J. Med. 279*: 524-531 (Sept. 5) 1968.

76. Sutherland, J. M. and Mohlman, Y. M.: Antimicrobial Therapy in the Newborn Infant, *Pediat. Clin. N. Am. 8*:1143-1160 (Nov.) 1961.

77. Lucey, J. F. and Dolan, R. C.: Hyperbilirubinemia of Newborn Infants Associated with Parenteral Administration of a Vitamin K Analogue to the Mothers, *Pediatrics 23*: 553-560 (Mar.) 1959.

78. Knowles, J. A.: "Drugs Excreted into Breast Milk," in Shirkey, H. C., ed., *Pediatric Therapy, op.cit.,* p. 175.

79. Bartig, D. and Cohon, M. S.: Excretion of Drugs in Human Milk, *Hosp. Formulary Management 4*:26-27 (Apr.) 1969.

80. Ritschel, W. A.: Biological Half-Lives of Drugs, *Drug Intelligence Clin. Pharm. 4*:332-347 (Dec.) 1970.

81. Wilmore, D. W. and Dudrick, S. J.: Growth and Development of an Infant Receiving All Nutrients Exclusively by Vein, *J. Am. Med. Assoc. 203*:860-864 (Mar. 4) 1968.

82. Wilmore, D. W., *et al.*: Total Parenteral Nutrition in Infants with Catastrophic Gastrointestinal Anomalies, *J. Pediat. Surg. 4*:181-189 (Apr.) 1969.

83. Dudrick, S. J., *et al.*: Can Intravenous Feeding as the Sole Means of Nutrition Support Growth in the Child and Restore Weight Loss in an Adult? *Ann. Surg. 169*:974-984 (June) 1969.

84. Filler, R. M., *et al.*: Long-Term Total Parenteral Nutrition in Infants, *New Engl. J. Med. 281*:589-594 (Sept. 11) 1969.

85. Belin, R. P.: Pediatric Surgeon, Univ. of Ky. Medical Center, Personal Communication.

86. Filler, R. M. and Eraklis, A. J.: Care of the Critically Ill Child: Intravenous Alimentation, *Pediatrics 46*:456-461 (Sept.) 1970.

87. Beargie, R. A.: Director of Nurseries, Univ. of Ky. Medical Center, Personal Communication.

88. Dudrick, S. J.: Rational Intravenous Therapy, *Am. J. Hosp. Pharm. 28*:82-91 (Feb.) 1971.

89. Babcock, K. B.: Standards for Hospital Accreditation, *Bull. Joint Comm. Accred. Hosp.,* No. 11, March, 1956.

90. Gleason, M. N., *op.cit.*

91. Dunphy, T. W. and Hart, L.L.: Clinical Pharmacist and Pharmacy Resident, Univ. of Ky. Medical Center, Personal Communication.

92. Appley, L. A.: The Nature of Management (movie), American Management Association, Gateway Production, Pittsburgh, Pa., 1968.

ACKNOWLEDGEMENT

The authors wish to express their sincere gratitude to the many people who helped make this chapter possible; to the editors who had the faith in the concept of emerging specialization such as pediatric pharmacy practice; to Paul Parker for his personal confidence and his role in creating the opportunity to practice; to Warren Wheeler and his staff in pediatrics, especially Robert Beargie and Vernon James for their counsel, guidence and confidence; to Charles Walton and John Oliver for their editorial counsel; and to Phyllis Moreman for her unselfish aid in preparation of the manuscript.

14

Pharmacy services in small hospitals, extended care facilities and nursing homes

by Fred M. Eckel and Don C. McLeod

There are approximately 7,200 hospitals in the United States. Many of these are small facilities, often in rural areas, without the services of a full-time hospital pharmacist. There are currently more than 13,000 licensed nursing homes with more than 762,000 beds and about 10,000 related facilities with more than 262,000 beds. Together there are more than 23,000 long-term care facilities supplying more than 1 million beds. Patients in small hospitals and nursing homes use many pharmaceuticals and there is an acute need for better controls over these agents. Modern pharmaceutical services now being performed by pharmacists can provide solutions to the many drug usage-related problems in health care institutions.

SOCIAL AND CLINICAL ASPECTS OF AGING

To provide optimal services to the elderly the pharmacist must understand the social and clinical implications of aging. The aging process is ever present and continuous in everyone. The first quarter century is manifested by the biological development and maturation of the individual and then a slow but inevitable decline begins. The aging process is both personal and public and involves the physical, mental and spiritual being. The aging process does not occur at the same rate or manifest itself equally in individuals. These citizens categorized as aged are generally 65 years or older and constitute about 10 percent of the population. Generalizations can be made about the more than 20 million aged citizens, but health practitioners must recognize that this is a collection of individuals each with unique and personal needs. The means and averages indicate trends and directions, but it is still the individual who must be treated.

The increased mobility of families, urbanization and the breakdown of family ties common in rural, agrarian communities have ushered the development of retirement towns, public housing for the elderly, old age homes and nursing homes. There are parallels to this in other societies. In the aboriginal Eskimo society food and goods were insufficient to support those incapable of performing vital work. When the old man could no longer hunt and the old woman's teeth could not chew and soften hides it was time to join their ancestors. The mores dictated their departure and the old and young accepted this with dignity and finality. The old were merely led away from the community and left on the ice to die a quick and peaceful death. This was necessary in order that the young have food and clothing and be able to rear their children. The institutions of isolation for the elderly in this nation in some ways offer a fate less humane than that of the old Eskimo. People are removed from the way of life and those they have lived with for decades. They are cloistered in a facility so that "normal" life can proceed at home. The young no longer experience the pleasures and agonies of their relatives growing old.

This is the social context in which the pharmacist must provide vital health care services for millions of people. He must be attuned to the social, economic and political forces at large as well as the needs of each patient. Particularly in the nursing home and hospital environment, the pharmacist must be cognizant of the clinical implications of aging if he is to properly advise other health practitioners and provide optimal services to the elderly. Diseases of aging, *i.e.*, atherosclerosis, cancer and prostatic hypertrophy, are increasing in prevalence as the longevity is extended. The management of degenerative and involutional changes related to aging is of utmost importance.

The skin and subcutaneous tissues undergo atrophy and develop fissures and wrinkles. Inelasticity results as changes occur in collagen and elastic fibers. Sweat glands are lost and the skin becomes very dry. Angiomas and keratoses develop as sebaceous glands are lost and balding occurs as hair follicles are lost. A propensity for decubitus ulcers occurs as subcutaneous tissue is lost and temperature regulatory ability is decreased.

In skeletal muscle there is a thinning of fibers, a loss of cross striations and a replacement with fibrous tissue. Ligaments, cartilaginous joints and vertebrae calcify and ossify and force many postural changes. Bones undergo demineralization and osteoporosis develops. Changes in the vertebrae, ribs and sternum can impair respiration.

Great changes are wrought in the nervous system and special senses. Reflexes become progressively slower and tactile discrimination diminishes. There is a loss of neural control of circulation and a greater susceptibility to shock results. The vision undergoes debilitating changes. Macular degeneration (corneal opacities), sclerosis and atrophy of the retina, cataracts and glaucoma all occur. Hearing is affected as a hearing loss begins in the higher frequencies and spreads to the lower. Brain lesions can cause dysphasia or aphasia in speech. Teeth loss, poor dentures and changes in the jaw muscles and joints cause lesser problems that are bothersome. Smell and taste are diminished and the patient loses his appetite. His food is not as good as it used to be. There is a loss of speed and accuracy in a variety of cognitive and psychomotor functions. There may be a narrowing of interests and the patient may become melancholy and pessimistic. There may be much mental confusion with intervening lucid periods. A state of senility is reached.

Cardiovascular diseases are the leading cause of death in the elderly accounting for about 65 percent of all fatalities. Cardiac cells atrophy, dry out and are not replaced. Arteriosclerosis, a hardening of the arteries, becomes pronounced with advanced age. Atherosclerosis, a process whereby serum phospholipids, triglycerides and cholesterol deposit as plaques on the lumen of arteries and arterioles, causes difficulty in many vital organs and tissues. These two processes result in hypertension and cause ischemia throughout the body. One of the earlier signs of ischemia is angina pectoris as the myocardium is inadequately perfused with blood and oxygen during periods of exertion. Coronaries become occluded finally with a myocardial infarction resulting. Intermittent claudication in the calves is a sign of peripheral vascular disease. In later life, perhaps 20 years or so after the onset of angina and other signs of ischemia, cerebral insufficiency will become pronounced with resulting changes in motor and cognitive skills. Reduced renal blood flow triggers the angiotensin-renin mechanism thus producing even more hypertension with inevitable damage to the liver and other vital organs. All of this may end with heart failure.

The efficiency of the respiratory system is greatly compromised in the elderly. The diaphram is weakened and there is diminished resiliency (elasticity) of the lungs. There is a thickening of the membrane between the alveoli causing poor gaseous exchange. Obesity and pulmonary artery changes compound these problems. In some, emphysema develops and terminates in death.

In the gastrointestinal tract there is reduced gastric motility, diminished peristalsis and achlorhydria causing poor digestion and constipation. Constipation is furthered by dehydration, anticholinergic drugs and antacids which raise *p*H levels in the intestines and kill off the lactobacilli flora. Hemorrhoids are painful and can worsen anemia. Calculi in the bile ducts (gallstones) occur quite frequently.

Urinary tract disease is very troublesome. Renal blood flow and glomerular filtration rate are diminished, often by as much as 50 percent. Tubular function is diminished resulting in even poorer diuresis. Prostatic enlargement is common in men and infections of the bladder and urethra are common in women. Urinary incontinence, *i.e.*, polyuria and nocturia, becomes a way of life for many.

Women undergo menopause with a decrease in estrogen production while men have a diminished level of anabolic hormones. The elderly cannot cope with a variety of stresses, *i.e.*, excess glucose and cold weather, as well as the young. There is a decreased function and reserve capacity of the hemopoietic system. Nutrition is often poor and there is altered metabolism. Due to changes in the intestines there is malabsorption of certain food components. The elderly develop a preference for sugars, the food they need least.

Many of these changes in body function are of paramount importance in drug therapy. Most of these conditions are treated with drugs as one consideration. As another, they can alter the absorption, distribution, metabolism and excretion of drugs. The elderly cannot be treated as the average adult when correct dosages of many drugs are being determined. Changes in gastric function may cause a drug to be poorly absorbed. Dehydration and loss of tissue mass alter the volume of drug distribution. Microsomal enzyme metabolism in the liver may be diminished and prolong the action of certain drugs. Reduced glomerular filtration rate may greatly increase the biological half-life of many drugs, *i.e.*, kanamycin. There are also changes in the reaction of drugs at receptor sites. A drug that once sedated a patient may now cause excitation. Side effects that once were not troublesome may now be dangerous, *i.e.*, hypotensive episodes induced by chlorpromazine.

With a proper understanding of the social and medical problems of the aged, the pharmacist will be a more effective provider of services to this increasing segment of the population. A thorough knowledge of the biomedical sciences is required in order to appreciate the finer aspects of rational drug therapy.

TYPES OF FACILITIES AND REGULATIONS GOVERNING THEM

Before discussing pharmacy services it is first necessary to define the types of facilities with which this chapter is concerned. Hospitals are health care facilities with the equipment and personnel needed to diagnosis and treat illness and injury on an inpatient basis. Due to the small size of many hospitals it may seem difficult to justify a full-time pharmacist. Many of these hospitals obtain their pharmacy service through a community pharmacist who is in the hospital only on a part-time basis.

Nursing homes play an important role in the nation's health care program. These facilities have had their greatest development since the 1950's when it became profitable for individuals and corporations to invest in their construction and operation. They provide skilled nursing care including nursing services and other specialized procedures requiring training, judgment, technical knowledge and skills. They provide care to the person who requires inpatient care but is not in need of continuous hospital services. The majority of persons using these facilities are elderly.

With the passage of the Medicare program the federal government gave additional emphasis to the nursing home's role in comprehensive patient care in the community. In order to insure quality patient care in these institutions the government developed minimum standards for their operation. These standards have been published as the *Conditions of Participation for Extended Care Facilities*. An extended care facility (ECF) is a nursing home which has met the standards of the *Conditions of Participation* and has been certified to participate in the Medicare program. Certification for Medicare participation is voluntary and must be requested by the nursing home. Although the extended care facility deals mainly with elderly patients, there is an increasing emphasis on patients of all ages recuperating from illness or surgery and who no longer require the extensive services provided by hospitals. For this reason, extended care facilities may be found in association with hospitals. The nursing home and extended care facility require the services of a pharmacist but usually not full-time. They provide an opportunity for the community pharmacist to expand his professional service in the community.

The pharmacist should be familiar with the related facilities in the community. Although service to these facilities will not be discussed here they need similar services from the pharmacist. One type of facility, the boarding home, developed during the late 1930's to provide shelter for the beneficiaries of Old Age Assistance of the Social Security Act of 1935. These facilities were usually small in nature and were often operated by widows or unemployed couples. Today many of these continue to exist although larger facilities sponsored by fraternal, church groups or local governments offer residential care consisting primarily of room and board with limited services such as laundry and help with correspondence and shopping.

Another large group of facilities are called rest homes or homes for the aged. As residents of boarding homes became older and less able to care for themselves it was necessary to provide them with more personal care. This level of care consists of room and board plus personal services such as help in walking and getting into and out of bed; assistance in bathing, dressing and feeding; preparation of a special diet; and supervision over medication that can be self-administered. With the attention being focused on the elderly and their needs, new types of facilities have been developed. Retirement villages, church-sponsored homes and so forth have developed to provide all three levels of care—skilled nursing care, personal care and residential care—in one setting.

Federal regulations have been promulgated creating standards for a facility called an Intermediate Care Facility (ICF) Type A and Type B. Type A facilities provide a minimum level of nursing care while Type B facilities provide only personal care. The standards for an ICF are to be incorporated into each state's licensure program for these facilities. This new facility has been developed to provide more uniformity in the terminology being used to describe the facilities and level of care in these related health care facilities.

All of the facilities described above require licensure. Standards vary by state as does the agency responsible for enforcing the licensure standards. Frequently the State Board of Health licenses hospitals and nursing homes and the State Department of Social Service (Welfare) licenses rest homes and boarding homes. The pharmacist must be familiar with the licensing standards particularly for pharmacy service before he begins to provide service. If the facility is certified for Medicare participation he should be familiar with the *Conditions of Participation* for Hospitals or for extended care facilities. These documents also specify standards for pharmacy service. Many hospitals and some nursing homes also participate in a voluntary accreditation program sponsored by the Joint Commission on Accreditation of Hospitals. The JCAH publishes accreditation standards which cover pharmacy services. The pharmacist should be familiar with them.

PHILOSOPHY OF SERVICE AND DRUG USE CONTROL

Today's drugs have been described as ballistic missiles with atomic war heads, yet they are prescribed, dispensed and administered as if they were bows and arrows. Certainly, this is the situation which exists in many small hospitals and nursing homes. That changes must be made in drug usage practices is becoming apparent. The pharmacist, the only member of the health team primarily concerned with drugs, is the logical person to initiate these improvements. He must understand the entire drug distribution and administration cycle, its weaknesses and strengths, before he can effectively initiate any changes. Many pharmacists have not recognized or accepted the fact that there are problems with the traditional system. Even when a pharmacist is aware of the scope of the problem, he often says that it is not his concern. Since he feels he cannot control the drug usage activity of the physician or the drug administration activity of the nurse he elects to leave their aspects of the drug usage system unchallenged.

The pharmacist must recognize that he is responsible for the safe and proper use of drugs throughout the entire institution. Although the extent of his involvement and responsibility might vary throughout the chain of events, he must be concerned about the safety of the entire cycle. Using diplomacy and tact he must be willing to challenge unsafe, inefficient or inadequate practices performed by any health professional wherever they might occur within the system.

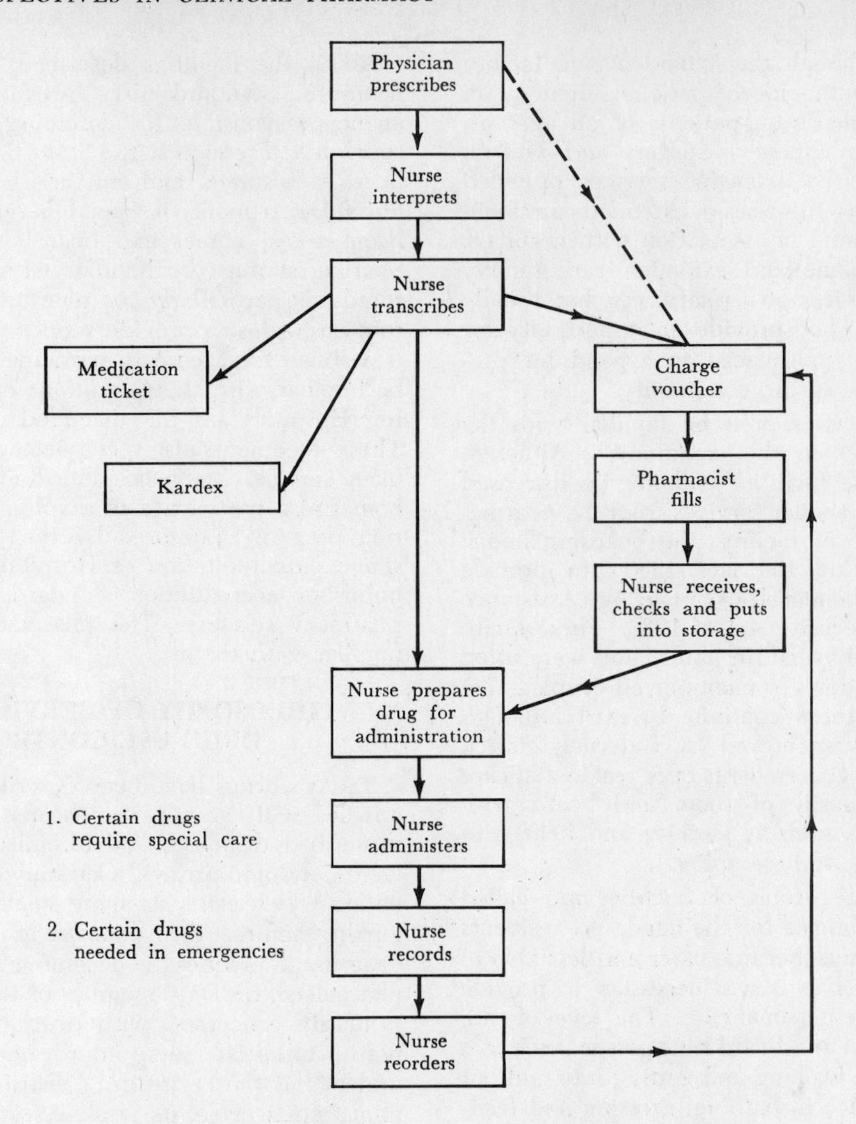

Figure 1. Flow of the drug order

The welfare of the patient must be the pharmacist's primary concern. Brodie has indicated that pharmacy's main responsibility is drug use control. He defined this as "that system of knowledge, understanding judgment, procedures, skills, controls, and ethics that assures optimal safety in the distribution and use of medication." He continues that "drug use control becomes a chain of events that extends ultimately to the bedside. Each link must contribute its maximal strength to the chain as a whole. When a break occurs at any one point and for whatever reason, drug use control is lost and patient welfare is held in jeopardy."[1] This is the attitude the pharmacist must possess to render adequate pharmacy service to hospitals and nursing homes.

Systems of Drug Use Control

It is beyond the scope of this chapter to describe the various drug distribution systems in use; however, a brief description of the traditional drug distribution system is needed for the pharmacist's understanding of his role. (Figure 1). This system operates within the overall policies regarding drugs developed by the pharmacy and therapeutics committee. The physician prescribes by specifying on the patient's chart the desired medication. The patient's chart serves as a document on which all services requested and all activities performed for a patient are recorded. The nurse or ward secretary then transcribes the medication order to a medication ticket, a nursing Kardex and frequently to a charge voucher. The medication ticket is used to tell the nurse when to administer the medication. The nursing Kardex provides the nurse with a record of the drugs and treatments a patient is to receive. The charge voucher is used to obtain the drug from the pharmacy. When the nurse receives the medication from the pharmacy, she checks it and stores it in the medication cabinet. Then relying on her medication ticket, the nurse administers the drug to the patient. She then records on the patient's chart the fact that she did administer the medication. As the supply of medication decreases it is reordered by completing another charge voucher. This system requires much paper work and medication errors are common. The disadvantages with the traditional system are numerous. Most can be eliminated with the unit dose distribution system. This system has been utilized in small hospitals and nursing homes with great success. The sample policy and procedure manual included in this chapter is based on the unit dose system.

When beginning to provide pharmacy service to a small hospital or nursing home it might not be feasible for the pharmacist to implement a unit dose distribution system. There are many programs he may initiate. Four that should receive first consideration are: (1) develop a procedure so that the pharmacist has the opportunity to review all original physician's drug orders, (2) develop a procedure to regularly inspect all drug storage areas, (3) review the entire drug administration program and (4) activate the pharmacy and therapeutics (P&T) committee. Oftentimes the pharmacist is the key to the activities of the P&T committee. The effectiveness of this committee frequently determines how meaningful the pharmacist's clinical role will be in the facility.

The first consideration in a drug distribution system is the origin of the drug order. In a nursing home environment, the physicians frequently write prescriptions for their patients' medications. Usually they also write this information on the patients' medication records. In some instances, the physician only writes the information on a medication chart; this order is then interpreted and relayed by nursing personnel to the pharmacist. When only a nurse interprets a physician's order, the possibility of a medication error increases since the nurse is not as familiar as the pharmacist with drug names. Methods should be developed to eliminate this source of error. Hospitals have been concerned about this problem and some have developed a special physician's order form. The feature of the form is a carbon copy of the physician's order made as he writes the original. This copy is then transmitted to the pharmacy. Thus, there is no need for a separate order to be written by the nurse or the physician. This mechanism permits a copy of the physician's order to be prepared for the pharmacist's direct interpretation without increasing the work of the physician. There are many forms which have been designed to meet particular needs.

The pharmacist should visit, for the purpose of inspection, all areas where medications are kept. This should occur at least monthly, and preferably more often. It is advisable to conduct the inspection in conjunction with the appropriate nursing personnel. There are many activities the pharmacist can perform during this inspection visit. An inspection form serves as a guide for the pharmacist and may be used as a written record of the inspection visit. The pharmacist should retain a copy for his files and may give one to the director of nursing as a record to be maintained by the facility. Whenever weaknesses are found in the medication control system, the pharmacist has the responsibility of enforcing their correction. The administrator of the facility and director of nursing must cooperate with the pharmacist to correct the problem.

One area of pharmacist assistance to the nursing home is enforcement of the automatic stop order policy. It is essential that some type of automatic stop orders for drugs be established to prevent the indiscriminate continuation of a patient's medication without checking with the physician. The pharmacist should develop these policies in conjunction with the medical staff. He should develop methods to enforce the automatic stop order policy once it has been established. One of the easiest ways to accomplish this is to maintain a patient drug profile. Once the pharmacist has all the information about the patient's drug therapy he can monitor drug usage. Of course, before the medication is stopped, the pharmacist should check with the prescribing physician.

Another area in which the pharmacist can assist the nursing home is in the development of an emergency drug kit for nursing home use. The purpose of such a container is to have available at the time of an emergency those drugs and supplies which might be of a life-saving nature. It is important that there be some guarantee that the needed drug is available. A written list to enable periodic checking serves as a minimum safeguard. An additional safeguard involves fitting the kit with a seal. It is important to use a seal that is easily broken as its function should not be that of a lock. When the seal is broken, it indicates that the kit has been entered and must be checked. The pharmacist and the physician should determine the drugs to be included in the kit. The pharmacist can assume responsibility for its upkeep and when notified that the kit has been entered, replace the drugs used, reseal the kit and issue a charge to the proper person.

Policies and Procedures

The function of a written policy and procedural manual in the proper operation of the pharmacy department has been suggested by the Medicare program. The pharmacist is required, under the *Conditions of Participation*, to develop and implement policies and procedures which will insure the safe and proper use of drugs at all times in the institution. Archambault states that to satisfy this requirement the pharmacist, in consultation with the medical, nursing and administrative staff, must develop and issue a policy and procedural manual.[2] Many pharmacists who provide a part-time service to a hospital or an extended care facility are interested in developing such a manual, but often they are not sure what it should contain nor even how to go about preparing it. Occasionally upon reviewing a policy and procedural manual it is evident that there has been some confusion between a policy and a procedure. Before undertaking the preparation of a manual the difference should be understood. A policy is a broad, general statement established to help personnel carry out the objectives of the organization. Departmental policies are, in a sense, rules and regulations, and are the basis of all activities of the department. A procedure tells how the policy or activity is to be accomplished. It starts at the beginning of a task and follows the activity until it is completed.

The pharmacy's policies and procedures should be integrated with those of other departments. The policy and procedural manual, although designed specifically for the pharmacy department, must be consistent with all other policies and procedures of the institution. Before attempting to prepare a manual the pharmacist should review all the policies and procedures of the facility. Since the policies and procedures for the pharmacy have an effect upon the personnel in other departments, the appropriate people should be consulted before any policy or procedure is developed. These individuals should also review the complete policies and procedures before they are implemented.

The policy and procedural manual should be developed for each specific institution. Model policy and procedural manuals have been developed. However, the use of a model manual verbatum should be avoided. A policy and procedural manual must be developed specifically for each institution to reflect the particular needs of that institution. What is an acceptable procedure in one facility might not work in another. Other policy and procedural manuals should only be used as guides. When used in this manner they can be quite helpful.

The policy and procedural manual can be used in court to determine what is reasonable to expect as to the competency of an average pharmacist or pharmaceutical service in an institution. Therefore, it has been suggested that the completed policy and procedural manual be reviewed by the institution's lawyer to be certain that every statement is legally sound. Because of the possible legal significance, it is essential that the policy and procedures in the manual conform to those currently being followed by the personnel of the institution. As policies or procedures change, the manual must reflect these changes.

There is no one format to follow in developing the manual. Because the completed manual is not a permanent document, it should follow a format which will simplify revision. One suggested format is to prepare a procedure for each activity (*e.g.*, emergency drug kit, labeling of inpatient orders). The policy should be the first sentence of the procedure. Each procedure is filed alphabetically, by title, in a loose-leaf notebook. When a procedure changes, it is then a simple matter to make the change in the policy and procedural manual.

As a general guide a sample policy and procedural manual for a unit dose drug distribution system in an extended care facility follows. With some modifications these policies and procedures are applicable in small hospitals.

Educational Activities

Pharmacists should participate in the educational activities of the facility. The pharmacist, because of his educational background and specialized knowledge of drugs, can contribute to the education of health professionals through participation in committee activities and inservice training programs. The pharmacist should serve as a member of the utilization review committee, pharmacy and therapeutics committee and infection committee. In smaller facilities all of these functions might be incorporated into one formal committee. Through his participation he can foster rational and economical drug therapy.

Inservice training programs are established as a necessary activity in these facilities. The main problem encountered with the inservice training program is planning a program and obtaining qualified speakers. Many problems involve drugs, their uses, toxicities, compatibilities and contra-indications. Other problems arise from the use of professional appliances and equipment. The pharmacist should be able to demonstrate and discuss such equipment with the employees of these facilities. Still other problems arise from a lack of knowledge or understanding of the over-all drug therapy of chronic diseases. The pharmacist has an understanding of drug therapy and can discuss it.

The advantages to the pharmacist of participating in the inservice training program are many. The personal satisfaction of participation in an educational program is in itself rewarding. Planning for each program forces the pharmacist into a continuing educational program which will be reflected in his daily practice of pharmacy. He will be forced to keep abreast of developments in pharmacy and medicine. It should improve his self-confidence in communicating with his patients about their health care problems and in discussing medical problems with the physician.

Pharmacists often have difficulty remembering their pharmacology training because they do not have the opportunity to see the clinical results of a drug. Although the physician may have less formal training in pharmacology than the pharmacist, he has a better working knowledge of the subject because he learns by association and clinical observation. In the small hospital and nursing home, the pharmacist has an excellent chance to become familiar with patients and actually see the results of drug therapy. This should enable him to gain a greater understanding and appreciation of the drugs he dispenses. As the pharmacist observes chronic disease, his understanding of such conditions should improve. This increased knowledge will be reflected in the pharmacist's understanding and concern for public health. As he becomes more versed on public health matters, his value to the community increases. He will be able to participate in community health planning committees, be a spokesman for various health education drives and, in general, be a community health leader. As the pharmacist expands his practice of pharmacy from the confines of his prescription department to the protection of the public health of the whole community and its individual needs, he will be fulfilling an important role in the community.

Reimbursement for Pharmacy Services

The pharmacist should be reimbursed adequately and fairly for the professional services rendered patients in a health care facility. Charges to the patient should be reasonable and based on accurate cost accounting. These two conditions are rather basic but have proven very difficult and illusive in application.

Hospitals have traditionally used income from drug charges to subsidize losses in other departments, *i.e.*, dietary and housekeeping. Since the advent of Medicare, many hospitals use cost accounting principles. Drug charges may be set at a level to recoup pharmacy expenses, to provide for needed capital improvement and to budget increases in the department. Hospitals may apply a fee rather than a percentage markup. Some hospitals have developed fee systems for drug charges but have calculated fees designed to provide the same level of income as the previous charging system. Most hospitals are still plodding along with a percentage markup on drugs. This is usually arbitrary and may even be chosen to correspond with normal retail prescription charges in the area.

Most hospital pharmacists are paid on a salary basis assuming a 40-hour work week. Others are paid wages on an hourly basis. Pharmacists serving small hospitals on a less than full-time basis are usually paid by one of these two methods. Many of these pharmacists find it easier to estimate the average number of hours required each month for their services and to derive a retainer fee based on what they feel their time and services are worth. Most pharmacists favoring the current concept of the fee system maintain that the difference between the cost of the drug to the pharmacist or hospital and the charge to the patient should be a fixed dollar amount or fee. This fee is applied on a per dose or per prescription basis and covers pharmacy salaries, both professional and nonprofessional, and overhead such as light, heat, janitorial services, supplies and equipment. Whitney, McLeod and Richards recommend that the professional fee be redefined to reflect only professional expenses — mainly the pharmacist's salary and educational expenses.[3] General overhead, technical and secretarial salaries would be recouped by adding a service fee to each dose or prescription. Professional expenses would be prorated as a daily charge to each patient regardless of the drugs used since professional services are unrelated to the costs or quantity of medication dispensed. Hennessey has applied this concept in a Detroit hospital.[4]

Another concept is that of a standard daily charge for drugs and professional services. An enormous amount of personnel time is consumed in documenting medication usage and posting charges for each patient. Many charges are unaccounted in some hospitals and it is difficult to summarize all expenses at the time of discharge. This daily charge could vary depending on the service, *i.e.*, maternity, surgery or medicine. This is really an extension of the insurance principle and would eliminate unusually large medication charges to any patient. This concept becomes particularly attractive as third parties assume a larger part of total hospital payments. The goal of management in this system is to document total expenses, determine where and why they occur and to minimize total costs.

The pharmacist is paid in a different manner in most nursing homes and extended care facilities. Although a few large facilities have their own pharmacy and employ a pharmacist, most pharmacists provide drugs from their own pharmacy and are reimbursed on the basis of prescriptions dispensed and the items sold to the facility. Some pharmacists, particularly those serving ECF's, receive a consultant fee in addition to the drug charges. This retainer fee is usually paid on a monthly basis.

There is now widespread controversy concerning reimbursement for pharmaceutical services in nursing homes and ECF's. The root of the problem is the pharmacist himself. Traditionally, pharmacy has been largely business-oriented rather than health care-oriented. The pharmacist priced drugs and his services as any other commodity in the marketplace. The public does not think in terms of paying for professional services when they have need of the pharmacist; they think in terms of paying for the drug. The pharmacist has taught the public to think in terms of discounts and cut rates because of his orientation to markups and common merchandising methods. It should therefore not be surprising that owners and administrators of nursing homes seek discounts or rebates on pharmacy charges in their facilities. Pharmacists, in fact, often approach the nursing home with an offer of a discount in order to secure the "account." After all, in the usual business sense one can offer a lower price when great volume is involved. The fundamental difference in the nursing home is that the patient pays the usual price, and in some cases a higher charge, while the nursing home profits from the so-called discount — more properly a rebate. This discount is commonly in the range of 10-25 percent of total drug charges. For example, if the total monthly drug charges in a nursing home are $2,000 and the discount rate is 25 percent, the patients are billed by the facility and the pharmacist is paid $1,500. The $500 is retained by the nursing home. It is obvious that this rebate tends to be inflationary since it is not passed to the payee. In the case of Medicare, it is supposed to be passed on to the federal government.

Most of the older, single-unit proprietary facilities were quite satisfied with a 10 percent rebate. Many of the nursing home chains are now requesting and receiving 20-25 percent rebates. This is very disturbing to the pharmacist desiring to provide a quality patient service within the framework of a professional fee system of reimbursement. An inordinately large fee is required assuming that the usual fee is based on sound accounting principles. The pharmacist charging a markup may have to increase the percentage in order to provide the service. The fact that the pharmacist is supplying a needed health care service tends to be lost somewhere in the percentage manipulations. One nursing home executive has intimated that his corporation seeks this percentage merely because it increases profits and it can be obtained. He further said that they would require it of physicians except that because of supply and demand physicians can successfully refuse to grant it. This chain receives rebates from physical therapists and other providers of service with the exception of physicians.

It must be recognized that the nursing home does incur expenses for the pharmacist's benefit. Most facilities collect from the patients and pay the pharmacist in one amount for all charges. The account may run two or three months in arrears but will be paid. Most credit card companies provide a similar service for about 5 percent and pay within a month. It is obvious that this service is not worth 10-25 percent in itself. It has been suggested that the nursing home deserves to profit from the pharmacist not merely to meet expenses, since it has created the environment whereby the pharmacist can practice and earn a livelihood.

It is clear that the pharmacist must soon rationalize his charges and develop a philosophy of practice and service which is understandable to third party payees, to the public and to other health care professionals. The business qualities that many pharmacists have taken pride in during the past may not sustain them in the future, if they are to be regarded as health care practitioners. The common wisdom of the mercantile world will reduce the pharmacist to a lowly pawn if he has not the professional philosophy and integrity to chart a new course. The winds are now carrying the ship aground; oarsmen not orators are desperately needed.

A compromise solution to pharmacy reimbursement in nursing homes which is satisfactory to the patient, the nursing home and the pharmacist must be reached.

The pharmacist's charges should be based on actual costs incurred and on what his services and time are worth. He should be reimbursed for these justifiable charges. If the nursing home provides the pharmacist a service, *i.e.*, collection and guaranteed payment, then it should be reimbursed accordingly. It is recommended that this be viewed as a service fee per monthly account collected and that it be clearly stated to the patient. For example, if a patient's total monthly charges were $20, the pharmacist submits a summary billing at the end of the month for that amount plus the collection fee of $1. The pharmacist is thus paid $21 and the nursing home would subsequently bill the pharmacist for the $1 collection charge. The patient knows what he is paying and there is no hidden rebate. If the nursing home feels it must "profit" from the pharmacist's services, then this profit, whether it be a percentage of a dollar amount, is added to the pharmacist's charges as an additional charge by the nursing home. It should be clear to the patient and fiscal intermediaries what the charge is and who is getting the money. The onus should not be on the pharmacist or any other health care provider to justify charges not really theirs. The question is not whether the nursing home is due a profit but whether the pharmacist is going to straighten his back and insist on an ethical and honest system of reimbursement. The burden is on the pharmacist to do this, not the nursing home industry. They are merely taking economic advantage of a vulnerable profession.

A short example of cost accounting used to determine a professional fee for unit dose services in a nursing home should be of value. The unit dose system is described in the policy and procedure section of this chapter. The following costs were calculated in 1970.

Unit Dose Cost Analysis
One Month's Pharmacy Services
52-Bed Nursing Home

Rent 100 sq. ft. @ $5/ sq. ft./yr.	$ 41.70
Inventory expenses $2,000 @ 10% investment return/yr.	16.66
Delivery 6 mile/day @ .15/mile	27.00
Bookkeeping 8 hrs. @ $2/hr.	16.00
Pharmacist's salary 55 hrs. @ $7/hr.	385.00
Social Security, Insurance, etc. approx.	30.00
	$516.36

Total number of prescriptions (each drug order = 1 Rx; only 1 Rx for a particular drug per month; aspirin given away - no charges)	273

$$\text{Fee per Rx/mo.} = \frac{\$516.36}{273} = \$1.89$$

Fee used to charge patients = $2.00
To offset $1.75 paid by Medicaid for about 1/3 of Rxs.

Acquisition drug costs for month plus packaging costs	$ 645.65
102 Medicaid Rxs at $1.75	178.50
171 Private pay Rxs at $2.00	342.00
Total of all patient charges for month	$1,166.15

It should be noted that technicians can perform activities consuming at least half of the above professional time, *i.e.*, filling medication cart and making delivery to nursing home. The inventory and rent costs could be easily lowered by servicing more patients from the pharmacy. There are other expenses such as library costs and equipment costs, but these are not great enough to appreciably alter the fee.

The costs presented could easily be recouped through a capitation system of payment. Dr. Francke, in his 1970 Remington Address, has suggested this form of payment for the pharmacist.[5] Wertheimer has also pointed out the advantages of such a system.[6] The following is a determination of a capitation fee using the previous cost figures:

Total Costs	$516.36
Number of Patients	52

$$\text{Capitation fee/patient/month} = \frac{\$516.36}{52} \approx \$10.00$$

The patient's charge per month then equals the capitation fee plus the acquisition cost of the drugs. This system removes the vested interest of the pharmacist in either cost of drugs used or the number of prescriptions dispensed. Such a system could help eliminate current reimbursement difficulties in nursing homes if third parties recognized this system of payment and reimbursed the pharmacist directly.

Considerable attention has been given to reimbursement in this chapter since a sound philosophy of reimbursement is intimately linked to the clinical and professional future of the pharmacist.

References

1. Brodie, D. C.: Drug-Use Control—Keystone to Pharmaceutical Service, *Drug Intelligence* 1:63-65 (Feb.) 1967.
2. Archambault, G. F.: Medicare and Pharmacy Services, *Hosp. Formulary Management* 2:23-29 (Jan.) 1967.

3. Whitney, H. A. K., Jr., McLeod, D. C. and Richards, J. W.: A New Definition of the Pharmacist's Fee, *Am. J. Hosp. Pharm. 25*:691-693 (Dec.) 1968.

4. Hennessy, N. B.: A Fee-Per-Patient-Per-Day Basis for Delivering Pharmaceutical Services to an Institution, *J. Am. Pharm. Assoc. NS9*:561-562 (Nov.) 1969.

5. Francke, D. E.: Medicines, Medical Care, Manpower and Mankind, *Am. J. Hosp. Pharm. 28*:410-421 (June) 1971.

6. Wertheimer, A. I.: The Pricing of Professional Services, *J. Am. Pharm. Assoc. NS11*:26-27 (Jan.) 1971.

7. Crawley, H. K., Eckel, F. M. and McLeod, D. C.: Comparison of a Traditional and Unit Dose Drug Distribution System in a Nursing Home, *Drug Intelligence Clin. Pharm. 5*:166-170 (June) 1971.

Additional References

Rawlings, J. L. and Mathieson, D. R.: Unit-Dose Packaging Spurs Optimum Therapy in "Project ECF," *Pharm. Times 36*:50-56 (Oct.) 1970.

McLeod, D. C. and Eckel, F. M.: Relationship Between Method of Reimbursement and Scope of Pharmacy Service in Nursing Homes, *J. Am. Pharm. Assoc. NS9*:62-64 (Feb.) 1969.

Anon.: *Working with Older People,* Vol. 1, The Practitioner and the Elderly, pub. 1459, U. S. Dept. of H. E. W., P. H. S. Division of Medical Care Administration, Adult Health and Aging Branch, Arlington, Va. (Aug.) 1966.

Eckel, F. M. and Latiolais, C. J.: An Analysis of Pharmaceutical Services in Forty-One Nursing Homes, *Am. J. Hosp. Pharm. 21*:351-360 (Aug.) 1964.

Pharmaceutical Policy and Procedure Manual (Name of Facility)

1.00 ORGANIZATION OF PHARMACEUTICAL SERVICES

Policies and procedures have been developed to insure the highest quality of pharmaceutical services to the patients of (name of facility). Attention has been given all aspects of the medication distribution and administration system so that drug therapy will be safe, rational and economical. These policies and procedures have been developed by the pharmacist(s) and have been approved by the medical and nursing staffs. These policies and procedures are official policy and constitute regulations of the facility.

All pharmaceutical services are provided by (names of pharmacists), pharmacists at (name and address of pharmacy). Pharmaceuticals are delivered daily to the facility by the pharmacy. The pharmacy is open according to the following schedule:

Figure 2. Pharmacy patient drug profile

PHARMACY PATIENT DRUG PROFILE
MONTH: YEAR:
ALLERGIES (in red): __________

PATIENT'S NAME:
PHYSICIAN:
METHOD OF PAYMENT:

DRUG - STRENGTH - ROUTE DIRECTIONS - TIMES	Rx NUMBER	BEGIN / STOP	1	2	3	4	5	6	7	8	9	10	11	12	13	14	15	16	17	18	19	20	21	22	23	24	25	26	27	28	29	30	31	#	@	COST

TOTAL COST __________

FEES __________

TOTAL BILL __________ (this sheet)

Form No. A-1697

Monday-Friday ______________
Saturday ______________
Sunday ______________
Holidays ______________

The order for any urgently needed medication not available in the facility should be telephoned to the pharmacist at once.

Pharmacy Telephone No. ______________
Home Telephone No. ______________

A schedule of the pharmacist on call each evening and weekend is posted in the facility.

The Pharmacy and Therapeutics Committee of the (name of facility) is organized to promote the safe and rational use of drugs in the facility and to establish official policies and procedures concerning the use and control of drugs.

The committee consists of the following:

Chairman (usually a physician)
Secretary (usually a pharmacist)
Other physicians
Director of Nursing
Administrator (usually ex officio)

2.00 PHYSICIANS' MEDICATION ORDERS

2.01 All medication orders should be written by the physician in the patient's chart on the physicians' order form. If the order is telephoned, only the charge nurse should take the verbal order. All verbal orders must be countersigned by the physician within 48 hours. The nurse receiving the order should record it on the physicians' order sheet followed by the name of the physician, the time received and the signature of the nurse. The order should be read back to the physician for confirmation.

2.02 The physician's orders should be written legibly and include (1) date and hour written, (2) name of medication, (3) dosage (metric system only), (4) route of administration, (5) frequency and times of administration, (6) duration of order and (7) signature of physician. The pharmacist and/or nurse should question the physician whenever orders are ambiguous or of doubtful efficacy.

2.03 An automatic stop order policy provides that after a predetermined time a drug order is stopped unless (1) the order indicates a specific number of doses to be given, (2) an exact period of time for the administration of the drug is indicated or (3) the attending physician reorders the drug. The following time intervals for the various drug classifications are in effect:

	Drug classification	Interval
1.	Narcotics	3 days
2.	Antibiotics	7 days
3.	Anticoagulants	7 days
4.	Anti-emetics	7 days
5.	Cold and cough preps	7 days
6.	Sulfonamides	7 days
7.	Antineoplastics	7 days
8.	Antihistamines	7 days
9.	Dermatologicals	7 days
10.	Hormones	7 days
11.	All others	30 days

(According to the Medicare regulations all drugs must be reordered every 30 days)

For orders not specifying the number of doses or the duration of administration, the pharmacist will dispense only until the specified stop order is reached. The physician should be notified before the last dose is given so that he may reorder the drug if necessary. It is not necessary to phone the physician at night. The pharmacist will keep patient medication records and can notify the physician and have the physician reorder or stop the drug in the nursing home. Cardiovascular, antidiabetic and anticonvulsant drugs are not to be stopped without approval of the physician, although the general 30 day limit will be used as a guideline for renewal of the orders by the physician.

2.04 (a) The pharmacist will daily check with appropriate nursing personnel to determine which patients have new medication orders. The pharmacist will routinely verify these orders in the patient's medical record.

(b) A direct copy (*i.e.*, photocopy, carbon copy or NCR-type copy) of all new medication orders shall be transmitted to the pharmacist.

3.00 PROCUREMENT AND DISPENSING OF MEDICATIONS

3.01 The pharmacist, with the assistance of the medical staff, shall determine the source of manufacture and supply of all stock medications, including intravenous and irrigating fluids, used in the nursing home.

3.02 The pharmacist shall select the brand or manufacturer whenever the basic drug prescribed is available from more than one source. The pharmacist is responsible for insuring that only quality products of known efficacy are used.

3.03 Drugs admitted with the patient or brought in by the family shall not be used unless labeled, packaged and approved by the pharmacist. Unneeded admission drugs will be disposed of by the pharmacist.

3.04 The pharmacist shall supervise all labeling of pharmaceuticals. Drugs and chemicals should not be transferred to other containers except when supervised by the pharmacist.

3.05 Drug samples are not to be used unless labeled, packaged and approved by the pharmacist.

3.06 Each medication container, including single unit packages, should be labeled with: (1) the official (generic) name of the drug, (2) the strength per unit (metric system), (3) a control number relating to the manufacturer's batch number, and (4) an expiration date if listed.

3.07 Drugs requiring dilution or reconstitution, other than those for immediate and complete use, should be labeled with: (1) name of patient, (2) amount of medication per unit volume, (3) name of nurse preparing dose, (4) date and time of preparation and (5) the expiration date. Whenever practical, all drugs requiring dilution or reconstitution will be prepared and properly labeled by the pharmacist.

3.08 Additives to intravenous solutions should be noted by labeling the bottle with: (1) names and amounts of drugs added, (2) date and time of preparation, (3) the expiration date if known, (4) the name of the person preparing the admixture and (5) the recommended flow rate of the solution. Whenever feasible, intravenous admixtures will be prepared and delivered by the pharmacy.

3.09 The physician must specifically request all drugs to be given a patient upon temporary or permanent discharge. These drugs will be dispensed by the pharmacist in quantities which serve as a convenience for the patient.

3.10 The pharmacy shall maintain a patient drug profile for each nursing home patient. This profile shall be used for dispensing, for monitoring drug therapy and for billing. (Figure 2.)

3.11 The pharmacy will dispense daily a 24-hour supply of medications in single unit packages. Each patient will have a drawer in the medication cart for the storage of his medications. (Each patient actually has two drawers – one at the pharmacy to be filled for the next day, and one in the medication cart being used.)

4.00 STORAGE AND SAFE ENVIRONMENT FOR DRUGS

4.01 The medication cart, which contains most patient medications, should be locked when not in use and stored in a secure place.

4.02 All medications requiring refrigeration will be kept in the medication refrigerator at the nursing unit. The temperature should be periodically checked by an enclosed thermometer.

4.03 Intravenous and irrigation solutions maintained as stock or for a patient shall be kept in a locked cabinet at the nursing station.

4.04 The following single unit packages of nonlegend medications are kept as stock and are stored in the bottom of the medication cart:

A. Milk of magnesia, 30 ml.
B. Cascara sagrada aromatic fluid extract, 5 ml.
C. Mineral oil, 30 ml.
D. Bisacodyl suppositories, 10 mg.
E. Magnesium-aluminum hydroxide gel, 30 ml.
F. Aspirin tablets, 300 mg.
G. Aspirin suppositories, 300 mg.

4.05 The following single unit packages of legend medications are kept in the bottom of the medication cart and are intended for stat orders that are urgent:

A. Ampicillin capsules, 250 mg. (4)
B. Ampicillin injection, 500 mg (2)
C. Diazepam tablets, 5 mg. (4)
D. Diphenhydramine capsules, 50 mg. (4)
E. Digoxin tablets, 0.125 mg (4)
F. Digoxin tablets, 0.25 mg. (4)
G. Hydrochlorothiazide tablets, 50 mg. (4)
H. Penicillin VK tablets, 250 mg. (4)
J. Tetracycline capsules, 250 mg. (4)

4.06 Disinfectants and cleansing agents should be stored in an area separate from all medications.

4.07 Alcoholic beverages should be stored in cabinets separate from medications and controlled by the professional staff. Alcohol has pharmacologic properties which justify a high degree of control, particularly when the patient is taking medications.

4.08 Only the charge nurse, or someone under her supervision, and the pharmacist should have a key to the medication storage areas.

4.09 Both the pharmacist and nurse are responsible for the storage and utilization of medications in the facility. They should jointly inspect, usually weekly, all storage areas and medication records. A written report of each inspection should be filed with copies going to the pharmacist and director of nursing. Remedial action on any deficiences should be initiated immediately.

5.00 DRUG ADMINISTRATION

5.01 Only qualified personnel may administer drugs. If nonprofessionals administer drugs they shall be supervised by the nurse (and pharmacist).

5.02 A loose-leaf notebook with a drug administration record for each patient is the basic medication document (Figure 3). This administration profile shall contain the following information on each ordered drug: (a) name of drug, (b) strength or amount, (c) route of administration, (d) frequency and times of administration and (e) stop order date if applicable. The administration is charted in this document and the orders should be regularly checked with the physicians' order sheet for accuracy.
(Note: This system eliminates the need for medication cards and a separate nursing Kardex containing medication orders. This one document is referred to at regular medication times and when prn drugs are need.)

5.03 Drugs will be administered according to the following schedule unless otherwise specifically ordered:

MEDICATION PERIODS:

INTERPRETATION:	6 am	10 am	2 pm	8 pm
Once a day		10 am		
Twice a day	6 am			8 pm
Three times a day	6 am		2 pm	8 pm
Four times a day	6 am	10 am	2 pm	8 pm
Before meals	6 am	10 am	2 pm	
After meals		10 am	2 pm	8 pm
(Unless excess G.I. irritation encountered - then give immediately with meal.)				
Bedtime				8 pm

5.04 At the above regularly scheduled dosage times, the person administering drugs pushes the medication cart from room to room. The patient drug records are arranged in the notebook according to the layout of patients' rooms. When the patient is located and identified, the drug record is observed and needed doses removed from the patient's cart

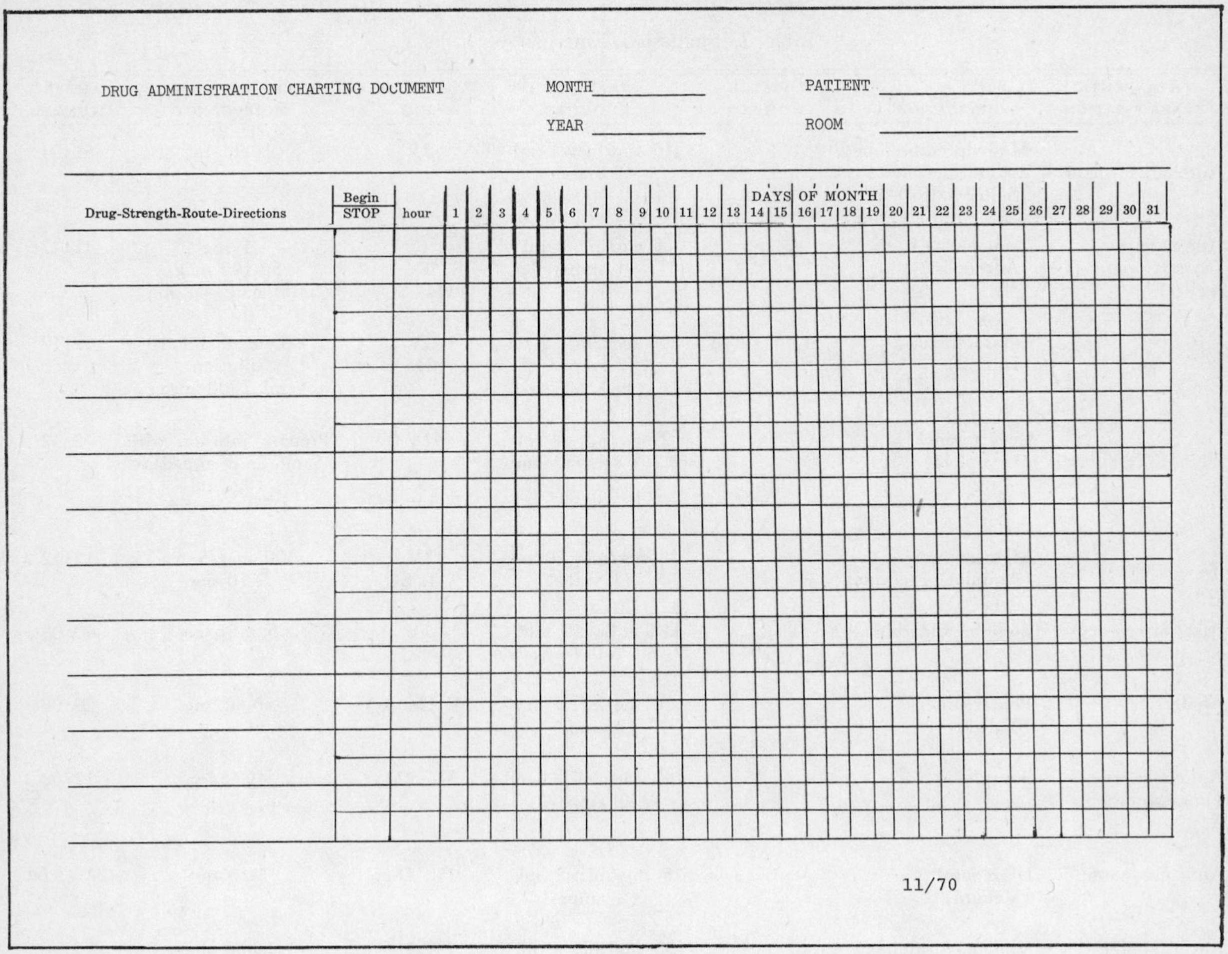

DRUG ADMINISTRATION CHARTING DOCUMENT MONTH_________ PATIENT ____________

YEAR _________ ROOM ____________

Drug-Strength-Route-Directions	Begin / STOP	hour	DAYS OF MONTH																														
			1	2	3	4	5	6	7	8	9	10	11	12	13	14	15	16	17	18	19	20	21	22	23	24	25	26	27	28	29	30	31

11/70

Figure 3. Drug administration charting document

drawer. The doses are checked against the drug record and the package opened only at the moment of administration. A dose opened but not administered for any reason should be placed back in the drawer and returned to the pharmacy.

5.05 As soon as medications are administered the person administering should chart the activity by placing his initials in the appropriate location in the drug record.

5.06 The apical pulse should be taken and recorded before digitalis glycosides are administered. If the pulse rate is below ......, the dose should be withheld.

5.07 Any dose removed from the stat drug supply should be logged on the inventory sheet provided as follows: (a) name of nurse, (b) name of patient, (c) drug, strength and amount and (d) date.

5.08 When all drug administration is completed at a particular time, the cart should be locked and stored in the designated place.

5.09 The medication cart key should be deposited with the charge nurse. The pharmacy also maintains a key.

5.10 The nurse must evaluate a patient's status and determine the need before prn medications are administered.

5.11 No drug shall be administered unless information concerning its actions, side effects, contraindications, etc. is available to the nurse.

5.12 Each nursing station or dosage preparation area should have posted a metric-apothecary conversion chart for both volume and weight measures. A list of standard medical-pharmaceutical abbreviations should be available to the nurses.

5.13 No medication should be kept at the bedside unless specifically ordered in writing by the physician. The quantities of drugs self-administered should be noted in the chart.

5.14 All medication errors shall be reported by completion of an incident report. The charge nurse shall be notified immediately, and depending on the severity of the error, the physician telephoned. The pharmacist also should be informed.

Whenever an adverse drug reaction is suspected all drugs should be stopped and the physician telephoned immediately. The reaction should be described in the nurses notes and the pharmacist informed.

In the case of an accidental poisoning or drug overdose the physician or pharmacist should be telephoned immediately. A poison antidote and drug counterdose chart is placed on each

Table 1. Suggested Emergency Drugs

THERAPEUTIC CLASSIFICATION	MEDICATION	LOCATOR NUMBER	STRENGTH AMOUNT	ROUTE ADM	USUAL DOSE EMERGENCY	AHFS** NUMBER
Adrenal Hormone	Methylprednisolone Sodium Succinate (Solu-Medrol)		40 mg/ml; 1 ml (2 vials)	IV	10-40 mg	68:04
Adrenergics (Sympathomimetics)	Epinephrine* (Adrenalin)		1 mg/ml; 1 ml (4 amps)	IC IV IM, SQ	1 mg 50-100 mcg 100 mcg - 1 mg	12:12
	Isoproterenol (Isuprel)		200 mcg/ml; 5 ml (2 amps)	IV IM	1-3 ml of a 1:10 dilution 1 ml (200 mcg)	12:12
	Levarterenol (Levophed)		2 mg/ml; 4 ml (0.2% soln) 2 amps	IV	Prepare infusion with 4 ml amp added to 1000 ml D5W or NS	12:12
	Metaraminol (Aramine, Pressonex)		10 mg/ml; 10 ml (1 vial)	IV IM, SQ	500 mcg-5 mg 2-10 mg	12:12
Alkalinizer	Sodium Bicarbonate*		44.6 mEq/50 ml 50 ml vial (4 vials)	IV	5 mEq/Kg	40:08
Analgesic	Pentazocine (Talwin)		30 mg/ml; 2 ml (2 amps)	IV, IM, SQ	30-60 mg	28:08
Anticholinergic (Parasympatholytic)	Atropine		400 mcg/ml; 1 ml (2 amps)	IV, IM	400 mcg	12:08
Anticonvulsant	Diazepam* (Valium)		5 mg/ml; 2 ml (2 amps)	IV, IM	5-10 mg	28:16.08
Antihistamine	Diphenhydramine* (Benadryl)		50 mg/ml; 1 ml (2 amps)	IV, IM	10-50 mg	4:00
Calcium Salt	Calcium Gluconate		100 mg/ml; 10 ml (2 amps)	IV	500 mg-2 g	68:24
Caloric Agent	Dextrose		500 mg/ml; 50 ml (50% soln) 1 vial	IV	50 ml (25 g)	40:20
Cardiac Drugs	Digoxin		250 mcg/ml; 2 ml (4 amps)	IV	500 mcg-1 mg	24:04
	Lidocaine*		10 mg/ml (1% soln)	IV	50 mg (5 ml)	72:00
	Procainamide (Pronestyl)		100 mg/ml; 10 ml (1 vial)	IV IM	200 mg-1 g 500 mg-1 g	24:04
	Quinidine Gluconate		80 mg/ml; 10 ml (1 vial)	IV IM	Dilute 10 ml to 50 ml with D5W; Infuse 1 ml/min. 600 mg	24:04
Spasmolytic	Aminophylline		25 mg/ml; 10 ml (2 amps)	IV	250-500 mg	86:00
Miscellaneous	Water for Injection		30 ml (1 vial)	—	——	—
	Dextrose 5% in Water (D5W)		1 Liter	IV	——	—
	Normal Saline		1 Liter	IV	——	—

*Available in prefilled, disposable syringes
**AMERICAN HOSPITAL FORMULARY SERVICE (Drug Information Source)

nursing station and, if necessary, appropriate first aid may be given by the charge nurse. For further information, contact the following poison control center:

Name, Address and Telephone number of Poison Control Center

6.00 EMERGENCY DRUG SUPPLY

6.01 The emergency drug supply is maintained in a sealed (not locked) kit at the nursing station. The contents of the kit have been approved by the medical staff.

6.02 An appropriate expiration date is placed on the kit by the pharmacist, and whenever this date is exceeded or the seal broken the kit is returned to the pharmacist for update and reissue.

6.03 These drugs may be administered only on the order of a physician.

6.04 The administration of an emergency drug should be recorded on the voucher form in the kit and on the medication record.

6.05 The following drugs and supplies shall be maintained in the kit (Table 1).

7.00 NARCOTICS AND CONTROLLED DRUGS

7.01 Drugs with abuse potential classified as controlled drugs shall be treated as other drugs in the unit dose system. Inventory by the nursing staff is unnecessary since the pharmacist issues these drugs in a 24-hour supply and checks their usage daily.

7.02 (a) Narcotics will be issued in single unit packages and treated as other drugs in the unit dose system. The pharmacist will closely monitor their usage on a daily basis.

(b) Narcotics will be issued to a patient in single unit packages in predetermined quantities and kept in a separate locked storage area. A daily inventory will be made by the nursing staff and an inventory sheet maintained on each prescription. This inventory sheet is updated after each dose is administered by noting the following: (1) nurse administering, (2) date, (3) amount given and (4) balance on hand.

(c) Those hospitals maintaining control drugs as ward stock will keep inventory sheets on each quantity of control drugs issued from the pharmacy.

7.03 If method 7.02b is used to control narcotics, any narcotic remaining because of a discontinued order or the death of the patient should be destroyed by the pharmacist in the presence of a nurse. This should be noted and countersigned in the medical record. These drugs may be returned to the regional BNDD office but federal law does not require this for narcotics issued on prescription to patients.

7.04 Unused narcotics left at the facility by a physician should be returned to that physician.

15

The clinical pharmacist in an interprofessional group practice

by Paul W. Lofholm

The essence of any clinical practice is direct patient care. Clinical medicine involves taking care of patients and their diagnosis; clinical pharmacy is taking care of patients and their treatment. This type of practice requires a knowledge of patients and their health. Pharmacists who provide patient-oriented care to those living at home are the clinically-oriented pharmacists who practice in the community. It is this type of practice I will describe, based on personal experiences with the Ross Valley Medical Clinic, Greenbrae, California.

The pharmacy practice is associated with a group medical practice which provides ambulatory services to the patients of Marin County, just north of San Francisco. At present, this health facility has eight medical specialties and 24 physicians, and provides the following services: clinical laboratory, diagnostic x-ray, physical therapy, optical and pharmacy. In effect, this facility provides one-stop ambulatory services under one roof. It is located adjacent to the county's largest hospital where back-up services can be provided.

The pharmacist is a recent addition to this group medical practice staff. I was asked to join the staff at the time when it was relocating in a new facility to be constructed which would include a pharmacy. It is interesting to note that the addition of pharmaceutical services was not based on economic considerations, but rather on professional considerations of what a pharmacist could contribute to the health team, and to the patient in the way of traditional services. However, the traditional service was to emerge as a clinical service.

The Pharmacist's Traditional Role

The traditional pharmacist's role is the storekeeper of drugs for the community. This concept is based on the inherent nature of drugs, *i.e.*, the public has had to obtain medication on the prescription of a physician, due to the danger of self-diagnosis and self-treatment. In addition to safeguarding the community's drug supply, the pharmacist assures the safety and purity of a prescribed drug and its dose for the patient. Furthermore, the pharmacist is expected to prepare extemporaneously those pharmaceuticals which are not commercially available or are too unstable to be prepared by the manufacturer in the ready-to-use state. The pharmacist by tradition individualizes the prescription to meet the needs of the patient. This traditional function provides efficient, accurate and reasonable service to the public and specifically to patients who frequent our Clinic.

Few health practitioners attempt to prevent disease. Few pharmacists have been concerned with what happens to drugs once they have been transformed into medication and they leave the pharmacy. Traditional pharmacy has been primarily concerned with in-pharmacy activities as they have related to the distributive function of selling restrictive commodities. In comparing traditional practice to clinical practice, pharmacy's traditional practice has been geared to meeting the requirements of the law, and providing an adequate inventory of pharmaceuticals to meet the prescriber's needs. The pharmacist's expertise has been in drug products, their availability, use and dosage, and in controlling prescribing practices. In addition, while some pharmacists have a strong tie with the patients they serve, acting as the patient's most accessible entry point to the health care system, other pharmacists never see the person to whom they provide service. In contrast, the clinically-oriented pharmacist has as a prerequisite the challenge to obtain knowledge about the patient before he can contribute in a meaningful way to the patient's health.

Emergence of a Clinical Role

Although these traditional thoughts were considered for the Clinic, there was, fortuitously, the thought not to foster a typical drug store. There is no commercial image. Sensing the opportunities to provide a new standard of care, the pharmacy was designed by the pharmacist to permit a maximum degree of communication between pharmacist and patient. The lack of a commercial image has been manifested by the absence of drugs on display. This point in itself is not necessarily a clinical concept, but the emphasis in knowledge-related services rather than commodity services, enjoys clinical repercussions. The clinical pharmacist primarily brings therapeutic knowledge to the health team and patient. He may or may not be associated with a dispensing function. The patient can be significantly influenced in this undistracting environment, and, the pharmacist need not spend his time on the promotion of a wide variety of assorted items typical of today's retailing. He can devote his full attention to promoting optimal health care delivery.

The clinically-oriented pharmacist is primarily concerned with patients. He only discovers that his customers are really patients when he communicates with them. However, in traditional ambulatory practice, it is possible that patients never see or talk with the pharmacist. The notion of the phantom pharmacist has been ascribed to this "count and pour" practice. Patients walk out bewildered amongst the retail jungle where someone has performed an act which cannot be seen or heard. It is essential, but they know not why. The clinical practice must encourage direct patient-pharmacist communication in its design.

Communications with the Patient and Physician

The Ross Valley Pharmacy provides several areas for patient communication. The patient may come to the dispensing area to discuss health problems with the pharmacist. The area is similar to a bank where the teller and customer come together. Without having to walk some distance, the pharmacist can directly interact with the patient. In addition, the patient may be seated at a desk for interview by the pharmacist. The barriers are minimal. There are no displays or glass windows to hide the pharmacist, yet essential drug security is maintained. In this environment, the patient and the pharmacist may interact.[1]

The clinically-oriented pharmacist does more than dispense drugs. He is interested in therapeutics — why the patient received the prescription, and what happens to the patient when he takes his drug. He is not to presuppose anything and is interested in knowing whether or not the patient takes his drugs. Some studies suggest that up to 50 percent of the patients who receive medications fail to take them.[2-4]

Patients in the community having acute illnesses may be forced to stay home from work or out of school. They may come to the doctor to obtain a cure, so that they can get back to their responsibilities and pleasures. No one likes to be sick. Therefore, questions in the mind of the patient must be answered. How long will it take to get better? When can I stop the medication? Is there anything I should know about this medication? Along with these legitimate demands are the questions of the prescriber, such as what should I use to treat this affliction? What is the best treatment available? What do I do when the patient has a medical complication in which therapy has to be compromised? Where do I go when a drug doesn't work and we have an apparent therapeutic failure? The tendency is usually to blame the drug's lack of effect on the patient's lack of response, rather than on an error in prescribing, dosing or the duration of therapy.[5] Likewise, side effects are often ascribed to the patient's changing condition rather than something that was likely predictable on pharmacologic grounds. Rational therapeutics is one goal of the clinically-oriented pharmacist, that is, to get the right drug for the right patient at the right time in sufficient quantity and dose to improve or maintain health.[6]

Ambulatory care must also deal with chronically ill patients. The problems of therapy are more complex; and the patient asks several additional questions. What happens if I forget to take this medicine? How can I get more of this medication? Likewise, the prescriber must carefully weigh the decision of whether or not to treat, and perhaps whether or not to commit the patient to a life-long course of therapy. Questions of safety and efficacy take on infinite proportions. Though the pharmacist does not make the diagnosis, he must understand it so that he can continually evaluate the patient and his response to therapy and can monitor the use of the drug. The second goal of clinical practice is recognized in chronic therapy *as a mainstream function* of the pharmacy — that is, drug-use control.

Drug-Use Control

Drug-use control is defined as the sum total of knowledge, understanding, judgments, procedures, skills, controls and ethics that assures optimal safety in the distribution and use of medication.[7] Drug-use control suggests that the pharmacist use all of his expertise to insure the effective and safe use of medication. It recognizes the patient for his total medication profile and adds the dimension of time to therapeutics. Whereas the traditional pharmacist has been primarily concerned with the effect of one drug on a patient at a specific time (only at the time of dispensing), the clinically-oriented pharmacist is concerned about the more complex issue, the effect of a drug interacting with other drugs during the total time a drug may manifest its effect. He assumes responsibility for monitoring and maintaining a continuum of therapy within the framework of the health team. He consults with the physician not only when it may be legally necessary, but more important, when it is therapeutically necessary. And, more often than not, he assumes the short-run management of therapy.

Drug-use control further suggests that the pharmacist does more than his traditional function in the drug delivery system, that he does more than distribute, stock, inventory and store drugs for the community, that he does more than compound or follow the traditional function of mixing medicines (a tradition which is more in the minds of the patient than the pharmacist). Drug-use control implies a guarantee to the patient that he will not only receive the right drug, but also the best drug.[8] Changing emphasis from a commodity orientation, with correctness and accuracy which dispensing demands, to an involvement with patients and their therapeutics — tailoring medications and usage regimens to best meet their needs — assumes certain background requirements. All pharmacists who are interested in patients practice to some degree clinically. The decision to practice 100 percent clinically is a matter of choice; that is, to involve oneself completely with the patient and his therapy, is basically a matter of choice.

Nature of Practice

As compared to traditional practice, what does clinical practice mean to the practicing pharmacist? It means that the pharmacist knows more about drugs than mere product information; that is, how the item comes, the strength, who makes it and its cost. He knows about the patient's condition and its significance, and he understands why each drug is being used. This kind of information comes from an interview with the patient. It also may come from the patient's chart, the pharmacist's past experiences or other pieces of information the pharmacist obtains in casual conversation with the patient. The pharmacist can make judgments about drug selection, having the diagnosis and pertinent medical and drug history, much to the improvement of patient care. His effectiveness in terms of rational prescribing is determined by how well he communicates his knowledge to the prescriber, the patient and associated pharmacists. Specifically, clinical pharmacy in group practice is denoted by the pharmacist's knowledge of ambulatory patients and how to treat their illnesses – such information being obtained through direct interaction with patients and physicians. For example: penicillin is the drug of choice to treat staphylococcal infections which are sensitive to this antibiotic.[9] What can the clinical pharmacist contribute to the selection and use of this antibiotic in practice? In oral therapy, phenoxymethyl penicillin (penicillin V) is usually used in preference to benzyl penicillin (penicillin G), because the absorption of penicillin V is more predictable, and for the same dose higher blood levels are obtained with penicillin V.[10-12] However, if the dose of penicillin G were doubled, comparable levels to penicillin V could be obtained. If the patient should be one of the 1 to 10 percent who are allergic to penicillin,[13-14] then the pharmacist must consider other antistaphylococcal antibiotics, such as erythromycin, lincomycin or clindamycin.[9] In addition, after weighing the factors concerning self-administration of antibiotics (*i.e.*, will the patient follow directions and completely use the prescribed medication?) and after considering cost the pharmacist can present the best judgment for the situation. So, it is more than who makes penicillin V, does it come in 80, 90, 100, or 110 ml sizes and how much will a five-day course cost to treat the patient with a staphylococcal infection. It is also what is the best way to treat the patient, and therefore what else should be considered when selecting drugs, including predisposed factors such as allergy to penicillin.

My contribution to our interprofessional group practice is to relate my experiences with drugs in therapeutics, to evaluate therapeutic decisions that are made regarding drugs prescribed and to educate both the patient and physician on how to obtain optimal drug usage. For example, to minimize the effect of food on antibiotics intended for systemic use and to reduce the incidence of diarrhea associated with high concentrations of antibiotics which have failed to be absorbed and lead to altered gastrointestinal flora, antibiotics should be taken on an empty stomach.[15,16] This means most antibiotics must be taken at least one-half hour before or two hours after meals (or one hour after meals for children as a compromise to not taking the prescribed drug at all). Furthermore, to reduce the potential for gastric irritation, all drugs should be taken with at least one-half glass of water. For those acquainted with the acute administration of alcohol, drug administration may be likened to the difference between the effect of a straight shot of whiskey on the stomach and the effect of a highball. If the drug has nothing into which it can dissolve, high local concentrations may produce irritation and nausea and lead to the patient's discontinuing his medication. The pharmacist has the responsibility to see to it that those patients who need drugs should have a successful experience in taking them, as well as to see to it that those who should not receive drugs do not obtain them (drug-use control).

Therapeutic contributions may take the form of new drug evaluations. The pharmacist must have knowledge of the disease, the prognosis, standard treatment methods and specific drugs which are employed. He must relate the pharmacology to the clinical management of the patient and be able to explain the drug's use, dosage, route, major metabolic pathways, dose responses and side effects including their occurrence and significance. For example: If a diagnosis of Parkinsonism were to be presented, could a clinical decision be made as to whether or not a patient should be placed on a drug? What is Parkinsonism? What are the symptoms? What is the current drug of choice? What are the benefits and risks of the new versus the older therapy? What happens from the physiologic, biochemical or pharmacologic standpoint? Which patients can benefit and for how long, considering Parkinsonism is a chronic disease? What side effects are likely to occur? What is the attitude of the patient toward his disease? Should this patient be committed to life-long therapy?

These are the decisions the pharmacist should help to make in order to practice 100 percent in the area of clinical pharmacy. From my experience as a clinical practitioner, these are some of the questions I have been asked. The patient, hearing of levodopa long before it was released for general use and before the basic research was complete, sought ways to obtain the drug, at any cost or risk. One must understand the extent to which Parkinsonism disables patients to appreciate the patient's compulsion to try "anything new." Physicians asked, will it work in tremor? What is the starting dose? What are the side effects, or can hypotension occur? To what extent, and so forth? Again, the pharmacist must do more than stock the drug; he must know how to use the drug, how to educate and advise the physicians on proper evaluations and how to prescribe for patients with Parkinsonism or any other disease.

Personal experience indicates the following points are important in pharmacist-physician interactions in group practice. The pharmacist joins the health team as an independent member, but informal relationships must be developed for the team to function effectively. There must be a mutual respect, a give and take. The less distance between the two, the greater the chance for interdependence. The relationship must develop horizontally, not vertically. The pharmacist must have direct access to the physician when the situation demands it. Communication is the skill which determines the overall level of patient care; therefore, this skill should receive priority for pharmacists seeking a clinical dimension.

Interaction of the health team with the patient ultimately requires communication if the patient's management is to be unified. No one member can continually provide all the services necessary to manage a patient. Hence, the institutionalization of the community's health resources into a mutually dependent health team. This interdependence is not new to traditional pharmacy, as the physician long ago gave up his dispensing role to the pharmacist; however, the pharmacist can contribute more to the team if he can communicate effectively about patients.

What can pharmacy do to more effectively communicate? In essence, the pharmacist must know about patients and about physicians and the way they think. The pharmacist must be in the right location. He must be motivated and committed to providing information which is patient-oriented. He must have available information sources to provide answers for therapeutic questions. What is available to treat a pulmonary Proteus infection at home? What is the drug of choice, route and dose, and can you document your answer? Some pharmacists present several choices of therapy when recommending treatment and establish their preference. To make these decisions, the pharmacist must have enough information about the patient to make a clinically acceptable answer. If an acceptable answer is not immediately forthcoming, do not guess, but return the physician's call with a documented answer or offer to research the problem. In limited situations, however, such as group medical practices or medical buildings, the pharmacist may go directly to the physician's office to confer or follow up on therapy. Some pharmacists find that a bulletin is a useful way to communicate about drugs and therapeutics, and provide prescribers with new knowledge.

Whatever the means of communication, there are some general points to think out before attempting to communicate. The physician is primarily a diagnostician and secondarily a therapist. He is incident-oriented rather than statistically-oriented when it comes to rational drug use. If he has had a bad experience with a drug, he may be unwilling ever to try that drug again regardless of its statistical virtue. He is more comfortable with a drug with which he is familiar; therefore, there may be some resistance to other equivalent therapeutic agents. However, the increased use of a closed formulary in hospitals or government programs has been successful although an unfamiliar agent may occasionally be used. In addition, the manufacturing industry has had little difficulty introducing new products to the medical community, even if the product is a molecular modification or another brand of ampicillin, suggesting that change is the rule rather than the exception.

When entering a new community, find out where and when continuing education meetings of the medical community are held. Hospital departments and large group medical practices often meet routinely. By inquiring, the pharmacist can attend these meetings and get a feel for the community's approach to therapeutic problems and, in turn, the physicians and pharmacists can become acquainted. The pharmacist must leave his four walls if he is going to develop clinically.

To understand therapeutic approaches, ask questions of the physician. What was the diagnosis? Why was this drug used? What has happened to the patient? To function together, the physician and pharmacist exchange therapeutic knowledge for diagnostic information.

Be aware of all current advertising, marketing and detailing practices, as they influence therapy. There is need for an unbiased viewpoint in the community. And one must be prepared to qualify a biased manufacturer's statement, as well as to evaluate critically the presented information. When given any opportunity, the pharmacist must demonstrate his expertise. The emerging clinical practice demands an aggressive performance of high quality.

At present, due to the distance between the prescribing step and the patient's subsequent interaction with a pharmacist, it is important for the pharmacist to "educate" the prescriber. Continuing education programs by pharmacists for physicians, such as in a group medical practice or interprofessional local association meetings, are useful. Evaluation of prescribing practices suggest topics of discussion. The entry of new physicians or other prescribers to the community is a stimulus for a clinical pharmacist's action to tap the potential for increasing change. Once a prescribing pattern is established for the community, the team will possess another common reference point to coalesce them. Patients will receive a uniform high level care as the result of a team effort. From the pharmacist's standpoint, all prescribers in the community will use a selected, well-known spectrum of pharmaceuticals. The dispensing pharmacist will have to stock fewer drugs than before, and can take advantage of cost savings through volume purchases.

Several observations can be made with respect to advertising. Repetition is the by-word of some manufacturers as there are many "me-too" drugs on the market. Advertising policies attempt to establish an exclusiveness for a given drug. Often small differences are emphasized when, in effect, the products of a given class are extremely similar.[17] Moreover, similarities between drugs of the same pharmacological class made by the same manufacturer are difficult to evaluate as the company directs its advertising and public information (and perhaps clinical research) to specific markets with specific drugs. Smith, Kline and French has approached numerous markets with its phenothiazine derivatives. It has been so successful that the prescriber may not know that chlorpromazine, prochlorperazine, trifluoperazine and trimeprazine are all chemically related as well as therapeutically related. Do we need thousands of drugs in the armamentarium?

When the communicative effort is initiated by the pharmacist, he should remember the positive approach. If the question is about a drug interaction which may occur, criticism of the prescriber should be avoided and clinical experiences should be available to back up your position. The overzealous pharmacist has frequently sounded the alarm when a drug interaction situation arose, only to find out that his source – the latest table – was incorrect or clinically insignificant. The usual response is for the physician to tell the pharmacist politely that he's been using the combination for some time, and don't bother him. Physicians are not likely to change overnight because suddenly a pharmacist appears on the scene and tells the physician how to use drugs wisely! It takes some time, perhaps a lifetime, to bury certain long-standing beliefs about drug usage (some physicians order, and nurses continue to give tetracycline with milk, or iron supplements, or antacids, or other inorganic cations). Each physician has his favorite drug for this or that condition. He has arrived at his choice by experience, in effect conducting his own clinical trial, controlled or otherwise. His choice may have stood the test of time, but it may not be *the* drug of choice today. Yet, in his hands, it could be his drug of choice. The pharmacist must carefully weigh this old therapy versus "improved" therapy with his own ability to communicate. Some therapeutic problems may be of low priority and it may not be worth pursuing until many other therapeutic issues are resolved. For example, the comparison between antihistamines may take a back seat to evaluations of antibiotics.

For those pharmacists who have doubts about relationships with other health team members, here is a case in point. In a telephone call to a physician, "Bill, I just told your patient that if he does not die from aplastic anemia from the phenylbutazone, he will surely bleed to death because he is already taking warfarin!" This kind of approach does a great deal to permanently end this team's season, and it is unlikely that the pharmacist will have a chance to operate with this physician again. And not because the pharmacist was incorrect, but because his approach was wrong. Communicate about the problem of phenylbutazone and warfarin interactions; do not act as a policeman, telling the physician not to use the combination, because the dosage of anticoagulant can be adjusted and titrated by performing serial prothrombin times.

At the current stage of development, the pharmacist must be prepared to answer the complex therapeutic questions rather than the simple ones. The good physician has an armamentarium of, perhaps, 30 drugs. He knows more about the therapeutics of those 30 drugs than the typical pharmacist. The pharmacist is unlikely to be consulted on the use of belladonna tincture, but the physician may want advice on the treatment of a fungal otitis externa. In other words, when the pharmacist's level of sophistication takes on the kind of problems which are not routinely seen, he is then recognized as truly a consultant. One must prepare for this level of competency.

Basic therapeutic information can be reviewed when new physicians request information. What is the treatment of choice for Parkinsonism? Select the drug of choice and the alternatives for patients with tremor, rigidity or akinesias. Formulary considerations may also provide discussions on basic therapeutic information as well as continuing education presentations. For example, at this time, trichlormethiazide appears to be the thiazide of choice, based on a comparison of effectiveness, safety and cost. If this is so, why is not more of it used? The clinically-oriented pharmacist can effect prescribing practices to the benefit of patient care when he communicates.

Likewise, from some unpublished reports, it appears that coated phenoxymethyl penicillin tablets (Abbott and Lilly) produce better dissolution characteristics than do uncoated products (Lederle, Wyeth and Robins).[18] Therefore, in the absence of conflicting data, it appears that coated tablets of phenoxymethyl penicillin should be dispensed in preference to uncoated tablets, on the assumption that a higher cure rate will be obtained. Presumably, more drug would reach the site of infection in those patients where effective concentration was marginal due to interference with absorption. In my opinion, about 5 percent of the patients who require penicillin would benefit. On the other hand, in liquid formulation, it would appear that any brand would deliver the label concentration to the absorption site because the drug is already in solution.

In the use of tetracycline, patients are often overdosed[19] but in the use of chloramphenicol, patients are often underdosed.[20] In brand selection, one has more latitude in selecting tetracycline for oral use. As long as the compendium standards are met and certain cations are kept out of the formulation, the brand makes little difference. However, the latitude with chloramphenicol is not as great and the condition of the patient is more critical. Only brands of proven merit should be selected. And, finally, cost is not a uniformly acceptable criterion for quality.[21]

Recently there have been statements made on the incidence of rash from various ampicillin products. It has been stated that there is less incidence of rash when the anhydrous form is used. The references suggest that the incidence is related to the contaminates in the trihydrate form.[22,23] If this is so, pharmacists should see to it that those patients who are prone to allergic reactions receive the anhydrous form. There are undoubtedly other factors which have clinical importance. The previous examples have been cited only as indications of how the pharmacist can, through effective communication, make a significant clinical contribution to improved patient care.

By changing the pharmacist's image from a commodity profile to a knowledge profile while simultaneously increasing his patient services, the patient will expect more. He will expect the pharmacist to have an understanding of his disease, personality, state of health and therapy. He will expect that his medication plan is safe and effective, tailored to his needs. The patient will, therefore, come to expect an individualized service from the pharmacist above and beyond the traditional "counting and pouring."

Patient Records

Historically, the pharmacist has kept records of his activities including prescription records, accounting records, drug acquisition records, drug inventory records and daily summary records of his prescription dispensing (Day Book). But few pharmacists have kept records specifically organized for patients, *i.e.*, patient records. There are significant benefits to patient health when patient records are kept. Moreover, the philosophy of the clinically-oriented pharmacist goes so far as to include this record as an essential component of practice.

The prescription blank is the vehicle of communication between physician and pharmacist. Since there may be a continuing need for the medicine, the prescription is filed. However, there are some shortcomings to the customary filing systems. The traditional numerical prescription filing system allows one to find a document primarily by number and secondarily by date. As a consequence, a patient who has lost his prescription number may not be able to have his prescription renewed again. Furthermore, patients may receive a number of prescriptions, but the pharmacist does not have a convenient or organized method to review the patient's drug usage *in toto*. The only partial clue may come from the pharmacist's accounting records. Furthermore, in pharmacies where more than one pharmacist may practice, a patient can have an identical prescription dispensed on consecutive days, while the pharmacists have no idea of this over-utilization of medication.

In this age of specialization, patients may see several physicians. Should the patient need medical services during the night or on weekends, an associate of his regular physician may see him. But, as opposed to the institutional setting, the physician in the community often will not have access to other physicians' records. Drug interactions or incompatibilities may arise. Though we may not have a means to comunicate medical information throughout the community as yet (a computerized medical record bank would provide this information to those with access), each pharmacy should be able to organize its records to assist the patient and physician when such circumstances arise. Patient records can provide this information.

Though patients are allergic or react untowardly to some medications, physicians may continue to prescribe these medications as an oversight, and pharmacists, trusting the physician's alacrity, may dispense the medication, and the patient learns of his misfortune only after it is too late. Unless the pharmacist has some historical record which documents the previous allergic reaction, such as the patient record, the patient will receive another antigenic challenge.

It should be evident that the serially-numbered prescription filing and retrieval system does nothing to protect patient welfare. It is organized for the convenience of the pharmacist and its associated legal requisites.[24] If the pharmacist is willing to promote patient safety and maintain documentation of efficacy, he should consider a reorganization of his records to meet the needs of the patient. Before considering the process, the pharmacist must recognize that he is taking responsibility not only for dispensing the right drug, as requested, but also he is taking the responsibility of making a judgment that the medication is safe for use in this patient, based on his knowledge and the standard of care in the community. It is a responsibility not to be taken lightly and for which there should be adequate compensation.

As a matter of philosophy, the patient record is not the ultimate, but it does provide historical information about the patient, his diseases and his drug usage. It is, or should be, an efficient means of recording relevant drug information about the patient; therefore, the patient record serves as a reference to review the patient's significant drug history. In time, these documents may serve to evaluate trends in drug utilization and to document the pharmacist's activity which has been directly applied to patient care, thus serving as a mechanism for improving therapeutic care in the community.

Cain discussed the patient record systems in 1964. He described the family record card to include the following: (1) full name and address of the patient; (2) age and other information including idiosyncrasies, adverse drug reactions and known chronic diseases; (3) date medication dispensed; (4) prescription order number; (5) name of physician; (6) drug, potency and quantity; and (7) fee.[25]

The pharmacist should enter the above information on the family record card, and review the patient's entire record before medications are dispensed, bearing in mind the philosophy: "Is there any reason why this patient should not receive this drug?" If the medication request is justified the medication is dispensed and the drug information is posted to the family's record. It is filed alphabetically and retrieved when needed again. This record is invaluable when one thinks in terms of the whole patient and what a particular medication will do to this patient. Other benefits have been identified in that the family can easily obtain a tax record by summing the fee column for a given year. For some pharmacists, this may be the motivating reason for utilizing the record.

From my experience, this record has some significant drawbacks. The family record, although it provides a patient orientation, is not designed for efficient use, nor for posting renewals. It lacks space necessary to enter clinically significant data. Specifically, drug data are posted, one line per drug. If one provides services for a family of four, the sorting out of who takes what is time-consuming, *i.e.*, when one is monitoring for drug interactions. Drug utilization, in terms of "are all drugs being taken when consistent for use,"[26] is difficult to assess quickly and one may have to go to the prescription order itself. Because enough space must be allotted for each member of an average family in order to record his age, allergies, etc., the card may have a limited space and hence, life span. Therefore, comparing the relatively insignificant cost of paper with the cost of a pharmacist trying to retrieve and use a family record in a meaningful way, the simpler, more complete patient record was designed.

The patient record card provides a health-oriented service offered by the pharmacist. Essentially, any factor which might affect therapy, cause allergy, rule-out therapy or improve therapy should be included and noted.[27-29] The record should be organized for efficient use by having a standard printed format. The pharmacist's patient record is analogous to the physician's office records or the hospitalized patient's chart.

Drug History

Ideally, the patient record is initiated by taking a drug history by the pharmacist. The history is a personal recount of the patient's experiences in the past with drugs and other factors which relate to therapeutics. At this time, patient identification information is obtained (*i.e.*, patient's full name, address, telephone number and accounting information). Any patient characteristics which might affect therapy are noted (sex, birthdate, weight, genetic background, occupation, hobbies, social habits and chronic medical conditions). It should be recognized by the pharmacist that exposure to environmental conditions may predispose a patient to some chemicals which are allergenic, or that work out of doors may limit the use of phototoxic or photoallergic drugs. Moreover, genetic differences may help to explain drug allergies or sensitivities in some patients (*e.g.*, Negroes and primaquine[30]), or differences in metabolic rates of handling some drugs (*e.g.*, INH and slow versus fast deactivators[31]). Patients who have narrow angle glaucoma should not receive anticholinergic drugs;[32] those with glucose-6 phosphate dehydrogenase deficiencies should not receive certain oxidant drugs (*e.g.*, primaquine, sulfonamides and salicylates[33,34]). Patients who work with some types of rubber may be sensitive to hydroxyquinoline derivatives found in bleaching creams.[35] Patients who develop their own photographs may have a contact dermatitis to certain drugs because of a cross-reaction with their developing chemicals. Patients with a history of tuberculosis usually should not have glucocorticoids.[36] Dietary tastes and allergy (*e.g.*, shell fish) may rule out the use of some drugs. Sensitivity due to iodine may exclude drugs like isopropamide iodide (Darbid, Ornade, Tuss-Ornade) from one's therapeutic list.

Previous untoward reactions should be documented by the pharmacist. The date of occurrence should be established. Drugs may have an untoward or allergic potential due to, among other things, the impurities in the product.[22] Product changes due to improvements in technology or for other reasons may have reduced this potential over time. This problem was said to have occurred with some of the early lots of chlorpromazine and since the patent has expired may occur again as other brands enter the market. Likewise, an impurity (a chloro derivative) has been incriminated in phenacetin-containing products, which can produce toxicity leading to kidney damage after chronic use.[37,38]

The kind of reaction should be obtained from the patient and from whoever made the diagnosis — a layman or professional. For example, if a patient is nauseated from a drug, he may express his reaction by stating that he is allergic to the drug, *i.e.*, he had an unpleasant reaction. But, if the drug is codeine, one can expect the drug is likely to cause nausea. The nausea is an *expected* reaction or side effect, and for future reference, this occurrence does not necessarily preclude the use of that drug again. This kind of patient response may also explain why some patients state they cannot take codeine, yet the structurally similar narcotic analogues do not cause any particular problem. No drug should be denied a patient because of the occurrence of an expected side effect especially if it is the only drug which is available. Side effects are undesired *expected* reactions seen in the majority of patients receiving a drug in its appropriate dosage.[39]

By carefully questioning a patient on drug effects and reactions, one also gains valuable insight as to how the patient considers drugs, their effects, and their usefulness. An assessment of a patient's reliability can also be made by the pharmacist. The patient's record should contain a statement as to the patient's overall respect for drugs, and ability and desire to take them. Allergies should be identified. They should be defined with respect to cause: food, drug or cosmetic. And a correlation between types of chemical agents and allergies produced should be attempted. The current drug therapy should be listed on the patient record. It should include prescription as well as non-prescription drug utilization. In some cases, it is also advisable to consider drugs recently taken especially in the last six months.

The record of pharmaceutical services on the patient-record should document the medication, its characteristics and utilization periods. If the record is legally complete, the pharmacist may actually dispense and renew prescription requests from this record, laws and practices permitting. The information data should include the following: the date or week of service, the prescriber's name and the drug name, strength, dosage form, quantity dispensed. The "Sig" or amount used per day, or prescription number (to permit referral back to the original document) should be recorded. It should be realized that the patient's illness or medication usage does not require a daily monitoring system like that system used in some hospitals; a weekly annotation is adequate. Furthermore, these patients will possibly require your services for some time; thus the problem of paper storage and life span should be considered in form design. Since the above material identifies the therapeutics prescribed for the patient akin to a prescription blank, it may be argued that one already has this information on the blank. But the purpose of the record is

Family Name | First Name | Telephone No. | Acct. No. | Year

Address - No. | Street | City | Weight - Date

Chronic Conditions
1.
2.
3.
4.

Birth Date

Sex

Physicians
1. M.D. 1350 S. Eliseo Dr. Greenbrae
2. M.D. 1350 S. Eliseo Dr. Greenbrae
3.

Remarks:

Drug Allergies
Drug | Reaction | Date

Ross Valley Pharmacy PATIENT RECORD © Day - Lofholm RVP 701

Rx No.	By	Fee	No.	D.F.	Drug Name & Strength	Week No. 1 5 10 15 20 25 30 35 40 45 50
Sig: 1 2 QOD QD 2X 3X 4X AC PC HS PRN					Ref: 1 2 3 4 5 ___ DATE	
Sig: 1 2 QOD QD 2X 3X 4X AC PC HS PRN					Ref: 1 2 3 4 5 ___ DATE	
Sig: 1 2 QOD QD 2X 3X 4X AC PC HS PRN					Ref: 1 2 3 4 5 ___ DATE	
Sig: 1 2 QOD QD 2X 3X 4X AC PC HS PRN					Ref: 1 2 3 4 5 ___ DATE	
Sig: 1 2 QOD QD 2X 3X 4X AC PC HS PRN					Ref: 1 2 3 4 5 ___ DATE	
Sig: 1 2 QOD QD 2X 3X 4X AC PC HS PRN					Ref: 1 2 3 4 5 ___ DATE	
Sig: 1 2 QOD QD 2X 3X 4X AC PC HS PRN					Ref: 1 2 3 4 5 ___ DATE	
Sig: 1 2 QOD QD 2X 3X 4X AC PC HS PRN					Ref: 1 2 3 4 5 ___ DATE	

Figure 1. Patient record form

to allow the pharmacist to monitor the patient's total drug regimen together with clinical information in a rather brief time period, rather than to retrieve each prescription and refer to it individually. The patient record organizes the pharmacist's activity for efficiency and ease of comprehension.

Other bits of information may also be useful. The fee for service information will summarize prescription activities, promote uniformity in charges and will reflect changes in wholesale costs when they occur. With some drugs, a cumulative figure of the quantity of a particular drug which has been taken is useful to minimize toxicity, *i.e.,* injectable kanamycin. In order to justify drug utilization patterns and promote optimal therapy, the diagnosis may be included on the prescription record. It would appear essential that the pharmacist have the diagnosis if he is to make his major contribution to the team. Furthermore, if the team is going to compete for the patient for optimal health care service, members must work together to achieve a healthy patient.

The patient record form used by the Ross Valley Pharmacy is illustrated (Figure 1). This record was designed by the author and Dr. Robert Day, University of California at San Francisco. It contains appropriate space for the information mentioned previously. It permits recording drug use and renewal dates by using the weeks of the year to chart such activity. The horizontal dimension provides space for information on the frequency of renewal, and the vertical axis provides a drug interaction dimension. To reduce the amount of time spent by the pharmacist in filling out the form, the patient may fill out all information above the heavy black line. The number of different drug entries and the average frequency of use should be considered in the design of the form. As a rule of thumb, the average patient receives four prescriptions per year, two of which are refills.[40,41] Therefore, this form should have several years of use provided it is printed on heavy enough paper. Finally, in the emerging pharmacies which provide patient-oriented services and which are dispensing prescriptions for a large number of patients, the pharmacist is limited by his maximum personal output. Therefore the patient record form should be designed so that it is easy to use, is efficient and still allows the necessary patient information to be studied and evaluated periodically.

Patient Interviews

Patient records in part depend upon a useful, relevant and effective patient interview. Pharmacists should be alerted to recognize problems in communicating with patients about their health and disease, and they should develop their own techniques to successfully elicit information from the patient. Patients must be approached in such a manner that they will cooperate and be comfortable. One should point out to the patient the benefits of recording drug allergies, and other drugs which are currently being used to minimize therapeutic misadventure. Patients are unaccustomed to having a pharmacist interview them but they will cooperate and confide if they understand the purpose of the interview. Finally, the interview should be conducted in a special area set aside for this purpose. Without a private environment, patients are often unwilling to discuss their personal health conditions or therapy.

Patients often forget what medicines they take, and this is a problem when a pharmacist attempts to interview them. The patient may take a drug infrequently. He may have taken a drug for so long that he associates it with food or something else, rather than medicine. He has completely accepted his condition and the medicine he takes for it. Likewise, women who take oral contraceptives may not associate or want to associate with the fact that these pills are drugs. Women of child-bearing age may have to be asked directly if they are taking birth-control pills. Therefore, to help patients remember what they do take, some interview format should be followed to discover the extent of drug use. The interviewer might ask the patient what drugs he is taking. Because of the connotation of the term "drug," the patient's response may be biased. Therefore, the terms "medicine," "medication," "pills" or "prescription" may be preferable to the term "drug." After noting the response, take a second line of questioning: "Do you take a specific kind of drug?" (*i.e.*, antibiotics, aspirin, antacids, heart medication, antihistamines, thyroid, tranquilizers, laxatives and so forth. The pharmacist can obtain drug history information by asking questions about specific dosage forms such as: "Do you use eye drops, nose drops, suppositories, ointments or powders?" Finally, the pharmacist may seek answers relating to symptoms or conditions: "What do you take when you have a cold, pain, cough, sore throat, or what do you use when you get cut?" In a questionnaire presented to patients participating in a study on the use of psychotropic agents in the United States, people were asked to respond to how recently they had taken the following types of pills:

1. Pills that help you sleep at night, such as Sleep-Eze, phenobarbital and the like.
2. Pills to calm you down and keep you from getting nervous and upset — pills that are often called tranquilizers, such as Equanil, Compoz and the like.
3. Pills that pep you up, help you stay awake, make you more alert and less tired, that help you to lose weight — pills that are often called stimulants, such as Dexedrine, Dexamyl, No-Doz, Preludin and the like.[42]

Some pharmacists who recognize the value of interviewing and patient records, will still not be motivated to undertake this service because they complain about a lack of time. Again, let me state that without interviewing and patient records, the potential to practice clinically is significantly blunted. If one wants to practice with a patient orientation, he must create the time necessary to spend with patients. Technological advances and the use of assistants to perform the manipulative skills currently performed by the pharmacist at the dispensing case will produce some change. Once the patient seizes upon the contribution a pharmacist has made in helping him better his therapy, he will seek those who provide this service.

Some pharmacists have already begun to innovate. They have the patient complete an information sheet for them, to be subsequently transcribed to a permanent record by a typist.[43] Or, the patient may fill out a portion of the record himself. Then the pharmacist can spend his time discussing pertinent therapeutic issues or historical events which the patient has identified for him.

All pharmacists who begin a clinical practice from a dispensing pharmacy should study and evaluate their dispensing systems and methods with respect to efficiency. If the time for dispensing can be lessened, they may spend more time with patients. Can the labeling activities and accounting activities be performed at the same time through the use of carbon paper?

Can new typing devices be used to semi-automate the renewal activities?[44,45] In other words, can the initial labeling work be captured on a paper tape or card to be used for renewal in an automated procedure? Can the dispensing case and drug storage areas be laid out better to save time and motion? Innovation is long overdue.

Drug Information

The clinical pharmacist in the community needs drug information which is characteristic of ambulatory patients. He needs information relating to the drug of choice, route and dosage, especially for biologicals, drugs outside of the physician's immediate specialty, new drugs, new indications and seldom used but therapeutically significant drugs. In addition, information relating to side effects and toxicity go hand in hand with any drugs used. The clinical pharmacist may inquire: has a reaction ever been reported before? What is the nature of the reaction? If severe, how do you treat the reaction? How often does this reaction occur? Should therapy be stopped? In the community there is some specialized information which is needed such as overdose data, poison identification information, first-aid measures, antidotes and supportive treatment. Other information includes the nature and treatment of photoallergic reactions, anaphylaxis, iatrogenic disease and the untoward effects of chronic therapy.

The frequently used sources of drug information of value to the community practitioner include the following:*

1. *American Hospital Formulary Service*
2. *APhA Handbook of Non-Prescription Drugs*
3. *Biochemistry Text*
4. *Clinical Toxicology of Commercial Products*
5. *Current Diagnosis and Treatment*
6. *Martindale's Extrapharmacopoeia*
7. *Medical Manual of Therapeutics*
8. *Merck Index*
9. *Nutrition Text*
10. *Perspectives in Clinical Pharmacy*
11. *The Pharmacological Basis of Therapeutics*
12. *Physicians' Handbook*

The journals to which clinically-oriented community pharmacists should subscribe include the following:*

1. *ClinAlert*
2. *Drug Intelligence and Clinical Pharmacy*
3. *FDA Abstracts*
4. *The Medical Letter*
5. *New England Journal of Medicine*
6. *Rational Therapeutics*

*Refer to Chapter 8 for more complete information.

Other drug information sources include key references on specific topics, such as drugs and pregnancy, drugs which cause photoallergic reactions, drugs which should not be used in impaired kidney or renal disease, penicillin or other drug allergy, drug interactions of clinical importance, drug interference with laboratory tests, antibiotics and superinfections and drug-induced hematological disease.[46] General educational materials include specific review articles, selected annual review articles and abstracts such as *International Pharmaceutical Abstracts (IPA)*. These and many other sources of information may be available from the local medical library (found at the medical society or in hospitals), a university library, a regional drug information service* and medical departments of pharmaceutical companies.

The pharmacist must be prepared to answer therapeutic questions posed to him by physicians; therefore, he must not only have adequate sources available to him but also he must be familiar with the sources to minimize retrieval time. This is to say, he must develop his own library as sort of a personalized collection of references, catalogued and retrieved to provide information and sources for hard copy, *i.e.*, Xeroxed copies for the individual requesting information. The pharmacist can learn from and support his opinions from this library.

The pharmacist with clinical training may find himself more and more evaluating the complications of therapy. He may screen the patient's therapy to determine its clinical significance; he may suggest treatment; or he may evaluate the complication in order to prevent its happening again. The patient may not communicate with the health team after treatment has been prescribed, even though therapy may continue for some time. The pharmacist should consider some form of followup for certain drugs, for certain patients and for certain diseases to provide optimal therapy. The followup is suggested to improve therapeutic success, to minimize the complications of therapy and to remind those patients who are on chronic therapy to maintain their therapy for this drug may be the only way that optimal health can be economically maintained. Chronic therapy must be reviewed with the patient. The patient should be educated about the potential length of time he will take medication. Patients who may receive drugs for the rest of their lives should be made aware of

* Consult American Society of Hospital Pharmacists for information regarding location of Drug Information Centers.

this possibility. If the drug has been previously prescribed and chronic therapy is necessary to maintain a level of health, then efforts should be made to continue the therapy. In summary, the pharmacist should provide drug and health information to the patient; likewise, he should contribute information about the patient to the health team, when appropriate.[47]

Principles of Therapy

A pharmacist interested in community clinical practice should master basic principles of therapy (*i.e.*, rational therapeutics). Any drug used should be the most effective drug for the indication and patient, yet it should have the least amount of side effects, minimal toxicity and be of reasonable cost. The drug should not significantly interrupt normal ambulatory functions, otherwise the patient may not continue therapy. There is no professional supervision of the patient in terms of drug administration, nor in terms of observance of debilitating side effects. In general, drugs are more innocuous as used in the community because of the limitations of self-administration. Oral therapy is used because of self-administration. Solids as dosage forms are preferred because they are less expensive and more stable than liquid forms, though they may take longer to go into solution and to act. Liquids are prescribed when patients cannot swallow solids due to age (pediatrics), disease (esophagitis) or personal preference. The rectal route is suggested when the oral route cannot be used, such as in severe nausea, or when local treatment is desired.

The pharmacist should consider the effect of food on the administration of drugs as previously explained. Food will alter the absorption of drugs either by delaying the absorption or by limiting the amount absorbed. Food delays the stomach's emptying time, prolonging the time for the drug to reach the absorption site, the intestine. However, for drugs acting locally in the gastrointestinal tract, administration with food or after meals may be advantageous.

It is generally known that *p*H conditions may affect the stability or absorption of drugs. Gastric acidity significantly destroys the activity of penicillin G, therefore penicillin V is usually recommended for susceptible infections. Those *p*H conditions which favor the formation of the salt form of acids and bases may limit the absorption of those drugs, since drugs must be in their unionized form to be effectively absorbed.

Drugs which lack water solubility are most susceptible to the technology of dosage formulation.[48,49] In these conditions, there is the greatest chance for lack of efficacy due to dosage form design. It behooves the pharmacist to select those brands which have demonstrated efficacy if the patient is to receive optimal care (an increasingly significant role). Clinical ramifications are ever present. On the other hand, the activity of water-soluble drugs are little influenced by dosage form design provided that they are not enteric coated and the current compendium standards are maintained.

Another principle of oral therapy recognizes that side effects, diseases, prior surgical procedures, toxicities or contraindications may limit this route. Obstruction, unconsciousness, nausea and vomiting are contraindications. Some drugs, such as steroids, reserpine, phenylbutazone, indomethacin, caffeine or aspirin, may be contraindicated because of the potential for gastrointestinal ulceration. Lack of patient cooperation, understanding or acceptance of responsibility to take medications may suggest other routes to be used. Finally, because of uncertainties of drug absorption, the oral route may be ruled out, especially when the patient is acutely ill.

Drugs which significantly affect the ambulatory patient and his life style should be recognized with hazards weighed against other available drugs. Drugs which depress the nervous system take away one of the body's defense mechanisms of survival. Sometimes the patient is not even aware of the drug's effects. Lethal situations occur when other depressants are taken concurrently, or when patients operate automobiles or other machines which require the reactions of a normal man.[50] Drugs producing orthostatic hypotension may adversely affect ambulatory patients. Unexpected drops in blood pressure may have a temporary leveling effect on patients. Some phenothiazines and antihypertensive medications are associated with this effect.

Drugs which alter perception or sensory function may limit the body's defense mechanisms. Here are a few examples: Parasympatholytics have blocked the sweating mechanism leading to a form of heat stroke.[51,52] Lysergic acid diethylamide has not produced toxicity by itself, but patient's perceptions have been so grossly distorted that colors run together and depth perception is impaired which may lead to walking out in front of traffic or walking through windows only to land several stories below on the ground.[53] Local anesthetics placed repeatedly into the eye of a patient with a flash burn or

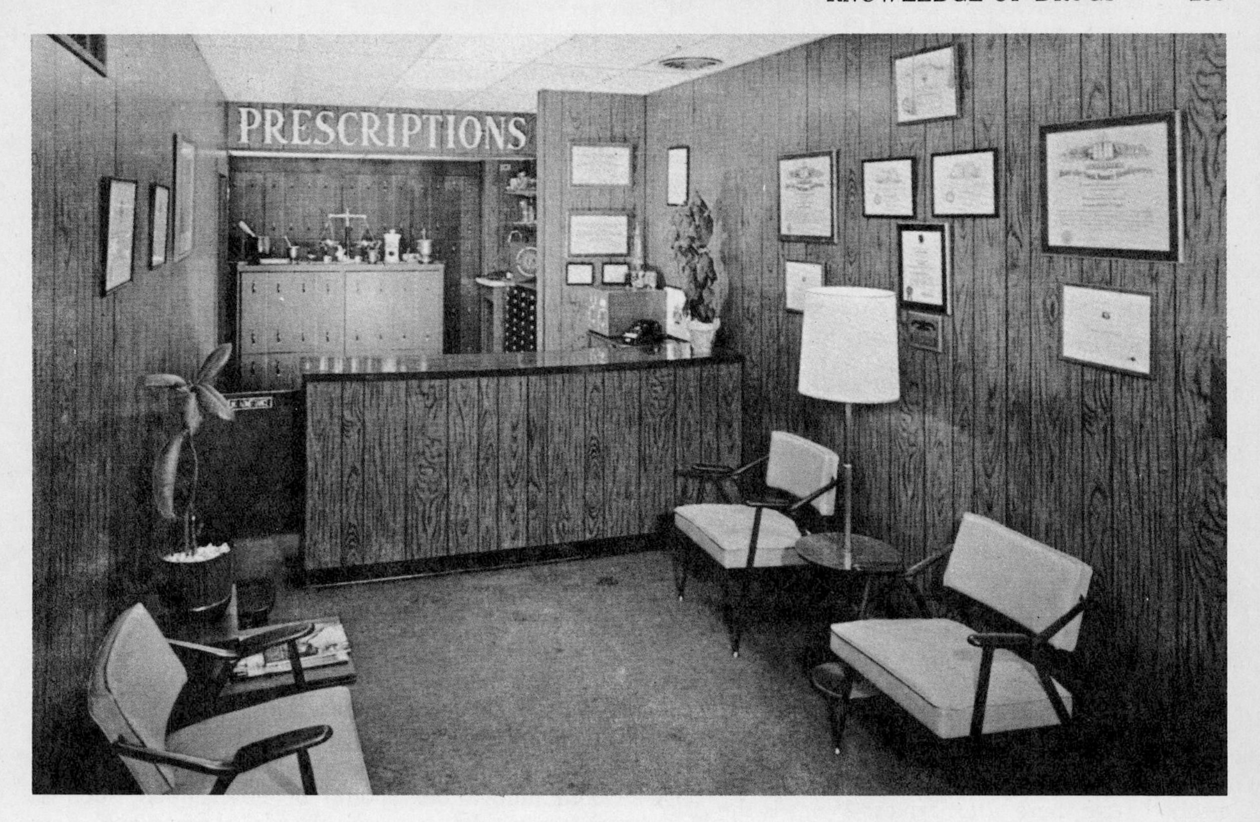

Figure 2. The pharmaceutical office of D'Angelos Pharmacy in East Rockaway, New York

minor injuries have led to a scratched cornea, severe keratitis and even permanent reduction of visual acuity because the patient could not feel what was going on.[54,55]

In setting up a program to develop the clinical discipline in the community, one must possess a working knowledge of the drugs, diseases and types of patients most commonly seen. For example, depending on the age of the local population, drugs may be prescribed mostly for geriatric patients with one or more chronic diseases, for well patients who seek chemical contraception or for children with acute problems such as streptococcal throat infections or acute otitis media. The condition may be high blood pressure in an elderly person or in a husband with a young family, with the treatment varying widely for the same condition because high blood pressure in the young patient carries a greater risk than that in the older patient. Some patients love to take drugs, as any hypochondriac knows. Other patients hate to take anything, especially unnatural, synthetic things. So you may have to recommend digitalis leaf over digoxin despite the fact that the natural product has more side effects. If the patient will not take his medication, it does no good to prescribe it. If the patient does not know how to take his medication, it does no good to dispense it. And if there are any other factors which can be controlled or complied with to achieve a therapeutic objective, one had better try it. For example, some patients associate a significance to red-colored medicine. Some patients state they cannot take capsules. Even the dosage form must be tailored to the patient's needs.

As an integral member of the health team, the pharmacist must recognize conditions unique to his community in terms of the resources and the customs in the delivery of health care. Can any barriers for the patient be overcome by the pharmacist's intervention? Can the pharmacist communicate with the prescriber to provide a basis for improved patient care? Can a dentist be found for the patient on a Saturday night? Is there a pharmacist available to provide a specialized product to which the patient can be referred? Can the pharmacist communicate with the physician to provide a more readily available product for the patient, rather than have the patient attempt his own "treasure hunt"? Who can provide the medical services which this patient apparently needs?

Drugs for pregnancy, the prevention of pregnancy, infections, rashes, glaucoma, heart disease, anxiety, obesity, ulcers, cramps, diarrhea, vomiting, epilepsy, hypertension, pain, sleep, hyperkinesis and a whole host of other conditions are initially prescribed and continued in the community, not in the hospital. Clinical practice is not unique to the institution or where the stress of life is most threatening. The question or issue is to direct problems to the clinically-oriented pharmacist. Furthermore, it must be understood that the health care system in the community has a much more difficult time caring for and observing its patients and documenting results. Therefore, the impact of the clinical pharmacist will take some time to recognize.

The clinical approach to care is organized by diseases of various types of patients in an effort to predict effects. There is a correlation between the disease and its prognosis, morbidity, mortality and potential for rehabilitation. In therapeutics, one must test, under controlled conditions, the effect of standard, experimental, placebo and no treatment on a patient with a specific disease.

The expected prognosis is summoned while taking into account the likelihood and effects of chronic therapy. And, as in all health care, the attitude of the patient toward his health is probed. Are there alternatives? What is the risk? The benefit? If the physician decides on therapy, it will directly or indirectly become the contribution of the clinical pharmacist to see that the patient receives rational therapy and optimal drug-use control in the therapeutic management of that patient.

Finally, there are some attributes of practitioners or those seeking the practice of pharmacy which determine just how each individual fits into the health care delivery system. Ability to cooperate and communicate about those knowledge-related services, performed by the health team, at the patient level are essential. The location of practice determines the volume and extent of utilization and its substructure. Imagination gives rise to new ways to solve complex problems. Confidence is the energy which propels the individual into new encounters. One must make the most of his time in the health delivery system because there are not enough of us. Training establishes the level of practice and the long-range contributions to practice. Resources provide the wherewithal to repeat scientific decisions which have been made in the past in like or similar situations. Acceptance is the outcome of a job done in a manner which is useful, and appreciated. The pharmacist must contribute in all ways to keep the health team in the running. The community pharmacist must take advantage of all opportunities to promote better patient care.

Conclusions

Rational therapy demands that community patients understand how, when and how long to take prescribed medications. Optimal drug-use control concepts activate clinical responses from pharmacists in the area of multiple drug use, under and over-utilization and self-medication, suggesting the need for patient records and a look at the total *therapy*.

Patient records promote better therapy and can prevent adverse therapy. They identify the patient for whom therapy has been suggested, noting those characteristics which individualize therapy, and these records document the use of a drug in a specific condition. From the record, it becomes apparent that the pharmacist must develop ways to obtain additional information as well as to give information to other members of the health team.

The nature of the community itself presents challenges to the community pharmacist. He has a more difficult time observing patients on a day-to-day basis, when his practice is compared to that of the institutional pharmacist. Some study and innovations should be entertained, such as patient followup and the development of new relationships between the patient and the pharmacist as they are related to therapy and its management. This relationship may be developed at the time of the drug history interview and at the time of dispensing. Furthermore, patient mobility challenges the imagination of the community pharmacist to establish the concept of one pharmacist for the patient where all medication records are kept, to allow for optimal patient monitoring and to facilitate the transfer of records between practitioners.

The community pharmacist must have the clinical training and experience relating to ambulatory patients to be effective in the health team, as envisioned. He must provide patients with services and contribute his knowledge to their welfare. It is not enough to dispense the right drug; the pharmacist must see to it that the best drug is prescribed.

References

1. Crosby, D. J.: Pharmacists in Splendid Isolation, *New Engl. J. Med. 281*:331-332 (Aug. 7) 1969.

2. Roth, H. P. and Berger, D. G.: Studies on Patient Cooperation in Ulcer Treatment, *Gastroenterology 38*:630-633 (Apr.) 1960.

3. Dunlop, D. M.: Drug Control and the British Health Service, *Ann. Internal Med. 71*:237-244 (Aug.) 1969.

4. Gordis, L., Markowitz, M. and Lilienfeld, A. M.: Inaccuracy in Using Interviews to Estimate Patient Reliability in Taking Medication at Home, *Med. Care* 7:49 (Jan.-Feb.) 1969.

5. Morelli, H.: Solving Problems of Treatment of the Hypertensive Patient Who Has a Myocardial Infarction (Drug Interaction), Presented at the Symposium on Drug Therapy, Continuing Education in Health Sciences, University of California at San Francisco, Jan. 14, 1971, p. 12, 19, 20.

6. Anon.: Task Force on Prescription Drugs: The Drug Prescribers, Pub. 327-018 U. S. Govt. Printing Office, Dec., 1968, p. 3.

7. Brodie, D. C.: The Challenge to Pharmacy in Times of Change, Am. Pharm. Assoc. and Am. Soc. Hosp. Pharmacists, Washington, D. C., 1966, p. 39.

8. Heller, W. M.: At the Frontier, *Am. J. Pharm. Educ. 32*:733-746 (Dec.) 1968.

9. Anon.: Antimicrobial Drugs of Choice, *Med. Letter Drugs Therap. 10*:79-84 (Oct. 4) 1968.

10. Griffith, R. S.: Comparison of Penicillin V and Penicillin G Blood Levels, *Antibiot. Med. Clin. Therapy 5*:44-45 (Jan.) 1958.

11. Peck, F.: *Antibiot. Ann. 1955-56,* p. 506.

12. Reilly, M. J. *et al.*, (eds.): *American Hospital Formulary Service,* Am. Soc. Hosp. Pharmacists, Washington, D. C. (Dec.) 1962, p. 8:12.16 (Penicillin, Phenoxymethyl).

13. Van Arsdel, P. P., Jr.: Allergic Reactions to Penicillin, *J. Am. Med. Assoc. 191*:238-239 (Jan. 18) 1965.

14. Anon.: Penicillin Allergy, *Med. Letter Drugs Therap. 10*:101 (Dec. 13) 1968.

15. Griffith, R. S. and Black, H. R.: Comparison of Low Doses of Potassium Penicillin V with Larger Quantities of Potassium Penicillin G, *Current. Therap. Res. 6*:253-260 (Apr.) 1964.

16. Griffith, R. S. and Peck, F. B., Jr.; Comparison of Oral Penicillin V with Injectable Procaine Penicillin, *Antibiot. Chemother. 8*:143-148 (Mar.) 1958.

17. Fekety, F. R., Jr.: Clinical Pharmacology of the New Penicillins and Cephalosporins, *Pharmacol. Physicians 1*:1-7 (Oct.) 1967.

18. Mok, J. and Lofholm, P. W.: Unpublished Studies on the Dissolution of Phenoxymethylpenicillin, Dec. 1968.

19. Pratt, R.: Personal Communication, 1963.

20. Best, W. R.: Chloramphenicol-Associated Blood Dyscrasias. *J. Am. Med. Assoc. 201*:184-188 (July 17) 1967.

21. Goyan, J. E.: Generic Equivalency and Therapeutic Efficacy Statement, read before the Subcommittee on Health, Education, and Welfare Services, Interim Committee on Ways and Means, Calif. State Assembly, Nov. 22, 1966.

22. Shapiro, S., *et al.*: Drug Rash with Ampicillin and Other Penicillins, *Lancet 2*:969-972 (Nov. 8) 1969.

23. Knudsen, E. T., Dewdney, J. M. and Trafford, J. A. P.: Reduction in Incidence of Ampicillin Rash by Purification of Ampicillin, *Brit. Med. J. 1*:469-471 (Feb. 21) 1970.

24. Hussar, D. A.: "The Prescription," in Osol, A. *et al.* (eds.), *Remington's Pharmaceutical Sciences,* ed. 14, Mack Publishing Co., Easton, Pa., 1970, p. 1814-1816.

25. Cain, R.: Patient Record Systems, *J. Am. Pharm. Assoc. NS4*:164-168 (Apr.) 1964.

26. Anon.: Pharmacy Rules and Regulations, California State Board of Pharmacy, Section 1717 (h), p. 88 (1971).

27. Lofholm, P. W.: Factors Which May Affect Drug Therapy, Symposium on Thoughts on Being a Pharmacist, Continuing Education in Health Sciences, University of California at San Francisco, Jan. 30 1969.

28. Weinstein, L. and Dalton, A. C.: Host Determinants of Response to Antimicrobial Agents, *New Engl. J. Med. 279*: 467-473 (Aug. 29), 524-531 (Sept. 5), 580-588 (Sept. 12) 1968.

29. Goldstein, A., Aronow, L. and Kalman, S.: *Principles of Drug Action,* Harper and Row, New York, N. Y. 1968, pp. 343-734.

30. Kellermeyer, R. W. *et al.*: Hemolytic Effect of Therapeutic Drugs, *J. Am. Med. Assoc. 180*:388-394 (May 5) 1962.

31. Evans, D. A. P., Manley, K. A. and McKusick, V. A.: Genetic Control of Isoniazid Metabolism in Man, *Brit. Med. J. 2*:485-491 (Aug. 13) 1960.

32. Havener, W. H.: *Ocular Pharmacology,* ed. 2, C. V. Mosby Co., St. Louis, Mo., 1970, pp. 192, 459-461.

33. Brewer, G. J., Tarlov, A. R. and Alving, A. S.: The Methemoglobin Reduction Test for Primaquine-Type Sensitivity of Erythrocytes, *J. Am. Med. Assoc. 180*:386-388 (May 5) 1962.

34. Beutler, E.: Drug-Induced Hemolytic Anemia, *Pharmacol. Rev. 21*:73-103 (Mar.) 1969.

35. Anon.: Triturations — Hydroquinones and Depigmenting Agents, *Bull. Peninsula Pharm. Soc. 5*:53 (Oct.) 1966.

36. Goodman, L. S. and Gilman, A.: *The Pharmacological Basis of Therapeutics,* ed. 4, The MacMillan Co., New York, N. Y., 1970, p. 1338.

37. Gault, M. A. *et al.*: Syndrome Associated with the Abuse of Analgesics, *Ann. Internal Med. 68*:906-925 (Apr.) 1968.

38. Harvald, B., Valdorf-Hansen, F. and Nielsen, A.: Effect on the Kidney of Drugs Containing Phenacetin, *Lancet 1*:303-305 (Feb. 6) 1960.

39. Koch-Weser, J.: Definition and Classification of Adverse Drug Reactions, *Drug Inform. Bull. 2*:72-78 (July-Sept.) 1968.

40. Anon.: Cost and Acquisition of Prescribed and Non-Prescribed Medicines — United States July 1964 to June 1965, PHS Publication No. 1000, Series 10-No. 33, U. S. Dept. of HEW, U. S. Govt. Printing Office, Oct., 1966, p. 7.

41. Brodie, D. C.: Drug Utilization and Drug Utilization and Control, Health Services and Mental Health Administration, Rockville, Md., Apr., 1970, p. 17.

42. Balter, M. B. and Levin, J.: The Nature and Extent of Psychotropic Drug Usage in the United States, *Psychopharmacol. Bull. 5*:3-13 (Oct.) 1969.

43. Miller, R. A.: Personal communication, University of California School of Pharmacy, San Francisco, Dec. 1969.

44. Stein, Stanley I.: Semi-Automating a Community Pharmacy, *J. Am. Pharm. Assoc. NS9*:522-524 (Oct.) 1969.

45. Itel Corporation (Palo Alto, Calif.), IBM, Friden (Flexowriter).

46. Miller, A.: Sources of Drug Information, Presented at Continuing Education Symposium for Pharmacists, University of California, Jan., 1970, p. 40.

47. Hansten, P. D.: Pharmacist's Role in Treatment, *New Engl. J. Med. 280*:565 (Mar. 6) 1969.

48. Sorby, D. L.: Symposium on 'Some Thoughts on Being a Pharmacist', A Guide to Selecting the Generic Product. Continuing Education in Health Sciences, University of California at San Francisco, Jan. 31, 1969.

49. Anon.: Task Force on Prescription Drugs, *op. cit.*, p. 24.

50. Perry, C. J. G. and Morgenstern, A. L.: Drugs and Driving, *J. Am. Med. Assoc. 195*:376-379 (Jan. 31) 1966.

51. Goodman, L. S. and Gilman, A.: *op. cit.*, p. 545.

52. Hofmann, W. W., and Hollister, L. E.: Pharmacotherapy for Parkinson's Disease: A New Era, *Pharmacol. Physicians 4*:1-8 (July) 1970.

53. Goodman, L. S. and Gilman, A.: *op. cit.*, p. 196-197.

54. Epstein, D. L. and Paton, D.: Keratitis from Misuse of Corneal Anesthetics, *New Engl. J. Med. 279*:396-399 (Aug. 22) 1968.

55. Vaughan, D., Cook, R. and Asbury, T.: *General Ophthalmology,* ed. 5, Lange Medical Publications, Los Altos Calif., 1968, p. 45.

Suggested Reading

1. Knapp, D. A. *et al.*: The Pharmacist as a Drug Advisor, *J. Am. Pharm. Assoc. NS9*:502-505, 543 (Oct.) 1969.

2. Knapp, D. A. and Knapp, D. E.: An Appraisal of the Contemporary Practice of Pharmacy, *Am. J. Pharm. Educ. 32*:747-758 (Dec.) 1968.

3. Rosner, M. M.: Attitudes Toward Maintaining Family Records on Drug Sensitivities, *J. Am. Pharm. Assoc. NS4*: 169-172, 175 (Apr.) 1964.

16

Biological half-lives and their clinical applications

by Wolfgang A. Ritschel

The term "half-life" or "half-time" is an expression used in isotope chemistry. It is the time required for half of the atoms of a radioactive substance present at the beginning to become disintegrated. Thus one-half of a given quantity of P^{32} is converted to S^{32} in 14.3 days. This half-life is independent of the amount used. With the half-life, half of the radioactive element A is transferred to the element B. It is a constant parameter for one and the same substance.

The term "biological half-life" means the same in principle but it is not a constant parameter for a given substance at any dose or administered in different dosage forms. The biological half-life is rather complex and depends on different factors. The biological half-life or half-life-time or elimination half-life was introduced into pharmacokinetics by Dost.[1] This term is indeed one of the most important pharmacokinetic parameters because it allows a schedule to ensure the maintenance of effective blood levels without excessive cumulation or danger of toxicity. Drugs having a long half-life need to be given at long dose intervals or smaller doses at less frequent intervals to maintain the therapeutic concentration. When the biological half-life is short, higher maintenance doses at shorter time intervals are required. As a general rule it may be said that blood and tissue levels are directly proportional to the absorbed dose at low dose levels and inversely proportional to the inactivation of drug. At higher doses there may be non-proportionality.

As defined in biopharmaceutics, biological half-life is the time required for the plasma, serum or whole blood drug concentration to drop to one-half its value following the establishment of the pseudo-equilibrium. The loss of drug from plasma, serum or whole blood is due to metabolism or excretion into urine or feces. Only those drugs which are absorbed have a biological half-life. Those drugs which act locally in the gastrointestinal tract, such as charcoal, kaolin and pectin, have therefore no biological half-life. Using the term biological half-life implies that the loss of unchanged drug follows a first-order reaction.

The biological half-life, expressed as $t_{1/2}$ or $t_{50\%}$ of a drug is a function of the magnitude of all the different volumes of body fluids and body tissues and all the rate constants of the system, including the rate constants for distribution. It depends on the drug transfer through and across the different membranes and barriers, the metabolism and the urinary excretion of the unchanged drug.[2]

DETERMINATION OF BIOLOGICAL HALF-LIFE

In a one-compartment model the drug is evenly distributed between the blood system and the tissues and other body fluids. In this case the whole body can be considered as one reaction container or one compartment. In a two-compartment model the drug is not evenly distributed between the blood system or central compartment and the tissues or other body fluids, which are called peripheral compartments. The drug leaves the central compartment and enters the peripheral compartment as characterized by the rate constant k_{12} and it leaves the peripheral compartment, entering the central compartment, as characterized by the rate constant k_{21}.

The biological half-life is most accurately calculated from blood level curves obtained upon intravenous administration of the drug. The drug concentration in blood, serum or plasma is plotted on semi-log paper versus time. The graphs are then used for mathematical or graphical determination of the biological half-life. Biological half-lives may also be obtained from blood level data after peroral or intramuscular administration.[3,4]

The concept of a one-compartment model and a two-compartment model is given in Figures 1 and 2.

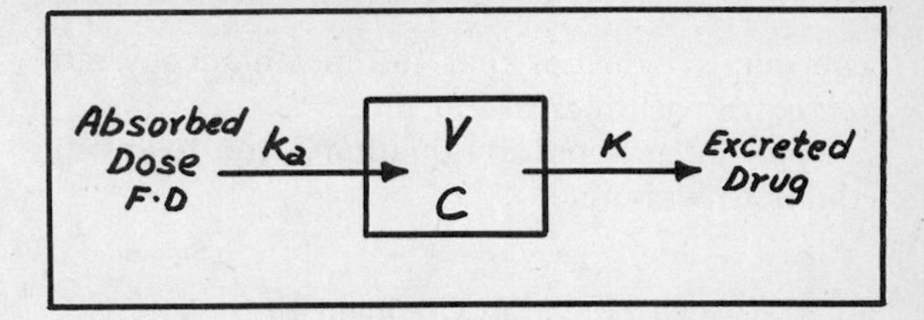

Figure 1. Open one-compartment model

V = volume of compartment
C = drug concentration in compartment
K = elimination rate constant
k_a = absorption rate constant

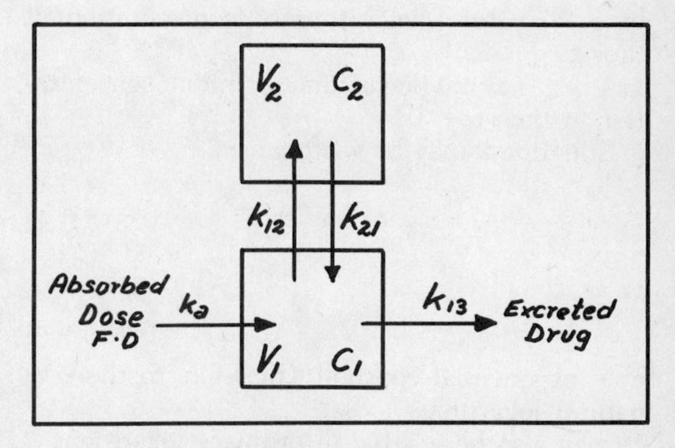

Figure 2. Open two-compartment model

V_1 = volume of central compartment
C_1 = drug concentration in central compartment
V_2 = volume of peripheral compartment
C_2 = drug concentration in peripheral compartment
k_{12} = rate constant for drug entering peripheral compartment (also termed as k_1)
k_{13} = elimination rate constant (also termed as k_{e1} or K or K_{e1})
k_{21} = rate constant for re-entering central compartment (also termed as k_{-1})
k_a = absorption rate constant

ONE COMPARTMENT MODEL

Mathematical Method

When the rate of a reaction is proportional to the first power of the concentration of a reactant and may be expressed mathematically in the form of Equation 1,

$$\frac{dc}{dt} = -k \cdot c \qquad \text{(Equation 1)}$$

the reaction is said to be of first order with respect to the reactant.

c = concentration, when t= O
k = proportionality constant (first-order rate constant)

Equation 1 indicates that the instantaneous rate of change of concentration (=dc/dt) is directly proportional to concentration c at time t.

The minus indicates that the instantaneous rate decreases with increase in time.

Upon integration of Equation 1 the following equation is obtained:

$$\ln c = \ln c_o - k \cdot t \quad \text{(Equation 2)}$$

ln = natural or Napierian logarithm
log = ordinary logarithm to the base 10

Both may be converted into each other by the following equation:

$$\ln x = 2.303 \cdot \log x \quad \text{(Equation 3)}$$

ln c = natural logarithm of concentration at time t
ln c_o = natural logarithm of initial concentration at time t = 0

Equation 2 may be written as:

$$\ln \frac{c}{c_o} = -k \cdot t \quad \text{(Equation 4)}$$

or as

$$c = c_o \cdot e^{-kt} \quad \text{(Equation 5)}$$

e = exponential constant (ln refers to the e of natural logarithms).
It may also be written in ordinary logarithms

$$\log c = \log c_o - k' \cdot t \quad \text{(Equation 6)}$$

or as

$$c = c_o \cdot 10^{-k' \cdot t} \quad \text{(Equation 7)}$$

whereby k' is:

$$k' = \frac{k}{2.303} \quad \text{(Equation 8)}$$

Both Equations 2 and 6 will be recognized as producing straight lines, if ln or log of the concentration is plotted on graph paper against the time t. This action is an identifying characteristic of reactions in which the rate of reaction is proportional to the concentration of single reactant, *i.e.*, of a first-order reaction.

How can the rate constant k be calculated?

If one considers for instance Equation 6, and writes instead of k' the equivalent k/2.303, the following equation may be obtained:

$$\log c = \log c_o - \frac{k}{2.303} \cdot t \quad \text{(Equation 9)}$$

On rearrangement it becomes:

$$k = \frac{2.303}{t} \cdot \log \frac{c_o}{c} \quad \text{(Equation 10)}$$

A modification of this equation, in which a is the initial amount of the drug, and x is the amount of drug that is eliminated (lost) at time t, one obtains:

$$k = \frac{2.303}{t} \cdot \log \frac{a}{a\text{-}x} \quad \text{(Equation 11)}$$

Equation 10 or 11 may be used to calculate k of first-order reactions, when both the concentrations at the beginning c_o and at elapsed time t are known. Sometimes c_o is either unknown or is not a suitable reference. This is the case in estimation of rate of elimination of drugs upon extravascular administration. The given dose divided by the volume of distribution must never be considered as the initial concentration except upon intravenous administration. In all other routes of administration the c_o depends on the actual amount being absorbed. In that case the concentration c_1 at time t_1 and c_2 at a later time t_2 are used to calculate k by the following modification:

$$k = \frac{2.303}{t_1 - t_2} \cdot \log \frac{c_1}{c_2} \quad \text{(Equation 12)}$$

Although reaction rates may be quantitatively expressed in terms of numerical values of k, for many purposes a more useful expression is in terms of the half-life. At half-life $t_{1/2}$ the concentration c is half of the initial concentration, *i.e.*, $c = c_o/2$.

If using Equation 10 one can calculate the following:

$$k = \frac{2.303}{t_{1/2}} \cdot \log \frac{c_o}{\frac{c_o}{2}} = \frac{2.303}{t_{1/2}} \cdot \log 2 \quad \text{(Equation 13)}$$

$$\log 2 = 0.301$$

$$k = \frac{2.303 \cdot 0.301}{t_{1/2}} = \frac{0.693}{t_{1/2}} \quad \text{(Equation 14)}$$

$$t_{1/2} = \frac{0.693}{k} \quad \text{(Equation 15)}$$

Or if one uses Equation 4, the following may be calculated:

$$\ln \frac{c}{c_o} = -k \cdot t \quad \text{(Equation 4)}$$

At the half-life the concentration is half of the original amount.

$$\ln \frac{c_o}{c} = 2.303 \cdot \log \frac{1}{2} = -2.303 \cdot \log 2 \quad \text{(Equation 16)}$$

$$-k \cdot t_{1/2} = -2.303 \cdot \log 2 \quad \text{(Equation 17)}$$

$$t_{1/2} = \frac{2.303}{k} \cdot \log 2 \quad \text{(Equation 18)}$$

$$t_{1/2} = \frac{0.693}{k} \quad \text{(Equation 19)}$$

And using k′ one obtains the following from Equation 18:

$$k' = \frac{k}{2.303} \quad \text{(Equation 8)}$$

$$k = k' \cdot 2.303 \quad \text{(Equation 20)}$$

$$t_{1/2} = \frac{2.303}{k' \cdot 2.303} \cdot \log 2 \quad \text{(Equation 21)}$$

$$t_{1/2} = \frac{\log 2}{k'} \quad \text{(Equation 22)}$$

$$t_{1/2} = \frac{0.301}{k'} \quad \text{(Equation 23)}$$

First-order reactions are apparent monomolecular reactions.[3,4]

Showing a practical example we use the plasma levels of proxyphylline [7-(2-hydroxypropyl) theophylline] after peroral administration of a solution of 490 mg proxyphylline in 10 ml of distilled water as given in Table 1.

The plasma values plotted on Cartesian graph paper are illustrated in Figure 3.

Table 1. Plasma Levels of Proxyphylline After Peroral Administration of a Solution of 490 mg Proxyphylline in 10 ml Distilled Water[5,6]

TIME IN HOURS	PROXYPHYLLINE PLASMA CONCENTRATION IN MCG/ML
0.25	3.2
0.5	4.7
1	7.3
1.5	9.5
2	8.8
4	6.2
6	4.5
10	2.4

In order to prove that drug elimination follows first-order reaction these data are transferred to semi-log paper as seen in Figure 4.

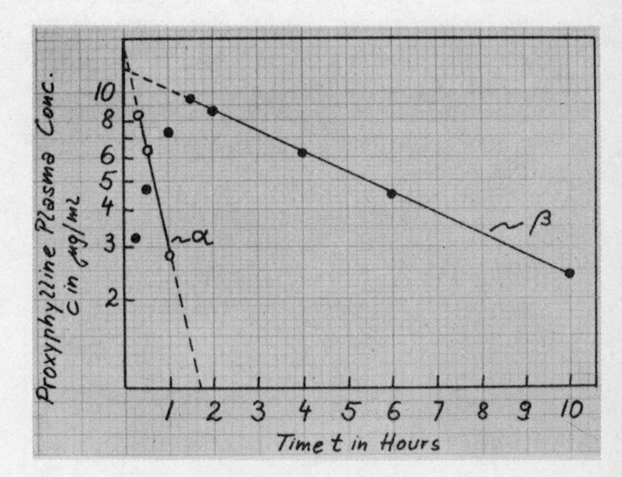

Figure 4. Calculation of elimination rate constant from a graph upon plotting proxyphylline plasma concentration values (see Table 1) on semi-log paper. The slope β is used for elimination rate constant calculation[8]

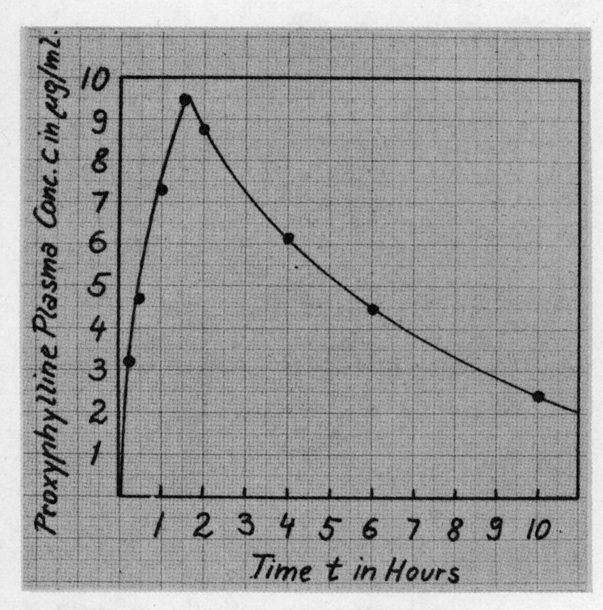

Figure 3. Plasma level of proxyphylline (upon peroral administration of 490 mg in solution) on Cartesian graph paper[5,6,7]

On extrapolation of the terminal mono-exponential decline of the curve to the y-axis, one obtains for c_o = 12. The concentration, for instance, at the time t = 10 hours, is 2.4. Taking the natural logarithm of the concentrations at 0 and 10 hours, and substituting in Equation 24, the elimination rate constant of 0.160 (hr^{-1}) is obtained.

$$k_{el} = \frac{2.303 \cdot (\log c_o - \log c_t)}{t_t - t_o} \quad \text{(Equation 24)}$$

$$= \frac{2.303 \cdot (\log 12 - \log 2.4)}{10.0} = 0.160\ [hr^{-1}] \quad \text{(Equation 25)}$$

Using Equation 26 we obtain:

$$t_{1/2} = \frac{\ln 2}{k} = \frac{0.693}{k} = \frac{0.693}{0.160} = 4.3 \text{ hr} \qquad \text{(Equation 26)}$$

Graphical Method

Using Figure 5, the biological half-life can be graphically determined. On the ordinate are two concentrations selected in the ratio 2:1. These must fall on the straight line on the slope of the semi-log graph, that is, for example, at the concentration of 9 and 4.5 mcg/ml, represented by the lines y_1 and y_2 or, in another example, at 8 and 4 mcg/ml, represented by the lines y_3 and y_4 or, in a third example, at the concentration of 6 and 3 mcg/ml, represented by the lines y_5 and y_6. Where these lines meet the elimination slope, the intersections give the time on the abscissa, at t_1 and t_2, or t_3 and t_4, or t_5 and t_6. Graphically, the biological half-life $t_{1/2}$ is calculated according to Equation 27, if two concentrations have been selected in the ratio 2:1.

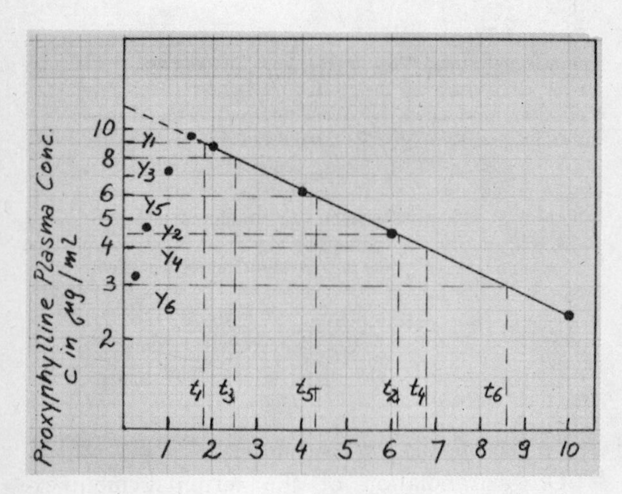

Figure 5. Graphical method for estimation of biological half-life[9]

$$t_{1/2} = t_b - t_a \qquad \text{(Equation 27)}$$

$$t_{1/2} = t_2 - t_1 = 6.1 - 1.8 = 4.3 \text{ (hrs)} \qquad \text{(Equation 28)}$$

$$t_{1/2} = t_4 - t_3 = 6.8 - 2.5 = 4.3 \text{ (hrs)} \qquad \text{(Equation 29)}$$

$$t_{1/2} = t_6 - t_5 = 8.6 - 4.3 = 4.3 \text{ (hrs)} \qquad \text{(Equation 30)}$$

In this case only those points of the curve have to be used which are on the straight line. This procedure is only applicable if $k_1 >> k_2$ which usually is the case.

The simplest method for the determination of the biological half-life is the direct graphical method.[10]

It shall be pointed out, that for correct calculation of biological half-life the tail end of the curve should be used. Many half-lives reported are incorrect because blood samples were not collected for a long enough period of time and the declining slope thus may be overlapped by a still ongoing absorption and distribution.

Two Compartment Models

In the case of a two compartment model the declining straight line is composed of elimination and back transport of drug from the peripheral compartment into the central compartment. In a two compartment model the blood level curve upon intravenous administration is plotted on semilog paper, as seen from Figure 6.[11]

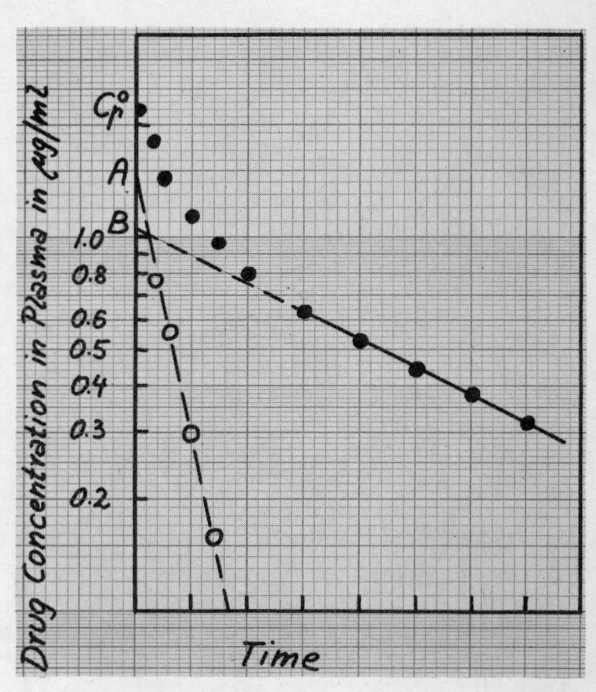

Figure 6. Calculation of elimination rate constant from a graph for a two compartment model[11]

The original plasma concentration is termed $C_p°$. The decline slope β is extrapolated to the ordinate. The intersection with the ordinate is called B. The differences between the extrapolated line and the actual plasma values are plotted on the same graph, yielding in the distribution slope α (drug distribution between plasma and tissue). The intersection of slope α with the ordinate is termed A.

The slopes α and β represent the three rate constants:

k_{12} = distribution rate constant from plasma to tissue
k_{21} = distribution rate constant from tissue to plasma
k_{13} = elimination rate constant

The calculation of elimination rate constant is done using Equation 31:

$$k_{13} = \frac{C_p^o}{A/\alpha + B/\beta} \quad \text{(Equation 31)}$$

The slopes α and β are determined by using Equations 32 and 33, where k_{el} is substituted by α and β respectively,

$$\alpha \text{ (or } \beta) = \frac{2.303}{t} \cdot \log \frac{A \text{ (or B)}}{c_t} \quad \text{(Equation 32)}$$

$$\alpha \text{ (or } \beta) = \frac{\ln A \text{ (or B)} - \ln c_t}{t_1 - t_o} \quad \text{(Equation 33)}$$

as rewritten from Equation 24 and Equation 25.

If the biological half-life of a drug is estimated from the β-slope of plasma levels after rapid intravenous injection under the assumption of the validity of a one compartment open model instead of a two compartment open model which applies to a particular drug, then it will be found that the estimated biological half-life will be greater than the true model half-life as estimated from k_{13}.[12]

USE OF BIOLOGICAL HALF-LIFE IN PRACTICE

Drug Poisoning

Plotting the concentration c versus the time for a reaction of first order, a concentration will be found at the end of each time interval which is always one-half of the value of c at the beginning of the interval. However, plasma concentration curves after very high doses, such as in poisoning cases, seldom exhibit a single exponential decline, but rather, it may take many hours after dosing to reach a pseudo-equilibrium state. Having the biological half-life for a substance, the remaining concentration of the drug in the body, or the amount of drug eliminated from the body, can be easily calculated at any time according to Table 2.

Table 2. Fraction of Original Drug Amount in the Body After Half-Lives Assuming First-Order Kinetics

FRACTION OF ORIGINAL DRUG AMOUNT REMAINING	PERCENT	CUMULATION OF HALF-LIVES
1	–	–
1/2	50	1
1/4	25	2
1/8	12.5	3
1/16	6.25	4
1/32	3.125	5
1/64	1.5625	6
1/128	0.78125	7
1/256	0.3906	8
1/512	0.195	9
1/1024	0.097	10

Suppose a drug has a half-life of 50 minutes and one wants to know when the drug concentration in the body will be less than 10 percent or, in other words, at what time 90 percent of the drug will be eliminated. In this case one has to consider 90 percent elimination of the absorbed drug, not of the amount administered, because the biological half-life is the amount reduced to one-half of the originally absorbed amount. From Table 2 the fractions of the initial amounts, 1/8 = 12.5 percent and 1/16 = 6.25 percent for the half-lives of 3 and 4 respectively, can be found. The half-life is then

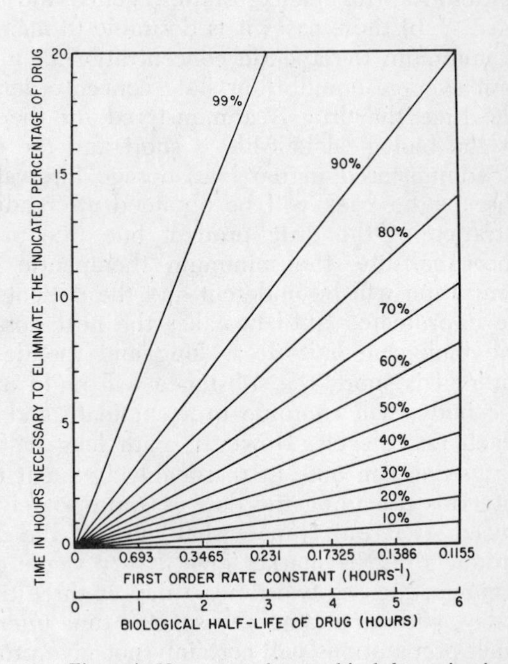

Figure 7. Nomogram for graphical determination of time necessary to eliminate a certain percentage of drug knowing either the elimination rate constant or the biological half-life[2]

multiplied by the cumulative numbers of half-lives. The half-life of 50 minutes multiplied by the cumulative numbers 3 and 4 yields 150 and 200, respectively, when 12.5 percent and 6.25 percent will still be present in the body.

Therefore, 10 percent will be approximately in the middle, so it can be said that after about 175 minutes approximately 90 percent of the absorbed drug will be eliminated. One can assume that any drug will be practically eliminated after 10 half-lives.

Wagner has given a nomogram (Figure 7) showing the time necessary to eliminate the indicated percentage of drug against the biological half-life of the drug after the drug has equilibrated with the various fluids and tissues of the body.[2]

Dosage Regimen Calculation

The importance of biological half-life in medicine and clinical pharmacy is primarily for calculation of proper dosage regimen. An exact dosage regimen calculation is necessary for all those drugs for which it is desired to maintain a minimum therapeutic concentration. This will certainly not be necessary for remedies to be given occasionally, such as preparations against headache, common cold or vitamin preparations. But it is necessary and can be vital for chemotherapeutic agents, such as sulfonamides and antibiotics, for cancerostatic agents and others.[13-17] In these cases it is desirable to maintain a minimum therapeutic concentration or a certain average equilibrium state concentration for the time the drug is administered for therapy. If the biological half-life is short and the drug is administered in too long dosage intervals, a therapeutic peak will be obtained after administration of the drug product but, due to the short half-life, the minimum therapeutic concentration will be undercut and the patient will be unprotected until he takes the next dose. If the biological half-life is long and the dosage interval is short, the substance will build up in the body, will continue to accumulate and will reach toxic levels. However, with long half-life drugs one can dose at reasonably frequent time intervals providing the dose is appropriately reduced. It is unfortunate that most of the drug products on the market give a very vague dose regimen, such as two times a day or three times a day, without stating any specific time interval. Such preparations will certainly not give protection to the patient at least overnight.

From clinical experience and also for mathematical reasons it has been found that the most suitable value of the dosing interval τ will be that which is nearly equal to the biological half-life $t_{½}$ of the drug.

If τ is equal to $t_{½}$, then the dose ratio R^* should be as given in Equation 34:

$$R^* = \frac{D^*}{D} = \frac{2}{1} \qquad \text{(Equation 34)}$$

R^* = Dose ratio
D^* = Loading or priming dose
D = Maintenance dose

If, for example, the maintenance dose D is therapeutically effective, then the loading dose D^* should be two times the maintenance dose given at the dosing interval equal to the half-life. When the loading dose D^* is already effective, then the maintenance dose D should be half of the loading dose, given in intervals equal to the biological half-life.

The clinical pharmacist is expected to be expert on drugs and drug products and to be advisor to the health team. But how can he take this responsibility if he does not receive the proper information? The pharmaceutical industry should be requested to give more information in the inserts of drug products on the biological half-life of the drug as well as the minimum therapeutic concentration. ($D_{Th.\ conc.}$ in [mg/kg]). This information would help the pharmacist to calculate the proper dose size and dosage regimen.

VARIATIONS IN BIOLOGICAL HALF-LIFE

It should be recognized that the biological half-life is not an absolute value for a given drug; it may have variations due to the following reasons:

(1) dosage size effects
(2) variations in urinary excretion due to fluctuating renal function
(3) inter-subject and intra-subject variations
(4) effect of age
(5) effect of other drugs
(6) protein binding of drugs
(7) disease (renal failure)

Dosage Size Effects

Many of the processes in the body such as active transport, metabolism and distribution of drugs may depend on the amount of drug present. Increasing the drug amount may result in saturation of one or more processes, as for instance the active transport of vitamin B_{12} is saturated in such a way so that not more than 1.5 mcg of vitamin B_{12} is absorbed, independent of higher doses. However absorption occurs by passive diffusion above such a point. If the processes are saturated the half-life of the drug will increase. Levy found that salicylic acid administered in a dose of 1 g has a half-life of approximately six hours.[18] But when the dose is increased to 10 g the half-life increases to about 19 hours because of the overloading of the metabolic processes.

Also for ephedrine and methylephedrine, a change in half-life was found due to different size doses. By increasing the dose of ephedrine by approximately 20 percent, the half-life increased in the same subject from 2.52 hours to 3.63 hours.[19]

Variations in Urinary Excretion

In urinary excretion a complex process exists in which glomerular filtration, active tubular excretion of ions and passive reabsorption of the un-ionized moiety of a drug are involved. Reabsorption depends on the amount of lipoid-soluble nonionized form present, which is dependent on the *p*H of the urine. Therefore, reabsorption will change by altering the urinary *p*H. With increased reabsorption of drugs there is increased recycling of the drug within the body producing an increase of half-life. The sulfonamide SETD (sulfaethidole) with a pKa of 5.5 has a half-life of 11.4 hours if the urine *p*H is kept between 4.8 and 5.2, but on alkalinization of the *p*H to approximately 8 the half-life is reduced to 4.2 hours.[20] This problem has been reviewed extensively by Beckett.[21] The urinary excretion rate may be controlled by adjusting the *p*H with simultaneous administration of ammonium chloride to acidify the urine, or by sodium bicarbonate to alkalinize it. Also the influence of probenecid on simultaneous administration with penicillin increases the half-life of penicillin probably due to competition for the transport in the kidney.

Inter-Subject Variations

Most of the half-life values given in the literature are mean values. The half-lives for individuals may vary widely even under highly standardized human populations. After administration of 15 mg of d-(+) amphetamine in solution to four different individuals, Beckett found half-lives of 4.32, 4.75, 4.93 and 5.2 hours respectively.[21] Working with sulfonamides Krüger-Thiemer found even twofold differences in the half-lives.[22] The reasons for the inter-subject variations are mainly hereditary, but may also be due to different diets, different amounts of water intake, physical activity and other factors.

Table 3. Biological Half-Lives in Newborn, Premature and Full-Term Infants in Comparison to Older Children and Adults

DRUG	SUBJECT	AGE	HALF-LIFE OF DRUG (HRS.)
Chloram-	Premature Infant	1 day	15-22
phenicol	Premature Infant	12-23 days	8-15
succinate	Children	5 years	4.0
	Adult	—	3.5-5.0
Streptomycin	Premature Infant	1.3 days	7.0
	Adult	—	2.2-3.2
Kanamycin	Premature Infant	< 48 hours	18
	Premature Infant	5-22 days	6
	Adult	—	2-4
Tetracycline-1-	Newborn Infant	1-2 days	16.2
methylene	Infants	3-7 months	9.8
lysine	Children	5-11 years	6.8
Ampicillin	Premature Infant	3-6 days	3.6
	Premature Infant	21-39 days	1.9
	Term Infant	< 24 hours	3.4
	Term Infant	4-5 days	2.2
	Adult	—	0.75-2.0
Methicillin	Premature Infant	4-5 days	3.3
	Premature Infant	4-7 days	2.4
	Premature Infant	13-15 days	2.0
	Premature Infant	17-33 days	1.4
	Premature Infant	26-30 days	1.4
	Term Infant	< 24 hours	3.3
	Term Infant	4-5 days	1.3
	Term Infant	8-30 days	0.9
	Adult	—	0.5
Oxacillin	Premature Infant	8-15 days	1.6
	Premature Infant	20-21 days	1.2
	Term Infants	1-6 days	1.5
	Term Infants	1 year	1.1
	Adult	—	0.7
Neomycin	Premature Infant	4-10 days	5.4
	Premature Infant	13-21 days	3.7
Colistimethate	Premature Infant	4 days	2.6
	Premature Infant	12-51 days	2.3
	Term Infants	1 day	9.0
	Term Infants	3-4 days	2.6
	Adult	—	1.5-2
Cephaloridine	Term Infant	1 day	5.4
	Term Infant	4 days	3.7
	Term Infant	10-14 days	2.1
	Term Infant	2-4 months	1.1
Oleandomycin	Term Infant	2-4 days	3.2
	Term Infant	10-15 days	3.0
	Adult	—	4.0
Sulfonamide	Term Infant	1-10 days	280.0
2-Sulfanilami-	Term Infant	11-30 days	136.8
do-3-methoxy-			
pyrazine	Term Infant	2 months	67.8
(sulfamethoxy-	Children	1-4 years	44.2
pyrazine)	Adults	—	71.1

adapted partly from Sereni, F and Prinicipi, N.[24] and Dost, F. H.[24,25]

The half-life of ephedrine administered in the same dose varied in three subjects from 2.52 to 3.26 hours, and at a higher dose in the same subjects from 2.77 to 3.63 hours, and for methylephedrine from 3.96 to 4.95 hours.[19]

Effect of Age

The reasons for differences in the biological half-life at different ages may be found in the differences in the metabolic capacity as well as in the total water economy at different ages. Premature children and very young infants have only a very small capacity to metabolize drugs. This results in significant prolongation of the biological half-life.[23] This is also the reason why most drugs are more toxic in very young children than in adults, and lower dosages have to be given than indicated by the weight. In the pediatric age range (2-16 years) higher mg/Kg doses are indicated, however. Similar is the case with aged adults where the metabolic processes are slowed down.

The differences in biological half-lives in antibiotics and sulfonamides in newborn, premature and full-term infants in comparison to older children and adults are shown in Table 3.

Effect of Other Drugs

The simultaneous administration of ammonium chloride and sodium bicarbonate for acidifying or alkalinization of the urine as well as probenecid for the prolongation of penicillin have already been discussed. Many drugs show a drug interaction with drugs given simultaneously or an increase or decrease of the metabolism of the other drugs. When acetaminophen (N-acetyl-p-aminophenol) is given simultaneously with hydrocortisone the hydrocortisone blood level increases yielding a longer half-life because the two drugs compete for the same metabolizing enzyme.[26] When the metabolism of one drug is increased by another drug a shortened half-life will result.

Many drugs stimulate their own metabolism as has been shown for phenylbutazone,[27,28,29] tolbutamide,[28,30] probenecid,[30] diphenhydramine[30,31] and other drugs.

Because antipyrine is completely metabolized and distributed evenly in body water it has been suggested that, by estimating changes in the biological half-life of this compound, information could be obtained concerning the relative activity of the drug metabolizing enzymes in an animal before and after chronic exposure. Using this method Welch and co-workers showed the effect of simultaneously administered drugs with antipyrine, with the resulting decrease of the antipyrine biological half-life, as seen in Table 4.[30]

Table 4. Effect of Drugs on Biological Half-Life of Antipyrine in Dogs[30]

DRUG PRE-TREATMENT	ANTIPYRINE HALF-LIFE IN MINUTES BEFORE DRUG PRE-TREATMENT	AFTER DRUG PRE-TREATMENT
Phenobarbital		58 ± 13
Phenylbutazone	110 ± 10	71 ± 10
Tolbutamide		68 ± 4

Antipyrine (100 mg/Kg) was administered intravenously and the biological half-life determined. One week later the dogs were treated perorally with either 10 mg/Kg of phenobarbital daily for 21 days, 100/Kg of phenylbutazone daily for 10 days or 100 mg/Kg of tolbutamide daily for 10 days. The half-life of antipyrine was redetermined 24 hours after the last dose of the drug had been given. The significantly lower half-life for antipyrine following the administration of the other drugs is shown in Table 4.

Protein Binding of Drugs

The interactions of drug molecules with plasma and tissue proteins are of great interest because binding may alter the biological activity and drug distribution within the body which, in turn, influence the biological half-life. Only that part of a drug not bound to plasma protein, the so-called free drug, is available for distribution to other compartments as well as for pharmacological action. If plasma-binding increases the biological half-life will increase. This is very important in regard to the biological half-life because in most cases the drug concentration in the total blood or in the plasma is determined chemically. By this method the total drug content is measured, rather than the free drug, which will therefore not give the true plasma concentration of a free drug. Blood levels of tetracyclines, as determined by chemical methods, were believed to differ markedly from blood levels determined by microbiological assays.[32] The difference in the results between the two methods was thought to be due to protein binding, but could not be verified. Unfortunately, protein binding is not a fixed parameter or absolute value because by increasing of drug concentration in the blood, the degree of binding will decrease in most cases due to a saturation of the available protein. This has been shown with sulfonamides. Normally, with an increase of the dose, there was a decrease of binding.[33] Rieder found in his study on 26 sulfonamides a decrease of binding occurred in all cases with increase of the concentration.[34] Some examples are given in Table 5.

Table 5. Binding of Sulfonamides to Human Plasma Protein Depending on Drug Concentration[34]

Sulfonamide	EPB VALUES SULFONAMIDE CONCENTRATION IN PLASMA μMOL/ML 0.16	0.4	1.0
Sulfanilamide	13.9	12.7	7.1
Sulfadiazine	48.7	45.1	37.8
Sulfamerazine	80.2	75.2	56.8
Sulfamethyldiazine	88.4	85.8	73.8
Sulfadimidine	82.6	78.6	66.0
Sulfadimethoxine	99.8	98.7	92.3
Sulfamethoxazole	72.1	67.8	59.0
Sulfisoxazole	94.5	89.6	76.5
Sulfathiazole	80.2	77.0	68.0
Sulfaethidole	98.4	98.3	94.3

The EPB values (Extent of Protein Binding) in Table 5 can be calculated according to Equation 35:

$$EPB = \frac{\text{concentration of drug bound to plasma protein}}{\text{total concentration of drug in plasma}} \times 100 \qquad \text{(Equation 35)}$$

Several drugs have been found which are able to displace other drugs from their protein binding. One example is ethyl biscoumacetate which replaces the protein-bound sulfonamides.[35]

Disease

Changes in physiological conditions (stress) and pathological conditions (disease) have a great influence on biological half-life. Renal failure especially may lead to a marked increase in biological half-life as seen from Table 6.

Table 6. Biological Half-Lives of Some Antibiotics at Normal and Decreased Kidney Function (Decompensated Retention)[36]

ANTIBIOTIC	BIOLOGICAL HALF-LIFE UNDER NORMAL KIDNEY FUNCTION	UNDER DECOMPENSATED RETENTION
Gentamicin	2 (h)	up to 12 (h)
Penicillin G	0.5-1 (h)	7 to 10 (h)
Ampicillin	1-2 (h)	4 to 6 (h)
Tetracycline	8 (h)	4 to 5 (days)
Chlortetracycline	5-6 (h)	7 to 11 (h)
Rolitetracycline	6-7 (h)	4 to 5 (days)
Streptomycin	2-3 (h)	2 to 5 (days)
Colistin	1.5-2 (h)	12 (h) and more
Kanamycin	4 (h)	4 to 5 (days)
Erythromycin	1-2 (h)	5 (h)
Chloramphenicol	2-4 (h)	2 to 4 (h)

The reason why the biological half-life of chloramphenicol is not prolonged in the presence of renal failure is due to the fact that the intact chloramphenicol molecule is not excreted via the kidneys but is completely metabolized in the liver. For those drugs which are significantly excreted via the kidneys their half-lives depend upon the extent of reduction of kidney function, since the rate constant for overall elimination is directly proportional to the endogenous creatinine clearance. In the case of liver diseases biological half-lives of those drugs which are primarily metabolized, usually will be prolonged.

During pregnancy biological half-life of a drug may be prolonged due to diminished blood flow through the kidney.[37] Drugs for which such a prolongation of biological half-lives has been found are gentamicin (normal $t_{½}$ = 1 to 1.5 [hrs.], during pregnancy $t_{½}$ = 2.4 [hrs.]) and nitrofurantoin (normal $t_{½}$ = 0.3 [hrs.], during pregnancy $t_{½}$ = 1.1 [hrs.]).

BIOLOGICAL HALF-LIVES IN MAN

Table 7 is a compilation of half-lives collected as library assignments to the senior students of the College of Pharmacy, University of Cincinnati, in the academic years 1969/70 - 1970/71. Data from 99 different journals were systematically retrieved. In the second year we obtained a MEDLARS search. Unfortunately, only a small percentage of the 1,981 computer print-outs checked brought relevant data. We are very thankful to the Medlars Center, Health Center Library, Ohio State University, Columbus, Ohio for its cooperation. The data collected by the students were randomly checked and verified by a graduate student, Mr. Anthony Serracino-Inglott, to whom I am very grateful.

In the process of compiling several hundred values it would not be unusual for some errors to creep in, especially when the compilation is made by pooling the efforts of many. Therefore, I would be most grateful to any readers who inform me of any mistakes noted in the compilation. I would also like to point out some of the limitations of the data collected.

In their calculation of the biological half-life some authors applied the open one compartment model where apparently the open two compartment model should have been used. Whenever possible, we recalculated the biological half-lives when either plasma values or blood level curves were published. Another error made by many authors is the fact that blood sampling was not done for a long enough period of time and the biological half-lives were wrongly calculated from the upper part of the declining curve (in those cases, where any other route of administration except I.V. was used) instead of the tail end. Hopefully, we will collect additional and more precise data for a future edition.

Table 7. Biological Half-Lives in Man, If Not Otherwise Indicated

SUBSTANCE	$t_{1/2}$ [h]	REMARKS	REFERENCES
Acetaminophen	1.62-2.83		Nelson, E. and Morioca, T.: *J. Pharm. Sci. 52*:864, 1963.
	1.95		
	>4	Liver damage suspected	Prescott, L. F., Roscoe, P., Wright, N. and Brown, S. S.: *Lancet 1*:519, 1971.
	2.0 ± 0.1	Healthy adults	
	2.9 ± 0.3	Patients without liver damage	
	7.6 ± 0.8	Patients with liver damage	
	16	Patients with hepatic coma (first 48 hours)	
	60	Patients with hepatic coma (after first 48 hours)	
Acetazolamide	1.58		Maren, T. H. and Robinson, B.: *Bull. Johns Hopkins Hosp. 106*:1, 1960.
	1.8	In dog	Maren, T. H.: *Bull. Johns Hopkins Hosp. 95*: 199, 1954.
	0.45	In rabbit	Wistrand, P. J., Rawls, J. A. and Maren, T. H.: *Acta Pharmacol. 17*:337, 1961.
Acetohexamide	1.3		Forist, A., Vecchio, T. and Smith, D. L.: *Pharmacologist 6*:208, 1964.
Acetohexamide (p-α-hydroxyethyl)	4.6 ± 0.9	Metabolite of acetohexamide	Forist, A., Vecchio, T. and Smith, D. L.: *Pharmacologist 6*:208, 1964.
	4-6		Smith, D. L., Vecchio, T. and Forist, A. A.: *J. Clin. Exptl. Metab. 14*:229, 1965.
Acetylsalicylic acid	20-30	Very large doses	Levy, G., Vogel, A. W. and Amsel, L. P.: *J. Pharm. Sci. 58*:503, 1969.
($t_{1/2}$ determined as salicylic acid)	<3	Doses of less than 4 mg/Kg body weight	
	2.5-4		Bedford, C., Cummings, A. J. and Martin, B. V.: *Brit. J. Pharmacol. Chemotherap. 24*: 418, 1965.
	5.8		Smith, P. K., ref. Wilbrandt, W.: *Schweiz. Med. Wochschr. 94*:737, 1964.
	6	Dose in the range of 0.5 g	Levy, G. and Sahli, B. A.: *J. Pharm. Sci. 51*:58, 1962.
	6.1		Brodie, B. B. and Burns, J. J.: *Med. Exptl. 1*: 290, 1959.
	5-6		Chapman, D. G., Shenoy, K. G. and Campbell, J. H.: *Can. Med. Assoc. J. 81*:470, 1959.
Actidil	4		Data obtained from Burroughs Wellcome.
Albumin	410		Volwiler, W., Fremont-Smith, K. and McMartin, M. P.: *J. Clin. Invest. 31*:686, 1952.
Aldosterone	0.63		Laragh, J. H. and Kelly, W. C., *Advan. Metab. Disorders, 1*:217, 1964.
5-Allyl-(2-bromo -2-cyclohexenyl) -2-barbituric Acid	<1	In dog	Brodie, B. B.: *J. Am. Med. Assoc. 202*:600, 1967.
Allopurinol	3		Data supplied by Burroughs Wellcome.
Alphaprodine HCl	2-3		Shore, M. F.: *Can. Pharm. J. 103*:358, 1970.
Amantadine HCl	9-15		Bludner, W. E.: *J. Pharmacol. Exptl. Therap. 150*:24, 1965.

SUBSTANCE	$t_{1/2}$ [h]	REMARKS	REFERENCES
4-Amino-antipyrine	2	In goldfish after administration of polysorbate 80	Levy, G.: *J. Pharm. Sci. 58*:721, 1969.
p-Aminohippuric acid	0.17		Bertram, D., *Dissertation,* Giessen, 1968.
Aminophenazone	3		Brodie, B. B. and Axelrod, J.: *J. Pharmacol. Exptl. Therap. 99*:171, 1950.
p-Aminosalicylic acid (PAS)	1		Bennett, W. M., Singer, I. and Coggins, C. H.: *J. Am. Med. Assoc. 214*:1468, 1970.
	0.75-1		Walter, A. M. and Heilmeyer, L.: *Antibiotica-Fibel,* 2nd ed., Stuttgart, 1965.
	1.6		Cohen, F.: *Diseases Chest 30*:1, 1956.
	4.5 5 6	Potassium salt Sodium salt Ascorbate	Fischer, H., Browning, R. H., Donnerberg, R. L., Pratt, T. C. and Atwell, R. J.: *Am. Rev. Tuberc. Pulmonary Diseases 76*:880, 1957.
	0.75		Kunin, C. M.: *Ann. Internal Med. 67*:151, 1967.
	0.57-1.03		Jenne, J. W., MacDonald, F. H. and Medoza, E.: *Am. Rev. Respirat. Diseases 84*:371, 1961.
	1.02		Dost, F. H.: *Der Blutspiegel,* Leipzig, 1953.
	1.9		Lauener, H., Hodler, J., Favez, G., Dettwiler, E. and Hadorn, L.: *Klin. Wochschr. 35*:393, 1957.
d-Amphetamine	12.5 11 13	Calculated from blood level data	Malcolm, R.: *J. Pharm. Sci. 57*:92, 1968.
	13.5 12 13.5	Calculated from urine level data	Malcolm, R.: *J. Pharm. Sci. 57*:92, 1968.
	4.4-13.8	Psychotic, dependent subjects; urinary *p*H 5.1-6.0	Änggård, E., Gunne, L. M., Jönsson, L. E. and Niklasson, F.: *Europ. J. Clin. Pharmacol. 3*:3, 1970.
	18.2-33.6	Psychotic, dependent subjects; urinary *p*H 6.7-7.6	
	4.6-13.3	Non-psychotic, dependent subjects; urinary *p*H 5.1-6.4	
	2.2-4.4	Drug-naive subjects; urinary *p*H 2.2-4.2	
	5.7-25.8	Drug-naive subjects; urinary *p*H 6.8-8.06	
	2.6-6.2	Drug-dependent subjects; urinary *p*H 4.8-6.2	
	17.9-26.0	Drug-naive subjects; urinary *p*H 7.24-7.73	
	4.3-5.2		Beckett, A. H. and Tucker, G.: *J. Mondial Pharm. 3*:181, 1967.
Amphotericin B	18-24		Walter, A. M. and Heilmeyer, L.: *Antibiotica-Fibel,* 2nd ed., Stuttgart, 1965.
	24		Bennett, W. N., Singer, I. and Coggins, C. H.: *J. Am. Med. Assoc. 214*:1468, 1970.
	24		Goodman, L. S. and Gilman, A.: *The Pharmacological Basis of Therapeutics,* 4th ed., MacMillan Co., New York, NY 1970, p. 1300.
Ampicillin	4	9 premature infants 2-7 days of age	Axline, S. G., Yaffe, S. J. and Simon, H. J.: *Pediatrics 39*:97, 1967.

SUBSTANCE	$t_{1/2}$ [h]	REMARKS	REFERENCES
	2.8	6 premature infants 8-14 days of age	
	1.7	11 premature infants 15-30 days of age	
	1.6	9 premature infants 31-68 days of age	
	3.4	Term infants less than 24 hours	Boe, R. W., Williams, C. P. S., Bennett, J. V. and Oliver, T.: *Pediatrics 39*:194, 1967.
	2.2	Term infants 4-5 days	
	3.6	Premature infants 3-6 days old	Sereni, F. and Principi, N.: *Ann. Rev. Pharmacol. 8*:453, 1968.
	1.9	Premature infants 21-31 days old	
	3.4	Term infants less than 24 hrs.	
	2.2	Term infants 4-5 days	
	11.8	During peritoneal dialysis in patients with renal failure	Back, A. and Cohen, S. L.: *J. Clin. Pathol. 21*:88, 1968.
	1.1	Calculated from k_{el}	Gibaldi, M. and Schwartz, M.: *Clin. Pharmacol. Therap. 9*:345, 1968.
	1.4	Calculated from k_{el}, probenecid also administered. Same values for I.V. and I.M. administration	
	1.5		Bennett, W. M., Singer, I., and Coggins, C. H.: *J. Am. Med. Assoc. 214*:1468, 1970.
	1-2		Walter, H. M. and Heilmeyer, L.: *Antibiotica-Fibel,* 2nd ed., Stuttgart, 1965.
	0.75		Naumann, P.: *Deut. Med. Wochschr. 90*: 1085, 1965.
	1.5		Bennett, W. M., Singer, I. and Coggins, C. H.: *J. Am. Med. Assoc. 214*:1468, 1970.
	1.8 2.6	Creatinine clearance 32.1	Kunin, C. M. and Finkelberg, Z.: *Ann. Internal Med. 72*:349, 1970.
	6.4	Creatinine clearance 13.5	
	8.8	Creatinine clearance 7.8	
	18.2	Creatinine clearance 4.5	
Ancillin	0.7	Calculated from k_{el}	Gibaldi, M. and Schwartz, M.: *Clin. Pharmacol. Therap. 9*:345 1968.
	0.8	Calculated from k_{el}, probenecid also administered	Gibaldi, M. and Schwartz, M.: *Clin. Pharmacol. Therap. 9*:345, 1968.
Antipyrine	11		Brodie, B. B. and Axelrod, J.: *J. Pharmacol. Exptl. Therap. 98*:97, 1950.
	12 1.8 1.7	 In monkey In dog	Burns, J. J.: *Ann. N.Y. Acad. Sci. 151*:959, 1968.
	1.87 1.18	In dog, after pretreatment with phenylbutazone	Welch, R. M., Harrison, Y. E. and Burns, J. J.: *Toxicol. Appl. Pharmacol. 10*:340, 1967.

SUBSTANCE	$t_{1/2}$ [h]	REMARKS	REFERENCES
	1.8 1.13	In dog, after pretreatment with tolbutamide	Welch, R. M., Harrison, Y. and Burns, J. J.: *Toxicol. Appl. Pharmacol. 10*:340, 1967.
	1.92 0.97	In dog, after pretreatment with phenobarbital	
	1.77	In dog	
	1.22	In dog, after pretreatment with chlordane	
	1.82	In monkey	
	0.53	In monkey, after pretreatment with phenobarbital	
Apomorphine	0.142	In mouse	Kaul, P. N., Brockmann-Hanssen, E. and Leong Way, E.: *J. Pharm. Sci. 50*:248, 1961.
D-Arabinose	1.26		Segal, St. and Foley, J. B.: *J. Clin. Invest. 38*:407, 1959.
L-Arabinose	1.7		Segal, St. and Foley, J. B.: *J. Clin. Invest. 38*:407, 1959.
Arabinosyl-6-mercaptopurine (ara-MP, NSC-406021)	1.68 ± .23	Ara-MP-S^{35} was used in the study	Loo, T. L. and Lu, K.: 118th Annual Meeting A.Ph.A. Acad. of Pharmaceutical Sciences San Francisco, California, March-April, 1971.
	0.95 ± 0.28	In dog	
Bacitracin	1.3		Eagle, H., Newman, E. V., Greif, R., Burkholder, T. M. and Goodman, S. C.: *J. Clin. Invest. 26*:919, 1947.
	1.5		Kunin, C. M.: *Ann. Internal Med. 67*:151, 1967.
Barbital	4.8		Louw, A. and Sonne, L. M.: *Lancet 2*:961, 1956.
Benzacyl	2.6		Schönholzer, G., Lauener, H. and Hurni, H.: *Schweiz. Med. Wochschr. 85*:222, 1955.
2-Benzene-sulfonamido-5(β-methoxy)-pyrimidine	3 24	Phase I Phase II	Gerhards, E. and Kolb, K. H.: *Arzneimittel-Forsch. 15*:1375, 1965.
Bilirubin	0.57		Bergmann, G. V.: *Klin. Wochschr. 5*:776, 1927.
			Otto, F. M. G.: *Monatsschr. Kinderheilk, 106*: 257, 1958.
Bishydroxycoumarin	27 ± 5		Solomon, H. M. and Schrogie, J.: *Clin. Pharmacol. Therap. 8*:66, 1967.
	2.4-5.7	Different liver weights, in rats	Levy, G.: *J. Pharm. Sci. 57*:1881, 1968.
	4.6-5.6	Different doses, in rats	
Bis-phenyl-(2-chlorophenyl)-l-imidazolylmethane (Bay b 5097)	3-5	In mice, rats, hamsters, dogs and cattle	Plempel, L., Bartmann, K. and Büchel, K. H.: *German Med. Monthly 14*:532, 1969.
Bradykinin, synthetic	0.17-0.36	In dog	McCarthy, D. A. and Potter, D.: *J. Pharmacol. Exptl. Therap. 148*:118, 1965.
Bromsulphthalein	0.092		Wichmann, H. M.: *Dissertation*, Giessen, 1967.
Caesium chloride	2616-3576		Rundo, J., Mason, J. I., Newton, D. and Taylor, B. T.: *Nature 200*:188, 1963.
Caffeine	3.5		Lockhart, E. E.: *J. Am. Med. Assoc. 187*:380, 1964.

SUBSTANCE	$t_{1/2}$ [h]	REMARKS	REFERENCES
Calcium	2.95		Krane, St. M., Brownell, G. L., Stanburg, J. B. and Corrigan, H.: *J. Clin. Invest. 35*:874, 1956.
Carbenicillin	1.5		Bennett, W. M., Singer, I. and Coggins, C. H.: *J. Am. Med. Assoc. 214*:1468, 1970.
	1 ± 0.25	2 g I.V., patients with normal renal function	Hoffman *et al.*: *Ann. Internal Med. 73*:173, 1970. through
	1.9 ± 0.6	Patients with severe hepatic dysfunction	Brown, H. S., Cariola, S. M., Eckel, F. M., McLeod, D. C., Pulliam, C. C. and Woodall, H. B.: *Drug Intelligence Clin. Pharm. 5*:12, 1971.
	15.75 ± 5.2	Patients with oliguria	Hoffman *et al.*: *Ann. Internal Med. 73*:173, 1970. through
	<4	Patients with creatinine clearance above 30 ml/min.	Brown, H., Cariola, S., Eckel, F., McLeod, D., Pulliam, C. and Woodall, H.: *Drug Intelligence Clin. Pharm. 5*:12, 1971.
Carbochromen	1		Schraven, E., Nitz, R. E. and Klarwein, M.: *Arzneimittel-Forsch. 20*:1905, 1970.
Carbochromen Acid	1-1.3		Schraven, E., Nitz, R. E. and Klarwein, M.: *Arzneimittel-Forsch. 20*:1905, 1970.
Cephalexin	5 2 2.5-3	Newborn Adults Infants (6-12 months)	Marget, V. W., and Daschner, F.: *Arzneimittel-Forsch. 19*:1956, 1969.
	0.9 11.1	Creatinine clearance 15.2	Kunin, C. and Finkelberg, Z.: *Ann. Internal Med. 72*:349, 1970.
	7.7	Creatinine clearance 13.5	
	10.8	Creatinine clearance 9.2	
	13.9	Creatinine clearance 4.0	
	0.55-1.21		O'Callaghan, C. H., Tootell, J. P. R. and Robinson, W. D.: *J. Pharm. Pharmacol. 23*:50, 1971.
Cephaloridine	0.83		Goodman, L. S. and Gilman, A., *The Pharmacological Basis of Therapeutics,* 4th ed., MacMillan Co., New York, NY, 1970, p. 1280.
	10.4	Mean half-life determined in 11 patients undergoing maintenance hemodialysis	Curtis, J. R. and Marshall, M.: *Brit. Med. J. 2*:149, 1970.
	5.25-16.0	Range determined in 11 patients undergoing hemodialysis	
	11.43	Mean half-life in anephric patients	
	8.75-16.0	Range of half-life in anephric patients	
	9.86	Mean half-life in patient with endogenous creatinine clearance of less than 5 ml/min.	
	5.25-14.5	Range of half-life in patients with endogenous creatinine clearance of less than 5 ml/min.	
	12.9	Patient No. 1, 12 months duration of maintenance hemodialysis	
	11.75	Patient No. 1, after 27 months duration of hemodialysis	

SUBSTANCE	$t_{1/2}$ [h]	REMARKS	REFERENCES
	7.7	Patient No. 2, 12 months duration of maintenance hemodialysis	
	5.25	Patient No. 2, 33 months duration of maintenance hemodialysis	
	16.0	Patient No. 3 (anephric) 9 months duration of maintenance hemodialysis	
	11.0	Patient No. 3, (anephric) 24 months duration of maintenance hemodialysis	
	13.6	Patient No. 4 (anephric) 9 months duration of maintenance hemodialysis	
	8.75	Patient No. 4 (anephric) 33 months duration of maintenance hemodialysis	
	14.5	Patient No. 5, pre-dialysis day	
	13.25	Patient No. 5, post-dialysis day	
	4	Patient No. 5, during dialysis	
	7.75	Patient No. 6, pre-dialysis day	
	9.2	Patient No. 6, post-dialysis day	
	4	Patient No. 6, during dialysis	
	10.0	Patient No. 7, (anephric) pre-dialysis day	
	9.25	Patient No. 7, (anephric) post-dialysis day	
	2.5	Patient No. 7 (anephric) during dialysis	
	1.5	Normal renal function	Benner, E. J.: *J. Infect. Diseases 122*:104, 1970.
	20-23	Impaired renal function	
	1.5	Normal renal function	Bennett, W. M., Singer, I. and Coggins, C. H.: *J. Am. Med. Assoc. 214*:1468, 1970.
	1.3	Calculated from k_{el}	Gibaldi, M. and Schwartz, M. A.: *Clin. Pharmacol. Therap. 9*:345, 1968.
	1.5	Probenecid is also administered. Calculated from k_{el}	
	14.1	Data taken during peritoneal dialysis	Buck, A. and Cohen, S. L.: *J. Clin. Pathol. 21*: 88, 1968.
	1.5	Normal patients	Kunin, C. M.: *Ann. Internal Med. 67*:151, 1967.
	20-23	Patients with oliguria	
Cephalothin	0.5-0.85	Normal patients	Kunin, C. M.: *Ann. Internal Med. 67*:151, 1967.
	2.9-8	Patients with oliguria	Kunin, C. M.: *Ann. Internal Med. 67*:151, 1967.
	0.5-0.85		Bennett, W. M., Singer, I. and Coggins, C. H.: *J. Am. Med. Assoc. 214*:1468, 1970.
	0.85	Normal renal function	Benner, E. J.: *J. Infect. Diseases 122*:104, 1970.
	2.9	Impaired renal function	
Chloramphenicol	2.5		Bennett, W. M., Singer, I. and Coggins, C. H.: *J. Am. Med. Assoc. 214*:1468, 1970.

SUBSTANCE	$t_{1/2}$ [h]	REMARKS	REFERENCES
	3.5-5		Spitzy, K. H.: *Arzneimittel-Forsch. 12*:172, 1962.
			Weiss, C. F., Glazko, A. J. and Weston, J. K.: *New Engl. J. Med. 262*:787, 1960.
	1.5-3.5		Goodman, L. S. and Gilman, A.: *The Pharmacological Basis of Therapeutics,* 4th ed., MacMillan Co., New York, NY, 1970, p. 1270.
	1.6-3.3 3.2-4.3	 Patients with oliguria	Kunin, C. M.: *Ann. Internal Med. 67*:151, 1967.
	2-4		Böhm, C.: *Nierfunktionsstorung und Antibiotika,* Bedeutung den Nierenfunktion Scripta Medica, Merck, Darmstadt.
Chlorcyclizine	12		Data obtained from Burroughs Wellcome
Chlordane	240	In dog	Welch, R. M., Harrison, Y. and Burns, J. J.: *Toxicol. Appl. Pharmacol. 10*:340, 1967.
Chlordiazepoxide	7-15		Data obtained from Roche Labs.
Chlorphenoxyiso-butyric acid	12		Solomon, H. M.: *Safer and More Effective Drugs,* by Goldstein, S. W., A.Ph.A. Academy of Sciences, Washington, D.C., 1968, p. 49.
Chlorphentermine	41		Hungwon, J. and Triggs, E. J.: *J. Pharm. Sci. 59*:306, 1970.
Chlorpromazine	2-31		Curry, H. S., Marshall, J. H. and Davis, J. H.: *Arch. Gen. Psychiat. 22*:209, 1970.
	6	Dose 10.9 mg/Kg	Curry, H. S.: *Agressologie 9*:115, 1968.
Chlorpropamide	24-36		Bennett, W. M., Singer, I. and Coggins, C. H.: *J. Am. Med. Assoc. 214*:1468, 1970.
	35		Bhatia, S. K., Hadden, D. R., Montgomery, D. A. D. and Weaver, J. A.: *Brit. Med. J. 2*: 570, 1970.
Chlortetracycline	2.3		Marshall, E. K.: *J. Pharmacol. Exptl. Therap. 92*:43, 1948.
	3.5		Brainerd, A. D., Bruyn, H. B., Meiklejohn, G. and O'Gara, L.: *Antibiot. Chemotherapia 1*: 447, 1951.
	5.6		Walter, A. M. and Heilmeyer, L.: *Antibiotica-Fibel,* 2nd ed., Stuttgart, 1965.
	5.6	Normal patients	Kunin, C. M.: *Ann. Internal Med. 67*:151, 1967.
	6.8-11.0	Patients with oliguria	
Cholesterol	192		London, D. and Rittenberg, D.: *J. Biol. Chem. 184*:687, 1950.
Cholesterol (free)	196.8 ± 12	In dog	Gudjarnasen, S.: *J. Pharmacol. Exptl. Therap. 161*:47, 1968.
	348 ± 24	Nicotine treated animals	
Cholesterol (esterified)	201.6 ± 28	In dog	Gudjarnasen, S.: *J. Pharmacol. Exptl. Therap. 161*:47, 1968.
	319.2 ± 26	Nicotine treated animals	
CL 11, 366	1		Travis, D. M.: *J. Pharmacol. Exptl. Therap. 151*:464, 1966.
	0.33	In dog	Travis, D. M.: *J. Pharmacol. Exptl. Therap. 143*:383, 1964.
	0.41	In rabbit	Wistrand, P. J., Rawls, J. A. and Maren, T. H.: *Acta Pharmacol. 17*:337, 1961.
Clindamycin	4.52 4.13-4.99		Novak, E., Wagner, J. G. and Lamb, D. J.: *Intern. J. Klin. Pharmakol. Therap. Toxik. 3*: 201, 1970.

SUBSTANCE	$t_{1/2}$ [h]	REMARKS	REFERENCES
	2.4		Cleocin (Upjohn) package insert
	2.38		Wagner, J. G., Novak, E., Patel, N., Chidester, C. G. and Lummis, W. L.: *Am. J. Med. Sci. 256*:25, 1968.
	1.5-3.54		
Clofibrate	12		Goodman, L. S. and Gilman, A.: *The Pharmacological Basis of Therapeutics,* 4th ed., MacMillan Co., New York, NY, 1970, p. 767.
Cloxacillin	0.8	Uremic patients	Rosenblatt, J. E., Brodie, J. L., Kind, A. and Kirby, W.: *Arch. Internal Med. 12*:345, 1968.
	0.42	Healthy patients	Beckett, A. and Cohen, S. L.: *J. Clin. Pathol. 21*:88, 1968.
	2.5	After dialysis	
	0.67	Calculated from plasma values	Modr, Z. and Dvoracek, K.: *Rev. Czechoslovak. Med. 69*:79, 1969.
	0.7	Calculated from urine values	
Colchicine	0.32 ± 0.12	Patients with miscellaneous disorders	Wallace, S. L.: *Am. J. Med. 48*:443, 1970.
	0.48 ± 0.2	Patients with gout	
	0.15 ± 0.01	Patients with chronic liver disease	
	0.67 ± 0.43	Patients with chronic renal failure	
	60	In leucocytes	Orr, J. S.: *Lancet 1*:88, 1971.
Colistin	1.5-2		Walter, A. M. and Heilmeyer, L.: *Antibiotica-Fibel,* 2nd ed., Stuttgart, 1965.
	1.6-2.7	Normal	Kunin, C. M.: *Ann. Internal Med. 67*:151, 1967.
	48-72	Patients with oliguria. Calculated from data presented in the literature	
	1.5-2		Böhm, C.: *Nierenfunktionsstörung und Antibiotika,* E. Merck A. G. Darmstadt, p. 32.
	2.4	In premature infants	Axline, S. F., Yaffe, S. J. and Simon, H. J.: *Pediatrics 39*:97, 1967.
	2.6	In 4-day-old infants	
	2.3	In 12-51-day-old infants	
	3	Normal men	Wright, W. and Welch, A.: *Antibiot. Ann. 60*:61, 1960.
	2		Bennett, W. M., Singer, I. and Coggins, C. H.: *J. Am. Med. Assoc. 214*:1468, 1970.
Colistimethate sodium	4.5	Normal renal function	Goodwin, N. J. and Friedman, E. A.: *Ann. Internal Med. 68*:984, 1968.
	4.75	Moderate renal insufficiency	
	12.75	Severe renal insufficiency	
	10.25	Negligible renal function	
Congo red	2.64		Schubert, R. and Wiegand, E.: *Klin. Wochschr. 25*:273, 1947.
Corticosterone	0.57	In dog	Knippers, F., Ely, R., Hughes, E. R. and Kelly, V. C.: *Proc. Soc. Exptl. Biol. Med. 95*:187, 1957.

SUBSTANCE	$t_{1/2}$ [h]	REMARKS	REFERENCES
	0.33	In dog	Chen, C., Freeman, S. and Willoughby, H. W.: *Endocrinology 65*:539, 1959.
Cortisone	0.38	In dog	Knipers, F., Ely, R. S., Hughes, E. R. and Kelly, V. C.: *Proc. Soc. Exptl. Biol. Med. 95*: 187, 1957.
	0.75	In dog	Silber, R. H. and Morgan, E. R.: *Clin. Chem.* 2:170, 1956.
Coumermycin A	5.06-8.77	Calculated from k_{13}	Kaplan, S. A.: *J. Pharm. Sci. 59*:309, 1970.
	14.8-46.3	As calculated by Kaplan	
Cyclophosphamide	4.1		Data obtained from Mead Johnson.
Cycloserine	10		Kunin, C. M.: *Ann. Internal Med. 67*:157, 1967.
	8-12	Peroral	Conzelman, G. M., Jr.: *Am. Rev. Tuberc. 74*:739, 1956.
Cystine	1032		Margen, S. and Tarver, H.: *J. Clin. Invest. 35*:1161, 1956.
Decamethonium	0.8		Christensen, C. B.: *Acta Pharmacol. Toxicol. 26*:461, 1968.
Demethylchlor-tetracycline	12.7		Rosenblatt, J. E.: *Antimicrob. Agents Chemotherap. 6*:134, 1966.
	11.8		Kunin, C. M. and Findland, M. N.: *New Engl. J. Med. 259*:999, 1958.
	12.7		Kunin, C. M., Dornbush, A. C. and Findland, M. N.: *J. Clin. Invest. 38*:1950, 1959.
	12.3		Kunin, C. M.: *Ann. Internal Med. 67*:151, 1967.
Desferrioxamine	1.3 ± 0.2	Nephrectomized dog	Peters, G., Schmid, K., Brunner, H. and Keberle, H.: *Biochem. Pharmacol. 15*:93, 1966.
Desipramine	33	Accumulation half-life for a particular patient	Van Rossum, J. M.: *J. Pharm. Sci. 57*:2164, 1968.
Deslanoside	36		Weissler, A. M., Snyder, J. R., Schoenfeld, C. D. and Cohen, S.: *Am. J. Cardiol. 17*:768, 1966.
Desmethyl-imipramine	7.5-52	Female psychiatric patients	Hammer, W., Marten, S. and Sjoquist, F.: *Clin. Pharmacol. Therap. 10*:44, 1969.
	1	Rabbit	Dingell, J. V., Sulser, F. and Gilette, J. R.: *J. Pharmacol. Exptl. Therap. 143*:14, 1964.
	9	Rat	
	0.84	Mouse	
Dexamethasone	3.34		Peterson, R. E.: *Ann. N.Y. Acad. Sci. 82*:846, 1959.
	1.0	In dog	Silber, R. H.: *Ann. N.Y. Acad. Sci. 82*:821, 1959.
Diazepam	2-3	During first 6 hours	Desilva, J. A., Koechlin, B. A. and Bader, G.: *J. Pharm. Sci. 55*:692, 1966.
	27-28	After first 24 hours	
Diazoxide	48-72		Calesnick, B., Katchen, K. and Black, J.: *J. Pharm. Sci. 54*:1277, 1965.
	22-31		Sellers, E. M. and Koch-Weser, J.: *New Engl. Med. 281*:1143, 1969.
Dicloxacillin	1.03	Uremic patients	Rosenblatt, J. E., Brodie, J. L., Kind, A. C. and Kirby, W. M. V.: *Arch. Internal Med. 121*:345, 1968.
	0.7	Healthy patients	

SUBSTANCE	$t_{1/2}$ [h]	REMARKS	REFERENCES
	0.96 ± 0.75		Modrk, Z. and Dvoracek: *Rev. Czekos. Med.* 1969.
	0.4	Normal	McCloskey, R. V. and Hayes, C. P.: *Antimicrob. Agents Chemotherap.* 1967.
	0.8	Phase I (normal)	
	0.5	Phase 2	
	1.6	During dialysis	
	0.67	Between dialysis (phase 1)	
	1.5	Between dialysis (phase 2)	
	0.9		Swintosky, J. V., Dittert, L. W. and Doluisio, J. T.: *Am. J. Hosp. Pharm. 26*:519, 1969.
Dicumarol	32.0		Brodie, B. B., Weiner, M., Burns, J. J., Simon, G. and Yale, R. K.: *J. Pharmacol. Exptl. Therap. 106*:453, 1952.
Digitoxin	102-112		Weissler, A. M., Snyder, J. R., Schoenfeld, C. D. and Cohen, S.: *Am. J. Cardiol. 17*: 768, 1966.
	72-144		Bennett, W. M., Singer, I. and Coggins, C. H.: *J. Am. Med. Assoc. 214*:1468, 1970.
Digoxin	36		Bennett, W. M., Singer, I. and Coggins, C. H.: *J. Am. Med. Assoc. 214*:1468, 1970.
Dihydrostreptomycin	0.33	As sulfate salt dose in water	Caldwell, H. C., Rednick, A. B., Scott, G. C., Yakatan, G. J. and Ziv, D.: *J. Pharm. Sci. 59*:1689, 1970.
	0.52	As sulfate salt dose in oil susp.	
	3.46	As pamoate salt dose in oil susp.	
Dimethyl-imipramine	1	In rabbit	Dingell, J. V., Sulser, F. and Gilette, J. R.: *J. Pharmacol. Exptl. Therap. 143*:14, 1964.
	9	In rat	
	0.84	In mouse	
Dimethyl-sulfoxide	6	In rat	Hucker, H. B., Ahmad, P. M. and Miller, E. A.: *J. Pharmacol. Exptl. Therap. 154*:176, 1966.
Diphenhydramine	1-1.16	In rat and dog	Welch, R. M., Harrison, Y. E. and Burns, J. J.: *Toxicol. Appl. Pharmacol. 10*:340, 1967.
Diphenylhydantoin	23.5 ± 11		Kater, R. M. H., Roggin, G., Tobon, G., Zieve, P. and Iber, F. L.: *Am. J. Med. Sci. 258*:35, 1969.
	16.3 ± 6.8	In alcoholic group	
	7.3 ± 1.2	In dog	Kopayi, T. and Auery, M. A.: *Clin. Pharmacol. Therap. 7*:252, 1966.
	15	Decreased in uremia	Bennett, W. M., Singer, I. and Coggins, C. H.: *J. Am. Med. Assoc. 214*:1468, 1970.
	12-29	Data from 5 subjects	Riegelman, S.: *Drug Inform. Bull. 3*:59, 1969.
	13		
	28	Chloramphenicol administered simultaneously	Visconti, J. A.: *Ann. Meeting Paper* (O.S.H.P.) Ohio, 5/1/70.
Doxycycline	15		Goodman, L. S. and Gilman, A.: *The Pharmacological Basis of Therapeutics,* 4th ed., MacMillan Co., New York, NY, 1970, p. 1256.

SUBSTANCE	$t_{1/2}$ [h]	REMARKS	REFERENCES
	18.5-23		Fabre, J., Pitton, J. J., Virieux, C., Laurencet, F. L., Bernhardt, J. P. and Godel, J. C.: *Schweiz. Med. Wochschr. 97*:915, 1967.
	15.1		Rosenblatt, J. E.: *Antimicrob. Agents Chemotherap. 6*:134, 1966.
Ephedrine	5.99	Average urinary *p*H = 6.30	Welling, P. G., Lee, K. P., Patel, J. A., Walker, J. E. and Wagner, J. G.: 118th Annual Meeting, A.Ph.A. Academy of Pharmaceutical Sciences, San Francisco, California, March-April 1971.
Epinephrine	0.04		Vensalu, A.: *Acta Physiol. Scand. Suppl. 173*: 49, 1960.
Erythromycin	1-2 1.4		Böhm, C.: *Nierenfunktionsstörung und Antibiotika,* E. Merck, A. G., Darmstadt, p. 32.
	4.8-5.8	In patients with oliguria	Kunin, C. M.: *Ann. Internal Med. 67*:151, 1967.
	1.5		Walter, A. M. and Heilmeyer, L.: *Antibiotica-Fibel,* 2nd ed., Stuttgart, 1965.
	1.6		Maple, F. M., O'Leary, B. and Kirby, W. M. M.: *Antibiot. Chemotherapia 3*:863, 1953.
	1.5		Bennett, W. M., Singer, I. and Coggins, C. H.: *J. Am. Med. Assoc. 214*:1468, 1970.
Erythromycin stearate	1.2		Chun, A. H. C. and Wiegand, R.: 118th Annual Meeting, A.Ph.A. Academy of Pharmaceutical Sciences, San Francisco, California, March-April, 1971.
Estradiol	0.084	In rat	Welch, R. M. and Levin, W.: *J. Pharmacol. Exptl. Therap. 160*:171, 1968.
Ethanol	4.33	In dog	Haggard, W. R. and Greenberg, L. A.: *J. Pharmacol. Exptl. Therap. 52*:167, 1934.
Ethionamide	2-4	Peroral	Walter, A. M. and Heilmeyer, L.: *Antibiotica-Fibel,* 2nd ed., Stuttgart, 1965.
Ethoxzolamide	0.417	In rabbit	Wistrand, P. J., Rawls, S. A. and Maren, T. H.: *Acta Pharmacol. 17*:337, 1961.
Ethylbis-coumacetate	2.4		Brodie, B. B., Weiner, M., Burns, J. J., Simon, G. and Yale, R. K.: *J. Pharmacol. Exptl. Therap. 106*:453, 1952.
Ethylene glycol salicylate	2.2 ± 0.2		Wurster, D. E. and Kramer, S. F.: *J. Pharm. Sci. 50*:288, 1961.
Ethyl salicylate	2.2 ± 0.2		Wurster, D. E. and Kramer, S. F.: *J. Pharm. Sci. 50*:288, 1961.
EXP 338 (5-imino-2,2,4,4, -tetracis-trifluomethyl-imidazolidine)	8		Levine, H., Jossman, P. and Friend, D. G.: *Clin. Pharmacol. Therap. 9*:448, 1968.
Factor I (Fibrinogen)	100		Smith, J. W.: *Manual of Medical Therapeutics,* 19th ed., Little Brown and Co., Boston, 1969, p. 274.
Factor II (Prothrombin)	50-72		Smith, J. W.: *Manual of Medical Therapeutics,* 19th ed., Little, Brown and Co., Boston, 1969, p. 274.
Factor V (Proaccelerin. Labile Factor)	20-40		Smith, J. W.: *Manual of Medical Therapeutics,* 19th ed., Little, Brown and Co., Boston, 1969, p. 274.
Factor VII (Proconvertin, Stable Factor)	4-6		Smith, J. W.: *Manual of Medical Therapeutics,* 19th ed., Little, Brown and Co., Boston, 1969, p. 274.
	6.2		Helleman, J.: *Brit. J. Haematol. 9*:506, 1963.

SUBSTANCE	$t_{1/2}$ [h]	REMARKS	REFERENCES
Factor VIII (Antihemophilic Factor, AHF	10-20		Smith, J. W.: *Manual of Medical Therapeutics,* 19th ed., Little, Brown and Co., Boston, 1969, p. 274.
Factor IX (Christmas Factor, Plasma Thromboplastin Component - PTC)	25-30		Smith, J. W.: *Manual of Medical Therapeutics,* 19th ed., Little, Brown and Co., Boston, 1969, p. 274.
	13.9		Helleman, J.: *Brit. J. Haematol. 9*:506, 1963.
Factor X (Stuart (-Power)-Factor)	16.5		Helleman, J.: *Brit. J. Haematol. 9*:506, 1963.
	25-50		Smith, J. W.: *Manual of Medical Therapeutics,* 19th ed., Little, Brown and Co., Boston, 1969, p. 274.
Factor XI (Plasma Thromboplastin Antecedent, PTA)	40-80		Smith, J. W.: *Manual of Medical Therapeutics,* 19th ed., Little, Brown and Co., Boston, 1969, p. 274.
Factor XII (Hageman Factor)	50		Smith, J. W.: *Manual of Medical Therapeutics,* 19th ed., Little, Brown and Co., Boston, 1969, p. 274.
Factor XIII (Fibrin-Stabilizing Factor, FSF)	100-150		Smith, J. W.: *Manual of Medical Therapeutics,* 19th ed., Little, Brown and Co., Boston, 1969, p. 274.
Fanasil	96-180	Infants and children	Vest, M.: *Schweiz. Med. Wochschr. 96*:920, 1966.
	340	Newborn	
	150-200		Greenberg, R. N.: *Brit. Med. J. 3*:649, 1967.
Flurazepam	1	In dog	Randall, R. O., *et al.*: *Arch. Intern. Pharmacodyn. 178*:224, 1969. through Brown, H. S., Cariola, S. M., Eckel, F. M., McLeod, D. C., Pulliam, C. C. and Woodall, H. B.: *Drug Intelligence Clin. Pharm. 5*:12, 1971.
Folic Acid	0.7		Spray, G. H. and Witts, L. J.: *Clin. Sci. 11*: 273, 1952.
			Spray, G. H. and Witts, L. J.: *Brit. Med. J. 2*:62, 1952.
Fusidinic Acid	4-6		Walter, A. M. and Heilmeyer, L.: *Antibiotica-Fibel,* 2nd ed., Stuttgart, 1965.
Gentamicin	1-1.5		Walter, A. M. and Heilmeyer, L.: *Antibiotica-Fibel,* 2nd ed., Stuttgart, 1965.
	1.8-10.1	Creatinine clearance range of 11.5 ml/min. to 98.5 ml/min.	Bergan, T., Brodwall, E. K. and Oyri, A.: *Acta Med. Scand. 189*:1, 1971.
	2.5		Bennett, W. M., Singer, I. and Coggins, C. H.: *J. Am. Med. Assoc. 214*:1468, 1970.
	2		Böhm, C.: *Nierfuntionsstörung und Antibiotika,* Merck A. G., Darmstadt, p. 32.
	2.3	Normal patients, prolonged in patients with oliguria	Kunin, C. M.: *Ann. Internal Med. 67*:151, 1967.
	1-1.5	Normal humans	Kobyletzki, D.: *Med. Welt. 19*:2010, 1968.
	2.4	Dose given pre-partem	
	4	Patients with normal glomerular filtration rate	Goodman, L. S. and Gilman, A.: *The Pharmacological Basis of Therapeutics,* 4th ed., MacMillan Co., New York, NY, 1970, p. 1298.
	45	Patients with uremia	Rodriguez, V., Stewart, D. and Bodey, G.: *Clin. Pharm. Therap. 11*:275, 1970.
	2		through *Biol. Abstr.* 115246.

SUBSTANCE	$t_{1/2}$ [h]	REMARKS	REFERENCES
Glibenclamide (HB 419)	6.6	During dynamic steady state	Christ, O. E., Heptner, W. and Rupp, W.: "Investigations on Absorption, Excretion and Metabolism in Man after Administration of C^{14}-Labeled HB 419," in *HB 419 - A New Oral Antidiabetic Drug,* by Levine, R. and Pfeiffer, E. F., Georg Thieme Verlag, Stuttgart, 1969, p. 51.
	0.38	Initially (Phase I)	
	5	Peroral	
	5-7		Bhatia, S. K., Hadden, D. R., Montgomery, D. A. D. and Weaver, J. A.: *Brit. Med. J. 2*: 570, 1970.
γ-Globulin	340		Havens, W. J., Jr., Kickensheets, J., Bierly, J. N. and Eberhard, J.: *J. Immunol. 73*:256, 1964.
			Dixon, F. J., Talmage, O. M., Maurer, P. H. and Deichmiller, M.: *J. Exptl. Med. 96*:313, 1952.
	192 158 113 129 45 508	In dog In monkey In rabbit In guinea pig In mouse In cattle	Dixon, F. J., Talmage, O. M., Maurer, P. H., and Deichmiller, M.: *J. Exptl. Med. 96*:313, 1952.
Globulins, total	180		Oeff, K.: *J. Exptl. Med. 123*:309, 1954.
Glucose	0.41		Mähr, G. through Dost, F. H.: *Grundlagen der Pharmakokinetik,* 2nd. ed., Stuttgart, p. 298, 1968.
Glutamic dehydrogenase	85		Rauen, H. M.: *Biochemisches Taschenbuch,* 2nd ed., Berlin, 1964.
Glutamic oxaloacetic transaminase	50-60		Rauen, H. M.: *Biochemisches Taschenbuch,* 2nd ed., Berlin, 1964.
Glutamic pyruvic transaminase	75-90		Rauen, H. M.: *Biochemisches Taschenbuch,* 2nd ed., Berlin, 1964.
Glutethimide	6.5	In rats	Goodman, L. S. and Gilman, A.: *The Pharmacological Basis of Therapeutics,* 4th ed., MacMillan Co., New York, NY, 1970, p. 129.
	10		Bütikofer, E., Cottier, P., Imhof, P., Keberle, H., Riess, W. and Schmid, K.: *Arch. Exptl. Pathol. Pharmakol. 244*:97, 1962.
Glycocoll	240 144	 In rats	Spermson, D. B. and Dittenberg, D.: *J. Biol. Chem. 184*:405, 1950.
Glycodiazine (glymidine sodium)	4.6	Mean half-life normal liver and kidney function	Held, H., Kaminski, B. and Oldershausen, V.: *Diabetologia 6*:386, 1970.
	3.1-5.6	Range of half-life in patients with normal liver and kidney function	
	12	During treatment with phenylbutazone	
	5.8-19.6	Range during treatment with phenylbutazone	
	7.5	During treatment with phenprocoumarol	
	4.3-15.7	Range during treatment with phenprocoumarol	
	7.6	During treatment with doxycycline	

SUBSTANCE	$t_{1/2}$ [h]	REMARKS	REFERENCES
	4.6-10.6	Range during treatment with doxycycline	
Griseofulvin	17.5		Rowland, M., Riegelman, S. and Epstein, W. L.: *J. Pharm. Sci. 57*:984, 1968.
	0.7-1.87	In rabbit	Fischer, L.: *Dissertation Abstr. 26*:5732, 1966. through *Intern. Pharm. Abstr.* 1966, 1255.
			Fischer, L. and Riegelman, S.: *J. Pharm. Sci. 54*:1571, 1965.
	18-24	Peroral dose	Walter, A. M. and Heilmeyer, L.: *Antibiotica-Fibel,* 2nd ed., Stuttgart, 1965.
Heparin	1.61 ± 0.07	Measured by the whole-blood clotting time test	Estes, J.: *J. Am. Med. Assoc. 212*:1492, 1970.
	1.72 ± 0.10	Measured by the whole-blood activated partial thromboplastin time test	
	1.34 ± 0.10	Measured by the activated plasma partial thromboplastin time test	
	1.32 ± 0.07	Measured by the partial thromboplastin time test	
Heroin	0.042	In mouse	Murphree, H.: *Clin. Pharmacol. Therap. 3*: 473, 1962.
Hexamethonium	1.5		Morrison, D. and Paton, W.: *Brit. Med. J. 1*: 1299, 1953.
Hexobarbital	0.32 1 2.17 4.33	In mouse In rabbit In rat In dog	Koppayi, T. and Auery, M. A., *Clin. Pharmacol. Therap. 7*:252, 1966.
9-α F-Hydrocortisone	0.97	In dog	Silver, R. H. and Morgan, E. R., *Clin. Chem. 2*:170, 1956.
Hydrocortisone	0.73	In dog	Knipers, F., Ely, R. S., Hughes, E. and Kelly, V. C.: *Proc. Soc. Exptl. Biol. Med. 95*:187, 1957.
	1.68		Melby, J. C. and Sprink, W. W.: *J. Clin. Invest. 37*:1791, 1958.
			Liddle, G. W.: *Clin. Pharmacol. Therap. 2*: 615, 1961.
	0.95	In dog	Bilka, P. J. and Melby, J. C.: *Minnesota Med. 41*:263, 1958.
	0.82		Dulin, W. E., Barnes, L. E., Glenn, E., Lyster, S. C. and Collins, E. J.: *Metabolism 7*:398, 1958.
Hydroxypropyl-theophylline	4.3		Ritschel, W. A. and Clotten, R.: *Arzneimittel-Forsch. 19*:221, 1969.
Imipramine	3.5		Greengard, P. and Wilbrandt, W.: *Schweiz. Med. Wochschr. 94*:37, 1964.
	2 2.5 0.84	In rabbit In rat In mouse	Dingell, J. V., Sulser, F. and Gilette, J. R.: *J. Pharmacol. Exptl. Therap. 143*:14, 1964.
Indomethacin	10 17.6	Probenecid pre-administered	Skeith, M. D., Simkin, P. A. and Healey, L. A.: *Clin. Pharm. Therap. 9*:89, 1968.
	1-2		Solomon, H. M.: in *Safer and More Effective Drugs,* by Goldstein, S. W., APhA Academy of Pharmaceutical Sciences, Washington, D.C., 1968, p. 49.

SUBSTANCE	t½ [h]	REMARKS	REFERENCES
	0.33-4	Varies in different species	Hucker, H. B., Zacchei, A. G., Cox, S. V., Brodie, D. A. and Cantwell, N. H. R.: *J. Pharmacol. Exptl. Therap. 153*:237, 1966.
Insulin	1-2	Reg. crystalline by subcutaneous route	Bennett, W. M., Singer, I. and Coggins, C. H.: *J. Am. Med. Sci. 214*:1468, 1970.
	0.67		Berson, S. A., Yalow, R. S., Bauman, H., Rothschild, M. A. and Newerly, K.: *J. Clin. Invest. 35*:170, 1956.
Insulin, Endogenous Serum Immunoreactive	0.15-0.24		Williams, R. F., Gleason, R. E. and Soeldner, J. S.: *Metab. Clin. Exptl. 17*:1025, 1968.
Inulin	0.53		Polster, H.: *Z. Kinderheilk. 79*:555, 1957.
	0.61		Dost, F. H.: *Der Blutspiegel,* Leipzig, 1953.
	1.17		Schachter, D., Freinkel, N. and Schwarzt, I. L.: *Am. J. Physiol. 160*:532, 1950.
o-Iodobenzoic Acid	7-9 8-11 >31	Younger people Elderly people People with kidney damage	Dohnalek, J. and Eysselt, M.: *Scripta Med. Fac. Med. Univ. Brun. 37*:189, 1966.
Iron	42	Calculated from graph	Huglands, S.: *Acta Med. Scand. 186*:487, 1969.
	1.2-2.4		Rind, H., Gladtke, E. and Dost, F. H.: *Deut. Med. Wochschr. 90*:1124, 1965.
Isoniazid (INH)	1.0-2.6		Walter, A. M. and Heilmeyer, L.: *Antibiotica-Fibel,* 2nd ed., Stuttgart, 1965.
	1.1 3.6	Rapid Slow	Kunin, C. M.: *Ann. Internal Med. 67*:151, 1967.
	2-4		Bennett, W. M., Singer, I. and Coggins, C. H.: *J. Am. Med. Assoc. 214*:1468, 1970.
	0.98 2.65	Rapid inactivation Slow inactivation	Bercea, O. and Bonciocat, V. N.: *Arzneimittel-Forsch. 20*:241, 1970.
	1.05 ± 0.23	Rapid inactivation	Jenne, J. W., McDonald, F. M. and Medoza, E.: *Am. Rev. Respirat. Diseases 84*:371, 1961.
	3.18 ± 0.28	Slow inactivation	
	1.42 ± 0.70	Rapid inactivation after prolonged therapy with PAS	
	3.82-1.23	Slow inactivators after prolonged therapy with PAS	
Isoproterenol	0.015-0.23	In dogs	Portman, G. A., Minatoya, H. and Landa, A. M.: *J. Pharm Sci. 54*:973 1965.
Isoxsuprine	1	In dogs	Data obtained from Mead Johnson.
Kallidin, synthetic	0.22-0.61	In dogs	McCarthy. D. A. and Potter, D. E.: *J. Pharmacol. Exptl. Therap. 148*:118, 1965.
Kanamycin	4		Walter, A. M. and Heilmeyer, L.: *Antibiotica-Fibel,* 2nd ed., Stuttgart, 1965.
			Cutler, R. E. and Orme, B. M.: *J. Am. Med. Assoc. 209*:539, 1969.
	2 18	 Premature infants <2 days	Goodman, L. S. and Gilman, A.: *The Pharmacological Basis of Therapeutics,* 4th ed., MacMillan Co., New York, NY, 1970, p. 1286.
	6	5-22 day old infants	
	3-4		Bennett, W. M., Singer, I. and Coggins, C. H.: *J. Am. Med. Assoc. 214*:1468, 1970.
	3.5 5 2-30	Patients of different age groups and sexes with serum creatinine (in the pertinent period) of 0.7-15 mg/100 ml.	Sorensen, A. W., Szabo, L., Pedersen, A. and Scharff, A.: *Postgrad. Med. J. (Suppl.) 43*: 37, 1967.

SUBSTANCE	$t_{1/2}$ [h]	REMARKS	REFERENCES
	3 72-96	In patients with oliguria	Kunin, C. M.: *Ann. Internal Med. 67*:151, 1967.
	4		Axline, S. G. and Simon, H. J.: *Antimicrob. Agents Chemotherap. 64*:135, 1964.
	35.5	In dialysis	Buck, A. C. and Cohen, S. L.: *J. Clin. Pathol. 21*:81, 1968.
Lactic dehydrogenase	50-60		Rauen, H. N.: *Biochemisches Taschenbuch,* 2nd ed., Berlin, 1964.
Lanoxin	33		Data supplied by Burroughs Wellcome.
	33		Weissler, A. M., Snyder, J. R., Schoenfeld, C. D. and Cohen, S.: *Am. J. Cardiol. 17*:768, 1966.
Lasix	0.2-0.25		Haussler, A. and Hajdu, P.: *Arzneimittel-Forsch. 14*:713, 1964, from Goodman, L. S. and Gilman, A., 4th ed., 1970, p. 860, 871.
Lead	1680		Kehoe, R. A., Thamann, F. and Cholak, J.: *J. Ind. Hyg. 15*:320, 1933.
Levothyroxine	156	Measured by disappearance of radioiodine (I^{131})	Package insert of Synthroid, Flint Lab., Illinois, U.S.A., May, 1967.
Lignocaine	25	Calculated from k_{el} (0.027)	Beckett, A. H., Boyes, R. N. and Appleton, P. J.: *J. Pharm. Pharmacol. 18*:76S, 1966 (Suppl)
Lincomycin	4.6-4.8		Wagner, J. G., Northem, J. I. and Solkolski, W. T.: *Nature 207*:201, 1970.
	4.4-4.7		Kunin, C. M.: *Ann. Internal Med. 67*:151, 1967.
	5-6	Almost doubled in patients with hepatic insufficiency (10 hr.)	Goodman, L. S. and Gilman, A.: *The Pharmacological Basis of Therapeutics,* 4th ed., MacMillan Company, New York, NY, 1970, p. 1296.
Lipoprotein lipase	0.222		Högstedt, B. and Lindquist, B.: *Acta Paediat. 52*:61, 1963.
Lithium	10	$t_{1/2}$ calculated from Figure 3; dose given as sustained released tablets	Amdisen, A. and Sjögren, J.: *Acta Pharm. Suecia 5*:465, 1968.
LSD-25	1.72	Based on model	Wagner, J. G., Aghajanian, G. K. and Bing, O. H.: *Clin. Pharmacol. Therap. 9*:635, 1968.
	3.0	Calculated from plasma concentration	
	1.66 2.16 0.11	Monkey Cat Mouse	Jacobson, E.: *Clin. Pharmacol. Therap. 4*: 480, 1963.
	2.816		Boissier, J. R.: Symposium of Hallucinogenic Drugs, 30th FIP Congress, Geneva, Switzerland, Sept. 1, 1970.
D-Lyxose	1.43		Segal, St. and Foley, J. B.: *J. Clin. Invest. 38*:407, 1959.
Marezine	36		Data obtained from Burroughs Wellcome.
Medazepam	1-2		Schwartz, M. A. and Carbone, J.: *Biochem. Pharmacol. 19*:343, 1970.
Mepacrine	120		Dost, F. H.: *Der Blutspiegel,* Leipzig, 1953.
Meperidine	5.5 1.2 0.9	 Monkey Dog	Burns, J. J.: *Ann. New York Acad. Sci. 151*: 959, 1968.
Meprobamate	6.4-16.6		Hollister, L. E. and Levy, G.: *Chemotherapia 9*:20, 1964.
Merbaphen	6.3		Sollmann, T., Schreiber, N. E. and Cole, H. N.: *Arch. Dermatol. Syphilis 32*:1, 1935.

SUBSTANCE	$t_{1/2}$ [h]	REMARKS	REFERENCES
Mercaptopurine	0.35	In children	Loo, T. L., Luce, S. K., Sullivan, M. P. and Frei, E., III, *Clin. Pharmacol. Therap. 9*: 180, 1968.
	0.78	In adults	
Mercurosal	6.3		Sollmann, T., Schreiber, N. E. and Cole, H. N.: *Arch. Dermatol. Syphilis, 32*:1, 1935.
Mersalyl	8.5		Sollmann, T., Schreiber, N. E. and Cole, H. N.: *Arch. Dermatol. Syphilis 32*:1, 1935.
Methacycline	14.3		Kunin, C. M.: *Ann. Internal Med. 67*:151, 1967.
	8-15		Goodman, L. S. and Gilman, A.: *The Pharmacological Basis of Therapeutics,* 4th ed., MacMillan Co., New York, NY, 1970, p. 1256.
Methaqualone	8		Data obtained from W. H. Rorer.
Methazolamide	0.88	In rabbit	Wistrand, P. J., Rawls, J. A. and Maren, T. H.: *Acta Pharmacol. 17*:337, 1961.
	2.5	In dog	Sisson, G. M. and Maren, T. H.: *Fed. Proc. 15*:484, 1956.
Methdilazine	1.5	In rats	*Toxicol. Appl. Pharmacol. 2*:68, 1960. Data obtained from Mead Johnson.
Methenamine mandelate	2		Bennett, W. M., Singer, I. and Coggins, C. H.: *J. Am. Med. Assoc. 214*:1468, 1970.
Methicillin	0.5		Bennett, W. M., Singer, I. and Coggins, C. H.: *J. Am. Med. Assoc. 214*:1468, 1970.
	0.5		Kunin, C. M.: *Ann. Internal Med. 67*:151, 1967.
	4	Patients with oliguria	
	0.5-1		Walter, A. M. and Heilmeyer, L.: *Antibiotica-Fibel,* 2nd ed., Stuttgart, 1965.
	3.3	Premature infants 4-5 days old	
	2.4	Premature infants 4-7 days old	
	2.0	Premature infants 13-15 days old	
	1.4	Premature infants 17-33 days old	
	1.4	Premature infants 26-30 days old	
	3.3	< 24 hr. term infant	
	1.3	Term infants 4-5 days old	
	0.9	Term infants 8-30 days old	
	0.5	Adult	
	2.4	Premature infants 4-7 days old	Boe, R. W., Williams, C. P. S., Bennett, J. V. and Oliver, T. K.: *Pediatrics 39*:194, 1967.
	1.8	Infants, 11-14 days old	
	1.4	Infants 17-33 days old	
	3.3	Premature infants 4-5 days old	
	2.0	Premature infants 13-15 days old	
	1.4	Premature infants 26-30 days old	
	3.3	Infants < 24 hours term	
	1.3	Term infants 4-5 days	
	0.9	Term infants 8-15 days	
	0.8	Term infants 26-30 days	
Methionine	1200		Margen, S. and Taraver, H.: *J. Clin. Invest. 36*:1161, 1956.
Methotrexate	1		Rees, R. B., *et al.*: *Arch. Dermatol. 95*:2, 1967.

SUBSTANCE	$t_{1/2}$ [h]	REMARKS	REFERENCES
	2.23 ± 0.35	3H labeled methoxtrexate used in the study (MTX-H)	Henderson, E. S., Adamson, R. H. and Oliverio, V. T.: *Cancer Res. 25*:1018, 1965.
p-Methoxy-cinnamate	0.4	In rabbit	Woo, W. S.: *J. Pharm. Sci. 57*:27, 1968.
Methyl-prednisolone	1.52	In dog	Bilka, P. J. and Melby, J. C.: *Minnesota Med. 41*:263, 1958.
	1.35	In dog	Dulin, W. E., Barnes, L. E., Glenn, E. M., Lyster, S. C. and Collins, E. J.: *Metabolism 7*:398, 1958.
6-Methyl-F-prednisolone	1.83	In dog	Dulin, W. E., Barnes, L. E., Glenn, E. M., Lyster, S. C. and Collins, E. J.: *Metabolism 7*:398, 1958.
5-Methylpyrazole-3-carboxylic acid	1 1.8 1.9	In rat In dog In man	Drug Actions, Interactions and Reactions, *Drug Intelligence 1*:353, 1967.
Methyl salicylate	2.2 ± 0.2		Wurster, D. E. and Kramer, S. F.: *J. Pharm. Sci. 50*:288, 1961.
3-Methyl salicylic acid	18		*Brit. J. Pharmacol. 25*:470, 1965.
α-MMT	500		Beckel, M. H.: *Drug Res. 11*:123, 1968.
MTPR (6-methylthiopurine ribonucleoside)	5 days	Plasma radioactivity	Loo, T. L., Luce, S. K., Sullivan, M. P. and Frei, E. III, *Clin. Pharmacol. Therap. 9*:180, 1968.
Nafcillin	0.55 1.08	Uremic patients	Kind, A. C., Tupasi, T. E., Standiford, H. C. and Kirby, W.: *Arch. Internal Med. 125*:685, 1970.
	1.1	Half-lives calculated from k_{el} values; probenecid also administered	Gibaldi, M. and Schwartz, M. A.: *Clin. Pharmacol. Therap. 9*:345, 1968.
Nalidixic Acid	8.25	Calculated from k_{el}	Moore, W. E., Portmann, G. A., Stander, H. and McChesney, E. W.: *J. Pharm. Sci. 54*: 36, 1965.
Neohydrin	0.83-1.33		Borghgraef, R. R. M., Kessler, R. H. and Pitts, R. F.: *J. Clin. Invest. 35*:1055, 1956.
Neomycin	5.4 3.7	Infants 4-10 days Infants 13-21 days	Stanton, G. A., Yaffe, S. J. and Simon, H. J.: *Pediatrics 39*:97, 1967.
Nitrofurantoin	0.3		Reckendorf, H. K., Castringius, R. and Spingler, H.: *Med. Welt 14*:816, 1963.
	0.5		Bennett, W. M., Singer, I. and Coggins, C. H.: *J. Am. Med. Assoc. 214*:1468, 1970.
	0.45-0.57		Data supplied by Eaton Labs.
	0.33		Kunin, C. M.: *Ann. Internal Med. 67*:151, 1967.
	0.3 1.1	 Pre-partem	Kobyletzki, V. D.: *Med. Welt 19*:2010, 1968.
Nitroglycerin	0.55		Ritschel, W. A. and Clotten, R.: *Arzneimittel-Forsch. 20*:1180, 1970.
Nor-chlorcyclizine	216		Data obtained from Burroughs-Wellcome
Nor-orphenadrine	25		Data obtained from Riker.
Nortriptyline	20-60		Hammer, W., Martens, S. and Sjoquist, F.: *Clin. Pharmacol. Therap. 10*:44, 1969.
Noscapine	0.15	In mouse and in rabbit	Gibaldi, M. and Werner, N. D.: *J. Pharm. Sci. 54*:769, 1965.
	0.147	In man	Nayak, K. P., Brockmann-Hanssen, E. and Way Leong, E.: *J. Pharm. Sci. 54*:191, 1965.

SUBSTANCE	$t_{1/2}$ [h]	REMARKS	REFERENCES
Novobiocin	2.26 ± 1.09		Hitzenberger, G. and Spitzy, K.: *Arzneimittel-Forsch.* 7:291, 1957.
	2.3		Kunin, C. M.: *Ann. Internal Med.* 67:151, 1967.
Oleandomycin	1		Walter, A. M. and Heilmeyer, L.: *Antibiotica-Fibel,* 2nd ed., Stuttgart, 1965.
Orphenadrine	14		Data obtained from Riker.
Ouabain	22		Weissler, A. M., Snyder, J. R., Schoenfeld, C. D. and Cohen, S.: *Am. J. Cardiol.* 17:768, 1966.
Oxacillin	1.1-1.5		Ruedy, J.: *Can. Med. Assoc. J.* 94:1343, 1966.
	1.6	Premature infants 8-15 days old	Sereni, F. and Principi, W.: *Ann. Rev. Pharmacol.* 8:453, 1968.
	1.2	Premature infants 20-21 days old	
	1.5	Infants, 1-6 days old	
	1.1	Infants, 1 year old	
	0.7	Adults	
	0.5	Uremic patients	Rosenblatt, J. E., Brodie, J. L., Kind, A. C. and Kirby, W. M.: *Arch. Internal Med.* 121: 345, 1968.
	0.383		
	0.40		Kind, A. C., Tupasi, T. E., Standiford, H. C. and Kirby, W. M.: *Arch. Internal Med.* 125: 685, 1970.
	1.23	Uremic patients	
	0.616	From urine conc. data	Modr, Z. and Dvoracek, K.: *Rev. Czech. Med.* 69:79, 1969.
	0.363	From serum conc. data	
	0.5		Kunin, C. M.: *Ann. Internal Med.* 67:151, 1967.
	2.0	Patients with oliguria	
Oxypurinol	17-42		Data obtained from Burroughs-Wellcome
Oxyphenylbutazone	27-64		Hammer, W., Martens, S. and Sjoquist, F.: *Clin. Pharmacol. Therap.* 10:44, 1969.
	0.5	In dog	Brodie, B. B., *J. Am. Med. Assoc.* 202:600, 1967.
	72		Burns, J. J.: *Ann. N.Y. Acad. Sci.* 151:959, 1968.
	8	In monkey	
	0.5	In dog	
Oxytetracycline	9.2		Walter, A. M. and Heilmeyer, L.: *Antibiotica-Fibel,* 2nd ed., Stuttgart, 1965.
	9.6		Kunin, C. M.: *Ann. Internal Med.* 67:151, 1967.
Ozafuradene	0.7	Solubilized I.V.	Conklin, D. and Buzard, J. A.: *J. Pharm. Sci.* 54:1770, 1965.
	0.94	Susp. I.V.	
	1.25-1.7	I.V.	
P2565	0.15		Beckel, M. H.: *Drug Res.* 11:123, 1968.
2 PAM (pralidoxine salts)	1.7·		Kondutzer, A.: *J. Pharm. Sci.* 57:1142, 1968.
Papavarine	1.67		Voltero, L. D.: *Pharmic-Rev.* 9:299, 1970.
Penicillin G	0.5		Bennett, W. M., Singer, I. and Coggins, C. H.: *J. Am. Med. Assoc.* 214:1468, 1970.
	0.40	Women under 50 years	Hansen, J. M., Kapman, J. and Laursen, H.: *Lancet* 1:1170, 1970.
	0.93	Women over 70 years	
	0.35	Men under 30 years	
	0.65	Men over 65 years	

SUBSTANCE	$t_{1/2}$ [h]	REMARKS	REFERENCES
	0.5-1		Buckland, F.: *Ref. Deut. Med. Wochschr. 71*: 121, 1946.
			Eagle, H., Fleischman, R. and Musselman, A. D.: *J. Bacteriol. 57*:119, 1949.
			Fleming, A., Young, M. Y., Suchet, J. and Rowe, A. J. E.: *Lancet 2*:621, 1944.
			McAdam, I. W. J., Duguid, J. P. and Challinor, S. W.: *Lancet 2*:336, 1944.
	7.2-10.5	Patients with oliguria	Kunin, C. M.: *Ann. Internal Med. 67*:151, 1967.
Pentaerythritol tetranitrate	6.3		Davidson, I. W. F., Miller, H. S. and DiCarlo, F. J.: *J. Pharm. Sci. 60*:274, 1971.
Pentazocine	2.5-6.0	Variation between subjects but independent of route of administration	Beckett, A. H., Taylor, J. F. and Kourounakis, P.: *J. Pharm. Pharmacol. 22*:123, 1970.
Pentobarbital	42		Brodie, B. B., Burns, J. J., Lester, C. M., Lief, P. A., Bernstein, E. and Papper, E. M.: *J. Pharmacol. Exptl. Therap. 109*:26, 1953.
Phenobarbital	24-48		"Evaluations of Drug Interactions," APhA, Washington, D. C., 1971, Chapter, "General Mechanisms Involved in Drug Interactions and Their Clinical Implications."
	48-144		Butler, T. C., Mahaffee, C. and Waddell, W. J.: *J. Pharmacol. Exptl. Therap. 111*:425, 1954.
Phenylbutazone	45		Burns, J. J., Rose, R. K., Chenkin, T., Goldman, A., Schulert, A. and Brodie, B. B.: *J. Pharmacol. Exptl. Therap. 109*:346, 1953.
			Burns, J. J., Yü, T. F., Dayton, P. G., Brodie, B. B. and Gutman, A. B.: *Proc. IV Europ. Congr. Istanbul 1959,* p. 802.
			Burns, J. J., Yü, T. F., Dayton, P. G., Gutman, A. B. and Brodie, B. B.: *Ann. N.Y. Acad. Sci. 86*:253, 1960.
			Herrmann, O.: *Med. Exptl. 1*:170, 1959.
	72		Burns, J. J.: *Ann. N.Y. Acad. Sci. 151*:959, 1968.
	6	In dog	Zbinden, G.: *Advan. Pharmacol. 2*:65, 1963.
	8	In monkey	Burns, J. J.: *Ann. N.Y. Acad. Sci. 151*:959, 1968.
	3 6 5	In rabbit In rat In guinea pig	Burns, J. J., Yü, T. F., Dayton, P. G., Gutman, A. B. and Brodie, B. B.: *Ann. N.Y. Acad. Sci. 86*:253, 1960.
	6 6	In horse In dog	Burns, J. J.: *Ann. N.Y. Acad. Sci. 151*:959, 1968.
	31-175	Data reported from different patients	Vessell, E.: *Science 159*:1479, 1968.
	3-6 72	In lab animals In man	Brodie, B. B.: *J. Am. Med. Assoc. 202*:600, 1967.
Phenylpropanol	3.9		Heimlich, K. R., McDonneill, D., Flanagan, T. L. and O'Brien, P.: *J. Pharm. Sci. 50*:232, 1961.
Plasma	648		Margen, S. and Taraver, H.: *J. Clin. Invest. 35*:1161, 1956.
Polymyxin B	14.3	In dialysis	Buck, L. C. and Cohen, S. L.: *J. Clin. Pathol. 21*:88, 1968.
	6	Calculated from data presented in the literature	Kunin, C. M.: *Ann. Internal Med. 67*:151, 1967.

SUBSTANCE	$t_{1/2}$ [h]	REMARKS	REFERENCES
	48-72	Calculated from data presented in the literature; patients with oliguria	
Pralidoxime (2PAM)			
—chloride	1.7		Kondritzer, A. A., Zvirblis, P., Goodman, A. and Paplanus, S. H.: *J. Pharm. Sci. 57*:1142, 1968.
—iodide	2.1		
—lactate	1.7		
—methane sulfonate	1.65		
—phosphate	1.4		
Prednisolone	3.34		Peterson, R. E.: *Recent Progr. Hormone Res. 15*:237, 1959.
	1	In dog	Knipers, F., Ely, R., Hughes, E. and Kelly, V.: *Proc. Soc. Exptl. Biol. Med. 95*:187, 1957.
	1.15	In dog	Bilka, P. J. and Melby, J. C.: *Minnesota Med. 41*:263, 1958.
	1.18		Silber, R. H.: *Ann. N.Y. Acad. Sci. 82*:821, 1959.
Prednisone	0.55		Silber, R. H. and Morgan, E. R.: *Clin. Chem. 2*:170, 1956.
Probenecid	6-12		Bennett, W. M., Singer, I. and Coggins, C. H.: *J. Am. Med. Assoc. 214*:1468, 1970.
	2-4		Jusko, W. J., Levy, G. and Leonards, J. R.: *J. Pharm. Sci. 59*:464, 1970.
Procaine hydrochloride	0.37	Calculated from blood level data	Wikinski, J. A., Usubiaga, J. E. and Wikinski, R. W.: *J. Am. Med. Assoc. 213*:621, 1970.
Propicillin	0.5-1		Walter, A. M. and Heilmeyer, L.: *Antibiotica-Fibel,* 2nd ed., Stuttgart, 1965.
Propionylerythromycin lauryl sulfate	1.6		Chun, A. H. C. and Wiegand, R. G.: 118th Annual Meeting A.Ph.A. Academy of Pharmaceutical Sciences, San Francisco, March-April, 1971.
Propranolol	2.3	I.V. administration	Shand, D. G., Nuckolls, E. M. and Oates, J. A.: *Clin. Pharmacol. Therap. 11*:112, 1970.
	3.2	Peroral administration	
Protein (total)	230		Volwiler, W., Fremont-Smith, K. and McMartin, M. P.: *J. Clin. Invest. 31*:686, 1952.
Prothrombin	41	In dog	Hellemans, J., *et al.*: *Brit. J. Haematol. 9*: 506, 1963.
Pseudoephedrine	7		Data obtained from Burroughs-Wellcome
	5	Urinary *p*H = 5.3	
	13	Urinary *p*H = 8	
Psicofuranine	2.33		Forist, A. A.: *J. Pharm. Sci. 54*:927, 1965.
	1.81		
Pyrazinamide	10-16		Walter, A. M. and Heilmeyer, L.: *Antibiotica-Fibel,* 2nd ed., Stuttgart, 1965.
Pyrazole	14	Alcohol also administered in rats	Lester, D. and Benson, G. D.: *Science 169*: 282, 1970.
2 Pyridine aldoxine methachloride	2.4		Sidell, F. R., Williams, A. G. and Ellin, R. I.: *J. Pharm. Sci. 58*:1093, 1969.
Pyrimethamine	360	In dog	Woolley, D. W.: *J. Clin. Pharmacol. Therap. 1*:556, 1960.
	36		Data obtained from Burroughs-Wellcome
Pyrrolidino-methyltetracycline	6-7		Böhm, C.: *Nierenfunktionsstörung und Antibiotica,* E. Merck A. G., Darmstadt, p. 32.
Quinine	4-6		Bennett, W. M., Singer, I. and Coggins, C. H.: *J. Am. Med. Assoc. 214*:1468, 1970.
Quinidine HCl	4.5	Calculated from blood level data	Rasmussen, S.: *Acta Pharmacol. Toxicol. 24*: 331, 1966.
Quinidine sulfate	7.5		Riegelman, S.: *Drug Inform. Bull. 3*:59, 1969.

SUBSTANCE	$t_{1/2}$ [h]	REMARKS	REFERENCES
	7.5		Goldberg, W. A. and Chalabarlic, S. G.: *Can. Med. Assoc. J. 91*:991, 1964.
Reserpine	0.4	$t_{1/4}$ quoted in text	Becuel, M. H.: *Drug Res. 11*:123, 1968.
Riboflavin	1.4	Rapid half-life	Levy, G. and Jusko, W. J.: *J. Pharm. Sci. 59*: 487, 1970.
	1.1		Levy, G. and Jusko, W. J.: *J. Pharm. Sci. 54*: 285, 1965.
	1.2		Levy, G. and Jusko, W. J.: *J. Pharm. Sci. 55*: 1322, 1966.
	5.1 4.8 1.5 2.2	5 day old male 5 day old female 5 day old male 6 day old female	Jusko, W. J., Khanna, N., Levy, G., Stern, L. and Yaffee, S.: *Pediatrics 45*:945, 1970.
D-Ribose	1.7		Segal, St. and Foley, J. B.: *J. Clin. Invest. 38*: 407, 1959.
Rifampin	7 1.5-5	In dog In rat, rabbit, monkey, man	Cohn, H. D.: *J. Clin. Pharmacol. 9*:118, 1969.
Rifamycin	1.46		Hitzengerger, G. and Spitzy, K. H.: *Arzneimittel-Forsch. 7*:291, 1957. Bergamini, N. and Fowst, G.: *Arzneimittel-Forsch. 15*:952, 1965.
Ristocetin	2-3		Walter, A. M. and Heilmeyer, L.: *Antibiotica-Fibel,* 2nd ed., Stuttgart, 1965.
RO4-1204	0.2		Beckel, M. H.: *Drug Res. 11*:123, 1968.
Rolitetracycline	4.5		Strauch, D. and Koch, E.: *Münch. Med. Wochschr. 100*:1, 1958.
Salicylic phenolic	0.7	In rats	Levy, G., Weintraub, L., Matjuzawa, T. and Oles, S. R.: *J. Pharm. Sci. 55*:1319, 1966.
Salicyluric acid	0.3	Approx. calculations	Levy, G., Amsel, L. P. and Howard, C. E.: *J. Pharm. Sci. 58*:7, 1969.
Serum protein	57.6	In rat	Oeff, K.: *Z. Exptl. Med. 123*:309, 1954.
Sodium salicylate	6.2		Gibaldi, M. and Kanig, J. L.: *J. Pharm. Sci. 54*:599, 1965.
Sodium thiosulfate	0.65		Gladtke, E.: Der Thiosulfatraum des Kindes, 54. Beiheft, Z. Arch. Kinderheilk, 1966.
Streptomycin	2.2-3.2		Kunin, C. M. and Finland, M.: *J. Clin. Invest. 38*:1509, 1959. Wechselberg, K. and Weidenbusch, E.: *Ergeb. Inn. Med. N.F. 2*:713, 1962.
	2.4-2.7 52-100	Normal patients Patients with oliguria	Kunin, C. M.: *Ann. Internal Med. 67*:151, 1967.
	2.72 ± 0.47 1.52 ± 0.14	 In dog	Boxer, G. E., Jelinek, V. C., Tompsett, R., Dubois, R. and Edison, A.: *J. Pharmacol. Exptl. Therap. 92*:226, 1948.
	2.5		Bennett, W. M., Singer, I. and Coggins, C. H.: *J. Am. Med. Assoc. 214*:1468, 1970.
	2-4	Adults and young children	Goodman, L. S. and Gilman,, A.: *The Pharmacological Basis of Therapeutics,* 4th ed., MacMillan Co., New York, N.Y. 1970, p. 767.
	100	BUN in range of 100-150 mg/100 ml	
	7	Premature infants	
Sulfacetamide	12.8		Krüger-Thiemer, E. and Bünger, P.: *Arzneimittel-Forsch. 11*:867, 1961.
	7		Rieder, J.: *Arzneimittel-Forsch. 13*:81, 1963.
Sulfachloro-pyridazine	4.6		Krüger-Thiemer, E. and Bünger, P.: *Arzneimittel-Forsch. 11*:867, 1961.

SUBSTANCE	$t_{1/2}$ [h]	REMARKS	REFERENCES
	8.0		Rieder, J.: *Arzneimittel-Forsch. 13*:81, 1963.
Sulfadiazine	16.8		Bünger, P., Diller, W., Führ, J. and Krüger-Thiemer, E.: *Arzneimittel-Forsch. 11*:247, 1961.
	8-16		Loop, W.: *Mat. Med. Nordmark 14*:1, 1955.
	16.7		Rieder, J.: *Arzneimittel-Forsch. 13*:81, 1963.
			Krüger-Thiemer, E.: *Klin. Wochschr. 40*:153, 1962.
	16.0		Dettli, L. and Spring, P.: *Regensb. Ärztl. Fortbild. 14*:17, 1966.
Sulfadimethoxine	41		Bünger, P., Diller, W., Führ, J. and Krüger-Thiemer, E.: *Arzneimittel-Forsch. 11*:247, 1961.
			Krüger-Thiemer, E.: *Klin. Wochschr. 40*:153, 1962.
	23		Dost, F. H., Gladtke, E. and Rind, H.: *Monatsschr. Kinderheilk. 110*:259, 1962.
	28-42		Fust, B., Böhni, E., Schnitzer, R. J., Rieder, J. and Struller, T.: *Antibiot. Chemotherapia 8*:32, 1960.
	33		DeLorenzo, W. F. and Schnitzer, R. J.: *Ann. N.Y. Acad. Sci. 82*:10, 1959.
	20.2		Schönfeld, H.: *Chemotherapia 4*:8, 1962.
	35		Rieder, J.: *Arzneimittel-Forsch. 13*:81, 1963.
	36		Dettli, L. and Spring, P.: *Regensb. Ärztl. Fortbild. 14*:17, 1966.
Sulfadimethyl-oxazole	10.6		Krüger-Thiemer, E. and Bunger, P.: *Arzneimittel-Forsch. 11*:867, 1961.
			Krüger-Thiemer, E.: *Klin. Wochschr. 40*:153, 1962.
			Rieder, J.: *Arzneimittel-Forsch. 13*:81, 1963.
	7.4		Schönfeld, H.: *Chemotherapia 4*:8, 1962.
	8.8		Kuemmerle, H. P. and Contzen, H.: *Chemotherapia 4*:535, 1962.
	4.4-5.5		Degen, R.: *Kinderärztl. Praxis 30*:391, 1962.
	6.8		Gladtke, E.: *Arch. Kinderheilk. 169*:133, 1963.
Sulfadricramide	7.3 ± 1.2	In dog	Koppayi, T. and Auery, M. A.: *Clin. Pharmacol. Therap. 7*:252, 1966.
Sulfaethidole	5.5-13.3		Swintosky, J. V., Bondi, A., Jr. and Robinson, M. J.: *J. Am. Pharm. Assoc. Sci. Ed. 47*:753, 1958.
	11.4 4.2	Urinary $pH = 5$ Urinary $pH = 8$	Portnoff, J. B., Kostenbauder, A. B. and Swintosky, J. V.: *J. Pharm. Sci. 51*:1084, 1962.
Sulfaethyl-pyrimidine	26.8		Bünger, P. and Koch, G., *Arzneimittel-Forsch. 11*:726, 1961.
Sulfaethyl-thiadiazole	10.5		Krüger-Thiemer, E. and Bünger, P., *Arzneimittel-Forsch. 11*:867, 1961.
	5.8		Schönfeld, H.: *Chemotherapia 4*:8, 1962.
	4.8		Rieder, J.: *Arzneimittel-Forsch. 13*:81, 1963.
Sulfalene	65		Martin, D. C. and Arnold, J. D.: *J. Clin. Pharmacol. J. New Drugs 9*:3, 1969.
Sulfamerazine	16-24		Loop, W.: *Mat. Med. Nordmark 14*:1, 1955.
	23.5		Krüger-Thiemer, E.: *Klin. Wochschr. 40*:153, 1962.
			Rieder, J.: *Arzneimittel-Forsch. 13*:81, 1963.

SUBSTANCE	$t_{1/2}$ [h]	REMARKS	REFERENCES
			Bünger, P., Diller, W., Führ, J. and Krüger-Thiemer, E.: *Arzneimittel-Forsch.* *11*:247, 1961.
Sulfamethapyrazine	65		Vandenbergh, E., Clement, J. and Woestijne, K. P., *Brit. J. Diseases Chest* *64*:58, 1970.
Sulfamethazine	5		Taraszka, M. J. and Delor, R. A.: *J. Pharm. Sci.* *58*:207, 1969.
	6-8		Krüger-Thiemer, E.: *Klin. Wochschr.* *40*:153, 1962.
			Loop, W.: *Mat. Med. Nordmark* *14*:1, 1955.
	7		Rieder, J.: *Arzneimittel-Forsch.* *13*:81, 1963.
Sulfamethoxine	36.6		Rieder, J.: *Arzneimittel-Forsch.* *13*:81, 1963.
			Krüger-Thiemer, E.: *Klin. Wochschr.* *40*:153, 1962.
			Gladtke, E. and Schmalz, C.: *Arzneimittel-Forsch.* *15*:927, 1965.
	11.7		Schönfeld, H.: *Chemotherapia* *4*:8, 1962.
	34.1		Kuemmerle, H. P. and Contzen, H.: *Chemotherapia* *4*:535, 1962.
	29.6		Rind, H. and Gladtke, E.: *Monatsschr. Kinderheilk.* *112*:239, 1964.
	36.0		Dettli, L. and Spring, P.: *Regensb. Ärztl. Fortbild.* *14*:17, 1966.
Sulfamethoxy-diazine	> 48		Vignoli, L., Defretin, J. P., Vassallo, J. M. and Cristan, B.: *Therapie* *20*:1491, 1965.
Sulfamethoxy-pyrazine	60		Dost. F. H.: *Grundlagen der Pharmakokinetik,* 2nd ed., Stuttgart, 1968, p. 298.
	63.3		Sereni, F. and Principi, N.: *Ann. Rev. Pharmacol.* *8*:453, 1968.
	36.0		Dettli, L. and Spring, P.: *Regensb. Ärztl. Fortbild.* *14*:17, 1966.
Sulfamethoxy-pyridazine	63		Dettli, L. and Spring, P.: *Regensb. Ärztl. Fortbild.* *14*:17, 1966.
	34.6		Krüger-Thiemer, E.: *Klin. Wochschr,* *40*:153, 1962.
			Bünger, P., Diller, W., Führ, J. and Krüger-Thiemer, E.: *Arzneimittel-Forsch.* *11*:247, 1961.
			Krüger-Thiemer, E. and Bünger, P.: *Arzneimittel-Forsch.* *11*:867, 1961.
	44		DeLorenzo, W. F. and Schnitzer, R. J.: *Ann. N. Y. Acad. Sci.* *82*:10, 1959.
	60		Linke, H.: *Deut. Gesundheitsw.* *18*:823, 1963.
	40		Rieder, J.: *Arzneimittel-Forsch.* *13*:81, 1963.
	71.5		Dettli, L., Spring, P., and Raeber, I.: *Intern. J. Clin. Pharmacol. Therap. Toxicol.* *2*:130, 1967.
Sulfamethyl-isoxazole	9-12		Krüger-Thiemer, E. and Bünger, P.: *Arzneimittel-Forsch.* *11*:867, 1961.
	11		Rieder, J.: *Arzneimittel-Forsch.* *13*:81, 1963.
	10		Bünger, P., Diller, W., Führ, J. and Krüger-Thiemer, E.: *Arzneimittel-Forsch.* *11*:247, 1961.
			Dettli, L. and Spring, P.: *Regensb. Arztl. Fortbild.* *14*:17, 1966.
			Krüger-Thiemer, E.: *Klin. Wochschr.* *40*:153, 1962.
	8.8		Gladtke, E.: *Arch. Kinderheilk.* *169*:133, 1963.

SUBSTANCE	$t_{1/2}$ [h]	REMARKS	REFERENCES
Sulfamethyl-pyrimidine	40.8		Krüger-Thiemer, E.: *Klin. Wochschr. 40*:153, 1962.
	31.9		Rieder, J.: *Arzneimittel-Forsch. 13*:81, 1963.
Sulfa-5-methyl-thiadiazole	1.5-1.6		Nelson, E. and Reilly, J.: *J. Pharm. Sci. 54*: 599, 1965.
Sulfamethopyrazine	50.3-111.8		Devriendt, A., Jansen, F. H. and Weemaes, I.: *Europ. J. Clin. Pharmacol. 3*:36, 1970.
Sulfamono-methoxine	30		Rieder, J.: *Arzneimittel-Forsch. 13*:81, 1963.
Sulfanilamide	8.8		Bünger, P., Diller, W., Führ, J. and Krüger-Thiemer, E.: *Arzneimittel-Forsch. 13*:81, 1963.
	5	In dog	Maren, T. H., Palmer, R. F. and Griffith, M. E.: *Biochem. Pharmacol. 6*:21, 1961.
	1.4	In rabbit	Wistrand, P. J., Rawls, J. A. and Maren, T. H.: *Acta Pharmacol. 17*:337, 1961.
	10		Frisk, A.: *Acta Med. Scand. Suppl. 142*:1, 1963.
4-Sulfanilamido-5,6-di-methoxy-pyrimidine	93		Rind, H. and Gladtke, E.: *Monatsschr. Kinderheilk. 112*:239, 1964.
	126		Schönfeld, H., *Chemotherapia 4*:8, 1962.
			Portwich, F. and Buttner, H.: *Klin. Wochschr. 42*:740, 1961.
5-Sulfanilamido-2-4-di-methyl-pyrimidine	30.5		Rieder, J.: *Arzneimittel-Forsch. 13*:81, 1963.
	32.7		Bünger, P., Diller, W., Führ, J. and Krüger-Thiemer, E.: *Arzneimittel-Forsch. 11*:247, 1961.
6-Sulfanilamido-2-meth-oxy-methyl-4-meth-oxypyrimidine	6.7		Rind, H. and Gladtke, E., *Monatsschr. Kinderheilk. 112*:239, 1964.
4-Sulfanilamido-3,6-meth-oxy pyrimidine	100		Dettli, L. and Spring, P.: *Regensb. Ärztl. Fortbild. 14*:17, 1966.
2-Sulfanilamido-5-methylpyrimidine	36.3-40.8	Peroral route	Krüger-Thiemer, E. and Eriksen, S. P.: *J. Pharm. Sci. 53*:1249, 1966.
	17.1	I.V. route	
Sulfaphenazole	11		Krüger-Thiemer, E. and Bünger, P.: *Arzneimittel-Forsch. 11*:867, 1961.
	9-10		DeLorenzo, W. F. and Schnitzer, R. J.: *Ann. N.Y. Acad. Sci. 82*:10, 1959.
	8.3		Schönfeld, H.: *Chemotherapia 4*:8, 1962.
	10		Dettli, L. and Spring, P.: *Regensb. Ärztl. Fortbild. 14*:17, 1966.
			Rieder, J.: *Arzneimittel-Forsch. 13*:81, 1963.
	8.6		Bünger, P., Diller, W., Führ, J. and Krüger-Thiemer, E.: *Arzneimittel-Forsch. 11*:247, 1961.
	8-12		Krüger-Thiemer, E.: *Klin. Wochschr. 40*:153, 1962.
Sulfapyridine	9.4		Krüger-Thiemer, E.: *Arzneimittel-Forsch. 11*: 867, 1961.
	6.5-9.4		Krüger-Thiemer, E.: *Klin. Wochschr. 40*:153, 1962.
Sulfasomidine (sulfa-dimethyl-pyrimidine)	7.4		Rieder, J.: *Arzneimittel-Forsch. 13*:81, 1963.
	6-8		Krüger-Thiemer, E.: *Klin. Wochschr. 40*:153, 1962.
			Loop, W.: *Mat. Med. Nordmark 14*:1, 1955.
	7.5		Gladtke, E. and Schmalz, C.: *Arzneimittel-Forsch. 11*:726, 1961.

SUBSTANCE	$t_{1/2}$ [h]	REMARKS	REFERENCES
Sulfasymazine	14.0		Dettli, L., Spring, P. and Raeber, I.: *Intern. J. Clin. Pharmacol. Therap. Toxicol.* *2*:130, 1967.
Sulfathiazole	3.5		Krüger-Thiemer, E. and Bünger, P.: *Arzneimittel-Forsch.* *11*:867, 1961.
	3.8		Rieder, J.: *Arzneimittel-Forsch.* *13*:81, 1963.
	3.4-3.6		Krüger-Thiemer, E.: *Klin. Wochschr.* *40*:153, 1962.
Sulfinpyrazone	8.8		Ogryzlo, M. A., Digby, J. W., Montgomery, D. B., Houpt, J. B., McKenzie, D. H. and Holmes, V.: *Minerva Med.* *1*:263, 1961.
Sulfisoxazole	3-4		Bennett, W. M., Singer, I. and Coggins, C. H.: *J. Am. Med. Assoc.* *214*:1468, 1970.
	6.1		Bünger, P., Diller, W., Führ, J., and Krüger-Thiemer, E.: *Arzneimittel-Forsch.* *11*:247, 1961.
			Krüger-Thiemer, E.: *Klin. Wochschr.* *40*:153, 1962.
	6-7		DeLorenzo, W. F. and Schnitzer, R.: *Ann. N.Y. Acad. Sci.* *82*:10, 1959.
	6.0		Rieder, J.: *Arzneimittel-Forsch.* *13*:81, 1963.
	4.7		Gladtke, E.: *Arch. Kinderheilk.* *169*:133, 1963.
	5-9		Data supplied by Roche Labs.
Symmetrel	20		Council on Drugs: *J. Am. Med. Assoc.* *201*: 34, 1967.
Taloximine	0.6	Phase I	Prime, F. J., Griffin, J. P., Turner, P., Ben-Dyke, R. and Pukering, R. W.: *Pharmacol. Clin.* *2*:155, 1970.
	2.7	Phase II	
			Edwards, G. and Griffin, J. P.: *Europ. J. Clin. Pharmacol.* *3*:18, 1970.
Testosterone	1.67		Sandberg, A. A. and Slaunwhite, W. R., Jr.: *J. Clin. Invest.* *35*:1331, 1956.
	1.99	As formate	James, K. C., Nicholls, P. J. and Roberts, M.: *J. Pharm. Pharmacol.* *21*:24, 1969.
	2.82	As formate	
	2.94	As acetate	
	3.75	As propionate	
	4.94	As butyrate	
	7.43	As valerate	
Tetracycline	6-8		Bennett, W. M., Singer, I. and Coggins, C. H.: *J. Am. Med. Assoc.* *214*:1468, 1970.
	2.87-10.3	For children 13-155 lbs. with novobiocin drops	Wagner, J. G.: *J. Pharm. Sci.* *56*:652, 1967.
	4.76	For children 37-120 lbs. with novobiocin drops	
	2.68-8.70	Range for above	
	5.31	For children 19-100 lbs. with tetracycline susp.	
	2.06-9.93	Range for above	
	4.99	For children 17-100 lbs. with tetracycline susp.	
	2.31-7.32	Range for above	
	7.08	Adults 120-204 lbs. with novobiocin granules	
	3.84-18	Range for above	
	6.28	Adults 116-220 lbs. HFC tetracycline 250 mg.	

SUBSTANCE	$t_{1/2}$ [h]	REMARKS	REFERENCES
	1.91-13.8	Range for above	
	8.5 57-108	Patients with oliguria	Kunin, C. M.: *Ann. Internal Med. 67*:151, 1967.
	8.5		Walter, A. M. and Heilmeyer, L.: *Antibiotica-Fibel,* 2nd ed., Stuttgart, 1965.
	6-8		Bennett, W. M., Singer, I. and Coggins, C. H.: *J. Am. Med. Assoc. 214*:1468, 1970.
	6.4		Swintosky, J. V., Dittert, L. W. and Doluisio, J. T.: *Am. J. Hosp. Pharm. 26*:519, 1969.
	6-8		Greenborg, P. A. and Sanford, J. P.: *Ann. Internal Med. 66*:465, 1967.
	29.5-78.7	7 ml/min. creatinine clearance	
	30-128	Patients with renal insufficiency undergoing peritoneal dialysis. Half-life during dialysis	
	64	Average for above range	
Tetraethylene-ammonium	0.67		Rennick, B. R., Moe, G. K., Lyons, R. H., Hoobler, S. W. and Neligh, R.: *J. Pharmacol. Exptl. Therap. 91*:210, 1947.
Thalidomide	3	In rat	Schumacher, H. and Blake, D. A.: *J. Pharm. Exptl. Therap. 160*:201, 1968.
Thioacetatone	8-12		Walter, A. M. and Heilmeyer, L.: *Antibiotica-Fibel,* 2nd ed., Stuttgart, 1965.
Thiopental	16		Lief, P. A., Bruns, J. J., Papper, E. M. and Brodie, B. B.: *Current Res. Anesthesia Analgesia 31*:147, 1952.
Thymian Oil	3.8		Pafrath, H. and Benecke, O.: *Arch. Exptl. Pathol. Pharmakol 176*:558, 1934.
Thyroxine (T_4)	> 168		Sterling, K., Bellabarba, D., Newman, E. S. and Brenner, M.; *J. Clin. Invest. 48*:1150, 1969.
Tolbutamide	7.5		Solomon, H. M. and Schrogie, J. J.: *Clin. Pharmacol. Therap. 8*:66, 1967.
	4		Bennett, W. M., Singer, I. and Coggins, C. H.: *J. Am. Med. Assoc. 214*:1468, 1970.
	7.8 ± 0.3 6-9	Probenecid also administered	Brook, R., Schrogie, J. and Solomon, A. H.: *Clin. Pharmacol. Therap. 9*:314, 1968.
	3.5-38	Range of half-lives quoted in the literature	
	5		Visconti, J. A.: Paper presented at the Annual Meeting of the Ohio Society of Hospital Pharmacists, 1970.
	15	Chloramphenicol also administered	
	2.75 ± 0.5 5.8 ± 2.2	In alcoholics	Kater, R. M. H., Roggin, G., Tobon, F., Zieve, P. and Iber, F. L.: *Am. J. Med. Sci. 258*:35, 1969.
	5.6		Bhatia, S. K., Hadden, D. R., Montgomery, D. A. D. and Weaver, J. A.: *Brit. Med. J. 2*: 570, 1970.
Tolonium (Toluidine Blue, seleno methionine, SE 75)	24-48		Diguillo, W. and Lindenaver, S. M.: *J. Am. Med. Assoc. 214*:2302, 1970.
Toxogonin	1.38		Sidell, F. R. and Groff, W. A.: *J. Pharm. Sci. 59*:793, 1970.
2,3,5-Triiodo-benzoic acid	395-403	In rat	Ice, R. D., Breckenridge, C. E., Jr. and Christian, J. E.: *J. Pharm. Sci. 55*:497, 1966.

SUBSTANCE	$t_{1/2}$ [h]	REMARKS	REFERENCES
Triamcinolone	5.0		Melby, J. C. and Dale, S. L.: *Med. Clin. N. Am. 45*:875, 1961.
	1.94 0.87	In dog In rat	Florini, J. R., Peets, E. A. and Buyske, D. A.: *J. Pharmacol. Exptl. Therap. 131*:187, 1961.
Triiodothyronine	31.2-33.6		Sterling, K., Bellabarba, D., Newman, E. S. and Brenner, M.: *J. Clin. Invest. 48*:1150, 1969.
L-Triiodothyronine (liothyronine sodium)	60		Prescribing information, Cytomel, S.K.F. Lab., Philadelphia, U.S.A., Oct. 1969.
Trimethoprim	16		Martin, D. C. and Arnold, J. D.: *J. Clin. Pharmacol. 9*:155, 1969.
	16.1 3.1	 In dog	Kaplan, S. H.: *J. Pharm. Sci. 59*:358, 1970.
Tryptophan	15.84		Tolckmitt, W.: *Habilitation*, Giessen, 1967.
Tubocurarine	0.217		Mahfouz, M.: *Brit. J. Pharmacol. 4*:295, 1949.
U18536	2.1 ± 0.2 3.0 ± 0.2	 Metabolite of U18536	Forist, A. A., Vecchio, T. J. and Smith D. L.: *Pharmacologist 6*:208, 1964.
Urea	1.17		Rehberg, P.: *Biochem. J. 20*:461, 1926.
Vancomycin	2-4		Walter, A. M. and Heilmeyer, L.: *Antibiotica-Fibel,* 2nd ed., Stuttgart, 1965.
	6 216	 Patients with oliguria (calculated from data presented in the literature)	Kunin, C. M.: *Ann. Internal Med. 67*:151, 1967.
	6		Goodman, L. S. and Gilman, A.: *The Pharmacological Basis of Therapeutics,* 4th ed., MacMillan Co., New York, NY, 1970, p. 1292.
	75	Calculated from serum level data of patients with kidney failure requiring regular hemodialysis	Eykyn, S., Phillips, I. and Evans, J.: *Brit. Med. J. 3*:80, 1970.
Viomycin	3-4		Walter, A. M. and Heilmeyer, L.: *Antibiotica-Fibel,* 2nd ed., Stuttgart, 1965.
Vitamin A	9.1		Beaumont, J. L. and Ardaillou, R.: *Rev. Franc. Etudes Clin. Biol. 4*:40, 1959.
Vitamin B_1	0.35		Dost, F. H.: *Der Blutspiegel,* Leipzig, 1953.
Vitamin B_{12}	123		Adams, J. F.: *Nature, 198*:200, 1963.
Vitamin C	384	In man, (study with C^{14} labeled L-ascorbic acid)	Burns, J. J.: *Ann. N.Y. Acad. Sci. 151*:959, 1968.
	96	In guinea pig	
Vitamin D	960		Warkany, J., Guest, G. M. and Grabill, F.: *J. Lab. Clin. Med. 27*:557, 1942.
Warfarin	41.0 26.5	 In alcoholics	Reidler, G.: *Thromb. Diath. Haemorrhag. 16*: 613, 1966. through Parker, W. J.: *J. Am. Pharm. Assoc. NS10*:664, 1970.
	47 ± 7 57	 Patient with hereditary resistence to peroral anticoagulants	O'Reilly, R.: *New Engl. J. Med. 282*:1448, 1970.
	47		Deykin, D.: *New Engl. J. Med. 282*:1486, 1970.
Water	0.93		Ther, L.: *Arch. Exptl. Pathol. Pharmakol. 205*:376, 1948.
Xylocaine	1.5		Data supplied by Astra Pharmaceutical Products from unpublished data.
D-Xylose	1.5		Segal, St. and Foley, J. B.: *J. Clin. Invest. 38*: 407, 1959.

References

1. Dost, F. H.: The Clearance, *Klin. Wochschr. 27*: 257-264 (Apr.) 1949 (in German).
2. Wagner, J. G.: Pharmacokinetics - 3. Half-Life and Volume of Distribution, *Drug Intelligence 2*:126-133 (May) 1968.
3. Ritschel, W. A.: Biological Half-Lives of Drugs, *Drug Intelligence Clin. Pharm. 4*:332-347 (Dec.) 1970.
4. Ritschel, W. A.: Symposium Lecture at 23rd Congress (General Assembly) of Federation International Pharmaceutique (FIP), Section Hospital Pharmacy, Geneva, (Sept. 1) 1970.
5. Ritschel, W. A. and Clotten, R.: Development of a Peroral Proxyphylline Retard Preparation I, *Arzneimittel-Forsch. 19*:221-225 (Mar.) 1969 (in German).
6. Ritschel, W. A. and Clotten, R.: Development of a Peroral Proxyphylline Retard Preparation, II, *Arzneimittel-Forsch. 19*:347-353 (Mar.) 1969 (in German).
7. Ritschel, W. A.: *Applied Biopharmaceutics* (A Continuing Education Program), University of Cincinnati College of Pharmacy, Cincinnati, Ohio, 1969. p. 217.
8. Ibid., p. 218.
9. Ibid., p. 264.
10. Dost, F. H.: *Grundlagen der Pharmakokinetik,* ed. 2, Georg Thieme Verlag, 1968. p. 275.
11. Ritschel, W. A.: *Applied Biopharmaceutics I,* op. cit., p. 259.
12. Wagner, J. G.: Biopharmaceutics - 9. Pharmacokinetic Concepts for the Clinician, Pharmacist and Nurse, *Drug Intelligence 3*:108-112 (Apr.) 1969.
13. Krüger-Thiemer, E.: Functional Relations Between Pharmacokinetic Properties and Dosage Schedule of Chemotherapeutic Agents, *Klin. Wochschr. 38*:514-520 (June) 1960 (in German).
14. Krüger-Thiemer, E.: Dosage Schedule and Pharmacokinetics in Chemotherapy, *J. Am. Pharm. Assoc. Sci. Ed. 49*:311-313, 1960.
15. Krüger-Thiemer, E.: Theory of Mechanism of Action of Bacteriostatic Chemotherapeutics. Quantitative Relation Between Dosage, *in vitro* Action, Pharmacokinetics and Distribution, *Jahresb. Borstel 5*:316-400, 1961 (in German).
16. Krüger-Thiemer, E. and Bünger, P.: The Role of the Therapeutic Regimen in Dosage Design. I, *Chemotherapia 10*:61-73, 1965 (in German).
17. Bünger, P., Diller, W., Führ, J. and Krüger-Thiemer, E.: Comparative Studies on Newer Sulfonamides, *Arzneimittel-Forsch. 11*:247-255, 1961 (in German).
18. Levy, G.: Pharmacokinetics of Salicylate Elimination in Man, *J. Pharm. Sci. 54*:959-967 (July) 1965.
19. Wilkinson, G. R. and Beckett, A. H.: Absorption, Metabolism, and Excretion of the Ephedrines in Man II, *J. Pharm. Sci. 57*:1933-1938 (Nov.) 1968.
20. Kostenbauder, H. B., Portnoff, J. B. and Swintosky, J. V.: Control of Urine *p*H and Its Effect on Sulfaethidole Excretion in Humans, *J. Pharm. Sci. 51*:1084-1089 (Nov.) 1962.
21. Beckett, A. H. and Tucker, G. T.: Problems in the *in Vivo* Evaluation of Drug Preparations and the Interpretation of *in Vivo* Data, *J. Mondial Pharm. 3*:181-202 (3) 1967.
22. Krüger-Thiemer, E. and Bünger, P.: Cumulation and Toxicity as Results of Wrong Dosage Schedule of Sulfonamides, *Arzneimittel-Forsch. 11*:867-874, 1961 (in German).
23. Dietel, V. and Walther, V.: Experimental Study on Elimination and Volume of Distribution of Sulfonamides in Premature Infants, *Z. Ges. Inn. Med. 16*:567-569 (July) 1961 (in German).
24. Sereni, F. and Principi, N.: Developmental Pharmacology, *Ann. Rev. Pharmacol. 8*:453-466, 1968.
25. Dost, F. H. and Gladtke, E.: Pharmacokinetics of 2-Sulfanilamido-3-Methoxypyrazine in the Child, *Arzneimittel-Forsch. 19*:1304-1307 (Aug.) 1969 (in German).
26. Corte, G. and Johnson, W.: Effect of N-Acetyl-para-Aminophenol on Plasma Levels of 17-Hydroxycorticosteroids, *Proc. Soc. Exptl. Biol. Med. 97*:751-755 (Apr.) 1958.
27. Conney, A. H., Davison, C., Gastel, R. and Burns, J. J.: Adaptive Increases in Drug Metabolism Enzymes Induced by Phenobarbital and Other Drugs, *J. Pharmacol. Exptl. Therap. 130*:1-8 (Sept.) 1960.
28. Remmer, H., Siegert, M. and Merker, H. J.: Increase of Drug Oxidizing Enzymes by Tolbutamide, *Arch. Exptl. Pathol. Pharmakol. 249*:71-84, 1964 (in German).
29. Burns, J. J., Rose, R. K., Chenkin, T., Goldman, A., Schulert, A. and Brodie, B. B.: The Physiological Disposition of Phenylbutazone (Butazolidin) in Man and a Method for Its Estimation in Biological Material, *J. Pharmacol. Exptl. Therap. 109*:346-357 (Nov.) 1953.
30. Welch, R. M., Harrison, Y. E. and Burns, J. J.: Implications of Enzyme Induction in Drug Toxicity Studies, *Toxicol. Appl. Pharmacol. 10*:340-351 (Mar.) 1967.
31. Burns, J. J., Conney, A. H. and Koster, R.: Stimulatory Effect of Chronic Drug Administration on Drug-Metabolizing Enzymes in Liver Microsomes, *Ann. N.Y. Acad. Sci. 104*:881-893, 1963.
32. Kunin, C. M. and Finland, M.: Clinical Pharmacology of the Tetracycline Antibiotics, *Clin. Pharmacol. Therap. 2*:51-69 (Jan.-Feb.) 1961.
33. Scholtan, W.: On the Protein-Binding of Long Acting Sulfonamides, *Chemotherapia 6*:180-195, 1963 (in German).
34. Rieder, J.: Physicochemical and Biological Studies on Sulfonamides, *Arzneimittel-Forsch. 13*:81-103 (Feb.) 1963 (in German).
35. Anton, A. H.: A Drug-Induced Change in the Distribution and Renal Excretion of Sulfonamides, *J. Pharmacol. Exptl. Therap. 134*:291-303 (Dec.) 1961.
36. Böhm, C.: *Nierenfunktionsstörung und Antibiotika,* E. Merck, Darmstadt, p. 32 (in German).
37. Kobyletzki, V. D.: Own Studies on Pharmacokinetics During Pregnancy and Lactation, *Med. Welt 19*:2010-2019 (Sept.) 1968 (in German).

17

pka values and some clinical applications

by Wolfgang A. Ritschel

INTRODUCTION

A drug must reach the receptor site to produce a drug interaction. Many drug interactions take place locally at the body surface or in deeper layers of the skin, in body cavities or they take place systematically in an inner organ after the blood carrying the drug reaches it.

If the drug is effective on the skin or mucosa surface only, then the drug is attached to the surface, to the epidermis, by means of ion-binding, hydrogen-binding or van der Waal's forces. This is called *adsorption.* If the drug goes into deeper layers of the skin or mucosa, it is called *penetration.* And if the drug passes the skin or mucosa or other lipid barriers and finally enters the blood stream or lymphatic stream and participates in metabolism, it is called *absorption.* Both terms, penetration and permeation, are summarized in the term *sorption.*[1]

Table 1. Terminology of Adsorption, Sorption and Absorption

TERM		LOCALIZATION
Adsorption		On the surface of cells
Sorption	Penetration	Into cells and tissue
Absorption	Permeation	Through cells and tissue and entering the blood and lymphatic system

Whether a drug is *ad*sorbed, penetrates or is *ab*sorbed depends on the physical and chemical properties of the drug such as water solubility, lipoid/water-partition coefficient, dissociation constant, chemical structure, molecular weight, etc. It depends further on the properties of the drug product or its formulation (*i.e.*, *p*H, selection of proper vehicle substances, etc.) and on the type of barrier (chemical composition of barrier, electrical charge, morphological structure, etc.).

At the site of absorption (paravenous, gastrointestinal, etc.) the drug molecule has to pass a lipoid barrier which might be a complex barrier such as the skin or tissues or the intestinal epithelium. There are different possibilities for crossing a membrane as follows: passive diffusion, convective absorption, active transport, facilitated diffusion, ion-pair absorption and pinocytosis.

The different pathways by which a solute may cross membranes can be summarized in three categories: (1) passive diffusion, in which the membrane is inert to the solute; (2) specialized transport, in which the membranes are actively involved in transporting a solute through the membrane; and (3) corpuscular transport, in which solid particles or lipoid droplets pass through a membrane by means of formation of vacuoles.

The absorption of a drug from the G.I. tract is the passage of this particular substance from the lumen into the blood stream. During this passage several membranes have to be crossed. In the first step the drug molecule permeates the epithelial membrane and enters the epithelial cell. On leaving the epithelial cell another membrane has to be crossed. Passing the basal membrane, the drug molecule enters the lamina propria of connective tissue, and passing further membranes it reaches the capillaries. From the capillaries the drug molecule is either carried with the blood stream via the portal vein or by the lymphatic system via the ductus thoracicus. In spite of the fact that not one but many membranes have to be passed, only the first membrane passage shall be dealt with because the crossing of the epithelial membranes is the first and apparently the rate-limiting step, once the drug is in solution in the luminal contents. It is further assumed that the structure of biological membranes is based on the unit membrane concept, so that the first step is representative for kinetic considerations of absorption.[1]

Most of the drugs are absorbed by passive diffusion[2] and to a small extent only by specialized transport systems.[3,4] The rate of permeation of organic nonelectrolytes through the lipid barrier depends largely on the lipoid/water partition coefficient. In the case of weak organic electrolytes the rate is also dependent on the *p*H and the resulting degree of dissociation, according to the theory of nonionic diffusion.

Passive diffusion is characterized by the rate of transfer of a substance across a membrane being directly proportional to the concentration gradient across the membrane. Both lipoid-soluble substances and lipoid-insoluble molecules of small size may cross the body membranes by passive or simple diffusion. In this specific case the membrane has only a passive role. Therefore the rate of absorption is determined by the physical and chemical properties of the dissolved substance, by the "solute" and by the concentration gradient. The technical term passive diffusion means the passing of lipid-soluble molecules from an aqueous fluid to the lipoid barrier, then through the lipoid barrier and from there into another aqueous phase, which might be the plasma, cerebrospinal fluid, milk or urine.

The biological membrane to be crossed by a solute is a lipoid barrier composed of layers of electrically charged macromolecules (lipids, proteins and mucopolysaccharides). These layers of electrically charged macromolecules attract or repel ions. The membrane structure consists of three layers, which all together have a thickness of approximately 75Å. The membrane thickness varies with the type of cells and the present state of function. The structure shows a double row of phospholipid molecules sandwiched between two layers of protein. The outer layer is covered with a carbohydrate complex. The phospholipids have their hydrophilic ends in contact with the protein and their hydrophobic ends abutting in the center of the membrane.[5-9] This process may be quantitated as outlined in Figure 1 and as described by Dettli and Spring.[10]

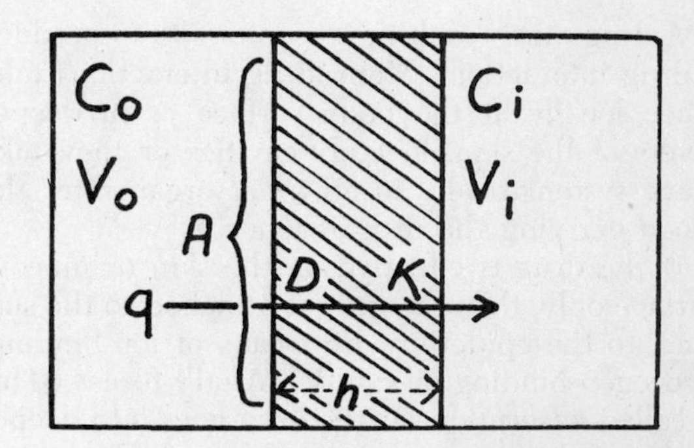

Figure 1. Passive diffusion of a solute through a membrane[11]

The passage of a solute depends on the difference of drug concentration between the outside of the membrane (c_o) and the inside of the membrane (c_i). In this case, the transport occurs through a *closed* membrane. The transport flux (q) is proportional to the partition coefficient (K) of the molecule type between the lipoid membrane and the solute in solution in the aqueous fluid. The amount of solute diffusing is proportional to the area of the membrane (A) and the thickness of the membrane (h). The diffusion constant (D) is the specific diffusibility of the molecule type in the membrane material. Only those molecules can penetrate which are soluble in the membrane material unless absorption occurs via water-filled pores or between cells. Therefore it is necessary that the molecule under consideration be water-soluble as well as lipoid-soluble. The diffusion follows the following mathematical equation:

$$\frac{dq}{dt} = D \cdot \frac{A}{h} \cdot K \cdot (c_o - c_i) \qquad \text{(Equation 1)}$$

In passive diffusion, during the transport of dissolved molecules, there is *no shifting* of the solvent.

In the case where the transport through the barrier is *rate-limiting* and the transfer is apparently *unidirectional*, Fick's first law of diffusion can be used which states that the amount of drug which diffuses per unit time through a cross sectional area of solvent is proportional to the cross-sectional area and the concentration gradient at this point.

$$dq = - D \cdot A \cdot \frac{dc}{dx} \cdot dt \qquad \text{(Equation 2)}$$

Initial drug transport by passive diffusion is proportional to the initial concentration in the lumen. If the drug concentration in the lumen is plotted versus the concentration of the absorbed amount at constant time of absorption, a straight line is obtained.

Plotting the amount of unabsorbed drug versus time, exponential curves are obtained which will, in most cases, give straight lines on semilog paper. In passive diffusion, absorption follows apparently first order reactions.

The permeation constant can be calculated from Equation 3.

$$\frac{dc_o}{dt} = - k \cdot c_o \qquad \text{(Equation 3)}$$

$\frac{dc_o}{dt}$ = concentration of drug diffusing from the outside compartment per unit time through the membrane

c_o = concentration in outside compartment (lumen)

k = permeation rate constant of drug

After integration with the limits of drug concentration c^o_o at time t_o and c_o at time t logarithmic transformation of ln in log Equations 4-8 are obtained for k:

$$\int_{c^o_o}^{c_o} \frac{dc_o}{c} = - k \int_{t_o}^{t} dt \qquad \text{(Equation 4)}$$

$$\ln c_o - \ln c^o_o = - k \cdot (t - t_o) \qquad \text{(Equation 5)}$$

$$\ln c_o - \ln c^o_o = - k \cdot t \qquad \text{(Equation 6)}$$

$$\log c_o - \log c^o_o = - \frac{k \cdot t}{2.303} \qquad \text{(Equation 7)}$$

$$k = \frac{2.303}{t} \cdot \log \frac{c^o_o}{c_o} \qquad \text{(Equation 8)}$$

This is the simplest form of absorption of a dissolved drug from one liquid compartment into another liquid compartment across a simple closed membrane and shows that this absorption obeys first order kinetics. In this consideration there are two criteria:[12]

(1) the drug concentration in the outside compartment of the membrane, which the drug leaves, must be constant

(2) the drug concentration in the inside compartment of the membrane, which the drug enters, must represent only the absorption process

Therefore, this simple Equation 3 can be used only for approximation of the absorption of a drug from the G.I. tract into the blood, because the drug concentration in the blood depends on other processes too, namely, distribution, metabolism, reabsorption and excretion. But this equation fits well to measure the transfer of a drug from the blood into cerebrospinal fluid, milk, ocular fluid, etc.

pKa and Degree of Ionization

Drugs may be classified into three categories according to their physical behavior in aqueous solution: (1) they may exist entirely as ions, such as K^+, Cl^- or NR^+_4 (strong electrolytes); (2) they may be undissociated, as with the steroids and the sugars (nonelectrolytes); or (3) they may be partially dissociated and exist in both an ionic and a molecular form, the relative concentrations of which will depend on the pKa of the agent and the *p*H of the medium (weak electrolytes).

Most of the drugs are either weak acids or weak bases. And because of the fact that most drugs are absorbed by passive diffusion of the *un-ionized* moiety, it is of great importance to what extent a drug is in the ionized and un-ionized form at a certain *p*H.[13-18] But *p*H, or to be more precise, hydrogen ion concentration, is of influence on the physical and chemical properties in connection with absorption, such as solubility of the drug, lipoid/water-partition coefficient, electrical membrane potential, permeability of the membrane and chemical reactivity.

At a certain *p*H the relative concentrations of the ionic and the molecular moieties of a drug are given by the Henderson-Hasselbach equation. For a weak acid HA, which ionizes according to Equation 9:

$$HA + H_2O = H_3O^+ + A^- \qquad \text{(Equation 9)}$$

the dissociation constant is given in Equation 10:

$$K_a = \frac{[H_3O^+] \cdot [A^-]}{[HA]} \qquad \text{(Equation 10)}$$

K_a = dissociation constant

$[A^-]$ = molar concentration of the acidic anion

$[H_3O^+]$ = molar concentration of the hydrogen ion

$[HA]$ = molar concentration of the undissociated acid

The Henderson-Hasselbach equation for weak acids is calculated from Equation 10 by taking the logarithm of both sides of the equation and multiplying both sides of the resultant equation by minus one. The relation as given in Equation 11 is obtained.

$$pH = \log \frac{[A^-]}{[HA]} + pKa \qquad \text{(Equation 11)}$$

As seen from Equation 11, the concentration of the ionic moiety of weak acids increases with increasing *p*H of the aqueous solution.

Acids are substances donating hydrogen ions, and bases are substances accepting hydrogen ions. If the acid BH^+, which is a conjugate of a weak base with a hydrogen ion, is in contact with water, an ionization or dissociation constant Ka can be obtained for the weak base, too.

$$BH^+ + H_2O = H_3O^+ + B \qquad \text{(Equation 12)}$$

The Henderson-Hasselbach equation for a weak base is therefore as follows:

$$pH = \log \frac{[B]}{[BH^+]} + pKa \qquad \text{(Equation 13)}$$

As seen from Equation 13, the concentration of the molecular (undissociated) moiety of a weak base increases with increasing *p*H of an aqueous solution.

Analogous to the *p*H (negative logarithm of hydrogen ion concentration) the ionization constant Ka is expressed as pKa:

$$pKa = -\log Ka \qquad \text{(Equation 14)}$$

From Table 2 it can be seen that for acidic drugs the lower the pKa the stronger the acid, while for basic drugs the higher the pKa the stronger the base.

Table 2. pKa Values for Some Acids and Bases

Acids	pKa	Bases	pKa
Strong ↑		Weak ↑	
Phenol red	strong	Urea	0.18
Sulfosalicylic acid	strong	Acetanilid	0.3
Picric acid	0.38	Caffeine	0.61
Saccharin	1.60	Theobromine	0.68
Phosphoric acid	2.12	Theophylline	0.7
5-Nitrosalicylic acid	2.3	Antipyrine	1.4
Benzylpenicillin	2.76	Benzocaine	2.78
Salicylic acid	3.0	Aniline	4.6
Tartaric acid	3.02	Aminopyrine	5.0
Citric acid	3.15	Papaverine	5.9
Probenecid	3.4	Reserpine	6.6
Aspirin	3.49	Philocarpine	6.8
Lactic acid	3.86	Apomorphine	7.0
Barbituric acid	3.98	Morphine	7.87
Benzoic acid	4.2	Physostigmine	7.88
Phenylbutazone	4.4	Codeine	7.9
Acetic acid	4.76	Strychnine	8.0
Carbonic acid	6.37	Chlorcyclizine	8.15
Sulfadiazine	6.48	Quinine	8.4
Sulfamerazine	7.06	Cocaine	8.41
Sulfathiazole	7.12	Procaine	8.8
Phenobarbital	7.41	Methapyrilene	8.85
Thiopental	7.60	Tripelennamine	8.95
Butalbital	7.68	Diphenhydramine	8.98
Barbital	7.91	Promethazine	9.08
Aprobarbital	7.91	Dextrorphan	9.2
Butethal	7.92	Ammonia	9.29
Secobarbital	8.08	Ephedrine	9.36
Pentobarbital	8.11	Atropine	9.65
Sulfapyridine	8.44	Quaternary Ammonium Compounds	strong
Boric acid	9.24		
Phenol	9.90		
α-D-Glucose	12.1		
↓ Weak		↓ Strong	

Using the Henderson-Hasselbach equation one can calculate the percentage of ionization of a monobasic weak acid or monoacidic weak base from the ratio of the concentration of the drug present in the ionic moiety to the total concentration of the drug present in the ionic and in the undissociated moiety, multiplied by 100:

$$\% \text{ ionization} = \frac{I \cdot 100}{I + U} \qquad \text{(Equation 15)}$$

I = ionized moiety
U = un-ionized moiety

On rearrangement Equation 16 is obtained:

$$\frac{U}{I} = \text{antilog (pKa} - \text{pH)} \qquad \text{(Equation 16)}$$

which can be solved for U:

$$U = I \cdot \text{antilog (pKa} - \text{pH)} \qquad \text{(Equation 17)}$$

Upon substitution of Equation 17 into Equation 15, the percentage of ionization for a weak acid is obtained:

$$\% \text{ ionization (acid)} = \frac{100}{1 + \text{antilog (pKa} - \text{pH)}} \qquad \text{(Equation 18)}$$

For a weak base the following Equation 19 is derived:

$$\% \text{ ionization (base)} = \frac{100}{1 + \text{antilog (pH} - \text{pKa)}} \qquad \text{(Equation 19)}$$

pH-Partition Hypothesis

Since membranes are more permeable to the un-ionized form of a given drug than to its ionized form because of the greater lipoid solubility of the un-ionized form, then passage through a membrane becomes a function of *p*H of the intestinal environment and the pKa value of the particular drug. Therefore, a weak acid will be more absorbed at low *p*H (stomach), because of low dissociation and therefore a high amount of un-ionized form. And weak bases will be more absorbed at higher *p*H values (intestines).

The concept of pKa is derived from the Henderson-Hasselbach equation:

for an acid:

$$\text{pKa} = \text{pH} + \log \frac{c_u}{c_i} \qquad \text{(Equation 20)}$$

for a base:

$$\text{pKa} = \text{pH} + \log \frac{c_i}{c_u} \qquad \text{(Equation 21)}$$

c_u = molar concentration of un-ionized molecules

c_i = molar concentration of ionized molecules

Table 3. Percent of Ionization at Known pKa and pH[19]

pKa − pH	Percent Ionized if anion (weak acid)	Percent Ionized if cation (weak base)
− 4	99.99	0.01
− 3	99.94	0.06
− 2	99.01	0.99
− 1	90.91	9.09
− 0.9	88.81	11.19
− 0.8	86.30	13.70
− 0.7	83.37	16.63
− 0.6	79.93	20.07
− 0.5	75.97	24.03
− 0.4	71.53	28.47
− 0.3	66.61	33.39
− 0.2	61.32	38.68
− 0.1	55.73	44.27
0	50.00	50.00
+ 0.1	44.27	55.73
+ 0.2	38.68	61.32
+ 0.3	33.39	66.61
+ 0.4	28.47	71.53
+ 0.5	24.03	75.97
+ 0.6	20.07	79.93
+ 0.7	16.63	83.37
+ 0.8	13.70	86.30
+ 0.9	11.19	88.81
+ 1	9.09	90.91
+ 2	0.99	99.01
+ 3	0.06	99.94
+ 4	0.01	99.99

For example, if one wants to know the degree of ionization of salicylic acid in plasma:

Known: pKa of salicylic acid = 3
pH of plasma = 7.4

$$\log \frac{c_u}{c_i} = \text{pKa} - \text{pH} = 3 - 7.4 = -4.4 \qquad \text{(Equation 22)}$$

The relation between un-ionized and ionized form is $1:10^{4.4}$; this means $\alpha \sim 1$, or that salicylic acid is practically 100 percent ionized.

In the stomach at *p*H 1:

$$\log \frac{c_u}{c_i} = 3 - 1 = 2 \qquad \text{(Equation 22)}$$

the ratio is therefore $10^2:1$, this means $\alpha \sim 0.01$ or that 1 percent is ionized.

It follows, further, from the Henderson-Hasselbach equation that when a substance is half ionized and half un-ionized at a certain *p*H, its pKa is equal to this *p*H. Or, in other words, at that *p*H which is equal to the pKa value half of the molecules of a drug are in ionized and half are in un-ionized form. The relation between ionization and *p*H is not linear, but is sigmoidal. A small change in *p*H will therefore have a great change in ionization, if *p*H and pKa values are close together.

Hogben, *et al.* considered that for weak electrolytes the un-ionized form, being more lipoid-soluble, would be preferentially absorbed across the membrane, say the intestinal epithelium, until an equilibrium is reached, when the concentration of the un-ionized form will be the same on both sides of the barrier, *i.e.*, in the gut and the plasma. They also calculated the *steady state* concentration of drugs between the gastrointestinal lumen and the plasma.[15] In their experiments drug solutions were injected intravenously and at the same time the gut was perfused. Administration was continued until there was no net transfer observed. It was found that at the steady state the concentration of acidic drugs was lower in the gut lumen than in the plasma. And the concentration ratio of a stronger acid was much lower than that of a weaker acid. The concentration of basic drugs was higher in the gut lumen than in plasma. And the concentration ratio of a stronger base was much higher than that of a weaker base.

Knowing the pKa value of a drug the theoretical equilibrium ratio can be calculated as follows: [14,20]

for weak acids:

$$R_a = \frac{c_g}{c_p} = \frac{1 + 10^{(pHg - pKa)}}{1 + 10^{(pHp - pKa)}} \quad \text{(Equation 23)}$$

or

$$R_a = \frac{1 + \text{antilog}\ (pH_g - pKa)}{1 + \text{antilog}\ (pH_p - pKa)} \quad \text{(Equation 24)}$$

for weak bases:

$$R_b = \frac{c_g}{c_p} = \frac{1 + 10^{(pKa - pHg)}}{1 + 10^{(pKa - pHp)}} \quad \text{(Equation 25)}$$

or

$$R_b = \frac{1 + \text{antilog}\ (pKa - pH_g)}{1 + \text{antilog}\ (pKa - pH_p)} \quad \text{(Equation 26)}$$

R_a = concentration ratio between gut and plasma for weak acids
R_b = concentration ratio between gut and plasma for weak bases
c_g = concentration in the gut lumen
c_p = concentration in the plasma

Shore and co-workers found that acidic drugs, being highly ionized in plasma, had c_g/c_p ratios between 0 and 0.6, and basic drugs, having little

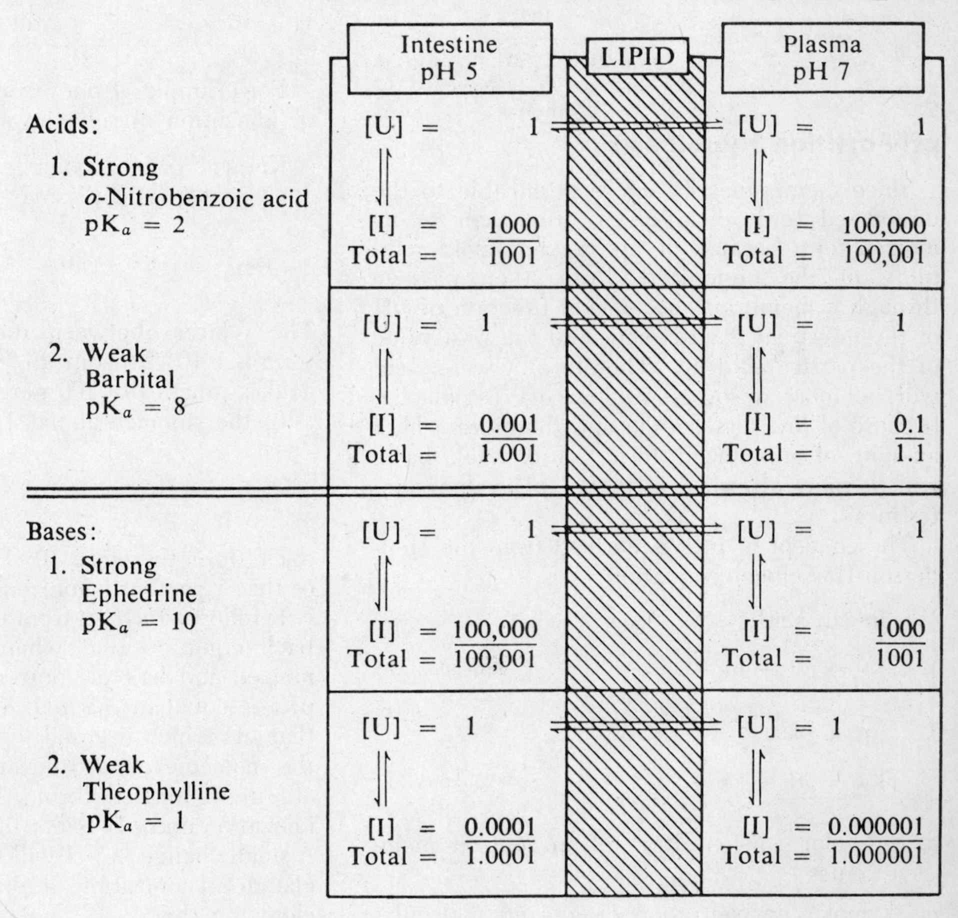

Figure 2. Theoretical distribution between the gastrointestinal tract and the plasma of organic acids and bases of various approximate pKa values. [U] and [I] represent concentrations of the un-ionized and the ionized moiety, respectively[21]

or no dissociation in plasma, showed c_g/c_p ratios between 1 and 40.[14] Hogben, *et al.* showed, furthermore, that the *p*H at the site of absorption in the jejunum is not necessarily identical with the *p*H of the intestinal content in the lumen. They calculated a "virtual" *p*H of 5.3 for the site of absorption at the intestinal membrane surface.[15]

If one considers two compartments separated by a membrane, some ions in the solution on one side of the membrane may be found which cannot cross to the other side. Such a situation results in the *Donnan distribution.* This is the case with erythrocytes, where the presence of hemoglobin anions affects the distribution of normally diffusible ions such as chloride. In this case there is a cell to plasma ratio of about 0.7 instead of 1.0. The distribution ratio of a cation then would be the reciprocal of the chloride ratio, namely 1.4. This phenomenon has to be separated from *unequal equilibrium distribution.* If one considers two liquid compartments with different *p*H values, separated by a membrane, selectively permeable to the un-ionized form, different drug concentrations may be found in the two compartments after steady state is reached, as seen in Figure 2.[21]

At the steady state in unequal equilibrium distribution, the concentration of the un-ionized form is the same in both compartments. But the concentrations of the ionized form are unequal to the difference in *p*H. Therefore, the total concentration of the solute (un-ionized and ionized form) on both sides of the membrane is a function of the *p*H of the two aqueous compartments as well as of the pKa of the solute.

But one has to be aware of the fact that very few if any drugs obey the *p*H-partition hypothesis as outlined above. It is possible that even an ionized drug might be sufficiently lipoid-soluble to permeate the membrane (G.I. barrier).[15] On the other hand the un-ionized form of a drug might not be sufficiently lipoid-soluble and therefore unable to cross the membrane. Furthermore one has to consider that this theory is not applicable where other transport mechanisms, such as active transport, are involved.

Regarding permeation of membranes it has been shown that the un-ionized form of a drug is important. But the drug-receptor-interaction in the biophase has not been considered. For this drug interaction with specific receptors a certain concentration of the ionized or un-ionized form of the drug is required. The degree of ionization in the biophase, in the plasma, having a *p*H of 7.4, can be calculated as outlined above.

CLINICAL APPLICATION OF pKa VALUES OF DRUGS AND pH OF ENVIRONMENTAL MEDIUM

Changes in Urinary pH

The urinary excretion of most drugs, which are either weak bases or weak acids, will be influenced by the urinary hydrogen ion concentration. Any alteration of the urinary *p*H, either done by simultaneous administration of ammonium chloride, sodium bicarbonate or acidic or alkaline drugs, such as the thiazides or acetazolamide, etc., or done unknowingly, will influence the activity of drugs.[22-24] As a general rule it can be assumed that weak electrolytes are excreted *p*H-dependent if the un-ionized fraction is lipoid-soluble and if the pKa values are within a range of 3.0 to 7.5 for weak acids and 7.5 to 10.5 for weak bases. When the urine is acidic the bases become concentrated in the urine and are excreted more rapidly. When the tubular urine is alkaline, weak bases become less concentrated in the urine than in the plasma and are excreted more slowly. This means that weak acids are excreted at a higher clearance in highly alkaline urine, while weak bases are excreted at higher clearance in acidic urine. Examples of drugs which are excreted *p*H-dependent include the weak acids such as barbiturates, nalidixic acid, nitrofurantoin, salicylic acid and sulfonamides. Weak bases include compounds such as amphetamine, amitriptyline, quinine, chloroquine, mepacrine, procaine, meperidine, levorphanol, nicotine and others.

The effect of *p*H change on tubular reabsorption is demonstrated in Figure 3.[25]

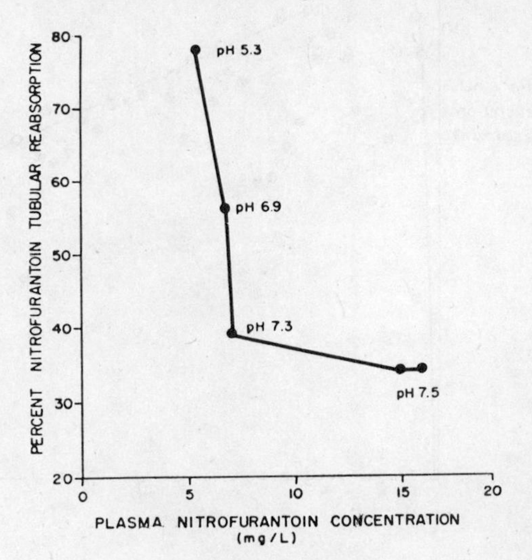

Figure 3. Effect of *p*H change on tubular reabsorption of nitrofurantoin[25]

Another example of pH-dependent excretion rates and increased or decreased drug activity is streptomycin, which is more rapidly excreted in alkaline urine, while the excretion of mecamylamine is reduced. Mercurial diuretics are more effective in acidic urine. A pH change is also done intentionally *i.e.*, it has been recommended that sodium bicarbonate be given along with several of the older sulfonamides to provide an alkaline urine in which the drugs are more soluble. In this way the possibility of crystalluria is reduced. Similarly, the analgesic effect of salicylic acid is prolonged with acidic urine. Consideration must also be given to the pH of urine in laboratory tests. In highly alkaline urine urobilinogen is excreted more than in acidic urine. In carrying out the urobilinogen test, this must be considered in order to avoid an error in diagnosis.

An effective technique to control urine pH for drug excretion studies in humans has been reported by Portnoff, Swintosky and Kostenbauder.[26] The pH range 4.5 to 5.0 is easily maintained constant to $\pm$ 0.1 pH by administering an initial dosage of approximately 3-4 g of ammonium chloride every hour for two to three hours until the desired pH has been attained. After that time smaller dosages at hourly intervals maintain the acidic urine pH. A constancy of approximately pH 8.0 is maintained by administering initial hourly doses of approximately 4 g of sodium bicarbonate, followed by smaller hourly doses after the desired pH has been attained. The total intake in the experiments was 10-15 g of ammonium chloride and 30-48 g of sodium bicarbonate.

Beckett and co-workers studied the influence of pH adjustment on excretion of basic and acidic drugs.[27-29] If using a basic drug, a smooth curve of rate of excretion against time can be obtained by rendering the urine acidic at about pH 5, or alkaline for an acidic drug. This method for pH adjustment will reveal a relation between drug re-absorption or excretion and the pH of urine. For those drugs which are relatively slowly metabolized in man and which are excreted in a high percentage into the urine in the unchanged form, an estimate can be made for duration of action under conditions of fluctuating urinary pH. From these studies it should be possible to predict the excretion pattern of the drug in subjects whose urinary pH is not controlled. In Figure 4 an example is given of urinary excretion of amphetamine, after oral administration under controlled and uncontrolled urinary pH. However, in poisoning cases acidifying for basic drugs

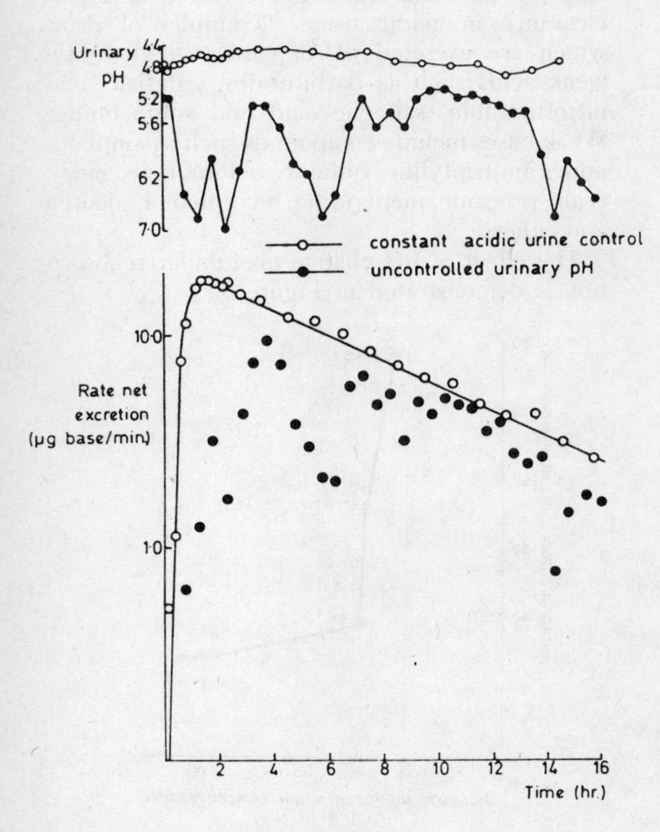

Figure 4. Urinary excretion of amphetamine after oral administration of 15 mg solution of D (+)-amphetamine sulfate[29]

or alkalinization for acidic drugs cannot be done unless the electrolyte balance of the patient has been checked, since high doses of NH_4Cl or $NaHCO_3$ may worsen the patient's condition.

Excretion of Drugs with Sweat

The epithelium of the sweat gland is preferentially permeable to the un-ionized form of drugs. Therefore acidic drugs attain sweat/plasma concentration ratios upon peroral or parenteral administration dependent on their pKa values. The lower the pKa values, the lower the ratio.[30-31] Sulfanilamide, with a pKa of 10.4, attains a ratio of approximately 0.7, sulfathiazole with a pKa of 8.4 attains a ratio of 0.6 and sulfathiazole with a pKa of 7.1 attains a ratio of 0.13. The acidic compound para-aminohippuric acid (PAH) with a pKa value of 3.8 attains a ratio of 0.02 only. These results are in close relation to the distribution of weak acids across a lipoid membrane separating plasma with a *p*H of 7.4 from a fluid (sweat) of somewhat lower *p*H.[30]

A substance which is known to be excreted via the sweat glands is vitamin B_1, or its metabolites.[32-34] Ritschel and Ritschel-Beurlin found in a field experiment during an expedition in the Ganges Delta that after a loading dose of 200-300 mg and a maintenance dose of 100 mg per day, the excretion of vitamin B_1, or its metabolites through the sweat was high enough to protect humans from mosquito stings.[35]

Mammillary Excretion of Drugs

Many drugs may pass from the plasma, from the blood, into the milk. The epithelium of the mammary gland behaves as a lipoid membrane, separating blood of *p*H 7.4 from milk with a *p*H of approximately 6.6. Various drugs administered intravenously to lactating cows and goats were studied by Rasmussen.[36-38] Basic drugs appear in the milk in a concentration greater than that in plasma and acidic compounds in a concentration lower than that in plasma. The basic compound erythromycin with a pKa value of 8.8 attains a milk/plasma concentration ratio of about 7, and the acidic drug benzylpenicillin G with a pKa value of 2.7 and some sulfonamides with pKa values between 7.1 and 7.4 attain ratios of less than 1. The lower the pKa value, the lower the ratio. Any completely un-ionized substance such as ethanol, urea and antipyrine distribute evenly between milk and plasma. Drugs which have been found to pass from blood into milk include thyreostatics, inhalation anesthetics, choral hydrate, barbiturates, antihistamines, salicylates, laxatives, caffeine and others.[39]

Nicotine passes readily into milk. This may even lead to nicotine poisoning of the child.[39] Penicillin and streptomycin pass into milk in concentrations much lower than the plasma concentrations of the maternal blood. This may lead to sensibilization against antibiotics or it may influence the intestinal flora of the suckling. The chloramphenicol concentration in the plasma of sucklings has been found to be approximately half of the maternal plasma concentration. Anticoagulants pass rapidly into milk and may attain higher concentration than in the maternal blood.[40] It is believed also that allergens may pass into milk. The concentration of erythromycin estolate is higher in the milk than in the maternal blood.[41]

Examples for Use of pKa of Drugs in Answering Clinical Questions

A. What is the approximate percent of ionization of aspirin (pKa = 3.49) in:
(a) stomach (*p*H 2) = 3.13
(b) duodenum (*p*H 5.6) = 99.23
(c) deeper small intestine (*p*H 7.2) = 99.98
(d) rectum (~ *p*H 7.8) = 99.99
(e) plasma (~*p*H 7.4) = 99.98

For calculating percent ionization of the weak acid aspirin, Equation 18 is used:

$$\% \text{ ionization (acid)} = \frac{100}{1 + \text{antilog (pKa} - \text{pH)}} \qquad \text{(Equation 18)}$$

From where will aspirin be primarily and most rapidly absorbed?
Answer: From the stomach but also intestine, since it has a high partition coefficient and a large surface area in the intestine, even though the percent unionized is low.

B. In a case of poisoning with phenobarbital, how could the drug be removed rapidly from the body?
Answer: Phenobarbital is a weak acid with a pKa 7.41. The degree of ionization according to Equation 18 in the cerebrospinal fluid (*p*H 7.3) is 43.7 percent, in plasma (*p*H 7.4) it is 49.42 percent.

If the *p*H gradient between two fluids is altered by changing the *p*H of plasma by acidifying with ammonium chloride or alkalization with sodium bicarbonate, those drugs which have a pKa in the range under consideration will have a significant change in ionization. The result will be that the cerebrospinal fluid/plasma concentration ratios will be changed. This principle is applicable for the distribution of phenobarbital between plasma and brain tissue. On lowering of the *p*H of plasma, the plasma level of phenobarbital decreases and the brain tissue level increases. If the plasma *p*H is raised the plasma level of phenobarbital increases and the brain tissue level decreases. If in this case $NaHCO_3$ is given I.V. until the plasma *p*H would be *p*H 8, then 79.55 percent would be ionized in plasma. Urinary *p*H will also become alkaline and the drug would be less reabsorbed, but excreted into urine.

C. A young mother asks her pharmacist whether there would be any chance that her child, who is breast fed, may get "yellow teeth" (due to deposition of tetracycline in the teeth) since she is on tetracycline hydrochloride for a severe infection.

Answer: In general basic drugs appear in the milk in a concentration greater than that in the maternal plasma and acidic compounds in a concentration lower than that in maternal plasma. Tetracycline is zwitterionic but has one pKa = 8.3. In the maternal plasma (*p*H 7.4) tetracycline is (according to Equation 18) 88.81 percent ionized, in the milk (*p*H 6.6) 98.04 percent ionized. The ratio of drug concentration in milk/plasma is calculated according to modified Equation 16.

$$R_b = \frac{1 + \text{antilog (pKa} - \text{pH (milk))}}{1 + \text{antilog (pKa} - \text{pH (plasma))}} \qquad \text{(Equation 27)}$$

$$= \frac{1 + 50.118}{1 + 7.943} = 5.71$$

Since the tetracycline concentration in the milk will be more than five times greater than the maternal plasma concentration, danger of deposition of tetracycline in the child's teeth exists and breast feeding should be discontinued for the period of tetracycline therapy.

D. Dr. Welby, a physician, asks a pharmacist whether he could make PAS (p-aminosalicylic acid) suppositories from PAS capsules, since his patient does not tolerate well peroral administration.

Answer: PAS is an acid with pKa 3.25 and is primarily absorbed from the stomach and upper intestine. For rectal administration an environmental *p*H of approximately 7.8 has to be considered. According to Equation 18, PAS is at *p*H 7.8 almost completely ionized, namely 99.997 percent. Rectal absorption is therefore unlikely and the drug should not be given rectally.

pKa Values

The following table is a compilation of pKa values collected as library assignments to the senior students of the College of Pharmacy, University of Cincinnati, in the academic year 1969/70 and as assignment to a Pharm.D. student, Mr. Mike Kavula in the Biopharmaceutics Seminar 1970. The data were collected from manuals, such as *Merck Index*, textbooks of physical and general chemistry, and systematic search in 99 different journals. Letters were written to more than 300 pharmaceutical companies asking for pKa values and pharmacokinetic data of their drugs. The industrial response was disappointing. The data collected were randomly checked and verified by Mr. Kavula, to whom I am very thankful.

In any compilation like this it is difficult not to overlook mistakes. The order of presentation was and is a problem. We would be very thankful if readers would inform us of any mistakes found and would supply pKa values of those drugs not listed in the following table.

Table 4. pKa Values for Drugs and Chemicals

NAME	PKA	REFERENCE
Abbott 29119	8.4	*Merck Index,* 8th ed., Merck and Co., Rahway, N.J., 1968, p. 1.
Acetamidine Hydrochloride	12.1	*Merck Index,* 8th ed., p. 1.
Acetanilid	1.0	Parrott, E. L.: *Pharmaceutical Technology, Fundamental Pharmaceutics,* Burgess Publishing Co., Minneapolis, Minn., 1970, p. 219.
Acetarsone	pKa_1 = 3.73 pKa_2 = 7.9 pKa_3 = 9.3	Hiskey, C. F. and Cantwell, F. F.: Ultraviolet Spectrum Correlations with the Conjugate Acid-Base Species of Acetarsone and Arsthinol, *J. Pharm. Sci. 75*:2105, 1968.
Acetazolamide	7.2	*Merck Index,* 8th ed., p. 6.
Acetic Acid	4.76	Parrott, E. L.: *Pharmaceutical Technology, Fundamental Pharmaceutics,* Burgess Pub. Co., Minneapolis, Minn., 1970, p. 215.
Acetic Acid m-Chlorophenyl	4.14	Beckett, A. H. and Moffat, A. C.: Kinetics of Buccal Absorption of Some Carboxylic Acids and the Correlation of the Rate Constants and n-Heptane:Aqueous Phase Partition Coefficients, *J. Pharm. Pharmacol. 22*:15, 1970.
Acetic Acid o-Chlorophenyl	4.07	Beckett, A. H. and Moffat, A. C.: Kinetics of Buccal Absorption of Some Carboxylic Acids and the Correlation of the Rate Constants and n-Heptane:Aqueous Phase Partition Coefficient, *J. Pharm. Pharmacol. 22*:15, 1970.
Acetic Acid p-Chlorophenyl	4.19	Beckett, A. H. and Moffat, A. C.: Kinetics of Buccal Absorption of Some Carboxylic Acids and the Correlation of the Rate Constants and n-Heptane:Aqueous Phase Partition Coefficients, *J. Pharm. Pharmacol. 22*:15, 1970.
Acetylcarnitine Hydrochloride	3.60	Yalkowsky, S. H. and Zografi, G.: Potentiometric Titration of Monomeric and Micellar Acylcarnitines, *J. Pharm. Sci. 59*:798, 1970.
Acetylcholine	4.5	Robson, J. M. and Stacey, R. S.: *Recent Advances in Pharmacology,* 4th ed., Little Brown and Co., Boston, 1968, p. 108.
N-Acetylhyalobiuronic Acid	3.3	*Merck Index,* 8th ed., p. 537.
Acetylsalicylic Acid	3.49	Parrott, E. L.: *Pharmaceutical Technology, Fundamental Pharmaceutics,* Burgess Publishing Co., Minneapolis, Minn., 1970, p. 215.
Aconitine	8.11	Parrott, E. L.: *Pharmaceutical Technology, Fundamental Pharmaceutics,* Burgess Publishing Co., Minneapolis, Minn., 1970, p. 219
	5.88	*Merck Index,* 8th ed., p. 15.
Acoric Acid	5.65	*Merck Index,* 8th ed., p. 15.
Actinobolin, acidic basic	8.8 7.5	*Merck Index,* 8th ed., p. 18.
		Merck Index, 8th ed., p. 15.
5′-Adenylic Acid	pK_1 = 3.8 pK_2 = 6.2	*Merck Index,* 8th ed., p. 21.
Adipic Acid	4.43	Parrott, E. L.: *Pharmaceutical Technology, Fundamental Pharmaceutics,* Burgess Pub. Co., Minneapolis, Minn., 1970, p. 215.
Akuammicine	7.45	*Merck Index,* 8th ed., p. 27.
Akuammine	7.5	*Merck Index,* 8th ed., p. 27.
α-Alanine	9.05	Parrott, E. L.: *Pharmaceutical Technology, Fundamental Pharmaceutics,* Burgess Pub. Co., Minneapolis, Minn., 1970, p. 215.
β-Alanine	pK_1 = 3.6 pK_2 = 10.19	*Merck Index,* 8th ed., p. 27.
DL-Alanine	pK_1 = 2.35 pK_2 = 9.87	*Merck Index,* 8th ed., p. 27.

NAME	pKa	REFERENCE
Alanosine	4.8	*Merck Index,* 8th ed., p. 27.
Aluminum Hydroxide	12.20	Parrott, E. L.: *Pharmaceutical Technology, Fundamental Pharmaceutics,* Burgess Pub. Co., Minneapolis, Minn., 1970, p. 215.
Allobarbital	7.79	Suzuki, A., Higuchi, W. I. and Ho, N. F. H.: Theoretical Model Studies of Drug Absorption and Transport in the Gastrointestinal Tract II, *J. Pharm. Sci. 59*:651, 1970.
Allopurinol	~9.0	Data by: Burroughs-Wellcome, Tuckahoe, N.Y. 10707
Allylamine	9.69	Hong, Wen-Hai and Connors, K. A.: Identification of Aliphatic Amines from Rates of Cinnamoylation, *J. Pharm. Sci. 57*: 1789, 1968.
Allylbenzyl Barbituric Acid	7.21	Parrott, E. L.: *Pharmaceutical Technology, Fundamental Pharmaceutics,* Burgess Pub. Co., Minneapolis, Minn., 1970, p. 216.
5-Allyl-5-Isobutylbarbituric Acid	7.63 ± 0.1	Maulding, H. V. and Zoglio, M. A.: pKa Determinations Utilizing Solutions of 7-(2-Hydroxypropyl) Theophylline, *J. Pharm. Sci. 60*:309, 1971.
	7.86	Fincher, J. H., Entrekin, D. N. and Hartman, C. W.: *J. Pharm. Sci. 55*:23, 1966.
Amicetin	10.4 7.0	*Merck Index,* 8th ed., p. 50.
Aminoacetic Acid (Glycine)	9.78	*Merck Index,* 7th ed., p. 490. Through: Brooke, D. and Guttman, D. E.: Complex Formation Rate IV, *J. Pharm. Sci. 57*:1677, 1968.
p-Aminobenzoic Acid	4.65 4.80	*Merck Index,* 8th ed., p. 53.
Aminocaproic Acid	pK_1 = 4.43 pK_2 = 10.75	*Merck Index,* 8th ed., p. 55.
(α-Aminoethyl) Dimethyl-Phenylsilane HCl	10.26	Fessenden, R. J. and Coon, M. D.: A Silicon Analog of a Sympathomimetic Amine, *J. Med. Chem. 7*:561, 1964. Through: *Intern. Pharm. Abstr. 1*:21, 1964.
p-Aminohippurate	3.8	Wagner, J. G.: *Drug Intelligence 2*:294, 1968.
2-Amino-4-methyl-4-phenylpentane	9.42	Garrett, E. R. and Chemburkar, P. B.: Evaluation, Control, and Prediction of Drug Diffusion Through Polymeric Membranes, *J. Pharm. Sci. 57*:1401, 1968.
3-Amino-1-phenylbutane sulfate	9.30	Garrett, E. R. and Chemburkar, P. B.: Evaluation, Control and Prediction of Drug Diffusion Through Polymeric Membranes, *J. Pharm. Sci. 57*:1401, 1968.
4'-Aminopropiophenone	2.42	Garrett, E. R. and Chemburkar, P. B.: Evaluation, Control and Prediction of Drug Diffusion Through Polymeric Membranes II, *J. Pharm. Sci. 57*:949, 1968.
Aminopterin	5.5	Baker, B. R. and Jordaan, H.: Analogs of Tetrahydrofolic Acid XXVIII. Mode of Pyrimidine Binding to Dihydrofolic Reductase pH Profile Studies, *J. Pharm. Sci. 54*:1740, 1965.
p-Aminosalicylic Acid	3.25	*Merck Index,* 8th ed., p. 62.
6-Amino-2-thiouracil	—	Garrett, E. R. and Weber, D. J.: Metal Complexes of Thiouracils I: Stability Constants by Potentiated Titration Studies and Structures of Complexes, *J. Pharm. Sci. 59*:1383, 1970.
Ammonium Hydroxide	9.26	Parrott, E. L.: *Pharmaceutical Technology, Fundamental Pharmaceutics,* Burgess Pub. Co., Minneapolis, Minn., 1970, p. 219.
Amobarbital	7.94	Suzuki, A., Higuchi, W. I. and Ho, N. F. H.: Theoretical Model Studies of Drug Absorption and Transport in the Gastrointestinal Tract II, *J. Pharm. Sci. 59*:651, 1970.
	8.5	Data by: Smith, Kline and French, Philadelphia, Pa. 19101
Amphetamine	9.77	Leffler, E. B., Spencer, H. M. and Burger, A.: *J. Am. Chem. Soc. 73*:2611,

NAME	PKA	REFERENCE
		Through: Beckett, A. H., Boyes, R. N. and Triggs, E. J.: Kinetics of Buccal Absorption of Amphetamines, *J. Pharm. Pharmacol. 20*:92, 1968.
	9.93	Data by: Smith, Kline and French, Philadelphia, Pa. 19101
Ampicillin	$pK_1 = 2.50$* $pH_2 = 7.20$* $pK_1 = 2.54$** $pK_2 = 7.22$**	Data by: Bristol Laboratories, Syracuse, N.Y. 13201 *Grant and Alburn, *J. Am. Chem. Soc., 86*:3870, 1964. **Bristol Laboratories (1965)
	$pK_1 = 2.66$ $pK_2 = 7.25$	Hou, J. P. and Poole, J. W.: The Amino Acid Nature of Ampicillin and Related Penicillins, *J. Pharm. Sci. 58*:1510, 1969.
	2.53	Rapson, H. D. C. and Bird, A. E.: *J. Pharm. Pharmacol. Suppl. 15*:222T, 1963. Through: Winningham, D. G., Nemoy, N. J. and Stamey, T. A.: Diffusion of Antibiotics from Plasma into Prostatic Fluid, *Nature 219*:139, 1968.
n-Amylamine	10.64	Hong, Wen-Hai and Conners, K. A.: Identification of Aliphatic Amines from Rates of Cinnamoylation, *J. Pharm. Sci. 57*:1789, 1968.
Anileridine	$pK_1 = 3.7$ $pK_2 = 7.5$	*Hagers Handbuch der Pharmazeutischen Praxis,* Vol. I, Allgemeiner Teil, Wirkstoffgruppen I, Springer-Verlag, 1967, p. 789.
Anserine	$pK_1 = 2.64$ $pK_2 = 7.04$ $pK_3 = 9.49$	*Merck Index,* 8th ed., p. 87.
Antazoline HCl	7.2	Robson, J. M. and Stacey, R. S.: *Recent Advances in Pharmacology,* 4th ed., Little Brown and Co., Boston, 1968, p. 108.
Apomorphine HCl	7.2	*Hagers Handbuch der Pharmazeutischen Praxis,* Vol. I, Allgemeiner Teil, Wirkstoffgruppen I, Springer-Verlag, 1967, p. 837.
	$pK_a = 8.92$ $pK_b = 7.0$	*Merck Index,* 8th ed., p. 96
Aporeine	6.1	*Merck Index,* 8th ed., p. 96
Aprobarbital	7.54	Fincher, J. H., Entrekin, D. N. and Hartman, C. W.: *J. Pharm. Sci. 55*:23, 1966.
Arecoline	5.3	Robson, J. M. and Stacey, R. S.: *Recent Advances in Pharmacology,* 4th ed., Little, Brown and Co., Boston, 1968, p. 108.
	7.16	Parrott, E. L.: *Pharmaceutical Technology, Fundamental Pharmaceutics,* Burgess Pub. Co., Minneapolis, Minn., 1970, p. 219.
	7.4 (HBr)	*Hagers Handbuch der Pharmazeutischen Praxis,* Vol. I, Allgemeiner Teil, Wirkstoffgruppen I. Springer-Verlag, 1967. p. 935.
	6.84	*Merck Index,* 8th ed., p. 99.
L-Arginine	12.48	Parrott, E. L.: *Pharmaceutical Technology, Fundamental Pharmaceutics,* Burgess Pub. Co., Minneapolis, Minn., 1970, p. 215.
Arginine	$pK_1 = 2.18$ $pK_2 = 9.09$ $pK_3 = 13.2$	*Merck Index,* 8th ed., p. 99.
Arsenic	2.30 7.08 9.22	Parrott, E. L.: *Pharmaceutical Technology, Fundamental Pharmaceutics,* Burgess Pub. Co., Minneapolis, Minn., 1970, p. 216.
Arsenious Acid	12.22	Parrott, E. L.: *Pharmaceutical Technology, Fundamental Pharmaceutics,* Burgess Pub. Co., Minneapolis, Minn., 1970, p. 216.
Arsthinol	9.5 ± 1	Hiskey, C. F. and Cantwell, F. F.: Ultraviolet Spectrum Correlations with the Conjugate Acid-Base Species of Acetarsone and Arsthinol, *J. Pharm. Sci. 57*:2105, 1968.

NAME	PKA	REFERENCE
Ascorbic Acid	$pK_1 = 4.17$ $pK_2 = 11.57$	*Merck Index,* 8th ed., p. 105.
	$pK_1 = 4.2$ $pK_2 = 11.6$	*Hagers Handbuch der Pharmazeutischen Praxis,* Vol. II, Wirkstoffgruppen II, Springer-Verlag, 1967, p. 721.
L-Aspartic Acid	3.86	Parrott, E. L.: *Pharmaceutical Technology, Fundamental Pharmaceutics,* Burgess Pub. Co., Minneapolis, Minn., 1970, p. 216.
Aspartic Acid	$pK^1_1 = 1.88$ $pK^1_2 = 3.65$ $pK^1_2 = 9.60$	*Merck Index,* 8th ed., p. 107.
Aspergillic Acid	5.95	*Merck Index,* 8th ed., p. 107.
Atropine	5.93	Medwick, T., Kaplan, G. and Weyer, L. G.: Measurement of Acidity and Equilibria in Glacial Acetic Acid with the Glass Calomel Electrode System, *J. Pharm. Sci. 58*:308, 1969.
	4.35	*Merck Index,* 8th ed., p. 110.
	9.65	Parrott, E. L.: *Pharmaceutical Technology, Fundamental Pharmaceutics,* Burgess Pub. Co., Minneapolis, Minn., 1970, p. 219.
Azaserine	8.55	*Merck Index,* 8th ed., p. 114.
6-Azathymine	7.6	*Merck Index,* 8th ed., p. 114.
Barbital	7.91	Suzuki, A., Higuchi, W. I. and Ho, N. F. H.: Theoretical Model Studies of Drug Absorption and Transport in the Gastrointestinal Tract II, *J. Pharm. Sci. 59*:651, 1970.
	7.90	Parrott, E. L.: *Pharmaceutical Technology, Fundamental Pharmaceutics,* Burgess Pub. Co., Minneapolis, Minn., 1970, p. 216.
Barbituric Acid	3.98	Parrott, E. L.: *Pharmaceutical Technology, Fundamental Pharmaceutics,* Burgess Pub. Co., Minneapolis, Minn., 1970, p. 216.
Benzimidazole	5.48	*Merck Index,* 8th ed., p. 131.
Benzimidazole 2-acetonitrile	4.20 ± 0.02 11.76 ± 0.02	Cohen, J. L. and Connors, K. A.: Stability and Structure of Some Organic Molecular Complexes in Aqueous Solution, *J. Pharm. Sci. 59*:1271, 1970.
Benzocaine	7.60	Medwick, T., Kaplan, G. and Weyer, L. G.: Measurement of Acidity and Equilibria in Glacial Acetic Acid with the Glass Calomel Electrode System, *J. Pharm. Sci. 58*:308, 1969.
	2.78	Parrott, E. L.: *Pharmaceutical Technology, Fundamental Pharmaceutics,* Burgess Pub. Co., Minneapolis, Minn., 1970, p. 219.
Benzoic Acid	4.21	Beckett, A. H. and Moffat, A. C.: Kinetics of Buccal Absorption of Some Carboxylic Acids and the Correlation of the Rate Conctants + n-Heptane: Aqueous Phase Partition Coefficients, *J. Pharm. Pharmacol. 22*:15, 1970.
	4.20	Parrott, E. L.: *Pharmaceutical Technology, Fundamental Pharmaceutics,* Burgess Pub. Co., Minneapolis, Minn., 1970, p. 216.
Benzoylecgonine	2.23	Parrott, E. L.: *Pharmaceutical Technology, Fundamental Pharmaceutics,* Burgess Pub. Co., Minneapolis, Minn., 1970, p. 219.
Benzylamine	9.34	Hong, Wen-Hai and Connors, K. A.: Identification of Aliphatic Amines from Rates of Cinnamoylation, *J. Pharm. Sci. 57*:1789, 1968.
D-(−)-Benzyllactic Acid	3.85	Randinitis, E. J., Barr, M., Wormser, H. C. and Nagwekar, J. B.: Kinetics of Urinary Excretion of D-(−)-Mandelic Acid and Its Homologs I: Mutual Inhibitory Effect of D-(−)-Mandelic Acid and Its Certain Homologs on Their Renal Tubular Secretion in Rats, *J. Pharm. Sci. 59*:806, 1970.
Benzylpenicillin Sodium	2.76	*Merck Index,* 8th ed., p. 141.

NAME	PKA	REFERENCE
		Parrott, E. L.: *Pharmaceutical Technology, Fundamental Pharmaceutics,* Burgess Pub. Co., Minneapolis, Minn., 1970, p. 216.
	2.7	*Hagers Handbuch der Pharmazeutischen Praxis,* Vol. I, Allgemeiner Teil, Wirkstoffgruppen I. Springer-Verlag, 1967, p. 995.
Benzylpenicillin	2.73	Rapson, H. D. C. and Bird, A. E.: *J. Pharm. Pharmacol. Suppl. 219*:222T, 1963.
		Through: Winningham, D. G., Nemoy, N. J. and Stamey, T. A.: Diffusion of Antibiotics from Plasma into Prostatic Fluid, *Nature, 219*:139, 1968.
Benzylpenicillinic Acid	2.74	*Merck Index,* 8th ed., p. 140.
Berbamine	7.33	*Merck Index,* 8th ed., p. 142.
Berberine	11.53	Parrott, E. L.: *Pharmaceutical Technology, Fundamental Pharmaceutics,* Burgess Pub. Co., Minneapolis, Minn., 1970, p. 219.
	2.47	*Merck Index,* 8th Edition, p. 142.
Betaine-L-Bromide	1.75	Bonkoski, S. and Perrin, J. H.: Measurement of the Apparent Dissociation Constants of Some Betaine Salts by Spectropolarimetry, *J. Pharm. Sci. 57*:1784, 1968.
Betaine-L-Chloride	1.75	Bonkoski, S. and Perrin, J. H.: Measurement of the Apparent Dissociation Constants of Some Betaine Salts by Spectropolarimetry, *J. Pharm. Sci. 57*:1784, 1968.
Biguanide	pK_1 = 11.52 pK_2 = 2.93	*Merck Index,* 8th ed., p. 148
3,6-Bis(dimethylamino-methyl)catechol • 2HCl	6.35 9.65	Kinget, R. D. and Schwartz, M. A.: Model Catalysts Which Simulate Penicillinase III, *J. Pharm. Sci. 57*:1916, 1968.
3,6-Bis(Morpholinomethyl) catechol HCl	pK_1 = 5.65 pK_2 = 7.32	Kinget, R. D. and Schwartz, M. A.: Model Catalysts Which Simulate Penicillinase III, *J. Pharm. Sci. 57*:1916, 1968.
4,6-Bis(Morpholinomethyl) pyrogallol 2HCl	pK_1 = 6.25 pK_2 = 7.66 pK_3 = 9.65	Kinget, R. D. and Schwartz ,M. A.: Model Catalysts Which Simulate Penicillinase III, *J. Pharm. Sci. 57*:1916, 1968.
Bithionol	pK_1 = 4.82 pK_2 = 10.50	*Merck Index,* 8th ed., p. 158.
Boric Acid	9.24	Parrott, E. L.: *Pharmaceutical Technology, Fundamental Pharmaceutics,* Burgess Pub. Co., Minneapolis, Minn., 1970, p. 216.
Bromcresol Green	4.7	*Merck Index,* 8th ed., p. 164.
	–0.85	Gupta, V. D. and Reed, J. B.: First pKa Values of Some Acid-Base Indicators, *J. Pharm. Sci. 59*:1683, 1970.
Bromcresol Purple	6.3	*Merck Index,* 8th ed., p. 164.
	–0.75	Gupta, V. D. and Reed, J. B.: First pKa Values of Some Acid-Base Indicators, *J. Pharm. Sci. 59*:1683, 1970.
Bromotiren	pK_1 = 2.17 pK_2 = 6.45 pK_3 = 7.60	*Merck Index,* 8th ed., p. 346.
Bromphenol Blue	4.0	*Merck Index,* 8th ed., p. 171.
	–0.95	Gupta, V. D. and Reed, J. B.: First pKa Values of Some Acid-Base Indicators, *J. Pharm. Sci. 59*:1683, 1970.
8-Bromotheophylline	5.45	Maulding, H. V. and Zoglio, M. A.: pKa Determinations Utilizing Solutions of 7-(2-Hydroxypropyl) Theophylline, *J. Pharm. Sci. 60*:309, 1971.
Bromothymol Blue	7.0	*Merck Index,* 8th ed. p. 171.
	–0.662	Gupta, V. D. and Cadwallader, D. E.: Determination of First pKa' Value and Partition Coefficients of Bromothymol Blue, *J. Pharm. Sci. 57*:2140, 1968.

NAME	PKA	REFERENCE
Brucine	7.95 2.3	Parrott, E. L.: *Pharmaceutical Technology, Fundamental Pharmaceutics,* Burgess Pub. Co., Minneapolis, Minn., 1970, p. 219.
	$pK_1 = 6.04$ $pK_2 = 11.7$	*Merck Index,* 8th ed., p. 171.
Butethal	8.10	Fincher, J. H., Entrekin, D. N. and Hartmen, C. W.: *J. Pharm. Sci. 55*:23, 1966.
n-Butylamine	10.60	Hong, Wen-Hai and Connors, K. A.: Identification of Aliphatic Amines from Rates of Cinnamoylation, *J. Pharm. Sci. 57*:1789, 1968.
sec-Butylamine	10.56	Hong, Wen-Hai and Connors, K. A.: Identification of Aliphatic Amines from Rates of Cinnamoylation, *PJ. Pharm. Sci. 57*:1789, 1968.
tert-Butylamine	10.82	Hong, Wen-Hai and Connors, K. A.: Identification of Aliphatic Amines from Rates of Cinnamoylation, *J. Pharm. Sci. 57*:1789, 1968.
Butylcarnitine Hydrochloride	3.56	Yalkowsky, S. H .and Zografi, G.: Potentiometric Titration of Monomeric and Micellar Acylcarnitines, *J. Pharm. Sci. 59*:798, 1970.
Butyl Chlorpromazine	9.7	Zografi, G. and Munshi, M.: Effect of Chemical Modification of the Surface Activity of Some Phenothiazine Derivatives, *J. Pharm. Sci. 59*:819, 1970.
n-Butyric Acid	4.82	Parrott, E. L.: *Pharmaceutical Technology, Fundamental Pharmaceutics,* Burgess Pub. Co., Minneapolis, Minn., 1970, p. 216.
Caffeine	0.61	Parrott, E. L.: *Pharmaceutical Technology, Fundamental Pharmaceutics,* Burgess Pub. Co., Minneapolis, Minn., 1970, p. 219.
Capreomycin	$pK_1 = 6.2$ $pK_2 = 8.2$ $pK_3 = 10.1$	*Merck Index,* 8th ed., p. 202.
Carbachol	4.8	Robson, J. M. and Stacey, R. S.: *Recent Advances in Pharmacology,* 4th ed., Little, Brown and Co., Boston, 1968, p. 108.
Carbinoxamine Maleate	8.1	Borodkin, S. and Yunker, M. H.: Interaction of Amine Drugs with a Polycarboxylic Acid Ion Exchange Resin, *J. Pharm. Sci. 59*:481, 1970.
5-Carboethoxy-2-thiouracil	6.43	Garrett, E. R. and Weber, D. J.: Metal Complexes of Thiouracils I: Stability Constants by Potentiometric Titration Studies and Structures of Complexes, *J. Pharm. Sci. 59*:1383, 1970.
Carbomycin	$pK_b = 7.2$ $pK_a = 6.8$	*Merck Index,* 8th ed., p. 207.
Carbonic Acid	6.37 10.25	Parrott, E. L.: *Pharmaceutical Technology, Fundamental Pharmaceutics,* Burgess Pub. Co., Minneapolis, Minn., 1970, p. 216.
5-Carboxy-2′-deoxyuridine	$pK_1 = 4.0$ $pK_2 = 9.8$	Nestler, H. J. and Garrett, E. R.: Prediction of Stability in Pharmaceutical Preparations XV, *J. Pharm. Sci. 57*:1117, 1968.
5-Carboxyuracil	$pK = 4.2$	Nestler, H. J. and Garrett, E. R.: Prediction of Stability in Pharmaceutical Preparations XV, *J. Pharm. Sci. 57*:1117, 1968.
Carbocromenum	8.3	Borodkin, S. and Yunker, M. H.: Interaction of Amine Drugs with a Polycarboxylic Acid Ion Exchange Resin, *J. Pharm. Sci. 59*:481, 1970.
Carnitine HCl	3.80	Yalkowsky, S. H. and Zografi, G.: Potentiometric Titration of Monomeric and Micellar Acylcarnitines, *J. Pharm. Sci. 59*:798, 1970.
Carnosine	$pK_1 = 2.64$ $pK_2 = 6.83$ $pK_3 = 6.83$	*Merck Index,* 8th ed., p. 212.

NAME	PKA	REFERENCE
Cephalothin Sodium	2.5	Winningham, D. G., Nemoy, N. J. and Stamey, T. A.: Diffusion of Antibiotics from Plasma into Prostatis Fluid, *Nature 219*:139, 1968.
Cevadine	8.85	Parrott, E. L.: *Pharmaceutical Technology, Fundamental Pharmaceutics,* Burgess Pub. Co., Minneapolis, Minn., 1970, p. 219.
Chloracetic Acid	2.86	Parrott, E. L.: *Pharmaceutical Technology, Fundamental Pharmaceutics,* Burgess Pub. Co., Minneapolis, Minn., 1970, p. 216.
p-Chlorobenzoic Acid	3.98	Parrott, E. L.: *Pharmaceutical Technology, Fundamental Pharmaceutics,* Burgess Pub. Co., Minneapolis, Minn., 1970, p. 216.
m-Chlorobenzoic Acid	3.82	Parrott, E. L.: *Pharmaceutical Technology, Fundamental Pharmaceutics,* Burgess Pub. Co., Minneapolis, Minn., 1970, p. 216.
o-Chlorobenzoic Acid	2.82	Parrott, E. L.: *Pharmaceutical Technology, Fundamental Pharmaceutics,* Burgess Pub. Co., Minneapolis, Minn., 1970, p. 216.
p-Chlorophenylacetic Acid	4.19	Parrott, E. L.: *Pharmaceutical Technology, Fundamental Pharmaceutics,* Burgess Pub. Co., Minneapolis, Minn., 1970, p. 216.
m-Chlorophenylacetic Acid	4.14	Parrott, E. L.: *Pharmaceutical Technology, Fundamental Pharmaceutics,* Burgess Pub. Co., Minneapolis, Minn., 1970, p. 216.
o-Chlorophenylacetic Acid	4.07	Parrott, E. L.: *Pharmaceutical Technology, Fundamental Pharmaceutics,* Burgess Pub. Co., Minneapolis, Minn., 1970, p. 216.
1-(p-Chlorophenyl)-4,6-diamino-2,2-dimethyl-1,2-dihydro-s-triazine	11.2	Baker, B. R. and Jordaan, J. H.: Analogs of Tetrahydrofolic acid XXVIII. Mode of Pyrimidine Binding to Dihydrofolic Reductase pH Profile Studies, *J. Pharm. Sci. 54*:1740, 1965.
5-(p-Chlorophenyl)-2,4-diamino-6-methylpyrimidine	7.7	Baker, B. R. and Jordaan, J. H.: Analogs of Tetrahydrofolic Acid XXVIII. Mode of Pyrimidines Binding to Dihydrofolic Reductase pH Profile Studies, *J. Pharm. Sci. 54*:1740, 1965.
5-(p-Chlorophenyl)-2,4-diamino-6-(trifluoromethyl) pyrimidine	2.8	Baker, B. R. and Jordaan, J. H.: Analogs of Tetrahydrofolic Acid XXVIII. Mode of Pyrimidines Binding to Dihydrofolic Reductase pH Profile Studies *J. Pharm. Sci. 54*:1740, 1965.
3-(p-Chlorophenyl)-5,6, dihydro-2-ethylimidazo (2,1-b) thiazole	9.30	Maulding, H. V. and Zoglio, M. A.: pKa Determinations Utilizing Solutions of 7-(2-Hydroxypropyl) Theophylline, *J. Pharm. Sci. 60*:309, 1971.
3-(p-Chlorophenyl)-2-ethyl-2,3,5,6-tetrahydro-imidazo (2,1-b) thiazol-3-ol	7.68	Maulding, H. V. and Zoglio, M. A.: pKa Determinations Utilizing Solutions of 7-(2-Hydroxypropyl) Theophylline, *J. Pharm. Sci. 60*:309, 1971.
Chloroquine	$pK'H_2A + 2 = 8.37$ $pK'HA^+ = 10.76$	Schill, G.: Photometric Determination of Amines and Quaternary Ammonium Compounds with Bromothymol Blue Part 5. Determination of Dissociation Constants of Amines, *Acta Pharm. Suecica 2*:99, 1965, through *Intern. Pharm. Abtsr. 2*:21, 1965.
8-Chlorotheophylline	5.5	Eichman, M. L., Guttman, D. E., VanWinkel, Q. and Guth, E. P.: *J. Pharm. Sci. 51*:66, 1962, through Brooke, D. and Guttman, D. E.: Complex Formation Influence on Reaction Rate IV, *J. Pharm. Sci. 57*:1677, 1968.
Chlorphenamine	9.3	Robson, J. M. and Stacey, R. S.: *Recent Advances in Pharmacology,* 4th ed., Little, Brown and Co., Boston, 1968, p. 108.
	8.3	Data by Smith, Kline and French, Philadelphia, PA 19101.
Chlorpromazine HCl	$pK'HA^+ = 9.32$	Schill, G.: Photometric Determination of Amines and Quaternary Ammonium Compounds with Bromothymol Blue, Part I, 5. Determination of Dissociation Constants of Amines, *Acta Pharm. Suecica 2*:99, 1965, through *Intern. Pharm. Abstr. 2*:21, 1965.

NAME	pKA	REFERENCE
	9.3 9.2	Zografi, G. and Munshi, M.: Effect of Chemical Modification of the Surface Activity of Some Phenothiazine Derivatives, *J. Pharm. Sci. 59*:819, 1970.
	9.9	Data by Smith, Kline and French, Philadelphia, PA. 19101.
	7.8	*Hagers Handbuch der Pharmazeutischen Praxis,* Zweiter Band, Wirkstoffgruppen II, Springer-Verlag, 1967. p. 380.
1-Chlorpromazine	9.4	Zografi, G. and Munshi, M.: Effect of Chemical Modification of the Surface Activity of Some Phenothiazine Derivatives, *J. Pharm. Sci. 59*:819, 1970.
3-Chlorpromazine	9.2	Zografi, G. and Munshi, M.: Effect of Chemical Modification of the Surface Activity of Some Phenothiazine Derivatives, *J. Pharm. Sci. 59*:819, 1970.
Cholate	4.95-4.98	Johns, W. H. and Bates, T. R.: Quantification of the Binding Tendencies of Cholestyramine I: Effect of Structure and Added Electrolytes on the Binding of Unconjugated and Conjugated Bile Salt Anions, *J. Pharm. Sci. 58*:179, 1969.
Cholic Acid	6.4	*Merck Index,* 8th ed., p. 254.
Cinchonamine	8.28	*Merck Index,* 8th ed., p. 262.
Cinchonidine	pK_1 = 5.80 pK_2 = 10.03	*Merck Index,* 8th ed., p. 262.
	8.20 3.97	Parrott, E. L.: *Pharmaceutical Technology, Fundamental Pharmaceutics,* Burgess Pub. Co., Minneapolis, Minn., 1970, p. 219.
Cinchonine	8.15 4.08	Parrott, E. L.: *Pharmaceutical Technology, Fundamental Pharmaceutics,* Burgess Pub. Co., Minneapolis, Minn., 1970, p. 219.
	pK_1 = 5.85 pK_2 = 9.92	*Merck Index,* 8th ed., p. 263.
Cinchophen	4.43	Perelman, Y. A. and Prudeus, L. P.: Potentiometric Titration of Organic Acid Mixture. Report 1. Methods for Quantitative Determination of Some Jointly Present Aromatic Acids and Barbiturates, *Aptechn. Delo 14*:37, 1965.
Cinnamic Acid (cis)	3.88	Parrott, E. L.: *Pharmaceutical Technology, Fundamental Pharmaceutics,* Burgess Pub. Co., Minneapolis, Minn., 1970, p. 216.
Cinnamic Acid (trans)	4.43	Parrott, E. L.: *Pharmaceutical Technology, Fundamental Pharmaceutics,* Burgess Pub. Co., Minneapolis, Minn., 1970, p. 216.
Citric Acid	3.06 4.74 5.40	Parrott, E. L.: *Pharmaceutical Technology, Fundamental Pharmaceutics,* Burgess Pub. Co., Minneapolis, Minn., 1970, p. 216.
Citrulline	pK_1 = 2.43 pK_2 = 9.41	*Merck Index,* 8th ed., p. 268.
Clindamycin	7.72 ± 0.04	Taraszka, M. J.: Absorption of Clindamycin from the Buccal Cavity, *J. Pharm. Sci. 59*:873, 1970.
Cloxacillin Sodium	2.90 ± 0.03	Data by: Bristol Laboratories, Syracuse, N.Y. 13201
Cocaine	5.59	*Merck Index,* 8th ed., p. 275.
	8.41	Parrott, E. L.: *Pharmaceutical Technology, Fundamental Pharmaceutics,* Burgess Pub. Co., Minneapolis, Minn., 1970, p. 219.
Codeine	6.05	*Hagers Handbuch der Pharmazeutischen Praxis,* Vol. I, Allgemeiner Teil, Wirkstoffgruppen I, Springer-Verlag, 1967, p. 840.
		Merck Index, 8th ed., p. 276.
	7.95	Parrott, E. L.: *Pharmaceutical Technology, Fundamental Pharmaceutics,* Burgess Pub. Co., Minneapolis, Minn., 1970, p. 219.

NAME	PKA	REFERENCE
Coenzyme A	9.6 (thiol) 6.4 (secondary phosphate) 4.0 (adenine NH_3^+)	*Merck Index,* 8th ed., p. 277.
Colchicine	1.65	Parrott, E. L.: *Pharmaceutical Technology, Fundamental Pharmaceutics,* Burgess Pub. Co., Minneapolis, Minn., 1970, p. 219.
	12.35	*Merck Index,* 8th ed., p. 278.
Coniine	10.9	Parrott, E. L.: *Pharmaceutical Technology, Fundamental Pharmaceutics,* Burgess Pub. Co., Minneapolis, Minn., 1970, p. 219.
	3.1	*Merck Index,* 8th ed., p. 282.
3-Acetyl-4-hydroxy-coumarin	4.26	Adachi, T. and Ejima, A.: On the pKa Value of 3-Acetyl-4-hydroxycoumarin and Dehydroacetic Acid, *Bull. Natl. Inst. Hyg. Sci. 81*:20, 1963, through *Intern. Pharm. Abstr.* Vol. 2; No. 14, July, 1965.
Coumermycin A	5.8-6.2	Newmark, H. L. and Berger, J.: Coumermycin A — Biopharmaceutical Studies, *J. Pharm. Sci. 59*:1246, 1970.
Cresol Red	8.3	*Merck Index,* 8th ed., p. 292.
	1.05	Gupta, V. D. and Reed, J. B.: First pKa Values of Some Acid-Base Indicators, *J. Pharm. Sci. 59*:1683, 1970.
Cupreine	7.43	Parrott, E. L.: *Pharmaceutical Technology, Fundamental Pharmaceutics,* Burgess Pub. Co., Minneapolis, Minn., 1970, p. 219.
	6.57	*Merck Index,* 8th ed., p. 299.
Cyclamate	2.28	Talmage, J. M., Chafetz, L. and Elefant, M.: Observations on the Instability of Cyclamate in Hydro-Alcoholic Solution, *J. Pharm. Sci. 57*:1073, 1968.
Cyclobarbital	7.50	Suzuki, A., Higuchi, W. I. and Ho, N. F. H.: Theoretical Model Studies of Drug Absorption and Transport in the Gastrointestinal Tract II, *J. Pharm. Sci. 59*:651, 1970.
Cyclohexylamine	10.64	Hong, Wen-Hai and Connors, K. A.: Identification of Aliphatic Amines from Rates of Cinnamoylation, *J. Pharm. Sci. 57*:1789, 1968.
5-Cyclohexen-1-yl-5-ethyl-1-methylbarbituric Acid	8.14	Suzuki, A., Higuchi, W. I. and Ho, N. F. H.: Theoretical Model Studies of Drug Absorption and Transport in the Gastrointestinal Tract II, *J. Pharm. Sci. 59*:651, 1070.
Cyclopentolate HCl	7.93	Wang, E. S. N. and Hammarlund, E. R.: Corneal Absorption Reinforcement of Certain Mydriatics, *J. Pharm. Sci. 59*:1559, 1970.
Cyclopentylamine	9.95	Hong, Wen-Hai and Connors, K. A.: Identification of Aliphatic Amines from Rates of Cinnamoylation, *J. Pharm. Sci. 57*:1789, 1968.
Cycloserine	$pK_1 = 4.5$ $pK_2 = 7.4$	Brunner, R. and Machek, G.: *Die Antibiotica,* Band II, Die Mittleren Antibiotica, 1965, p. 132.
Cysteine	$pK_1 = 1.71$ $pK_2 = 8.33$ $pK_3 = 10.78$	*Merck Index,* 8th ed., p. 317.
Cystine (L)	$pK_1 = 1.0$ $pK_2 = 2.1$ $pK_3 = 8.02$ $pK_4 = 8.71$	*Merck Index,* 8th ed., p. 317.
	8.00 10.25	Parrott, E. L.: *Pharmaceutical Technology, Fundamental Pharmaceutics,* Burgess Pub. Co., Minneapolis, Minn., 1970, p. 216.
Cytidine	pKa (amino cationic) = 4.22 pKa (sugar anionic) = 12.5	*Merck Index,* 8th ed., p. 218.

NAME	pKA	REFERENCE
2′-Cytidylic Acid	pKa_1 = 0.8 pKa_2 = 4.36 pKa_3 = 6.17	*Merck Index,* 8th ed., p. 318.
3′-Cytidylic Acid	pKa_1 = 0.8 pKa_2 = 4.28 pKa_3 = 6.0	*Merck Index,* 8th ed., p. 318.
Cytisine	pK_1 = 6.11 pK_2 = 13.08	*Merck Index,* 8th ed., p. 318.
	7.92 0.92	Parrott, E. L.: *Pharmaceutical Technology, Fundamental Pharmaceutics,* Burgess Pub. Co., Minneapolis, Minn., 1970, p. 219.
Cytosine	pK_1 = 4.60 pK_2 = 12.16	*Merck Index,* 8th ed., p. 319.
Dapsone	1.0 (pK_b = 13.0)	*Merck Index,* 8th ed., p. 321.
Decylcarnitine HCl	3.65	Yalkowsky, S. H. and Zografi, G.: Potentiometric Titration of Monomeric and Micellar Acylcarnitines, *J. Pharm. Sci. 59*:798, 1970.
Dehydroacetic Acid	5.12	Adachi, T. and Ejima, A.: On the pKa Value of 3-Acetyl-4-Hydroxycoumarin and Dehydroacetic Acid, *Bull. Natl. Inst. Hyg. Sci. 81*:20, 1963, through *Intern. Pharm. Amstr.* Vol. 2 No. 14 30 July 65.
Dehydrocholic Acid	4.91	Johns, W. H. and Bates, T. R.: Quantification of the Binding Tendencies of Cholestyramine II: Mechanism by Interaction with Bile Salts and Fatty Acid Salt Anions, *J. Pharm. Sci. 59*: 329, 1970.
Deoxycholate	4.97-5.17	Johns, W. H. and Bates, T. R.: Quantification of the Binding Tendencies of Cholestyramine I: Effect of Structure and Added Electrolytes on the Binding of Unconjugated and Conjugated Bile Salt Anions, *J. Pharm. Sci. 58*:179, 1969.
Deoxycholic Acid	6.58	*Merck Index,* 8th ed., p. 328.
2′-Deoxyuridine	pK_1 = 9.3	Nestler, H. J. and Garrett, E. R.: Prediction of Stability in Pharmaceutical Preparations XV, *J. Pharm. Sci. 57*:1117, 1968.
Deserpidine	6.68	*Merck Index,* 8th ed., p. 331.
Desoxyephedrine HCl	9.5	Borodkin, S. and Yunker, M. H.: Interaction of Amine Drugs with a Polycarboxylic Acid Ion Exchange Resin, *J. Pharm. Sci. 59*:481, 1970.
Dextroamphetamine Sulfate	10.05	Data by: Smith, Kline and French, Philadelphia, Pennsylvania, 19101.
Dextromethorphan HBr	8.25	Garrett, E. R. and Chemburkar, P. B.: Evaluation, Control and Prediction of Drug Diffusion through Polymeric Membranes III, *J. Pharm. Sci. 57*:1401, 1968.
Diallylbarbituric Acid	7.78	Parrott, E. L.: *Pharmaceutical Technology, Fundamental Pharmaceutics,* Burgess Pub. Co., Minneapolis, Minn., 1970, p. 216.
5,5-Diallyl-1-methyl-barbituric Acid	8.06	Suzuki, A., Higuchi, W. I. and Ho, N. F. H.: Theoretical Model Studies of Drug Absorption and Transport in the Gastrointestinal Tract II. *J. Pharm. Sci. 59*:651, 1970.
1,10-Diaminodecane	$pK'H_2A + 2 = 10.7$ $pK'HA^+ = 11.2$	Schill, G.: Photometric Determination of Amines and Quaternary Ammonium Compounds with Bromothymol Blue Part 5. Determination of Dissociation Constants of Amines, *Acta Pharm. Suecica 2*:99, 1965, through *Intern. Pharm. Abstr. 2*:21, 1965.
Dibenzylamine	—	Hong, Wen-Hai and Connors, K. A.: Identification of Aliphatic Amines from Rates of Cinnamoylation, *J. Pharm. Sci. 57*:1789, 1968.
Dichloracetic Acid	1.3	Parrott, E. L.: *Pharmaceutical Technology, Fundamental Pharmaceutics,* Burgess Pub. Co., Minneapolis, Minn., 1970, p. 216.

NAME	PKA	REFERENCE
2,5-Dichloroaniline	9.17	Medwick, T., Kaplan, G. and Weyer, L. G.: Measurement of Acidity and Equilibria in Glacial Acetic Acid with the Glass-Calomel Electrode System, *J. Pharm. Sci. 58*:308, 1969.
Dicloxacillin Sodium	2.67	Hou, J. P. and Poole, J. W.: The Amino Acid Nature of Ampicillin and Related Penicillins, *J. Pharm. Sci. 58*:1510, 1969.
Diethylamine	10.98	Hong, Wen-Hai and Connors, K. A.: Identification of Aliphatic Amines from Rates of Cinnamoylation, *J. Pharm. Sci. 57*:1789, 1968.
	10.11	*Merck Index,* 8th ed., p. 357.
Diethylthiambutene	8.90	*Hagers Handbuch der Pharmazeutischen Praxis,* Erster Band, Allgemeiner Teil, Wirkstoffgruppen I, Springer-Verlag, 1967, p. 876.
N,N-Diethylaniline	5.56	Medwick, T., Kaplan, G. and Weyer, L. G.: Measurement of Acidity and Equilibria in Glacial Acetic Acid with the Glass-Calomel Electrode System, *J. Pharm. Sci. 58*:308, 1969.
Dihydroergocornine	6.76 ± 0.02	Maulding, H. V. and Zoglio, M. A.: Physical Chemistry of Ergot Alkaloids and Derivatives I: Ionization Constants of Several Medicinally Active Bases, *J. Pharm. Sci. 59*:700, 1970.
Dihydroergocriptine	6.74 ± 0.02	Maulding, H. V. and Zoglio, M. A.: Physical Chemistry of Ergot Alkaloids and Derivatives I: Ionization Constants of Several Medicinally Active Bases, *J. Pharm. Sci. 59*:700, 1970.
Dihydroergocristine	6.74 ± 0.02	Maulding, H. V. and Zoglio, M. A.: Physical Chemistry of Ergot Alkaloids and Derivatives I: Ionization Constants of Several Medicinally Active Bases, *J. Pharm. Sci. 59*:700, 1970.
Dihydroergotamine	6.75 ± 0.03	Maulding, H. V. and Zoglio, M. A.: Physical Chemistry of Ergot Alkaloids and Derivatives I: Ionization Constants of Several Medicinally Active Bases, *J. Pharm. Sci. 59*:700, 1970.
Dihydroergotamine Mesylate	8.0	Robson, J. M. and Stacey, R. S.: *Recent Advances in Pharmacology,* 4th ed., Little, Brown and Co., Boston, 1968, p. 108.
3,4-Dihydro-1-hydroxy-3-oxo-1H-1,2-benziodoxin	7.54	Wolf, W., Chen, J. C. and Hsu, L.: Chemistry and Biochemistry of Polyvalent Iodine Compounds V, *J. Pharm. Sci. 55*:68, 1966.
1,3-Dihydro-1-hydroxy-3-oxo-1,2-benziooxole	7.35	Wolf, W., Chen, J. C. and Hsu, L.: Chemistry and Biochemistry of Polyvalent Iodine Compounds V, *J. Pharm. Sci. 55*:68, 1966.
1,6-Dihydroxyphenazine	$pKNH^+ = 1.52$ pKOH(1st) = 6.38 pKOH(2nd) = 8.80	Machida, T., Shiota, H., Hujioka, N. and Yamaguchi, R.: Determination of Ionization Constants of 1,6-Dihydroxyphenazine and Molar Ratio of its Metal Chelates, *Ann. Rept. Hoshi. Coll. Pharm. 38*:15, 1964, through *Intern. Pharm. Abstr.*
3,5-Diiodotyrosine	$pK_1 = 2.12$ $pK_2 = 6.48$ $pK_3 = 7.82$	*Merck Index,* 8th ed., p. 370.
Diiodo-L-tyrosine	6.48	Parrott, E. L.: *Pharmaceutical Technology, Fundamental Pharmaceutics,* Burgess Pub. Co., Minneapolis, Minn., 1970, p. 216.
Diisoamylamine	10.94	Hong, Wen-Hai and Connors, K. A.: Identification of Aliphatic Amines from Rates of Cinnamoylation, *J. Pharm. Sci. 57*:1789, 1968.
Diisobutylamine	10.68	Hong, Wen-Hai and Connors, K. A.: Identification of Aliphatic Amines from Rates of Cinnamoylation, *J. Pharm. Sci. 57*:1789, 1968.
Diisooctylamine	—	Hong, Wen-Hai and Connors, K. A.: Identification of Aliphatic Amines from Rates of Cinnamoylation, *J. Pharm. Sci. 57*:1789, 1968.
Dimethylamphetamine	8.16	Leffler, E. B., Spencer, H. M. and Burger, A.: *J. Am. Chem. Soc. 73*:2611, through Beckett, A. H., Boyes, R. N. and Triggs, E. J.: Kinetics of Buccal Absorption of Amphetamines, *J. Pharm. Pharmacol. 20*:92, 1968.

NAME	pKA	REFERENCE
2,4-Dimethylbenzoic Acid	4.28	Beckett, A. H. and Moffat, A. C.: Kinetics of Buccal Absorption of Some Carboxylic Acids and the Correlation of the Rate Constants + n-Heptane: Aqueous Phase Partition Coefficients, *J. Pharm. Pharmacol. 22*:15, 1970.
2,5-Dimethylbenzoic Acid	4.05	Beckett, A. H. and Moffat, A. C.: Kinetics of Buccal Absorption of Some Carboxylic Acids and the Correlation of the Rate Constants + n-Heptane: Aqueous Phase Partition Coefficients, *J. Pharm. Pharmacol. 22*:15, 1970.
3,5-Dimethylbenzoic Acid	4.31	Beckett, A. H. and Moffat, A. C.: Kinetics of Buccal Absorption of Some Carboxylic Acids and the Correlation of the Rate Constants + n-Heptane: Aqueous Phase Partition Coefficients, *J. Pharm. Pharmacol. 22*:15, 1970.
5,6-Dimethyl-2-thiouracil	8.08	Garrett, E. R. and Weber, D. J.: Metal Complexes of Thiouracils I: Stability Constants by Potentiometric Titration Studies and Structures of Complexes, *J. Pharm. Sci. 59*:1383, 1970.
Dimethylthiambutene	8.95	*Hagers Handbuch der Pharmazeutischen Praxis,* Vol. I, Allgemeiner Teil, Wirkstoffgruppen I, Springer-Verlag, 1967, p. 877.
N,N-Dimethyltryptamine	8.68	*Merck Index,* 8th ed., p. 379.
2,4-Dinitroaniline	18.46	*Merck Index,* 8th ed., p. 330.
Diphenhydramine HCl	7.7 (apparent)	Robson, J. M. and Stacey, R. S.: *Recent Advances in Pharmacology,* 4th ed., Little. Brown and Co., Boston, 1968, p. 108.
	8.98	Ritschel, W. A.: *Applied Biopharmaceutics I,* Hamilton, IL, 1969, p. 169.
5,5-Diphenylbarbituric Acid	7.52	Maulding, H. V. and Zoglio, M. A.: pKa Determinations Utilizing Solutions of 7-(2-Hydroxypropyl) Theophylline, *J. Pharm. Sci. 60*:309, 1971
Dipyridamole	6.4	Data by: Geigy Pharmaceuticals, Ardsley, New York 10502.
2,6-Di-tert-butyl-pyridine	3.58	*Merck Index,* 8th ed., p. 348.
Doxycycline	3.4 7.7 about 9.7	*Merck Index,* 8th ed., p. 398.
Ecgonine	11.11	*Merck Index,* 8th ed., p. 402.
	2.78	Parrott, E. L.: *Pharmaceutical Technology, Fundamental Pharmaceutics,* Burgess Pub. Co., Minneapolis, Minn., 1970, p. 219.
Emetine	$pK_1 = 5.77$ $pK_2 = 6.64$	*Merck Index,* 8th ed., p. 407.
	8.23 7.36	Parrott, E. L.: *Pharmaceutical Technology, Fundamental Pharmaceutics,* Burgess Pub. Co., Minneapolis, Minn., 1970, p. 219.
Enteromycin	4.3	*Merck Index,* 8th ed., p. 409.
Ephedrine (Base)	9.5	Borodkin, S. and Yunker, M. H.: Interaction of Amine Drugs with a Carboxylic Acid Ion Exchange Resin, *J. Pharm. Sci. 59*:481, 1970.
Epinephrine	5.5 (apparent)	Robson, J. M. and Stacey, R. S.: *Recent Advances in Pharmacology,* 4th ed., Little, Brown and Co., Boston, 1968, p. 108.
Epinephrylborate	$pK_1 = 10.00$ $pK_2 = 8.8$ $pK_3 = 2.6$	Data by: Barnes-Hind Pharmaceuticals, Inc., Sunnyvale, California 94086.
Ergonovine	6.8	*Merck Index,* 8th ed., p. 415.
Ergostine	6.30 ± .04	Maulding, H. V. and Zoglio, M. A.: Physical Chemistry of Ergot Alkaloids and Derivatives I: Ionization Constants of Several Medicinally Active Bases, *J. Pharm. Sci. 59*:700, 1970.
Ergotamine	6.25	Maulding, H. V. and Zoglio, M. A.: Physical Chemistry of Ergot Alkaloids and Derivatives I: Ionization Constants of Several Medicinally Active Bases, *J. Pharm. Sci. 59*:700, 1970.

NAME	PKA	REFERENCE
Ergotaminine	6.72	Maulding, H. V. and Zoglio, M. A.: Physical Chemistry of Ergot Alkaloids and Derivatives I: Ionization Constants of Several Medicinally Active Bases, *J. Pharm. Sci. 59*:700, 1970.
Erythromycin	$pK_1 = 8.8$	*Merck Index,* 8th ed., p. 419.
Erythromycin Lactobionate	8.8	McGuire, J. M., Bunch, R. L., Anderson, R. C., Boaz, H. E., Flynn, E. H., Powell, H. M. and Smith, J. W.: *Antibiot. Chemotherap. 2*:281, 1952, through Winningham, D. G., Nemoy, N. J. and Stamey, T. A.: Diffusion of Antibiotics from Plasma into Prostatic Fluid, *Nature 219*:139, 1968.
Ethacrynic Acid	$pK' = 3.50$	*Merck Index,* 8th ed., p. 425.
Ethanolamine	9.44	Parrott, E. L.: *Pharmaceutical Technology, Fundamental Pharmaceutics,* Burgess Pub. Co., Minneapolis, Minn., 1970, p. 219.
Ethyl Chlorpromazine	8.6	Zografi, G. and Munshi, M.: Effect of Chemical Modification on the Surface Activity of Some Phenothiazine Derivatives, *J. Pharm. Sci. 59*:819, 1970.
N-Ethyl-cyclohexylamine	11.3	Hong, Wen-Hai and Conners, K. A.: Identification of Aliphatic Amines from Rates of Cinnamoylation, *J. Pharm. Sci. 57*:1789, 1968.
Ethyldilvasene	4.4	Robson, J. M. and Stacey, R. S.: *Recent Advances in Pharmacology,* 4th ed., Little, Brown and Co., Boston, 1968, p. 115.
Ethylisopropylbarbituric Acid	8.01	Parrott, E. L.: *Pharmaceutical Technology, Fundamental Pharmaceutics,* Burgess Pub. Co., Minneapolis, Minn., 1970, p. 216.
5-Ethyl-5-isopentyl-1-methyl-barbituric Acid	8.31	Suzuki, A., Higuchi, W. I. and Ho, N. F. H.: Theoretical Model Studies of Drug Absorption and Transport in the gastrointestinal Tract II, *J. Pharm. Sci. 59*:651, 1970.
2-Ethylmercapto-4-hydroxy-pyrimidine	7.01	Garrett, E. R. and Weber, D. J.: Metal Complexes of Thiouracils I: Stability Constants by Potentiometric Titration Studies and Structures of Complexes, *J. Pharm. Sci. 59*:1383, 1970.
Ethyl-1-methylbutyl-barbituric Acid	8.11	Parrott, E. L.: *Pharmaceutical Technology, Fundamental Pharmaceutics,* Burgess Pub. Co., Minneapolis, Minn., 1970, p. 216.
Ethylmorphine	7.88	Parrott, E. L.: *Pharmaceutical Technology, Fundamental Pharmaceutics,* Burgess Pub. Co., Minneapolis, Minn., 1970, p. 219.
α-Ethylphenethylamine	9.30	Garrett, E. R. and Chemburkar, P. B.: Evaluation, Control and Prediction of Drug Diffusion Through Polymeric Membranes, *J. Pharm. Sci. 57*:1401, 1968.
4-Ethyl-4-phenyl-glutaramic acid	4.6	Agarwal, S. P. and Blake, M. I.: Determination of Glutethimide, Aminoglutethimide, and Bemegride by Nonaqueous Titration, *J. Pharm. Sci. 54*:1668, 1965, through *Intern. Pharm. Abstr.* Vol. 3 No. 10, 30 May 66.
Etioporphyrin	18.0	*Merck Index,* 8th ed., p. 443.
Filicinic Acid	5.8	*Merck Index,* 8th ed., p. 458.
Folic Acid	2.5	Baker, B. R. and Jordaan, J. H.: Analogs of Tetrahydrofolic Acid XXVIII. Mode of Pyrimidine Binding to Dihydrofolic Reductase pH Profile Studies, *J. Pharm. Sci. 54*:1740, 1965.
Folinic Acid	3.1 4.8 10.4	*Merck Index,* 8th ed., p. 468.
Formic Acid	3.75	Parrott, E. L.: *Pharmaceutical Technology, Fundamental Pharmaceutics,* Burgess Pub. Co., Minneapolis, Minn., 1970, p. 216.
Fumaric Acid	3.75 3.03	Parrott, E. L.: *Pharmaceutical Technology, Fundamental Pharmaceutics,* Burgess Pub. Co., Minneapolis, Minn., 1970, p. 216.

NAME	pKA	REFERENCE
Funtumine	9.18	*Merck Index,* 8th ed., p. 474.
Furosemide	3.65	Hajdu, Von P. and Haussler, A.: Untersuchungen mit dem Salidiureticum 4-Chlor-N-(2-furylmethyl) - 5-sulfamylantranil-saure, *Arzneimittel-Forsch. 14*:709, 1964.
Furtrethonium	4.8 (apparent)	Robson, J. M. and Stacey, R. S.: *Recent Advances in Pharmacology,* 4th ed., Little, Brown and Co., Boston, 1968, p. 108.
Fusidic Acid	5.35	*Merck Index,* 8th ed., p. 478.
GABA (Gamma-Amino Butyric Acid)	4.01	Yalkowsky, S. H. and Zografi, G.: Potentiometric Titration of Monomeric and Micellar Acylcarnitines, *J. Pharm. Sci. 59*: 798, 1970.
Gallic Acid	4.40	Parrott, E. L.: *Pharmaceutical Technology, Fundamental Pharmaceutics,* Burgess Pub. Co., Minneapolis, Minn., 1970, p. 216.
Garryine	8.70	*Merck Index,* 8th ed., p. 483.
GBB $(H_3)_3N^+CH_2CH_2CH_2COOH$	4.02	Yalkowsky, S. H. and Zografi, G.: Potentiometric Titration of Monomeric and Micellar Acylcarnitines, *J. Pharm. Sci. 59*: 798, 1970.
Gelsemine	7.75	*Merck Index,* 8th ed., p. 484.
Gibberellic Acid	4.0	*Merck Index,* 8th ed., p. 489.
Gladiolic Acid	4.4	*Merck Index,* 8th ed., p. 491.
D-Glucoascorbic Acid	pK_1 = 4.26 pK_2 = 11.58	*Merck Index,* 8th ed., p. 493.
α-Glucose-1-phosphate	pK_1 = 1.11 pK_2 = 6.13	*Merck Index,* 8th ed., p. 495.
L-Glutamic Acid	4.07 9.47	Parrott, E. L.: *Pharmaceutical Technology, Fundamental Pharmaceutics,* Burgess Pub. Co., Minneapolis, Minn., 1970, p. 216.
Glutamic Acid	pK_1 = 2.19 pK_2 = 4.25 pK_3 = 9.67	*Merck Index,* 8th ed., p. 497.
Glutamine	pK_1 = 2.17 pK_2 = 9.13	*Merck Index,* 8th ed., p. 497.
Glutaric Acid	4.34	Parrott, E. L.: *Pharmaceutical Technology, Fundamental Pharmaceutics,* Burgess Pub. Co., Minneapolis, Minn., 1970, p. 217.
Glutathione	pK_1 = 2.12 pK_2 = 3.53 pK_3 = 8.66 pK_4 = 9.12	*Merck Index,* 8th ed., p. 497.
Glutethimide	9.2	Agarwal, S. P. and Blake, M. I.: Determination of Glutethimide, Aminoglutethimide, and Bemegride by Nonaqueous Titration, *J. Pharm. Sci. 54*:1668, 1965, through *Intern. Pharm. Abstr.* Vol 3 No. 10 30 May 66.
Glycerophosphoric Acid	1.47 6.19	Parrott, E. L.: *Pharmaceutical Technology, Fundamental Pharmaceutics,* Burgess Pub. Co., Minneapolis, Minn., 1970, p. 217.
Glycine	2.35 9.78	Parrott, E. L.: *Pharmaceutical Technology, Fundamental Pharmaceutics,* Burgess Pub. Co., Minneapolis, Minn., 1970, p. 217.
	pK_1 = 2.34 pK_2 = 9.60	*Merck Index,* 8th ed., p. 500.
Glycocholate	2.78-4.35	Johns, W. H. and Bates, T. R.: Quantification of the Binding Tendencies of Cholestyramine I: Effect of Structure and Added Electrolytes on the Binding of Unconjugated and Conjugated Bile Salt Anions, *J. Pharm. Sci. 58*:179, 1969.
Glycocholic Acid	4.4	*Merck Index,* 8th ed., p. 500.

NAME	pKa	REFERENCE
Glycodeoxycholate	2.46-3.98	Johns, W. H. and Bates, T. R.: Quantification of the Binding Tendencies of Cholestyramine I: Effect of Structure and Added Electrolytes on the Binding of Unconjugated and Conjugated Bile Salt Anions, *J. Pharm. Sci. 58*:179, 1969
N-Glycylglycine	$pK_1 = 3.12$ $pK_2 = 8.17$	*Merck Index,* 8th ed., p. 501.
Gnoscopine	7.8	*Merck Index,* 8th ed., p. 503.
Goitrin	10.5	*Merck Index,* 8th ed., p. 503.
Haloperidol	8.3	*Hagers Handbuch der Pharmazeutischen Praxis,* Vol. II, Wirkstoffgruppen II, Springer-Verlag, 1967, p. 397.
Harman	6.10	*Merck Index,* 8th ed., p. 517.
Heptoxime	$pK_1 = 10.65 \pm 0.2$ $pK_2 = 12.21 \pm 0.2$	*Merck Index,* 8th ed., p. 524.
Heptylpenicillin Sodium	2.66	*Merck Index,* 8th ed., p. 524.
Hexanoic Acid	4.85	Ekwall, P., Rosendahl, T. and Lofman, N.: *Acta Chem. Scand. 11*:590, 1960, through Yalkowsky, S. H. and Zografi, G.: Potentiometric Titration of Monomeric and Micellar Acylcarnitiness, *J. Pharm. Sci. 59*:798, 1970.
Hexobarbital	8.34	Suzuki, A., Higuchi, W. I. and Ho, N. F. H.: Theoretical Model Studies of Drug Absorption and Transport in the Gastrointestinal Tract II, *J. Pharm. Sci. 59*:651, 1970.
n-Hexylamine	10.64	Hong, Wen-Hai and Connors, K. A.: Identification of Aliphatic Amines from Rates of Cinnamoylation, *J. Pharm. Sci. 57*:1789, 1968.
Histamine	5.1 (apparent)	Robson, J. A. and Stacey, R. S.: *Recent Advances in Pharmacology,* 4th ed., Little, Brown and Co., Boston, 1968, p. 108.
L-Histidine	9.18	Parrott, E. L.: *Pharmaceutical Technology, Fundamental Pharmaceutics,* Burgess Pub. Co., Minneapolis, Minn., 1970, p. 217.
	$pK_1 = 1.78$ $pK_2 = 5.97$ $pK_3 = 8.97$	*Merck Index,* 8th ed., p. 532.
Hippuric Acid	3.64	Parrott, E. L.: *Pharmaceutical Technology, Fundamental Pharmaceutics,* Burgess Pub. Co., Minneapolis, Minn., 1970, p. 217.
Homatropine	7.4 (apparent)	Robson, J. M. and Stacey, R. S.: *Recent Advances in Pharmacology,* 4th ed., Little, Brown and Co., Boston, 1968, p. 108.
Homocystine	$pK_1 = 1.59$ $pK_2 = 2.54$ $pK_3 = 8.52$ $pK_4 = 9.44$	*Merck Index,* 8th ed., p. 535.
HON (2-Amino-5-hydroxy-levulinic Acid)	2.91	*Merck Index,* 8th ed., p. 536.
Hyalobiuronic Acid	$pK_1 = 2.6$ $pK_2 = 7.1$	*Merck Index,* 8th ed., p. 537.
Hydrastine	7.8	*Merck Index,* 8th ed., p. 539.
	6.23	Parrott, E. L.: *Pharmaceutical Technology, Fundamental Pharmaceutics,* Burgess Pub. Co., Minneapolis, Minn., 1970, p. 220.
Hydrastinine	2.62	*Merck Index,* 8th ed., p. 539.
	11.38	Parrott, E. L.: *Pharmaceutical Technology, Fundamental Pharmaceutics,* Burgess Pub. Co., Minneapolis, Minn., 1970, p. 220.
Hydrochinine	8.67	Parrott, E. L.: *Pharmaceutical Technology, Fundamental Pharmaceutics,* Burgess Pub. Co., Minneapolis, Minn., 1970, p. 220.
Hydrochlorothiazide	7.9 9.2	*Merck Index,* 8th ed., p. 541.

NAME	pKa	REFERENCE
Hydrocodone Bitartrate	8.3	*Hagers Handbuch der Pharmazeutischen Praxis, Vol. I, Allgemeiner* Teil, Wirkstoffgruppen I, Springer-Verlag, 1967, p. 815.
	8.8-9.0	Data by: Endo Laboratories, 1000 Stewart Ave., Garden City, NY, 11530
Hydrocyanic Acid	9.14	Parrott, E. L.: *Pharmaceutical Technology, Fundamental Pharmaceutics,* Burgess Pub. Co., Minneapolis, Minn., 1970, p. 217.
Hydroflumethiazide	$pK_1 = 8.9$ $pK_2 = 10.7$	*Merck Index,* 8th ed., p. 543.
Hydroquinine	$pK = 5.33$	*Merck Index,* 8th ed., p. 547.
β-Hydroxy-ammonium butyric Acid	3.80	Yalkowsky, S. H. and Zografi, G.: Potentiometric Titration of Monomeric and Micellar Acylcarnitines, *J. Pharm. Sci. 59*: 798, 1970.
4-(2-Hydroxy-3-isopropyl-aminopropoxy) indole	9.65 ± 0.1	Maulding, H. V. and Zoglio, M. A.: pKa Determinations Utilizing Solutions of 7-(2-Hydroxypropyl) Theophylline, *J. Pharm. Sci. 60*:309, 1971.
D-(−)-4-Hydroxy-4-phenylbutanoic Acid	4.70	Randinitis, E. J., Barr, M., Wormser, H. G. and Nagwekar, J. B.: Kinetics of Urinary Excretion of D-(−)-Mandelic Acid and Its Homologs I: Mutual Inhibitory Effects of D-(−)-Mandelic Acid and Its Tubular Secretion in Rats, *J. Pharm. Sci. 59*:806, 1970.
p-Hydroxybenzylpenicillin Sodium	2.62	*Merck Index,* 8th ed., p. 548.
Hydroxyglutamic Acid	$pK_1 = 2.09$ $pK_2 = 4.18$ $pK_3 = 9.20$	*Merck Index,* 8th ed., p. 550.
Hydroxyproline	$pK_1 = 1.82$ $pK_2 = 9.65$	*Merck Index,* 8th ed., p. 555.
Hydroxy-L-proline	12.08	Parrott, E. L.: *Pharmaceutical Technology, Fundamental Pharmaceutics,* Burgess Pub. Co., Minneapolis, Minn., 1970, p. 217.
Hygromycin	8.9	*Merck Index,* 8th ed., p. 557.
Hygromycin B	7.1 8.8	*Merck Index,* 8th ed., p. 557.
Hyoscyamine	9.3 (apparent)	Robson, J. M. and Stacey, R. S.: *Recent Advances in Pharmacology,* 4th ed., Little, Brown and Co., Boston 1968, p. 108.
Hypochlorous Acid	7.46	Parrott, E. L.: *Pharmaceutical Technology, Fundamental Pharmaceutics,* Burgess Pub. Co., Minneapolis, Minn., 1970, p. 217.
Hypoxanthine	8.50 ± 0.06	Cohen, J. L. and Connors, K. A.: Stability and Structure of Some Organic Molecular Complexes in Aqueous Solution, *J. Pharm. Sci. 59*:1271, 1970.
	5.30 ($pK_b = 8.7$)	*Merck Index,* 8th ed., p. 559.
Ibogaine	8.1	*Merck Index,* 8th ed., p. 559.
Iodic Acid	0.78	Parrott, E. L.: *Pharmaceutical Technology, Fundamental Pharmaceutics,* Burgess Pub. Co., Minneapolis, Minn., 1970, p. 217.
Iodinin	12.5	*Merck Index,* 8th ed., p. 570
Iminodiacetic Acid	$pK_1 = 2.98$ $pK_2 = 9.89$	*Merck Index,* 8th ed., p. 562.
Indolacetic Acid	4.75	*Merck Index,* 8th ed., p. 565.
p-Iodophenylacetic Acid	4.18	Parrott, E. L.: *Pharmaceutical Technology, Fundamental Pharmaceutics,* Burgess Pub. Co., Minneapolis, Minn., 1970, p. 217.

NAME	PKA	REFERENCE
Inosinic Acid	$pK_1 = 2.4$ $pK_2 = 6.4$	*Merck Index,* 8th ed., p. 567.
Isoamylamine	10.6	Hong, Wen-Hai and Connors, K. A.: Identification of Aliphatic Amines from Rates of Cinnamoylation, *J. Pharm. Sci. 57*:1789, 1968.
Isobutamide	$pK_1 = 7.1$ $pK_2 = 8.6$	*Merck Index,* 8th ed., p. 580.
Isobutylamine	10.72	Hong, Wen-Hai and Connors, K. A.: Identification of Aliphatic Amines from Rates of Cinnamoylation, *J. Pharm. Sci. 57*:1789, 1968.
Isobutyric Acid	4.81	Parrott, E. L.: *Pharmaceutical Technology, Fundamental Pharmaceutics,* Burgess Pub. Co., Minneapolis, Minn., 1970, p. 217.
L-Isoglutamine	$pK_1 = 3.81$ $pK_2 = 7.88$	*Merck Index,* 8th ed., p. 584.
Isoleucine	$pK_1 = 2.27$ $pK_2 = 9.62$	*Merck Index,* 8th ed., p. 585.
DL-Isoleucine	9.76	Parrott, E. L.: *Pharmaceutical Technology, Fundamental Pharmaceutics,* Burgess Pub. Co., Minneapolis, Minn., 1970, p. 217.
Isolysergic Acid	3.44	*Merck Index,* 8th ed., p. 585.
Isopilocarpine	6.83	Parrott, E. L.: *Pharmaceutical Technology, Fundamental Pharmaceutics,* Burgess Pub. Co., Minneapolis, Minn., 1970, p. 220.
Isoprenaline	8.64	*Merck Index,* 8th ed., p. 591.
Isopropylamine	10.63	Hong, Wen-Hai and Connors, K. A.: Identification of Aliphatic Amines from Rates of Cinnamoylation, *J. Pharm. Sci. 57*:1789, 1968.
N-Isopropyl-cyclohexylamine	11.3	Hong, Wen-Hai and Connors, K. A.: Identification of Aliphatic Amines from Rates of Cinnamoylation, *J. Pharm. Sci. 57*:1789, 1968.
Isoproterenol	8.64	*Merck Index,* 8th ed., p. 591.
Isoquinoline	5.4	Parrott, E. L.: *Pharmaceutical Technology, Fundamental Pharmaceutics,* Burgess Pub. Co., Minneapolis, Minn., 1970, p. 220.
Isovaleric Acid	3.84	Parrott, E. L.: *Pharmaceutical Technology, Fundamental Pharmaceutics,* Burgess Pub. Co., Minneapolis, Minn., 1970, p. 217.
Itaconic Acid	3.84 5.55	Parrott, E. L.: *Pharmaceutical Technology, Fundamental Pharmaceutics,* Burgess Pub. Co., Minneapolis, Minn., 1970, p. 217.
Kanamycin Sulfate	7.2	Winningham, D. G., Nemoy, N. J. and Stamey, T. A.: Diffusion of Antibiotics from Plasma into Prostatic Fluid, *Nature 219*:139, 1968.
Kinetin	$pK_1 = 2.7$ $pK_2 = 9.9$	*Merck Index,* 8th ed., p. 601.
Lactic Acid	3.86	Parrott, E. L.: *Pharmaceutical Technology, Fundamental Pharmaceutics,* Burgess Pub. Co., Minneapolis, Minn., 1970, p. 217.
	3.83	*Merck Index,* 8th ed., p. 604.
	3.87	*Hagers Handbuch der Pharmazeutischen Praxis,* Vol. II, Wirkstoffgruppen II, Springer-Verlag, 1967. p.
L-Lactic Acid	3.79	*Merck Index,* 8th ed., p. 605.
Lauric Acid	4.92	Johns, W. H. and Bates, T. R.: Quantification of the Binding Tendencies of Cholestyramine II: Mechanism of Interaction with Bile Salts and Fatty Acid Salt Anions, *J. Pharm. Sci. 59*: 329, 1970.

NAME	pKA	REFERENCE
DL-Leucine	9.74	Parrott, E. L.: *Pharmaceutical Technology, Fundamental Pharmaceutics,* Burgess Pub. Co., Minneapolis, Minn., 1970, p. 217.
	$pK_1 = 2.36$ $pK_2 = 9.60$	*Merck Index,* 8th ed., p. 616.
Leucomycin	5.69	*Merck Index,* 8th ed., p. 617.
Leucovorin	3.1 4.8 10.4	*Merck Index,* 8th ed., p. 468.
Levarterenol	5.5 (apparent)	Robson, J. M. and Stacey, R. S.: *Recent Advances in Pharmacology,* 4th ed., Little, Brown and Co., Boston, 1968, p. 108.
Lidocaine	7.86	Data by: Astra Pharmaceutical Products, Inc., 7 Neponset St., Worcester, MA 01606
Lincomycin (free base)	**7.6**	*Merck Index,* 8th ed., p. 620.
Lincomycin HCl	7.5	Morozowich, W., Lamb, D. J., Karnes, H. A., Mackellar, F. A., Lewis, C., Stern, K. F. and Rowe, E. L.: Synthesis and Bioactivity of Lincomycin-2-Phosphate, *J. Pharm. Sci. 58*: 1485, 1969.
Linoleic Acid	5.10	Johns, W. H. and Bates, T. R.: Quantification of the Binding Tendencies of Cholestyramine II: Mechanism of Interaction with Bile Salts and Fatty Acid Salt Anions, *J. Pharm. Sci. 59*: 329, 1970.
Liothyronine Sodium	8.45	Data by: Smith, Kline and French, Philadelphia, Pa. 19101.
Lithium Acetate	6.82	Medwick, T., Kaplan, G. and Weyer, L. G.: Measurement of Activity and Equilibria in Glacial Acetic Acid with the Glass-Calomel Electrode System, *J. Pharm. Sci. 58*:308, 1969.
Lithocholic Acid	4.99	Johns, W. H. and Bates, T. R.: Quantification of the Binding Tendencies of Cholestyramine II: Mechanism of Interaction with Bile Salts and Fatty Acid Salt Anions, *J. Pharm. Sci. 59*:329, 1970.
Lochnericine	4.2	*Merck Index,* 8th ed., p. 625.
Lochneridine	5.5	*Merck Index,* 8th ed., p. 625.
Lysergic Acid	3.44	*Merck Index,* 8th ed., p. 632.
Lysine	$pK_1 = 2.20$ $pK_2 = 8.90$ $pK_3 = 10.28$	*Merck Index,* 8th ed., p. 633.
L-Lysine	10.53	Parrott, E. L.: *Pharmaceutical Technology, Fundamental Pharmaceutics,* Burgess Pub. Co., Minneapolis, Minn., 1970, p. 217.
Maleic Acid	2.00 6.26	Parrott, E. L.: *Pharmaceutical Technology, Fundamental Pharmaceutics,* Burgess Pub. Co., Minneapolis, Minn., 1970, p. 217.
Malic Acid	3.40 5.05	Parrott, E. L.: *Pharmaceutical Technology, Fundamental Pharmaceutics,* Burgess Pub. Co., Minneapolis, Minn., 1970, p. 217.
Malonic Acid	2.85 6.10	Parrott, E. L.: *Pharmaceutical Technology, Fundamental Pharmaceutics,* Burgess Pub. Co., Minneapolis, Minn., 1970, p. 217.
Mandelic Acid	3.37	Parrott, E. L.: *Pharmaceutical Technology, Fundamental Pharmaceutics,* Burgess Pub. Co., Minneapolis, Minn., 1970, p. 217.
D-(—)-Mandelic Acid	3.35	Randinitis, E. J., Barr, M., Wormser, H. C. and Nagwekar, J. B.: Kinetics of Urinary Excretion of D-(—)-Mandelic Acid and Its Homologs I: Mutual Inhibitory Effect of D-(—)-Mandelic Acid and Its Certain Homologs on Their Renal Tubular Secretion in Rats, *J. Pharm. Sci. 59*:806, 1970.
Mefenamic Acid	4.2	*Merck Index,* 8th ed., p. 648.

NAME	PKA	REFERENCE
Meperidine (Pethidine)	8.7	*Hagers Handbuch der Pharmazeutischen Praxis,* Vol. I. Allgemeiner Teil, Wirkstoffgruppen I, Springer-Verlag, 1967, p. 786.
	7.5	Data by: Winthrop Laboratories, N.Y.
Mercaptopurine	7.6	Data by: Burroughs-Wellcome, Tuckahoe, NY 10707.
Metaphanine	6.76	*Merck Index,* 8th ed., p. 667.
Metharbital	8.17	Suzuki, A., Higuchi, W. I. and Ho. N. F. H.: Theoretical Model Studies of Drug Absorption and Transport in the Gastrointestinal Tract II, *J. Pharm. Sci. 59*:651, 1970.
Methapyrilene HCl	8.8	Borodkin, S. and Yunker, M. H.: Interaction of Amine Drugs with a Polycarboxylic Acid Ion Exchange Resin, *J. Pharm. Sci. 59*:481, 1970.
Methazolamide	7.30	*Merck Index,* 8th ed., p. 672.
DL-Methionine	9.21 3.21	Parrott, E. L.: *Pharmaceutical Technology, Fundamental Pharmaceutics,* Burgess Pub. Co., Minneapolis, Minn., 1970, p. 217.
Methionine	pK_1 = 2.28 pK_2 = 9.21	*Merck Index,* 8th ed., p. 675.
Methylamphetamine	9.87	Keffler, E. B., Spencer, H. M. and Burger, A.: *J. Am. Chem. Soc. 73*:2611, through Beckett, A. H., Boyes, R. N. and Triggs, E. J.: Kinetics of Buccal Absorption of Amphetamines, *J. Pharm. Pharmacol. 20*:92, 1968.
N-Methyl-cyclohexylamine	10.9	Hong, Wen-Hai and Connors, K. A.: Identification of Aliphatic Amines from Rates of Cinnamoylation, *J. Pharm. Sci. 57*:1789, 1968.
Methyldesorphine	9.3	*Hagers Handbuch der Pharmazeutischen Praxis,* Vol. I, Allgemeiner Teil, Wirkstoffgruppen I, Springer-Verlag, 1967, p. 809.
Methyldilvasene	5.0	Robson, J. M. and Stacey, R. S.: *Recent Advances in Pharmacology,* 4th ed., Little, Brown and Co., Boston, 1968, p. 115.
Methyldopa	pK_1 = 2.218 (carboxyl) pK_2 = 9.157 (phenolic) pK_3 = 10.629 (amino) pK_4 = 12.00	Halmekoski, J. and Lukkari, S.: Ionization Constants of Pharmaceuticals Part 2. -Methyl-3,4-Dihydroxyphenylalanine (Aldomet), *Farm. Aikakauslehti 74*:173, 1965, through *Intern. Pharm. Abstr.* Vol 3 No. 2.
Methylergonovine	6.65 ± .03	Maulding, H. V. and Zoglio, M. A.: Physical Chemistry of Ergot Alkaloids and Derivatives I: Ionization Constants of Several Medicinally Active Bases, *J. Pharm. Sci. 59*:700, 1970.
Methylfurtrethonium	5.5-6.0	Robson, J. M. and Stacey, R. S.: *Recent Advances in Pharmacology,* 4th ed., Little, Brown and Co., Boston, 1968, p. 115.
α-Methylphenethylamine HCl	9.07	Garrett, E. R. and Chemburkar, P. B.: Evaluation, Control and Prediction of Drug Diffusion Through Polymeric Membranes III, *J. Pharm. Sci. 57*:1401, 1968.
Methyphenobarbital	7.70	Suzuki, A., Higuchi, W. I. and Ho, N. F. H.: Theoretical Model Studies of Drug Absorption and Transport in the Gastrointestinal Tract II, *J. Pharm. Sci. 59*:651, 1970.
1-Methyl-5-phenylpentyl-amine	9.50	Garrett, E. R. and Chemburkar, P. B.: Evaluation, Control and Prediction of Drug Diffusion Through Polymeric Membranes, *J. Pharm. Sci. 57*:1401, 1968.
Methylprednisolone-21-phosphate	pK_1 = 2.55 pK_2 = 6.04	Flynn, G. L. and Lamb, D. J.: Factors Influencing Solvolysis of Corticosteroid-21-phosphate Esters, *J. Pharm. Sci. 59*:1433, 1970.
Methyl Red	pK_1 = 2.5 pK_2 = 9.5	*Merck Index,* 8th ed., p. 691.
n-Methylsulfanilamide	10.8	Wagner, J. G.: Biopharmaceutics 7, *Drug Intelligence 2*:294, 1968.
5-Methyl-2-thiouracil	7.71	Garrett, E. R. and Weber, D. J.: Metal Complexes of Thiouracils I: Stability Constants by Potentiometric Titration. Studies and Structures of Complexes, *J. Pharm. Sci. 59*:1383, 1970.

NAME	pKA	REFERENCE
6-Methyl-2-thiouracil	7.73	Garrett, E. R. and Weber, D. J.: Metal Complexes of Thiouracils I: Stability Constants by Potentiometric Titration. Studies and Structures of Complexes, *J. Pharm. Sci. 59*:1389, 1970.
Methysergide	6.62 ± .02	Maulding, H. V. and Zoglio, M. A.: Physical Chemistry of Ergot Alkaloids and Derivatives I: Ionization Constants of Several Medicinally Active Bases, *J. Pharm. Sci. 59*:700, 1970.
Methicillin Sodium	3.01 ± 0.5	Data by: Bristol Laboratories, Syracuse, N.Y. 13201.
Methymycin	pK = 8.3 (pK_b = 5.7)	*Merck Index,* 8th ed., p. 693.
Moperone HCl	8.3	*Hagers Handbuch der Pharmazeutischen Praxis,* Vol. II, Wirkstoffgruppen II, Springer-Verlag, 1967, p. 397.
Moroxydine HCl (ABOB)	$pK'H_2A + 2$ = 2.51 $pK'HA^+$ = 13.2	Schill, G.: Photometric Determination of Amines and Quaternary Ammonium Compounds with Bromothymol Blue, Part 5. Determination of Dissociation Constants of Amines, *Acta Pharm. Suecica 2*:99, 1965, through *Intern. Pharm. Abstr. 2*: 21, 1965.
Morphine	pK_a = 9.85 pK_b = 6.13	*Hagers Handbuch der Pharmazeutischen Praxis,* Vol. I, Allgemeiner Teil, Wirkstoffgruppen I, Springer-Verlag, 1967, p. 827.
	7.87	Parrott, E. L.: *Pharmaceutical Technology, Fundamental Pharmaceutics,* Burgess Pub. Co., Minneapolis, Minn., 1970, p. 220.
Morpholine	4.39 pK_b = 9.61	*Merck Index,* 8th ed., p. 703.
	8.70	Hong, Wen-Hai and Connors, K. A.: Identification of Aliphatic Amines from Rates of Cinnamoylation, *J. Pharm. Sci. 57*:1789, 1968.
3-Morpholinomethyl catechol · HCl	pK_1 = 6.75 pK_2 = 9.66	Kinget, R. D. and Schwartz, M. A.: Model Catalysts Which Simulate Penicillinase III, *J. Pharm. Sci. 57*:1916, 1968.
Mycobacidin	5.1	*Merck Index,* 8th ed., p. 707.
NADP	pK_1 = 3.9 pK_2 = 6.1	*Merck Index,* 8th ed., p. 711.
Nafcillin Sodium	2.65	Hou, J. P. and Poole, J. W.: The Amino Acid Nature of Ampicillin and Related Penicillins, *J. Pharm Sci. 58*:1510, 1969.
Nalidixic Acid, Sodium	6.0	Winningham, D. G., Nemoy, N. J. and Stamey, T. A.: Diffusion of Antibiotics from Plasma into Prostatic Fluid, *Nature 219*:139, 1968.
α-Naphthonic Acid	3.70	Parrott, E. L.: *Pharmaceutical Technology, Fundamental Pharmaceutics,* Burgess Pub. Co., Minneapolis, Minn., 1970, p. 217.
β-Naphthonic Acid	4.16	Parrott, E. L.: *Pharmaceutical Technology, Fundamental Pharmaceutics,* Burgess Pub. Co., Minneapolis, Minn., 1970, p. 217.
Narceine	9.3	*Merck Index,* 8th ed., p. 720.
	3.3	Parrott, E. L.: *Pharmaceutical Technology, Fundamental Pharmaceutics,* Burgess Pub. Co., Minneapolis, Minn., 1970, p. 220.
Narcotine	6.18	Parrott, E. L.: *Pharmaceutical Technology, Fundamental Pharmaceutics,* Burgess Pub. Co., Minneapolis, Minn., 1970, p. 220.
Nicotine	8.07	Beckett, A. H. and Taylor, J. F.: Blood Concentration of Pethidine and Pentazocine in Mother and Infant at Time of Birth, *J. Pharm. Pharmacol. Suppl. 19*:50, 1967.
	pK_1 = 6.16 pK_2 = 10.96	*Merck Index,* 8th ed., p. 730.
	7.85 3.04	Parrott, E. L.: *Pharmaceutical Technology, Fundamental Pharmaceutics,* Burgess Pub. Co., Minneapolis, Minn., 1970, p. 220.

NAME	PKA	REFERENCE
Nicotinic Acid	4.87	Parrott, E. L.: *Pharmaceutical Technology, Fundamental Pharmaceutics,* Burgess Pub. Co., Minneapolis, Minn., 1970, p. 217.
	4.76	*Merck Index,* 8th ed., p. 730.
6-Nitrobenzimidazole	2.89 ± .03 10.69 ± .05	Cohen, J. L. and Connors, K. A.: Stability and Structure of Some Organic Molecular Complexes in Aqueous Solution, *J. Pharm. Sci. 59*:1271, 1970.
Nitrofurantoin	7.2	Data by: Eaton Laboratories, Norwich, NY 13815
8-Nitrotheophylline	3.55 ± 0.05	Cohen, J. L. and Connors, K. A.: Stability and Structure of Some Organic Molecular Complexes in Aqueous Solution, *J. Pharm. Sci. 59*:1271, 1970.
Nitrous Acid	3.40	Parrott, E. L.: *Pharmaceutical Technology, Fundamental Pharmaceutics,* Burgess Pub. Co., Minneapolis, Minn., 1970, p. 217.
Noracetylcholine	3.5	Robson, J. M. and Stacey, R. S.: *Recent Advances in Pharmacology,* 4th ed., Little, Brown and Co., Boston, 1968, p. 115.
Norcarnitine HCl	3.81	Yalkowsky, S. H. and Zografi, G.: Potentiometric Titration of Monomeric and Micellar Acylcarnitines, *J. Pharm. Sci. 59*: 798, 1970.
Norformicin	9.4	*Merck Index,* 8th ed., p. 745.
Normethadone HCl	9.23	*Hagers Handbuch der Pharmazeutischen Praxis,* Vol. I, Allgemeiner Teil, Wirkstoffgruppen I., Springer-Verlag, 1967, p. 883.
Norvaline	$pK_1 = 2.36$ $pK_2 = 9.72$	*Merck Index,* 8th ed., p. 750.
Noscapine HCl	6.2	*Hagers Handbuch der Pharmazeutischen Praxis,* Vol. I, Allgemeiner Teil, Wirkstoffgruppen I, Springer-Verlag, 1967, p. 857.
Novobiocin	$pK_1 = 4.3$	Brunner, R. and Machek, G.: *Die Antibiotica,* Vol. II, Die Mittleren Antibiotica 1965, p. 547.
	$pK_2 = 9.1$	*Merck Index,* 8th ed., p. 750.
n-Octylamine	10.65	Hong, Wen-Hai and Connors, K. A.: Identification of Aliphatic Amines from Rates of Cinnamoylation, *J. Pharm. Sci. 57*:1789, 1968.
Octylcarnitine HCl	3.60	Yalkowsky, S. H. and Zografi, G.: Potentiometric Titration of Monomeric and Micellar Acylcarnitines, *J. Pharm. Sci. 59*:798, 1970.
Oleandomycin Phosphate	8.5	Celmer, W. O., Els, H. and Murai, K.: *Antibiotics Ann.* 476, 1957-58, through Winningham, D. G., Nemoy, N. J. and Stamey, T. A.: Diffusion of Antibiotics from Plasma into Prostatic Fluid, *Nature 219*:139, 1968.
		Brunner, R. and Machek, G.: *Die Antibiotica,* Vol. II, Die Mittleren Antibiotica, 1965, p. 52.
Oleic Acid	5.35	Johns, W. H. and Bates, T. R.: Quantification of the Binding Tendencies of Cholestyramine II: Mechanism of Interaction with Bile Salts and Fatty Acid Salt Anions, *J. Pharm. Sci. 59*: 329, 1970.
Ornithine	$pK_1 = 1.94$ $pK_2 = 8.65$	*Merck Index,* 8th ed., p. 767.
Oxacillin Sodium	2.88 ± .03	Data by: Bristol Laboratories, Syracuse, N.Y. 13201 (1968).
Oxalic Acid	1.19 4.21	Parrott, E. L.: *Pharmaceutical Technology, Fundamental Pharmaceutics,* Burgess Pub. Co., Minneapolis, Minn., 1970, p. 217.
Oxapropanium Iodide	3.3	Robson, J. M. and Stacey, R. S.: *Recent Advances in Pharmacology,* 4th ed., Little, Brown and Co., Boston, 1968, p. 115.
Oxipurinol (active metabolite of allopurinol)	7.7	Data by: Burroughs-Wellcome, Tuckahoe, NY 10707

NAME	PKA	REFERENCE
Oxycodone HCl	8.8-9.0	Data by: Endo Laboratories.
Oxymorphone	pK_1 = 8.50 pK_2 = 9.33	Data by: Endo Laboratories.
Oxyphenbutazone	4.7	Data by: Geigy Pharmaceuticals, Ardsley, New York 10502 (6-70)
Oxytetracycline HCl	3.5 7.6 9.2	Stephens, C. R., Murai, K., Brunings, K. J. and Woodward, R. B.: *J. Am. Chem. Soc. 78*:4155, 1956, through Winningham, D. G., Nemoy, N. J. and Stamey, T. A.: Diffusion of Antibiotics from Plasma into Prostatic Fluid, *Nature 219*: 139, 1968.
Papaverine	8.07	*Merck Index,* 8th ed., p. 782.
	5.90	Parrott, E. L.: *Pharmaceutical Technology, Fundamental Pharmaceutics,* Burgess Pub. Co., Minneapolis, Minn., 1970, p. 220.
Papaverine HCl	6.4	*Hagers Handbuch der Pharmazeutischen Praxis,* Vol. I, Allgemeiner Teil, Wirkstoffgruppen I, Springer-Verlag, 1967, p. 867.
Pelargonic Acid	4.96	Johns, W. H. and Bates, T. R.: Quantification of the Binding Tendencies of Cholestyramine II: Mechanism of Interaction with Bile Salts and Fatty Acids Salt Anions, *J. Pharm. Sci. 59*: 329, 1970.
Pelletierine	9.25	Parrott, E. L.: *Pharmaceutical Technology, Fundamental Pharmaceutics,* Burgess Pub. Co., Minneapolis, Minn., 1970, p. 220.
Penicillamine	carboxyl = 1.8 α-amino = 7.9 β-thiol = 10.5	*Merck Index,* 8th ed., p. 789.
1,5-Pentanediamine	pK_1 = 10.25 pK_2 = 9.13	*Merck Index,* 8th ed., p. 794.
Pentanoic Acid	4.80	Ekwall, P., Rosendahl, T. and Lofman, N.: *Acta Chem. Scand. 11*:590, 1960, through Yalkowsky, S. H. and Zografi, G.: Potentiometric Titration of Monomeric and Micellar Acylcarnitines, *J. Pharm. Sci. 59*:798, 1970.
2-Pentenylpenicillin Sodium	2.87	*Merck Index,* 8th ed., p. 795.
Pentobarbital	8.11	Suzuki, A., Higuchi, W. I. and Ho, N. F. H.: Theoretical Model Studies of Drug Absorption and Transport in the Gastrointestinal Tract II, *J. Pharm. Sci. 59*:651, 1970.
	8.17	Fincher, J. H. and Entrekin, D. N. and Hartman, C. W.: *J. Pharm. Sci. 55*:23, 1966.
Perchloric Acid	5.82	Medwick, T., Kaplan, G. and Weyer, L. G.: Measurement of Acidity and Equilibria in Glacial Acetic Acid with the Glass Calomel Electrode System, *J. Pharm. Sci. 58*:308, 1969.
Periodic Acid	1.64	Parrott, E. L.: *Pharmaceutical Technology, Fundamental Pharmaceutics,* Burgess Pub. Co., Minneapolis, Minn., 1970, p. 217.
Perivine	7.5	*Merck Index,* 8th ed., p. 799.
Perusitin	6.2 6.2	Lang, Hui-ying and Sun, Nan-jun: Studies on the Cardiac Glycosides of Thevetia Peruviana Merr. Syn. Thevetia Neriifolia Juss. II. Isolation and Identification of Cerberin, Ruvoside, and a New Cardiac Glycoside-Perusitin, *Acta Pharm. Sinica 11*:464, 1964, through *Intern. Pharm. Abstr.* Vol. 2 No. 3 15 Feb. 65.
Phaseolin	9.13	*Merck Index,* 8th ed., p. 802.
Phenadoxone HCl	6.7	*Merck Index,* 8th ed., p. 803.
Phenethicillin Potassium	2.82	Data by: Bristol Laboratories, Syracuse, NY, 13201 (1962)

NAME	pKA	REFERENCE
Phenobarbital	7.41	Suzuki, A., Higuchi, W. I. and Ho, N. F. H.: Theoretical Model Studies of Drug Absorption and Transport in the Gastrointestinal Tract II, *J. Pharm. Sci. 59*:651, 1970.
Phenol	9.89	Parrott, E. L.: *Pharmaceutical Technology, Fundamental Pharmaceutics,* Burgess Pub. Co., Minneapolis, Minn., 1970, p. 217.
	10.0	*Merck Index,* 8th ed., p. 810.
Phenolphthalein	9.70	Parrott, E. L.: *Pharmaceutical Technology, Fundamental Pharmaceutics,* Burgess Pub. Co., Minneapolis, Minn., 1970, p. 217.
Phenol Red	1.03	Gupta, V. D. and Reed, J. B.: First pKa Values of Some Acid-Base Indicators, *J. Pharm. Sci. 59*:1683, 1970.
Phenolsulfonphthalein	7.9	Data by: Hynson, Westcott and Dunning, Pharmaceutical Laboratory, Baltimore, Maryland 21201
		Merck Index, 8th ed., p. 810.
Phenoxypropazine	6.9	*Hagers Handbuch der Pharmazeutischen Praxis,* Vol II, Wirkstoffgruppen II, Springer, Verlag, 1967, p. 407.
Phentolamine	7.7 (apparent)	Robson, J. M. and Stacey, R. S.: *Recent Advances in Pharmacology,* 4th ed., Little, Brown and Co., Boston, 1968, p. 108.
Phenylacetic Acid	4.31	Parrott, E. L.: *Pharmaceutical Technology, Fundamental Pharmaceutics,* Burgess Pub. Co., Minneapolis, Minn., 1970, p. 217.
Phenylalanine	$pK_1 = 2.58$ $pK_2 = 9.24$	*Merck Index,* 8th ed., p. 815.
DL-Phenylalanine	9.24	Parrott, E. L.: *Pharmaceutical Technology, Fundamental Pharmaceutics,* Burgess Pub. Co., Minneapolis, Minn., 1970, p. 218.
Phenyl Biguanide	$pK_1 = 10.76$ $pK_2 = 2.13$	*Merck Index,* 8th ed., p. 815.
Phenylbutazone	4.5	Data by: Geigy Pharmaceuticals, Ardsley, New York 10502
		Merck Index, 8th ed., p. 815.
	4.70 ± 0.2	Maulding, H. V. and Zoglio, M. A.: pKa Determinations Utilizing Solutions of 7-(2-Hydroxypropyl) Theophylline, *J. Pharm. Sci. 60*:309, 1971.
α-Phenylcinnamic Acid (cis form)	6.1	*Merck Index,* 8th ed., p. 816.
α-Phenylcinnamic Acid (trans form)	4.8	*Merck Index,* 8th ed., p. 816.
β-Phenethylamine	9.83	Hong, Wen-Hai and Connors, K. A.: Identification of Aliphatic Amines from Rates of Cinnamoylation, *J. Pharm. Sci. 57*:1789, 1968.
Phenylethylbarbituric Acid	7.41	Parrott, E. L.: *Pharmaceutical Technology, Fundamental Pharmaceutics,* Burgess Pub. Co., Minneapolis, Minn., 1970, p. 216.
DL-Phenyllactic Acid	3.80	Randinitis, E. J., Barr, N., Wormser, H. C. and Nagwekar, J. B.: Kinetics of Urinary Excretion of D-(−)-Mandelic Acid and Its Homologs I: Mutual Inhibitory Effect of D-(−)-Mandelic Acid and Its Secretion in Rats, *J. Pharm. Sci. 59*:806, 1970.
Phenylpropanolamine HCl	9.4	Borodkin, S. and Yunker, M. H.: Interaction of Amine Drugs with a Carboxylic Acid Ion Exchanfie Resin, *J. Pharm. Sci. 59*:481, 1970.
Phenyltoloxamine Citrate	9.1	Data by: Endo Laboratories, Garden City, N.Y. 11530.
Phenyramidol	5.85	*Merck Index,* 8th ed., p. 821.

NAME	PKA	REFERENCE
Phenytoin	8.31-8.33	Agarwal, S. P. and Blake, M. I.: Determination of the pKa Value for 5,5-Diphenylhydantoin, *J. Pharm. Sci. 57*:1434, 1968.
Phosphocreatine	4.6	*Merck Index,* 8th ed., p. 823.
Phosphoric Acid	2.12 7.21 12.32	Parrott, E. L.: *Pharmaceutical Technology, Fundamental Pharmaceutics,* Burgess Pub. Co., Minneapolis, Minn., 1970, p. 218.
Phosphorous Acid	1.80 6.15	Parrott, E. L.: *Pharmaceutical Technology, Fundamental Pharmaceutics,* Burgess Pub. Co., Minneapolis, Minn., 1970, p. 218.
Phthalic Acid	2.89 5.51	Parrott, E. L.: *Pharmaceutical Technology, Fundamental Pharmaceutics,* Burgess Pub. Co., Minneapolis, Minn., 1970, p. 218.
Physostigmine	pK_1 = 6.12 pK_2 = 12.24	*Merck Index,* 8th ed., p. 828.
	7.88 1.76	Parrott, E. L.: *Pharmaceutical Technology, Fundamental Pharmaceutics,* Burgess Pub. Co., Minneapolis, Minn., 1970, p. 220.
Picric Acid	0.38	Parrott, E. L.: *Pharmaceutical Technology, Fundamental Pharmaceutics,* Burgess Pub. Co., Minneapolis, Minn., 1970, p. 218.
Pilocarpine HCl	pK_1 = 6.8 pK_2 = 1.3	Data by: Barnes-Hind Pharmaceuticals, Inc.
	6.85 1.43	Parrott, E. L.: *Pharmaceutical Technology, Fundamental Pharmaceutics,* Burgess Pub. Co., Minneapolis, Minn., 1970, p. 220.
Pilocarpine	5.2	Robson, J. M. and Stacey, R. S.: *Recent Advances in Pharmacology,* 4th ed., Little, Brown and Co., Boston, 1968, p. 115.
	pK_1 = 7.15 pK_2 = 12.57	*Merck Index,* 8th ed., p. 833.
Piperidine	11.22	Hong, Wen-Hai and Connors, K. A.: Identification of Aliphatic Amines from Rates of Cinnamoylation, *J. Pharm. Sci. 57*:1789, 1968.
	2.80	*Merck Index,* 8th ed., p. 838.
Piperazine Adipate	pK_1 = 5.7 pK_2 = 9.8	*Hagers Handbuch der Pharmazeutischen Praxis,* Vol. I, Allgemeiner Teil, Wirkstoffgruppen I. Springer-Verlag, 1967, p. 961.
Piperine	12.22	*Merck Index,* 8th ed., p. 838.
Piperylon	pK_1 = 5.90 pK_2 = 9.15	*Merck Index,* 8th ed., p. 839.
Platyphylline Hydrotartrate	5.95	Perelman, Ra. M.: Potentiometric Titration of Platyphylline Hydrotartrate in Aqueous and Nonaqueous Solutions. *Aptechn. Delo 14*:44, 1965, through *Intern. Pharm. Abstr.* Vol. 2 No. 20, 30 Oct. 65.
Polymyxin B sulfate	8-9	Winningham, D. G., Nemoy, N. J. and Stamey, T. A.: Diffusion of Antibiotics from Plasma into Prostatic Fluid, *Nature 219*:139, 1968.
Potassium Acetate	6.37	Medwick, T., Kaplan, G. and Weyer, L. G.: Measurement of Acidity and Equilibria in Glacial Acetic Acid with the Glass-Calomel Electrode System, *J. Pharm. Sci. 58*:308, 1969.
Prilocaine	7.89	Data by: Astra Pharmaceutical Products, Inc., Worcester, Mass. 01606
Probarbital	8.01	Suzuki, A., Higuchi, W. I. and Ho, N. F. H.: Theoretical Model Studies of Drug Absorption and Transport in the Gastrointestinal Tract II, *J. Pharm. Sci. 59*:651, 1970.
Procaine	8.85	Parrott, E. L.: *Pharmaceutical Technology, Fundamental Pharmaceutics,* Burgess Pub. Co., Minneapolis, Minn., 1970, p. 220.

NAME	PKA	REFERENCE
Prochlorperazine	8.1 7.5	Zografi, G. and Munshi, M.: Effect of Chemical Modification of the Surface Activity of Some Phenothiazine Derivatives, *J. Pharm. Sci. 59*:819, 1970.
	8.1	Data by: Smith Kline and French, Philadelphia, Pa. 19101
L-Proline	10.6	Parrott, E. L.: *Pharmaceutical Technology, Fundamental Pharmaceutics,* Burgess Pub. Co., Minneapolis, Minn., 1970, p. 218.
Promazine HCl	pK'HA+ = 9.40	Schill, G.: Photometric Determination of Amines and Quaternary Ammonium Compounds with Bromothymol Blue Part 5. Determination of Dissociation Constants of Amines, *Acta Pharm. Suecica 2*:99, 1965, through *Intern. Pharm. Abstr. 2*: 21 15 Nov. 65.
	9.4 9.5	Zografi, G. and Munshi, M.: Effect of Chemical Modification of the Surface Activity of Some Phenothiazine Derivatives, *J. Pharm. Sci. 59*:819, 1970.
Promethazine HCl	9.1	Zografi, G. and Munshi, M.: Effect of Chemical Modification of the Surface Activity of Some Phenothiazine Derivatives, *J. Pharm. Sci. 59*:819, 1970.
Propionic Acid	4.87	Parrott, E. L.: *Pharmaceutical Technology, Fundamental Pharmaceutics,* Burgess Pub. Co., Minneapolis, Minn., 1970, p. 218.
Di-n-propylamine	11.00	Hong, Wen-Hai and Connors, K. A.: Identification of Aliphatic Amines from Rates of Cinnamoylation, *J. Pharm. Sci. 57*:1789, 1968.
n-Propylamine	10.53	Hong, Wen-Hai and Connors, K. A.: Identification of Aliphatic Amines from Rates of Cinnamoylation, *J. Pharm. Sci. 57*:1789, 1968.
6-n-Propyl-2-thiouracil	7.76	Garrett, E. R. and Weber, D. J.: Metal Complexes of Thiouracils I: Stability Constants by Potentiometric Titration Studies and Structures of Complexes, *J. Pharm. Sci. 59*:1383, 1970.
Pseudoephedrine HCl	9.7	Borodkin, Saul and Yunker, Martin H.: Interaction of Amine Drugs with a Polycarboxylic Acid Ion Exchange Resin, *J. Pharm. Sci. 59*:481,1970.
Pseudotropine	10.20	Parrott, E. L.: *Pharmaceutical Technology, Fundamental Pharmaceutics,* Burgess Pub. Co., Minneapolis, Minn., 1970, p. 220.
Pyrethamine	4.2	Robson, J. M. and Stacey, R. S.: *Recent Advances in Pharmacology,* 4th ed., Little, Brown and Co., Boston, 1968, p. 115.
Pyrimethamine	7.2	Data by: Burroughs-Wellcome, Tuckahoe, NY 10707
Pyromucic (furoic) Acid	3.15	Parrott, E. L.: *Pharmaceutical Technology, Fundamental Pharmaceutics,* Burgess Pub. Co., Minneapolis, Minn., 1970, p. 218.
Pyrophosphoric Acid	0.85 1.96 6.68 9.39	Parrott, E. L.: *Pharmaceutical Technology, Fundamental Pharmaceutics,* Burgess Pub. Co., Minneapolis, Minn., 1970, p. 218.
Pyrotartaric Acid	4.07	Parrott, E. L.: *Pharmaceutical Technology, Fundamental Pharmaceutics,* Burgess Pub. Co., Minneapolis, Minn., 1970, p. 218.
Pyrrolo-Pyrimidines R = $C_6H_3N_3$-CH_3 a = NHC_2H_5 b = NHC_3H_7 c = NHC_5H_{11} d = NC_5H_{10}	a = 5.64 b = 5.52 c = 5.66 d = 5.28	Hammer, R. H.: Pyrrolo (2,3-d) Pyrimidines, *J. Pharm. Sci. 57*:1616, 1968.
Quinidine	8.6 4.0	Parrott, E. L.: *Pharmaceutical Technology, Fundamental Pharmaceutics,* Burgess Pub. Co., Minneapolis, Minn., 1970, p. 220.

NAME	PKA	REFERENCE
Quinidine Sulfate	8.8	Borodkin, S. and Yunker, M. H.: Interaction of Amine Drugs with a Polycarboxylic Acid Ion Exchange Resin, *J. Pharm. Sci. 59*:481, 1970.
Quinine	8.0 4.11	Parrott, E. L.: *Pharmaceutical Technology, Fundamental Pharmaceutics,* Burgess Pub. Co., Minneapolis, Minn., 1970, p. 220.
Quinoline	4.5	Parrott, E. L.: *Pharmaceutical Technology, Fundamental Pharmaceutics,* Burgess Pub. Co., Minneapolis, Minn., 1970, p. 220.
Reserpine	6.6	*Hagers Handbuch der Pharmazeutischen Praxis,* Vol. II., Wirkstoffgruppen II, Springer-Verlag, 1967, p. 372. *Merck Index,* 8th ed., p. 912.
Riboflavin Monophosphate	$pK_1 = 2.5$ $pK_2 = 6.5$ $pK_3 = 10.3$	*Hagers Handbuch der Pharmazeutischen Praxis,* Vol. II, Wirkstoffgruppen II, Springer-Verlag, 1967, p. 682.
Saccharin	1.60	Parrott, E. L.: *Pharmaceutical Technology, Fundamental Pharmaceutics,* Burgess Pub. Co., Minneapolis, Minn., 1970, p. 218.
Salicylamide	8.2	Bates, T. R., Lambert, D. A. and Jones, W. H.: Correlation Between the Rate of Dissolution and Absorption of Salicylamide from Tablet and Suspension Dosage Forms, *J. Pharm. Sci. 58*:1468, 1969.
Salicylic Acid	2.97	Parrott, E. L.: *Pharmaceutical Technology, Fundamental Pharmaceutics,* Burgess Pub. Co., Minneapolis, Minn., 1970, p. 218.
Sarcosine	2.26	Parrott, E. L.: *Pharmaceutical Technology, Fundamental Pharmaceutics,* Burgess Pub. Co., Minneapolis, Minn., 1970, p. 220.
Scopolamine	8.7	Robson, J. M. and Stacey, R. S.: *Recent Advances in Pharmacology,* 4th ed., Little, Brown and Co., Boston, 1968, p. 108.
DL-Serine	9.15	Parrott, E. L.: *Pharmaceutical Technology, Fundamental Pharmaceutics,* Burgess, Pub. Co., Minneapolis, Minn., 1970, p. 218.
Serotonin	6.6	Robson, J. M. and Stacey, R. S.: *Recent Advances in Pharmacology,* 4th ed., Little, Brown and Co., Boston, 1968, p. 115.
Sodium Acetate	6.56	Medwick, T., Kaplan, G. and Weyer, L.: Measurement of Acidity and Equilibria in Glacial Acetic Acid with the Glass-Calomel Electrode System, *J. Pharm. Sci. 58*:308, 1969.
Sodium Perchlorate	5.54	Medwick, T., Kaplan, G. and Weyer, L. G.: Measurement of Acidity and Equilibria in Glacial Acetic Acid with the Glass-Calomel Electrode System, *J. Pharm. Sci. 58*:308, 1969.
Solanine	7.34	Parrott, E. L.: *Pharmaceutical Technology, Fundamental Pharmaceutics,* Burgess Pub. Co., Minneapolis, Minn., 1970, p. 220.
Sparteine	11.76 4.54	Parrott, E. L.: *Pharmaceutical Technology, Fundamental Pharmaceutics,* Burgess Pub. Co., Minneapolis, Minn., 1970, p. 220.
Stearic Acid	5.75	Johns, W. H. and Bates, T. R.: Quantification of the Binding Tendencies of Cholestyramine II: Mechanism of Interaction with Bile Salts and Fatty Acid Salt Anions, *J. Pharm. Sci. 59*: 329, 1970.
Streptovitacin A (acid catalyzed dehydration products)	10.8	Notari, R. E. and Caiola, S. M.: Catalysis of Streptovitacin A Dehydration: Kinetics and Mechanisms, *J. Pharm. Sci. 58*: 1203, 1969.
Strychnine	8.0 2.3	Parrott, E. L.: *Pharmaceutical Technology, Fundamental Pharmaceutics,* Burgess Pub. Co., Minneapolis, Minn., 1970, p. 220.
Succinic Acid	4.19 5.57	Parrott, E. L.: *Pharmaceutical Technology, Fundamental Pharmaceutics,* Burgess Pub. Co., Minneapolis, Minn., 1970, p. 218.

NAME	pKA	REFERENCE
Sulfabenz	10.94	*Merck Index,* 8th ed., p. 994.
Sulfacarbamide	1.8 5.5	Struller, Th.: Progress in Sulfonamide Research, *Prog. Drug Res. 12*:402, 1968.
Sulfacetamide	pK = 1.78	Suzuki, A., Higuchi, W. I. and Ho, N. F. H.: Model Studies of Drug Absorption and Transport in the Gastrointestinal Tract II, *J. Pharm. Sci. 59*:655, 1970.
Sulfachlorpyridazine	5.9	Struller, Th., Progress in Sulfonamide Research. *Progress in Drug Research, 12*:404, 1968.
Sulfadiazine	pK_1 = 2.00 pK_2 = 6.48	Suzuki, A., Higuchi, W. I. and Ho, N. F. H.: Theoretical Model Studies of Drug Absorption and Transport in the Gastrointestinal Tract II, *J. Pharm. Sci. 59*:665, 1970.
	6.37	Yoshioka, M., Hamamoto, K. and Kubota, T.: *Yakugaku Zasshi 84*:90, 1964.
Sulfadicramide	5.4	Struller, Th.: Progress in Sulfonamide Research, *Prog. Drug Res. 12*:402, 1968.
Sulfadimethoxine	pK_1 = 2.02 pK_2 = 6.70	Suzuki, A., Higuchi, W. I. and Ho, N. F. H.: Theoretical Model Studies of Drug Absorption and Transport in the Gastrointestinal Tract II, *J. Pharm. Sci. 59*:651, 1970.
	5.98	Yoshioka, M., Hamamoto, K. and Kubota, T.: *Yakugaku Zasshi 84*:90, 1964.
Sulfadimidine (sulfamethazine)	pK_1 = 2.36 pK_2 = 7.38	Suzuki, A., Higuchi, W. I. and Ho, N. F. H.: Theoretical Model Studies of Drug Absorption and Transport in the Gastrointestinal Tract II, *J. Pharm. Sci. 59*:655, 1970.
	7.4	Struller, Th.: Progress in Sulfonamide Research, *Prog. Res. 12*:402, 1968.
		Wagner, John G.: Biopharmaceutics 7, *Drug Intelligence 2*: 294, 1968.
Sulfaethidole	pK_1 = 1.93 pK_2 = 5.60	Suzuki, A., Higuchi, W. I. and Ho, N. F. H.: Theoretical Model Studies of Drug Absorption and Transport in the Gastrointestinal Tract II, *J. Pharm. Sci. 59*:651, 1970.
Sulfafurazol	pK_1 = 1.55 pK_2 = 5.10	Suzuki, A., Higuchi, W. I. and Ho, N. F. H.: Theoretical Model Studies of Drug Absorption and Transport in the *Gastrointestinal Tract II, J. Pharm. Sci. 59*:655, 1970.
	4.79	Yoshioka, M., Hamamoto, K. and Kubota, T.: *Yakugaku Zasshi 84*:90, 1964.
Sulfalene	6.1	Struller, Th.: Progress in Sulfonamide Research, *Prog. Drug Res. 12*:404, 1968.
Sulfamerazine	pK_1 = 2.26 pK_2 = 7.06	Suzuki, A., Higuchi, W. I. and Ho, N. F. H.: Theoretical Model Studies of Drug Absorption and Transport in the Gastrointestinal Tract II, *J. Pharm. Sci. 59*:655, 1970.
	6.85	Yoshioka, M., Hamamoto, K. and Kubota, T.: *Yakugaku Zasshi 84*:90, 1964.
	6.7	Struller, Th.: Progress in Sulfonamide Research, *Prog. Drug Res. 12*:403, 1968.
Sulfameter	6.8	*Merck Index,* 8th ed., p. 996.
Sulfamethizole	pK_1 = 2.00 pK_2 = 5.45	Suzuki, A., Higuchi, W. I. and Ho, N. F. H.: Theoretical Model Studies of Drug Absorption and Transport in the Gastrointestinal Tract II, *J. Pharm. Sci. 59*:655, 1970.
	5.22	Yoshioka, M., Hamamoto, K. and Kubota, T.: *Yakugaku Zasshi 84*:90, 1964.
	5.45	*Merck Index,* 8th ed., p. 996.
Sulfamethoxazole	pK_1 = 1.76 pK_2 = 5.80	Suzuki, A., Higuchi, W. I. and Ho, N. F. H.: Theoretical Model Studies of Drug Absorption and Transport in the Gastrointestinal Tract II, *J. Pharm. Sci. 59*:655, 1970.
	5.72	Yoshioka, M., Hamamoto, K. and Kubota, T.: *Yakugaku Zasshi 84*:90, 1964.

NAME	pKA	REFERENCE
Sulfamethoxypyridazine	$pK_1 = 2.06$ $pK_2 = 7.00$	Suzuki, A., Higuchi, W. I. and Ho, N. F. H.: Theoretical Model Studies of Drug Absorption and Transport in the Gastrointestinal Tract II, *J. Pharm. Sci. 59*:655, 1970.
	7.17	Yoshioka, M., Hamamoto, K. and Kubota, T.: *Yakugaku Zasshi 84*:90, 1964.
	6.7	*Merck Index,* 8th ed., p. 996.
Sulfamethylphenazole	5.69	*Merck Index,* 8th ed., p. 997.
Sulfamethomidine	6.1	Struller, Th.: Progress in Sulfonamide Research, *Prog. Drug Res. 12*:1968.
Sulfametoyl	4.9	Struller, Th.: Progress in Sulfonamide Research, *Prog. Drug Res. 12*:402, 1968.
Sulfamonomethoxine	$pK_1 = 2.00$ $pK_2 = 5.90$	Suzuki, A., Higuchi, W. I. and Ho, N. F. H.: Theoretical Model Studies of Drug Absorption and Transport in the Gastrointestinal Tract II, *J. Pharm. Sci. 59*:651, 1970.
Sulfamoxole	7.4	Struller, Th.: Progress in Sulfonamide Research, *Prog. Drug Res. 12*:404, 1968.
Sulfanilamide	$pK_1 = 3.36$ $pK_2 = 10.43$	Suzuki, A., Higuchi, W. I. and Ho, N. F. H.: Theoretical Model Studies of Drug Absorption and Transport in the Gastrointestinal Tract II, *J. Pharm. Sci. 59*:655, 1970.
	10.4	Wagner, J. G.: Biopharmaceutics 7, *Drug Intelligence 2*:294, 1968.
n-Sulfamilyl-3,4-xylamide	4.37	Yoshioka, M., Hamamoto, K. and Kubota, T.: *Yakugaku Zasshi 84*:90, 1964.
Sulfaphenazole	$pK_1 = 1.9$ $pK_2 = 6.50$	Suzuki, A., Higuchi, W. I. and Ho, N. F. H.: Theoretical Model Studies of Drug Absorption and Transport in the Gastrointestinal Tract II, *J. Pharm. Sci. 59*:651, 1970.
	5.89	Yoshioka, M., Hamamoto, K. and Kubota, T.: *Yakugaku Zasshi 84*:90, 1964.
Sulfaproxyline	4.9	Struller, Th.: Progress in Sulfonamide Research. *Prog. Drug Res. 12*:403, 1968.
Sulfapyridine	$pK_1 = 2.58$ $pK_2 = 8.43$	Suzuki, A., Higuchi, W. I. and Ho, N. F. H.: Theoretical Model Studies of Drug Absorption and Transport in the Gastrointestinal Tract II, *J. Pharm. Sci. 59*:655, 1970.
	8.56	Yoshioka, M., Hamamoto, K. and Kubota, T.: *Yakugaku Zasshi 84*:90, 1964.
Sulfaguanidine	$pK_1 = 2.75$ $pK_2 = 12.05$	Suzuki, A., Higuchi, W. I. and Ho, N. F. H.: Theoretical Model Studies of Drug Absorption and Transport in the Gastrointestinal Tract II, *J. Pharm. Sci. 59*:655, 1970.
Sulfathiazole	$pK_1 = 2.36$ $pK_2 = 7.12$	Suzuki, A., Higuchi, W. I. and Ho, N. F. H.: Theoretical Model Studies of Drug Absorption and Transport in the Gastrointestinal Tract II, *J. Pharm. Sci. 59*:655, 1970.
	7.23	Yoshioka, M., Hamamoto, K. and Kubota, T.: *Yakugaku Zasshi 84*:90, 1964.
Sulfathiourea	4.8	Struller, Th.: Progress in Sulfonamide Research, *Prog. Drug Res. 12*:401, 1968.
Sulfinpyrazone	2.8	Data by: Geigy Pharmaceuticals, Ardsley, New York 10502.
Sulfisomidine	$pK_1 = 2.36$ $pK_2 = 7.5$	Suzuki, A., Higuchi, W. I. and Ho, N. F. H.: Theoretical Model Studies of Drug Absorption and Transport in the Gastrointestinal Tract II, *J. Pharm. Sci. 59*:655, 1970.
	7.49	Yoshioka, M., Hamamoto, K. and Kubota, T.: *Yukagaku Zasshi 84*:90, 1964.
Sulfobromophthalein	8.8	Data by: Hynson, Westcott and Dunning Pharmaceutical Laboratory, Baltimore, Maryland 21201.
Sulformethoxine	6.1	Struller, Th.: Progress in Sulfonamide Research, *Prog. Drug Res. 12*:404, 1968.

NAME	PKA	REFERENCE
Tartaric Acid	3.02 4.54	Parrott, E. L.: *Pharmaceutical Technology, Fundamental Pharmaceutics,* Burgess Pub. Co., Minneapolis, Minn., 1970, p. 218.
L-Tartaric Acid	$pK_1 = 2.93$ $pK_2 = 4.23$	*Merck Index,* 8th ed., p. 1014.
Taurine	$pK^1_1 = 1.5$ $pK^1_2 = 8.74$	*Merck Index,* 8th ed., p. 1015.
Taurocholate	1.56-3.33	Johns, W. H. and Bates, T. R.: Quantification of the Binding Tendencies of Cholestyramine I: Effect of Structure and Added Electrolytes on the Binding of Unconjugated and Conjugated Bile-Salt Anions, *J. Pharm. Sci. 58*:179, 1969.
Taurocholic Acid	1.4	*Merck Index,* 8th ed., p. 1015.
Tetracycline HCl	8.3	*Merck Index,* 8th ed., p. 1024.
1,3,4,5-Tetrahydro-1-hydroxy-3-oxo-1,2-benziodoxepin	7.37	Wolf, W., Chen, J. C. and Hsu, L.: Chemistry and Biochemistry of Polyvalent Iodine Compounds V, *J. Pharm. Sci. 55*:68, 1966.
2,3,5,6-Tetramethylbenzoic Acid	3.49	Beckett, A. H. and Moffat, A. C.: The Influence of Alkyl Substitution in Acids on Their Performance in the Buccal Absorption Test, *J. Pharm. Pharmacol. Suppl. 20*:239, 1968.
Tetramethylpyrimodo-pteridinetetrone	-0.55 ± 0.10	Higuchi, T. and Kristiansen, H.: Binding Specificity between Small Organic Solutes in Aqueous Solution: Classification of Some Solutes into Two Groups According to Binding Tendencies, *J. Pharm. Sci. 59*:1601, 1970.
Thebain	6.05	*Hagers Handbuch der Pharmazeutischen Praxis,* Vol. I, Allgemeiner Teil, Wirkstoffgruppen I, Springer-Verlag, 1967, p. 874.
	7.95	Parrott, E. L.: *Pharmaceutical Technology, Fundamental Pharmaceutics,* Burgess Pub. Co., Minneapolis, Minn., 1970, p. 220.
Theobromine	0.12	Parrott, E. L.: *Pharmaceutical Technology, Fundamental Pharmaceutics,* Burgess Pub. Co., Minneapolis, Minn., 1970, p. 220.
Theophylline	8.75	Maulding, H. V. and Zoglio, M. A.: pKa Determinations Utilizing Solutions of 7-(2-Hydroxypropyl) Theophylline, *J. Pharm. Sci. 60*:309, 1971.
THF amino-alcohol	4.73 $pK_b = 9.27$	*Merck Index,* 8th ed., p. 552.
Thiamine Mononitrate	4.8	Gupta, V. Das, Cadwallader, D. E., Herman, H. B. and Honigberg, I. L.: Effect of pH and Dye Concentration on the Extraction of a Thiamine Dye Salt by an Organic Solvent, *J. Pharm. Sci. 57*:1199, 1968. *Merck Index,* 8th ed., p. 1037.
Thiamylal	7.48	Suzuki, A., Higuchi, W. I. and Ho, N. F. H.: Theoretical Model Studies of Drug Absorption and Transport in the Gastrointestinal Tract II, *J. Pharm. Sci. 59*:651, 1970.
Thiopental	7.45	Suzuki, A., Higuchi, W. I. and Ho, N. F. H.: Theoretical Model Studies of Drug Absorption and Transport in the Gastrointestinal Tract II, *J. Pharm. Sci. 59*:651, 1970.
2-Thiouracil	7.46	Garrett, E. R. and Weber, D. J.: Metal Complexes of Thiouracils I: Stability Constants by Potentiometric Titration Studies and Structures of Complexes, *J. Pharm. Sci. 59*:1383, 1970.
m-Toluic Acid	4.24	Beckett, A. H. and Moffat, A. C.: Kinetics of Buccal Absorption of Some Carboxylic Acids and the Correlation of the Rate Constants and n-Heptane: Aqueous Phase Partition Coefficients, *J. Pharm. Pharmacol. 22*:15, 1970.
o-Toluic Acid	3.92	Beckett, A. H. and Moffat, A. C.: Kinetics of Buccal Absorption of Some Carboxylic Acids and the Correlation of the Rate Constants and n-Heptane: Aqueous Phase Partition Coefficients, *J. Pharm. Pharmacol. 22*:15, 1970.

NAME	PKA	REFERENCE
p-Toluic Acid	4.33	Beckett, A. H. and Moffat, A. C.: Kinetics of Buccal Absorption of Some Carboxylic Acids and the Correlation of the Rate Constants and n-Heptane: Aqueous Phase Partition Coefficients, *J. Pharm. Pharmacol. 22*:15, 1970.
Tranylcypromine Sulfate	8.2	Data by: Smith, Kline and French, Philadelphia, Pa. 19101.
Triacetyloleandomycin	6.6	*Merck Index,* 8th ed., p. 1064.
Triamterene	6.2	Data by: Smith, Kline and French, Philadelphia, Pa. 19101.
Triazenoimidazole	7.4	James, R. H., Sternglanz, P. D. and Shealy, Y. F.: 5(Or 4)-(3,3-Bis(2-chlorethyl)-1-triazemo) imidazole-4 (or 5)-carboxamide: A Titrimetric Determination of Its v-Traizolinium Transformation Product and Studies of Its Stability, *J. Pharm. Sci. 58*:1195, 1969.
Tribenzylamine	4.87	Medwick, T., Kaplan, G. and Weyer, L. G.: Measurement of Acidity and Equilibria in Glacial Acetic Acid with the Glass-Calomel Electrode System, *J. Pharm. Sci. 58*:308, 1969.
Trichloracetic Acid	0.89	Parrott, E. L.: *Pharmaceutical Technology, Fundamental Pharmaceutics,* Burgess Pub. Co., Minneapolis, Minn., 1970, p. 218.
Trifluoperazine	8.1, 8.4	Zografi, G. and Munshi, M.: Effect of Chemical Modification on the Surface Activity of Some Phenothiazine Derivatives, *J. Pharm. Sci. 59*:819, 1970.
	8.1	Data by: Smith, Kline and French, Philadelphia, Pa. 19101.
5-Trifluromethyl-2′-deoxyuridine	pK = 7.85	Nestler, H. J. and Garrett, E. R.: Prediction of Stability in Pharmaceutical Preparations XV, *J. Pharm. Sci. 57*:1117, 1968.
5-Trifluoromethyluracil	pK_1 = 7.4 pK_2 = 12.6	Nestler, H. J. and Garrett, E. R.: Prediction of Stability in Pharmaceutical Preparations XV, *J. Pharm. Sci. 57*:1117, 1968.
Triflupromazine HCl	9.2	Zografi, G. and Funshi, M.: Effect of Chemical Modification of the Surface Activity of Some Phenothiazine Derivatives, *J. Pharm. Sci. 59*:819, 1970.
Trimethoprim	7.2	Kaplan, S. A., Weinfeld, R. E., Cotler, S., Abruzzo, C. W. and Alexander, K.: Pharmacokinetic Profile of Trimethoprim in Dog and Man, *J. Pharm. Sci. 59*:358, 1970.
2,4,6-Trimethylbenzoic Acid	3.56	Beckett, A. H. and Moffat, A. C.: The Influence of Alkyl Substitution in Acids on Their Performance in the Buccal Absorption Test, *J. Pharm. Pharmacol. Suppl. 20*:239, 1968.
Tripelennamine HCl	8.3	Robson, J. M. and Stacey, R. S.: *Recent Advances in Pharmacology,* 4th ed., Little, Brown and Co., Boston, 1968, p. 108.
Triphenylguanidine	5.71	Medwick, T., Kaplan, G. and Weyer, L. G.: Measurement of Acidity and Equilibria in Glacial Acetic Acid with the Glass-Calomel Electrode System, *J. Pharm. Sci. 58*:308, 1969.
3,4,6-Tris(dimethylamino-methyl) catechol • 3 HCl	pK_1 = 4.95 pK_2 = 7.10 pK_2 = 10.35	Kinget, R. D. and Schwartz, M. A.: Model Catalysts Which Simulate Penicillinase III, *J. Pharm. Sci. 57*:1916, 1968.
3,4,6-Tris(morpholino-methyl) catechol • 3 HCl	pK_1 = 3.75 pK_2 = 5.80 pK_3 = 7.90	Kinget, R. D. and Schwartz, M. A.: Model Catalysts Which Simulate Penicillinase III, *J. Pharm. Sci. 57*:1916, 1968.
Tromethamol	6.06	Medwick, T., Kaplan, G. and Weyer, L. G.: Measurement of Acidity and Equilibria in Glacial Acetic Acid with the Glass-Calomel Electrode System, *J. Pharm. Sci. 58*:308, 1969.
Tromethamine	8.10	Bruice, T. C. and York, J. L.: *J. Am. Chem. Soc. 83*:1382, 1961, through Brooke, D. and Guttman, D. E.: Complex Formation Influence on Reaction Rate IV, *J. Pharm. Sci. 57*: 1677, 1968.
Tropacocaine	4.32	
	4.32	*Merck Index,* 8th ed., p. 1083.
	9.68	Parrott, E. L.: *Pharmaceutical Technology, Fundamental Pharmaceutics,* Burgess Pub. Co., Minneapolis, Minn., 1970, p. 220.

NAME	PKA	REFERENCE
DL-Tropic Acid	4.20	Randinitis, E. J., Barr, M., Wormser, H. C. and Nagekar, J. B.: Kinetics of Urinary Excretion of D-(—)-Mandelic Acid and Its Homologs I: Mutual Inhibitory Effect of D-(—)-Mandelic Acid and Its Certain Homologs on Their Renal Tubular Secretion in Rats, *J. Pharm. Sci. 59*:806, 1970.
Tryptophan	9.39	Parrott, E. L.: *Pharmaceutical Technology, Fundamental Pharmaceutics,* Burgess Pub. Co., Minneapolis, Minn., 1970, p. 218.
L-Tyrosine	9.11	Parrott, E. L.: *Pharmaceutical Technology, Fundamental Pharmaceutics,* Burgess Pub. Co., Minneapolis, Minn., 1970, p. 218.
Uracil	pK_1 = 9.0 pK_2 = 13.	Nestler, H. J. and Garrett, E. R.: Prediction of Stability in Pharmaceutical Preparations XV, *J. Pharm. Sci. 57*:1117, 1968.
Urea	0.18	Parrott, E. L.: *Pharmaceutical Technology, Fundamental Pharmaceutics,* Burgess Pub. Co., Minneapolis, Minn., 1970, p. 220.
Uric Acid	3.89	Parrott, E. L.: *Pharmaceutical Technology, Fundamental Pharmaceutics,* Burgess, Pub. Co., Minneapolis, Minn., 1970, p. 218.
Valeric Acid	4.81	Parrott, E. L.: *Pharmaceutical Technology, Fundamental Pharmaceutics,* Burgess Pub. Co., Minneapolis, Minn., 1970, p. 218.
DL-Valine	9.72	Parrott, E. L.: *Pharmaceutical Technology, Fundamental Pharmaceutics,* Burgess Pub. Co., Minneapolis, Minn., 1970, p. 218.
Viomycin Sulfate	pK_1 = 2.8 pK_2 = 5.87 pK_3 = 13.4	Dyer, J. R., Hayes, H. B. and Miller, Jr., E. G.: Chemistry of Viomycin, Presented at the Third Interscience Conference on Antimicrobial Agents and Chemotherapy, Washington, (Oct. 28-30) 1963.
Warfarin	5.05	Data by: Endo Laboratories, Garden City, N.Y. 11530.
Wy-4508	pK_1 = 2.68 pK_2 = 7.50	Hou, J. P. and Poole, J. W.: The Amino Acid Nature of Ampicillin and Related Penicillins, *J. Pharm. Sci. 58*:1510, 1969.
Wy-7953	pK_1 = 2.62 pK_2 = 7.60	Hou, J. P. and Poole, J. W.: The Amino Acid Nature of Ampicillin and Related Penicillins, *J. Pharm. Sci. 58*:1510, 1969.
Wy-8542	pK_2 = 7.65	Hou, J. P. and Poole, J. W.: The Amino Acid Nature of Ampicillin and Related Penicillins, *J. Pharm. Sci. 58*:1510, 1969.
Xanthine	9.95	Cohen, J. L. and Connors, K. A.: Stability and Structure of Some Organic Molecular Complexes in Aqueous Solution, *J. Pharm. Sci. 59*:1970.
Xylocaine	7.86	Beckett, A. H. and Taylor, J. F.: Blood Concentrations of Pethidine and Pentazocine in Mother and Infant at time of Birth, *J. Pharm. Pharmacol. Suppl. 19*:50, 1967.
Yohimbine	6.7 (apparent)	Robson, J. M. and Stacey, R. S.: *Recent Advances in Pharmacology,* 4th ed., Little, Brown and Co., Boston, 1968, p. 108.

References

1. Korn, E. D.: Structure of Biological Membranes, Science *153*:1491-1498 (Sept.) 1966.

2. Vogt, W.: Absorption of Drugs by Diffusion, *Arch. Exptl. Pathol. Pharmakol. 250*:210-231 (Feb.) 1965 (in German).

3. Schanker, L. S.: Passage of Drugs Across Body Membranes, *Pharmacol. Rev. 14*:501-530 (Dec.) 1962.

4. Rummel, W. and Forth, W.: Active Transport and Enteral Absorption, *Pharm. Ztg. 109*:1053-1054, 1964 (in German).

5. Ganong, W. F.: *Review of Medical Physiology,* 4th ed., Lange 1969.

6. Danielli, J. F., in Kitching, J. A.: *Recent Developments in Cell Physiology,* Academic Press, New York 1954.

7. Robertson, J. D., in Locke, M.: *Cellular Membranes in Development I,* Academic Press, New York, 1964.

8. Höber, R.: *Physical Chemistry of Cells and Tissue,* Blakiston, Philadelphia, 1945, pp. 1-676.

9. Bungenberg de Jong, H. G. and Bonner, J.: Phosphatide-Complex Coacervates as Ionic Systems and Their Relation to the Protoplasmic Membrane, *Proc. Royal Acad. Amsterdam 38*:797-866, 1935.

10. Dettli, L. and Spring, P.: 23rd International Congress of Pharmaceutical Sciences, Münster (W. Germany) 1963, Govi-Verlag, Frankfurt, 1964, p. 85.

11. Ritschel, W. A.: *Applied Biopharmaceutics I,* University of Cincinnati College of Pharmacy, Cincinnati, Ohio, 1969, p. 130.

12. Doluisio, J. T. and Dittert, L. W.: Biopharmaceutical Parameters, *Am J. Pharm. Educ. 32*:895-910 (Dec.) 1968.

13. Cammarata, A. and Martin, A. N.: "Physical and Biological Activity," in Burger, A.: *Medical Chemistry,* ed. 3, Part I, Wiley-Interscience, New York, London, Sydney, Toronto, 1970, p. 140.

14. Shore, P. A., Brodie, B. B. and Hogben, C. A. M.: The Gastric Secretion of Drugs — a *p*H Partition Hypothesis, *Therapy 119*:361-369 (Mar.) 1957.

15. Hogben, C. A. M., Tocco, D. J., Brodie, B. B. and Schanker, L. S.: On the Mechanism of Intestinal Absorption of Drugs, *J. Pharmacol. Exptl. Therap. 125*:275-282 (Apr.) 1959.

16. Schanker, L. S., Shore, P. A., Brodie, B. B. and Hogben, C. A. M.: Absorption of Drugs from the Stomach: I. The Rat, *J. Pharmacol. Exptl. Therap. 120*:528-539 (Aug.) 1957.

17. Hogben, C. A. M., Schanker, L. S., Tocco, D. J. and Brodie, B. B.: Absorption of Drugs from the Stomach II. The Human, *J. Pharmacol. Exptl. Therap. 120*:540-545 (Aug.) 1957.

18. Schanker, L. S., Tocco, D. J., Brodie, B. B. and Hogben, C. A. M.: Absorption of Drugs from the Rat Small Intestine, *J. Pharmacol. Exptl. Therap. 123*:81-88 (May) 1958.

19. Münzel, K.: The Influence of Formulating on the Response of Drug Products, *Progr. Drug Res. 10*:204-359, 1966 (in German).

20. Jacobs, M. H.: Some Aspects of Cell Permeability to Weak Electrolytes, *Cold Spr. Harbor Symp. Quant. Biol. 8*: 30-39, 1940.

21. Korolkovas, A.: *Essentials of Molecular Pharmacology,* Wiley-Interscience, New York, London, Sydney, Toronto, 1970, p. 31.

22. Schanker, L. S.: "Physiological Transport of Drugs," in Harper, N. J. and Simmonds, A. B.: *Advances in Drug Research,* Academic Press, London, New York, 1964, p. 100.

23. Kostenbauder, H. B., Portnoff, J. B. and Swintosky, J. V.: Control of Urine *p*H and Its Effect on Sulfaethidole Excretion in Humans, *J. Pharm. Sci. 51*:1084-1089 (Nov.) 1962.

24. Milne, M. D.: Influence of Acid-Base Balance on Efficacy and Toxicity of Drugs, in Symposium on Clinical Effects of Interaction Between Drugs, *Proc. Roy. Soc. Med. 58*:961-963 (Nov.) 1965.

25. Woodruff, M. W., Malvin, R. L. and Thompson, I. M.: The Renal Transport of Nitrofurantoin. Effect of Acid-Base Balance upon Its Excretion, *J. Am. Med. Assoc. 175*:1132-1135 (April) 1961.

26. Portnoff, J. B., Swintosky, J. V. and Kostenbauder, H. B.: Control of Urine *p*H and Its Effect on Drug Excretion in Humans, *J. Pharm. Sci. 50*:890 (Oct.) 1961.

27. Beckett, A. H., Boyes, R. N. and Tucker, G. T.: Use of the Analogue Computer to Predict the Distribution and Excretion of Drugs under Conditions of Fluctuating Urinary *p*H, *J. Pharm. Pharmacol. 20*:277-282 (Apr.) 1968.

28. Beckett, A. H., Boyes, R. N. and Tucker, G. T.: Use of the Analogue Computer to Examine the Quantitative Relation Between Urinary *p*H and Kidney Reabsorption of Drugs Partially Ionized at Physiological *p*H, *J. Pharm. Pharmacol. 20*:269-276 (Apr.) 1968.

29. Beckett, A. H. and Tucker, G. T.: Symposium on "The Influence of Formulation on the Absorption of Drugs." 27th FIP Congress, Montpellier, Sept. 4th, 1967, *J. Mondial Pharm. 10*:181 (Jul.-Sept.) 1967.

30. Schanker, L. S.: "Physiological Transport of Drugs" in Harper, N. J. and Simmonds, A. B.: *Advances in Drug Research,* Academic Press, London, New York, 1964, p. 97.

31. Thaysen, J. H. and Schwartz, I. L.: The Permeability of Human Sweat Glands to a Series of Sulfonamide Compounds, *J. Exptl. Med. 98*:261-268 (Sept.) 1953.

32. Anon.: (editorial): *Deut. Apotheker-Ztg. 102*:1546, 1962 (in German).

33. Eder, H. L.: Flea Bites. Prevention and Treatment with Thiamine Chloride, *Archiv Paediat. 62*:300-301 (July) 1945.

34. Müting, D.: *Med. Klin. 53*:1023, 1958.

35. Ritschel, W. A. and Ritschel-Beurlin, G.: Sunderbans Expedition, *Deut. Apotheker-Ztg. 103*:1098-1103, 1963 (in German).

36. Rasmussen, F.: Mammary Excretion of Sulphonamides, *Acta Pharmacol. Toxicol. 15*:139-148, 1958.

37. Rasmussen, F.: Mammary Excretion of Benzylpenicillin, Erythromycin, and Penethamate Hydroiodide, *Acta Pharmacol. Toxicol. 16*:194-200, 1959.

38. Rasmussen, F.: Mammary Excretion of Antipyrine, Ethanol and Urea, *Acta Vet. Scand. 2*:151-156, 1961.

39. Ritschel, W. A.: Drugs and Drug Products Which Should Not Be Administered During Pregnancy, Lactation and to Newborns, *Deut. Apotheker-Ztg. 102*:1601-1606, 1962 (in German).

40. Weiss, W.: *Subsidia Med. 12*:119, 1960.

41. Kobyletzki, D. V.: Own Studies on Pharmacokinetics During Pregnancy and Lactation, *Med. Welt. 19*:2010-2019 (Sept.) 1968 (in German).

18

Formulation of non-sterile dosage forms

by Gerald E. Schumacher

The role of dosage form design in the clinical practice of pharmacy is twofold. An understanding of the physical, chemical and preparative principles which influence the choice of dosage forms is requisite knowledge for the clinical pharmacist engaged in consultative functions involving the selection of dosage forms and the factors which influence their performance. This chapter will examine some theory of dosage form design and develop a "building block" technique for formulating preparations. The latter method is not employed in the pharmaceutical literature although one major[1] and three secondary[2,3,4] references are available.

Since the clinical pharmacist is most likely to encounter the extemporaneous design and preparation of nonsterile solutions, suspensions and emulsions, these dosage forms will be covered in this chapter. Parenterals are commented on only briefly since they are the subject of the following chapter. Tablets, aerosol and suppository theory is well treated in the literature.[1,4]

Choice of Dosage Form

Three general factors influence the choice of dosage form, assuming that patient preference is not a consideration:

(1) The solubility of the drug in the vehicle.
(2) The stability of the drug in the vehicle.
(3) The absorption or penetration characteristics of the drug in the vehicle.

Most drugs are weak organic acids or bases with limited aqueous solubility. To prepare the drug in solution form, it is necessary to determine that the total solubility desired can be achieved in water or a mixture of water and co-solvents. If this is not possible, then it will be necessary to employ a suspension as the dosage form. Alternately, it may be desirable to dissolve the drug in a nonpolar solvent followed by emulsification of the solvent in water.

The solution is the most practical and efficacious dosage form from a preparative point of view but this benefit must be weighed against the comparative stability of the drug in solution, suspension, emulsion and dry powder forms. Drugs in solution generally degrade by first and second order kinetic processes while drugs in suspension usually follow zero order kinetics. Since first and second order degradations generally proceed more rapidly than zero order degradations, it may be necessary to prepare the drug in suspension, or even dry form, if stability is a critical factor.

The absorption of drugs following oral, subcutaneous, intramuscular and rectal administration, or drug penetration after topical administration, is a function of drug solubility in the vehicle and physiological fluids as well as many other factors. In the case of poorly soluble drugs, the choice of vehicle which maximizes absorption may outweigh aqueous solubility and stability as factors. This consideration also applies to situations in which control of the absorption or penetration rate is desired.

Role of Solubility

For weakly acidic or basic drugs two components, the undissociated plus the dissociated forms of the drug, comprise the total solubility in solution. For any given situation the concentration desired in the dosage form may be defined as the total solubility required. Of the two species in solution, the undissociated form has the limiting solubility, which is a constant for a given solution composition and temperature and is designated in reference sources as the solubility of the drug. This aqueous solubility is often less than the total solubility desired in the dosage form.

Two procedures are commonly used to improve the total solubility of the drug: (1) increase the concentration of the dissociated species by ionization and (2) increase the solubility of the undissociated species by modifying the composition of the vehicle.

The solution process follows the scheme, undissolved drug ⇌ dissolved undissociated drug (UD) ⇌ dissolved dissociated species (D). Assume that a sufficient quantity of the drug is added to solution until the limiting solubility of UD is achieved. At this point an equilibrium is established between UD and D and the solution is saturated with respect to UD but not with respect to the more soluble D. If the total solubility required in the dosage form exceeds the combined limiting solubility of UD plus the concentration of D, then it is possible to increase the total solubility by altering the *p*H of the solution to yield a greater concentration of D. This process drives the above solution reaction to the right by converting UD, which has the fixed solubility, to D which possesses greater solubility due to ion-dipole interaction with aqueous and other polar solvents. It is now possible to add more drug to the solution, replenishing the concentration of UD, up to the limiting solubility of the species. The end result of altering the *p*H of the solution is to enhance the total solubility by increasing the concentration of D, the dissociated component, while maintaining the concentration of UD, the undissociated component.

The second approach to increasing total solubility is to enhance the solubility of the undissociated species of the drug by altering the polarity of the solvent through the use of semipolar co-solvents.[5-8] These procedures are summarized in Figure 1.

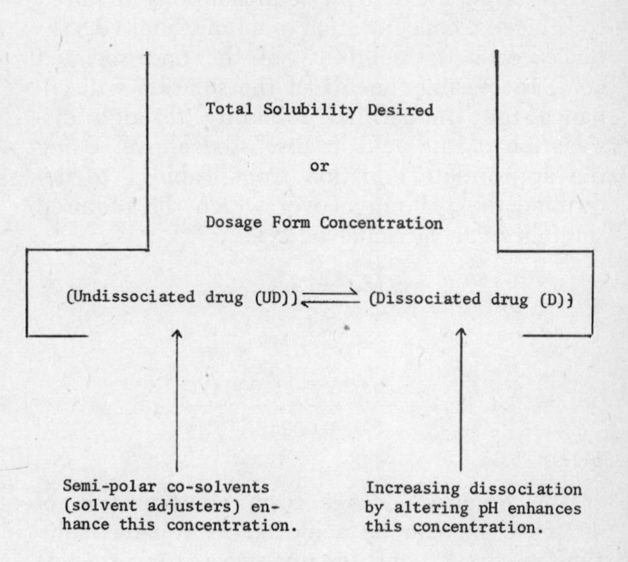

Figure 1. Total solubility considerations in dosage form design

Other methods of improving the total solubility by increasing the solubility of the undissociated form have been infrequently employed. The use of surfactants to solubilize UD by micellar solubilization has been successful.[9-10] This technique also has biopharmaceutical implications in altering the absorption characteristics of drugs.[11] Increased solubility through complexation with a variety of organic compounds has been utilized.[12-14] These techniques will not be expanded in this chapter.

Table 1 summarizes some equations useful in dosage form design which result from the dissociation behavior of weak acids and bases. Derivations appear in the literature.[15-16] These equations allow the formulator to predict the total solubility of a drug at a given *p*H or, conversely, the *p*H at which a given total solubility will precipitate from solution. To illustrate the use of these equations, and to demonstrate the influence of solubility on the choice of dosage form, assume that an oral preparation of the weak acid amobarbital is desired at a concentration of 44 mg/5 ml.[17] The total solubility required is then 0.88 percent. The choice of free acid or its sodium salt is undetermined at this point. The following data are obtained or calculated from the literature:

$pK_a = 7.4$
$K_a = 4.0 \times 10^{-8}$
Molecular weight of acid = 226
Molecular weight of salt = 248
Solubility of acid = S_a = 0.77 g/1000 ml = 0.0034 moles/liter
Total solubility required = S_t = 8.8 g/1000 ml = 0.036 moles/liter

It is apparent that the total solubility required to achieve a concentration of 44 mg/5 ml (0.88%) far exceeds the solubility of the undissociated acid. Increasing the *p*H of the solution will enhance the amobarbital solubility through dissociation of the acid as discussed above. Using the appropriate equation from Table 1 to determine the *p*H range over which the required solubility can be achieved:

$$pH = pK_a + \log \frac{(S_t - S_a)}{(S_a)}$$

$$= 7.4 + \log \frac{(0.036 - 0.0034)}{0.0034}$$

$$pH = 8.3$$

The required dosage form concentration of 44 mg/5 ml can be achieved in aqueous solutions of *p*H 8.3 and greater. Decreasing the *p*H below 8.3 will result in precipitation of the undissociated form of amobarbital. It should be noted that the pK values obtained from the literature for use in the equations of Table 1 are usually dissociation constants for drugs in pure water. Since the completed dosage form will contain other solutes which may alter the dissociation constant and drug solubility, the calculated values for the *p*H range and the total solubility may vary somewhat from those calculated for pure water. The equations do serve as good approximations, however.

The formulator may choose to prepare the oral amobarbital solution at a *p*H above 8.3. In this case the choice of the free acid or the sodium salt is not critical since the ultimate solubility is a function of the dissociation equilibria between the undissociated and dissociated species of amobarbital. Use of the salt will only speed the solution process.

Table 1. Total Solubility Relationships and Dissociation Equations in Dosage Form Design

(1) (Total Solubility (S_t)) = (Undissociated (S_a or S_b) + (Dissociated)

(2) $HA + H_2O \rightleftharpoons H_3O^+ + A^-$ (Acids)
$B + H_2O \rightleftharpoons OH^- + BH^+$ (Bases)

(3) For Acids: $S_t = S_a \left(1 + \frac{K_a}{(H_3O^+)}\right)$

$$pH = pK_a + \log \frac{(\text{dissociated})}{(\text{undissociated})} = pK_a + \log \frac{(S_t - S_a)}{(S_a)}$$

For Bases: $S_t = S_b \left(1 + \frac{K_b (H_3O^+)}{K_w}\right)$

$$pH = pK_w - pK_b + \log \frac{(\text{undissociated})}{(\text{dissociated})} = pK_w - pK_b + \log \frac{(S_b)}{(S_t - S_b)}$$

Where S_a or S_b = Molar solubility of undissociated acid or base.
S_t = Total molar solubility.
K_a or K_b = Dissociation constant of acid or base.
K_w = Dissociation constant of water.
*p*H = *p*H below which the acidic drug precipitates from solution or *p*H above which the basic drug precipitates from solution.

Preparing the oral amobarbital solution within the acceptable alkaline *p*H range may be undesirable for reasons of stability or palatability. Assume that *p*H 5 is chosen for the preparation as a result of these considerations. The use of another equation from Table 1 will predict the total solubility which can be achieved at this *p*H, keeping the limitations stated above in mind:

$$S_t = S_a \left(1 + \frac{K_a}{(H_3O^+)}\right)$$

$$= 0.0034 \left(1 + \frac{4.0 \times 10^{-8}}{1 \times 10^{-5}}\right)$$

$$S_t = 0.0034 \text{ moles/liter} = 0.077\%$$
$$= 3.85 \text{ mg/5 ml}$$

At *p*H 5 a total solubility of 3.85 mg/5 ml can be obtained. This is an unreasonable concentration for an oral dosage form of amobarbital so it will be necessary to increase the total solubility of the undissociated species. This is the only recourse since increasing the *p*H, for purposes of this example, has been ruled out previously.

A number of empirical observations have demonstrated that the undissociated form of many drugs exhibits a maximum solubility for a given drug in a given solvent system at one or more specific dielectric constants which are then denoted as the "dielectric requirement(s)" of the drug.[18,19] If the solvent system is altered, the quantitative measure of the solubility may vary but the dielectric requirement at maximum solubility is qualitatively unchanged. Since the dielectric constant is an index of the polarity of a solute or solvent, and most weak acids and bases will show a dielectric requirement considerably below the dielectric constant of water, it is possible to blend semi-polar co-solvents with water to decrease the polarity of the vehicle and increase the solubility of the undissociated species. These co-solvents can be designated as solvent adjusters.

The use of dielectric requirements has limitations, however. Solubility can only be correlated with the dielectric constant when the solvents used in the vehicle exhibit similar bonding characteristics. Furthermore, as mentioned above, the absolute solubility of a solute at a given dielectric requirement will vary from one solvent system to another. Nonetheless, blending solvent adjusters such as ethyl alcohol, propylene glycol and glycerin with water to decrease the polarity of the vehicle and, consequently, increase the solubility of the undissociated form of many drugs has been quite successful.[20,22] For the clinical pharmacist, it is generally unnecessary to determine the dielectric requirement of a drug. It is necessary to determine from the literature, or more often by personal study, the concentration of some reference solvent adjuster which must be blended with water to achieve the total solubility of drug required over the 5-30°C. temperature range.

Employing these concepts in the determination of a suitable solvent system for the amobarbital solution, ethyl alcohol is considered as a possible solvent adjuster for increasing the solubility of undissociated amobarbital since the drug is 20 percent soluble in alcohol. Assume that 40 percent ethyl alcohol in water is shown to maintain the required total solubility of 0.88 percent amobarbital at *p*H 5, and 5-30°C. The equation for calculating the apparent dielectric constant (ADC) of the vehicle is given in Table 2:[20]

$$ADC = \frac{\Sigma(\% \text{ solvent} \times \text{DC solvent})}{100}$$

Since ethyl alcohol and water have dielectric constants (DC) of approximately 25 and 80 at room temperature, respectively, the ADC of the 40 percent ethyl alcohol vehicle may be determined:

$$ADC = \frac{(40\% \times 25) + (60\% \times 80)}{100} = 58$$

A blend of 40 percent ethyl alcohol in water exhibits an apparent dielectric constant of 58 and this value maintains 44 mg/5 ml of amobarbital in solution at *p*H 5. Since at this *p*H all of the amobarbital is already present in the undissociated form, it is safe to recognize that this blend will insure the total solubility at lower *p*H values also. Furthermore, the formulator is generally assured of maintaining the total solubility with blends exhibiting dielectric constants which vary 5 percent from the calculated value. Thus an apparent dielectric range of 55-61 is probably suitable.

Other ingredients in the formulation may also lower the apparent dielectric constant of the vehicle, if they are present in substantial concentration, so it is possible to reduce the quantity of ethyl alcohol as a result of the contribution of other ingredients. Assume that 40 percent sorbitol (DC of 60) and 20 percent sucrose (DC of 60) are chosen as sweeteners to be used in the ethyl alcohol-water vehicle.

The final concentration of ethyl alcohol can be calculated:

$$58 = \frac{(E\% \times 25)+((40 - E\%)\times 80)+(40\% \times 60)+(20\% \times 60)}{100}$$

E = 18% = Ethyl alcohol
40 − E = 22% = Water

A vehicle composed of 40 percent sorbitol, 20 percent sucrose, 18 percent ethyl alcohol and 22 percent water should maintain the required total solubility of amobarbital. Naturally, other solvent adjusters such as propylene glycol or glycerin may replace some or all of the alcohol and the required concentrations can be calculated as above.

When solvent adjusters are used in solutions, it is appropriate to use the free acid or base form of the drug as opposed to a salt because the solution process is accelerated. The drug is dissolved in the solvent adjuster before it is added to the rest of the solution. It is important to reassert the empirical nature of the relationship between solubility and the apparent dielectric constant. The presence of high concentrations of sorbitol and sucrose, for instance, may change the anticipated solubility of amobarbital as predicted from the simple ethyl alcohol-water system by altering intermolecular bonding between drug and solvent. Yet, this technique is a useful first approximation for the formulator. Dielectric constant values are available in the literature.[23,24] A few useful values are included in Table 2.

Table 2. Approximate Dielectric Constant of Some Pharmaceutical Ingredients at Room Temperature

Compound	*Approximate Dielectric Constant*
Water	80
Sorbitol	60
Sucrose	60
Glycerin	43
Propylene glycol	32
Ethyl alcohol	25
PEG 400	19
Mineral oil	2-4

$$ADC = \frac{\Sigma\ (\%\ \text{Solvent} \times \text{DC Solvent})}{100}$$

ADC = Apparent dielectric constant of solvent blend.
DC = Dielectric constant of solvent.

Summarizing the procedures for determining the suitability of the solution as a dosage form based on solubility considerations alone:

(1) Compare the total solubility of the drug required in the dosage form to the solubility of the undissociated form of the drug. If the total solubility is in excess, then consider altering the solution *p*H to increase solubility through dissociation. Calculate the *p*H range over which the total solubility may be achieved.

(2) If the *p*H range is unsatisfactory, then consider increasing the total solubility by enhancing the solubility of the undissociated form of the drug. Determine the apparent dielectric constant of an ethyl alcohol-water blend which achieves the desired total solubility. Modify the concentration of alcohol or replace it if desired by noting the influence of other ingredients in the final formulation on the dielectric constant of the vehicle.

It is important to note that all additions of solvent adjusters such as ethyl alcohol are not dictated by solubility considerations; therapeutic, palatability and stability factors can contribute to the need for semi-polar co-solvents.

The clinical pharmacist may be called upon to recommend or formulate a dosage form for an investigational drug whose dissociation constant is not known. The equations of Table 1, as well as the biopharmaceutical considerations of absorption and penetration, demonstrate the need for this value. An approximation of the dissociation constant which is suitable for preliminary formulation considerations may be obtained by the following method:

(1) Determine the acidic or basic nature of the drug by noting whether total solubility improves upon increasing or decreasing the *p*H, respectively.

(2) Assuming that the drug is an acid, the appropriate equation from Table 1 is:

$$pH = pK_a + \log \frac{(\text{dissociated})}{(\text{undissociated})}$$

Prepare a very dilute solution of the drug. Add enough base such as sodium hydroxide to half-neutralize the acidic drug. At this point, the concentration of dissociated and undissociated species is equal, the log term drops out of the equation and the observed *p*H of the solution equals the pK_a of the drug. This method yields only a rough approximation of the dissociation constant because the thermodynamic activity of the drug has been neglected. But the technique is a useful tool in lieu of the more sophisticated methods presented in the literature.[25,26]

From a solubility point of view, the drug is prepared as the suspension dosage form when *p*H alteration or solvent adjusters or both fail to provide the total solubility required. This often happens with polyvalent, inorganic salts and with some very weakly acidic or basic drugs for which dissociation is too small to yield an appreciable increase in solubility. Aluminum hydroxide and griseofulvin are disparate examples of drugs which demonstrate poor solubility in aqueous solutions as well as in semi-polar solvents. Altering solution *p*H would negate the therapeutic utility of aluminum hydroxide while little dissociation of griseofulvin is possible. Suspensions are appropriate considerations.

The emulsion as a dosage form is useful for (1) drugs which are soluble in nonpolar solvents but poorly soluble in semi-polar and polar solvents, (2) nonpolar liquid drugs which are immiscible with water or water-solvent adjuster blends and (3) topical preparations.

For oral dosage forms, the drug is dissolved in a vegetable oil prior to emulsification while hydrocarbons are generally used for topical formulations. Since the nonpolar solvent is employed, except in the case of topical preparations, for the purpose of maintaining the solubility of drugs which are poorly soluble in water it is necessary to choose a nonpolar solvent which displays a favorable distribution coefficient against water. In dilute concentrations, the distribution coefficient (K^o_w) is a measure of the ratio of concentrations of drug in nonpolar solvent and water at equilibrium.

Assume that a 50:50 emulsion (oil-in-water) of a nonpolar solvent and water is desired as the vehicle for a dosage form containing an acidic drug. The total solubility (S_t) required in the vehicle is 0.05 molar while the aqueous solubility of the undissociated drug (S_a) is 0.002 molar. Two different nonpolar solvents, A and B, are considered for use. Both are capable of accommodating the desired total solubility of the drug. The distribution coefficients of A and B against water which has been acidified to assure no dissociation of the drug are 100 and 10, respectively. At equilibrium, the total solubility of 0.05 mole of drug per 1000 ml of emulsion is distributed between the 500 ml each of the nonpolar and aqueous phases as follows:

A

$$K^o_w = \frac{100}{1}$$

$$= \frac{0.0495 \text{ mole in A}}{0.0005 \text{ mole in water}}$$

$$= \frac{0.990 \text{ mole/liter in A}}{0.001 \text{ mole/liter in water}}$$

B

$$K^o_w = \frac{10}{1}$$

$$= \frac{0.0455 \text{ mole in B}}{0.0045 \text{ mole in water}}$$

$$= \frac{0.091 \text{ mole/liter in B}}{0.009 \text{ mole/liter in water}}$$

It is apparent from these calculations that the relationship between the distribution coefficient and the aqueous solubility of the undissociated form of the drug is critical. In this example the choice of nonpolar solvent B is unwise because the distribution coefficient is not great enough to sufficiently deplete the drug from the aqueous phase. The equilibrium concentration of drug in water exceeds the aqueous solubility (S_a) by more than fourfold. Of course, if the *p*H of the aqueous phase were increased, the water solubility would be enhanced through dissociation. In the example above, however, in which dissociation is suppressed, solvent A is the appropriate choice.

Thus, solubility exerts an important influence on the choice of dosage form. Preparations are aqueous when the total solubility desired can be achieved at the *p*H of interest. Dosage forms are hydro-alcoholic, or contain other solvent adjusters, if the addition of these semi-polar solvents converts an insoluble dose to a soluble one. When this technique fails, the formulator seeks the suspension or the emulsion form.

Role of Stability

Drug stability often becomes the dominant consideration in dosage form design. The principles of drug stability evaluation are discussed in other chapters of this book. Furthermore, many excellent reviews of the subject appear in the literature.[27-30] A few observations pertinent to the role of stability in the choice of dosage form will be treated here.

The stability of drugs in liquid media is influenced by (1) *p*H, (2) solvent, (3) buffers, (4) temperature, (5) metals, (6) oxygen and (7) light. Drugs in solution generally degrade by first and second order kinetic mechanisms. In these processes the rate of degradation of the drug is proportional to the concentration of reactants; the rate is more rapid in the initial stages of the reaction and decreases with time as the reactants are depleted. On the other hand, drugs in suspension usually degrade by zero order kinetics; the rate is constant with time and is independent of reactant concentration. These observations suggest that the suspension dosage form is usually more stable than the solution form. Table 3 summarizes the equations used for predicting the degradation rate and fractional life expectancy of zero and first order reactions.

To demonstrate the stability of solutions as compared to suspensions, assume that an aspirin solution and suspension are prepared and buffered at *p*H 2.5 and 25°C. The following data are obtained for the aspirin solution:[31,22]

$pK_a = 3.49$
$S_t = 3.68$ Gm/liter
$k_{(1)} = 0.0488$ day^{-1}

Using the half-life expression from Table 3:

$$t_{0.5} = \frac{0.693}{k_{(1)}} = \frac{0.693}{0.0488} = 14.2 \text{ days}$$

The time required to deplete one-half of the original concentration of aspirin in solution (3.68 g/liter) is 14.2 days.

Table 3. Integrated Rate Equations and Fractional-Life Relationships

(1) Zero Order Degradations

$$k_{(o)} = \frac{(A_o) - (A)}{t}$$

$$t_{0.9} = \frac{(A_o)}{10\ k_{(o)}}$$

$$t_{0.5} = \frac{(A_o)}{2\ k_{(o)}}$$

(2) First Order Degradations

$$k_{(1)} = \frac{2.3 \log ((A_o)/(A))}{t}$$

$$t_{0.9} = \frac{0.104}{k_{(1)}}$$

$$t_{0.5} = \frac{0.693}{k_{(1)}}$$

Where $k_{(o)}$ and $k_{(1)}$ = Zero and first order rate constants, respectively.

(A_o) and (A) = Initial concentration and concentration at a given time, respectively.

$t_{0.9}$ and $t_{0.5}$ = Time at which 90 percent and 50 percent of the initial concentration of drug remains, respectively.

Now prepare the aspirin in suspension form in a concentration of 0.35 g/5 ml or 70.0 g/liter, buffered to *p*H 2.5, at 25°C. Since in suspension form, some of the drug is in solution to the limit of saturation, while the remaining drug is undissolved, the rate constant for the zero order reaction, $k_{(o)}$, represents the product of the first order rate constant for the solution, $k_{(1)}$ and the solubility of the drug at the *p*H of interest S_t. The following data are obtained for the aspirin suspension:[33]

Initial concentration of suspension = A_o = 70 g/liter

$k_{(o)} = k_{(1)}\ (S_t) = (0.0488$ day$^{-1})$ (3.68 g/
Using the half-life expression from Table 3:

$$t_{0.5} = \frac{A_o}{2k_{(o)}} = \frac{70}{(2)\ (0.18)} = 194 \text{ days}$$

The time required to deplete one-half of the original concentration of aspirin in suspension is 194 days. The suspension form prolongs the half-life of the aspirin by nearly fourteenfold over the half-life in solution. While it is true that pharmaceutical preparations are rarely permitted to degrade to one-half their initial concentration before discarding them, and that one-tenth to one-quarter degradation is more realistic, the same types of equations may be applied for any fractional life degradation, as shown in Table 3, and the same trend will develop. Thus, when stability in solution is too short to be practical, it is often necessary to resort to preparing the suspension to enhance the stability of the product.

Now assume that the aspirin solution is prepared at *p*H 5 and 25°C. When the *p*H of the solution was 2.5, an inspection of the pK_a (3.49) suggests that the total solubility observed was essentially that of the undissociated aspirin (S_a). At a *p*H of 5, the drug is almost completely ionized, the total solubility which can be achieved is much greater (85.2 g/L) and the suspension dosage form cannot be prepared in the usual dosage range (70.0 g/L) due to the high solubility. The following data are obtained from the literature:[31]

$S_t = 85.2$ g/L
$k_{(1)} = 0.314$ day^{-1}

Using the half-life expression from Table 3:

$$t_{0.5} = \frac{0.693}{k_{(1)}} = \frac{0.693}{0.314} = 2.2 \text{ days}$$

Increasing the *p*H of the solution from 2.5 to 5.0 has decreased the half-life of aspirin in solution more than sixfold.

This example points up the complexities of dealing with drug stabilities. Altering *p*H of the aspirin solution from *p*H 2.5 to 5.0 changed three factors which influence stability: (1) the relative concentrations of undissociated and dissociated forms of aspirin were changed; (2) the relative concentrations of hydronium ion and hydroxyl ion, two species which can often catalyse drug degradation, were changed; and (3) the relative concentrations of the components of the buffer solution, which may themselves have degradation potential, were changed.

Some or all of these factors contribute to the stability of aspirin as well as most drugs. By studying the stability of a drug over an extended *p*H range and in different buffers, a stability *vs.* *p*H profile is generated which aids the formulator in choosing the *p*H and buffer system required for optimum stability. The aspirin example also demonstrated the relationships between *p*H, solubility and stability. If the suspension is desired for maximizing stability, then a *p*H must be chosen which suppresses solubility. This can be determined by using the equation of Table 1.

The relationship between the first order rate constant and temperature is as follows:

$$k_{(1)} = Ae^{-Ea/RT}$$

where A = a constant related to the number of molecular collisions occurring per unit time and the molecular configuration during collision.

Ea = the activation energy which is related to the fraction of molecules which possess sufficient energy, upon collision, to lead to a degradation of reactants.

Stating the equation in logarithmic form and noting the first order relationship of $k_{(1)}$ and $t_{0.5}$ from Table 3:

$$\log k_{(1)} = \log A - \frac{E_a}{2.3\ RT}$$

$$\log t_{0.5} = \log \frac{0.693}{A} + \frac{E_a}{2.3\ RT}$$

These equations demonstrate that stability decreases with increases in temperature. Furthermore, a plot of log $t_{0.5}$ against the reciprocal of the absolute temperature (1/T) generates a straight line. This observation suggests the procedure for studying stability at elevated temperatures, to conveniently shorten the degradation time and then to extrapolate the linear plot to room temperature. In this manner room temperature stability data, as well as data for other important temperatures, can be obtained. These procedures are discussed in the literature.[27-29, 34-36]

When metals, oxygen and light contribute to the instability of drugs, it is often possible to diminish their effect by using chelating agents, antioxidants and proper packaging, respectively. These techniques are treated at length in the literature.[27-30, 37] Other, more sophisticated, stability considerations such as the ionic strength and dielectric constant of the solution will not be discussed here. They are covered in the references cited above.

THE FORMULATION OF SOLUTIONS

The general formula for oral solutions is as follows:

Active ingredients
Solvent adjusters, if needed
Buffer, if needed
Sweeteners
Miscellaneous palatability enhancers, if needed
Flavors
Color
Preservatives
Distilled water

Solvents

The selection of solvents represents the initial consideration in developing the formula. As discussed above, the solvent is chosen on the basis of solubility, stability and palatability data. When a solvent adjuster is required to enhance the total solubility desired in solution, the adjuster for oral preparations is usually chosen from ethyl alcohol, propylene glycol, glycerin or mixtures of these solvents. Phenobarbital 0.4 percent, for example, which approximates the concentration in the official elixir, requires about 30 percent ethyl alcohol to maintain the total solubility.[38] Using the data of Table 2, an apparent dielectric constant of approximately 63 for the blend is calculated. Similar calculations suggest that 35 percent propylene glycol or 50-55 percent glycerin in water should also maintain the 0.4 percent phenobarbital concentration.

The official preparation blends ethyl alcohol 12.5 percent, glycerin 45 percent and water. Other mixtures have proven effective.[38] Propylene glycol, for instance, is often used to decrease the required concentration of ethyl alcohol when high concentrations of the latter diminish palatability or are contraindicated.

Buffers

Buffers are used to suppress solubility and to maintain solutions within the *p*H range of maximum stability, as discussed above. Buffer concentrations generally do not exceed 0.1 molar although this depends on the molarity of the active ingredients. Since buffer systems often possess the ability to accelerate drug degradation (general acid-base catalysis), and this potential varies with the buffer used, it is desirable to investigate two or three systems and to use the minimum concentration necessary to maintain the desired *p*H.

Sweeteners

The sweetening system is the heart of oral liquid preparations and is evaluated after the choice of solvents. Two considerations are involved: (1) the specific character of sweeteners and (2) the vague and subjective quality of "body" and "mouthfeel." Taken together, these components contribute to the palatability of the preparation.

Three general types of sweetener systems are frequently used in dosage form design:[1,3,39] (1) sucrose *and* sorbitol with or without synthetic sweeteners; (2) sucrose *or* sorbitol with or without synthetic sweeteners; and (3) miscellaneous natural sweeteners, alone or in combination, with or without synthetic sweeteners.

Little work has been published on the relative efficacy of sucrose, sorbitol and their combinations in enhancing the palatability of oral solutions.[39-42] But evidence to date suggests that the most palatable syrup preparations are achieved by combining the natural sugar sucrose with the polyol sorbitol and then enhancing the sweetness with synthetic sweeteners if needed. Sucrose or sorbitol employed alone is usually less acceptable. Sweetening with synthetics alone, such as saccharin or cyclamate, when the procedure is unnecessary, is not recommended because sucrose and/or sorbitol contribute needed body. While many formulations believe that a combination of sucrose and sorbitol in the sweetener system is preferable to the use of either agent alone, the choice of sucrose or sorbitol as the major component of the blend is unresolved at present. A combination of the sweeteners appears to reduce the crystallization and "cap-locking" characteristics of the sugars; an undesirable effect which can be suppressed even more by adding 2-3 percent glycerin to the vehicle.[41-42]

The sweetener system can be classified as contributing medium-light or medium-heavy "body" to the solution. Two starter blends, alternating the major sweetening component, are offered in each category:

Medium-Light Body

Sorbitol Solution USP	33%	Syrup USP	27%
Syrup USP	12%	Sorbitol Solution USP	12%
Distilled Water qs		Distilled Water qs	

Medium-Heavy Body

Sorbitol Solution USP	50%	Syrup USP	40%
Syrup USP	18%	Sorbitol Solution USP	20%
Distilled Water qs		Distilled Water qs	

It is convenient to equate the sweetening capacity of the various sweeteners although the taste character and capacity of each agent varies with concentration, *p*H and temperature. Acknowledging these limitations, the "sucrose equivalency" of the various sweeteners is summarized in Table 4 and used as a "rule-of-thumb" for preliminary formulations. The medium-light body vehicles listed above possess approximately 30 percent sucrose equivalent and contribute 40-45 percent solids to the solutions. The medium-heavy vehicles produce approximately 45 percent sucrose equivalent and contribute 60-70 percent solids to the solution.

The use of glycerin in oral preparations has declined in recent years. Glycerin contributes sweetness and body to vehicles in addition to its role as a solvent adjuster. But since concentrations above 10 percent are distasteful and its capacity as a solvent adjuster is inferior to propylene glycol, the use of glycerin for solvency, sweetness and body has largely been replaced with combinations of propylene glycol and sorbitol.[3]

The major synthetic sweeteners include sodium and calcium saccharin, sodium and calcium cyclamate and cyclamic acid. At this writing, the future of the cyclamates, cyclamic acid

Table 4. Sucrose Equivalents of Various Sweeteners

Sweetener	*Sucrose Equivalent*[a]
Sorbitol crystals	0.5
Sorbitol Solution USP[b]	0.5
Syrup USP[c]	0.9
Sucrose	1.0
Cyclamate	30.0
Cyclamic acid	30.0
Cyclamate-saccharin as 10-1	60.0
Saccharin	300.0

[a]Interpreted as 1 Gm of saccharin contributing the same sweetening capacity as 300 Gm of sucrose, 10 Gm of cyclamate, etc.

[b]Sorbitol Solution USP is 91% w/v.

[c]Syrup USP is 85% w/v.

and saccharin is unsettled. The cyclamates will be included in this chapter, however, in the interest of completeness. In the absence of their use, formulators are urged to replace cyclamates with one-tenth the quantity of saccharin, as an initial trial, as suggested in Table 4.

Most people favor the palatability of unmedicated cyclamate-saccharin (10:1) sweetened solutions over cyclamate or saccharin solutions alone. But this preference becomes less clear-cut when synthetics are added to vehicles sweetened with either sucrose or sorbitol or both because the taste of the latter agents predominates. The preference is even less precise when medicated ingredients are added to the solution or syrup. In most formulations, there is probably no substantial palatability difference in equivalent concentrations of cyclamate, saccharin or their combinations when added to enhance the sweetness of existing medicated syrups.[3] The use of cyclamic acid contributes a tart-sour taste to vehicles in addition to sweetness. For example, a 2 percent cyclamic acid solution is simulated by a solution of 2 percent sodium cyclamate plus 2.5-3.0 percent citric acid.

The sweetness of vehicles may be classified, for the purpose of this chapter, as follows:

(1) Lightly-sweetened; contains less than 50 percent sucrose equivalent in sweeteners and is generally used for medications with little to no distaste, elixirs, suspensions and emulsions.

(2) Moderately-sweetened; contains 50-100 percent sucrose equivalent in sweeteners and is the range used for most medicated solutions.

(3) Heavily-sweetened; contains more than 100 percent sucrose equivalent in sweeteners and is used for medications with great distaste.

In the initial stages of the formulation, it is usually advisable to try a medium-light body sweetener vehicle as presented above. If this blend produces sufficient body but insufficient sweetness, 0.1 percent increments of saccharin or cyclamate-saccharin (10:1) or 1 percent increments of cyclamate may be added until a satisfactory response is achieved. If the medium-light body vehicle does not produce the desired viscosity or "mouthfeel" then a medium-heavy body sweetener vehicle is the next consideration. Synthetics may again be added if necessary. It is generally inadvisable to exceed the sucrose-sorbitol concentrations recommended above for medium-heavy body vehicles because greater concentrations lead to palatability, flow, crystallization and medicament solubility problems.

Consider the following two sweetener systems as an amplification of the above discussion:

(1)	Sorbitol Solution USP	33.0%
	Syrup USP	12.0%
	Sodium Saccharin	0.2%
	Distilled Water qs	
(2)	Sorbitol Solution USP	50.0 %
	Syrup USP	18.0 %
	Sodium Saccharin	0.15%
	Distilled Water qs	

These two vehicles, using the data of Table 4, both possess 85-90 percent sucrose equivalent and should be similar in sweetness although the body of the solutions differ. Solution (1) is a medium-light body, moderately-sweetened vehicle while solution (2) is medium-heavy body and moderately-sweetened.

Miscellaneous Palatability Enhancers

The palatability of some medicaments, notably those that elicit bitter and salty tastes, is often enhanced by the addition of an acidifying agent. Citric acid is the most common additive and is used in concentrations of 0.25 to 1.0 percent. The greatest application of acidifiers is in diminishing the salty taste of electrolytes and in enhancing the taste of some fruit flavors.

Somewhat apart from acidification is the palatability enhancement which is sometimes achieved by the inclusion of 0.25-0.5 percent sodium chloride in solutions which are highly sweetened. Whether the "salt effect" is useful in a given medicated syrup formulation depends upon trial and error. The "salt effect" is usually contraindicated in hydroalcoholic solutions.

Flavors

Flavors make a significant contribution to the palatability of dosage forms. Since flavoring is more an art than a science and palatability is often subject to individual preference, no rules for flavoring will be stated in this chapter. A good background in flavor technology can be achieved by reading the literature.[43-45] In addition, two manuals on flavoring are available from manufacturers.[46,47]

A flavor library including cherry, chocolate, mint, orange and raspberry is often adequate to solve most common flavoring problems.[43] As generalizations, salty tasting drugs often respond well to citrus flavors fortified with 0.25-1.0 percent citric acid, butterscotch and maple. Sour tasting drugs are also improved by citrus flavors. Bitter tasting medicaments are often masked by chocolate, some citrus and mint flavors. The anesthetic properties of mint flavors may be quite effective for some after tastes. But mints are commonly contraindicated with salty tasting medicaments because they markedly accentuate the salty taste.[3]

The major problems in flavoring include (1) improper flavoring due to careless or rigid choice of flavors, (2) excessive flavoring and (3) failure to compensate for after taste. Trial and error, the judicious use of two and three component flavor blends and observation of the flavor and concentration recommendations of the individual flavor manufacturers are good advice in this area of formulation.

Colors

The color of oral solution dosage forms should complement the flavors used in the formulation. For external preparations the color is often associated with use.

Three classes of dyes are available: (1) F D & C dyes for food, drug and cosmetic use; (2) D & C dyes for drug and cosmetic use; and (3) external D & C dyes for non-oral drug and cosmetic use.

All water-soluble F D & C dyes are anionic. Although the possibility exists for interaction of these dyes with cationic drugs and ingredients, this interaction is uncommon since the usual concentration range for dyes is 0.001-0.01 percent. The major incompatibilities of the dyes are their susceptibility to *p*H changes, oxidizing agents, reducing agents and light, all of which can lead to color changes or precipitation. F D & C Red No. 2 is a good choice in most instances. F D & C Yellow No. 5 is also fairly stable except in the presence of reducing agents. F D & C Green No. 1 demonstrates general purpose utility in acidic media but it should be used with caution in alkaline solutions and in the presence of oxidizing agents. Detailed information on dyes is available in the literature.[48]

The concentration of dye used can be critical. Inadequate concentrations produce shades which are difficult to produce from batch to batch. Passing the solutions through filter media may lead to batch variation if dyes are adsorbed onto the filter material. On the other hand, excessive concentrations may result in staining of containers as well as ionic interactions.

Preservatives

The topic of preservatives includes:

(1) Preservatives for protection against microbial growth.
(2) Antioxidants against oxidative degradation.
(3) Chelating agents for complexing trace metal catalysts.

Methylparaben and propylparaben are the most popular antimicrobial preservatives for general purpose use. They are effective over the *p*H range of 1-11 although activity drops off markedly above *p*H 9. The two parabens are usually employed in combination, in this way inhibiting bacterial, mold and yeast growth, in a total concentration of 0.1-0.2 percent. A common concentration is methylparaben and propylparaben as 0.1 and 0.02 percent, respectively. The aqueous insolubility of the parabens presents difficulties which are overcome by dissolving in (a) boiling water or (b) semi-polar solvents such as propylene glycol and ethyl alcohol.

Benzoic acid and its sodium salt are often employed as antimicrobial agents in acidic preparations in concentrations of 0.1-0.2 percent. Since antimicrobial activity resides in the undissociated form of the molecule, due to greater efficiency of traversing the lipid-like cell membrane, the use of benzoic acid and its salts above *p*H 5 is discouraged.

In hydroalcoholic solutions, an ethanol concentration of 20 percent or more is generally considered to be an effective preservative strength.

The most popular antioxidants for aqueous systems are the sodium salts of metabisulfite, bisulfite and sulfite.[49] These salts are used in concentrations of 0.05-0.5 percent. Examples of drugs which are stabilized against oxidative degradation by antioxidants include dextrose, streptomycin, neomycin, penicillin, some salicylates, some steroids and some alkaloids.[50] The use of antioxidants for investigational drugs, in the absence of stability information, must be regarded as empirical; they may be used prophylactically unless they are shown to accelerate degradation.

Chelating or sequestering agents are used to enhance the activity of antioxidants by forming soluble complexes with trace amounts of heavy metal ions which could otherwise catalyse oxidative degradation.[49] The salts of EDTA, of which disodium edetate is official, are frequently used chelating agents. In concentrations of 0.01-0.05 percent in aqueous media, edetate effectively sequesters most common metal ions.

Developing the Formulation

The various ingredients of the general formulation may be classified as objective and subjective components:

(1) Objective components: chemical form of

ingredients, solvent adjusters, buffers and preservatives.

(2) Subjective components: sweeteners, flavors, colors and nonspecific palatability enhancers.

Objective components are stipulated by the concentration desired in the dosage form, stability considerations and preparative techniques. Subjective components, on the other hand, are more flexible and are best assessed by using a palatability or taste panel. This technique is well described in the literature.[39, 41, 51]

To demonstrate the utilization of the various components of the general formulation, consider the design of an antihistamine-decongestant solution. Designate the antihistamine as "A" and the decongestant as "D". Both drugs are basic amine-containing drugs. Then assume that the dosage concentration is stipulated by the formulator and the remaining data are obtained from the literature, from the manufacturer or by personal experiment:

	A	*D*
Dosage concentration	5 mg/5 ml	10 mg/5 ml
Total solubility desired (S_t)	0.005 molar	0.02 molar
Molecular weight	200	100
Aqueous solubility of base (S_b)	0.01 molar	0.01 molar
K_b	10^{-5}	10^{-6}
Susceptibility to oxidative degradation	No	Yes
Range of *p*H stability	3-8	2-7

Using the above data and the equations of Table 1, suggests that solubility is not a consideration for drug "A" since S_b already exceeds S_t. Drug "D", however, requires dissociation to obtain the desired S_t and this is achieved below *p*H 7.5. Since stability is good in mildly acidic solutions and palatability is also best in this range, the total solubility of both drugs can be obtained at acidic *p*H, which makes the use of solvent adjusters unnecessary.

Using a *p*H range of 4-6 as acceptable for this product, the choice of chemical form of the drugs merits consideration. Drug "A" can obviously be used as the free base but drug "D" requires acidification to achieve its total solubility. If the free base form of drug "D" is used, then the *p*H should be acidified or buffered within the *p*H 4-6 range. On the other hand, these drugs are weak bases, so using salts of the drugs which are composed of a strong acid and the weak base will produce solutions which are probably already in the desired *p*H range. In this case, acidification or buffering may not be necessary. Assume that the maleate salt of drug "A" is used in conjunction with the hydrochloride salt of drug "D".

A medium-light body, moderately-sweetened solution is a good vehicle for initial trial. Either of the two vehicles recommended above is appropriate. If it proves necessary to enhance palatability by adding synthetic sweeteners, then the use of saccharin or cyclamate-saccharin (10:1) in 0.05 percent increments is considered.

Most amines respond well to fruit flavors.[46] The use of cherry, strawberry, raspberry, etc., or combinations, in concentrations recommended by the manufacturer, may be evaluated. Citric acid in concentrations of 0.25-0.75 percent may be considered with citrus flavors or for general palatability enhancement. Sometimes 3-5 percent ethyl alcohol is used in the formulation to incorporate the flavor oils and to enhance their solubility. Concentrations of alcohol up to 5 percent are generally indistinguishable in highly sweetened viscous vehicles. Above this concentration, palatability may decrease.

To correlate flavor with color, F D & C Red No. 2, in concentrations of 0.001 percent and up, should be considered. The final choice and concentrations of sweeteners, flavors, palatability enhancers, and colors should be the result of palatability panel testing.

The parabens may be effectively employed as preservatives in a combination of 0.1 and 0.02 percent for methyl and propylparabens respectively. Sodium bisulfite should be added to suppress the oxidative lability of drug "D" and EDTA may be considered as a precautionary measure. With these factors in mind, a trial formulation which may survive taste panel and stability analysis could be:

Antihistamine-Decongestant Syrup

"A" maleate	0.10%
"B" hydrochloride	0.20%
Citric acid monohydrate	0.50%
Sodium bisulfite	0.10%
Disodium edetate	0.05%
Methylparaben	0.10%
Propylparaben	0.02%
Saccharin sodium	0.05%
Sorbitol Solution USP	33.00%
Syrup USP	12.00%
Strawberry imitation flavor	qs
F D & C Red No. 2	qs
Distilled water qs ad	100.00%

It is easy to appreciate that many different formulations could be generated by altering the variables or that this formulation may be unsatisfactory in some respects. Palatability and stability are variables which must be evaluated. Other formulation techniques are discussed in the literature.[3,52]

THE FORMULATION OF SUSPENSIONS

The design of good suspensions is more difficult than that of liquids because of the complexities of suspension technology. Dispersed systems are subject to a number of influences including thermodynamics, electrokinetics, and interfacial, sedimentation and rheological properties. Each of these characteristics can affect suspension stability. Space does not allow for a detailed presentation of suspension theory and technology. Nonetheless, the formulator is urged to acquire this background from the literature.[53-59] A capsule summary of pertinent theory is presented here.[58]

From a thermodynamic viewpoint, when particles are reduced in size during preparation of a suspension, the total surface area of the particles is increased which leads to an increase in the free energy associated with the surface. The particles will attempt to reduce this surface free energy by decreasing the total surface area through particle association and aggregation. When the particles are dispersed, they acquire a surface charge by a variety of means. The surface charge attracts a concentrated layer of ions of opposite charge about the particle which partially neutralizes the original charge on the particle. The well known zeta potential measures the electrical potential of the particle at the concentrated layer. The greater the zeta potential, the greater the repulsion between particles, which promotes diminished particle association. Decreasing the zeta potential by further neutralizing the surface charge leads to a loose association of particles through flocculation or a more rigid association through aggregation, depending on the degree of neutralization. Stoke's law predicts that the sedimentation of dispersed particles with time is inevitable and that the velocity of sedimentation can be suppressed by decreasing particle size or by increasing vehicle viscosity or both.

The formulation of suitable suspensions requires that the product should redisperse readily prior to administration and that it should flow easily from the container. If the suspended particles sediment individually or as tightly bound aggregates, they will frequently cake as a solid mass at the bottom of the container. But if the dispersed particles are induced to associate by Van der Waal's forces in loose, open structures known as floccules, as opposed to tightly bound aggregates, the floccules will settle but they do not cake. These settled clusters may be redispersed quite readily. But even this sedimentation can be decreased by using a viscosity enhancing agent. These observations are the basis of the controlled flocculation method of preparing suitable suspensions.[60]

Another approach to suspension formulation utilizes the rheological properties which can be built into suspensions by the proper choice of suspending agents. Good suspensions result from vehicles which exert maximum resistance to sedimentation while at rest but minimum resistance to flow upon agitation. It is often difficult to find these two properties combined in a suspension that employs a single suspending agent. Using two suspending agents is often the answer. Maximum resistance to sedimentation by the suspended particles when the preparation is at rest can be conferred by a thixotropic, plastic type of suspending agent such as Veegum, bentonite, microcrystalline cellulose or Carbopol. Ready flow upon agitation can be contributed by pseudoplastic agents such as the celluloses and alginates. This method of producing a stable suspension may be called the "combined rheologies" method and may also owe part of its efficacy to inducing some degree of flocculation in the system.[61]

Two common methods of flocculating suspended particles are (1) adding electrolytes to the system which partially neutralizes the surface charge on the particles and (2) using polymers, like many of the common protective colloids cited above, which are capable of absorbing part of their structure on the suspended particles while linking other particles in loose association with other parts of their structure. It is then possible to combine some aspects of both methods, controlled flocculation and combined rheologies, by using pseudoplastic and plastic protective colloids which contribute some capacity to flocculate particles in addition to enhancing the viscosity of the suspension.

In summary, the most important factors to consider in routinely preparing suspensions are to (1) decrease particle size with appropriate dispersing equipment, (2) partially flocculate the suspended particles to minimize caking, (3) build sufficient viscosity into the system to suppress the sedimentation of the flocculated aggregates and (4) balance the viscosity and rheological characteristics of the suspension so that the preparation flows readily from the container upon moderate agitation.

The general formula for oral suspensions is as follows:

Active ingredients
Buffer, if needed
Sweeteners
Acidifiers, if needed
Flavors
Color
Preservatives
Protective colloids
Distilled water

For many of these components, the principles of their use in suspensions are merely a modification of their use in solutions.

Buffers are used, if needed, to suppress solubility and to enhance stability. Acidifiers are sometimes used in suspensions to alter *p*H for maximum performance of suspending agents, to improve stability and to enhance preservative potential but infrequently to improve palatability.

The color of suspensions is often that of the suspended ingredients. When color is desired for oral products, the same rules of association with flavor apply as for solutions. Terpeneless mint flavors are popular for antacid suspensions. Smooth, bland flavors such as butterscotch, custard, chocolate, vanilla and some fruit flavors are also used.

Since suspensions usually possess body in themselves, it is not advisable to use concentrations of sucrose or sorbitol which exceed 20-25 percent. If this does not provide sufficient sweetness, then saccharin may be added in increments of 0.01 percent. Suspension sweetness rarely exceeds 50 percent sucrose equivalent. In fact, 5-20 percent sucrose equivalent is common.

Preservatives such as the parabens have been observed to interact with macromolecules like the protective colloids to form complexes which reduce the "free," active concentration of preservative in solution.[62,63] It is a good precaution to at least double the preservative concentration in formulating suspensions.

A number of protective colloids are used in suspensions to enhance viscosity and to suppress the sedimentation and caking potential of the dispersed drugs. Common ingredients include the celluloses, alginates, tragacanth, Veegum, bentonite and Carbopol. The formulator is urged to become familiar with their properties.[64-67] Only two agents will be discussed here as prototypes, the plastic hydrocolloid Veegum and the pseudoplastic hydrocolloid carboxymethylcellulose.

Veegum is a very useful and versatile form of colloidal magnesium aluminum silicate which is similar in properties to bentonite. It is available in many grades, is anionic, effective over the *p*H range of 4-11, but is affected by moderate concentrations of electrolytes.[66,68,69]

Carboxymethylcellulose (CMC) is the sodium salt of a cellulose polymer in which some of the hydroxyl groups of the polymer are converted to carboxymethyl groups. CMC is available in a number of viscosity grades, is effective over the *p*H range of 4-11 and demonstrates intolerance to some electrolytes in moderate concentrations.

The viscosity and rheological characteristics contributed by protective colloids are influenced by (1) the dispersing equipment used in preparing the suspensions, (2) the solution temperature employed for hydrating the suspending agents, (3) the hydration time employed and (4) the other ingredients in the suspension. Batch to batch uniformity calls for precise and reproducible preparative techniques.[3]

Developing the Formulation

Assume that an antacid-demulcent suspension is being developed which contains the insoluble drugs, aluminum hydroxide and magnesium trisilicate. In designing the suspending system, the formulator strives to build suitable viscosity into the preparation, to form a structured network which traps or supports the dispersed particles and to partially flocculate the particles through particle linking or, less frequently, through partial neutralization of the surface charge.

If the active ingredients are suspended in water alone, the particles quickly sediment to a cake which is not redispersible upon shaking. Employing a single suspending agent such as CMC at the maximum concentration which still allows pouring upon agitation, does not suppress caking. Using Veegum alone may minimize caking but it does not prevent sedimentation and the appearance of a supernatant layer. Blending CMC and Veegum in appropriate concentrations, however, yields a suspension with little to no supernatant formation and no caking.[58] This technique, which is a variant of the "combined rheologies" method, is often successful in preparing suitable suspensions. The general approach is to begin with 0.5 percent of each suspending agent varying the respective concentrations by 0.2 percent increments until optimum performance is achieved.

Since aluminum hydroxide and magnesium trisilicate are insoluble over the useful *p*H range and stability is not a problem, there is no need for including a buffer in the formulation. Nor is an antioxidant, chelating agent, acidifier or color indicated. Sometimes, however, a surfactant is added to the formulation to aid in dispersing drugs which are not easily wetted. The effect is to reduce the interfacial tension between solid and liquid. This technique is not needed in this example.

For sweetening, the pleasing taste of sorbitol in low concentrations can be considered. Generally, suspensions are lightly sweetened. If this component needs to be intensified, a synthetic sweetener is added. A blend of mint and bland flavors may be effective. Lastly, the parabens, at twice the solution concentration, can be effective antimicrobial agents.

The completed formulation, suitable for initial palatability and stability trials, is as follows:

Antacid-Demulcent Suspension

Aluminum hydroxide	4.00%
Magnesium trisilicate	12.00%
Carboxymethylcellulose (low viscosity grade)	1.00%
Veegum regular	0.50%
Sorbitol Solution USP	20.00%
Methylparaben	0.20%
Propylparaben	0.04%
Peppermint flavor	qs
Vanilla flavor	qs
Distilled water qs ad	100.00%

Once again, the variables, such as protective colloids, flavors and sweeteners, are apparent. Other sample formulations appear in the literature.[3,67,69,70]

THE FORMULATION OF EMULSIONS

Space does not allow for a thorough treatment of the physical principles underlying emulsion design. The topic is well covered in the literature.[71-76]

Just as the particles of a suspension attempt to reduce free surface energy by decreasing the total surface area of the particles, so it is that after two immiscible liquids are agitated together and one is then temporarily dispersed within the other, the liquids rapidly revert into two layers. Dispersing the liquid forming the internal, or dispersed, phase has created a greatly enlarged surface area and a concomitant increase in surface free energy. Since the increase in total surface area is inevitable in emulsification, the globules of the dispersed phase will coalesce in order to minimize the thermodynamic instability. A surfactant can be added to maintain a dispersed phase, attributed in part to lowering the interfacial tension by minimizing the energy gain. Yet, the lowering of interfacial tension is often not sufficient in itself to deter coalescence. Stable emulsions require surfactants which not only lower interfacial tension but also form a mechanical barrier about the globules which protects them from coalescence.[74] The nature of this mechanical barrier, in the case of oil-in-water emulsions, is probably a viscous, highly-ordered layer of water molecules which surround the surfactant and create a film shield between globules.[72]

Far more emulsifying agents are available than any formulator can become familiar with. Many systems have been developed for relating the emulsifying characteristics of various agents. The most popular system, and the one with the greatest utility, is the HLB or "Hydrophile-Lipophile Balance" system. The formulator should become acquainted with its use.[3,71,77,78]

In brief, the HLB system assigns values to each of the oil phase components of emulsion systems which indicate their relative lipophilic or hydrophilic character. The higher the HLB value, the more hydrophilic the ingredient is. Since HLB values are additive, it is possible to compute the HLB requirement of the oil phase of an emulsion. Then, knowing the HLB value of an emulsifying agent, it is possible to determine the most effective emulsifiers for a given emulsion by matching the requirement of the emulsion to the value of the emulsifier. Water-in-oil emulsions are usually formed when using emulsifiers within the HLB range of 3-6 while oil-in-water systems form within the HLB range of 8-18.

To demonstrate an HLB calculation, although a detailed study of the system is recommended, assume that an oil-in-water lotion is to contain 30 percent mineral oil, 2 percent anhydrous lanolin and 2 percent cetyl alcohol. These three components comprise the oil phase of the emulsion and constitute 34 percent of the lotion. Of the oil phase, 88 percent is mineral oil, 6 percent is lanolin and 6 percent is cetyl alcohol. Multiplying each of these percentages (as decimals) by the appropriate HLB requirement (0.88 x 10, 0.06 x 12, 0.06 x 15) as shown in Table 5 and taking the sum yields the average HLB requirement of the emulsion. Choosing an emulsifier or a blend of emulsifiers near this HLB requirement, which in this case is 10.4, should produce a satisfactory emulsion.

The HLB system was developed by Atlas Chemical Industries to meet the characteristics of their emulsifiers. The performance of non-Atlas emulsifiers may not conform to the predictions of the HLB system. Nonetheless, the use of this technique for all emulsifiers yields a good starting point for emulsion formulation.

Emulsion systems in pharmacy include lotions, creams, absorption bases, bath oils, oral, parenteral and aerosol emulsions. Space allows for a treatment of only oil-in-water lotions and creams. Formulations and techniques for other emulsions are available in the literature.[3,76,79,80]

The general formula for topical oil-in-water emulsions is as follows:

Oil Phase
Active ingredients
High melting point waxes, if needed
Emollient-lubricants
Emulsifiers
Antioxidant, if needed
Perfume, if needed

Aqueous Phase
Water-soluble ingredients
Humectant-application enhancer
Preservatives
Color, if needed
Distilled water

As mentioned early in the chapter, if an emulsion is being prepared due to greater solubility and/or stability in the oil phase as compared to the aqueous phase, then the oil phase must be chosen so that the drug effectively partitions and remains in the oil. If, instead, the emulsion is chosen for reasons of cosmetic efficacy, then the above considerations are not pertinent.

High melting point waxes are added to emulsions to thicken lotions and to solidify creams and ointments. Generally, concentrations of cetyl alcohol or stearyl alcohol from 5-10 percent will convert aqueous liquids to creams.[3]

Emollient-lubricants enhance the pliability of the skin, suppress moisture loss, alter emulsion texture and viscosity and serve as the vehicle for appropriately soluble ingredients. Mineral oil, isopropyl myristate and lanolin fractions are used in concentrations of 10-40 percent.

Antioxidants such as propyl gallate, butylated hydroxyanisole, butylated hydroxytoluene, and tocopherol, protect unsaturated oils and labile drugs from oxidative degradation in the oil phase when used in concentrations of 0.01-0.03 percent.

The choice of emulsifiers is vast. In choosing an appropriate emulsion, the following factors must be considered: (1) ionic nature of the emulsifier, (2) chemical type of emulsifier, (3) concentration of the emulsifier required to yield a stable emulsion.

Cationic emulsifiers are effective over the *p*H range of 3-7. They are used in emulsions containing cationic medicaments, high concentrations of electrolytes and high acidity. Anionic emulsifiers are used at *p*H 8 and above. They are employed for anionic medicaments, alkaline detergents and shampoos. Nonionic emulsifiers are the most versatile agents, effective over the *p*H range of 3-10 and are not markedly affected by electrolytes or the ionic nature of the medicaments.[3]

Nonionic emulsifiers are the only agents to be discussed here; the Spans and Tweens of Atlas Chemical Industries are prototypes. The most effective emulsions are prepared by blending lipophilic (Spans) and hydrophilic (Tweens) emulsifiers to match the required HLB of the oil phase of the emulsion. Blending emulsifiers in this manner leads to a more coherent and tightly packed emulsifier film coating the globules of the dispersed phase. This, in turn, provides a greater barrier to coalescence. Table 6 provides a few HLB values of emulsifiers. More complete tables appear in the literature or in the brochures of emulsifier manufacturers.[3,71,76,77] Even when the optimum HLB value has been calculated, it is possible that different chemical types of emulsifiers at similar HLB values will yield varying emulsion stabilities. This is a trial and error procedure. Nonionic emulsifiers are generally used in concentrations of 10-20 percent of the oil phase. Ionic emulsifiers usually require a considerably smaller concentration.

A different type of nonionic emulsifier can be classified as an emulsifying wax. Glyceryl monostearate, nonionic self-emulsifying (GMS-SENI), is a prototype in this category. In this form, glyceryl monostearate imparts emulsification, thickening and emolliency to emulsions. With its use, the need for other high melting point waxes may be decreased or omitted. For some applications then, self-emulsifying glyceryl monostearate can replace a blend of emulsifiers and some or all of the high melting point wax in a formulation.

Glyceryl monostearate alone is a high melting point wax. In self-emulsifying form, it is available in cationic, anionic and nonionic forms. Concentrations above 15 percent convert lotions to creams.

In the aqueous phase, humectant-application enhancers like sorbitol, glycerin and propylene glycol in concentrations of 5-10 percent decrease evaporation, increase lubricity and ease of application, and enhance the texture and feel of the product upon application.

The interaction of some preservatives, such as the parabens, with nonionic emulsifiers and perhaps ionic emulsifiers, reduces the concentration of "free," active preservative in the aqueous phase. A 5 percent Tween 80 emulsion, for instance, can reduce "free" methylparaben and propylparaben to 20 percent and 5 percent of their initial concentrations, respectively.[62] This is probably the result of micellar solubilization or some other form of complexation between preservative and emulsifier.[81] Furthermore, most preservatives distribute themselves between the oil and water phases of the emulsion which enhances the depletion of "free" preservative from the aqueous phase. As a rule of thumb, for each 1 percent of nonionic emulsifier, it is wise to include an additional 0.05 percent methylparaben and 0.01 percent propylparaben to the initial concentration.[3] If the partitioning and complexation data are known for the preservative, then equations are available for calculating the exact preservative concentration required.[81]

Developing the Formulation

The simplest form of an oil-in-water lotion includes:

Mineral oil	10%
Emulsifiers	2-10%
Distilled water qs ad	100%

Blending Tween 80 and Span 80, using the data of Tables 5 and 6 to achieve the required HLB of 10 for mineral oil, completes the formulation:

Mineral oil	10.0%
Span 80	4.7%
Tween 80	5.3%
Distilled water qs ad	100.0%

Table 5. O/W HLB Requirements of Some Ingredients

Ingredient	*HLB* (±1)
Cetyl alcohol	15
Stearic acid	15
Stearyl alcohol	14
Lanolin, anhydrous	12
Mineral oil	10
Beeswax	9
Petrolatum	8

Table 6. HLB Values of Some Emulsifiers

Emulsifier	*HLB*
Glyceryl monostearate	3.8
Sorbitan monooleate (Span) 80	4.3
Sorbitan monostearate (Span) 60	4.7
Glyceryl Monostearate, nonionic self-emulsifying	11.0
Polysorbate (Tween) 60	14.9
Polysorbate (Tween) 80	15.0

This thin lotion can develop enhanced emolliency and viscosity by increasing the mineral oil concentration to a maximum of 40 percent. Alternately, enhanced viscosity can be achieved by adding 2-5 percent cetyl or stearyl alcohol or 5-10 percent of GMS-SENI. If the latter ingredient is used, then the emulsifiers and the alcohol are decreased or eliminated. Using cetyl alcohol, stearyl alcohol or GMS-SENI to replace part or all of the mineral oil also decreases emolliency and the oily residue while substituting a drier, less greasy film.

Emollient-lubricants such as a 5-20 percent isopropyl myristate or liquid lanolin fraction may be desired for enhanced emolliency and/or solvency potential. A humectant such as 5-10 percent sorbitol may be considered.

After adding preservatives, the rudimentary formula has become more complex and probably more efficacious:[3]

Mineral oil	10.0%
Liquid lanolin fraction	10.0%
Cetyl alcohol	2.5%
Span 80	3.4%
Tween 80	6.6%
Sorbitol Solution USP	10.0%
Methylparaben	0.5%
Propylparaben	0.1%
Distilled water qs ad	100.0%

Note the change in emulsifier ratio to meet the new HLB requirements of 11.4 for the oil phase. Many formula variations are apparent.

Creams can also be produced, depending on the desired texture and application properties, by modifying lotion formulas. A rudimentary oil-in-water cream formula follows:

Petrolatum	40.0%
Emulsifiers	5.0%
Distilled water qs ad	100.0%

Replacing the pertrolatum with 5-15 percent cetyl or stearyl alcohol confers a dry, non-greasy texture to the cream. Glyceryl monostearate is also suitable, after deleting or decreasing the emulsifiers, in concentrations of 15-25 percent.

Upon adding emollient-lubricants, a humectant-application enhancer and preservatives, two possible formulations with different textures may emerge:[3]

Cetyl alcohol	10.0%
Mineral oil	10.0%
Liquid lanolin fraction	10.0%
Span 80	1.2%
Tween 80	3.6%
Sorbitol Solution USP	5.0%
Methylparaben	0.5%
Propylparaben	0.1%
Distilled water qs ad	100.0%

Cetyl alcohol	7.50%
Mineral oil	7.50%
GMS-SENI	7.50%
Sorbitol Solution USP	7.50%
Methylparaben	0.20%
Propylparaben	0.04%
Distilled water qs ad	100.0 %

Countless variations of these mineral oil-based creams can be developed.

When a non-greasy, vanishing type of cream is desired, a stearic acid-based preparation is developed. Vanishing creams differ from mineral oil-based creams in (1) reducing the concentration of the oil phase, (2) minimizing the concentration of emollient-lubricants and (3) decreasing the concentration of emulsifiers, which should be blended to HLB 9-10. A typical vanishing cream formulation follows:[3]

Stearic acid, triple-pressed	20.00%
Mineral oil	2.00%
Span 60	2.00%
Tween 60	1.50%
Sorbitol Solution USP	5.00%
Methylparaben	0.20%
Propylparaben	0.04%
Distilled water qs ad	100.00%

Additional formulations for various emulsion dosage forms appear in the literature.[3,76,79,80] These formulations, as well as those recommended by various emulsifier manufacturers, should be consulted so that the formulator acquaints himself with the characteristics and applications of many surfactants.

THE FORMULATION OF PARENTERAL PREPARATIONS

The design of parenteral preparations follows the same procedures for solubility, stability and ingredient choice as employed for nonsterile preparations. Much of the preceding discussion is directly applicable to this dosage form.

Parenteral preparations differ from the formulation of nonsterile solutions, suspensions and emulsions in the following manner:

(1) The preparation must be sterile and nonpyrogenic.
(2) Isotonicity of the preparation may be a factor depending on the site of injection and the volume of solution administered.
(3) Some vehicles are applicable for parenterals but not for oral preparations.
(4) Since, as discussed early in the chapter, there is an inverse relationship between stability and temperature, autoclaving of parenteral preparations places some new demands on the formulation.
(5) Ingredients which contribute to palatability in the general formulations are obviously absent from parenteral preparations.

The formulator is urged to consult the excellent reviews of parenteral product technology in the literature.[82-86]

Although the formulator may prepare large volume intravenous fluids, irrigating solutions and small volume injectables, he will probably be required most frequently to formulate small volume, single or multiple dose vials.

The formulation of parenteral preparations containing suspensions and emulsions is covered in a fine review article.[85] Considering only the small volume parenteral solution in this chapter, the general formulation is as follows:

Active ingredients
Buffer, if needed
Preservatives, if needed
Tonicity contributors, if needed
Solvents

As suggested earlier, two factors make the choice of ingredients and their purity more critical for parenteral solutions than for nonsterile products.

(1) The high temperature encountered in the autoclaving process, if this procedure can be tolerated, enhances the potential for hydrolytic, oxidative, trace metal and acid-base catalysis when these processes are applicable. To minimize this potential, materials of highest purity are always used and buffers, antioxidants and chelating agents may be indicated although they may not have been required for the same product in nonsterile form.
(2) The sterility and nonpyrogenicity of parenteral products is mandatory. In addition, particulate matter must be minimized, even particles too small for visual detection, since foreign matter may have a deleterious effect in capillaries and other small vessels.[88]

The choice of the chemical form of the active ingredients and the appropriate buffer system, if needed, follows the same considerations as discussed for nonsterile solutions. The buffer capacity should be great enough to serve its chemical role but low enough so that the body buffers and fluids can rapidly neutralize the *p*H, to minimize discomfort, upon injection. Preservatives follow the same indications as for nonsterile solutions except that it is not uncommon to double the concentration of antimicrobial agents since sterility must be maintained throughout the life of the preparation. The parabens or benzyl alcohol (1-2 percent) are frequently used. Chelating agents such as EDTA are a good precaution but antioxidants are only used when indicated.

Adjusting the solution near isotonicity is not a universally accepted procedure. Nonetheless, hypotonic or hypertonic solutions can often contribute to discomfort upon administration.

The variety of solvents employed for parenteral solutions exceeds the selection suitable for oral administration; water for injection, propylene glycol, polyethylene glycol, dimethylacetamide, ethyl oleate and fixed oils such as corn, cottonseed, peanut and sesame oils are examples.[86] The choice of solvents depends, as before, on solubility and stability considerations.

Two types of small volume parenteral solutions are prepared:

(1) Single dose preparations which are intended for one dose only and contain no antimicrobial preservatives. They are packaged in glass vials which meet U.S.P. and N.F. specifications and the vials are capped with a rubber diaphragm and a metal closure designed for one use only.

(2) Multiple dose preparations which are intended to contain more than one dose, require antimicrobial preservatives and are limited in size to 30 ml. Glass vials for these preparations also meet official specifications while the rubber diaphragm and metal closure are designed for multiple puncture and entry.

When sterile solutions must be prepared but autoclaving leads to excessive degradation, then it is necessary to prepare solutions by aseptic techniques. For this purpose, laminar flow hoods and bacterial retentive filtration techniques are employed. The clinical pharmacist is urged to acquire these techniques from the literature.[89]

Two formulations are presented to clarify some of the considerations outlined above:

ATROPINE INJECTION
(Multiple Dose Vial)

Atropine sulfate	0.04%
Citric acid	1.00%
Sodium citrate	1.00%
Sodium bisulfite	0.10%
EDTA	0.01%
Mannitol	1.00%
Benzyl alcohol	1.00%
Water for injection USP qs ad	100.00%

In this formulation the citrate buffer system is fixed at pH 3.5-4.0 to maximize stability and to insure solubility of the basic drug. The antioxidant and chelating agent are precautionary additives. Mannitol furnishes tonicity adjustment; sodium chloride also can be used for this purpose. Benzyl alcohol is an antimicrobial preservative which also contributes a slight local anesthetic activity. If the preparation were intended for single dose only, then the benzyl alcohol could be eliminated.

PENTOBARBITAL INJECTION (85)
(Multiple Dose Vial)

Pentobarbital sodium	15.0%
Propylene glycol	60.0%
Benzyl alcohol	2.0%
Water for injection USP qs ad	100.0%

Propylene glycol is used as a solvent adjuster in this case to enhance the solubility of pentobarbital and to decrease hydrolysis during autoclaving. If the pentobarbital acid is used, then the pH should be adjusted to alkalinity.

The formulation and preparation of parenteral solutions is a complex endeavor. The reader is again urged to consult the literature.[82-87]

Limitations of This Chapter

This chapter contains general information which is intended to alert the reader to some considerations in dosage form design as well as to guide him to more sophisticated and specific coverage in the literature. The "building block" approach to formulation has been emphasized.

Space limitations and chapter focus have conferred some restrictions on the presentation:

(1) Generalizations and brevity have been emphasized. This technique always invites a false sense of security and dulls the awareness of the individual considerations which must attend each dosage formulation.
(2) Preparative methods have not been included. These procedures are available in the literature.[1,3]
(3) Few examples of formulations have been included. Reference citations have been noted for each dosage form.
(4) An appendix of ingredient and equipment suppliers, as well as manufacturer's literature, has not been included but may be found in the literature.[3]
(5) The mechanisms of drug degradation and the biopharmaceutical implications which influence the choice and formulation of the dosage form have not been included.
(6) The quality control techniques which are requisite to any program of formulation and production have not been included. An excellent chapter appears in the literature.[90]
(7) Dosage forms such as tablets, capsules, aerosols and suppositories are not included. Good coverage of these topics may be found in the literature.[1,4]

Despite these limitations, the primary goal of this chapter is intact: a general treatment of some of the underlying principles in dosage form design. Hopefully, this information provides the clinical pharmacist with another packet of knowledge which he should acquire to fulfill the consultative component of his practice.

References

1. Lachman, L., Lieberman, H. A. and Kanig, J. L., ed.: *The Theory and Practice of Industrial Pharmacy,* Lea & Febiger, Philadelphia, 1970.

2. Macek, T. J.: "Formulation," in Osol, A. *et al.,* eds: *Remington's Pharmaceutical Sciences,* ed. 14, Mack Publishing Co., Easton, Pennsylvania, 1970, p. 1463-1477.

3. Schumacher, G. E.: The Bulk Compounding Technology of Liquids and Semi-Solids, *Am. J. Hosp. Pharm. 26*:70-99 (Feb.) 1969.

4. Osol, A. *et al.,* ed.: *Remington's Pharmaceutical Sciences,* ed. 14, Mack Publishing Co., Easton, Pennsylvania, 1970.

5. Martin, A. N., Swarbrick, J. and Cammarata, A.: *Physical Pharmacy,* ed. 2, Lea & Febiger, Philadelphia, 1969, p. 312.

6. Lachman, L.: *op. cit.,* p. 437.

7. Krause, G. M. and Cross, J. M.: Solubility of Phenobarbital in Alcohol-Glycerin-Water Systems, *J. Am. Pharm. Assoc. Sci. Ed. 40*:137-142 (Mar.) 1951.

8. Edmonson, T. D. and Goyan, J. E.: The Effect of Hydrogen Ion and Alcohol Concentration on the Solubility of Phenobarbital, *J. Am. Pharm. Assoc. Sci. Ed. 47*: 810-812 (Nov.) 1958.

9. Swarbrick, J.: Solubilized Systems in Pharmacy, *J. Pharm. Sci. 54*:1229-1237 (Sept.) 1965.

10. Mulley, B. A.: "Solubility in Systems Containing Surface Active Agents," in Bean, H. S., Beckett, A. H. and Carless, J. E., ed.: *Advances in Pharmaceutical Sciences,* Academic Press, Inc., New York, 1964, vol. 1, p. 87-194.

11. Gibaldi, M. and Feldman, S.: *J. Pharm. Sci. 59*:579, 1970.

12. Martin, A. N.: *op. cit.,* p. 342.

13. Lachman, L.: *op. cit.,* p. 442.

14. Higuchi, T. and Lach, J. L.: Investigations of Some Complexes Formed in Solution by Caffeine, *J. Am. Pharm. Assoc. Sci. Ed. 43*:349-354 (June), 524-530 (Sept.) 1954.

15. Martin, A. N.: *op. cit.,* p. 310.

16. Lachman, L.: *op. cit.,* p. 440.

17. Schumacher, G. E.: Ionic Equilibria, *p*H and Choice of Solvents, *Am. J. Hosp. Pharm. 26*:354-356 (June) 1969.

18. Paruta, A., Sciarrone, B. and Lordi, N.: Correlation Between Solubility Parameters and Dielectric Constants (Letters), *J. Pharm. Sci. 51*:704-705 (July) 1962.

19. Lordi, N. *et al.*: Dielectric Constants and Solubility (Letters), *J. Pharm. Sci. 53*:463-464 (Apr.) 1964.

20. Moore, W. E.: The Use of an Approximate Dielectric Constant to Blend Solvent Systems, *J. Am. Pharm. Assoc. Sci. Ed. 47*:855-857 (Dec.) 1958.

21. Moore, W. E.: Use of an Approximate Dielectric Constant in Solubility Studies, *J. Pharm. Sci. 51*:391-392 (Apr.) 1962.

22. Gorman, W. G. and Hall, G. D.: Dielectric Constant Correlations with Solubility and Solubility Parameters, *J. Pharm. Sci. 53*:1017-1020 (Sept.) 1964.

23. Martin, A. N.:*op. cit.,* p. 129.

24. Weast, R. C. *et al.,* eds.: *Handbook of Chemistry and Physics,* ed. 51, Chemical Rubber Company, Cleveland, Ohio, 1970, p. E-61.

25. Martin, A. N.: *op. cit.,* p. 281.

26. Parke, T. V. and Davis, W. W.: Use of Apparent Dissociation Constants in Qualitative Organic Analysis, *Anal. Chem. 26*:642-645 (Apr.) 1954.

27. Lachman, L.: *op. cit.,* p. 669-710.

28. Martin, E. W. and Hoover, J. E., eds.: *Husa's Pharmaceutical Dispensing,* ed. 6, Mack Publishing Co., Easton, Pennsylvania, 1966, p. 440-463.

29. Parrot, E.: *Pharmaceutical Technology,* Burgess Publishing Company, Minneapolis, 1970, p. 250-273.

30. Martin, A. N.: *op. cit.,* p. 389.

31. Garrett, E. R.: The Kinetics of Solvolysis of Acyl Esters of Salicylic Acid, *J. Am. Chem. Soc. 79*:3401-3408 (July 5) 1957.

32. Garrett, E. R.: Prediction of Stability in Pharma-

ceutical Preparations, *J. Am. Pharm. Assoc. Sci. Ed. 46*:584-586 (Oct.) 1957.
33. Martin, E. W.: *op. cit.,* p. 445.
34. Parrott, E.: *op. cit.,* p. 257.
35. Martin,A. N.: *op. cit.,* p. 374, 396.
36. Lin, S.: *Bull. Parenteral Drug Assoc. 23*:269, 1969.
37. Martin, A. N.: *op. cit.,* p. 387.
38. Peterson, C. F. and Hopponen, R. E.: Solubility of Phenobarbital in Propylene Glycol-Alcohol-Water Systems, *J. Am. Pharm. Assoc. Sci. Ed. 42*:540-572 (Sept.) 1953.
39. Schumacher, G. E.: Formulation Technology, *Am. J. Hosp. Pharm. 27*:762-765 (Sept.) 1970.
40. Schumacher, G. E.: Bulk Compounding Technology, *Am. J. Hosp. Pharm. 25*:154-155 (Mar.) 1968.
41. Ward, D. R., Lathrop, L. B. and Lynch, M. J.: Taste and Cap-Locking Behavior of Pharmaceutical Syrups, *Drug Cosmetic Ind. 99*:48-53, 157 (July) 1966.
42. *Bulletin LS-100,* Atlas Chemical Laboratories, 1968.
43. Wesley, F.: Flavor and the Modern Pharmaceutical, *J. Am. Pharm. Assoc. 18*:674-677 (Nov.) 1957.
44. Wesley, F.: Flavoring Lessons, *J. Am. Pharm. Assoc. NS1*:292,294 (May) 1961.
45. Wesley, F.: Problems in Masking Modern Pharmaceuticals, *Drug Cosmetic Ind. 89*:580-581, 636, 642-645 (Nov.) 1961.
46. Wesley, F.: *Pharmaceutical Flavor Guide,* Fritzsche Bros. Inc., 6 Ninth Avenue, New York, New York, 10011, 1957.
47. PFC Index, Foote and Jenks, Inc., Jackson, Michigan 49204.
48. Martin, E. W.: *op. cit.,* p. 759.
49. Lachman, L.: Antioxidants and Chelating Agents as Stabilizers in Liquid Dosage Forms, *Drug Cosmetic Ind. 102*:36-40, 146-148 (Jan.); 43-45, 146-149 (Feb.) 1968.
50. Schroeter, L. C.: Sulfurous Acid Salts and Pharmaceutical Antioxidants, *J. Pharm. Sci. 50*:891-901 (Nov.) 1961.
51. Schumacher, G. E. and Crowell, W. J.: Palatability of Some Potassium Salts in Flavored Vehicles, *Am. J. Hosp. Pharm. 21*:226-229 (May) 1964.
52. Formulary of Liquid Oral Products, Bulletin LD-94, Atlas Chemical Industries, Inc., Wilmington, Delaware 19899.
53. Ecanow, B., Gold, B. and Ecanow, C.: Newer Aspects of Suspension Theory, *Am. Perfumer Cosmetics 84*:27-30 (Nov.) 1969.
54. Hiestand, E. N.: Theory of Coarse Suspension Formulation, *J. Pharm. Sci. 53*:1-18 (Jan.) 1964.
55. Nash, R. A.: The Pharmaceutical Suspension, *Drug Cosmetic Ind. 97*:843-846, 939, 942-954 (Dec.) 1965.
56. Sprowls, J. B. and Beal, H. M., eds.: *American Pharmacy,* ed. 6, J. B. Lippincott Co., Philadelphia, 1966, p. 180-236.
57. Martin, A. N.: *op. cit.,* p. 515-548.
58. Schumacher, G. E.: Bulk Compounding Technology, *Am. J. Hosp. Pharm. 26*:548-550 (Sept.) 1969.
59. Schumacher, G. E.: Bulk Compounding Technology, *Am. J. Hosp. Pharm. 26*:650-652 (Nov.) 1969.
60. Martin, A. N.: Physical Chemical Approach to the Formulation of Pharmaceutical Suspensions, *J. Pharm. Sci. 50*:513-517 (June) 1961.
61. Samyn, J. C.: An Industrial Approach to Suspension Formulation, *J. Pharm. Sci. 50*:517-522 (June) 1961.
62. Patel, N. K. and Kostenbauder, H. B.: Interaction of Preservatives with Macromolecules, *J. Am. Pharm. Assoc. Sci. Ed. 47*:289-293 (Apr.) 1958.
63. Patel, N.: *Can. J. Pharm. Sci. 2*:97, 1967.
64. Martin, E. W.: *op. cit.,* p. 203-222.
65. Patel, B. N.: Hydrocolloids in Cosmetic Pharmaceutical Dispersions, *Drug Cosmetic Ind. 95*:337, 451 (Sept.) 1964.
66. Barr, M.: General Characteristics and Applications of the Montmorillonite Hydrocolloids, *Am. Perfumer Cosmetics 78*:37-48 (Feb.) 1963.
67. Avicel Applications Bulletin, FMC Corporation, Marcus Hook, Pennsylvania 19061.

68. Schumacher, G. E.: The Use of Veegum in Suspensions and Creams, *Am. J. Hosp. Pharm. 25*:661-662 (Nov.) 1968.
69. Veegum Applications, Bulletins No. 44, 56, R. T. Vanderbilt Co., 230 Park Avenue, New York, New York 10017.
70. Lachman, L.: *op. cit.,* p. 517-537.
71. Becher, P.: *Emulsions—Theory and Practice,* ed. 2, Reinhold Publishing Corp., New York, 1965, p. 49-208.
72. Davies, J. T. and Rideal, E. K.: *Interfacial Phenomena,* ed. 2, Academic Press, Inc., New York, 1963, p. 343-450.
73. Garret, E. R.: Stability of Oil-in-Water Emulsions, *J. Pharm. Sci. 54*:1557-1570 (Nov.) 1965.
74. Schumacher, G. E.: Bulk Compounding Technology—Emulsions, *Am. J. Hosp. Pharm. 27*:64-66 (Jan.) 1970.
75. Sherman, P.: *Emulsion Science,* Academic Press, Inc., New York, 1968, p. 1-75.
76. Lachman, L.: *op. cit.,* p. 463-490.
77. Griffin, W. C., Lynch, M. J. and Lathrop, L. B.: Emulsions, *Drug Cosmetic Ind. 101*:41-45, 170-175 (Oct.) 1967.
78. The Atlas HLB Systems, Bulletin LD-97, Atlas Chemical Industries, Wilmington, Delaware 19899.
79. Atlas Cosmetic Formulary, LD-125, LD-132, Atlas Chemical Industries, Wilmington, Delaware 19899.
80. Lachman, L.: *op. cit.,* p. 491-516.
81. Kostenbauder, H.: *Developments in Industrial Microbiology,* Plenum Press, New York, 1962, vol. 3, p. 286.
82. Lachman, L.: *op. cit.,* p. 563-604.
83. Osol, A.: *op. cit.,* p. 1519-1544.
84. Martin, E. W.: *op. cit.,* p. 398-419.
85. Macek, T. J.: Preparation of Parenteral Dispersions, *J. Pharm. Sci. 52*:694-699 (July) 1963.
86. Spiegal, A. J. and Noseworthy, M. M.: Use of Nonaqueous Solvents in Parenteral Products, *J. Pharm. Sci. 52*: 917-927 (Oct) 1963.
87. Parrott, E.: *op. cit.,* chap. 10.
88. *Safety of Large Volume Parenteral Solutions,* Food and Drug Administration, Washington, D. C. 20204.
89. Lamy, P. P., Davies, W. L. and Kitler, M. E.: Contamination Control with Laminar Flow Hoods, *Hosp. Pharm. 3*:12-19 (July) 1968.
90. Lachman, L.: *op. cit.,* p. 711-749.

19

Principles of formulation of parenteral dosage forms

by Anthony P. Simonelli and David S. Dresback

The injection of sterile dosage forms of drugs through or into the skin offers many advantages in drug therapy. Thus it is imperative that the clinical pharmacist thoroughly understands the principles behind the design of parenteral dosage forms, the rationale of parenteral therapy, and the methods of preparation. The pharmacist must have an adequate background in physiology, physical pharmacy, microbiology, chemistry, and biopharmaceutics in order to properly prepare parenteral dosage forms or, for that matter, to properly handle parenterals in the hospital. Thus it is seen that the study of parenteral preparations successfully brings together nearly all of the disciplines of the undergraduate pharmacy curriculum.

It is not the purpose of this chapter to present a complete preparation manual for parenteral production nor to discuss the organization of a parenteral production area. There are many excellent sources for this information and a number of these are listed in the bibliography.[1-5] In addition these references will be referred to in the text at the appropriate times. The purpose of this chapter, on the other hand, is to present and discuss important physico-chemical principles in order to form a firm foundation for the understanding of the design, the preparation, and the use of parenteral preparations. As compared to the other dosage forms, parenteral dosage forms offer numerous advantages in drug therapy. They can provide an immediate blood level of a given drug which is invaluable in many emergency situations; they are useful in administering medication to the unwilling, nauseous, or comatose patient; they provide blood levels which are usually predictable and thus they are invaluable in clinical investigation as well as in other forms of therapy that require accurate dosage control. Parenteral dosage forms are usually of a liquid nature and therefore can be easily used to accurately administer varied dosages to the patient. The accuracy of dosages given parenterally is enhanced by the fact that usually the drug is administered by a professional in a controlled hospital setting. In addition, parenteral therapy is the only way that is presently available to the physician to increase the blood volume of a patient. Finally, it is also possible to alter parenteral dosage forms in such a way that the blood levels and duration of action obtained from them can be markedly changed to suit the purpose of the physician. This last advantage, coupled with the many routes of administration available for parenteral products, has provided the major impetus for the development of the wide range of applications of parenteral products that exists today.

Unfortunately, there also are disadvantages in the preparation and the use of parenteral dosage forms. Since the medication is injected directly into the body any type of patient reaction or toxicity is greatly increased and very difficult to reverse. Moreover, the preparation of parenterals presents a number of problems not common to other dosage forms in that they must be sterile, pyrogen free, and free from particulate matter.

MODIFICATION OF THE BLOOD CONCENTRATION vs TIME PROFILE

The pharmacist is often called upon to prepare a formulation that will provide either a very rapid or a prolonged therapeutic response. In practice there are a number of ways available to achieve control of the therapeutic response and they include the following:

1. the choice of the route of administration;
2. the choice of an adjunct drug therapy;
3. the choice of a specific drug analog or combination of analogs; and
4. the choice of the specific ingredients and quantities to be included in the formulation.

Before discussing the techniques that can be utilized to alter the onset and duration of blood concentration profiles of drugs, it would be appropriate to first describe a biological model which will be useful in subsequent discussions. The model illustrated in Figure 1, is applicable to a drug that is administered at a non-therapeutic site and is transported via the blood stream to the therapeutic site of action. Figure 1 schematically shows the pathway of a drug for these conditions from the time it is released from the dosage form to the time it reaches the site of its pharmacological activity. This model or a part of it with minor modifications is applicable to all types of medication regardless of the route of administration or dosage form. The model shows that the drug first must be released from its dosage form (compartment I) to the biological fluid (compartment II) at the site of administration. The biological fluid, for example, would be the gastric fluid for a drug taken orally or the rectal fluid for a drug inserted via a suppository. Of course, the formulation can be a member of any class of preparation, for example, a solution, an emulsion or a suspension. After its release from the administered dosage form, the drug must be transported through the biological fluid to the barrier (compartment III) which separates the biological fluids from the blood stream. This barrier obviously will not be

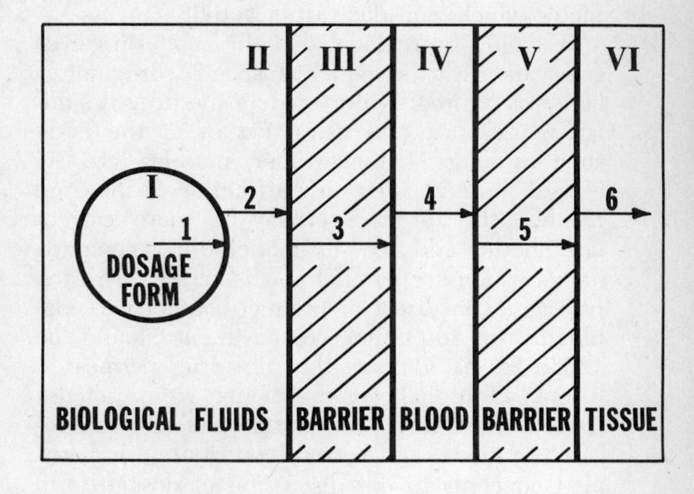

Figure 1: A schematic of a model depicting the transport of drug from its dosage form to the site of action.
Step 1: Release of drug from its dosage form (I) to the biological fluid (II)
Step 2: Transport of drug from dosage form interface to the biological barrier (III)
Step 3: Permeation of drug through the barrier to the blood (IV)
Step 4: Transport of drug through the blood to the biological barrier (V)
Step 5: Transport of drug through the biological barrier
Step 6: Transport of drug from the barrier interface to the site of action

the same for all sites of administration and for this reason it will be left ambiguous. The barrier, however, does include all tissues between the biological fluids and the blood and therefore consists of membranes, fluids, walls, etc. After the drug permeates this barrier into the blood (compartment IV), it is transported via the bloodstream to all parts of the body. Before the drug can reach the desired site of action (compartment VI), it must first permeate another barrier (compartment V) which again can consist of a combination of membranes, fluids, walls, etc. The above model clearly shows that the route of administration can significantly affect the blood concentration profile of a drug as each route would involve different components in each of the compartments. It is generally safe to assume that an increase in concentration of the drug in the blood will result in an increase in the driving force for the transport of drug to the site of action. Thus, in the subsequent discussion it will be assumed that an increase in blood concentration will result in an increase in drug activity and vice versa. For the drugs in which an increase in blood concentration does not affect the biological activity, the absorption rate is not important. Therefore, in the latter case, the alteration of the dosage form is not a factor which can affect drug activity.

It should be realized that this model involves only the tissue in which a specific drug interaction is desired. Unfortunately the drug is similarly transported to many tissues of the body such as lungs, kidneys, liver, muscles, etc. As a result in most cases only a fraction of the drug reaches the target site. To be more correct one should add to this model other compartments which are parallel and in series with each other, and in direct or indirect contact with the blood. An additional compartment should be added for each tissue that the drug permeates. These additional compartments were not included since they would unnecessarily complicate the model and yet not contribute any pertinent concepts to our discussion of dosage form design.

Parenteral Routes of Administration

The most rapid onset of drug activity obviously would be achieved by direct administration to the site of action since all of the compartments, I through V, in Figure 1 are circumvented. Examples of this approach are many and include intrathecal, intracisternal, direct cardiac injection, intradermal injections and intravenous injections when the target site is a component of the blood. Direct administration to the site of action often must be utilized when the barriers imposed by compartments III or V severely prevent the drug from reaching a therapeutic concentration at the desired site. An example of this is the brain barrier. Many drugs do not pass through this barrier to an appreciable extent and therefore these drugs must be injected directly into the cerebro-spinal cavity.

Direct injections to the desired site of action are not always possible, and in these cases an intravenous injection is generally used when rapid onset of activity is desired. These injections are made directly into the blood stream and thereby circumvent compartments I through III. For intramuscular or subcutaneous injections, on the other hand, the drug must be transported through all the compartments shown in Figure 1. As a result, when compared to intravenous injections, these injections usually do not provide a rapid onset but do produce a longer duration of drug activity. Thus by varying the route of administration, one can significantly alter the onset and duration of therapeutic activity of a drug administered

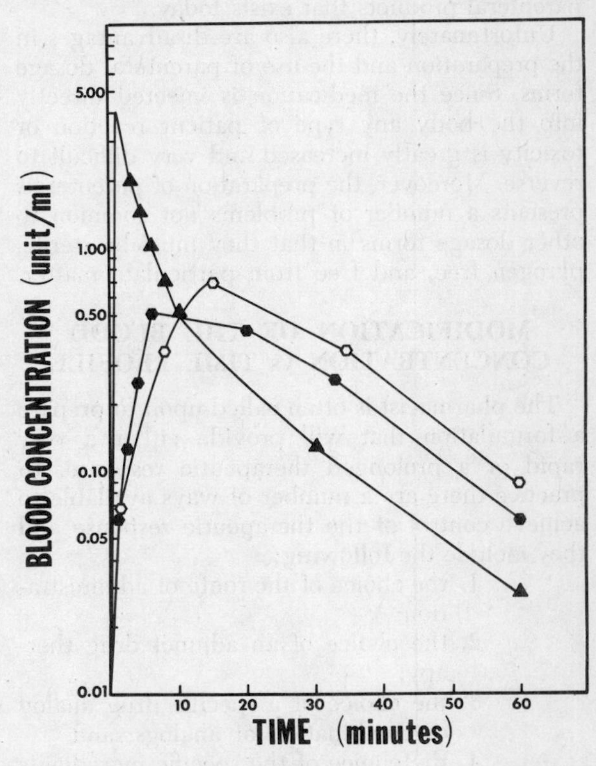

Figure 2: The effect of the route of administration on blood concentration of penicillin as a function of time following the injection of 15,000 units. Taken from reference 6.
▲ Intravenous
○ Subcutaneous
● Intramuscular

parenterally. This is illustrated by Figure 2 which shows the blood concentration as a function of time for penicillin administered by the various parenteral routes.[6] These data confirm that intravenous injections provide maximum blood concentrations more rapidly than either intramuscular or subcutaneous injections.

Adjunct Drugs

Adjunct drug therapy can also be utilized to alter the response of a given drug. An adjunct drug is one that is not the principal therapeutic agent but merely modifies the overall pharmacological activity of the primary drug. The administration of probenicid during penicillin therapy provides an excellent example of the use of this method to alter the drug blood concentration of the therapeutic agent. In this case the probenicid has been shown to compete with penicillin in the biochemical mechanism responsible for penicillin excretion by the kidney tubules.[7] As a result the penicillin blood levels are higher and of longer duration for a given dose of penicillin if administered to a patient who has been treated with probenicid than if given to a patient who has not been treated with probenicid. It seems reasonable to assume that higher blood levels for longer periods of time should also result in higher and longer tissue concentrations since the driving force (difference in concentration) of the drug through compartment V of the model shown in Figure 1 is greater and of longer duration. The use of probenicid to increase blood levels and thus minimize the dose needed was an important one during the early development of penicillin therapy when penicillin was extremely expensive. Another example which is more prevalent today is the concurrent administration of epinephrine with local anesthetics. The local vasoconstriction caused by the use of epinephrine provides a longer anesthetic activity.[7] Figure 1 can again be used to illustrate. It shows that the drug should remain at the site of injection for a longer period of time if the rate of transport through compartment III is decreased, thereby resulting in longer local anesthesia. Hyaluronidase[8] has been used in the past as an adjunct drug to cause the therapeutic drug to permeate the tissues of compartment III more rapidly, thus resulting in more rapid absorption.

Drug Analogs

There are a number of examples reported in the literature which illustrate the altering of the drug response by the use of drug analogs. Drug analogs are compounds which are obtained by altering the substituents of a parent compound. Barbiturates illustrate this principle very well. The onset, duration, and the degree of activity of barbituric acid is markedly affected by the use of different substituents and, in fact, these differences are the very basis of barbiturate classification.[7] The sulfa drugs make up another class of drugs which, although not normally injected parenterally, should be included in this discussion. A change in the substituents of the parent sulfa compound can cause the excretion rate, metabolism, and even the site of activity to change drastically.[9] As seen in Table 1, the biological half-life of these sulfa derivatives is considerably altered by changes of the parent compound.

Table 1. Biological Half-Life ($t_{1/2}$) in Man[9]

DRUG	$t_{1/2}$ (HR)
Sulfamethylthiadiazole	2
Sulfaethidole	8
Sulfisoxazole	8
Sulfamethoxypyridazine	34

Although the above methods can be utilized to control the blood level profile of a drug, these methods are severely limited by the clinical situation, physician requirements, etc. Alteration of the formulation, however, can provide a number of ways to control the blood level profile and is relatively independent of the biological process of absorption. In addition, this approach offers the added advantage that the release rate of the drug from the dosage form can often be correlated to *in vitro* experiments and to *a priori* predictions using physico-chemical fundamentals. For this reason our attention will be directed to the alteration of the formulation as a means to control blood levels of drugs.

PARENTERAL FORMULATIONS

Intravenous Injection Formulations

The intravenous injection of a drug is the administration technique of choice when the maximum blood level of a drug must be achieved as rapidly as possible. The blood concentration reaches a maximum very quickly after an intravenous injection since the injected drug solution rapidly mixes with the blood. This time of mixing is approximately four minutes. It would be expected that the duration of a single intravenous injection would be a function of the dose administered because a higher initial drug concentration in the blood would logically result in a longer duration of drug presence. The specific effect that the dose has on the duration of the blood level depends upon the mechanism responsible for the removal of the drug from the bloodstream. The rate of disappearance of a drug from the blood will be controlled by biological processes such as excretion, metabolism, degradation, tissue uptake and so forth. For most drugs the overall elimination process is first order, which means that in a given time a certain fraction of the drug in the blood stream will disappear regardless of the initial concentration. The time required for one half of the drug to disappear from the blood is called the "biological half-life" of the drug and can differ widely from one drug to another. For example, the biological half-life ($t_{1/2}$) of sulfaethidole is 8 hours and that of sulfamethoxypyridazine is 34 hours.[9] Since the elimination process is generally first order it should be noted that increasing the dose by a given factor does not necessarily increase the duration of drug activity by the same factor. This can be illustrated with the aid of Figure 3 which shows the serum concentration resulting from intravenous injections containing different concentrations of penicillin.[10] If we assume that 0.03 units of penicillin per ml of serum is necessary for antimicrobial activity, it is seen that an increase in the doses illustrated in Figure 3 does not uniformly increase the duration of activity by the same proportion.

If the elimination process is first order a rule of thumb can be stated as follows: "The doubling of a dose injected intravenously does not double the duration but merely extends it one half-life." Similarly, quadrupling the dose extends the duration only two half-lives. Finally by increasing the dose of the drug eight times the duration of activity will be extended by only three half-lives. The application of the above half-life rule can be illustrated by data previously reported for penicillin injections.[11] The experimental points and the solid line curve shown in Figure 4 were reproduced from the article. Using other data reported in the same article, one can estimate the biological half-life to be one hour. This half-life and the above half-life rule of thumb were used to calculate the theoretical curve of the corresponding duration for the doses shown in Figure 4. The theoretical curve represented by the linear dotted line shows excellent agreement with the experimentally observed data and therefore confirms the validity of this rule. This concept indicates that the use of an increased dose for an intra-

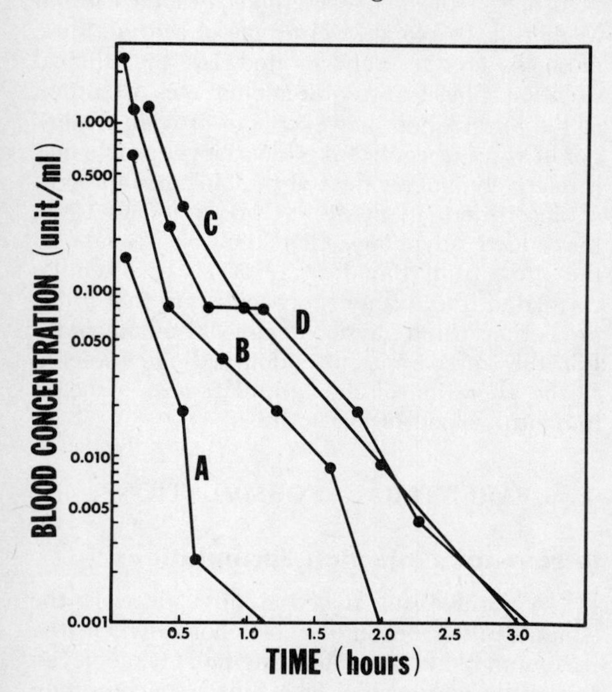

Figure 3: The effect of the dose on blood concentration of penicillin as a function of time following intravenous injection. Taken from reference 10.
A = 5,000 units
B = 10,000 units
C = 20,000 units
D = 40,000 units

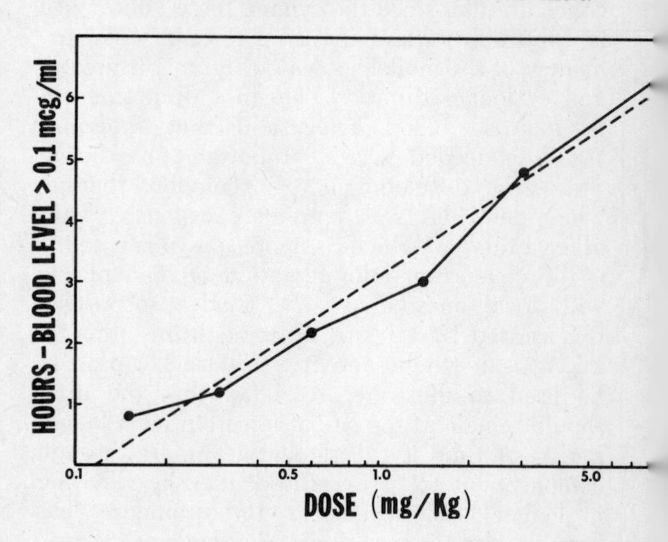

Figure 4. Time for which various doses of penicillin G administered intramuscularly provided serum concentrations in excess of 0.1 microgram/ml. Taken from reference 11.
● Experimental data points taken from reference
——— Curve shown in reference
- - - - - Theoretical curve calculated using a half-life of one hour

venous injection for the purpose of increasing the duration of drug activity is not very fruitful, since an increased duration of activity generally would be only desirable for drugs with a rather short biological half-life which require prohibitively high doses to significantly change the duration of activity. In order to obtain a sustained blood concentration by the intravenous method the physician must resort to other techniques such as continuous intravenous drip or frequent injections. It is possible that protein binding, complexation, prodrugs and so forth can be used to provide prolonged drug activity. These methods, however, require extensive research to perfect and are normally not available to the clinical pharmacist.

Intramuscular and Subcutaneous Injection Formulations

An intramuscular or subcutaneous injection, on the other hand, always provides a much longer, although lower, blood level than an intravenous injection for a given dose. This is shown by the data illustrated in Figure 2. The reason for this is evident since the biological model shown in Figure 1 shows that, opposed to intravenous injections, compartments I, II, and III are now operative, thus decreasing the rate of absorption. Another important difference between intramuscular or subcutaneous injections and intravenous injections is that the dosage forms intended for intramuscular or subcutaneous use can be altered in order to control the blood level as a function of time. However, the use of these changes can be successful only in systems in which the slowest step in the absorption process is the release of drug from the formulation and not in which the slowest step is the transport of drug through the biological tissues or fluids. This fact follows from the rule that states: *a process which follows a series of consecutive steps will proceed at the rate of the slowest step.* The slowest step of the process is usually referred to as the "rate determining" or "rate limiting step" of the process. The application of this principle can be illustrated using Figure 5.

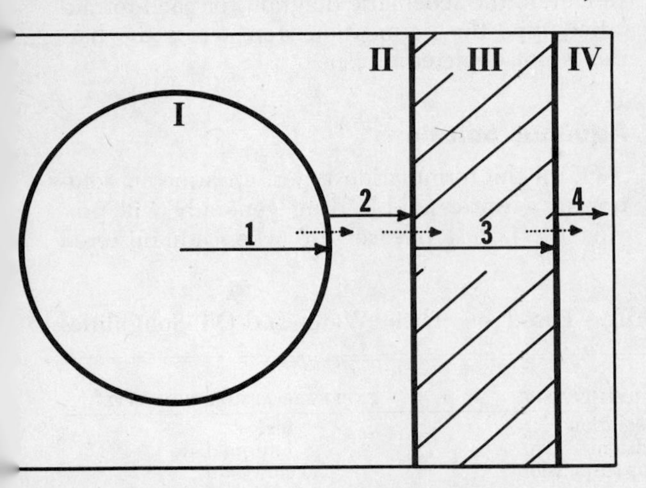

Figure 5: A schematic of a model depicting transport of drug from its dosage form to the blood.
Step 1: Transport of drug from within the dosage form (I) to its interface with the biological fluid (II)
Step 2: Transport through the fluid to the biological barrier (III)
Step 3: Transport through the barrier to the barrier-blood interface
Step 4: Transport through the blood
(•••>) Dotted arrows represent transfer processes from one compartment to another

The model shown in Figure 5 is an expanded and more detailed representation of a part of the model previously shown in Figure 1. Figure 5 will be more useful than Figure 1 at this point since it focuses our attention on the release of drug from the dosage form to the fluid at the site of administration. It is intuitive that the rate of appearance of drug in the blood stream will be a function of the rate of transfer of drug across the barrier (III) and the rate of release of drug from the dosage form. Since the process of absorption is made up of consecutive steps, the slowest step will control the rate of absorption. If the rate of absorption from the biological fluids is relatively rapid with respect to the rate of release from the dosage form, then the release rate from the dosage form will be the rate determining step. With this in mind it is easily seen that there are many ways available for the control of the release rate of drugs from either subcutaneous or intramuscular injections. For example, one can use solutions, suspensions, or even solid implants. Subsequent material will indicate that often the release rate from a dosage form either is or can be made the rate limiting step of the drug absorption process.

In the discussion that follows there will be no differentiation of dosage forms intended for either intramuscular or subcutaneous use. The principles that will be discussed are similar since essentially the same model is applicable for both (Figure 5). It should be kept in mind, though, that a given dosage form given by the intramuscular route will not provide the same release profiles if given by the subcutaneous route. As previously explained, the components of the compartments in Figure 1 would be different for the two routes.

There are various ways to classify the approaches which have been used in parenteral dosage form design. The rate of release of the drug from any intramuscular or subcutaneous dosage form will depend on the chemical and physical properties of the drug. For example, the effect on the absorption rate of a pH change in the vehicle will depend on the drug type (*i.e.*, acid, base or neutral). This suggests that one method of discussing these dosage forms could be based upon the physical-chemical properties of the drug.

One physical property which provides a convenient classification scheme is the solubility of the drug. Solubility data are usually easy to obtain (*e.g.*, from the *Merck Index*) and will allow the formulator to determine the type of formulations that are available to him for the particular drug in question. Table 2 lists the type of formulations that can be used for each of the solubility types of drugs. One should recall that often a drug can exist either as a water-soluble salt or as the non-ionized species which is usually water-insoluble. As discussed in the previous chapter, the ratio of the above two species will be dependent on the pH and the characteristic pKa of the drug. Thus it is seen that by proper pH adjustment it may be possible for a drug to be classified in either the water-soluble or water-insoluble class depending on the dosage form needed.

Although the classification listed in Table 2 indicates the formulation types that are available for a given drug solubility type, its usefulness to the formulator is limited. One must first understand the physico-chemical principles involved in the release of a drug from each formulation type before he can successfully design formulations to fit given drug release needs. For a better understanding of these principles the discussion in this chapter will follow a classification based on the type of formulation. Starting with the system containing the minimum possible number of rate determining steps (an aqueous solution), the discussion will proceed to the most complex system (an oleaginous suspension). With this in mind the formulation types will be discussed in the following order.

1. Aqueous solutions
2. Aqueous suspensions
3. Oleaginous solutions
4. Oil-in-water emulsions
5. Water-in-oil emulsions
6. Oleaginous suspensions

The fate of each type of formulation upon injection will be illustrated by a schematic diagram showing the physical situation at the injection site at the time of injection ($t=0$) as well as a diagram representing the physical situation at some time later ($t=t$). As the discussion proceeds from one system to another, new processes will be progressively introduced which may or may not affect the rate or the duration of drug activity. Although occasionally the rate of transfer across the barrier (compartment III in Figure 5) is the rate limiting step, it should be re-emphasized that the following discussion will involve only those situations in which the rate of release from the dosage form is rate limiting. In fact, in the schematic diagram for each formulation type the permeation step across the barrier is not depicted.

Aqueous Solutions

Of all the formulation types, an aqueous solution of a water-soluble drug generally will provide the fastest release rate when administered

Table 2. Parenteral Formulations Available for Drugs—Based on Their Water-and-Oil Solubilities

	SOLUBILITY			
	WATER	OIL	FORMULATION TYPE	EXPECTED ABSORPTION RATE*
(1)	yes	no	aqueous solution w/o emulsion oleaginous suspension	fastest intermediate slowest
(2)	no	yes	o/w emulsion oleaginous solution aqueous suspension	fastest intermediate slowest
(3)	no	no	aqueous suspension oleaginous suspension	fastest slowest
(4)	yes	yes	aqueous solution oleaginous solution	fastest slowest

*No doubt there are many exceptions to these predictions, but these predictions will serve as the first estimate if no other information is available. In general, the formulation that provides the faster drug release would provide a shorter duration of drug activity, while the slow release formulation will result in a longer duration of activity.

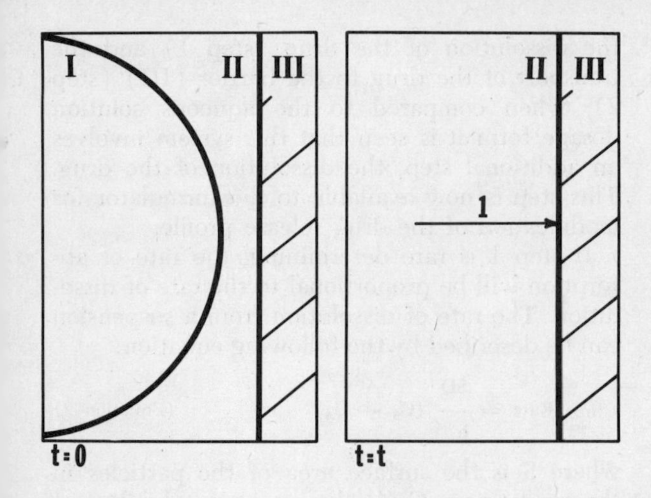

Figure 6: A schematic of a model depicting release of drug from an intramuscular or subcutaneous injection of an aqueous solution.
t = 0: Exact time of injection (no mixing has occurred)
t = t: Situation at some later time. All release processes are participating
Step 1: Transport of drug through the biological fluid (II) to the biological barrier (III)

by the intramuscular or subcutaneous route. The physical situation at the site of injection for this dosage form is illustrated by Figure 6. At t = 0 the schematic shows the system at the exact time the aqueous solution is injected, and at t = t the schematic shows the system after sufficient time has passed so that the injected fluid has mixed with the biological fluid and all of the transport processes involved in the absorption process are participating. Note that the dosage form (I) itself is no longer depicted at t = t because the injection fluid has readily mixed with the biological fluid of the tissues to produce a homogeneous solution. Thus there are only two processes occurring at this time which are necessary for absorption. The first process involves drug transport from the bulk of the solution (II) at the injection site (II) to the barrier (III), step 1 in Figure 6. The second process involves the permeation of the drug through the biological barrier, and thereby be rate determining. Of course, either step may be rate determining. It is possible, for example, that in a resting patient the transport of drug through the biological fluid may occur by a slower process than the permeation of drug through the barrier and thereby be rate determining. In an active patient the turbulence caused by the continuous flexing of the tissue at the injection site may cause the drug to be rapidly transported through the biological fluid. In this case the rate of permeation of the drug through the barrier may be slower than the transport process, and thus the rate of barrier permeation may be rate limiting.

It was reported that intramuscular injections of penicillin given at 9 p.m. to hospitalized patients gave consistently higher blood levels after 12 and 24 hours when compared to the same dose given at 9 a.m.[12] These results were explained by a decreased activity at the injection sites of the resting patients.[12] Thus these results are in good agreement with the above model.

The transport of drug to the barrier (step 1) is the only process in this dosage form which can be altered by the clinical pharmacist. For a diffusion controlled process the rate of transport can be shown to be:

$$\text{Rate} = \frac{DA}{h}(C_A - C_B) \qquad \text{(Equation 1)}$$

where D is the aqueous diffusion coefficient for the drug; A is the cross sectional surface area of the interface between the biological fluids and the so-called biological barrier; h is the width of the aqueous diffusion layer through which the drug is diffusing; C_A is the concentration in the bulk of the biological fluids; and C_B is the drug contentration at the interface. When the transport process is rate determining, the concentration at the barrier interface, C_B, generally will be zero since the drug is removed rapidly from the barrier interface by the faster permeation process. In addition, A and h will be constant. The above equation will then reduce to the following equation: Rate = k DC_A where k is the constant A/h. This equation shows that there are two variables, the bulk concentration and the diffusion coefficient, which can be altered by the clinical pharmacist in order to control the absorption rate of the drug. Although the aqueous diffusion coefficient can be altered by changing the viscosity of the medium at the injection site, this approach is not useful in this system because the final viscosity is independent of that belonging to the dosage form. At t = t the dosage form has been greatly diluted by the biological fluid, thus the viscosity of the fluid at the injection site has remained essentially unchanged.

The rate of absorption of a drug is directly proportional to the resultant concentration of drug in the biological fluid after injection. This resultant concentration is a function of the amount of drug injected. Consequently, the rate of absorption can be altered by changing either the concentration or volume of a given injection. Unfortunately both approaches are limited. The volume of injection is often limited by patient tolerance and drug concentration is limited by solubility of the drug. The solubility of a compound, however, often can be increased by the use of various salts, complexes or solvents. In summary, an aqueous solution provides the formulator with a very limited number of variables than can be used to increase the rate of absorption and no variable that can be used to effectively control the duration of biological activity.

Aqueous Suspensions

The duration of release obtained after the intramuscular or subcutaneous administration of an aqueous suspension is longer than that obtained when the aqueous solution of the drug is administered. In addition, a suspension must occasionally be utilized in order to administer a required dose of a poorly soluble drug.

The model illustrating the release of drug from this dosage form is seen in Figure 7. At t = t, it is seen that the aqueous vehicle of the dosage form (I) has mixed with the biological fluid (II) at the injection site causing the original (t = 0) dosage form interface to disappear. This model illustrates the steps which must occur in order for the drug to reach the biological barrier (III). These steps include

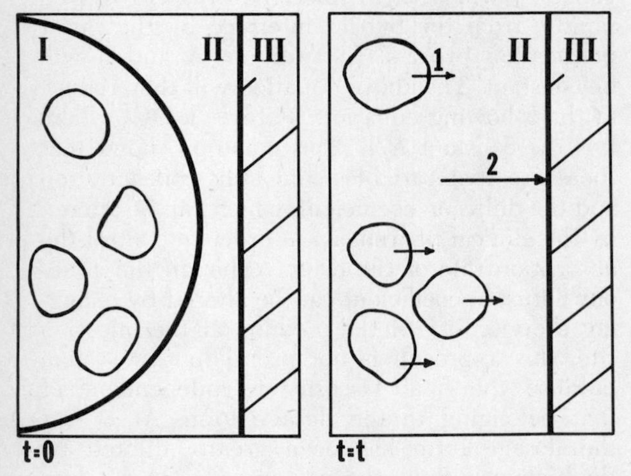

Figure 7: A schematic of a model depicting release of drug from an intramuscular or subcutaneous injection of an aqueous suspension.
t = 0: Exact time of injection (no mixing has occurred)
t = t: Situation at some later time. All release processes are participating
Step 1: Release of drug (dissolution)
Step 2: Transport of drug through the biological fluid (II) to the biological barrier (III)

the dissolution of the drug (step 1) and the transport of the drug to the barrier (III) (step 2); when compared to the aqueous solution dosage form it is seen that this system involves an additional step, the dissolution of the drug. This step is now available to the formulator for modification of the drug release profile.

If step 1 is rate determining, the rate of absorption will be proportional to the rate of dissolution. The rate of dissolution from a suspension can be described by the following equation:

$$\text{Rate} = \frac{SD}{h}(C_S - C_A) \qquad \text{(Equation 2)}$$

where S is the surface area of the particles in the suspension, C_S is the aqueous solubility of the drug, and the variables C_A, D and h have the same meaning as in Equation 1. For the same reasons previously given for aqueous solutions, D and h are not useful in the control of release profiles. Equation 2 shows that the alteration of surface area of the particles and solubility of the drug, on the other hand, can be very useful when step 1 is rate determining. The alteration in the solubility of a drug will be discussed briefly in a subsequent section of this chapter and a more thorough discussion will be found in the previous chapter.

By examining Equation 2, it is seen that the release rate is directly proportional to the surface area of the particles. The total surface area of a given amount of drug in suspension can be significantly increased by decreasing the size of the particles suspended. This permits one to control the release rate of the drug from the dosage form. It should be understood, however, that doubling the surface area of the particles for a given dose of a suspension may double the rate of drug release, but in doing so, it obviously will decrease the duration of drug release by the same factor.

Suspended particles of drugs will often undergo Ostwald Ripening, which is the growth of large crystals at the expense of small ones. This process will drastically alter the surface area of the particles as a function of time, and will result in unpredictable release profiles. It has been reported that steroid suspension particles, for example, can undergo alterations of size with time and thus give inconsistent blood levels when injected.[13] Obviously, it must be ascertained that the particles in a formulated suspension do not change their particle size distribution as a function of time. When particle size changes do occur, the use of peptizing agents can sometimes eliminate the problem.

The total surface area of suspended particles also can be increased by increasing the amount of drug suspended. The total surface area of the suspended particles, and hence the absorption rate of the drug, will be directly proportional to the amount suspended if the particle size is constant and step 1 is rate determining. It should be noted that under these conditions the duration of drug absorption does not change.

The effect of these changes will be different if step 2 is rate determining since Equation 1 will be controlling the release profile rather than Equation 2. Equation 1 shows that the rate of diffusion in the biological fluid, and hence the absorption rate of the drug under these conditions, is a function of the solubility of the drug but independent of the surface area of the particles.

It should be noted, however, that increasing the amount of drug suspended in a given dose volume, when step 2 is rate determining, can significantly increase the duration of drug release without causing a significant increase in the rate of release. This is true since the rate of drug release does not increase with an increase in the amount suspended. This is important in situations when the duration must be increased without an increase in rate. For example, an increase in rate would not be indicated for drugs exhibiting side effects or toxicity since increased peak blood levels would be undesirable. This increase in duration can be explained in the following way: as soon as the drug is removed from the biological fluid it is replaced by the drug which is dissolving. As a result, the concentration of drug in the fluid is constant even though the processes involved are not in equilibrium. This condition is called the "steady state" condition. The duration of this steady state condition for the suspension will depend on the amount of drug originally suspended. Since the concentration of the drug in solution during this time is constant, the rate remains unchanged. It is seen that the duration of drug release, when step 2 is rate determining, can be altered independently of the rate of drug release by simply adjusting the amount of drug suspended.

It would be worthwhile at this point to summarize the above discussion in a way which will permit the clinical pharmacist to make better use of the concepts presented in this section. Tables 3 and 4 tabulate the ways that an aqueous suspension formulation type can be changed for the two rate limiting conditions in order to achieve a desired result. Table 3 is useful when the rate of solution of the drug is so slow that this process becomes the rate determining step of the release process. If the dissolution rate is sufficiently increased, however, so that it is much faster than the rate of transport to the membrane, the transport step will then become the rate determining step and Table 4 will be applicable. The variables of this dosage form are the solubility of the drug in the medium, the size of the suspended particles, and the amount of drug suspended.

Table 3 shows that if the rate determining step is the rate of solution of the suspended drug particles, then the rate of absorption of the drug from an injected aqueous suspension can be increased by increasing the solubility of the drug in the medium, by decreasing particle size, and

Table 3. The Comparison of the Effects of Several Variables Upon the Rate and Duration of Drug Release from Either Oil or Aqueous Suspensions When the Rate Determining Step Is the Rate of Solution (Step 1, Figures 7 and 10)

FORMULATION VARIABLE			EFFECT ON RELEASE	
SOLUBILITY[a]	PARTICLE SIZE	TOTAL AMOUNT[b] OF DRUG	RATE	DURATION[c]
constant	constant	increase	increase	unchanged
constant	constant	decrease	decrease	unchanged
constant	decrease	constant	increase	decrease
constant	increase	constant	decrease	increase
increase	constant	constant	increase	decrease
decrease	constant	constant	decrease	increase

(a) Solubility in water for an aqueous suspension, solubility in oil for an oleaginous suspension.
(b) Includes the total amount of drug per dose; both suspended and in solution.
(c) The duration of absorption will be equal to the duration of release for the stated conditions. The duration of drug activity, however, is a function of tissue distribution, mechanism of elimination, biodegradation, etc. and thus is not necessarily equal to the duration of drug release.

Table 4. The Comparison of the Effects of Several Variables Upon the Rate and Duration of Drug Release from an Aqueous Suspension When the Rate Determining Step Is the Rate of Drug Transport to the Barrier (Step 2, Figure 7)

FORMULATION VARIABLE			EFFECT OF RELEASE	
AQUEOUS SOLUBILITY	PARTICLE SIZE	TOTAL AMOUNT OF DRUG[a]	RATE	DURATION[b]
constant	constant	increase	unchanged	increase
constant	constant	decrease	unchanged	decrease
constant	decrease	constant	unchanged	unchanged
constant	increase	constant	unchanged	unchanged
increase	constant	constant	increase	decrease
decrease	constant	constant	decrease	increase

(a) Includes the total amount of drug per dose, both suspended and in solution.
(b) The duration of absorption will be equal to the duration of release for the stated conditions. The duration of drug activity, however, is a function of tissue distribution, mechanism of elimination, biodegradation, etc., and thus is not necessarily equal to the duration of drug release.

by increasing the amount of drug suspended per dose. The rate of absorption can be decreased by the opposite adjustment of these variables, singly or in combination. It should be noted, however, that if the solubility or particle size is used to adjust the rate, the duration of release of the drug will also be affected by the same factor but in an inverse manner. The duration of release, on the other hand, is not changed when the amount of drug suspended is used to adjust the rate of release. One can also use a combination of these changes to obtain a particular release profile. For example, the particle size or solubility can be used to adjust the duration of release and the amount suspended can be used to alter the rate of release. To illustrate further, if the solubility of the drug is reduced by a factor of 2, the rate of release will be decreased by a factor of 2 and the duration of release will be increased by a factor of 2. If the amount of drug suspended is simultaneously increased by a factor of 4, both the rate as well as duration of release will be doubled.

Table 4, on the other hand, shows the effect of the above variables upon the rate and duration of drug release when the rate determining step is the rate of transport to the membrane. For example, reducing the particle size in this case will not affect either the rate or duration of drug release. Here the rate is seen to be directly proportional to solubility while duration is inversely proportional to solubility. It is interesting to note that the amount of drug injected has no effect on the rate but can be used to alter the duration of release. A combination of solubility and amount suspended can be used in this situation to obtain a desired profile. For example, if the solubilty is doubled and the amount suspended quadrupled, both the rate and duration of release will be doubled. When the rate of drug transport is rate limiting, it is seen that the situation is the same as that for an aqueous solution except for one important difference, *i.e.*, the suspended particles act as a reservoir and increase the duration of activity.

In conclusion it is seen that the clinical pharmacist can enjoy a relatively firm control of the release profile of a drug suspended in a vehicle since both the maximum blood level and duration of blood levels of a drug can be controlled by the formulation design.

Oleaginous Solutions

Often an oleaginous solution is preferred for a water-insoluble drug since this eliminates any concern for the physical instability inherent in suspension type formulations, such as particle size or polymorphic transitions, chemical instability of drugs in water, or difficulties which arise during the preparation of a particular suspension. The model depicting the injection site for this dosage form is shown in Figure 8. At $t = 0$ the model appears to be the same as the model used for the aqueous solution shown in Figure 6, but at a later time the oleaginous model involves more processes due to the immiscibility of the oil and biological fluid. It is this situation that provides additional means to control drug release. Figure 8 shows that the drug must be transported across the oleaginous phase (I) to the oil interface, must be extracted into the biological fluid (II), and then must be transported to the biological barrier (III). When the last step (the rate of transport through the biological fluids) to the barrier is rate determin-

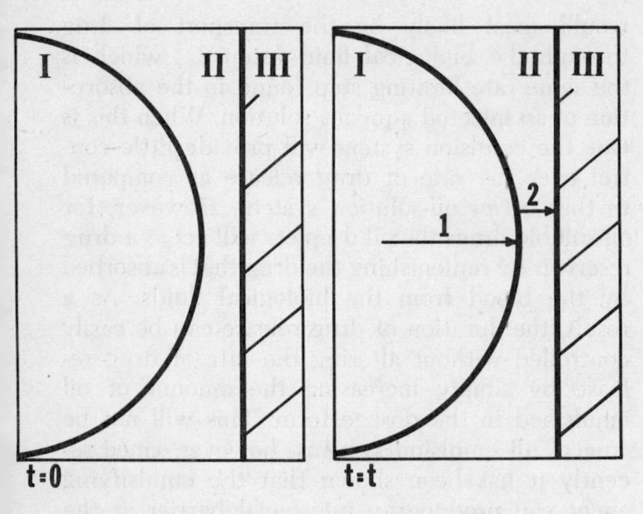

Figure 8: A schematic of a model depicting release of drug from an intramuscular or subcutaneous injection of an oleaginous solution
t = 0: Exact time of injection (no mixing has occurred)
t = t: Situation at some later time. All release processes are participating
Step 1: Transport of drug through the oil phase to the oil-biological fluid (II) interface
Step 2: Transport of drug through the biological fluid (II) to the biological barrier (III)

ing, little control of the rate or duration of the drug release can be obtained by changes in the formulation. The previous discussion (aqueous solutions) of this step applies equally well in this case. Fortunately, due to the different viscosity and the different diffusional pathways existing in the oil and the biological fluid, the rate of transport through the biological fluids generally will not be the rate determining step. The transfer of drug from the oil to the biological fluid is generally very rapid and therefore not expected to be the rate determining step of the release process. The partition coefficient, however, will predict the concentration of drug in the aqueous phase at the interface for a given concentration of drug in the oleaginous phase. Not being rate determining, this step is not useful for the control of drug release.

For injections of oleaginous solutions, the rate determining step generally will be the first step, the rate of transport of the drug through the oleaginous phase. Equation 1, presented in the discussion of aqueous solutions, also applies to the diffusion of a drug in oleaginous media providing the proper constants are introduced. It should be noted that in this system the area, A, of Equation 1 would be that of the oleaginous surface rather than that of the biological barrier. As opposed to aqueous solutions, the viscosity of the oleaginous phase can influence the rate of release. In this case the viscosity of the dosage form vehicle is not influenced by the biological fluid since the oil and tissue fluids are immiscible. Since the rate of diffusion is inversely proportional to the viscosity, the release rate of the drug can be decreased by increasing the viscosity of the oil. Again it should be recognized that if the amount of drug incorporated in the dosage form is kept constant and if the rate is increased then the duration will be decreased by the same factor.

Equation 1 also shows that the rate of drug release from injections of oleaginous solution will be proportional to the concentration of drug in the dosage form. In this case, however, the duration of drug release will remain constant because the amount of drug incorporated will be proportional to the concentration of drug in the oil if the volume of injection is kept constant.

For a solution of a given concentration, the rate of release will be a function of the volume injected but it may not be directly proportional to the volume. Equation 1 indicates that the rate will be directly proportional to the surface area of the oil injection, but the surface area may not be directly proportional to the volume. The relationship between surface area and volume depends upon the shape of the oil globule after injection, and, of course, this shape is unknown. However, if a spherical or cubical shape is assumed then the surface area is proportional to the two-thirds power of the volume injected. For example, increasing the volume (and therefore the dose) by a factor of 8 will only increase the rate by a factor of 4; whereas, increasing the total dose by a factor of 27 will only increase the rate by a factor of 9. Since the increase in the rate of release from the dosage form is less than the increase in dose, the duration of release must also increase with an increase in dose. The duration will be proportional to the volume of the dose to the one-third power.

In summary, the release profile of a drug resulting from an injection of an oleaginous solution can be adjusted by changes in the drug concentration, the viscosity and the volume of the injection. However, it should be recognized that in practice, the magnitude of the changes of these variables is rather limited due to factors

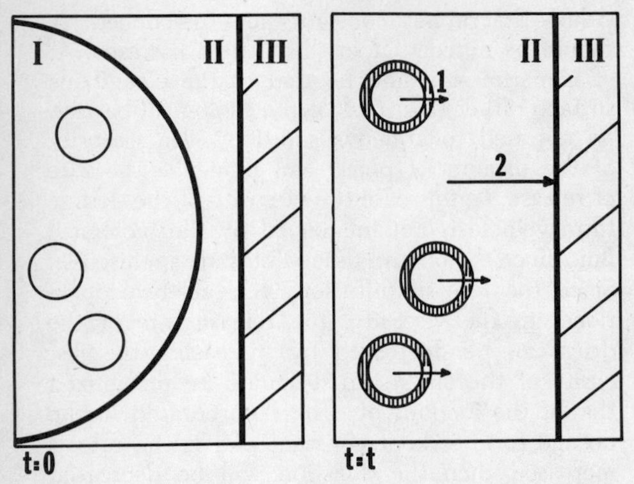

Figure 9: A schematic of a model depicting release of drug from an intramuscular or subcutaneous injection of an oil in water emulsion
t = 0: Exact time of injection (no mixing has occurred)
t = t: Situation at some later time. All release processes are participating
Step 1: Release of drug from the oil globules to the biological fluid (II)
Step 2: Transport of drug through the biological fluid (II) to the biological barrier (III)

such as a patient tolerance of large volumes of injections, limited drug solubility in oil, or inadequate syringeability of a highly viscous solution. Therefore, the release profiles can be only adjusted to a limited degree in this system.

Oil-in-Water Emulsions

Although the use of an oil-in-water emulsion for parenteral therapy is rare, the discussion of this dosage form is included here for the purposes of continuity. As seen in Figure 9, the aqueous phase of the dosage form (I) will be miscible with the biological fluid (II) and thereby lose its identity after injection. Superficially, it would appear that the release process is identical to that described for the oleaginous solution, but there are two important differences that cause the emulsion and oleaginous solution systems to behave differently. The diffusion layer thickness of emulsion globules is small compared to that of the oleaginous solution, and the total surface area of the emulsion oil globules is much larger. Thus according to Equation 1, the release rate of the drug from the oleaginous phase is much more rapid in the emulsion system than in the oil-solution system. This would indicate that for emulsions the rate determining step would most likely be the transport of drug through the biological fluid (step 2), which is the same rate limiting step found in the absorption of an injected aqueous solution. When this is true the emulsion system will provide little control over the rate of drug release as compared to that of an oil-solution system. However, for oil-soluble drugs the oil droplets will act as a drug reservoir by replenishing the drug that is absorbed by the blood from the biological fluids. As a result, the duration of drug release can be easily controlled without altering the rate of drug release by simply increasing the amount of oil emulsified in the dosage form. This will not be true of all emulsion systems, however, since recently it has been shown that the emulsifying agent can produce an interfacial barrier at the oil-water interface.[14] For example, properly formulated gelatin emulsions can inhibit drug transfer from the oleaginous phase to the aqueous phase by factors as large as 10,000.[14] It also was shown that the introduction of certain surfactants to this gelatin emulsion can greatly alter this rate of transfer.[15] Of course, if this rate of release were slowed significantly then the rate of drug release from the oil would possibly become the rate determining step. This would then give the formulator control over the release profile. However, it is not suggested here that the clinical pharmacist should attempt to control the rate of release by altering the emulsion system since a great deal of research is necessary to obtain a useful product.

In summary, oil-in-water emulsion systems are not often used for intramuscular or subcutaneous injection. This is probably due to the limited control of drug release that they afford and to the large amount of developmental research that is necessary.

Water-in-Oil Emulsions

As in the case of the oil-in-water emulsion system, the water-in-oil emulsion system is included in this discussion for purposes of continuity. This system is illustrated in Figure 10. After injection, the external phase of the emulsion dosage form (I) does not mix with the biological fluid (II), and as a result, it retains its identity after injection. When compared to the oil solution (Figure 8) at t = t, it is seen that this emulsion system has introduced a new release process, that is, the release of the drug from the aqueous globules to the external oleaginous medium of the dosage form. Of course, an interfacial barrier of an emulsifying agent or some

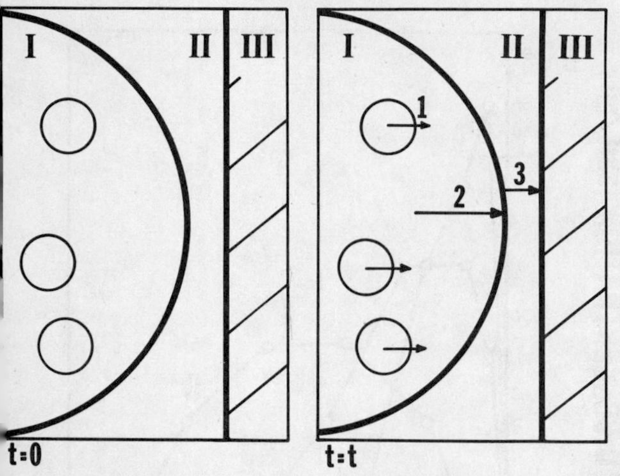

Figure 10: A schematic of a model depicting release of drug from an intramuscular or subcutaneous injection of an oleaginous suspension or a water-in-oil emulsion.

t = 0: Exact time of injection (no mixing has occurred)

t = t: Situation at some later time. All release processes are participating

Step 1: Release of drug from either water globules or solid particles (dissolution) to the oil phase

Step 2: Transport of drug through the oil to the oil-biological fluid interface

Step 3: Transport of drug through the biological fluid (II) to the biological barrier (III)

other additive can exist at the water-oil interface of the water globules in this emulsion system and can markedly alter absorption characteristics. For purposes of this discussion, it will be assumed that an interfacial barrier is not existing in the system. The possible effects of this system on blood profile data will depend upon the solubility characteristics of the drug. If the drug is oil-soluble almost all of the drug in the emulsion system would be in the oil phase, and as a result, the dosage form would behave much like the simple oleaginous solution. In this case the emulsion system should offer few new advantages. If the drug is water-soluble it would concentrate in the internal phase of the emulsion, the water phase, and this possibly would result in a longer duration of drug activity. It is likely that this dosage form system has not been utilized because the oleaginous suspension system, which will be discussed next, offers a more controllable formulation.

Oleaginous Suspensions

Contrasted to the emulsion systems, oleaginous suspensions have been widely used to control the release profile of drugs injected intramuscularly or subcutaneously. The schematic diagram used for the water-in-oil emulsion system (Figure 10) can be used to describe the release of drug from the oleaginous suspension system as well. The release of the drug from the dosage form and its transport to the barrier involve the following steps: step 1, the drug dissolves in the oil—its rate of solution being given by Equation 2; step 2, the drug diffuses through oleaginous media—its rate of diffusion being given by Equation 1; step 3, the drug partitions from the oil into the biological fluids and is transported to the biological barrier—the rate of transport being governed by Equation 1. Each of these steps offers several possibilities to the clinical pharmacist for the control of the release profile of the drug. Of course, Equation 2 is applicable only if the aqueous constants are replaced by those of the oleaginous system. As previously discussed under the topic of aqueous suspensions, there are a number of variables that can be used to control the dissolution rate and these include the alteration of the total surface area of the solid drug and the oil solubility of the drug. Another similarity to the aqueous suspension system is that the duration of activity can be increased under certain conditions by increasing the amount of suspended drug in the oil. The last variable in this system is the viscosity of the oleaginous media. This variable is found in the oleaginous solutions, but is absent in aqueous suspensions. Thus oleaginous suspensions seem to offer the advantages of both the aqueous suspension and the oleaginous solution system.

If the dissolution of the drug (step 1) is rate determining, then this dosage form will have the same release characteristics as an aqueous suspension with step 1 rate determining. Thus the rate of release can be altered by changing the particle size of the drug, by changing the solubility of the drug in oil, or by changing the amount of drug suspended. It should be noted, however, that if the particle size is increased excessively the particles may settle to the edge of the oleaginous-biological fluid interface and the drug then may be directly leached out by the biological fluid. This could result in an increase rather than the expected decrease in release rate. This change in mechanism will be a function of the particle size and the viscosity of the media. If the transport of the drug through the oil (step 2) is rate determining, then the release profile can be changed by the same variables described under oleaginous solutions as well as the variables discussed under aqueous suspensions in which the rate of transport is rate determining. For example, the release profile could be altered by changing viscosity of the media. This is often done by the addition of wax or some other ingredient to the oil. Another method to change the release profile would be to alter the length of the pathway that the drug must take through the oil. This can be achieved by the addition of inert insoluble particles to the oleaginous vehicle. As previously discussed under oleaginous solutions, step 3 is seldom rate limiting and therefore will not be discussed further.

Tables 3 and 5 tabulate the formulation variables which can be changed by the clinical pharmacist and the resultant effect of these changes on the release profile. When step 1 is rate determining it is seen that the same tabulation applies to an oleaginous suspension that applied to an aqueous suspension. Therefore, the previous discussion in this chapter covering aqueous suspensions relating to Table 3 is equally applicable to the oleaginous suspensions.

Table 5 tabulates the changes of the formulation variables and the effect of these changes upon the release profile when the rate of transport of the drug through the oleaginous media is rate determining. Comparison to Table 4 shows that the variables and their effects in Table 5 are the same as Table 4 with the exception of the new variable, viscosity. Again, the previous discussion relating to Table 4 under aqueous suspensions regarding the common variables applies here. The effect of viscosity upon oleaginous transport of drug has also been previously discussed under oleaginous solutions. It should be clear to the reader at this point that the oleaginous suspension system provides the greatest control of the release profile

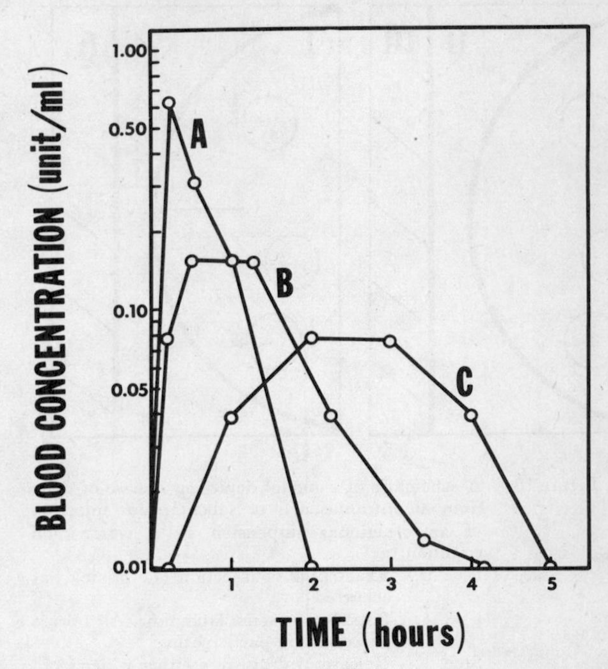

Figure 11: The effect of formulation on blood concentration of penicillin as a function of time following intramuscular injection. Adapted from reference 16.
A. Sodium penicillin G in normal saline solution 45,000 units
B. Sodium penicillin G in peanut oil 33,200 units
C. Calcium penicillin G in peanut oil with 1% beeswax 66,400 units

by combining the advantages of all the other systems. Thus, it is not surprising that oleaginous suspensions are widely used in parenteral therapy.

Applications

The above concepts must be considered whenever a parenteral dosage form is being developed.

Table 5. The Comparison of the Effects of Several Variables Upon the Rate and Duration of Drug Release from an Oleaginous Suspension When the Rate Determining Step Is the Rate of Drug Transport to the Biological Fluid-Oil Interface (Step 2, Figure 10)

FORMULATION VARIABLES				EFFECT ON RELEASE	
OLEAGINOUS VISCOSITY	OLEAGINOUS SOLUBILITY	PARTICLE SIZE	AMOUNT SUSPENDED[a]	RATE	DURATION[b]
constant	constant	constant	increase	unchanged	increase
constant	constant	constant	decrease	unchanged	decrease
constant	constant	decrease	constant	unchanged	unchanged
constant	constant	increase	constant	unchanged	unchanged
constant	increase	constant	constant	increase	decrease
constant	decrease	constant	constant	decrease	increase
increase	constant	constant	constant	decrease	increase
decrease	constant	constant	constant	increase	decrease

(a) Includes the total amount of drug per dose, both suspended and in solution.
(b) The duration of absorption will be equal to the duration of release for the stated conditions. The duration of drug activity, however, is a function of tissue distribution, mechanism of elimination, biodegradation, etc., and thus is not necessarily equal to the duration of drug release.

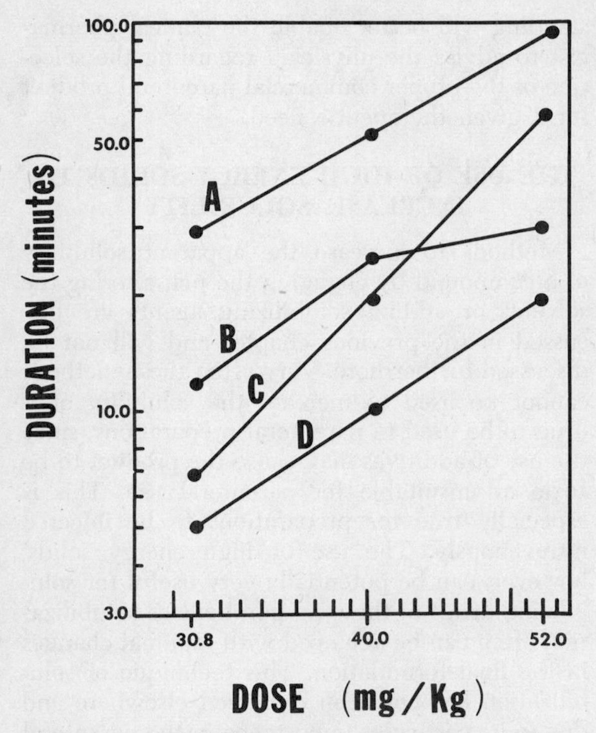

Figure 12: The duration of sleep in mice as a function of dose after injection of barbiturates as an aqueous solution and as an O/W emulsion. Taken from reference 17.
A. Pentobarbital O/W emulsion
B. Sodium pentobarbital aqueous solution
C. Thiopental O/W emulsion
D. Sodium thiopental aqueous solution

In addition, these concepts often can be used to predict blood level profiles that will result from an injection of a given dosage form. A few examples will be cited to illustrate satisfactorily these concepts. Figure 11 shows the blood levels as a function of time obtained when intramuscular doses of three different dosage forms of penicillin were given.[16] The peak concentration obtained from the three dosage forms is seen to be inversely proportional to the duration of drug presence in the blood. Starting with the highest peak blood level and smallest duration, the order is seen to be aqueous solution > oleaginous suspension > oleaginous suspension with beeswax. These findings are in agreement with the theoretical predictions made in earlier discussions.

The duration of sleep in mice when given various intravenous doses of barbiturates as an aqueous solution and as an oil-in-water emulsion is shown in Figure 12.[17] The authors indicated that the longer duration of the emulsion systems was due to the emulsion droplets acting as a drug reservoir.[17]

Buckwalter and Dickison found that suspensions of procaine penicillin G in sesame oil with 1 to 5 percent beeswax produced varied blood profiles as a function of the particle size of the procaine penicillin G particles.[18] As expected, the large particle formulation was absorbed rather slowly and had a longer duration than the small particle formulation.

The use of additives to alter the release pattern of a drug from an oleaginous suspension was mentioned previously and in Figure 11 the effect of added beeswax upon the release of penicillin is seen. Figure 13 shows that there is little difference in release profiles between oleaginous suspensions of sodium penicillin G in sesame oil with either beeswax or aluminum monostearate, but the release of procaine penicillin from suspensions in oil is markedly prolonged by the use of aluminum monostearate while there is little change with procaine penicillin suspensions con-

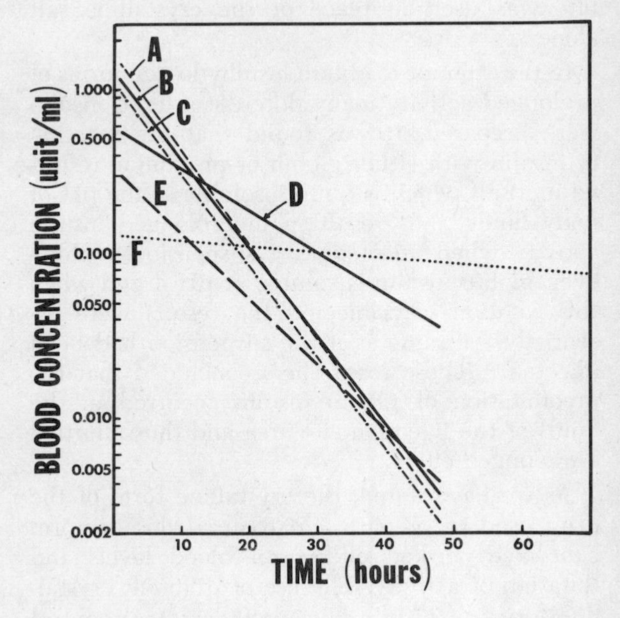

Figure 13: Average penicillin blood concentrations as a function of time after administration of six repository penicillin preparations, administered as a single intramuscular injection, 300,000 units each. Taken from reference 18.
A. Sodium penicillin G in peanut oil with 4.8% (w/v) white beeswax
B. Sodium penicillin G in peanut oil with 2% (w/v) aluminum monostearate
C. Procaine penicillin G in oil
D. Procaine penicillin G in peanut oil with 2% (w/v) aluminum monostearate (large particles)
E. Aluminum penicillin in peanut oil with 2% (w/v) aluminum monostearate
F. Procaine penicillin G in peanut oil with 2% (w/v) aluminum monostearate (small particles)

taining beeswax.[18] It should also be noted in Figure 13 that the large particle procaine penicillin product gave a higher peak concentration and shorter duration of blood concentration than the small particle product. This result may be possibly explained by the settling phenomenon discussed under the topic of oleaginous suspensions.

As shown in Figure 13 procaine penicillin G in oil with 2% w/v aluminum monostearate provided penicillin blood levels of long duration, but the peak blood levels were rather low. In an effort to obtain higher peak levels crystalline potassium penicillin G was added, but unfortunately, the aluminum monostearate inhibited the absorption of the crystalline salt as well as the procaine penicillin.[19] It was found that the use of a coprecipitate of crystalline penicillin G with pectin caused rapid absorption of drug from the oil suspension and thus much higher peak blood levels were attained when the coprecipitate was used in place of the crystalline salt alone.[20]

In the attempt to obtain insulin dosage forms of prolonged activity many different salts of insulin were prepared. It was found that the reaction of insulin with either globin or protamine resulted in a salt which is quite insoluble at the pH of body fluids, thus resulting in prolonged insulin activity when injected as a suspension.[21] However, globin insulin is soluble at pH 4 and when this solution was injected the results were essentially the same as if the suspension had been injected.[21] These researchers concluded that the precipitation of globin insulin occurred in the fluids of the injection site area and thus afforded a prolonged effect.

As we have noted, the crystalline form of the drug used to prepare a parenteral dosage form can have marked effects on blood levels and duration of activity. The use of different crystalline forms of insulin zinc provides great control over the duration of insulin activity. The amorphous form of insulin zinc particles is called semilente and provides hypoglycemic activity up to 16 hours while the crystalline form (ultralente) gives activity up to 30 hours or more.[22] Mixtures of these two forms of insulin zinc in suspension allow clinicians control over the duration of insulin activity.

It should be strongly emphasized that a thorough understanding of the concepts presented in this section will allow the clinical pharmacist to properly design and prepare a parenteral dosage form. In addition, this understanding will better enable the clinical pharmacist to advise the physician regarding the selection of the proper commercial parenteral product for a given therapeutic need.

THE USE OF HIGH ENERGY SOLIDS TO INCREASE SOLUBILITY

Methods to increase the apparent solubility of a compound by changing the pH, altering the solvent, or adding solubilizing agents are discussed in the previous chapter and will not be discussed further here. Very often these methods cannot be used to increase the solubility of a drug to be used in parenteral preparations, since the use of additives may cause the product to be toxic or unsuitable for parenteral use. This is especially true for preparations to be injected intravenously. The use of high energy solids, however, can be potentially very useful for solubilizing drugs in these preparations as solubilization often can be achieved with minimal changes in the final formulation. This technique of solubilization has not been discussed elsewhere and due to its particular importance in the parenteral area this procedure will be briefly covered in this chapter. Although it has been recognized for some time that high energy solids will provide higher solubilities and higher dissolution rates than the corresponding low energy solids of the same drug, relatively little has been done to utilize this phenomenon in drug formulation. The reason for this is not only due to the difficulties encountered in the production of the higher energy forms, but is also due to the difficulties encountered in the prevention of the transformation of the high energy form to the low energy form upon standing. Nevertheless, it is felt that it would be worthwhile to include a discussion of this phenomenon in this section since the method potentially can be very useful. It is also possible that a clinical pharmacist may be able to utilize a high energy form of a drug even though it reverts to the lower energy form if the preparation is used immediately.

For the above reasons, the clinical pharmacist should be prepared to investigate the use of high energy forms of drugs when the need arises. In addition, the principles involved often can explain unusual absorption behavior of solid containing dosage forms.

Polymorphism

When a solid drug can exist in more than one crystalline form, it is said to be polymorphic. Generally a drug, when crystallizing from a vapor, melt, or supersaturated solution, will form its lowest energetic crystal. This is called its stable crystalline form. Depending on the kinetic conditions imposed on the system, however, the drug may form a higher energetic crystal instead of the low energy crystal. The higher energetic crystalline forms are called unstable crystalline forms. The unstable crystalline forms generally will exhibit lower melting points, higher vapor pressures, higher solubilities and faster dissolution rates. Obviously, when the absorption of a drug is dependent on its dissolution rate, the unstable crystalline forms will yield faster absorption rates. The reason for the higher activity is related to the lattice energy of the drug. The higher energetic crystalline forms (unstable forms) require less energy to disrupt their structures. It should be stressed that the stable and unstable crystalline forms of a drug are identical in their chemical properties. For example, a solution prepared using an unstable crystalline form of a drug cannot be distinguished from a solution prepared using its stable crystalline form. Unstable crystalline forms can sometimes be prepared by rapid freezing of the drug melt, by sublimation, or by recrystallization of the drug from a solvent that inhibits the crystal growth and nucleation of the lower energy crystalline form but does not inhibit crystal growth and nucleation of the higher energy crystalline form. A number of examples can be given. Sulfathiazole appears as crystalline form I when recrystallized from water but appears as crystalline form II when recrystallized from normal propyl alcohol or s-butyl alcohol.[23] The aqueous solubility of the unstable crystalline form of sulfathiazole was found to be 1.7 times higher than the stable crystalline form.[24] Methylprednisolone appears as crystalline form I when recrystallized from acetone but as crystalline form II when recrystallized from t-butyl alcohol.[23] The solubility of the unstable crystalline form was found to be 1.8 times higher than the stable crystalline form.[25]

If one is to utilize polymorphs one must be able to identify them. There are a number of methods to distinguish between polymorphs and these methods include infrared absorption spectra, x-ray diffraction patterns, microscopic examination, and dissolution rates (if transformation does not occur during dissolution). Dissolution rates appear to be the most sensitive when examining systems made up of a mixture of crystalline forms, but the other methods are more reliable and reproducible for systems containing one alone.

Once the high energy form is obtained, its usefulness will depend upon the success of preventing its reversion to the low energy form prior to its use. This can possibly be achieved in a number of ways. The proper choice of solvent can prevent reversion. For example, the use of the solvent which was used to prepare the high energy form would prevent reversion. Of course, the suitability of any solvent for parenteral use must be determined. The addition of the polymer polyvinylpyrrolidone prevents the reversion of higher energy forms of sulfathiazole.[24,26,27] If information about specific reversion inhibitors is not available, it is recommended that one try the addition of various polymers, suspending agents, surfactants, dyes, or known crystal growth poisons of known safety.

Amorphous Drugs

When the solid form of the drug is non-crystalline, it is called amorphous. It should be emphasized that the amorphous form is not a polymorph since polymorphs are crystalline. Having no crystalline structure, the amorphous form of a drug would be of higher energy than any of its polymorphs and would therefore be more desirable. Since it has a higher energy, it is much more difficult to prepare and stabilize the amorphous form of a given drug as compared to any of the polymorphic forms.

The classical method to prepare the amorphous form of a compound is to freeze very rapidly a melt of the compound. It is believed that the molecules are prevented from reorienting before freezing and therefore they retain the structure of the melt. Unfortunately the amorphous form of a drug is very unstable and because of its high energy, reverts to a crystalline form rapidly. For this reason drugs are normally marketed in a stable crystalline form.

It has recently been shown that an amorphous form of a drug often can be prepared by coprecipitating it with a polymer such as polyvinylpyrrolidone.[24,26] It was shown that the polymer not only plays an important role in the formation of the high energy amorphous form but also acts as an inhibitor to prevent reversion to the low energy form.[24,26] These coprecipitates can be prepared by a number of methods. The drug and coprecipitating agent can be melted together and then quickly frozen;[28] the drug and coprecipitating agent can be dissolved together in a volatile solvent and the solvent can be removed by flash evaporation; or the two can be dissolved together in an aqueous solution and then freeze-dried. It has been shown that the dissolution rate and apparent solubility of a drug can be greatly increased by this method.[24,26,28-31]

STABILITY CONSIDERATIONS

There are many situations in which the pharmacist must know the effect of various conditions upon a product's shelf life. The precise methods for calculating the extent of these effects are presented in chapters 18 and 20. Unfortunately, the clinical pharmacist generally is not in a position to perform these rigorous calculations for one or more of the following reasons: the calculations take a great deal of time; time may be needed to conduct literature surveys; or, most importantly, the pharmacist may not know the exact conditions to which the drug has been subjected and thus an extremely accurate value may be impossible to obtain. It would be useful if there were a relatively simple and fast method of calculation for predicting the effect of temperature conditions upon shelf life. It will be shown that these methods exist and, in fact, do not require an extensive mathematical background or a great knowledge of kinetics.

This discussion of stability is especially important to the parenteral formulator since most parenteral dosage forms will contain water and thus degradation will be more likely to occur as compared to dry solid dosage forms. Also, many parenteral products are sterilized by autoclaving and the effects of this process must be estimated. Finally, a large number of commercially available products for parenteral use must be reconstituted prior to use. These reconstituted products usually have a rather short shelf life and the usability of these products greatly depends upon the storage conditions after reconstitution. The stability of the drug often dictates the method of sterilization, storage condition, shelf life, and even the method of preparation.

There are essentially four times when stability is important to the clinical pharmacist. During the preparation of the product the clinical pharmacist must be concerned about stability. For example, using heat to dissolve a drug may degrade it, or the use of heat during the final stages of lyophilization may have deleterious effects upon the drug. He also must be concerned about the stability of the drug during sterilization. This knowledge about the drug's stability may dictate, for example, that autoclaving cannot be used. Stability must also be considered in the determination of the proper storage conditions of the finished preparation and its projected shelf life. The fourth situation in which stability considerations are important is not as well defined as the above situations. In this case the pharmacist is asked to predict the remaining shelf life of a product which has been stored at a temperature other than the recommended storage temperature for which the shelf life is known. For example, consider a drug solution which has a refrigerated shelf life of one week but is accidentally stored at room temperature for three days. What is the refrigerated shelf life remaining? Does it have to be discarded immediately? Unfortunately, all too often these questions are not answered on the basis of scientifically sound principles but instead by intuitive guesses. Fortunately, this need not be the case.

It will be shown that the rate of degradation of a drug at autoclave temperature in relation to the rate of degradation at either room or refrigerator temperature can be calculated exactly and from this relationship the effect of autoclaving upon the shelf life at either room or refrigerator temperatures can be accurately calculated. In addition, a method will be presented which will allow the pharmacist to accurately and easily estimate the shelf life remaining after a product has been heated to any given temperature for any given period of time. The value of this latter method must be emphasized. One of the most common problems of stability which arises in the hospital pharmacy (or in the community pharmacy, for that matter) occurs when a product of known shelf life at one temperature is inadvertently stored at another temperature. Any method of calculation which can accurately predict the remaining shelf life in this situation is a powerful method indeed!

Approach to the Stability Problem

There are several ways to obtain information about the stability of a drug. First, if the drug in question is available commercially, then the brochures included with the drug should give some indication of shelf life. If this approach is not practical then the literature can be surveyed. For example, one can refer to the *Chemical Abstracts Index* under the proper topic or one can utilize the formula index of *Chemical Abstracts* to locate potentially useful articles. In the event one is unable to locate any information regarding the specific compound in question, it can be extrapolated from the data available dealing with structurally similar compounds. Often a basic organic chemistry textbook can be useful. Lastly, a kinetic study can be carried out in which the degradation of the drug is followed as a function of time at the various conditions in question. Of course, this method requires a great deal of time and equipment and is not a practical method of stability determination for the average pharmacist. The principles of kinetics have been discussed in the previous chapter and the rigorous calculations utilizing literature data will be made in the next chapter.

Few research papers involving kinetics include stability data at all of the temperatures which interest the pharmacist, such as room temperature, refrigerator temperature, autoclave temperature, etc. Hence, the pharmacist must extrapolate from the reported data to the temperatures in question and the rigorous methods of doing this are shown in the above named chapters. However, it will be shown that if the pharmacist can obtain from the literature only the heat of activation (ΔH^*) for the degradation reaction, then he will be able to make many predictions regarding stability without using difficult mathematical equations.

The material which will follow utilizes the concept of the Arrhenius Equation (see Chapters 18 and 20) to calculate the ratio of the degradation rates at two different temperatures for specific values of the heat of activation, ΔH^*. It is stressed that this factor is a ratio, that is, it is the rate at one temperature divided by the rate at another temperature. Thus, if the shelf life of a drug is known at one temperature, and if the ΔH^* for the degradation reaction is known, one will be able to easily calculate the effect of any other temperature on the drug's stability.

Effect of Autoclaving upon Shelf Life

The possible degradation of a drug in solution during autoclaving is a common and important problem in the parenteral formulation area. A method will be presented by which simple calculations can be made to predict the effect of autoclaving on the shelf life of a drug. For our calculations it is assumed that in autoclaving, the product is essentially at 121°C for thirty minutes. Tables 6 and 7 can be conveniently used to make accurate predictions of the effect of autoclaving on the shelf life of a drug at room or refrigeration temperature if the heat of activation of the degradation reaction is known. The factor of $k_{121°C}/k_{27°C}$ was rigorously calculated using the Arrhenius Equation at the temperatures of 121°C and 27°C where k is the rate constant of the degradation reaction at the given temperature. This factor is also equal to the number of times faster that the drug degrades at autoclave temperature as compared to room temperature. The factor $k_{121°C}/k_{5°C}$ is the corresponding factor for the refrigerator temperature of 5°C. For example, from the literature and from a package insert the pharmacist finds that the ΔH^* of the degradation reaction

Table 6. The Comparison of the Rate of Degradation at 121°C and the Rate of Degradation at 27°C, and the Loss of Room Temperature Shelf Life After Autoclaving for ½ Hour.[a] Both Are Shown as a Function of the Heat of Activation, ΔH^*

ΔH^* (KCAL/MOLE)	k_{121}/k_{27}[b]	LOSS OF ROOM TEMPERATURE SHELF LIFE
10	55	27.5 hours
12	123	3.2 days
15	407	8.5 days
20	3,002	9.0 weeks
25	22,400	15.3 months
30	174,000	10.3 years
35	1,230,000	7.0 decades
40	9,120,000	5.2 centuries
100	2.51 x 10^{17}	10^{11} centuries[c]

(a) Assume ½ hour effective time at 121°C.
(b) Ratio of rate constants at 121°C to 27°C. This is also the ratio of the rates of degradation at the two temperatures if all of the variables (except temperature) in the two systems are the same.
(c) The magnitude of this number is difficult to comprehend. This period of time, 10^{11} centuries, is approximately 10,000 times the lifetime of earth!

Table 7. The Comparison of the Rate of Degradation at 121°C and the Rate of Degradation at 5°C, and the Loss of Refrigerator Temperature Shelf Life After Autoclaving for ½ Hour.[a] Both Are Shown as a Function of the Heat of Activation, ΔH^*

ΔH^* (KCAL/MOLE)	k_{121}/k_5[b]	LOSS OF REFRIGERATOR TEMPERATURE SHELF-LIFE
10	204	102 hours
12	598	12.5 days
15	2,960	8.8 weeks
20	41,600	2.4 years
25	603,000	34.7 years
30	8,720,00	5 centuries
35	123,000,000	70 centuries
40	1,780,000,000	10^3 centuries
100	1.26 x 10^{23}	7 x 10^{16} centuries[c]

(a) Assume ½ hour effective time at 121°C.
(b) Ratio of rate constants at 121°C to 5°C. This is also the ratio of the rates of degradation at the two temperatures if all of the variables (except temperature) in the two systems are the same.
(c) The magnitude of this number is difficult to comprehend. This period of time, 7 x 10^{16} centuries, is approximately 10,000,000,000 times the lifetime of earth!

is 15 Kcal/mole and that the shelf life under refrigeration is six months. By referring to Table 7 it is seen that while the drug is at 121°C it is degrading 2,960 times faster than it would degrade if it were at 5°C. In addition, the degradation occurring in one-half hour at 121°C would be equivalent to the degradation occurring in approximately two months at 5°C. Hence, there would be approximately four months of refrigeration shelf life remaining. The loss of shelf life is expressed in the tables in terms of refrigerator and room temperature shelf life since usually the brochures and package inserts of commercially available products contain this data. It is seen that by simply knowing the ΔH^* of the reaction and the shelf life of the product at either room temperature or refrigerator temperature, the clinical pharmacist can easily calculate the extent of degradation and the shelf life remaining after autoclaving.

Estimating the Effect of Storage at Any Temperature Upon the Shelf Life of a Drug

The previous discussion presented exact methods of calculations for determining the shelf life remaining or the amount of degradation when a parenteral solution is autoclaved. Of course, the exact calculations may be made in a similar manner for any temperature which one may encounter and these methods of calculation can be found in Chapters 18 and 20. Since these calculations are rather lengthy, it would be worthwhile to discuss the use of simple rules of thumb which often will suffice under certain conditions. For example, the rule, "the reaction rate is doubled for every ten degree rise in temperature and halved for every ten degree decrease," is often invoked. The rule will usually give a useful figure for the degradation rate if one is involved with a hydrolysis reaction at room temperature. The factor of two, however, does not apply to all reactions at all temperatures. This factor, the ratio of the two rates of reaction at two temperatures separated by 10°C, is often referred to as R_{10} and is a function of the heat of activation, ΔH^*. Rather than use the factor of two, it would be far better to use the proper R_{10} for the given reaction and this can be easily determined by using the proper heat of activation (ΔH^*) which is normally reported for kinetic studies. The values of R_{10} for a number of heat of activations are reported in Table 8. It is seen that an R_{10} value of two is applicable to a heat of activation of 12 Kcal per mole for a 10°C decrease in temperature at room temperature while for a 10°C increase in temperature from room temperature the R_{10} value is 1.91. It should be noted that when using the table one should use the proper R_{10} value depending upon the temperatures being studied. If the heat of activation is greater than 15 Kcal per mole the use of an R_{10} value of two can lead to appreciable errors. It should also be noted that the R_{10} value is also a function of the specific temperatures used in calculation and that the R_{10} value decreases as the temperatures used increase. This dependence is clearly shown by Table 9 which lists the R_{10} values as a function of the temperatures used in the calculation. The values at 30 Kcal per mole show that this change with temperature can be very significant. This table also shows that the change of R_{10} values is a function of the heat of activation since the change is larger for larger heats of activation. The R_{10} rule of thumb, however, is useful for a "ball park figure" and is generally safe to use as it tends to predict a rate of degradation that is too fast at the higher temperatures rather than too slow; hence, the degree of degradation will not be underestimated if compared to room temperature. It should be cautioned that the reverse process of predicting room temperature shelf life from high temperature data would result in overestimating the shelf life by the same factor. However, it should be noted that one is seldom called upon to predict low temperature shelf life from high temperature data since usually drug brochures list only refrigerator or room temperature shelf life data and the pharmacist is generally concerned with the estimation of the effect of higher temperatures on the product.

This method of calculation using the R_{10} rule

Table 8. R_{10} Values as a Function of the Heat of Activation (ΔH^*) at Room Temperature (27°C)

ΔH^* (KCAL/MOLE)	$R_{10}\left(\frac{27°C}{17°C}\right)^a$	$R_{10}\left(\frac{37°C}{27°C}\right)^b$
3	1.19	1.18
10	1.78	1.72
12	2.00	1.91
15	2.38	2.24
20	3.16	2.95
25	4.24	3.92
30	5.66	5.07
35	7.55	6.65
40	10.00	8.72
50	17.80	15.13
100	389.00	224.00

(a) ratio; the rate at 27°C divided by the rate at 17°C
(b) ratio; the rate at 37°C divided by the rate at 27°C

Table 9. R_{10} Values as a Function of the Temperature Ratio at Heat of Activation, ΔH^*, of 12 and 30 Kcal Per Mole

TEMPERATURE RATIO	R_{10} AT 12 KCAL/MOLE = ΔH^*	30 KCAL/MOLE = ΔH^*
17°C/7°C	2.10	6.40
27°C/17°C	2.00	5.66
37°C/27°C	1.92	5.06
47°C/37°C	1.84	4.57
57°C/47°C	1.77	4.07
67°C/57°C	1.72	3.84
77°C/67°C	1.66	3.55
87°C/77°C	1.62	3.31
97°C/87°C	1.57	3.10
107°C/97°C	1.53	2.92
117°C/107°C	1.50	2.77
127°C/117°C	1.47	2.63

will be illustrated by several examples. It is assumed that the drug in question in all of the examples has a shelf life of one week (168 hours) at refrigerator temperature. The value of 7°C. was taken as refrigerator temperature in order to simplify calculations. In addition the heat of activation (ΔH^*) for the degradation reaction is assumed to be 12 Kcal/mole.

Example 1: Effect of room temperature (27°C) storage.

This is probably the most useful calculation to be presented since this stability question commonly arises in the practice of pharmacy at all levels. The increase in rate of degradation at room temperature as compared to refrigerator temperature must first be calculated. This involves three steps:

Step 1: Determine R_{10}.
From Table 8 R_{10} is seen to be 2.0 for this drug.

Step 2: Number of 10°C increments.
The number of 10°C increments between room temperature (27°C) and refrigerator temperature (7°C) is calculated as follows:

$$X = \frac{27°C - 7°C}{10°C} = 2$$

Step 3: Increase in rate of degradation.
$(R_{10})^X$ (where X is the number of 10°C increments between the two temperatures) is the number of times faster that the drug degrades at room temperature as compared to refrigerator temperature. In this case this factor is seen to be:

$$(2.0)^2 = 4$$

Thus the drug degrades 4 times faster at room temperature compared to refrigerator temperature.

There are two situations in which the above factor is useful. The first situation is when the shelf life of the drug at room temperature must be determined. If the drug degrades $(R_{10})^X$ faster at a given temperature as compared to refrigerator temperature, then the shelf life at the given temperature is $\frac{1}{(R_{10})^X}$ of the refrigerator temperature shelf life. In this case:

$$\frac{1}{(2.0)^2} \times 7 \text{ days} \times \frac{24 \text{ hours}}{\text{day}} = 42 \text{ hours}$$

Therefore, the product could only be stored for 42 hours at room temperature.

This method can also supply the answer to the second situation in which the product is accidentally left at room temperature for a period of time and the refrigerator temperature shelf life remaining must be determined. For example, what is the remaining refrigerator shelf life if the above product is stored at room temperature for one day?

$$\left[\begin{matrix}\text{4 times faster at} \\ \text{room temperature}\end{matrix}\right] \times 1 \text{ day} = 4 \text{ days}$$

Therefore, one day's storage at room temperature is equivalent to four days of storage at refrigerator temperature and hence the remaining shelf life of the product under refrigeration would be 3 days (7-4 days).

Example 2: The effect of heating the product at 87°C.

The calculations presented here would apply to cases in which the drug is heated significantly above room temperature. Examples would include excessively high temperature storage conditions or the use of heat to increase the rate of solution. Again, the calculation involves three steps:

Step 1: Determine R_{10}.
From Table 8 R_{10} is seen to be 1.91. Note the temperature condition is greater than room temperature and thus an R_{10} value of 1.91 is used instead of 2.00.

Step 2: Number of 10°C increments.

$$X = \frac{87°C - 7°C}{10°C} = 8$$

Step 3: Increase in rate of degradation.

$$(R_{10})^X = (1.91)^8 = 178$$

Therefore the drug degrades 178 times faster while at 87°C than it would degrade at refrigerator temperature.

Again, there are two situations in which this factor is useful. If the drug product were heated at this temperature for 57 minutes it would not be usable. This is calculated as follows:

$$7 \text{ days} \times \frac{24 \text{ hours}}{\text{day}} \times \frac{60 \text{ min.}}{\text{hour}} \times \frac{1}{178} = 57 \text{ min.}$$

If it were heated at 87°C for 13 minutes, its remaining shelf life at refrigerator temperature would be only 129 hours (about 5 days).

$$\begin{pmatrix}178 \text{ times}\\ \text{faster}\end{pmatrix} \times (13 \text{ min.}) \times \left(\frac{1 \text{ hour}}{60 \text{ min.}}\right) = 39 \text{ hrs.}$$

Thus 39 hours of refrigerator temperature shelf life are lost. The refrigerator shelf life remaining = 168 hours − 39 hours = 129 hours.

Example 3: Effect of Autoclaving.

If the drug were at autoclave temperature (121°C) for 30 minutes the product would not be usable since the rate of degradation would be $(1.91)^{11}$ or 1,231 times faster and thus less than 9 minutes at this temperature would be equivalent in degradation to its total refrigerator temperature shelf life. This is calculated as follows:

$$168 \text{ hours} \times \frac{60 \text{ min.}}{\text{hour}} \times \frac{1}{1{,}231} = 8.1 \text{ minutes}$$

This method, although convenient, does introduce some error. For example, exact calculations using the Arrhenius Equation for a heat of activation of 12 Kcal per mole would yield different values of shelf life when compared to R_{10} method. (See Table 10.) However, considering the convenience and time saved, the R_{10} rule is very useful for obtaining a value of the correct order of magnitude and is surprisingly accurate if the temperature variation is small. In addition it should be stressed that although the results in Table 10 appear to be significantly different it is seen that the R_{10} rule does give an overestimation of the degree of degradation. Therefore, without having to make extensive and difficult calculations, the rule informs the clinical pharmacist just what he is permitted to do and at what "price." For the drug described in Table 10 he would know, for example, that if his technicians heated his preparation for 13 minutes at 87°C he need not discard it if he were assured it would be utilized in a very short time, or it would permit him to label the preparation with a safe expiration date such as "5 days at refrigerator temperature." Table 10 also indicates that either method of calculation clearly shows that the preparation cannot be autoclaved.

It is seen that the clinical pharmacist needs only a value for the heat of activation of the degradation of the drug in question in order to generate a great deal of information regarding stability and shelf life. If this heat of activation is available from the literature then the use of the R_{10} (ratio of two reaction rates separated by 10°C) rule is useful and quite accurate particularly if the temperatures in question are rather close together. Fortunately, many stability problems which may arise in practice involve rather small temperature changes (for example, in the region of refrigerator and room temperature). Thus, the R_{10} rule will yield excellent predictions for most problems. If information is required for systems involving large temperature changes then the R_{10} rule is still useful but unfortunately introduces error. Of course, exact calculations can be made in this case from the Arrhenius Equation. For the specific case in which the effect of autoclaving on product shelf life is needed, Tables 6 and 7 should be consulted.

If the heat of activation of the degradation reaction is not available then there are two alternatives left open to the pharmacist. First, the literature can be surveyed in order to find a drug similar in structure to the drug in question. Often these drug analogs will degrade in a similar manner and then a rough estimate of ΔH^* can be obtained. Finally, if there are no data reported at all for the drug or its analogs, then the pharmacist must assume that vigorous heating will markedly degrade the compound. Thus autoclaving should definitely not be carried out and great care should be taken in using heat to dissolve the substance.

ISOTONICITY

In general, a preparation which is to be administered directly to tissues, blood and so forth should be made isotonic with respect to the tissue with which it will come in contact. Preparations that are not isotonic with the tissue can be painful to the patient and can even be deleterious to the tissue (e.g., hemolysis of red blood cells). Occasionally the adjustment of isotonicity will not be needed. This occurs, for example, when a very small volume of solution is to be administered intravenously. The critical concentration and volume at which adjustment of isotonicity is needed is not clear cut and thus, when in doubt, the safest procedure is to prepare an isotonic solution. Under certain conditions the adjustment of the tonicity of the solution is mandatory, for example, when a large volume of solution is to be injected. Since little effort is needed to make a solution isotonic, the adjustment of isotonicity should be made unless there are more important reasons for not doing so.

The average pharmacist has been introduced to the principles of the adjustment of isotonicity in relation to the preparation of ophthalmic solutions. Since these principles also apply to parenteral preparations, it would be worthwhile to review some aspects of these principles.

Osmotic Pressure

If two solutions of different concentrations are separated by a membrane through which the solutes cannot pass, then the solvent will attempt to equalize the two concentrations and the solvent will flow from the area of low solute concentration across the membrane to the area of high solute concentration. This process is called osmosis. The above membrane is then called a semipermeable membrane since it allows passage of the solvent but does not allow the passage of the solute.

If the volumes of the two solutions are fixed and the solvent is attempting to pass from one side of the membrane (low concentration) to the other side (high concentration), then an outward pressure on the side of the membrane from the high concentration side will result. If the membrane is flexible then we would expect it to stretch or even burst if the pressure became great enough.

Table 10. Comparison of R_{10} Method and Arrhenius Equation Predictions of Degradation for a Drug with Refrigerated Shelf Life[a] of 1 Week and a Heat of Activation of 12 Kcal Per Mole

CONDITIONS	EFFECTIVE PRODUCT LIFE[b] R_{10} METHOD[c]	ARRHENIUS METHOD[d]
at room temperature	42 hours	42 hours
heating at 87°C	57 minutes	81.7 minutes
at autoclave temperature	$<$9 minutes	17.1 minutes
at refrigerated temperature after heating at 87°C for 13 minutes	129 hours	141.8 hours

(a) Length of time preparation can be stored before it must be discarded.
(b) Time product can be exposed to the described condition before it must be discarded.
(c) Calculated using the $(R_{10})^X$ method.
(d) Calculated using the Arrhenius Equation (see Chapters 18 and 20.

Two solutions are said to be isosmotic when osmotic pressures (measured against a membrane permeable to solvent only) are equal. In general, this osmotic pressure is proportional to the number of molecules in solution. This means that any physical property that depends on the number of molecules in solution can be used to calculate osmotic pressure as a function of concentration. These physical properties, called colligative properties, include vapor pressure lowering, boiling point elevation and freezing point depression. Since the direct measurement of osmotic pressure is experimentally difficult, this concept permits one to calculate the osmotic pressure indirectly from a measurement of any one of the other colligative properties. These principles are equally applicable to biological systems when dealing with a biological membrane which is impermeable to a given solute.

When injecting solutions into the blood, it is important that the parenteral fluid does not cause a change in the "tone" of the red blood cells, *i.e.*, does not cause the size of the cell to change. If the size of the cell does not change, then the solution is said to be isotonic with respect to blood. Although isotonicity, with respect to other tissues of the body, cannot be described as explicitly as it is for blood, isotonicity can be defined in general terms. If there is no net transfer of solvent when any biological tissue is exposed to a solution, the solution is said to be isotonic with respect to that tissue.

It has been found that a 0.9 percent solution of sodium chloride in water is isotonic with respect to red blood cells and that red blood cells expand and sometimes burst (hemolysis) if placed in sodium chloride concentrations significantly lower (hypotonic) than 0.9 percent. On the other hand, the cells shrink (crenation) if placed in sodium chloride concentrations significantly higher (hypertonic) than 0.9 percent. The generally accepted explanation of these phenomena is that the cell wall membrane is acting as a semipermeable membrane in being impermeable to the solute. When the total solute concentration outside the cell is different than that inside, solvent passes across the membrane to equalize the solute concentration thus causing the cell to expand or contract. Thus osmosis is occurring and can explain both hemolysis and crenation. It should be noted that this explanation is based on an important assumption, *i.e.*, that only solvent is permeating the membrane. Unfortunately, biological membranes do not always exclude all solutes.

Isotonicity and Osmoticity

This brings to our attention a very important point. In many pharmaceutical references the terms isosmotic and isotonic are used interchangeably in relation to ophthalmic preparations. However, in dealing with parenteral products the difference between these terms should be clearly understood. Many investigators have concluded that by simply preparing solutions isosmotic with 0.9% NaCl solution (determined from freezing point depression measurement or some other colligative property), one can prepare a solution isotonic with respect to red blood cells. As long as the cell membrane is impermeable to the solute in question, then the terms isotonic and isosmotic can be used interchangeably. However, if the membrane is permeable to any of the solutes, the solute will cross the membrane into the cell causing the solution in contact with the cell to be hypotonic. This, in turn, will cause water to enter the cell and in so doing will usually cause hemolysis. Thus if a drug can pass across the cell membrane, an isosmotic solution of the drug will not be isotonic.

A large amount of data has been tabulated giving the concentrations of drugs which are either isosmotic or isotonic with blood.[1] When using the reference sources to obtain isotonicity parameters for an intravenous formulation, a formulator should use care to determine whether the given information was based upon values obtained from physical observations or from actual experiments with red blood cells. Usually the listed "isotonicity" values in a reference are obtained from suitable physical methods, such as freezing point depression, and thus are actually isosmoticity values. Whether these values can be used as isotonicity values depends upon the permeation characteristics of the drug across the membrane. For example, one reference lists percent-hemolysis at a so-called "isotonicity" concentration.[1] Ascorbic acid will be used as an example to illustrate the foregoing discussion.

Ascorbic acid is reported to be isosmotic with blood at a concentration of 5.05 percent.[1] However, an ascorbic acid solution of this concentration was shown to cause 100 percent hemolysis of red blood cells[1] and, thus, is by no means isotonic with respect to blood. Although there is a lack of definite data there is no reason to believe that a 5.05 percent solution of ascorbic acid would not be isotonic with respect to the corneal membrane. This indicates that the term isotonicity has real meaning only in relation to a specifically named cell or body tissue.

Another example is the effect of dextrose solutions on red blood cells. Five percent dextrose in water is usually considered to be isotonic but it has been reported that with respect to human erythrocytes the isotonic concentration is approximately 10 percent or twice the isosmotic concentration.[32] It would seem that the cell membrane is perhaps partially permeable to dextrose.[32] It is interesting to note that the same group found that dextrose in solution also markedly increases the resistance of the red blood cell wall to rupturing such that the cell can attain volumes in hypotonic dextrose solutions which are twice the volumes at which hemolysis usually occurs.

Isotonicity Calculations

Unfortunately very little data are available which present the effect of drug solutions on various tissues, so the pharmacist must generally rely upon the isosmoticity parameter to estimate isotonicity. The sodium chloride equivalent method is a popular method and tables are available giving that weight of sodium chloride which is osmotically equivalent to a unit weight of drug.[1] For example, if the sodium chloride equivalent of a drug was 0.2, then 0.2 gram of sodium chloride would be osmotically equivalent in solution to 1.0 gram of the drug in an equal volume of solution, or 0.2 grain of sodium chloride would be equivalent to 1 grain of the drug in an equal volume of solution. In practice one multiplies all of the quantities of all the components of the dosage form by the corresponding sodium chloride equivalents. Adding all of these products will yield the total sodium chloride equivalent for the components in solution. Subtracting this total equivalent sodium chloride from the quantity of sodium chloride that would make an equivalent volume of water isosmotic yields the amount of sodium chloride that must be added to the dosage form. An example calculation follows:

1. Formulation

(a) Dibucaine HCl	0.5 g
(b) NaH_2PO_4	0.2 g
(c) $Na_2HPO_4 \cdot 2H_2O$	0.045 g
Water qs 120 ml	Make isotonic with sodium chloride and prepare sterile solution for 2 ml single use ampuls.

2. Sodium chloride equivalents

	Wt. Component	×	NaCl Equiv.[1]	=	g NaCl equiv. to drug
(a)	0.5 g	×	0.14	=	0.07
(b)	0.2 g	×	0.50	=	0.1
(c)	0.045 g	×	0.44	=	0.02
					0.19 g

Therefore all the ingredients are equivalent to a total of 0.19 g of NaCl.

3. NaCl needed to make 120 ml of distilled water isosmotic

$$\frac{0.9 \text{ g NaCl}}{100 \text{ ml solution}} = \frac{X}{120} \text{ so } X = 1.08 \text{ g of NaCl}$$

4. NaCl that must be added

$$1.08 \text{ g} - 0.19 \text{ g} = 0.89 \text{ g}$$

Therefore 0.89 g of NaCl must be added to render the product isosmotic.

Another method preferred by many pharmacists which can be conveniently used to prepare isotonic solutions is called the V method. From the sodium chloride equivalents one can calculate the amount of water which can be added to a given quantity of drug which will result in a solution that is isosmotic with blood. These calculations have been made and the values presented in tables.[1] In these tables the proper quantity of water (V value) is listed which must be added to 0.3 gram of drug in order to prepare a solution of the desired isosmoticity. For example, if the V value for a drug is 23, then if 23 milliliters of water are added to 0.3 gram of the drug the resulting solution is isosmotic with blood.

Example Calculation:

1. Formulation

Dibucaine HCl	0.5 g
Water qs	120 ml

Prepare sterile isotonic solution with NaCl. Buffer pH 6.0.

2. Water needed for components of formulation

$$\text{g component}/0.3 \times \text{V factor}^{1} = H_2O \text{ needed}$$
$$0.5/0.3 \times 4.3 = 7.15 \text{ ml}$$

Thus 0.5 g of dibucaine HCl dissolved in 7.15 ml of water is isosmotic

3. Simply dilute the above isosmotic solution (7.15 ml) to 120 ml with an isotonic buffer at pH 6.0.

This method is convenient since one can quickly calculate and prepare an isotonic solution of all components and then can bring the solution to any volume with any isotonic fluid, (such as normal saline or buffered isotonic solution). The use of the E method to calculate the isotonicity of buffered solutions is tedious as one must calculate the NaCl equivalents for all the species of the buffer as well as drug. For salts, weakly ionized bases, and acids this also requires the calculation of fraction ionized for each of the species.

A combination of the two methods can be used if one is accustomed to the sodium chloride method but wishes to use isotonic buffered vehicles. After the total sodium chloride equivalent of a preparation has been calculated one can, at this point, calculate (using a proportion) the amount of water needed to make all the ingredients isotonic. For example, if the total sodium chloride equivalent of all the ingredients is equal to 0.19 g (see above, first example, step 2 in above), then the amount of water needed can be obtained by the following method:

$$\frac{0.9 \text{ g NaCl}}{100 \text{ ml of solution}} = \frac{0.19 \text{ g of NaCl Equivalent}}{X \text{ ml of } H_2O}$$

Therefore 21.1 milliliters of water added to all the weighed ingredients will produce an isosmotic solution. Any volume of an isotonic vehicle can be added to the solution without changing its isosmoticity. In the example given, the final volume would be adjusted to 120 milliliters.

The last method to be reviewed here is one which allows the formulator to estimate isotonic parameters of drugs even if there are no data available for the particular drug in question. The last two methods of calculation which were discussed were based on the weight of the drug used. As a result, the different molecular weights of compounds do not allow easy extrapolation from one compound to another. The use of a parameter based on molar concentrations circumvents this problem since equal molar concentrations of the same type of compounds should contain the same concentration of particles in solution and therefore the same parameter should apply for large groups of compounds. The experimental literature has been surveyed and average values of this molar parameter (called the L value) for each class of compounds are presented in tables.[1,33]

From this parameter one can calculate the NaCl equivalent by:

$$E = \frac{17L}{\text{Molecular Weight}}$$

and the V value by:

$$V = \frac{(567)\ L}{\text{Molecular Weight}}$$

Example calculation:

(1) Na_2R has a molecular weight of 300 where R is an anionic organic moiety. Na_2R is considered to be a 2-1 (uni-divalent) salt type and its molar parameter is 4.3.

(2) $E = \frac{(17)\ (4.3)}{300} = 0.244$

(3) $V = \frac{(567)\ (4.3)}{300} = 8.1$ ml

E and V values calculated in this manner for dibucaine HCl (uni-univalent) L = 3.4, m.w. = 379) are 0.153 and 6.45 ml respectively. These values are in rather close agreement with the values for E and V obtained in the tables which were used in the two previous formulation examples.

PREPARATION

The preparation of parenterals is perhaps the most challenging of all pharmaceutical procedures. A great deal of technique is needed in addition to the application of the pharmacist's training. Each parenteral product which one is asked to prepare should receive a large amount of study before work is begun, since there are large numbers of seemingly trivial problems which can result in an unacceptable product. There is no room for lack of foresight in the preparation of parenteral dosage forms.

The route and site of administration of the parenteral dosage form will usually have been chosen in accordance with principles outlined previously in this chapter. However, often the ideal mode of administration will not be attainable due to reasons involving the chemical or physical nature of the drug. Sometimes solubility will not allow the desired dosage form or concentration to be used. For example, attempts to obtain a water-soluble form of the drug may be unsuccessful and thus an intravenous injection will not be allowed.

The proper choice of a vehicle can often solve some of the aforementioned problems, *e.g.*, instability, insolubility and so forth. There are various vehicles used for parenterals and the pharmacist should know their uses well. If a drug degrades rapidly in aqueous media then perhaps an intramuscular preparation of an oil solution or suspension will be acceptable. Occasionally, glycols are used in small amounts to increase solubility of certain drugs. The *USP* and *NF* list the many strict requirements relating to the use of vehicles, particularly nonaqueous ones, and these sources should be consulted. Readily obtainable parenteral solutions such as Sodium Chloride Injection USP and Dextrose Injection USP are the vehicles of choice and are particularly useful as vehicles for drugs which will be administered at low concentration. At higher drug concentrations, problems of insolubility and hypertonicity may necessitate the use of other vehicles.

Many so-called "problems" of solubility can be solved with proper use of the principles of equilibria. The pharmacist should have a working knowledge of the use of pH and pK values to predict the solubility and the possible interactions of drugs. It should be noted that drugs in solution when injected intravenously may precipitate in the blood if they are not soluble at the physiologic pH. This insight into equilibria is not only needed for parenteral formulation but is invaluable to the pharmacist in the I.V. additive area. In this area the pharmacist is frequently asked to prepare intravenous solutions containing combinations of drugs. Usually there is little data describing the physical and chemical compatibility of these combinations and, unfortunately, many pharmacists respond only on the basis of visual observation of precipitates rather than predicting possible interactions on the basis of equilibria and pH considerations. The dependence on visual observations can be dangerous since reaction products are not necessarily water-insoluble. In addition, there often may be a time lag before a water-insoluble component is observed. It should be noted that these problems may be caused by the presence of impurities in additives and therefore nontherapeutic substances such as bacteriostatic agents, agents to render the solution isotonic, suspending agents, buffers, and antioxidants obviously must be of maximum purity.

The use of bacteriostatic agents is rather widespread in multidose parenteral dosage forms and often oversimplified. It is all too easy to consider a given preservative as a "universal" preservative to be used for all parenterals. There are many variables which may affect the choice of preservative. The preservative may be incompatible with the therapeutic agent, may modify drug activity, may not be effective against all organisms, may be an irritant, may unfavorably alter the pH, or may be too slow in its reaction with the organism (important in multiple dose vials). The proper choice of a preservative requires study of the available agents in relation to the proposed dosage form. It also should be mentioned that in an emergency situation in the I.V. additive area a pharmacist may be called upon to prepare a preparation for intravenous use containing a massive dose of a drug available only in multidose vials. The pharmacist should be aware in this case of the relatively large dose of preservative (or any other ingredient in the formulation for that matter) which is going to be administered, and if it is deemed necessary, should notify the physician.

The use of buffers in parenteral formulations intended for intravenous use is not recommended unless absolutely necessary to control problems such as stability and solubility. Of course, there is less concern if the dose is to be administered by the intramuscular or subcutaneous route. However, in this latter case a buffered solution at a pH noticeably different from the physiological pH can cause severe discomfort when injected. When buffers are to be used they should be of the lowest buffer capacity possible so that there will be minimal changes occurring in the biological system after injection. For example, if a small dose volume is to be diluted to a large volume and administered intravenously over a long period of time, then the effect of the buffer will not be particularly important. This is not true, however, if a large dose volume is to be given directly.

Severe limitations are often imposed on parenteral formulations and in turn on parenteral therapy by existing stability problems. The stability of the drug in the proposed vehicle will affect the method of sterilization, the method of preparation, and recommended storage conditions of the finished product. The problem of drug stability can sometimes be overcome by the use of drug stabilizers such as antioxidants, complexing agents, chelating agents, and buffers.

As with any additive, one must seriously consider the possible interactions of each additional component with the other ingredients of the formulation. An important method that is widely used to overcome stability problems involves the use of preparations which are reconstituted prior to administration by the addition of a solvent to the solid ingredients. The solid ingredients are usually prepared by lyophilization, or freeze drying. A solution of the ingredients to be lyophilized is prepared and sterilized by appropriate means. The sterile solution in vials or ampuls is then placed in the freeze dryer and brought to a very low temperature (*e.g.*, $-40°C$); when a vacuum is applied the water present will sublime and be removed in this way. These conditions are maintained for a long period of time until a sterile dry "button" remains. The product is usually stable in this dry form and thus has a long shelf life. Lyophilized solids normally dissolve very rapidly and therefore are easily reconstituted when needed.

Many of the above stability problems can be significantly aggravated by the presence of ingredients which can be introduced unknowingly by the use of poor technique, low quality chemicals, containers, etc. Obviously, everyone is agreed that chemicals must be of maximum purity, yet, the practice of using chemicals for parenteral compounding which were specifically bought for bulk compounding is widespread. Often, due to cost considerations and no demonstrated need for the highest quality chemicals for bulk compounding, a lower grade chemical will be purchased. The chemicals for the parenteral area should be only of the highest quality and for this reason a separate stock should be maintained.

Another important aspect of parenteral formulation that must be seriously considered is the method used to sterilize the product. Sterilization methods can be classified into two broad groups, "hot" and "cold" methods. The hot methods include steam sterilization and dry heat sterilization, while the cold methods include sterilization by filtration and gas.

The hot methods are suitable for sterilization of products which are not heat labile, and these methods have the distinct advantage of usually being the final step in the formulation process. Thus, there is negligible chance of recontamination after sterilization. Steam sterilization in the conventional autoclave is certainly the most rapid of the two hot methods but it requires certain safeguards. It is imperative that steam vapor reach the item to be sterilized, therefore wrapping of items must be done with care. The operation of the autoclave must be monitored in order to ascertain that the proper temperature and pressure is obtained for a sufficient period of time. The time of sterilization must be altered to fit the needs of the load of materials. For example, a two liter volume of material should require a longer sterilization time than a one milliliter volume of the same material. The details of autoclave sterilization can be found in suitable references and will be omitted here.[1]

The dry heat method of sterilization is useful for sterilization of items which cannot tolerate steam. Thus, solutions of drugs in fixed oils are often sterilized by this method. This method, unfortunately, requires a long sterilization time at a high temperature and many heat labile drugs, which are sufficiently stable for autoclaving, cannot be sterilized in this manner. The proper period of sterilization depends upon the size of the load and upon the volume in each container. Again, the process should be monitored to insure sterilization. For both steam and dry heat sterilization test strips containing nonpathogenic microorganism spores are available which can be placed with the load. These strips are then cultured to determine if proper sterilization has occurred.

The so-called cold methods of sterilization include sterilization by filtration and gas. Gas sterilization is popular in many hospitals for the sterilization of surgical garments, equipment, and other items through which the gas can penetrate. However, this technique is not particularly useful for the preparation of parenterals. The sterilizing gases obviously do not readily permeate closed parenteral containers and open solutions. Gas sterilization techniques can be used to sterilize thin layers of drug powders which will be subsequently used to prepare a sterile suspension. The questions of whether the gas is able to reach and interact with all of the microorganisms present in the solid, and the possible unknown reaction of the gas with the drug, show the gas sterilization technique of drug powders to be of doubtful value. Spore test strips are also used in gas sterilization to ascertain the success of sterilization.

The filtration methods of sterilization offer an extremely valuable procedure for preparing sterile parenteral solutions. These techniques allow sterilization of drug solutions which degrade significantly when autoclaved. In addition, these methods are rather rapid and easy to perform. Unfortunately, there are some disadvantages. Filters can adsorb drug from the solution. In addition, non-sterile products often result from this technique unless great care is exercised. Sterilization by filtration of large volumes of liquid usually requires a container to hold the bulk sterile solution, and final transfer from this container then must be made into clean sterile vials—the final dosage form. This transfer of the solution presents a possibility of recontamination, and, for this reason, the procedure requires excellent technique. It should be emphasized that this disadvantage is an important one and that terminal sterilization methods are preferred when they are permissible.

There are two types of filtration commonly in use, depth filtration and screen filtration. Unglazed porcelain filters, fritted glass filters, and various fibrous filters are depth filters. When properly manufactured they are suitable for sterilization procedures. Recently, screen filters have come into use and can be made of thin sheets of cellulose esters. The mechanisms of filtration for the two types of filters are quite different. Depth filters remove particles primarily by adsorption and physical entrapment as the particles travel through many tortuous pathways; thus, depth filters exhibit certain disadvantages. If operated for a prolonged period of time there is a possibility that a bacterium could find its way through the filter. If a solution is being passed through a depth filter at a given pressure and the operator increases the pressure in order to increase the flow rate, bacteria that were previously trapped can be "blown" through and contaminate the solution. In addition, the porcelain and glass filters are extremely difficult to clean and sometimes can only be cleaned by ignition. The operator is always faced with the possibility of not knowing that the filter is faulty. It is recommended after each sterilization operation with a depth filter that a run be made using a suspension of a nonpathogenic organism such as *Serratia marcescens* and that the filtrate be cultured. Depth filters can also introduce particulate matter since particles of the fibrous type of filter are constantly breaking off and then migrating through the filter.

Screen filtration, as the name implies, traps particles according to size. The size of the particle trapped is determined by the pore size rating given with the filter. Filtration through these filters progresses at a rapid rate and these filters provide none of the disadvantages listed above for depth filters. A major disadvantage of the cellulose ester screen filters is that they plug rather easily and are subject to heat damage in autoclave cycles if caution is not used.

A major consideration in the preparation of parenterals is the elimination of pyrogens from the final product. The source of water used for parenteral manufacture is of paramount importance in avoiding pyrogens, and the water should never be retained for more than twenty-four hours. Freshly washed glassware should be dried immediately since bacteria can thrive in the film of water that remains on the sides of the glassware after rinsing and this can ultimately result in pyrogen contamination. Fortunately, pyrogens are not volatile, hence, proper distillation will result in pyrogen free water. It should be noted, however, that a faulty still can produce pyrogen contaminated water. In preparations involving final filtration it is easy to relax one's guard in the preliminary procedures assuming that the final filtration will remove all bacteria, particulate matter, and pyrogens. However, as a rule, pyrogens are not filterable, and if once introduced in the process, will ultimately end up in the final product. Thus, the only approach to pyrogen control is extreme caution and care throughout the preparation procedure. In fact, it will be found that if this care is used, then it is also unlikely that particulate matter or sterility problems will arise. A more detailed treatment of pyrogens is beyond the scope of this presentation but can be found in the literature.[1,34]

All materials which will come into contact with the final solution must be of the highest quality. The various types of containers which are allowed for parenteral preparations are tabulated and discussed in the *USP* and *NF*. Careful thought must accompany any introduction of a new material or piece of equipment into a parenteral preparation procedure. For example, certain types of rubber tubing will decompose and "bleed" during certain autoclave cycles. When any type of nonaqueous solvent is added to a parenteral, the type of stopper to be used must be reconsidered. Vial stoppers which are satisfactory for an intended use with one solvent can drastically release components to another solvent.

The proper cleaning and preparation of the equipment to be used in a procedure is most important and often the presence of contaminants in a product can be attributed to this step. Vials, rubber stoppers and rubber tubing, as supplied by the manufacturer, are extremely dirty and careful washing is necessary. The handling of these items after washing is also quite important since particulate matter, bacteria, and pyrogens can be reintroduced at this time. After final rinsing of an item, direct open contact with the air should be minimized and the item should be readied for sterilization and sterilized as soon as possible. The transfer of materials from one location to another should be minimized. All equipment used in the manufacture of parenterals should be used exclusively for parenterals.

Occasionally, a parenteral formulator finds that his product passes all sterility and pyrogen tests but that a rather large number of vials contain visual particulate matter of unknown origin. The determination of the source of this contamination can often take a great deal of time, and usually the problem will be found to be a subtle breakdown in technique. A few examples are: a new brand of sterile disposable gloves was found to introduce large quantities of talc during the sterile transfer operation; new laboratory coats were found to introduce large amounts of lint to the atmosphere. These examples may seem trivial, but many breakdowns in technique in the parenteral formulation area can be attributed to the smallest unexpected sources.

The environment in which parenterals are produced is an important factor in the successful manufacture of parenterals. The area must be cleaned daily. If at all possible the "sterile" room, the room where the actual sterilization processes (*i.e.*, sterile filtration, sterile transfer and so forth) are performed, should be separated from the room where initial cleaning tasks and preparations are conducted. This sterile room ideally should be under positive pressure with filtered air. The sterile production area should be so located that traffic through the area is kept at a strict minimum. Any lint or fiber producing sources, such as certain types of cloth or paper, should not be allowed in the sterile work area. Ultraviolet lights are often used to reduce the bacteria count in the sterile area; however, it should be recognized that these lights are only effective over short distances.

For sterile transfer operations a laminar flow hood is extremely useful and has become a necessity in many hospitals. These hoods, passing sterilized air out directly towards the operator, afford a sterile work area in which the operator has a great deal of freedom; however, improper use or poor maintenance of these hoods can decrease their effectiveness. A contaminated object near the source of air flow can contaminate all objects in the flow path on the "down wind" side. For this reason, extreme care must be taken when working in these hoods. For the protection of the operator vertical flow hoods are available for projects involving the preparation of toxic agents, such as allergenic preparations. The older type of enclosed hoods, still found in many hospitals, is also well suited for the formulation of toxic agents. Ultraviolet radiation is often used in these hoods.

Parenteral dosage forms require the strictest

of quality controls. The following operations should be completed prior to release of the finished product: sterility and pyrogen testing should be carried out in accordance with the *USP*; analytical work must be carried out to determine the strength of the product; every individual dosage form should be checked visually for particulate matter; and ampuls should be tested for proper sealing by available means, such as immersion of the sealed ampuls in a hot dye solution and then allowing the immersed ampuls to cool.[1]

Undoubtedly, the most important factor in successful parenteral formulation is the knowledge and technique of the pharmacist carrying out the task. It has been proven that although methods are available for successful parenteral formulation the individual operator must make the methods work. Whenever the parenteral formulator does not concentrate on the project at hand, it is highly likely that a breakdown in the process will occur. Since the formulation of a parenteral product usually requires many hours to complete, small trivial errors causing the ruin of the product cannot be tolerated. Of greater importance is the fact that these trivial errors may lead to the administration of a toxic or ineffective product. Thorough planning and excellent technique cannot be overemphasized.

References

1. Osol, A. *et al.* eds.: *Remington's Pharmaceutical Sciences,* ed. 14, Mack Publishing Co., Easton, Pennsylvania, 1970.

2. Scigliano, J. A.: Preparation of Small Volume Injections, *Bull. Am. Soc. Hosp. Pharm. 13*:108-114 (Mar.-Apr.) 1956.

3. Macek, T. J.: Preparation of Parenteral Dispersions, *J. Pharm. Sci. 52*:694-699 (July) 1963.

4. Avis, K. E., Carlin, H. S. and Flack, H. L.: Preparation of Injectables — Philosophy and Master Procedures, *Am. J. Hosp. Pharm. 18*:223-233 (Apr.) 1961.

5. Gershenfeld, L.: The Hospital Pharmacist's Responsibilities in the Production of Parenterals, *Am. J. Pharm. 129*: 163 (1957).

6. Fleming, A. *et al.*: Penicillin Content of Blood Serum after Various Doses of Penicillin by Various Routes, *Lancet 2*:621 (1944).

7. Goodman, L. S. and Gilman, A. eds.: *The Pharmacological Basis of Therapeutics,* ed. 4, The MacMillan Co., New York, N. Y., 1970.

8. Schou, J.: Absorption of Drugs from Subcutaneous Connective Tissue, *Pharmacol. Rev. 13*:441 (1961).

9. Swintosky, J. V.: Biologic Half-Life and Tissue Concentrations, *Proc. Am. Assoc. Coll. Pharm. Teachers Seminar 13*:140 (1961).

10. Rammelkamp, C. H. and Keefer, C. S.: The Absorption, Excretion, and Distribution of Penicillin, *J. Clin. Invest. 22*:427 (1943).

11. Eagle, H., Fleischman, R. and Musselman, A. D.: The Serum Concentration of Penicillin G in Mice, Rabbits, and Men After Its Intramuscular Injection in Aqueous Solution, *J. Bacteriol. 57*:119 (1949).

12. Tucker, H. A. and Eagle, H.: Serum Concentrations of Penicillin G in Man Following Intramuscular Injection in Aqueous Solution and in Peanut Oil-Beeswax Suspension, *Am. J. Med. 4*:343 (1948).

13. Levy, G. and Nelson, E.: Pharmaceutical Formulation and Therapeutic Efficacy, *J. Am. Med. Assoc. 177*:125 (1961).

14. Ghanem, A., Higuchi, W. I. and Simonelli, A. P.: Interfacial Barriers in Interphase Transport — Retardation of the Transport of Diethylphthalate Across the Hexadecane-Water Interface by an Adsorbed Gelatin Film, *J. Pharm. Sci. 58*:165-174 (Feb.) 1969.

15. Ghanem, A., Higuchi, W. I. and Simonelli, A. P.: Interfacial Barriers in Interphase Transport II — Influence of Additives upon the Transport of Diethylphthalate Across the Hexadecane-Gelatin-Water Interface, *J. Pharm. Sci. 59*: 232-237 (Feb.) 1970.

16. Romansky, M. J. and Rittman, G. E.: A Method of Prolonging the Action of Penicillin, *Science 100*:196 (1944).

17. Ljungberg, S. and Jeppsson, R.: Intravenous Injection of Lipid Soluble Drugs, *Acta Pharm. Suecica 7*:435 (1970).

18. Buckwalter, F. H. and Dickison, H. L.: The Effect of Vehicle and Particle Size on the Absorption by the Intramuscular Route of Procaine Penicillin G Suspensions, *J. Am. Pharm. Assoc. Sci. Ed. 47*:661 (1958).

19. Buckwalter, F. H. and Dickison, H. L.: A New Absorption Delaying Vehicle for Penicillin, *J. Am. Pharm. Assoc. Sci. Ed. 37*:472 (1948).

20. Welch, H. *et al.*: Procaine Penicillin in Oil with Aluminum Monostearate and Pectin Treated Potassium Penicillin, *Antibiot. Chemotherapia 1*:245 (1951).

21. Reiner, L., Searle, D. S. and Lang, E. H.: On the Hypoglycemic Activity of Globin Insulin, *J. Pharmacol. Exptl. Therap. 67*:330 (1939).

22. Nabarro, J. D. N. and Stowers, J. M.: The Insulin Zinc Suspensions, *Brit. Med. J. 2*:1027 (1953).

23. Higuchi, W. I., Bernardo, P. D. and Mehta, S. C.: Polymorphism and Drug Availability II, *J. Pharm. Sci. 56*:200-207 (Feb.) 1967.

24. Simonelli, A. P., Mehta, S. C. and Higuchi, W. I.: Solubility Studies of the Polymorphic and High Energy PVP Coprecipitates of Sulfathiazole in Aqueous Solutions, *J. Pharm. Sci.,* to be published.

25. Higuchi, W. I. *et al.*: Polymorphism and Drug Availability, *J. Pharm. Sci. 52*:150-152 (Feb.) 1963.

26. Simonelli, A. P., Mehta, S. C. and Higuchi, W. I.: Dissolution Rates of High Energy Polyvinylpyrrolidone (PVP) - Sulfathiazole Coprecipitates, *J. Pharm. Sci. 58*:538-548 (May) 1969.

27. Simonelli, A. P., Mehta, S. C. and Higuchi, W. I.: Inhibition of Sulfathiazole Crystal Growth by Polyvinylpyrrolidone, *J. Pharm. Sci. 59*:633-637 (May) 1970.

28. Goldberg, A. H., Gibaldi, M. and Kanig, J. L.: Increasing Dissolution Rates and Gastrointestinal Absorption of Drugs *via* Solid Solutions and Eutectic Mixtures I, *J. Pharm. Sci. 54*:1145-1148 (Aug.) 1965.

29. Mehta, S. C., Simonelli, A. P. and Higuchi, W. I.: Solubility and Dissolution Behavior of High Energy Polymer Drug Coprecipitates, *J. Pharm. Sci.,* to be published.

30. Mayersohn, M. and Gibaldi, M.: New Method of Solid-State Dispersion for Increasing Dissolution Rates (communications), *J. Pharm. Sci. 55*:1323-1324 (Nov.) 1966.

31. Chiou, W. L. and Riegelman, S.: Preparation and Dissolution Characteristics of Several Fast-Release Solid Dispersions of Griseofulvin, *J. Pharm. Sci. 58*:1505-1510 (Dec.) 1969.

32. Setnikar, I. and Temelcou, O.: Osmotic Concentration and Osmotic Pressure in Injectable Solutions, *J. Am. Pharm. Assoc. Sci. Ed. 48*:628 (1959).

33. Wells, J. M.: Rapid Method for Calculating Isotonic Solutions, *J. Am. Pharm. Assoc. Pract. Ed. 5*:99 (1944).

34. Varney, R. F.: The Intruders — Pyrogens, *Bull. Parenteral Drug Assoc. 16*:6 (1962).

20

Predicting drug stability of parenteral admixtures

by Norman F. H. Ho

Centralized intravenous solution additive programs are wide-spread realities in pharmacy practice. Pharmacists are concerned about the compatibility and stability of parenteral admixtures they prepare. Concern and awareness of these problems are not sufficient. There are needs for general and specific information. However, when one searches the literature, he will undoubtedly conclude:

1. There is no specific information about the drug stability and incompatibility of drug X in dextrose 5 percent in water or drugs X and Y in Ringer's solution;

2. The information is in the classified files of the pharmaceutical manufacturer;

3. The pharmacist does not recognize that the information before him can be further interpreted; and

4. The available information is scattered in the literature, but when collected and evaluated together will yield answers to specific problems.

SCOPE

This chapter is intended to deal with the prediction of pharmaceutical stability of parenteral solutions from a kinetic point of view. Some of the important features will be pointed out but it will not be possible to discuss these in great detail. Although the topic of the physical and chemical incompatibility of drugs is highly relevant here, it is not proposed to discuss these problems. One might wonder if this is another treatise on chemical kinetics. What can it offer that is new? The author would agree that there isn't anything new one can add to the discussion of basic chemical kinetics which is adequately presented in varying degrees of sophistication in many places.[1-3] Then the novelty of this chapter is, perhaps, a matter of presentation.

Figure 1 shows that the prediction of the stability of drugs in parenteral solutions having clinical importance may be approached from two directions. The first approach is an indirect one and utilizes the stability data from basic kinetic studies such as those found in the *Journal of Pharmaceutical Sciences, Journal of Pharmacy and Pharmacology* and so forth. The other approach utilizes the kinetic stability data of the parenteral solution admixture itself in which commercially available parenteral drug products are employed. The choice of these approaches depends principally on the information available for the drug under environmental conditions, such as solvent, drug additives, temperature, pH and other factors, within which the stability of the drug is to be predicted.

STABILITY OF PARENTERAL SOLUTIONS OF CLINICAL SIGNIFICANCE

Stability Data of Drug(s) from Basic Research Study	Stability Data of Drug(s) in I.V. Solutions
Advantages:	*Advantages*:
a. Clinically relevant when judiciously and scientifically extrapolated	a. Clinically relevant
b. Basic understanding of the stability	b. Easily understood by pharmacists
c. Easily computerized	
d. Predicts the dependence of pH, temperature, solvent, buffer and other drugs in the mixture	
Disadvantages:	*Disadvantages*:
a. Solvent system and condition not generally clinically relevant	a. Generally, too specific to predict pH and temperature dependence
b. Not easily understood by pharmacists	b. Information not readily available
c. Requires physico-chemical and mathematical judgment	c. Information not readily computerized
Literature Source:	*Literature Source*:
J. Pharm. Sci., J. Pharm. Pharmacol.	Am. J. Hosp. Pharm., Drug Intelligence & Clin. Pharm., Intern. Pharm. Abstr., foreign journals, drug inserts

Figure 1. Schematic representation of the approaches to predicting drug stability in parenteral solutions of clinical significance

In regard to the first approach, it will be explained how one may look at the kinetic data of a drug in the scientific literature and judiciously extrapolate the results, determined under ideal conditions, to predict the stability of the drug in real solutions of clinical importance. To strengthen one's confidence in this theoretical approach, the theoretical predictions will be compared with experimentally determined values for some examples of simple parenteral solutions having clinical importance. In other words, it is desired to demonstrate the relevancy of theory to practice.

Perhaps many pharmacists will ask the question: "Why should we expend time and energy going through the scientific exercise of obtaining kinetic data of drugs and then making stability predictions?" First, it is significant, considering a lapse of as much as two to ten years between first appearance of fundamental kinetic data in the scientific literature and later publications on the stability of drug products in specific clinical parenteral preparations, that many stability problems could have been solved while awaiting verification. Can pharmacists or their patients afford to wait? Second, although many stability reports on clinical preparations are highly useful to the clinical pharmacist, they are restricted to specific conditions of the solvent, pH and temperature.[4-9] Once pharmacists are confident of the theoretical approach, the use of pertinent equations can extend the prediction of stability to include the variations of pH and temperature in the admixture. This is an important extension in view of the fact that it is sometimes desirable to refrigerate or freeze reconstituted injections for future administration, and to account for the batch to batch and supplier to supplier variation in pH of dextrose, electrolyte and other bulk intravenous fluids. It is conceivable that progressive I.V. additive and drug information centers will utilize equations, pre-evaluated and programmed on magnetic cards for small desk computers, to generate quantitative estimates of drug stability.

SOME THEORETICAL BACKGROUND CONSIDERATIONS

Interpretation of the Literature on Kinetic Studies

There are some important questions to be asked as to the kind of information needed to predict the stability of a drug in the many kinds of intravenous fluids at various pH, temperature and dilutions.

1. What is the mechanism of the reaction? Does it occur by hydrolysis, photochemical degradation or oxidation?

2. Does the reaction follow a first order kinetic process?

3. What is the effect of temperature on the reaction rate? The effect of pH? The effect of the kind of chemical species and concentration of salts, including buffers? The effect of the solvent system and the dielectric properties of the solvent?

4. What is the dissociation constant, K_a, of the drug? The solubility of the nonionized drug species and the salt form?

5. What are the pertinent equations describing the stability?

6. How does the solvent system in which the kinetic studies were carried out compare with clinical preparations containing the drug product in various bulk intravenous solutions?

Kinetics of Drug Decomposition

Generally, the decomposition of a drug in solution may be described by an apparent first order process. The term "first order" is used in the mathematical sense to describe a differential equation of the form:

$$\frac{dC}{dt} = -k_{app}\, C \qquad \text{(Equation 1)}$$

Physico-chemically, the expression means that the rate of change in the concentration of drug is proportional to the concentration of nondecomposed drug remaining. The general solution is found by integrating Equation 1 so that:

$$\int_{C_o}^{C} \frac{dC}{C} = -k_{app} \int_{0}^{t} dt \qquad \text{(Equation 2)}$$

which leads to:

$$\log \frac{C}{C_o} = -\frac{k_{app}}{2.303}\, t \qquad \text{(Equation 3)}$$

or:

$$\log C = \log C_o - \frac{k_{app}}{2.303}\, t \qquad \text{(Equation 4)}$$

where:

C = concentration of nondecomposed drug remaining at any time
C_o = initial concentration
C/C_o = fraction of nondecomposed drug remaining at any time
t = time
k_{app} = apparent first order rate constant in time^{-1}

As an illustration of the predictive nature of the theory, if one is interested in knowing the time at which one-half of the initial nondecomposed drug remains, then by Equation 3:

$$t_{0.5} = -\frac{2.303}{k_{app}} \log 0.5 \qquad \text{(Equation 5)}$$

All that remains to solve this problem is the knowledge of the rate constant, k_{app}, at constant environmental conditions of interest.

Many drugs of clinical importance undergo hydrolysis by general acid-base catalysis. Accordingly, the apparent first order rate constant may be further described by the general expression:

$$k_{app} = k_o + k_H\,[H^+] + k_{OH}\,[OH^-] + k_{HA}\,[HA] + k_A\,[A^-] + \cdots = k_o + \Sigma k_i C_i \qquad \text{(Equation 6)}$$

Here, k_i is the second order catalytic constant, in liter/mole/time of the respective catalytic species of concentration C_i, and k_o is the rate constant of the spontaneous reaction. It is important to note that through Equation 6 one can relate the rate of hydrolysis of a drug to the pH of the solution, the effect of buffer agents, such as the usual acetate and phosphate buffers, and the effect of drug additives and other drugs. It is implicit that the activity coefficient correction to concentration be taken to be unity. However, this parameter, which is related to the ionic strength of the solution, may be an important omission in view of the fact that many drugs are added to parenteral electrolyte solutions. If the hydrolysis involves principally specific hydrogen and hydroxyl ion catalysis, Equation 6 reduces to:

$$k_{app} = k_o + k_H\,[H^+] + k_{OH}\,\frac{K_w}{[H^+]} \qquad \text{(Equation 7)}$$

with the ion product of water $K_w = [H^+]\,[OH^-]$. Since K_w is a function of the temperature, T:

$$-\log K_w = pK_w = \frac{4470.99}{T} + 0.01706T - 6.0875 \qquad \text{(Equation 8)}$$

so that pK_w is 14.941 at 0° C and 14.0 at 25° C and 12.8 at 70°C.

To find the apparent first order rate constant $k_{app,1}$ at temperature T_1 from $k_{app,2}$ at T_2, the well-known Arrhenius relation is utilized in the following form:

$$\log k_{app,1} = \log k_{app,2} + \frac{\Delta H_a}{2.303R}\left(\frac{1}{T_2} - \frac{1}{T_1}\right)$$

(Equation 9)

where:

ΔH_a = apparent activation energy of the reaction in calories/mole

R = Universal gas constant of 1.99 cal/degree/mole

T = °C + 273.15, absolute temperature

CLINICAL RELEVANCE OF PREDICTING DRUG STABILITY FROM BASIC KINETIC STUDIES

To demonstrate the relevancy of theory to practice, the stability of parenteral solutions of methicillin sodium will be considered in a stepwise manner. It is the intent of the author by this method to acquaint those pharmacists who have not had a formal course in chemical kinetics, to refresh the memory of recent graduates in pharmacy and to stimulate all practitioners, particularly those engaged in intravenous admixture and drug information centers.

Reported Stability of Sodium Methicillin Preparations of Clinical Significance

Buffered sodium methicillin injection is provided as a sterile powder for reconstitution to a solution. Each 1.0 gram vial contains:

Methicillin sodium[a]	1.0 g
Sodium citrate	50.0 mg
Methylparaben	0.9 mg
Propylparaben	0.1 mg

[a] 1.0 g of sodium methicillin is equivalent to 0.9 g of the acid.

The recommended diluent is 1.5 ml of Sterile Water for Injection, USP or Sodium Chloride Injection, USP yielding a resultant pH of 6 to 6.6 for the reconstituted solution. The solution is considered stable for 24 hours at room temperature or four days under refrigeration.[10]

The stability of sodium methicillin in various bulk intravenous solutions has been reported in the literature.[4-10] Maximum 24 hour stability at 25° C occurs at pH 5.5-8.0 and the decomposition proceeds rapidly in increasingly acidic solutions. The correlation of stability determinations among investigators was good. However, one group erroneously reported that sodium methicillin solutions decomposed 8 percent after 24 hours at room temperature and pH 4.6 and 50 percent at pH 3.6 and pH 2.7 after 13 hours and 1.5 hours.[6] Upon recalculation of their data, the author found that at pH 4.6 there was 8 percent decomposed after 5.43 hours, and at pH 3.6 and pH 2.7 there was 50 percent decomposed after 4.57 hours and 0.56 hours, respectively; approximately a difference of a factor of three. The corrected estimates of stability agreed with the findings of other investigators and the data are summarized in Table 1.

Table 1. Decomposition of Sodium Methicillin Solutions at Room Temperature as Originally Reported and Later Corrected

pH	Decomposition in Percent	Hours (Initial Report)[5]	Hours (Corrected)
4.6	8	24	5.43
3.6	50	13	4.57
2.7	50	1.5	0.56

Interpretation of the Basic Kinetic Study of Sodium Methicillin

Whenever one wants to use the experimental findings of a fundamental study presented in the literature for a practical situation, there is often a dilemma of selecting pertinent information. Admittedly, herein lies the danger of extrapolating data derived from relatively ideal conditions to the present problem. Table 2 shows the general comparison of some of the important conditions of the study by Schwartz and coworkers with those conditions usually found for real parenteral admixtures.[11]

Table 2. Comparison of the Conditions of the Basic Kinetic Study and Parenteral Admixtures of Sodium Methicillin

Kinetic Study by Schwartz *et al.*[11]	Parenteral Admixture
SODIUM METHICILLIN:	
4.2 mg/ml	2 to 200 mg/ml
SOLVENT SYSTEM:	
Water plus buffers	Water plus dextrose, electrolytes, alcohol, buffers and/or other drugs
IONIC STRENGTH:	
0.5	0.03 to 0.158
TEMPERATURE:	
35 and 75°C	−15 to 25°C
pH:	
Variable	4.5 to 7.0

In this report kinetic studies were carried out with sodium methicillin in various aqueous buffer solutions at constant ionic strength of 0.5 at various temperatures. All the rates were apparent first order with respect to methicillin concentration.[11] Thus, Equations 1-4 apply here. Decomposition occurred by hydrolysis involving hydrogen and hydroxyl ion catalysis. The carbonate, citrate and acetate buffers had no effect on the degradation rates of methicillin; however, the phosphates had a catalyzing effect. Accordingly, the apparent (or observed) first order rate constant was described by

$$k_{app} = k_1 [H^+] f_{HP} + k_2 [H^+] f_P + k_{OH} [OH^-] + k_o + k_4 [P_T] f_{HPO_4} \qquad \text{(Equation 10)}$$

where k_1 and k_2 are the second order rate constants in acid solution, k_{OH} and k_4 are the second order rate constants for hydroxyl ion and phosphate catalysis, respectively, and k_o is the first order constant of the spontaneous hydrolysis. The f_{HP} is the fraction of the methicillin existing in the nonionized form and f_P, the fraction ionized; the f_{HPO_4} is the fraction of the HPO_4^{-2} species with respect to the total phosphate concentration, $[P_T]$. The catalysis by other phosphate species in the pH range of 5.9 to 8.1 was found to be insignificant. With the use of the expression for the dissociation constant K_a of methicillin

$$K_a = \frac{[H^+]\,[P^-]}{[HP]} = 1.83 \times 10^{-3} \qquad \text{(Equation 11)}$$

then

$$f_{HP} = \frac{[HP]}{[HP] + [P^-]} = \frac{[H^+]}{[H^+] + K_a} \qquad \text{(Equation 12)}$$

and

$$f_P = \frac{[P^-]}{[HP] + [P^-]} = \frac{K_a}{[H^+] + K_a} \qquad \text{(Equation 13)}$$

Table 3. Rate Constants[11]

Specific Constants	Units	Rate Constants at Various T°C	
		35°C	75°C
k_1	liter/mole/hr	600	($600<k_1<2\times10^4$)
k_2	liter/mole/hr	3200	(1.486×10^5)
k_o	hr^{-1}	(<0.032)	0.032
k_{OH}	liter/mole/hr	(<8000)	8000
k_4	liter/mole/hr	(<2.0)	2.0

In a likewise manner, one can obtain

$$f_{HPO_4} = \frac{1}{\dfrac{[H^+]^2}{K_2K_1} + \dfrac{[H^+]}{K_2} + \dfrac{K_3}{[H^+]} + 1} \qquad \text{(Equation 14)}$$

where K_1, K_2 and K_3 are the dissociation constants of phosphoric acid.[12] The pKa of methicillin at ionic strength 0.5 and 25° C is 2.74 ± 0.03 and is in agreement with other investigators.[13] The rate constants are listed in Table 3 for 35° and 75° C. Since Schwartz did not list all of the constants, the magnitude of the constants is indicated in parentheses and k_2 has been calculated at 75° C from the basic data.

A few comments on Equation 10 and Table 3 are worthwhile. The first order rate constants have units of time,$^{-1}$ the second order rate constants in moles liter^{-1} time^{-1} and the concentrations of catalytic species in moles liter.$^{-1}$ In the absence of phosphate buffers, Equation 10 reduces to

$$k_{app} = k_1 [H^+] f_{HP} + k_2 [H^+] f_P + k_{OH} [OH^-] + k_o \qquad \text{(Equation 15)}$$

and, in turn, at high alkaline pH

$$k_{app} \cong k_{OH} [OH^-] + k_o \qquad \text{(Equation 16)}$$

or at low acid pH

$$k_{app} \cong k_1 [H^+] f_{HP} + k_2 [H^+] f_P + k_o \qquad \text{(Equation 17)}$$

One can immediately write Equations 16 and 17 from 15 from his chemical and physical intuition or arrive at these limiting equations mathematically, for example, by selecting an acid pH, calculating k_{app} by Equation 15 and then observing that the term for alkaline hydrolysis, *i.e.*, $k_{OH} [OH^-]$, is an insignificant contribtuion to k_{app}. One of the lessons that the above example should convey is the feeling for the relative significance of numbers. It is from this lesson and also from the fact that most intravenous admixtures of sodium methicillin are in the pH range of 4 to 6.5 that the stability prediction of sodium methicillin preparations can be considered now, although Schwartz did not provide all of the rate constants (Table 3). This lack of explicit information in the literature is to be generally expected, but one can overcome this apparent difficulty through a chemical sense, knowledge of physical theory and use of mathematics.

Thus far, the basic study in the literature has provided us with some kinetic equations and constants at 35° and 75° C. To extend the data

Table 4. Calculated Values of Observed First Order Rate Constants at Various Temperatures and pH Including the Heats of Activation*

pH	k_{app} in hr^{-1} at Various T°C 35°C	75°C	ΔH_a in kcal $Mole^{-1}$
3.6	0.7241	32.779	20.3049
4.0	0.3065	14.1180	20.4067
4.5	0.0998	4.6318	20.4421
5.0	0.03182	1.510	20.560
6.0	0.0037	0.182	20.7623

*See Addendum I for method of calculation.

to other temperatures, one utilizes the Arrhenius relationship in the form of

$$\log k_{app} = \log A - \frac{\Delta H_a}{2.303R} \cdot \frac{1}{T} \quad \text{(Equation 18)}$$

where A is a constant, and the other terms have been defined before. According to Equation 18, a plot of log k_{app} *versus* 1/T yields a straight line with a negative slope of $\Delta H_a/2.303$ R and an intercept of log A. From the data in Table 3 and Equation 15, the observed first order rate constants at two temperatures and various pH were calculated and are shown in Table 4. Figure 2 shows the Arrhenius plots of the generated data in Table 4. It is evident that the plots are

Table 5. Comparison of Theoretical Predictions with Experimental Data on the Stability of Sodium Methicillin in Various Intravenous Solutions*

	Experimental					Theoretically
REFERENCE	pH of Mixture	T°C	Diluent	Time in Hours	Percent Drug Remaining	Predicted Percent Drug Remaining
5	2.7	25	Dextrose 5% or NaCl 0.9%	0.561	50	57.1
5	3.6	25	Dextrose 5% or NaCl 0.9%	4.57	50	37.0
9	4.0	25	Dextrose 5%	24	20	11.5
9	4.5	25	Dextrose 5%	24	53	48.7
5	4.6	25	Dextrose 5% or NaCl 0.9%	5.432	92	87.0
9	4.9	25	Dextrose 5% in lactated ringers	24	90	74.25
9	5.0	25	Dextrose 5%	24	86	80.2
9	5.2	25	Normosol-M —D5 (Abbott)	24	96	86.2
9	6.0	25	Dextrose 5%	24	100	97.5
9	6.15	25	Normosol-R (Abbott)	24	100	~100
9	6.3	25	Dextrose 5%	24	100	~100
9	6.3	25	Ringers	24	100	~100
10	6.0-6.6	25	Water or NaCl 0.9%	24	not given	97.5-100
10	6.0-6.6	10	Water or NaCl 0.9%	96	not given	97.5-100

*See Addendum II for method of calculation.

Table 6. Comparison of Theoretical Predictions with Experimental Data on the Stability of Sodium Methicillin in Various Intravenous Solutions*

	Experimental					
REFERENCE	pH of Mixture	T°C	Diluent	Percent Drug Remaining	Time in Hours	Theoretically Predicted Time in Hours
5	2.7	25	Dextrose 5% or NaCl 0.9%	50	0.561	0.578
5	3.6	25	Dextrose 5% or NaCl 0.9%	50	4.57	3.151
9	4.0	25	Dextrose 5%	20	24.0	17.887
9	4.5	25	Dextrose 5%	53	24.0	20.489
5	4.6	25	Dextrose 5% or NaCl 0.9%	92	5.432	3.412
9	5.0	25	Dextrose 5%	86	24.0	15.416
9	6.0	25	Dextrose 5%	90	not given	91.519

*See Addendum II for method of calculation.

restricted to the acid pH ranges and derived from a minimum of two calculated points. This is unavoidable because of the lack of data at other temperatures and in the alkaline range. The ΔH_a appears to be relatively constant within pH 4-6. Once the first order rate constant at one temperature and ΔH_a is provided, the rate constant at any desirable temperature may be readily determined on the assumption that the Arrhenius relationship holds throughout the temperature range. This is shown by Equation 9:

$$\log \frac{k_{app,2}}{k_{app,1}} = \frac{\Delta H_a}{2.303R} \cdot \frac{(T_2 - T_1)}{(T_2 T_1)} \quad \text{(Equation 9)}$$

Comparison of Theoretical Predictions with the Experimentally Evaluated Stability Data of Preparations

Tables 5 and 6 show a rather good agreement between the theoretically predicted and experimentally derived stability data of some sodium methicillin solutions of clinical importance. At a given time, pH and temperature, the theoretical predictions tend to underestimate the amount of drug remaining by 3 to 10 percent in comparison with the experimental findings (Table 5). Stated in another way, at a constant pH and temperature, the theoretical approach underestimates the time for a given degree of hydrolysis (Table 6). However, this is not surprising since it is well known that the rate of reaction is influenced by the ionic strength of the system such that the

Figure 2. A semilog plot of the Arrhenius relationship between the apparent first order rate constants and the temperatures as a function of pH of the solution. Data based on Table 4

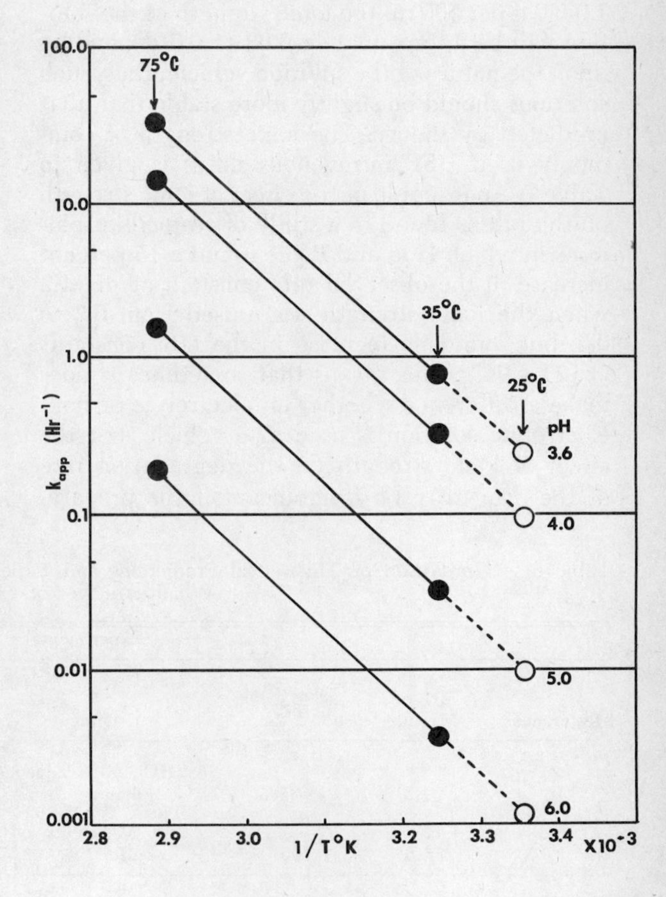

Table 7. pH Range and Ionic Strength of USP XVI Injections Generally Used for Bulk Intravenous Administration*

Official Injections	Acceptable pH range	Ionic Strength μ
Dextrose	3.5-6.5	---
Dextrose and sodium chloride	3.5-6.0	0.034 (NaCl 0.2%)
Lactated potassic saline	6.7-7.5	0.156
Lactated Ringer's	6.0-7.0	0.138
Ringer's	5.0-7.5	0.158
Sodium chloride	4.5-7.0	0.154 (NaCl 0.9%)
Sodium lactate†	6.0-7.3	0.144 ($NaC_3H_5O_3$ 1/6M)
Water	none listed	---

*See Addendum IV for method of calculating the ionic strength.
†When diluted, if necessary, to 0.2 M.

rate constant increases with increasing ionic strength.[14] As mentioned previously, the theoretical approach is based on kinetic data of an aqueous solvent system with constant 0.5 ionic strength. In the clinical situation in which sodium methicillin preparations range from 1.0-6.0 g per 500 ml the ionic strength of the solution will be approximately 0.03 to 0.3 depending upon the nature of the solution vehicle; thus, such solutions should be slightly more stable than that predicted by theory. The ionic strength of commonly used USP intravenous fluids is given in Table 7. An example of the effect of ionic strength on the rate is found in a study of ampicillin solutions in which Hou and Poole found a 15 percent increase in the observed rate constant at pH 1.2 when the ionic strength was raised from 0.2 to 0.5, but found no increase in the rate constants at pH 4.94.[15] This means that sometimes it does make a difference whether an electrolyte or nonelectrolyte solution is used as a vehicle, but the effect of ionic strength on the degradation rate of the drug may be insignificant if the preparation is administered within a reasonable amount of time.

The theoretical prediction was also extended to sodium methicillin in solution systems which are not of clinical importance (Table 8). It is interesting to observe that the experimentally determined stability of a 50 percent alcoholic solution was greater than the theoretically determined stability of an aqueous solution. Depending upon the nature of the reacting molecules, a decrease in the dielectric constant of the solvent may increase or decrease the rate process.[14] For example, the rate of glucose decomposition in acidic solutions is increased in solvents with decreasing dielectric constants. In contrast, the rate of ampicillin degradation in solution at pH 1.2 decreases linearly with increasing concentrations of ethanol, *i.e.*, decreasing dielectric constant of the solvent.[15] Thus, the role of the solvent on the rate is dependent upon its dielectric constant and ionic strength, among other factors.

Theoretical Predictions of Sodium Methicillin Solutions Containing Phosphates

So far, no stability predictions have been made when sodium methicillin is under the catalyzing influence of phosphates. In making incompatibility and stability charts the compiler would simply indicate an "X" for sodium methicillin and phosphate combinations. Is it really that absolute? If it is so, one would not be justified in adding hydrocortisone sodium succinate injection (Solu-Cortef, Upjohn) which contains 0.8 mg NaH_2PO_4 and 8.76 mg Na_2HPO_4 as buffer per 100 mg vial, or in using Travert 5% Electrolyte No. 2 (Baxter Laboratories) which contains 12.5 mEq HPO_4^{-2} per liter as electrolyte replacement. According to Equations 10 and 14, the extent of the catalyzing effect of phosphates will vary with the pH of the solution and total phosphate concentration.

Table 8. Comparison of Theoretical Predictions and Experimental Data on the Stability of Methicillin Preparations Which Are Not of Clinical Importance

Experimental						
Reference	pH of Mixture	T°C	Diluent	Percent Drug Remaining	Time in Minutes	Theoretically Predicted Time in Minutes
16	1.3	35	HCl, 50% aqueous ethanol	50	2-3	1.2
17	4.5	100	0.1 M acetate buffer	7.4	30	37

Table 9. Effect of Biphosphate Ion Catalysis on the Observed Rate Constant at 35°C as a Function of pH and Total Phosphate Concentration*†‡

pH	k'_{app} (hr^{-1})	Constant for HPO_4^{-2} Effects				Percent Increase in k'_{app} by Catalyzing Effect of HPO_4^{-2}
		k_4	f_{HPO4}	$[P_T]$	k_4f_{HPO} $[P_T]$	
5.0	3.182×10^{-2}	10^{-1}	6.153×10^{-3}	6.387×10^{-5}	3.93×10^{-8}	$\sim 1 \times 10^{-4}$
				1×10^{-2}	6.153×10^{-6}	$\sim 2 \times 10^{-2}$
6.0	3.7×10^{-3}	10^{-1}	5.837×10^{-2}	6.387×10^{-5}	3.728×10^{-7}	$\sim 1 \times 10^{-2}$
				1×10^{-2}	5.837×10^{-5}	~ 1.6

*Results generated from Equations 10-14 using data from Table 3.
†k'_{app} is the observed rate constant without effect of phosphate from Equation 15 and Table 4.
‡See Addendum II for method of calculation.

If sodium methicillin is added to a liter of normal saline containing 100 mg Solu-Cortef or a liter of Travert 5% Electrolyte No. 2 at 35° C and the pH of the mixture is 5 or 6, can the influence of phosphates on the stability be predicted? In the first case there is 6.387×10^{-5} M total phosphate and in the second case, approximately 1×10^{-2} M. Accounting only for the effect of specific hydrogen, hydroxyl and biphosphate ion catalysis, the predictions on the observed first order rate constants are shown in Table 9. As the pH is raised from 5 to 6, the $f_{HPO_4^{-2}}$ increases about ten-fold and, consequently, the effect of HPO_4^{-2} ion catalysis will increase for any given total phosphate concentration. In the solution containing Solu-Cortef, the rate of methicillin degradation will not increase more than 0.01 percent at pH 5-6 and 35°C. Likewise, in the other solution containing a higher phosphate concentration, the increase will not be more than 1.6 percent.

Comparison of the Theoretically Predicted and Experimental Solubility of Sodium Methicillin in Clinical Preparations

While many pharmacists, including drug information specialists, are concerned with the incompatibility and instability of intravenous drug admixtures, they frequently overlook among other things, the physical chemical phenomena of solubility as influenced by pH. This phenomena is amply treated by Martin.[18] In several instances sediment of crystals has been reported when 1.0 g of buffered sodium methicillin injection was added to 50 ml of 5 percent dextrose injection.[19] Upon using different lots of sodium methicillin and dextrose injections, sedimentation was not subsequently observed. Unfortunately, there was no serious experimental follow-up to identify the crystals and determine the pH of the solution.

However, one could possibly explain the phenomena on the basis of pH-solubility relationships. According to the theory, when salts of weak acids or bases are dissolved in water, the ionized (dissociated) and un-ionized (undissociated) species exist in equilibrium with each other. In the specific case of sodium methicillin, it follows that:

$$HP \leftrightarrows H^+ + P^-$$

The relative concentration of each kind of species is governed by the dissociation constant of the drug and the pH of the solution through the well-known Henderson-Hasselbach relationship.[12] When the pH conditions are such that the concentration of the un-ionized species exceeds its solubility, precipitation will occur.

The pH *below* which the salt of a weak acid precipitates from solution as the un-ionized acid at a constant temperature, *i.e.*, $pH_{P,acid}$, is expressed by:

$$pH_{P,acid} = pK_a + \log \frac{S - S_o}{S_o} \quad \text{(Equation 19)}$$

Table 10. Influence of pH on the Solubility of Sodium Methicillin in Commonly Prescribed Concentrations*

Total Volume of Solution in ml	$pH_{P,acid}$ for Various Concentrations of Sodium Methicillin at 25°C		
	1.0 g	4.0 g	6.0 g
2	5.83	--	--
8	--	5.83	--
12	--	--	5.83
50	4.43	5.04	5.21
500	3.34	4.02	4.20
1000	2.91	3.69	3.88

*See Addendum III for method of calculation.

Table 11. Manufacturer's Recommended Directons for Reconstitution of Buffered Sodium Methicillin Injection[10]

Vial	Volume (ml) of Water or NaCl Injection to be Added	Final Volume (ml)
1.0 g	1.5	2
4.0 g	5.7	8
6.0 g	8.6	12

Whereas, the pH *above* which the salt of a weak base precipitates from the solution as the un-ionized base is:

$$pH_{P,base} = pK_w - pK_b + \log \frac{S}{S - S_o} \quad \text{(Equation 20)}$$

Thus, the $pH_{P,acid}$ or $pH_{P,base}$ is dependent upon the initial molar concentration of salt added, S; the molar solubility of the free acid or base, S_o; and the pK of the acid, base and water.

Table 10 illustrates the application of Equation 19 to predict the pH below which sodium methicellin begins to precipitate as the undissociated methicillin acid. The concentrations chosen, 1.0 g/2 ml, 1.0 g/50 ml and so forth, represent the usual final concentrations that are used in therapy or those recommended by the manufacturer after reconstitution of the injectable product (Table 11). It is evident that the critical pH for the precipitation of the acidic drug increases as the concentration of sodium methicillin increases.

Figure 3. Stability of penicillin G potassium (1 million units/L) in dextrose 5% at 24 hours at 25°C and various pH. (Redrawn from reference 20)

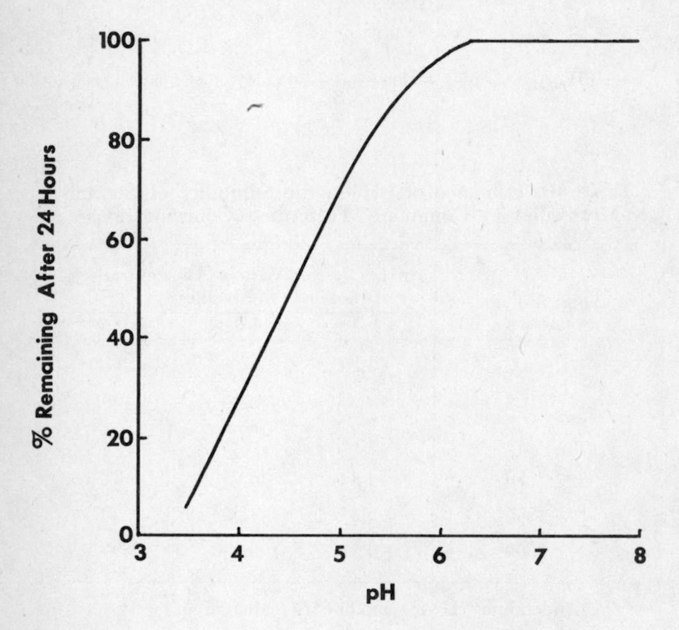

In practice this means that the chance of precipitating the drug is less when the concentration is low or when the pH of the solution is much greater than the $pH_{P,acid}$. Since the pH of a sodium methicillin parenteral solution depends upon the final concentration and dissociability of each ingredient in the admixture, the choice of the diluting solution becomes important from the viewpoint of stability and solubility of the drug. It is well-known that the USP injections which are used as diluting solvents and the large volume intravenous fluids have a wide pH range of acceptance (Table 7). In consideration of the problem of solubility alone, dextrose and dextrose/sodium chloride injections are not particularly desirable solvents for the primary reconstitution of sodium methicillin, unless their pH is at the official maximum pH of acceptance or the dilution is sufficiently high.

PREDICTING DRUG STABILITY FROM KINETIC STUDIES OF CLINICALLY IMPORTANT SOLUTIONS

It is intended to show in this section how one can use and extend the information available on the stability of clinically important parenteral drug solutions. Usually, this type of information is found in *Drug Intelligence and Clinical Pharmacy, American Journal of Hospital Pharmacy, International Pharmaceutical Abstracts* and similar publications. However, when one makes a reasonable literature search, he will find a paucity of data on specific parenteral admixtures. Furthermore, when there are data on a specific admixture, he will find (a) that it is presented in such a manner that is not particularly explicit to answer the kind of questions often asked, and (b) that it is not sufficiently comprehensive to relate the various situations such as pH, temperature and vehicle. There are two obvious reasons for this. First, it takes time, effort, initiative and reasonable scientific ability for a research-oriented pharmacist to find a reliable analytical method and then to study the kinetics of decomposition of the drug under varying conditions. Secondly, the presentation of the data in a manner that can be understood and utilized by others to whom the study is intended may vary.

Variations on a Method of Predicting Stability from Reports on Clinically Important Parenteral Preparations

Using a similar approach as before, the information available on the stability of clinically important parenteral solutions will be presented, and it will be shown explicitly how one can calculate and extend the prediction. In pointing out the limitations, one should recognize that it is not the intention of this author to detract from the value of the type of information given and the service it provides to the professional practitioner. Nor is it to criticize the efforts of the investigators, but rather it is to use the information given as a teaching example in what it can and cannot do in practice.

Case A:

One of the typical examples of presenting stability data is illustrated in Figure 3, in which the percent of the initial concentration remaining after 24 hours *versus* solution pH of penicillin G potassium in dextrose 5 percent in water at 25° C was given.[20] The first two columns of Table 12 give some pH values and the corresponding stability. Thus far, the information is specific and therefore self-limiting. For example, 49.23 percent of the initial concentration remains after 24 hours at 25° C and pH 4.5, 70 percent after 24 hours at pH 5.0, and 100 percent at pH 7-8.

If it is necessary to know, for some reason, how much remains after 48 hours at pH 5.0, or how long an expiration date should be specified for a solution at pH 5.0, can the answers be provided accurately? Unfortunately, the usual final answers given by pharmacists are "more than 70 percent remaining" and "less than 24 hours" to the first and second questions, respectively. However, re-interpreting the information from Figure 3, it is possible to be more precise. It is assumed, with the information available in Figure 3, that the decomposition of penicillin is apparently first order. As it turns out, a further search of the literature shows that this assumption is correct.[21,22] Regardless of this verification, it should be noted that the first order assumption is generally a rather good one for about one-half life of a drug, *i.e.*, the time at which 50 percent of the nondecomposed drug remains. From the viewpoint of calculations it is more convenient to convert the stability data in the second column of Table 12 to a suitable common parameter, the apparent first order rate constant k_{app}. A sample calculation follows.

Example: To convert 49.23 percent drug remaining after 24 hours at 25° C and pH 4.5 to k_{app}.

Rearranging Equation 3,

$$k_{app} = -\frac{2.303}{t} \log \frac{C}{C_o}$$

$$= -\frac{2.303}{24} \log 0.4923$$

$$= 0.02953 \text{ hr}^{-1}$$

Table 12. Interpretation of Literature Stability Data in Terms of Rate Constants for Case A

Literature Data		Extension of Literature Data by Theory		
pH	Percent Remaining After 24 Hours	k_{app} (hr^{-1})	$t_{0.9}$ (hr)*	$t'_{0.9}$ (hr)+
3.9	20.40	6.624×10^{-2}	1.59	
4.0	27.69	5.351×10^{-2}	1.97	1.77
4.35	40.30	3.787×10^{-2}	2.78	
4.5	49.23	2.953×10^{-2}	3.57	3.21
4.9	60.70	2.080×10^{-2}	5.07	
5.0	70.0	1.486×10^{-2}	7.09	6.38
5.1	70.5	1.457×10^{-2}	7.23	
5.5	88.46	0.511×10^{-2}	20.62	18.56
5.7	90.2	0.430×10^{-2}	24.5	
5.8	90.4	0.421×10^{-2}	25.1	
6.0	96.5	0.164×10^{-2}	60.24	54.22
7.0	100.0	---	>24.0	>24.0
8.0	100.0	---	>24.0	>24.0

*$t_{0.9}$ is the time in which 90 percent of nondecomposed drug is remaining.
+$t'_{0.9}$ allows for a 10 percent overestimation of the predicted $t_{0.9}$.

Table 13. Stability of Penicillin G Potassium (1 Million Units per Liter) in Various I.V. Fluids[25]

Diluent	pH	Percent Initial Pen. G-K Content Remaining: 6 Hours	24 Hours
Alcohol 5%, dextrose 5%	5.1	93.8	66.1
Dextrose 5% in water	4.9	94.0	54.2
Multi-electrolyte	7.3	93.9	90.5
Sodium chloride	5.7	97.4	86.3
Water for parenterals	5.8	100.0	89.8

Since k_{app} is now known, the fraction remaining at a given time can be calculated from Equation 3 and vice versa. A sample calculation is given below.

Example: To calculate the expiration date of penicillin G potassium in dextrose 5 percent in water at pH 5.0 and 25° C. The time for 10 percent decomposition to take place is generally taken as the maximum limit of shelf-life. Thus, it is necessary to solve $t_{0.9}$ when $C/C_o = 0.9$, the fraction of drug remaining. Rearranging Equation 3:

$$t = -\frac{2.303}{k_{app}} \log \frac{C}{C_o}$$

$$t_{0.9} = -\frac{2.303}{0.01486} \log 0.9$$

$$= 7.09 \text{ hr}$$

Table 12 summarizes some of the literature data, rate constant and predicted $t_{0.9}$. To account for experimental error within the stability data and the uncertainties in determining the stability values from Figure 3 in addition to the tendency to be conservative because of concern with a patient's well-being, an arbitrary 10 percent overestimation of the predicted time as indicated by $t'_{0.9}$ has been allowed.

Several limitations can be cited on the type of information given in Figure 3 and the extension of stability prediction in Table 12:

1. The temperature dependence of the rate of decomposition cannot be predicted.

2. The solvent effect on the rate through the ionic strength and dielectric properties of the vehicle is unknown. However, as a first approximation, the stability of a drug in dextrose solutions may be taken to be the same as those in water and electrolyte solutions (see Case B).

3. When the stability is not constant within a pH range, for example, pH 3-6 in Figure 3, accurate predictions can be made only when the penicillin is in a buffered solution so that the pH remains fairly constant. Predicting unbuffered penicillin solutions becomes hazardous.[23]

4. Although it is known that penicillin decomposes at pH 6-8,[24] extending the predictions cannot be done since the only apparent information shows there is no significant decomposition within 24 hours.

Case B:

Another typical example of a presentation of stability data is illustrated in Table 13 which gives the stability of penicillin G potassium in various common I.V. fluids at the initial *in situ* pH of the admixture.[25]

Based on Equation 3, a semilog plot of the percent remaining *versus* the time was applied. Equation 3 predicts a straight line with a negative slope equal to $k_{app}/2.303$. As we carefully scrutinize Figure 4, it is noticed that the data points do not indicate a linear curve. In other words, the stability is significantly less at 24 hours than would be predicted at six hours. Two immediate reasons may be postulated: (1)

Figure 4. Semilogarithmic plot of penicillin G potassium in various I.V. fluids at *in situ* pH. Based on data in Table 13

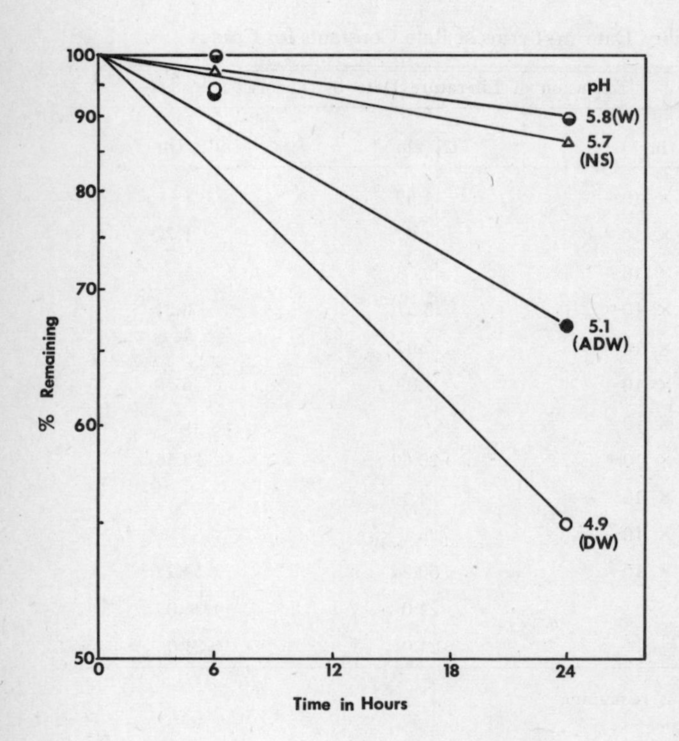

the changes in the pH of the admixture over a period of time as a result of the low total buffer capacity from the dilution effect of the buffered penicillin injection and the inherently low buffer capacity of the vehicle;[26] and, consequently, (2) the increasing autocatalytic activity of the admixture with time, according to a general acid-base catalysis reaction.[23]

Finding oneself in this situation, what should be done? Proceeding on, one could draw the best straight line by observation or least squares analysis. But, one should be ultraconservative for the sake of the patient and accept the line as drawn in Figure 4. This enables an estimation of the rate constants (see the example below). The rate constants and $t_{0.9}$ are summarized in Table 14.

Example: To calculate k_{app} for penicillin in an alcohol 5 percent, dextrose 5 percent solution at pH 5.1 from the slope in Figure 4 and to calculate $t_{0.9}$.

Rearranging Equation 1:

$$k_{app} = -\frac{1}{C}\frac{dC}{dt} = -2.303\frac{d \log C}{dt}$$

$$= -2.303\frac{\Delta \log C}{\Delta t}$$

Choosing any two points on the straight line:

$$k_{app} = -\frac{2.303 (\log 100 - \log 66.1)}{0 - 24}$$

$$= 0.01725 \text{ hr}^{-1}$$

Table 14. Interpretation of Literature Stability Data in Terms of Rate Constants for Case B

Diluent	pH	k_{app} (hr^{-1})	$t_{0.9}$ (hr)
Dextrose 5% in water	4.9	2.552×10^{-2}	4.13
Alcohol 5%, dextrose 5%	5.1	1.725×10^{-2}	6.11
Sodium chloride	5.7	0.614×10^{-2}	17.2
Water for parenterals	5.8	0.448×10^{-2}	23.5
Multi-electrolyte	7.3	0.416×10^{-2}	25.3

Thus, as before:

$$t_{0.9} = -\frac{2.303}{k_{app}} \log 0.9$$

$$= -\frac{2.303}{0.01725} \log 0.9 = 6.11 \text{ hr.}$$

Case C:

Table 15 represents the third example of data presentation. Here it is assumed that the addition of another drug product to the penicillin-dextrose solution does not result in incompatibility; rather, the activity of the penicillin and even the other drug additive is affected by the pH of the admixture through a general acid-base catalytic mechanism.

After following through as before in Case B, that is, obtaining first order plots of the data in Table 15 and then calculating the rate constants from the slope, the results of the calculations are obtained (Table 16).

Table 15. Stability of Penicillin G-K (10^6 units/L) with Various Additives in Dextrose 5% (25°C)[20]

Additive	Conc./L	Admixture pH	Activity (units/ml) After Mixing 0 hrs	6 hrs	24 hours
Aminophyllin (Searle)	500 mg	8.7	940	730	525
Aramine bitartrate	100 mg	4.35	850	790	350
Bejectal w/C	10 ml	3.9	920	580	127
Benadryl hydrochloride	50 mg	6.5	870	860	870
Compazine edisylate	10 mg	6.45	870	890	888
Gantrisin ethanolamine	4 g	7.4	900	870	868
Heparin sodium (Abbott)	20,000 units	6.65	920	900	965
Nembutal sodium	500 mg	9.0	920	760	535
Sodium bicarbonate (Abbott)	3.75 g	8.1	900	930	663
Sodium iodide (Abbott)	1 g	6.8	860	870	904

Table 16. Interpretation of Literature Stability Data in Terms of Rate Constants for Case C

Additive	Admixture pH	k_{app} (hr^{-1})	$t_{0.9}$ (hr)
Bejectal w/C	3.9	8.282×10^{-2}	1.27
Aramine bitartrate	4.35	3.695×10^{-2}	2.85
Gantrisin ethanolamine	7.4	0.153×10^{-2}	69.1
Sodium bicarbonate (Abbott)	8.1	1.272×10^{-2}	8.28
Nembutal sodium	9.0	2.555×10^{-2}	4.67
All others	6.45-6.8	---	>24.0

Comparison of the Results of Cases A, B and C

It is useful to compare the results in Tables 12, 14 and 16 for Cases A, B, and C, respectively. Whether penicillin G in dextrose solutions is more stable than that in electrolyte solutions at the same admixture pH is not quite clear, although there is an apparent tendency for less stability in electrolyte solutions from an ionic strength effect. To resolve this question, a further search in the literature on the basis of kinetic behavior of penicillin G is required.

When comparing Tables 12 and 16, evidence may be found that the addition of certain drug products, for example, Gantrisin Ethanolamine and Bejectal w/C, to penicillin in dextrose solution does appear to enhance the rate of decomposition of penicillin. With no immediate information available, nothing can be said about the corresponding stability of the added drug. However, which ever drug decomposes the fastest would determine the expiration date of the admixture.

From a practical point of view and hindsight, the time for 90 percent activity of penicillin remaining in the various I.V. fluids (Table 14) and in dextrose solutions with added drugs (Table 16) could have been estimated just from the predicted $t_{0.9}$ for penicillin in dextrose solution at constant pH in Table 12. This is a highly useful first approximative method since one needs only to know the pH of the admixture. Even though some of the rate constants are different, this first approximation will be reasonably good only when restricted to the prediction of time for low levels of decomposition or vice versa. In this manner, advantage is taken of the fact that "the margin of error becomes less significant as the target is less distant."

As pointed out by Parker,[21] a great deal of penicillin would be inactivated during the one to six hours it takes to administer the parenteral admixture, not counting the period it remains in storage after preparation in the central I.V. additive laboratory, unless the penicillin admixture is at pH 6-7.

CONCLUSIONS

In the previous section on the "Relevance of Predicting Drug Stability," the relevance of using the results of basic kinetic studies in the literature with the accompanying mathematics to predict the stability of drugs in clinically significant parenteral solutions was demonstrated. As an example, the stability of sodium methicillin in parenteral solutions was calculated from a theoretical approach. It is significant that the agreement with the experimental stability of methicillin solutions of clinical importance was good. Furthermore, by utilizing the example of sodium methicillin with substantiating references, a significant effort has been made to point out that, in general, the clinical pharmacists must not be lulled into thinking that there are no problems with the so-called "one I.V. additive admixture." Is it really just one drug additive to water? The contribution of electrolytes, sugars and alcohol to the physical chemistry of the solvent effect on the stability and solubility of the principal drug(s) via the pH, ionic strength, dielectric constant and specific ion catalysis also must be evaluated. However, given the necessary basic kinetic data, the pharmacist can make a quantitative approximation of the solvent effect on drugs in clinically important preparations.

In the final section an attempt has been made to show how the pharmacist could consolidate and interpret the current literature on the stability of clinically significant parenteral admixtures. The collected studies of Parker on the stability of penicillin G potassium admixtures were used as examples. Consolidation of the information was achieved by reducing the data, presented in a variety of ways, to a common parameter, that is, the first order rate constant. This enabled rapid calculations to be made based on theory and stability predictions to be refined as to the degree of chemical activity available in the solution at any time and vice versa. Further, it permitted the data to be interpreted and translated into practice more easily.

The underlying objective of this chapter was to improve the scientific performance of the pharmacist in the area of drug stability. The kinds of approaches demonstrated here are not unique. Physical and chemical scientists utilize the theoretical approach routinely as a first approximation to predict quantitatively what might happen to a system. One should realize that to be able to predict the stability of clinical parenteral preparations on this *a priori* basis is a powerful application of the theory, just as it is also powerful to predict *a priori* the incompatibility of intravenous admixtures on the basis of chemical structure alone. Among the subjects within the physical, chemical and biological sciences, chemical kinetics is one that is highly relevant and provides the scientific support, so badly needed, to daily professional practice in pharmacy.

Although it is realized that many hospital pharmacists, who are engaged in centralized I.V. admixture and drug information programs and have had formal academic education in pharmaceutics, feel these techniques are beyond their immediate comprehension and mathematical ability, this level of scientific sophistication in chemical kinetics and other areas is needed and contributes toward the total scientific uniqueness of the professional pharmacist. The premise that "the pharmacist should be the logical expert person to become involved in this or that by reason of his unique and sophisticated training" is quite meaningless unless he is committed to the challenge and demonstrates his commitment through performance.

References

1. Martin, A. N., Swarbrick, J. and Cammarata, A.: *Physical Pharmacy,* ed. 2, Lea and Febiger, Philadelphia, Pa., 1969, Chapter 14.
2. Frost, A. A. and Pearson, R. G.: *Kinetics and Mechanism,* ed. 2, John Wiley and Sons, New York, 1961.
3. Laidler, K. J.: *Chemical Kinetics,* ed. 2, McGraw-Hill, New York, 1965.
4. Granatek, A. P. and Buckwalter, F. H.: Stability of Sodium Dimethoxyphenylpenicillin, *J. Am. Pharm. Assoc. 54*:560 (Sept.) 1961.
5. Galleli, J. F.: Stability Studies of Drugs Used in Intravenous Solutions I., *Am. J. Hosp. Pharm. 24*:425 (Aug.) 1967.
6. Stolar, M. H., Carlin, H. S. and Blake, M. I.: Effect of Freezing on the Stability of Sodium Methicillin Injection, *Am. J. Hosp. Pharm. 25*:32 (Jan.) 1968.
7. Carlin, H. S. and Perkins, A. J.: Predicting Pharmaceutical Incompatibilities of Parenteral Medications, *Am. J. Hosp. Pharm. 25*:271 (June) 1968.
8. Galleli, J. F., MacLowry, J. D. and Skolaut, M. W.: Stability of Antibiotics in Parenteral Solutions, *Am. J. Hosp. Pharm. 26*:630 (Nov.) 1969.
9. Parker, E. A.: Compatibility Digest, *Am. J. Hosp. Pharm. 27*:67 (Jan.) 1970.
10. Package Insert, "Staphcillin — Buffered for Injection," Bristol Laboratories, Syracuse, New York.
11. Schwartz, M. A., Bara, E., Rubycz, I. and Granatek, A. P.: Stability of Methicillin, *J. Pharm. Sci. 54*:149 (Jan.) 1965.
12. Martin, A. N.: *Physical Pharmacy,* ed. 1, Lea and Febiger, Philadelphia, Pa., 1960, Ch. 9.
13. Rapson, H. D. C. and Bird, A. E.: Ionization Constants of Some Penicillins and of Their Alkaline and Penicillinase Hydrolysis Products, *J. Pharm. Pharmacol. 15*:222T (Dec.) 1963.
14. Martin, A. N.: *Physical Pharmacy,* ed. 1, ibid., p. 488.
15. Hou, J. P. and Poole, J. W.: Kinetics and Mechanism of Degradation of Ampicillin in Solution, *J. Pharm. Sci. 58*:447 (Apr.) 1969.
16. Doyle, F. P., Long, A. A., Nayler, J. H. and Stove, E. R.: New Penicillins Stable Towards Both Acid and Penicillinase, *Nature 192*:1183 (Dec. 23) 1961.
17. Narasimhachari, N. and Rao, G. R.: Physico-Chemical Studies on the Stability of Penicillin Salts III. Stability Studies on Some Newer Penicillins — A Note on the Spectrophotometric Estimation of 2,6 Dimethoxyphenyl Penicillin, *Hindustan Antibiot. Bull. 6*:114 (Feb.) 1964.
18. Martin, A. N.: *Physical Pharmacy,* ed. 1, ibid., p. 369.
19. Personal communication with Drug Information Center, Pharmacy Dept., University of Michigan Medical Center, Ann Arbor.
20. Parker, E. A.: Compatibility Digest, *Am. J. Hosp. Pharm. 26*:543 (Sept.) 1969.
21. Parker, E. A., Boomer, R. J. and Bell, S. C.: Parenteral Incompatibilities — Past, Present and Future, *Bull. Parenteral Drug Assoc. 21*:197 (Nov.-Dec.) 1967.
22. Effect of pH of the Medium on the Stability of Penicillin in Aqueous Solution, *Chem. Abstr. 53*:2538, 1959.
23. Macek, T. J., Hanus, E. J. and Feller, B. A.: The Stability of Penicillin G Solution in Aqueous Solution, *J. Am. Pharm. Assoc. Sci. Ed. 36*:322 (Aug.) 1948.
24. Brodersen, R.: Stability of Penicillin G in Aqueous Solution as a Function of Hydrogen Ion Concentration and Temperature, *Acta Pharmacol. 3*:345, 1947.
25. Parker, E. A.: Solution Additive Chemical Incompatibility Study, *Am. J. Hosp. Pharm. 24*:434 (Aug.) 1967.
26. Lundgren, P. and Landersjö, L.: Studies on the Stability and Compatibility of Drugs in Infusion Fluids I. pH and Buffer Capacity of Infusion Fluids, *Acta Pharm. Suecica 7*:407 (Sept.) 1970.
27. Ho, N. F. H. and Goeman, J. A.: Prediction of Pharmaceutical Stability of Parenteral Solutions I., *Drug Intelligence Clin. Pharm. 4*:69 (Mar.) 1970.
28. Gill, A. W., Severson, R. W. and Ho, N. F. H.: Prediction of Pharmaceutical Stability of Parenteral Solutions II., *Drug Intelligence Clin. Pharm. 4*:243 (Sept.) 1970.
29. Ho, N. F. H.: Prediction of Pharmaceutical Stability of Parenteral Solutions III., *Drug Intelligence Clin. Pharm. 5*:47 (Feb.) 1971.

Addendum I. Calculation of k_{app} at Various Temperatures Including ΔH_a.

Calculation of (a) k_{app} at 35°C and 75°C for pH = 5.0 conditions without phosphates, and (b) the ΔH_a, assuming that the Arrhenius relationship is valid.

With Equations 15, 12 and 13:

$$k_{app} = \frac{k_1\,[H^+]^2}{[H^+] + K_a} + \frac{k_2\,[H^+]\,K_a}{[H^+] + K_a} + k_{OH}\frac{K_w}{[H^+]} + k_o$$

Note that the ion product of water K_w varies with the absolute temperature and may be calculated by Equation 8:

$$-\log K_w = \frac{4470.99}{T} + 0.01706T - 6.0875$$

Assume K_a is independent of temperature since its temperature-dependency is unknown; however, this is not a serious error. Use the data in Table 3.

At 75°C:

$$k_{app} = \frac{(\sim 2 \times 10^4)(1 \times 10^{-5})^2}{10^{-5} + 1.83 \times 10^{-3}} + \frac{1.486 \times 10^5 \times 10^{-5} \times 1.83 \times 10^{-3}}{10^{-5} + 1.83 \times 10^{-3}} + \frac{(8 \times 10^3)(2.202 \times 10^{-13})}{10^{-5}} + 3.2 \times 10^{-2}$$

$$\cong 1.51 \text{ hr}^{-1}$$

At 35°C:

$$k_{app} = \frac{(6 \times 10^2)(1 \times 10^{-5})^2}{10^{-5} + 1.83 \times 10^{-3}} + \frac{3.2 \times 10^3 \times 10^{-5} \times 1.83 \times 10^{-3}}{10^{-5} + 1.83 \times 10^{-3}} + \frac{(<8 \times 10^3)(2.1 \times 10^{-14})}{10^{-5}} + (<3.2 \times 10^{-2})$$

$$\cong 0.03182 \text{ hr}^{-1}$$

ΔH_a can be calculated from the slope of a plot of Equation 18 or from Equation 9. Then, by Equation 9:

$$\Delta H_a = 2.303\, R \frac{(T_2 T_1)}{(T_2 - T_1)} (\log k_{app,2} - \log k_{app,1})$$

where T = °C + 273.15:

$$\Delta H_a = \frac{2.303 \times 1.99 \times 348.15 \times 308.15}{(348.15 - 308.15)} \times (\log 1.51 - \log 0.03182)$$

$$= 2.056 \times 10^4 \text{ cal/mole}$$

$$= 20.56 \text{ kcal/mole}$$

Addendum II. Prediction of Stability

A. Calculation of the percent of drug remaining at pH 5.0 and 25°C in 24 hours.

1. From the Arrhenius plot in Figure 2, derived from computations found in Addendum I and summarized in Table 4, $k_{app} = 0.0092 \text{ hr}^{-1}$ at 25°C. Utilizing Equation 3:

$$\log \frac{C}{C_o} = -\frac{k_{app}}{2.303} t$$

$$\log \frac{C}{C_o} = -\frac{0.0092 \times 24}{2.303} = -0.09587$$

$$\frac{C}{C_o} = 0.802$$

Percent drug remaining = 80.2%

2. Depending upon the data provided, one can solve the problem in an alternative way. From Table 4, $k_{app,35°C} = 0.03182$ and $\Delta H_a = 20.56$ kcal mole^{-1} at pH 5.0 To calculate $k_{app,25°C}$, we use Equation 9; thus:

$$\log k_{app,25°C} = \log k_{app,35°C} + \frac{\Delta H_a}{2.303R}\left(\frac{T_{25} - T_{35}}{T_{25}T_{35}}\right)$$

$$\log k_{app,25°C} = \log 0.03182 + \frac{2.056 \times 10^4}{2.303 \times 1.99}\left(\frac{298.15 - 308.15}{298.15 \times 308.15}\right)$$

$$= -1.9856$$

$$k_{app,25°C} = 1.033 \times 10^{-2}$$

Utilizing Equation 3:

$$\log \frac{C}{C_o} = -\frac{0.01033 \times 24}{2.303} = -0.10765$$

$$\frac{C}{C_o} = 0.781$$

Percent drug remaining = 78.1%

B. Calculation of the time at which there is 86 percent of drug remaining at pH 5.0 and 25°C.

In the previous problem it was shown that $k_{app} = 0.0092 \text{ hr}^{-1}$ at 25°C. Utilizing Equation 3:

$$t = -\frac{2.303 \log C/C_o}{k_{app}}$$

$$t = -\frac{2.303 \log 0.86}{0.0092}$$

$$= 16.42 \text{ hrs}$$

C. Calculation of the effect of phosphate on the k_{app} at 35°C when sodium methicillin is added to a liter of intravenous solution containing 100 mg Solu-Cortef and the pH of the total solution is 5.0.

In one liter of solution a 100 mg vial of Solu-Cortef will contribute 0.8 mg NaH_2PO_4 and 8.76 mg Na_2HPO_4. This is equivalent to 6.387 8.76 mg Na_2HPO_4. This is equivalent to 6.387×10^{-5} moles per liter total phosphate concentration. From Table 4 the calculated $k'_{app} = 0.03182\ hr^{-1}$ at 35°C when there is no phosphate present. By Equation 10, it follows that:

$$k_{app} = k'_{app} + k_4\ [P_T]\ f_{HPO_4}$$

where k_4 is less than 2 but will be in the order of 0.1 liter $mole^{-1}\ hr^{-1}$ from Table 3. With Equation 14 at pH 5.0:

$$f_{HPO_4} = \frac{1}{\frac{(10^{-5})^2}{(6.2 \times 10^{-8})(7.5 \times 10^{-3})} + \frac{10^{-5}}{6.2 + 10^{-8}} + \frac{2.13 \times 10^{-13}}{10^{-5}} + 1}$$

$$= 6.153 \times 10^{-3}$$

Therefore:

$$k_4\ [P_T]\ f_{HPO_4} = 10^{-1} \times 6.378 \times 10^{-5} \times 6.153 \times 10^{-3}$$

$$= 3.93 \times 10^{-8}\ hr^{-1}$$

The effect of phosphate represents an increase in the rate by:

$$\frac{k_4\ [P_T]\ f_{HPO_4}}{k'_{app}} \times 100 \cong 1 \times 10^{-4}\ \%$$

Addendum III. Prediction of Solubility as Influenced by pH. Calculation of $pH_{P,acid}$ for Sodium Methicillin Solution 1.0 g/2 ml at 25°C.

Pertinent constants: Solubility of methicillin acid, $\sim 10^{-3}$ M; M.W. of sodium salt, 402.42; pKa = 2.74 ± 0.03.

$$S = \frac{500\ g/liter}{402.42} = 1.2425\ M$$

Using Equation 19:

$$pH_{P,acid} = 2.74 + \log \frac{(1242.5 - 1.0) \times 10^{-3}}{1 \times 10^{-3}}$$

$$= 5.834$$

If $pH_{solution} < pH_{P,acid} = 5.834$, precipitation is predicted.

Addendum IV. Determination of Ionic Strength

A. Calculation of the ionic strength of Injection Sodium Chloride 0.9 percent solution.

The ionic strength μ is given by

$$\mu = 1/2 \cdot \Sigma c_i z_i^2$$

where $\Sigma c_i z_i^2$ is the product of the concentration of all ionic species in moles/liter and the square of the respective valence. The M.W. of NaCl is 58.5.

$$\frac{9\ g/liter}{58.5} = 0.154\ moles/liter\ NaCl$$

$$\mu = 1/2\ [(0.154 \times 1^2) + (0.154 \times 1^2)]$$

$$= 0.154$$

B. Calculation of the ionic strength of Ringer's Injection.

NaCl	8.6 g	0.147 moles/liter
KCl	0.3 g	0.0040 moles/liter
$CaCl_2 \cdot 2H_2O$	0.33 g	0.0022 moles/liter
Purified Water to make	1 liter	

$$\mu_{total} = \mu_{NaCl} + \mu_{KCL} + \mu_{CaCL_2}$$

$$= 1/2\ [(0.147 \times 1^2) + (0.147 \times 1^2)$$

$$+ (0.004 \times 1^2) + (0.004 \times 1^2)$$

$$+ (0.002 \times 2^2) + (0.0044 \times 1^2)]$$

$$= 0.158$$

21

Incompatibilities of drugs for intravenous administration

by Warren R. Kramer, Anthony S. Inglott and Robert J. Cluxton, Jr.

One of the most important types of drugs which require compounding is that for injection. In order to perform an I.V. additive service, the pharmacist must have reliable incompatibility literature available. Much has already been published on incompatibilities and this chapter combines these reports into a comprehensive and easily readable table.

The concentrations of the drugs used in the experimental work, the vehicles in which the tests were carried out and the volume of vehicle used are not included in the table. For these reasons, this table must be used only as a guide to potential incompatibilities. The two drugs listed may be incompatible in one vehicle or at one concentration, but this may change under other conditions. For example, calcium gluconate and magnesium sulfate can be combined in the same solution provided the calcium sulfate, which results from the combination, does not reach a concentration which exceeds its solubility.

The *p*H of various commercially available intravenous solutions used as vehicles for drugs added to them is shown in Table 1 because the *p*H of a solution may, at times, be important. The *p*H's of special solutions are easily obtained from the manufacturer's literature.

Column 1 of Table 2 lists in alphabetical order the nonproprietary names of drugs for intravenous administration. Only those drugs which are approved for intravenous use by the United States Food and Drug Administration are included in this column. Trade names are excluded from this column in order to keep the table as simple as possible. The *p*H which is shown under the nonproprietary name is the U.S.P.[1] or N.F.[2] standard. However, if the drug is unofficial, other references[14,20] were used to obtain this information. Frazier[3] published "Administration Routes of Parenteral Injections" earlier in *Drug Intelligence & Clinical Pharmacy*, which was the primary source of information as to the route of administration. However, the *American Hospital Formulary Service*[30] and the manufacturers' package inserts were also consulted.

The drugs listed in Column 2 are potentially incompatible with the corresponding drug in Column 1 and appear in alphabetical order according to the nonproprietary name. If there is a reference source directly behind the name, the literature does not indicate the brand name, On the other hand, when a trade name is recorded in the literature, this name appears in parentheses after the nonproprietary name, followed by the reference source in parentheses. Some of the drugs which appear in Column 2 are mentioned in the literature both by nonproprietary and trade names. In these instances each name is followed by at least one reference source. If only one reference is recorded in the table, this does not mean that this is the only reference reporting the potential incompatibility. Although not always possible, an attempt was made to use primary reference sources.

The nature of potential incompatibilities appears under each drug if such information was reported. Several of the references did not provide this information and therefore each drug does not have a corresponding comment.

It is not necessary to check in Column 1 both drugs which are being combined unless one is concerned as to which proprietary drugs were used in the experimental work, or if the *p*H is in question. The potential incompatibilties appear under each drug separately. For example, aminophylline is reported to be incompatible with hydralazine HCl. This can be seen by looking under either of the two drugs.

We hope that this table will be of assistance to those who have an I.V. additive program in operation, to those who are considering such a program and to those who may be conducting studies in this area.

Table 1. Comparison of *p*H's of Some Large Volume Solutions

NAME OF SOLUTION	U.S.P.	N.F.	ABBOTT	BAXTER	CUTTER	MCGAW
Dextrose 2.5% in Water	3.5-6.5		4.7	4.0	4.8	3.5-6.5
Dextrose 5% in Water	3.5-6.5		4.4	4.0	5.0	3.5-6.5
Dextrose 10% in Water	3.5-6.5		4.2	4.0	4.7	3.5-6.5
Dextrose 20% in Water	3.5-6.5		4.0	4.0	4.7	3.5-6.5
Dextrose 50% in Water	3.5-6.5		4.2	4.0	4.1-4.7	3.5-6.5
Dextrose 5% in ¼ N.S.	3.5-6.0		4.7	4.0	4.8	3.5-6.0
Dextrose 2.5% in ½ N.S.	3.5-6.0		4.8	4.5	5.0	3.5-6.0
Dextrose 5% in ½ N.S.	3.5-6.0		4.3	4.0	4.8	3.5-6.0
Dextrose 2.5% in N.S.	3.5-6.0		4.2	4.5	4.6	3.5-6.0
Dextrose 5% in N.S.	3.5-6.0		4.6	4.0	4.8	3.5-6.0
Dextrose 10% in N.S.	3.5-6.0		4.0	4.0	4.5	3.5-6.0
Dextrose 5% in ⅓ N.S.	3.5-6.0		4.5	4.0	4.8	3.5-6.0
Sodium Chloride 0.9%	4.5-7.0		5.4	5.5	6.1	4.5-7.0
Sodium Chloride ½ Strength	4.5-7.0		5.3	5.5	6.0	4.5-7.0
Sodium Chloride 5%	4.5-7.0		5.6	5.5	5.9	4.5-7.0
Sodium Chloride 3%				5.5	6.0	4.5-7.0
Protein Hydrolysate	4.0-7.0		5.3	5.5	5.4	5.2-5.6
Protein Hydrolysate w/D5W			5.3	5.0	5.2	
Fructose 10% in N.S.		3.0-6.0	3.7	4.0	3.4	
Fructose 10% in Water		3.0-6.0	3.8	4.0	3.5	3.0-6.0
Invert Sugar 5% in Water			4.1	4.0	3.8	3.9-5.1
Invert Sugar 10% in Water			4.0	3.7	3.9	3.9-5.1
Invert Sugar 5% in N.S.			4.1	4.0	3.8	3.9-5.1
Invert Sugar 10% in N.S.			3.9	3.7	3.8	3.9-5.1
Alcohol 5% in Dextrose 5%			4.5	4.5	4.4	3.5-6.0
Lactated Ringer's	6.0-75.		6.5	6.5	6.6	6.1-6.3
Ringer's	5.0-7.5		5.4	5.5	5.9	5.0-7.0
Dextrose 5% in Lactated Ringer's			4.9	5.0	4.9	4.9-5.2
Dextrose 2.5% in ½ L.R.			5.0	5.5	4.8	5.0-6.0
Lactated Potassic Saline Injection		6.5-7.5	6.5	6.5	6.6	6.5-7.5
Sodium Bicarbonate 5%			7.8	8.0	7.6	8.0-8.8
Water for Injection			5.5	6.0	5.8	5.5-7.3

Table 2. Potential Physical Incompatibilities of Drugs

Name of Drug	Drug Incompatibility [Nonproprietary (Trade)]
Albumin, Human Administer slow I.V.	Protein Hydrolysate (4) (5) Combined use not recommended due to the complex nature of the ingredients
Aminophylline *p*H 8.0 to 9.0 Aminophylline is not stable if the *p*H is significantly below 8. Theophylline crystals will form (10) Administer slow I.V. I.M.	Strong Acid Solutions (6) Precipitate forms (6) Anileridine HCl (Leritine) (9) Ascorbic Acid (9) Cephalothin Na (6) Precipitation (6) Chlorpromazine HCl (11) Immediate precipitate (11) Codeine Phosphate (9) Corticotropin (26) Dimenhydrinate (Dramamine) (8) Particulate matter observed (8) Diphenylhydantoin Na (Dilantin) (8) Particulate matter observed (8) Erythromycin Gluceptate (Ilotycin) (10) The antibiotic loses activity because it goes outside *p*H of 6.0 to 7.5 (10) Hydralazine HCl Yellow color produced (11) Hydroxyzine HCl (Vistaril) (8) Particulate matter observed (8) Insulin (10) Levorphanol Bitartrate (Levo-Dromoran) (9) Meperidine HCl (Demerol) (9) Methadone HCl (9) Morphine Sulfate (5) Oxytetracycline HCl (Terramycin) (9) Papaverine HCl (6) Precipitate forms (6) Penicillin G Potassium (22) Penicillin inactivation tends to occur in solutions with *p*H greater than 8.0. Aminophylline tends to raise the *p*H above this figure (22) Phenobarbital Na (7) Procaine HCl (9) Prochlorperazine Mesylate (11) (Compazine) (8) Particulate matter observed (8) Promazine HCl (11) (Sparine) (8) Particulate matter observed (8) Promethazine HCl (11) (Phenergan) (8) Particulate matter observed (8) Tetracycline HCl (Achromycin) (10) Aminophylline is not stable if *p*H is significantly below 8.0. No precipitate was seen in 12 hours, but the solution darkened and a faint ammonia-like odor was detected (10) Vancomycin HCl (Vancocin) (8) Particulate matter observed (8) Vitamin B Complex with C (6) (Berocca-C) (13) (Folbesyn) (9) High *p*H destroys vitamin activity (6)
Ammonium Chloride *p*H 4.5 to 6.0 Administer I.V.	Anileridine HCl (Leritine) (9) Chlortetracycline HCl (12) Codeine Phosphate (9) Dimenhydrinate (9) Levorphanol Bitartrate (Levo-Dromoran) (9) Methadone HCl (9) Nitrofurantoin Na (Furadantin) (5) Sulfadiazine Na (5) Sulfisoxazole (Gantrisin) (9) Warfarin Na (Panwarfarin) (12)
Amobarbital Sodium *p*H 9.6 to 10.4 Administer I.V. (cautiously) I.M.	Anileridine HCl (Leritine) (9) Cephalothin Na (Keflin) (5) Codeine Phosphate (9) Dimenhydrinate (Dramamine) (9) Diphenhydramine HCl (9) Hydrocortisone Succinate (9) (Solu-Cortef) (5) Hydroxyzine HCl (Vistaril) (9) Insulin (9) Levarterenol Bitartrate (Levophed) (9) Levorphanol Bitartrate (Levo-Dromoran) (9) Meperidine HCl (Demerol) (9) Methadone HCl (9) Methylphenidate HCl (5) Morphine Sulfate (5) Penicillin G Potassium (22) Penicillin inactivation tends to occur in solutions with *p*H greater than *p*H 8.0. Amobarbital tends to raise the *p*H above this figure (22) Phytonadione (4) Precipitate forms (4) Procaine HCl (9) (14) Streptomycin Sulfate (9) Tetracycline HCl (9) Vancomycin HCl (Vancocin) (9)
Amphotericin B *p*H 5.0 Administer slow I.V. infusion Intrathecal	Calcium Chloride (11) Haze developing over 3 hours (11) Calcium Gluconate (11) Haze developing over 3 hours (11) Calcium Disodium Versenate (11) Haze developing over 3 hours (11) Carbenicillin (11) Haze developing over 3 hours (11) Chlorpromazine HCl (11) Immediate precipitate (11) Chlortetracycline HCl (Aureomycin) (5) Diphenhydramine HCl (Benadryl) (5) Haze developing over 3 hours (11) Gentamicin Sulfate (11) Haze developing over 3 hours (11) Kanamycin Sulfate (11) Haze developing over 3 hours (11)

NAME OF DRUG	DRUG INCOMPATIBILITY [NONPROPRIETARY (TRADE)]
Amphotericin B (continued)	Metaraminol Bitartrate (11) Haze developing over 3 hours (11) Methyldopate HCl (11) Haze developing over 3 hours (11) Nitrofurantoin Na (Furadantin) (7) Normal Saline (5) Do not dilute with normal saline or water for injection containing preservative. Protect infusion bottle from light after dilution (5) Oxytetracycline HCl (11) (Terramycin) (5) Haze developing over 3 hours (11) Penicillin G Potassium (22) Penicillin inactivation tends to occur in solutions with *p*H greater than 8.0 This antibiotic tends to raise the *p*H above this figure (22) Polymixin B Sulfate (11) Haze developing over 3 hours (11) Potassium Chloride (11) Haze developing over 3 hours (11) Prochlorperazine Mesylate (11) Haze developing over 3 hours (11) Tetracycline HCl (12) (Achromycin) (7)
Ampicillin Sodium *p*H 8.5 to 10.0 Administer dilute I.V. I.M.	Do not mix with other medicaments (4) Additional drugs may change the *p*H and affect stability or compatibility of the solution (5)
Anileridine Hydrochloride *p*H 2.0 to 2.5 Administer slow dilute I.V. I.M. S.C.	Aminophylline (5) Ammonium Chloride (5) Amobarbital Na (Amytal) (5) Chlorothiazide Na (Diuril) (5) Heparin Na (9) Methicillin Na (5) (Dimocillin) (9) Nitrofurantoin Na (Furadantin) (5) Novobiocin Na (Albamycin) (5) Pentobarbital Na (Nembutal) (5) Phenobarbital Na (Luminal) (5) Secobarbital Na (Seconal) (9) Sodium Bicarbonate (5) Sodium Iodide (5) Sulfadiazine Na (9) Sulfisoxazole (Gantrisin) (5) Thiopental Na (Pentothal) (5)
Arginine Glutamate *p*H 5.8 Administer I.V. infusion	Thiopental Na (Pentothal) (5)
Ascorbic Acid (Vitamin C) *p*H 5.5 to 7.0 Administer I.V. I.M. S.C.	Alkaline Solutions (6) Decomposition occurs (6) Oxidizing Solutions (6) Decomposition occurs (6) Salts of Heavy Metals (6) Decomposition occurs (6) Aminophylline (9) Chloramphenicol Na Succinate (12) Chlordiazepoxide HCl (12) Conjugated Estrogens (12) Cyanocobalamin (6) (Rubramin) (9) Precipitate forms (6) Dextran (9) Epinephrine (6) Decomposition (6) Precipitate forms (6) Levarterenol (6) Decomposition occurs (6) Penicillin G Potassium (5) Phytonadione (5) Sulfonamides (6) Vitamin K_1 (Aqua-Mephyton) (9)
Atropine Sulfate *p*H 3.5 to 6.5 Administer slow I.V. I.M. S.C.	Alkaline Solutions (6) Decomposition occurs (6)
Blood *p*H 6.0 to 6.8 Administer I.V.	Avoid Mixing (6) American Association of Blood Banks recommends that no medication be added prior to, or during a transfusion except for A or B substances or both (5)
Calcium Chloride *p*H 6.0 to 8.2 Administer slow I.V.	Amphotericin B (11) Haze develops (11) Cephalothin Na (12) (Keflin) (4) Chlorpheniramine Maleate (14) (Chlor-Trimeton) (5) Chlortetracycline (14) (6) Should not be given with Ca (6) Folic Acid (6) Precipitate forms (6) Nitrofurantoin Na (Furadantin) (5) Oxytetracycline HCl (Terramycin) (6) Inactivation due to complex formation (6) Sodium Bicarbonate (4) Precipitate forms (4) Tetracycline HCl (4) (Achromycin) (6) Inactivation due to complex formation (6)
Calcium Disodium Versenate *p*H 6.5 to 8.0 Administer I.V.	Metal Salts (6) Complex formation (6) Amphotericin B (11) Haze develops over 3 hours (11) Dextrose (4) Hydralazine HCl (11) Yellow color produced (11) Oxytetracycline HCl (Terramycin) (6) Inactivation due to complex formation (6) Tetracycline HCl (Achromycin) (6) Inactivation due to complex formation (6)
Calcium Glucoheptonate Administer I.V.	Cephalothin Na (Keflin) (12) Oxytetracycline HCl (Terramycin) (6) Inactivation due to complex formation (6) Tetracycline HCl(Achromycin)(6)(4) Inactivation due to complex formation (6)

Name of Drug	Drug Incompatibility [Nonproprietary (Trade)]
Calcium Gluconate *p*H 6.0 to 8.2 Administer slow I.V. I.M. (adults only)	Amphotericin B (11) Haze develops over 3 hours (11) Cephalothin Na (6) (Keflin) (4) (7) Magnesium Sulfate (9) Novobiocin Na (Albamycin) (5) Oxytetracycline HCl (Terramycin) (6) Inactivation due to complex formation (6) Prednisolone-21-Phosphate (14) (Hydeltrasol) (8) Particulate matter observed (8) Prochlorperazine Edisylate (Compazine) (5) Promethazine HCl (Phenergan) (9) Sodium Bicarbonate (5) (4) Precipitate forms (4) Streptomycin Sulfate (5) Tetracycline HCl (6) (Achromycin) (8) Inactivation due to complex formation (6)
Carbenicillin *p*H 5.9 to 6.9 Administer slow I.V. I.V. infusion I.M.	Amphotericin B (11) Haze develops over 3 hours (11) Oxytetracycline HCl (11) Haze develops over 3 hours (11) Tetracycline HCl (11) Haze develops over 3 hours (11)
Cephalothin Sodium *p*H 5.2 Administer dilute I.V. deep I.M. Intraperitoneal	Change of *p*H to below 4 or above 7 (10) Not advised (10) **Aminophylline (6)** **Precipitation (6)** Amobarbital Na (6) (Amytal) (5) Precipitate forms (6) Calcium Chloride (12) Calcium Gluceptate (5) Calcium Gluconate (12) (7) Chlorpromazine HCl (Thorazine) (5) Chlortetracycline HCl (12) (Aureomycin) (5) Colistimethate Na (12) Diphenhydramine (4) Diphenylhydantoin Na (14) (Dilantin) (9) Erythromycin Gluceptate (5) Erythromycin Lactobionate (12) **Hydrocortisone (6)** **Precipitation (6)** Kanamycin Sulfate (12) (Kantrex) (5) Normal Saline (12) Oxytetracycline HCl (6) (Terramycin) (5) Penicillin G Sodium (9) Penicillin G Potassium (9) Pentobarbital Na (6) Precipitate forms (6) Phenobarbital Na (5) Polymyxin B Sulfate (12) Prochlorperazine Edisylate (Compazine) (5) Tetracycline HCl (12) Thiopental (6) Precipitate forms (6) Vitamin B Complex with C (5) Compatible with Betalin Complex with C according to manufacturer (5)
Chloramphenicol Sodium Succinate *p*H 6.0 to 7.5 Generally incompatible when the *p*H of the solution goes outside the range of 5.5 to 7.0 (12) Administer I.V.	Ascorbic Acid (12) Chlorpromazine HCl (11) Haze or precipitate forms (11) Chlortetracycline HCl (Aureomycin) (5) Diphenylhydantoin Na (Dilantin) (8) Particulate matter observed (8) Erythromycin Glucoheptonate (Ilotycin) (8) Particulate matter observed (8) Erythromycin Lactobionate (Erythrocin) (4) Precipitate forms (4) Hydrocortisone Na Succinate (4) Hydroxyzine HCl (Vistaril) (8) Particulate matter observed (8) Novobiocin Na (Albamycin) (9) Oxytetracycline HCl (Terramycin) (8) Particulate matter observed (8) Polymyxin B (4) Precipitate forms (4) Procaine HCl (12) (5) Prochlorperazine Edisylate (Compazine) (8) Particulate matter observed (8) Promazine HCl (Sparine) (8) Particulate matter observed (8) Promethazine HCl (Phenergan) (8) Particulate matter observed (8) Sulfadiazine Na (12) Tetracycline HCl (4) (Achromycin) (8) Precipitate forms (4) Tripelennamine HCl (Pyribenzamine) (8) Particulate matter observed (8) Vancomycin HCl (Vancocin) (8) Particulate matter observed (8) Vitamin B Complex (6) Vitamin B Complex with C (4) Precipitate forms (4) The riboflavin in vitamin B complex rapidly diminishes the potency of antibiotics (4)
Chlordiazepoxide Hydrochloride Administer slow I.V. deep I.M.	Ascorbic Acid (12) Diphenylhydantoin Na (12) Heparin Na (12) Pentobarbital Na (12) Promethazine HCl (12) Secobarbital Na (12)
Chlorothiazide Sodium Administer dilute I.V.	Anileridine HCl (Leritine) (9) Chlorpromazine HCl (11) Immediate precipitate (11) Codeine Phosphate (9) Hydralazine HCl (11) Yellow color with precipitate developing over 3 hours (11) Insulin (9) Levarterenol Bitartrate (Levophed) (9) Levorphanol Tartrate (Levo-Dromoran) (9) Methadone HCl (9) Morphine Sulfate (9) Polymyxin B Sulfate (11) Yellow color (11) Procaine HCl (9) Prochlorperazine Mesylate (11) Haze or precipitate (11)

Name of Drug	Drug Incompatibility [Nonproprietary (Trade)]
	Promazine HCl (11) (Sparine) (9) Immediate precipitate (11) Promethazine HCl (11) (Phenergan) (9) Immediate precipitate (11) Protein Hydrolysate (17) Haze or precipitate (17) Streptomycin Sulfate (9) Tetracycline HCl (Achromycin) (9) Vancomycin HCl (Vancocin) (9)
Chlorpheniramine Maleate *p*H 4.0 to 5.2 Administer I.V. I.M. S.C.	Calcium Chloride (9) Levarterenol Bitartrate (Levophed) (9) Pentobarbital Na (9) (Nembutal) (5)
Chlorpromazine Hydrochloride *p*H 3.0 to 5.0 Administer I.V. I.M.	Aminophylline (11) Immediate precipitate (11) Amphotericin B (11) Immediate precipitate (11) Benzylpenicillin (11) Haze developing over 3 hours (11) Cephalothin Na (Keflin) (5) Chloramphenicol (11) Haze or precipitate (11) Chlorothiazide (11) Immediate precipitate (11) Cloxacillin Na (11) Haze developing over 3 hours (11) Cyanocobalamin (12) Dexamethasone (6) Precipitate or inactivation (6) Dimenhydrinate (6) Precipitate or inactivation (6) Ethamivan (11) Immediate precipitate (11) Heparin Na (6) Precipitate or inactivation (6) Kanamycin (6) Manufacturer lists as incompatible (6) Methicillin Na (11) Haze developing over 3 hours (11) Paraldehyde (5) (12) Penicillin G Potassium (9) Precipitate forms (4) Pentobarbital Na (12) (Nembutal) (18) Phenobarbital Na (11) Immediate precipitate (11) Secobarbital Na (12) Sodium Bicarbonate (12) Sulfadiazine Na (11) Immediate precipitate (11) Thiopental Na (Pentothal) (18) Vitamin B Complex (6) Precipitate forms or inactivation occurs (6) Vitamin B Complex with C (12)
Chlortetracycline Hydrochloride *p*H 8.5 Administer dilute I.V. I. M.	Ammonium Chloride (12) Amphotericin B (5) Calcium Chloride (12) Should not be given with tetracyclines (4) Calcium Glucoheptonate (4) Should not be given with tetracyclines (4) Calcium Gluconate (4) Should not be given with tetracyclines (4) Cephalothin Na (12) (Keflin) (5) Chloramphenicol (5) Heparin (5) Hydrocortisone (5) Methicillin (5) Polymyxin B Sulfate (12) Promazine HCl (Sparine) (15) Physically incompatible (15)
Codeine Phosphate *p*H 3.0 to 6.0 Administer I.V. (very seldom) I.M. S.C.	Aminophylline (14) Ammonium Chloride (14) Amobarbital Na (14) (Amytal) (5) Chlorothiazide Na (Diuril) (5) (9) Diphenylhydantoin Na (14) Heparin Na (14) Methicillin Na (14) (Dimocillin) (9) Nitrofurantoin Na (Furadantin) (9) Novobiocin Na (Albamycin) (9) Pentobarbital Na (14) (Nembutal) (5) Phenobarbital Na (14) (Luminal) (9) Secobarbital Na (14) (Seconal) (9) Sodium Bicarbonate (14) Sodium Iodide (14) Sulfadiazine Na (14) Sulfisoxazole (Gantrisin) (9) Thiopental Na (Pentothal) (9)
Conjugated Estrogens *p*H 6.8 to 7.4 Administer I.V. I.M.	Ascorbic Acid (12)
Corticotropin (ACTH) *p*H 3.0 to 7.0 Administer I.V. I.M. S.C.	Novobiocin Na (Albamycin) (9) Sodium Bicarbonate (9)
Cyanocobalamin (Vitamin B-12) *p*H 4.0 to 5.5 Administer slow I.V. I.M. S.C.	Alkaline Solutions (6) Decomposition and inactivation (6) Reducing Solutions (6) Decomposition and inactivation (6) Ascorbic Acid (13) Chlorpromazine HCl (12) Vitamin B Complex with C (Folbesyn) (9) Vitamin K (Aqua-Mephyton) (9) Vitamin K Diphosphate (13) Warfarin Na (Panwarfarin) (15) Physically incompatible (15)
Deslanoside *p*H 5.5 to 7.0 Administer I.V. I.M.	Should not be mixed with fluids for infusion, but may be injected through Y-tube administration set (5)
Desoxyephedrine Hydrochloride Administer I.V. I.M. S.C.	Use in infusion is contraindicated (5)

Name of Drug	Drug Incompatibility [Nonproprietary (Trade)]
Dexamethasone-21-Phosphate *p*H 6.5 to 7.0 Administer I.V. infusion I.M. Intrasynovial	Chlorpromazine (6) Precipitation or Inactivation (6) Prochlorperazine Edisylate (Compazine (8) Particulate matter observed (8) Vancomycin HCl (Vancocin) (8)
Diazepam *p*H 6.2 to 6.9 Administer slow I.V. deep I.M.	Do not mix with any medications (6)
Digitoxin Administer I.V. I.M.	Should not be mixed with fluids but may be injected through Y-tube of administration set (5)
Digoxin Administer I.V. I.M.	Should not be mixed with fluids but may be injected through Y-tube of administration set (5)
Dimenhydrinate *p*H 6.0 Administer slow I.V. I.M.	Aminophylline (8) Particulate matter observed (8) Ammonium Chloride (9) Amobarbital Na (9) Chlorpromazine HCl (6) Precipitate forms or inactivation occurs (6) Diphenylhydantoin Na (Dilantin) (8) Particulate matter observed (8) Heparin (6) Hydrocortisone Na Succinate (Solu-Cortef) (8) Particulate matter observed (8) Hydroxyzine HCl (Vistaril) (8) Particulate matter observed (8) Pentobarbital Na (Nembutal) (18) Phenobarbital Na (Luminal) (8) Particulate matter observed (8) Prochlorperazine Edisylate (Compazine) (8) Particulate matter observed (8) Promazine HCl (Sparine) (8) Particulate matter observed (8) Promethazine HCl (Phenergan) (8) Particulate matter observed (8) Streptomycin (6) Thiopental Na (Pentothal) (18) Trifluoperazine HCl (12)
Diphenhydramine Hydrochloride Administer dilute I.V. deep I.M.	Amobarbital Na (9) (Amytal) (5) Amphotericin B (5) Cephalothin Na (Keflin) (4) Precipitate forms (4) Diphenylhydantoin Na (Dilantin) (8) Particulate matter observed (8) Pentobarbital Na (4) (Nembutal) (5) Precipitate forms (4) Phenobarbital Na (Luminal) (8) Particulate matter observed (8) Prednisolone-21-Phosphate (Hydeltrasol) (8) Particulate matter observed (8) Secobarbital Na (Seconal) (9) Thiopental Na (Pentothal) (9)
Diphenylhydantoin Sodium *p*H 10.0 to 12.3 Administer I.V. I.M.	Do not mix with other medications (4)
Ephedrine Sulfate *p*H 4.5 to 7.0 Administer dilute I.V. I.M. S.C.	Hydrocortisone Na Succinate (Solu-Cortef) (5) Pentobarbital Na (9) (Nembutal) (5) Phenobarbital Na (5) (Luminal) (9) Secobarbital Na (Seconal) (9) Thiopental Na (5) (Pentothal) (18)
Epinephrine Hydrochloride *p*H 2.5 to 5.0 Administer slow dilute I.V. I.M. S.C.	Ascorbic Acid (6) Decomposition (6) Hyaluronidase (Wydase) (9) Use all mixtures immediately (6) Mephentermine (12) (Wyamine) (13) Novobiocin Na (Albamycin) (9) Trifluoperazine HCl (12) Warfarin Na (Panwarfarin) (15)
Ergonovine Maleate *p*H 2.7 to 3.5 Administer I.V. I.M.	Should not be mixed with fluids for infusions but may be injected through Y-tube of administration set (5)
Erythromycin Gluceptate *p*H 6.5 to 7.5 Solutions having a *p*H above 7.5 or below 6.0 will deteriorate (10) Administer dilute I.V.	Cephalothin Na (Keflin) (5) Concentration of erythromycin greater than 10 mg/ml found to produce incompatibility (5) Chloramphenicol Na Succinate (Chloromycetin) (9) (5) Diphenylhydantoin Na (Dilantin) (4) Precipitate forms (4) Heparin Na (9) Novobiocin Na (9) Pentobarbital Na (4) (Nembutal) (5) Precipitate forms (4) Phenobarbital Na (4) (Luminal) (5) Precipitate forms (4) Prochlorperazine Edisylate (Compazine) (8) Manufacturer lists two drugs incompatibile (8) Secobarbital Na (9) Streptomycin Sulfate (9) Tetracycline HCl (9)
Erythromycin Lactobionate *p*H 6.5 to 7.5 Addition of this antibiotic to admixtures possessing a final *p*H less than 5.0 appears inadvisable (27) Administer I.V. deep I.M.	Aminophylline (10) Antibiotic loses activity (10) Cephalothin Na (12) (Keflin) (4) Not recommended by manufacturer (4) Precipitate occurs after 3 to 4 hours (19) Chloramphenicol Na Succinate (4) Colistimethate Na (Colymycin) (19) Precipitate within 1 hour (19) Heparin Na (4) (Panheparin) (19) Precipitate within 1 hour (19) Tetracycline HCl (4) Resulting *p*H will cause decomposition of both antibiotics (4)

Name of Drug	Drug Incompatibility [Nonproprietary (Trade)]
	Thiopental Na (4) Vitamin B Complex with C (4) Resulting *p*H will cause decomposition (4)
Ethamivan Administer I.V.	Chlorpromazine HCl (11) Immediate precipitate (11) Hydralazine HCl (11) Yellow color which develops into a precipitate in 3 hours (11) Prochlorperazine Mesylate (11) Immediate precipitate (11) Promazine HCl (11) Immediate precipitate (11) Promethazine HCl (11) Immediate precipitate (11)
Fibrinogen Administer dilute I.V.	Metaraminol Bitartrate (Aramine) (15) Promazine HCl (Sparine) (15) Whole Blood (12)
Fibrinolysin Administer dilute I.V.	Oxytocin (Pitocin) (15) Promazine HCl (Sparine) (15) Thiopental Na (Pentothal) (15)
Folic Acid *p*H 8.0 to 11.0 Administer I.V. I.M. S.C.	Calcium Salts (6) Precipitate forms (6) Iron Sulfate (6) Precipitate forms (6) Sulfonamides (6) Precipitate forms (6)
Furosemide *p*H 8.8 to 9.3 Administer I.V. I.M.	Acid Solutions (6)
Gentamicin Sulfate Administer slow I.V. infusion I.M.	Amphotericin B (11) Haze develops over 3 hours (11) Heparin (11) Immediate precipitate (11) Sulfadiazine Na (11) Crystalline precipitate (11)
Heparin Sodium *p*H 5.0 to 7.5 Administer I.V. I.M. deep S.C.	Anileridine HCl (Leritine) (5) Chlordiazepoxide (12) Chlorpromazine (6) Precipitate forms (6) Chlortetracycline HCl (5) Codeine Phosphate (5) Dimenhydrinate (Dramamine) (8) Particulate matter observed (8) Erythromycin Gluceptate (Ilotycin) (8) Particulate matter observed (8) Erythromycin Lactobionate (23) Precipitate forms within 1 hour (23) Gentamicin Sulfate (11) Immediate precipitate (11) Hyaluronidase (6) Complex formation (6) Hydrocortisone Sodium Succinate (Solu-Cortef) (5) Hydroxyzine HCl (Vistaril) (8) Particulate matter observed (8) Kanamycin Sulfate (11) (Kantrex) (23) Immediate precipitate (11) Levorphanol Bitartrate (Levo-Dromoran) (5) Meperidine HCl (Demerol) (5) Methadone HCl (5)
	Morphine Sulfate (5) Novobiocin Na (12) (Albamycin) (5) Oxytetracycline HCl (Terramycin) (5) Penicillin G Potassium (4) Precipitate forms (4) Manufacturer lists as incompatible (4) Polymycin B Sulfate (11) (6) Haze or precipitate (11) complex formation (6) Procainamide HCl (Pronestyl) (8) Particulate matter observed (8) Prochlorperazine Edisylate (Compazine) (8) Particulate matter observed (8) Promazine HCl (Sparine) (8) Particulate matter observed (8) Promethazine HCl (Phenergan) (8) Particulate matter observed (8) Protamine (6) Complex formation (6) Streptomycin Sulfate (11) (6) Immediate precipitate (11) complex formation (6) Tetracycline HCl (6) (Achromycin) (8) Precipitate forms (6) Vancomycin HCl (Vancocin) (8) Viomycin Sulfate (11) Immediate precipitate (11)
Hydralazine Hydrochloride Administer I.V. I.M.	Aminophylline (11) Yellow color produced (11) Calcium Disodium Versenate (11) Yellow color produced (11) Chlorothiazide (11) Yellow color and then precipitate forms in 3 hours (11) Ethamivan (11) Yellow color and then precipitate forms in 3 hours (11) Hydrocortisone Na Succinate (11) Yellow color produced (11) Mephentermine Sulfate (11) Yellow color produced (11) Phenobarbital Na (11) Yellow color and then precipitate forms in 3 hours (11) Sulfadiazine (11) Yellow color forms in 3 hours (11)
Hydrocortisone Sodium Succinate *p*H 7.0 to 8.0 The optimum *p*H is 7.0-8.0, but drug is stable at *p*H 6.0 for 72 hours and at *p*H 5.0 for 12 hours. It will precipitate in more acid solutions (10) Administer slow I.V. I.M.	Amobarbital Na (9) (Amytal) (5) Cephalothin Na (6) Precipitation (6) Chloramphenicol Na Succinate (Chloromycetin) (4) Precipitate forms (4) Chlortetracycline HCl (5) Colistimethate Na (12) Dimenhydrinate (Dramamine) (8) Particulate matter observed (8) Ephedrine Sulfate (9) Heparin Sodium (9) Hydralazine HCl (11) Yellow color produced (11) Kanamycin Sulfate (Kantrex) (8) Particulate matter observed (8) Metaraminol Bitartrate (Aramine) (24) Precipitate forms within 1 hour (24) Methicillin Na (Dimocillin) (9) Novobiocin Na (Albamycin) (9) Oxytetracycline HCl (Terramycin) (8) Particulate matter observed (8)

Name of Drug	Drug Incompatibility [Nonproprietary (Trade)]
	Pentobarbital Na (9) Phenobarbital Na (9) Prochlorperazine Maleate (9) (Compazine) (5) Promazine HCl (Sparine) (8) Particulate matter observed (8) Promethazine HCl (Phenergan) (8) Particulate matter observed (8) Secobarbital Na (Seconal) (9) Tetracycline HCl (Achromycin) (8) Particulate matter observed (8) Vancomycin HCl (Vancocin) (8) Particulate matter observed (8) Vitamin B Complex with C (Folbesyn) (8)
Insulin, Aqueous *p*H 2.5 to 3.5 Inactivated in alkaline range above 7.5 (10) Administer slow dilute I.V. S.C.	Aminophylline (10) Amobarbital Na (9) (Amytal) (5) Chlorothiazide Na (Diuril) (5) Diphenylhydantoin Na (9) (Dilantin) (5) Nitrofurantoin Na (Furadantin) (9) Novobiocin Na (Albamycin) (9) Pentobarbital Na (9) (Nembutal) (5) Phenobarbital Na (Luminal) (9) Secobarbital Na (Seconal) (9) Sodium Bicarbonate (9) Sulfadiazine Na (9) Sulfisoxazole (Gantrisin) (9) Thiopental Na (Pentothal) (9)
Kanamycin Sulfate *p*H 4.5 Administer I.V. infusion I.M. I.P. instillation directly into abscesses	Amphotericin B (11) Haze developing over 3 hours (11) Cephalothin Na (11) (Keflin) (5) Precipitate forms (6) Chlorpromazine HCl (4) Manufacturer lists as incompatible (4) Colistimethate Na (Coly-Mycin) (5) Dextrose (5) Diphenylhydantoin Na (9) (Dilantin) (8) Precipitate forms (4) Heparin Na (11) (8) (Panheparin) (23) Immediate precipitate (11) Hydrocortisone Na Succinate (Solu-Cortef) (8) Particulate matter observed (8) Methacillin Na (6) (Dimocillin) (8) (Staphcillin) (4) Precipitate forms (6) Manufacturer states rapid inactivation occurs (4) Nitrofurantoin Na (12) (Furadantin) (5) Pentobarbital Na (4) Precipitate forms (6) Phenobarbital Na (6) (Luminal) (8) Precipitate forms (6) Polymyxin B (12) Prochlorperazine Edisylate (Compazine) (8) No particulate matter observed, but manufacturer lists as incompatible (8) Secobarbital Na (6) Precipitate forms (6) Sulfadiazine Na (11) Immediate precipitate (11)

Name of Drug	Drug Incompatibility [Nonproprietary (Trade)]
	Sulfisoxazole (Gantrisin) (8) Particulate matter observed (8)
Levallorphan Tartrate *p*H 4.0 to 4.5 Administer I.V. I.M. S.C.	Diphenylhydantoin Na (Dilantin) (8) Particulate matter observed (8) Methicillin Na (Dimocillin) (8) Particulate matter observed (8) Prochlorperazine HCl (12) Sulfisoxazole (Gantrisin) (6) (8) Precipitate forms (6) Trifluoperazine HCl (12)
Levarterenol Bitartrate *p*H 3.0 to 4.5 Solutions of levarterenol in the 5.5 *p*H range should be used immediately (27) Alkaline solutions cause decomposition (6) Administer dilute I.V. Intracardiac	Amobarbital Na (9) (Amytal) (5) Ascorbic Acid (6) Decomposition occurs (6) Chlorothiazide Na (Diuril) (9) Chlorpheniramine Maleate (9) (Chlor-Trimeton) (5) Diphenylhydantoin Na (9) (Dilantin) (5) Nitrofurantoin Na (Furadantin) (9) Novobiocin Na (Albamycin) (9) Oxytocin (12) Pentobarbital Na (9) (Nembutal) (5) Phenobarbital Na (Luminal) (9) Secobarbital Na (Seconal) (9) Sodium Bicarbonate (9) Sodium Iodide (9) Streptomycin Sulfate (9) Sulfadiazine Na (9) Sulfisoxazole (Gantrisin) (9) Thiopental Na (Pentothal) (9)
Levorphanol Bitartrate *p*H 3.4-4.0 Administer I.V. I.M. S.C.	Aminophylline (5) Ammonium Chloride (5)(9) Amobarbital Na (Amytal) (5) Chlorothiazide Na (Diuril) (5) Heparin (5)(9) Methicillin (5) Nitrofurantoin Na (Furadantin) (5) (9) Novobiocin Na (Albamycin) (5) (9) Pentobarbital Na (Nembutal) (5) Phenobarbital Na (Luminal) (5) Sodium Bicarbonate (5)(9) Sodium Iodide (5)(9) Sulfadiazine Na (5) (9) Sulfisoxazole (Gantrisin) (5) Thiopental Na (Pentothal) (5)
Lidocaine Hydrochloride *p*H 6.0 to 7.0 Administer I.V. intracardiac nerve block	Alkaline Solutions (6) Precipitates (6)
Lincomycin Hydrochloride Administer I.V. infusion I.M.	Diphenylhydantoin Na (Dilantin) (5) Penicillin G Potassium (9) Penicillin G Sodium (9) Sulfadiazine Na (11) Crystals produced (11)
Magnesium Sulfate *p*H 5.5 to 7.0 Administer I.V. I.M. S.C.	Calcium Gluconate (9) Novobiocin Na (Albamycin) (9) Procaine HCl (9) Sodium Bicarbonate (9)

Name of Drug	Drug Incompatibility [Nonproprietary (Trade)]
Mannitol *p*H 4.5 to 7.0 Administer I.V. infusion	Strong Acidic and Alkaline Solutions (6) Blood (5) Possible agglutination and irreversible crenation (5)
Menadione Sodium Bisulfite *p*H 2.0 to 4.0 Should not be mixed with fluids for infusions but may be injected through Y-tube of administration set (5) Administer slow I.V. I.M. S.C.	Diphenylhydantoin Na (Dilantin) (8) Particulate matter observed (8) Promazine HCl (Sparine) (8) Particulate matter observed (8)
Meperidine Hydrochloride *p*H 3.5 to 6.0 Should not be mixed with fluids for infusions but may be injected through Y-tube of administration set (5) Administer slow I.V. (cautiously) I.M. S.C.	Aminophylline (9) Amobarbital Na (9) (Amytal) (5) Diphenylhydantoin Na (9) (Dilantin) (5) Heparin Na (9) Methicillin Na (Dimocillin) (9) Nitrofurantoin Na (Furadantin) (9) Pentobarbital Na (9) (Nembutal) (18) Phenobarbital Na (Luminal) (9) Secobarbital Na (12) Sodium Bicarbonate (9) Sodium Iodide (9) Sulfadiazine Na (9) Sulfisoxazole (Gantrisin) (9) Thiopental Na (Pentothal) (18)
Mephentermine Sulfate *p*H 4.0 to 6.5 Administer slow I.V. I.M.	Epinephrine HCl (12) Hydralazine HCl (11) Yellow color produced (11)
Metaraminol Bitartrate *p*H 3.5 to 4.5 Administer I.V. with caution I.M. S.C.	Amphotericin B (11) Haze developing over 3 hours (11) Diphenylhydantoin Na (9) (Dilantin) (8) Particulate matter observed (8) Fibrinogen (15) Hydrocortisone Na Succinate (9) (12) (Solu-Cortef) (24) Precipitate forms within 1 hour (24) Methicillin Na (Dimocillin) (8) Particulate matter observed (8) Morphine Sulfate (9) Nitrofurantoin Na (Furadantin) (10) Brown precipitate forms which may be caused by parabens in the anti-infective (10) Penicillin G Potassium (8) Penicillin G Sodium (9) Sulfadiazine Na (11) Crystals produced (11) Thiopental Na (Pentothal) (9) Warfarin Na (Panwarfin) (9)
Methamphetamine Hydrochloride *p*H 6.0 Administer I.V. I.M. S.C.	Thiopental Na (Pentothal) (18)
Methicillin Sodium *p*H 7.0 to 8.0 Administer I.V. deep I.M.	Acidic Solutions (6) Rapid inactivation (6) Anileridine HCl (Leritine) (9) Chlorpromazine HCl (6) Precipitation (6) Chlortetracycline HCl (5) Codeine Phosphate (9) Hydrocortisone Na Succinate (9) Kanamycin Sulfate (4)(6)(8) Rapid inactivation (6) Levallorphan (Lorfan) (6) Precipitation (6) Levorphanol Bitartrate (Levo-Dromoran) (9) Meperidine HCl (Demerol) (5) Metaraminol Bitartrate (Aramine) (8) Particulate matter observed (8) Methadone (9) Morphine Sulfate (9) Oxytetracycline HCl (11) (Terramycin) (4) Haze (11) or precipitate (4) forms Prochlorperazine Maleate (9) (Compazine) (8) Particulate matter observed (8) Promethazine HCl (Phenergan) (8) Particulate matter observed (8) Sodium Bicarbonate (9) Sulfadiazine Na (11) Crystals produced (11) Tetracycline HCl (4) Precipitate (4) Vancomycin HCl (Vancocin) (8) Particulate matter observed (8)
Methyldopate Hydrochloride *p*H 3.5 to 4.2 Administer I.V. infusion	Amphotericin B (11) Haze developing over 3 hours (11) Sulfadiazine Na (11) Crystals produced (11) Tetracycline HCl (11) Crystals produced (11)
Methylphenidate Hydrochloride Administer I.V. I.M. S.C.	Strong Alkaline Solutions (5) Barbiturates (5) Diphenylhydantoin Na (Dilantin) (8) Particulate matter observed (8) Phenobarbital Na (Luminal) (8) Particulate matter observed (8)
Methylprednisolone Sodium Succinate *p*H 7.0 to 8.0 Administer slow I.V. I.M.	Promethazine HCl (12)

Name of Drug	Drug Incompatibility [Nonproprietary (Trade)]
Morphine Sulfate *p*H 3.0 to 6.0 Should not be mixed with fluids for infusions but may be injected through Y-tube of administration set (5) Administer slow dilute I.V. I.M. S.C.	Aminophylline (5) Amobarbital Na (Amytal) (5) Chlorothiazide Na (Diuril) (5) Heparin (5) Meperidine HCl (Demerol) (5) Metaraminol Bitartrate (9) Methicillin (5) Nitrofurantoin Na (Furadantin) (5) Novobiocin Na (Albamycin) (5) Pentobarbital Na (9) Phenobarbital Na (Luminal) (5) Sodium Bicarbonate (5) Sodium Iodide (5) Sulfadiazine (5) Sulfisoxazole (Gantrisin) (5) Thiopental Na (Pentothal) (18)
Nafcillin Sodium *p*H 6.0 to 6.5 Nafcillin tends to precipitate as a fine flocculus at a *p*H of less than 5.6 (29) Administer I.V. infusion deep I.M.	Vitamin B Complex with C (12)
Nicotinamide *p*H 6.0 to 6.5 Administer slow I.V. I.M. S.C.	Alkaline Solutions (6) Decomposition occurs (6)
Nitrofurantoin Sodium *p*H 7.7 to 9.8 Administer dilute I.V.	Ammonium Chloride (5) Amphotericin B (4) Precipitate forms (4) Anileridine HCl (Leritine) (9) Calcium Chloride (5) Codeine Phosphate (9) Cresol (10) Tendency to precipitate drug (10) Insulin (9) Kanamycin Sulfate (Kantrex) (5) Precipitate forms (4) Levarterenol Bitartrate (Levophed) (9) Levorphanol Bitartrate (Levo-Dromoran) (9) Meperidine HCl (Demerol) (5) Metaraminol Bitartrate (Aramine) (10) Brown precipitate forms which may be caused by parabens in the anti-infective (10) Methadone HCl (9) Methylparaben (12) Morphine Sulfate (9) Para-Aminobenzoic Acid (12) Phenol (10) Polymyxin B Sulfate (4) Precipitate forms (4) Procaine HCl (9) Prochlorperazine Maleate (9) (Compazine) (5) Promethazine HCl (Phenergan) (9) Propylparaben (12) Streptomycin Sulfate (9) Tetracaine HCl (Pontocaine) (5) Tetracycline HCl (15) Physically incompatible (15) Vancomycin HCl (Vancocin) (9) Vitamin B Complex (6) Vitamin B Complex with C (4) Precipitate forms (4)
Novobiocin Sodium *p*H 7.4 to 8.5 Precipatates when mixed with any solution with *p*H below 6 (4) Administer dilute I.V. I.M. with caution	Amino Acids (6) Electrolytes (6) Anileridine HCl (Leritine) (5) Calcium Gluconate (9) Chloramphenicol Na Succinate (9) Codeine Phosphate (9) Corticotropin Aqueous (9) (ACTH) (5) Dextrose (9) Epinephrine HCl (12) (Adrenalin) (9) Erythromycin Glucoheptonate (9) Heparin Na (9) Hydrocortisone Succinate (9) Insulin (9) Levarterenol Bitartrate (Levophed) (9) Levorphanol Bitartrate (Levo-Dromoran) (5) Magnesium Sulfate (9) Methadone (9) Morphine Sulfate (9) Procaine HCl (9) Streptomycin Sulfate (9) Tetracycline HCl (9) Tetracyclines (6) Vancomycin HCl (Vancocin) (9) Vitamin B Complex with C (Folbesyn) (9)
Oleandomycin Administer I.V. infusion I.M.	Riboflavin (6)
Oxytetracycline Hydrochloride *p*H 8.5 Administer I.V. I.M.	Some inorganic ions (Ca, Mg, Mn, Fe) (6) Inactivation due to complex formation (6) Aminophylline (25) Amphotericin B (5) (11) Haze developing over 3 hours (11) Carbenicillin (11) Haze developing over 3 hours (11) Cephalothin Na (Keflin) (25) Precipitate forms within 1 hour (25) Chloramphenicol Na Succinate (9) (Chloromycetin) (8) Particulate matter observed (8) Cloxacillin Na (11) Haze developing over 3 hours (11) Diphenylhydantoin Na (9) (Dilantin) (8) Particulate matter observed (8) Heparin (5) Hydrocortisone Na Succinate (9) (Solu-Cortef) (8) Particulate matter observed (8) Iron Dextran (11) Haze developing over 3 hours (11) Methicillin Na (4) (11) Precipitate forms (4) Penicillin G Potassium (21) (4) Inactive after 24 hours (21) Precipitate forms (4) Pentobarbital Na (9) (Nembutal) (5)

Name of Drug	Drug Incompatibility [Nonproprietary (Trade)]
Oxytetracycline Hydrochloride (continued)	Phenobarbital Na (9) (Luminal) (8) Particulate matter observed (8) Polymyxin B (5) Prochlorperazine Edisylate (Compazine) (8) Manufacturer lists as incompatible (8) Sodium Bicarbonate (4) Sulfadiazine Na (11) Immediate precipitate (11) Sulfisoxazole (Gantrisin) (8) Particulate matter observed (8) Vitamin B Complex with C (Berocca C) (10) Out of *p*H range for vitamin to remain stable (10)
Oxytocin *p*H 2.5 to 4.5 Administer dilute I.V. I.M. S.C.	Fibrinolysin (15) Levarterenol Bitartrate (12) Warfarin Na (Panwarfin) (15) Physically incompatible (15)
Ouabain Administer slow I.V. I.M. (painful)	Should not be mixed with fluids for infusions but may be injected through Y-tube of administration set (5)
Papaverine Hydrochloride *p*H 3.0 to 4.5 Administer slow I.V. I.M. S.C.	Alkaline Solutions (6) Precipitate forms (6) Phenobarbital Na (6) Precipitate forms (6)
Paraldehyde Administer slow dilute I.V. I.M.	Chlorpromazine HCl (12) (Thorazine) (5)
Penicillin G Potassium *p*H 5.0 to 7.5 Penicillin is most stable at a *p*H of 7 (10) Penicillin inactivation tends to occur in solutions with *p*H greater than 8.0 (22) Administer I.V. infusion I.M. S.C. Intrathecal	Aminophylline (22) Amphotericin B (12) (Fungizone) (22) Precipitate forms within 1 hour (22) Ascorbic Acid (5) Cephalothin Na (Keflin) (9) Chlorpromazine HCl (12) (Thorazine) (4) Precipitate forms (4) Diphenylhydantoin Na (Dilantin) (8) Particulate matter observed (8) Heparin Na (4) Manufacturer lists as incompatible (4) Precipitate forms (4) Hydroxyzine HCl (Vistaril) (8) Particulate matter observed (8) Lincomycin HCl (Lincocin) (9) Metaraminol Bitartrate (Aramine) (8) Particulate matter observed (8) Oxytetracycline HCl (12) (Terramycin) (4) Precipitate forms (4) Prochlorperazine Edisylate (Compazine) (8) Particulate matter observed (8) Promazine HCl (Sparine) (8) Particulate matter observed (8) Promethazine HCl (Phenergan) (8) Particulate matter observed (8) Sodium Bicarbonate (22) Sodium Salts of Barbituric Acid Derivatives (22) Tetracycline HCl (12) (Achromycin) (8) Particulate matter observed (8) Thiopental Na (Pentothal) (15) Physically incompatible (15) Tromethamine (THAM) (22) Vancomycin HCl (Vancocin) (8) Particulate matter observed (8) Vitamin B Complex with C (27) Acid causes deactivation of antibiotic (27) Activity is rapidly lost at *p*H below 5.5. In most instances, the presence of the citrate buffer is sufficient to negate the slight acidity of most I.V. fluids (22)
Penicillin G Sodium Administer I.V. infusion I.M. S.C. Intrathecal	Cephalothin Na (Keflin) (9) Diphenylhydantoin Na (Dilantin) (9) Hydroxyzine HCl (Vistaril) (9) Lincomycin HCl (Lincocin) (9) Metaraminol Bitartrate (Aramine) (9) Prochlorperazine Edisylate (5) (Compazine) (9) Promazine HCl (Sparine) (9) Promethazine HCl (Phenergan) (9) Tetracycline HCl (Achromycin) (9) Thiopental Na (Pentothal) (9) Vancomycin HCl (Vancocin) (9)
Pentobarbital Sodium *p*H 10.0 to 10.5 Administer I.V. with caution I.M.	Anileridine HCl (Leritine) (5) Cephalothin Na (12) (Keflin) (4) Precipitate forms (6) Chlordiazepoxide (12) Chlorpheniramine Maleate (9) (Chlor-Trimeton) (5) Chlorpromazine HCl (4) (Thorazine) (5) Listed by manufacturer as incompatible (4) Codeine Sulfate (5) Dimenhydrinate (Dramamine) (9) Diphenhydramine HCl (Benadryl) (4) Precipitate forms (4) Diphenylhydantoin Na (Dilantin) (5) Ephedrine Sulfate (5) Erythromycin Gluceptate (5) Hydrocortisone Na Succinate (Solu-Cortef) (5) Hydroxyzine HCl (Vistaril) (5) Insulin (5) Levarterenol Bitartrate (Levophed) (5) Levorphanol Bitartrate (Levo-Dromoran) (5) Meperidine HCl (12) (Demerol) (5) Methadone HCl (9) Methylphenidate HCl (Ritalin) (5) Morphine Sulfate (9) Oxytetracycline HCl (Terramycin) (5) Phytonadione (Aqua-Mephyton) (4) Precipitate forms (4) Prochlorperazine Edisylate (12) (Compazine) (4) Listed by manufacturer as incompatible (4) Promazine HCl (Sparine) (5)

Name of Drug	Drug Incompatibility [Nonproprietary (Trade)]
	Promethazine HCl (12) (Phenergan) (5) Sodium Bicarbonate (5) Streptomycin (5) Succinylcholine Chloride (5) Tetracycline (5) (Achromycin) (9) Triflupromazine HCl (12) Vancomycin HCl (Vancocin) (5)
Pentylenetetrazol *p*H 6.0 to 8.5 Administer I.V. I.M. S.C.	Isoniazid (6) Prochlorperazine Edisylate (Compazine) (5)
Phenobarbital Sodium *p*H 8.5 to 10.0 Administer slow I.V. I.M. S.C.	Acidic Solutions (6) Precipitate forms (6) Aminophylline (7) Anileridine HCl (Leritine) (9) Cephalothin Na (6) Precipitate forms (6) Chlorpromazine HCl (6) (Thorazine) (4) Precipitate forms (6) Codeine Phosphate (9) Codeine Sulfate (5) Dimenhydrinate (Dramamine) (8) Particulate matter observed (8) Diphenhydramine HCl (Benadryl) (8) Particulate matter observed (8) Diphenylhydantoin Na (Dilantin) (8) Particulate matter observed (8) Ephedrine Sulfate (9) Erythromycin Gluceptate (Ilotycin) (8) Particulate matter observed (8) Hydralazine HCl (11) Yellow color and then precipitate forms in 3 hours (11) Hydrocortisone Succinate (9) (Solu-Cortef) (5) Hydroxyzine HCl (11) (Vistaril) (8) Particulate matter observed (8) Insulin (9) Kanamycin Sulfate (6) (Kantrex) (8) Precipitate forms (6) Levarterenol Bitartrate (Levophed) (9) Levorphanol Bitartrate (Levo-Dromoran) (9) Meperidine HCl (Demerol) (5) Methadone HCl (9) Methylparaben (12) Methylphenidate HCl (5) Morphine Sulfate (5) Oxytetracycline HCl (Terramycin) (8) Particulate matter observed (8) Papaverine (6) Precipitate forms (6) Para-Aminobenzoic Acid (12) Penicillin G Potassium (22) Penicillin inactivation tends to occur in solutions with *p*H greater than 8.0. This barbiturate tends to raise the *p*H above this figure (22) Phytonadione (4) Precipitate forms (4) Procaine HCl (5) Prochlorperazine Mesylate (11) (Compazine) (8) Particulate matter observed (8) Promazine HCl (11) (Sparine) (8) Particulate matter observed (8) Promethazine HCl (11) (Phenergan) (8) Particulate matter observed (8) Propylparaben (12) Sodium Bicarbonate (9) Streptomycin Sulfate (9) Succinylcholine Chloride (6) (9) Precipitate forms (6) Tetracycline HCl (4) (Achromycin) (8) Particulate matter observed (8) Tripelennamine HCl (Pyribenzamine) (8) Particulate matter observed (8) Vancomycin HCl (Vancocin) (9)
Phenylephrine Hydrochloride *p*H 3.0 to 6.5 Administer dilute I.V. I.M. S.C.	Diphenylhydantoin Na (Dilantin) (8) Particulate matter observed (8)
Phytonadione *p*H 5.0 to 7.0 Administer slow I.V. I.M. S.C.	Barbiturates (4) Precipitate forms (4) Ascorbic Acid (5) Diphenylhydantoin Na (Dilantin) (8) Particulate matter observed (8) Pentobarbital Na (4) Precipitate forms (4) Phenobarbital Na (4) Precipitate forms (4)
Potassium Chloride	Amphotericin B (11) Haze developing over 3 hours (11)
Procainamide Hydrochloride *p*H 4.0 to 6.0 Administer I.V. I.M.	Diphenylhydantoin Na (Dilantin) (8) Particulate matter observed (8)
Procaine Hydrochloride *p*H 3.0 to 5.5 Administer slow I.V.	Alkaline Solutions (6) Aminophylline (9) Amobarbital Na (9) (Amytal) (5) Chloramphenicol Na Succinate (12) (Chloromycetin) (5) Chlorothiazide Na (Diuril) (12) Diphenylhydantoin Na (Dilantin) (9) Magnesium Sulfate (9) Nitrofurantoin Na (Furadantin) (9) Novobiocin Na (Albamycin) (9) Phenobarbital Na (Luminal) (9) Secobarbital Na (Seconal) (9) Sodium Bicarbonate (9) Sodium Iodide (9) Streptomycin (6) Decomposition occurs (6) Sulfadiazine Na (9) Sulfisoxazole (Gantrisin) (9) Thiopental Na (Pentothal) (18)

NAME OF DRUG	DRUG INCOMPATIBILITY [NONPROPRIETARY (TRADE)]
Prochlorperazine	Aminophylline (4)
Edisylate	Precipitate forms (4)
Administer	Amobarbital Na (Amytal) (5)
I.V.	Amphotericin B (11)
I.M.	Haze produced over 3 hours (11)
	Calcium Gluconate (9)
	Chloramphenicol Na Succinate (Chloromycetin) (4)
	Precipitate forms (4)
	Chlorothiazide Na (Diuril) (5)
	Cyanocobalamin (Rubramin) (5)
	Dexamethasone Na Phosphate (Decadron) (4)
	Precipitate forms (4)
	Dimenhydrinate (Dramamine) (4)
	Precipitate forms (4)
	Diphenylhydantoin Na (Dilantin) (4)
	Precipitate forms (4)
	Erythromycin Gluceptate (Ilotycin) (4)
	Manufacturer lists as incompatible (4)
	Ethamivan (11)
	Immediate precipitate (11)
	Heparin Na (4)
	Precipitate forms (4)
	Hydrocortisone Na Succinate (Solu-Cortef) (5)
	Kanamycin Sulfate (Kantrex) (4)
	Manufacturer lists as incompatible (4)
	Levallorphan (12)
	Meralluride (Mercuhydrin) (5)
	Methacillin Na (5) (Dimocillin) (4)
	Precipitate forms (4)
	Nitrofurantoin Na (Furadantin) (5)
	Oxytetracycline HCl (Terramycin) (4)
	Manufacturer lists as incompatible (4)
	Paraldehyde (5)
	Penicillin G Potassium (4)
	Precipitate forms (4)
	Penicillin G Sodium (5)
	Pentobarbital Na (4) (Nembutal) (5)
	Precipitate forms (4)
	Pentylenetetrazol (Metrazol) (5)
	Phenobarbital Na (4) (Luminal) (5)
	Precipitate forms (4)
	Prednisolone-21-Phosphate (8) (Hydeltrasol) (8)
	Particulate matter observed (8)
	Sulfadiazine (11)
	Haze or precipitate (11)
	Sulfisoxazole (Gantrisin) (4)
	Precipitate forms (4)
	Tetracycline HCl (Achromycin) (4)
	Manufacturer lists as incompatible (4)
	Thiopental Na (Pentothal) (5)
	Vancomycin HCl (Vancocin) (4)
	Manufacturer lists as incompatible (4)
	Vitamin B Complex with C (4)
	Precipitate forms (4)
Promazine	Aminophylline (11)
Hydrochloride	Immediate precipitate (11)
*p*H 4.0 to 5.5	Chloramphenicol Na Succinate (Chloromycetin) (8)
Administer	Particulate matter observed (8)
I.V.	Chlorothiazide Na (11) (Diuril) (5)
I.M.	Immediate precipitate (11)
	Chlortetracycline HCl (Aureomycin) (9)
	Dimenhydrinate (Dramamine) (8)
	Particulate matter observed (8)
	Diphenylhydantoin Na (Dilantin) (8)
	Particulate matter observed (8)
	Ethamivan (11)
	Immediate precipitate (11)
	Fibrinolysin (15)
	Heparin Na (8)
	Particulate matter observed (8)
	Hydrocortisone Na Succinate (Solu-Cortef) (8)
	Particulate matter observed (8)
	Menadione Na Bisulfite (8) (Hykinone) (4)
	Precipitate forms (4)
	Penicillin G Potassium (8)
	Particulate matter observed (8)
	Penicillin G Sodium (9)
	Pentobarbital Na (9) (Nembutal) (5)
	Phenobarbital Na (11) (Luminal) (8)
	Particulate matter observed (8)
	Prednisolone-21-Phosphate (Hydeltrasol) (8)
	Particulate matter observed (8)
	Sodium Bicarbonate (15)
	Physically incompatible (15)
	Sulfisoxazole (Gantrisin) (8)
	Particulate matter observed (8)
	Thiopental Na (Pentothal) (9)
	Vitamin B Complex with C (Folbesyn) (8)
	Particulate matter observed (8)
	Warfarin Na (Panwarfin) (15) (Coumadin) (5)
	Physically incompatible (15)
Promethazine	Aminophylline (11)
Hydrochloride	Immediate precipitate (11)
*p*H 4.0 to 5.5	Calcium Gluconate (9)
Administer	Chloramphenicol Na Succinate (Chloromycetin) (8)
I.V.	Particulate matter observed (8)
I.M.	Chlordiazepoxide HCl (12)
	Chlorothiazide Na (11) (Diuril) (9)
	Immediate precipitate (11)
	Codeine Sulfate (12)
	Dimenhydrinate (Dramamine) (8)
	Particulate matter observed (8)
	Diphenylhydantoin Na (Dilantin) (8)
	Particulate matter observed (8)
	Ethamivan (11)
	Immediate precipitate (11)
	Heparin Na (8)
	Particulate matter observed (8)
	Hydrocortisone Na Succinate (9) (Solu-Cortef) (8)
	Particulate matter observed (8)
	Methicillin Na (9) (Dimocillin) (8) (Staphcillin) (4)
	Particulate matter observed (8)
	Methylprednisolone (12)
	Nitrofurantoin Na (Furadantin) (9)
	Penicillin G Potassium (8)
	Particulate matter observed (8)
	Penicillin G Sodium (9)
	Pentobarbital Na (12) (Nembutal) (18)
	Phenobarbital Na (11) (Luminal) (8)
	Haze or precipitate forms (11)

Name of Drug	Drug Incompatibility [Nonproprietary (Trade)]
	Prednisolone-21-Phosphate (Hydeltrasol) (8) Particulate matter observed (8) Secobarbital Na (12) Sulfisoxazole (Gantrisin) (8) Particulate matter observed (8) Thiopental Na (12) (Pentothal) (18) Vitamin B Complex with C (Folbesyn) (8) Particulate matter observed (8)
Protamine Sulfate *p*H 3.0 Administer slow I.V.	Change of *p*H (6) Heparin (6) Complex formation (6)
Pyridoxine Chloride (Vitamin B-6) *p*H 3.0 to 4.0 Administer slow I.V. I.M.	Alkaline Solutions (6) Iron Salts (6) Oxidizing Solutions (6)
Riboflavin (Vitamin B-2) *p*H 4.5 to 7.0 Administer slow I.V. I.M.	Alkaline Solutions (6) Reducing Solutions (6) Decomposition occurs (6) Metals (6) Actinomycin B (6) Oleandomycin (6) Streptomycin (6) Tetracycline (6)
Secobarbital Sodium *p*H 9.7 to 10.5 Administer I.V (cautiously) I.M.	Anileridine HCl (Leritine) (9) Chlordiazepoxide (12) Chlorpromazine HCl (12) Codeine Phosphate (9) Diphenhydramine HCl (Benadryl) (9) Diphenylhydantoin Na (Dilantin) (9) Ephedrine Sulfate (9) Erythromycin Gluceptate (9) Hydrocortisone Na Succinate (9) (Solu-Cortef) (5) Insulin (9) Levarterenol Bitartrate (9) (Levophed) (5) Levorphanol Bitartrate (Levo-Dromoran) (9) Meperidine HCl (12) Methadone HCl (9) Methylphenidate HCl (5) Penicillin G Potassium (22) Penicillin inactivation tends to occur in solutions with *p*H greater than 8.0 (22) Phytonadione (4) Precipitate forms (4) Procaine HCl (9) Prochlorperazine (12) Promethazine HCl (12) Streptomycin Sulfate (9) Tetracycline HCl (9) Vancomycin HCl (9) (Vancocin) (5)
Sodium Bicarbonate *p*H 7.0 to 8.0 Administer slow dilute I.V.	Anileridine HCl (Leritine) (9) Calcium Chloride (4) Precipitate forms (4) Calcium Gluconate (4) Precipitate forms (4) Chlorpromazine HCl (12) Codeine Phosphate (9) Corticotropin (9) Dihydromorphinone HCl (9) Insulin (9) Levarterenol Bitartrate (Levophed) (9) Levorphanol Bitartrate (Levo-Dromoran) (9) Magnesium Sulfate (9) Meperidine HCl (Demerol) (5) Methadone HCl (9) Methicillin Na (5) (Dimocillin) (9) Morphine Sulfate (9) Oxytetracycline HCl (12) (Terramycin) (4) Precipitate forms (4) Penicillin G Potassium (22) Penicillin inactivation tends to occur in solutions with a *p*H greater than 8.0 (22) Pentobarbital Na (9) (Nembutal) (5) Phenobarbital Na (9) Procaine HCl (9) Promazine HCl (Sparine) (15) Streptomycin Sulfate (9) Tetracycline HCl (Achromycin) (9) Thiopental Na (Pentothal) (18) Vancomycin HCl (Vancocin) (9) Vitamin B Complex with C (Folbesyn) (9)
Sodium Iodide *p*H 7.5 to 9.0 Administer slow I.V.	Anileridine HCl (Leritine) (9) Codeine Phosphate (9) Levarterenol Bitartrate (Levophed) (9) Levorphanol Bitartrate (Levo-Dromoran) (9) Meperidine HCl (Demerol) (5) Methadone HCl (9) Morphine Sulfate (9) Procaine HCl (9)
Succinylcholine Chloride *p*H 3.0 to 4.5 Administer I.V.	Alkaline Solutions (6) Pentobarbital Na (9) (Nembutal) (5) Incompatible (9) Thiopental Na (12) (Pentothal) (9) Incompatible (9)
Sulfadiazine Sodium *p*H 8.5 to 10.5 Administer dilute I.V. dilute I.M. S.C.	Ammonium Chloride (5) Anileridine HCl (Leritine) (9) Chlorpromazine HCl (11) Immediate precipitate (11) Codeine Phosphate (9) Gentamicin Sulfate (11) Crystals produced (11) Hydralazine HCl (11) Yellow color forming a precipitate in 3 hours (11) Insulin (9) Iron Dextran (11) Crystals produced (11) Kanamycin Sulfate (11) Immediate precipitate (11) Levarterenol Bitartrate (Levophed) (9) Levorphanol Bitartrate (Levo-Dromoran) (9) Lidocaine HCl (11) Crystals produced (11) Lincomycin HCl (11) Crystals produced (11) Meperidine HCl (Demerol) (5) Metaraminol Tartrate (11) Crystals produced (11)

Name of Drug	Drug Incompatibility [Nonproprietary (Trade)]
Sulfadiazine Sodium (continued)	Methadone HCl (9) Methicillin Na (11) Crystals produced (11) Methyldopate HCl (11) Crystals produced (11) Methylparaben (12) Morphine Sulfate (9) Oxytetracycline HCl (11) Immediate precipitate (11) Para-Aminobenzoic Acid (12) Procaine HCl (9) Prochlorperazine Mesylate (11) Haze or precipitate formed (11) Propylparaben (12) Streptomycin Sulfate (11) Crystals produced (11) Tetracycline HCl (11) (Achromycin) (9) Immediate precipitate (11) Vancomycin HCl (Vancocin) (9)
Sulfisoxazole Diethanolamine *p*H 7.3 to 7.8 Administer slow I.V. I.M. dilute S.C.	Acidic Solutions (6) Precipitation occurs (6) Ammonium Chloride (9) Anileridine HCl (Leritine) (9) Codeine Phosphate (9) Diphenylhydantoin Na (9) (Dilantin) (8) Particulate matter observed (8) Hydroxyzine HCl (Vistaril) (8) Particulate matter observed (8) Insulin (9) Kanamycin Sulfate (Kantrex) (8) Particulate matter observed (8) Levallorphan Tartrate (6) (Lorfan) (8) Precipitate forms (6) Levarterenol Bitartrate (Levophed) (9) Levorphanol (Levo-Dromoran) (9) Meperidine HCl (Demerol) (5) Methadone HCl (9) Morphine Sulfate (9) Oxytetracycline HCl (Terramycin) (8) Particulate matter observed (8) Polybrene (8) Particulate matter observed (8) Procaine HCl (9) Prochlorperazine Maleate (9) (Compazine) (8) Particulate matter observed (8) Promazine HCl (Sparine) (8) Particulate matter observed (8) Promethazine HCl (Phenergan) (8) Particulate matter observed (8) Streptomycin Sulfate (9) Tetracycline HCl (Achromycin) (8) Particulate matter observed (8) Thiopental Na (Pentothal) (15) Vancomycin HCl (Vancocin) (8) Particulate matter observed (8) Vitamin B Complex with C (Berocca C) (10) Outside *p*H range for stability of vitamin product (10)
Tetracaine Hydrochloride Administer I.V. I.M.	Nitrofurantoin Na (Furadantin) (5)
Tetracycline Hydrochloride *p*H 1.8 to 2.8 The ascorbic acid stabilizer becomes inactive when diluted in large volume parenterals, therefore solution must be used immediately after preparation. Darkening of solutions indicates formation of degradation product (10) Administer I.V. I.M.	Aminophylline (10) No precipitate seen but solution darkened and faint ammonia-like odor was observed in 12 hours (10) Amobarbital Na (9) (Amytal) (25) Amphotericin B (11) (Fungizone) (25) Haze developing over 3 hours (11) Calcium Salts (6) Inactivation due to complex formation (6) Carbenicillin (11) Haze developing over 3 hours (11) Cephalothin Na (Keflin) (25) Precipitate forms within 1 hour (25) Chloramphenicol Na Succinate (9) (Chloromycetin) (8) Particulate matter observed (8) Chlorothiazide Na (Diuril) (5) Cloxacillin (11) Haze developing over 3 hours (11) Diphenylhydantoin Na (9) (Dilantin) (8) Particulate matter observed (8) Erythromycin (6) Gluceptate (9) Precipitate forms (6) Erythromycin Lactobionate (4) Resulting *p*H will cause decomposition of both antibiotics (4) Heparin Na (8) Particulate matter observed (8) Hydrocortisone Na Succinate (9) (Solu-Cortef) (8) Particulate matter observed (8) Methicillin Na (Staphcillin) (4) Methyldopate HCl (11) Crystals produced (11) Nitrofurantoin Na (Furadantin) (6) Precipitate forms (6) Novobiocin Na (Albamycin) (9) Penicillin G Potassium (8) Particulate matter observed (8) Penicillin G Sodium (9) Pentobarbital Na (9) (Nembutal) (5) Phenobarbital Na (Luminal) (8) Particulate matter observed (8) Polymyxin B Sulfate (12) Prochlorperazine Edisylate (Compazine) (8) Manufacturer lists as incompatible (8) Riboflavin (6) Secobarbital Na (Seconal) (9) Sodium Bicarbonate (9) Sulfadiazine Na (11) Immediate precipitate (11) Sulfisoxazole (Gantrisin) (8) Particulate matter observed (8) Thiopental Na (Pentothal) (15) Vitamin B Complex (4) Riboflavin inactivates tetracycline (4) Warfarin Na (Panwarfin) (15) (Coumadin) (5)

NAME OF DRUG	DRUG INCOMPATIBILITY [NONPROPRIETARY (TRADE)]
Thiamine (Vitamin B-1) *p*H 3 to 4 Administer slow I.V. I.M.	Increase of *p*H to neutral or alkaline (6) Decomposition occurs (6) Reducing Solutions (6) Iron Salts (6)
Thiopental Sodium *p*H 10 to 11 Incompatible with acidic solutions (12) Administer diulte I.V.	Anileridine HCl (Leritine) (9) Arginine Glutamate (Modumate) (12) Precipitate within 1 hour (23) Cephalothin (6) Precipitate forms (6) Chlorpromazine HCl (Thorazine) (18) Codeine Phosphate (9) Dihydromorphinone HCl (9) Dimenhydrinate (Dramamine) (18) Diphenhydramine HCl (Benadryl) (18) Ephedrine Sulfate (18) Fibrinolysin (15) Insulin (9) Levarterenol Bitartrate (Levophed) (9) Levorphanol Bitartrate (Levo-Dromoran) (9) Meperidine HCl (Demerol) (18) Metaraminol Bitartrate (Aramine) (24) Precipitate within 1 hour (24) Methadone HCl (9) Methamphetamine HCl (Desoxyn) (18) Methylparaben (12) Morphine Sulfate (18) Para-Aminobenzoic Acid (12) Penicillin G Potassium (23) Precipitate within 1 hour (23) Penicillin G Sodium (9) Procaine HCl (18) Prochlorperazine Edisylate (Compazine) (18) Promazine HCl (Sparine) (9) Precipitate within 1 hour (23) Promethazine HCl (Phenergan)(18) Protein Hydrolysate (23) Visual precipitate forms (23) Propylparaben (12) Sodium Bicarbonate (9) Succinylcholine Chloride (9) Sulfisoxazole (Gantrisin) (9) Precipitate within 1 hour (23) Tetracycline HCl (Achromycin) (9) Precipitate within 1 hour (23) Incompatible with acidic solutions (12)
Trimethaphan Camsylate *p*H 4.9 to 5.6 Administer I.V. infusion	Alkaline Solutions (6)
Tripelennamine Hydrochloride *p*H 6.2-7.8 Administer slow I.V. I.M. S.C.	Chloramphenicol Na Succinate (Chloromycetin) (8) Particulate matter observed (8) Diphenylhydantoin Na (Dilantin) (8) Particulate matter observed (8) Pentobarbital Na (4) Precipitate forms (4) Phenobarbital Na (Luminal) (8) Particulate matter observed (8)
Tromethamine Administer I.V.	Penicillin G Potassium (22) Penicillin inactivation tends to occur in solutions with *p*H greater than 8.0. This drug tends to raise the *p*H above this figure (22)
Vancomycin Hydrochloride *p*H 2.4 to 4.5 Alkaline solutions produce a precipitate (6) Administer I.V.	Aminophylline (8) Particulate matter observed (8) Amobarbital Na (9) (Amytal) (4) Chloramphenicol Na Succinate (Chloromycetin) (8) Particulate matter observed (8) Chlorothiazide Na (Diuril) (4) Dexamethasone (6) (Decadron) (8) Precipitate forms (6) Diphenylhydantoin Na (Dilantin) (8) Particulate matter observed (8) Heparin Na (6) Precipitate forms (6) Hydrocortisone Na Succinate (Solu-Cortef) (8) Particulate matter observed (8) Methicillin Na (Dimocillin) (8) Particulate matter observed (8) Nitrofurantoin Na (Furadantin) (9) Novobiocin Na (Albamycin) (9) Penicillin G Potassium (6)(9) Precipitate forms (6) Penicillin G Sodium (9) Pentobarbital Na (9) Phenobarbital Na (Luminal) (9) Prochlorperazine Edisylate (Compazine) (4) Manufacturer lists as incompatible (4) Secobarbital Na (9) Sodium Bicarbonate (9) Sulfadiazine Na (9) Sulfisoxazole (Gantrisin) (8) Particulate matter observed (8) Vitamin B Complex with C (Folbesyn) (8) Particulate matter observed (8)
Vitamin B Complex *p*H 4 to 5 Administer I.V. I.M.	Alkaline Solutions (6) Chloramphenicol (6) Chlorpromazine (6) Erythromycin (6) Nitrofurantoin (6) Tetracycline (6)
Vitamin B Complex with C *p*H 3.0 to 6.5 Administer I.V. I.M.	Aminophylline (9) Cephalothin Na (12) (Keflin) (5) Manufacturer states that it is compatible with Betalin Complex with C (5) Chloramphenicol Na Succinate (Chloromycetin) (4) The riboflavin contained in vitamin B complex injections rapidly diminishes potency of antibiotics (4) Chlorpromazine HCl (12) Cyanocobalamin (Rubramin) (9)

NAME OF DRUG	DRUG INCOMPATIBILITY [NONPROPRIETARY (TRADE)]
Vitamin B Complex with C (continued)	Diphenylhydantoin Na (Dilantin) (8)
	Erythromycin Lactobionate (12)
	Hydrocortisone Na Succinate (Solu-Cortef) (8)
	Hydroxyzine HCl (Vistaril) (8)
	Nafcillin Na (12)
	Nitrofurantoin Na (12) (Furadantin) (5)
Warfarin Sodium *p*H 7.2 to 8.3 Administer I.V. I.M.	Ammonium Chloride (12)
	Cyanocobalamin (15) (Rubramin) (9)
	Physically incompatible (15)
	Dextrose (9)
	Epinephrine HCl (Adrenalin) (15)
	Metaraminol Bitartrate (Aramine) (15)
	Oxytocin (Pitocin) (15)
	Promazine HCl (Sparine) (15)
	Tetracycline HCl (Achromycin) (15)
	Vitamin B Complex with C (12)

References

1. United States Pharmacopeial Convention: *United States Pharmacopeia,* Eighteenth Revision, Mack Printing Company, Easton Pennsylvania, 1970.
2. American Pharmaceutical Association: *National Formulary,* Twelfth Edition, Mack Printing Company, Easton, Pennsylvania, 1970.
3. Frazier, Walter M.: Administration Routes of Parenteral Injections, *Drug Intelligence 3*:42-55 (Feb.) 1969.
4. Fowler, Thomas: Some Incompatibilities of Intravenous Admixtures, *Am. J. Hosp. Pharm. 24*:450-457 (Aug.) 1967.
5. Pelissier, Normand and Burgee, Sydney: Guide to Incompatibilities, *Hosp. Pharm. 3*:15-32 (Jan.) 1968.
6. Kochel, F.: Inkompatibilitaten Bei Mischungen Intravenoser Losungen, *Section Des Pharmaciens Des Hopitaux,* Federation Internationale Pharmaceutique, Sept. 3-4, 1968, pp 57-70.
7. Williams, Jon and Moravec, Daniel: *Intravenous Therapy,* Clissold Publishing Company, 1967.
8. Misgen, Richard: Compatibilities and Incompatibilities of Some Intravenous Solution Admixtures, *Am. J. Hosp. Pharm. 22*:92-94 (Feb.) 1965.
9. Patel, Jayant and Phillips, George: A Guide to Physical Compatibility of Intravenous Drug Admixtures, *Am. J. Hosp. Pharm. 23*:409-411 (Aug.) 1966.
10. Edward, Sister Mary: *p*H — An Important Factor in the Compatibility of Additives in Intravenous Therapy, *Am. J. Hosp. Pharm. 24*:440-449 (Aug.) 1967.
11. Riley, Brian: Incompatibilities in Intravenous Solutions, *J. Hosp. Pharm. 28*:228-240 (Aug.) 1970.
12. Lemberg, Herman: Compilation of Pharmaceutical Incompatibilities, *Hosp. Pharm. 2*:19-25 (Aug.) 1967.
13. Bogash, Robert: Compatibilities and Incompatibilities of Some Parenteral Medication, *Bull. Am. Soc. Hosp. Pharm. 12*:445-448 (July-Aug.) 1955.
14. Webb, John: A *p*H Pattern for I.V. Additives, *Am. J. Hosp. Pharm. 26*:31-35 (Jan.) 1969.
15. Dunworth, Robert and Kenna, Regis: Preliminary Report: Incompatibility of Combinations of Medications in Intravenous Solutions, *Am. J. Hosp. Pharm. 22*:190-191 (Apr.) 1965.
16. Riffkin, Charles: Incompatibilities of Manufactured Parenteral Products, *Am. J. Hosp. Pharm. 20*:19-22 (Jan.) 1963.
17. Kirkland, W. D., Jones, R. W., Ellis J. R. and Schultz, C. G.: Compatibility Studies of Parenteral Admixtures, *Am. J. Hosp. Pharm. 18*:694-699 (Dec.) 1961.
18. Jones, R. W., Stanko, G. L. and Gross, H. M.: Pharmaceutical Compatibilities of Pentothal and Nembutal, *Am. J. Hosp. Pharm. 18*:700-704 (Dec.) 1961.
19. Parker, E. A.: Compatibility Digest, *Am. J. Hosp. Pharm. 28*:412-413 (July) 1969.
20. Stetcher, Paul (Ed): *The Merck Index,* Eighth Edition, Merck and Company, Rahway, New Jersey 1968.
21. Dancey, John and Carew, David: The Availability of Antibiotics in Combination with Other Additives in Intravenous Solutions, *Am. J. Hosp. Pharm. 23*:543-551 (Oct.) 1966.
22. Parker, E. A.: Compatibility Digest, *Am. J. Hosp. Pharm. 26*:543-544 (Sept.) 1969.
23. Parker, E. A.: Compatibility Digest, *Am. J. Hosp. Pharm. 26*:653-655 (Nov.) 1969.
24. Parker, E. A.: Compatibility Digest, *Am. J. Hosp. Pharm. 27*:672-673 (Aug.) 1970.
25. Parker, E. A.: Compatibility Digest, *Am. J. Hosp. Pharm. 72*:327-329 (Apr.) 1970.
26. Parker, E. A.: Compatibility Digest, *Am. J. Hosp. Pharm. 27*:67-69 (Jan.) 1970.
27. Parker, Eugene: Parenteral Incompatibilities, *Hosp. Pharm. 4*:14-22 (Aug.) 1969.
28. Parker, Eugene: Compatibility Digest, *Am. J. Hosp. Pharm. 27*:492 (June) 1970.
29. Anon.: *The Medical Letter 11*:35 (Apr. 18) 1969.
30. ....: *American Hospital Formulary Service,* Am. Soc. Hosp. Pharm., Washington, D.C.

22

Dialysis of poisons and drugs

by George E. Schreiner

The dosage, absorption, metabolism, distribution, excretion and toxicology of drugs and environmental poisons has, in the past, been in the exclusive realm of the pharmacologists and the toxicologists. The expanded use of sedatives, tranquilizers, analgesics, antibiotics and other therapeutic agents, as well as alcohols, household chemicals and various environmental poisons, has led to the increasing availability of a steadily increasing variety of chemicals involved in clinical poisoning.

In England, where comprehensive incidence figures are more available, the rate of hospital admission of self-poisoned patients increased in Oxford by 63 percent between 1962 and 1965, and in Sunderland by 235 percent between 1962 and 1967.[1]

The poisoning of human beings by drugs or chemicals may be accidental, suicidal, homicidal or, "God forbid," as an instrument of chemical warfare. Twenty years ago it occurred to us that since most drugs and chemicals are transported via the bloodstream from the site of absorption or injection to the target site of drug action or metabolism, it would seem a rather basic and simple concept that the same bloodstream could be used in the reverse direction to transport the material away from its site of biological activity. To reverse this direction, it is obviously necessary to lower the blood concentration as rapidly as feasible and, therefore, decrease the tissue to blood gradient in a manner that would promote movement of the molecule from the tissue site of action toward the bloodstream. Abel, Roundtree and Turner[2] in their original laboratory experiments with a crude artificial kidney, experimented with the removal of salicylates from the bloodstream of a laboratory animal. Thus they presaged this new use of artificial and biologic membranes for the treatment of drug intoxication, in addition to the more familiar and proper use of the artificial "kidney" for the treatment of acute and chronic renal failure. In these past 20 years, an enormous clinical and laboratory experience has been recorded on the dialytic removal of drugs and poisons. Dialysis has not only proved to be an effective clinical treatment for the overdose of commonly employed medicinal agents and for the rapid removal of some environmental poisons, but it has also proved itself as a fundamental research tool to give a substantial insight into some of the problems of drug transport and distribution. Nephrologists, artificial organists and membrane scientists have easily been able to cope with the kinetics of acute and chronic drug overdosage because the uremic syndrome itself partakes of many of the features of an intoxication or poisoning.

Negative critics of dialytic therapy have tended to reiterate the same and all too familiar logical flaws: the use of too small a series; the swamping of important clinical results by including large numbers of mild to moderate intoxications; the description of "conservative" therapy including good nursing care, maintenance of an airway, monitoring of physiologic function, support of the respiration, support of the circulation, use of an intensive care unit or use of forced diuresis, as measures which are competitive with, rather than truly complementary to, the use of dialysis in the treatment of poisons. So that these straw men may remain recumbent, I would like to state our beliefs in clear and simple terms. We do not believe that all patients who have been exposed to an overdose of a drug or poison should be dialyzed. We do not believe that dialysis is a substitute for an airway or nursing care. We enthusiastically support all developments in conservative care which in some cases may eliminate and in all cases will enhance the clinical effectiveness of dialytic therapy. Our collective experience tells us, however, that there will always be one group of patients whose intoxication is so severe that maintenance of a good airway and support of the circulation, however effective, will not suffice. There will always be another group of patients with clinical poisoning for whom the morbidity and danger of prolonged coma or the intoxication of specific organ systems presents a risk that is no longer necessary to take. For these two groups of patients, we feel it is a simple truth to state that the best treatment is removal of the poison, all other things being equal, by the most rapid and efficient method available to that clinician working on that patient in that medical setting at that time. Moreover, certain agents are metabolized within the body to substances more noxious than the parent chemical (*e.g.*, methanol to formaldehyde, ethylene glycol to oxalic acid). In such instances, early rapid removal dialysis will be advisable and the treatment of choice. Dialysis then becomes not only therapeutic for the parent chemical but preventive therapy for the metabolite with considerable leverage in the physiologic equation. If the metabolite, for example, is 30 times as toxic as the parent substance, then removal of one unit of the ingested drug by dialysis will prevent 30 units of subsequent intoxication.

The standard criteria for judging the applicability of dialysis and the removal of drugs were formulated by Schreiner.[3]

1. Molecules should diffuse through the dialyzing membrane, such as cellophane or peritoneum, from plasma water and have a reasonable removal rate or dialysance.

2. The drug must be distributed in plasma water or accessible body fluid compartments, or readily equilibrate with the circulating volume. Tight protein or tissue binding limits dialysis. This limitation is diminished if the bound or loculated portion can equilibrate with plasma water during the usual time of clinical dialysis.

3. There should be a relationship between the blood concentration, the duration of the body's exposure to the chemical and its ultimate clinical toxicity. This has been termed the "time-dose-cytotoxic relationship."

4. The amount of poison dialyzed should constitute a significant addition to the normal body mechanisms for dealing with the particular poison under the physiologic circumstances which may be encountered under clinical conditions of intoxication. The mechanisms include metabolism, conjugation, enzyme induction, pharmacologic antagonism and elimination of the substance by bowel and kidney. The physiologic circumstances may include shock, oliguria and poor liver perfusion. Metabolic rates may not be extrapolated from the normal dog to the sick patient.

The development of low resistance, low priming volume dialyzers makes practical the presentation of large surface areas of membrane for the removal of poisons. These may have to be specially constructed for poison cases, may be approached by multiplication of layers or units, or by the operation of more than one dialyzer in parallel or sequence. Developments in membrane polymer chemistry reported elsewhere in the *Transactions* may also affect the efficiency and the rapidity by which poisons can be removed in particular clinical circumstances.

Table 1. Currently Known Dialyzable Poisons

Barbiturate*	Alcohols	Metals	Miscellaneous Substances
Barbital	Ethanol*	Arsenic	Thiocyanate*
Phenobarbital	Methanol*	Copper	Aniline
Amobarbital	Isopropanol	Calcium	Sodium chlorate
Pentobarbital	Ethylene glycol	Iron	Potassium chlorate
Butabarbital		Lead	Eucalyptus oil
Secobarbital		Lithium	Boric acid
Cyclobarbital		Magnesium	Potassium dichromate
	Analgesics	Mercury	Chromic acid
Glutethimide*	Acetylsalicylic acid*	Potassium	Digoxin
	Methylsalicylate	Sodium	Sodium citrate
Depressants, Sedatives and	Acetophenetidin	Strontium	Dinitro-ortho-cresol
Tranquilizers	Dextropropoxyphene		Amanita phalloides
Diphenylhydantoin	Paracetamol	Halides	Carbon tetrachloride
Primidone		Bromide*	Ergotamine
Meprobamate		Chloride*	Cyclophosphamide
Ethchlorvynol*		Iodide	5-Fluorouracil
Ethinamate	Antibiotics	Fluoride	Methotrexate
Methyprylon	Streptomycin		Camphor
Diphenhydramine	Kanamycin	Endogenous Toxins	Trichlorethylene
Methaqualone	Neomycin	Ammonia	Carbon monoxide
Heroin	Vancomycin	Uric acid*	Chlorpropamide
Gallamine triethiodide	Penicillin	Tritium*	Quinine
Paraldehyde	Ampicillin	Bilirubin	
Chloral hydrate	Sulfonamides	Lactic acid	
Chlordiazepoxide	Cephalothin	Schizophrenia	
	Cephaloridine	Myasthenia gravis	
Antidepressants	Chloramphenicol	Porphyria	
Amphetamine	Tetracycline	Cystine	
Methamphetamine	Nitrofurantoin	Endotoxin	
Tricyclic secondary amines	Polymyxin	Hyperosmolar state*	
Tricyclic tertiary amines	Isoniazid	Water intoxication	
Monoamine oxidase inhibitors	Cycloserine		
Tranylcypromine			
Pargyline			
Phenelzine			
Isocarboxazid			

*Kinetics of dialysis thoroughly studied and/or clinical experience extensive

The permeability of different membranes for solutes can be measured as stated by Renkin:[4]

$$P = \frac{\text{mol./min. diffusing}}{\text{mol./min. gradient}} \times \text{cm.}^2$$

Dialysance or the rate of removal of a solute from the blood/unit concentration difference between arterial blood and bath fluid can be expressed integrating Fick's Law to the length of dialysis:[4]

$$D = a(1 - e^{\frac{-PS}{a}})$$

where D is dialysance, a is blood flow, e the natural logarithm bearing the exponent of the product of membrane permeability (P), times surface area (S), divided by blood flow. As in peritoneal dialysis, the expression has the same dimensions as clearance *i.e.*, ml/minute.

Previous reviews[5,6] have provided a detailed bibliography for investigators and clinicians who wish to follow the details of a specific case. This search has been aided by MEDLARS and augmented by personal communications from members of the Society yielding unpublished data. In addition to dialysis, the removal of poisons may be accomplished by the use of gastric lavage, chelates, forced diuresis, dialysis, charcoal hemoperfusion[7] or perfusion through a resin column.[8] Diuresis, using mannitol,[9] urea[10] or saluretic agents should be maintained at 500 ml/hour, if tolerated. Peritoneal dialysis is less effective, particularly when hypotension is present, but is more widely available. Additives to increase peritoneal clearance of certain solutes include hypertonic glucose,[11] streptokinase,[12] albumin,[13] THAM[14] and lipids.[15]

Those drugs and poisons for which there is definite or presumptive evidence of significant removal by dialysis are listed in Table 1. They are grouped in the order in which they appear in the discussion. Clinical experience and experimental data are limited for some chemicals. Table 2 summarizes the clinical experience of the Renal Division at Georgetown University Hospital with 164 intoxicated patients treated by dialysis during a 20-year period.

Barbiturates

Barbiturate overdosage continues to be the common denominator for patients with depression and suicidal tendencies. In many countries, including our own, this has become a major public health problem. There are now over 600 poison control centers in the major population areas and a clearing house of information for poison control centers which, in 1967 received 100,000 case reports. Poisoning now represents more than half of childhood accidents.

In 1964 there were 478 recorded deaths due to barbiturate poisoning representing over 20 percent of deaths due to acute poisoning.[16] Because of the prejudicial effect on insurance settlements and the still prevalent social stigmata, there are many cases of barbiturate poisoning which go unreported in official records on causes of death. Recent reports suggest younger people are now involved in barbiturate poisoning[17,18] and one report includes infants under one year of age.[19]

Alkalinization of the urine increases excretion of phenobarbital, but not of short-acting barbiturates which have a higher pK.[20,21] Forced diuresis greatly increases the excretion of phenobarbital but this effect is slight with short-acting drugs, whereas the metabolites of the latter are excreted to a larger extent.[21] Clearances of short-acting barbiturates increase to about 5 ml/minute with forced diuresis[20] while phenobarbital clearance may reach 17 ml/minute.[22]

Depending on the specific drug involved, hemodialysis removes barbiturates 10 to 30 times faster than diuresis.[13,20,23] Clinical experience with dialysis now numbers over 300 reported patients and includes several detailed studies.[3,20,23-28] Maximal dialysance ranges from 65 ml/minute for secobarbital to 100 ml/minute for phenobarbital.[21] Removal of short-acting barbiturates by diuresis is limited by protein binding and by sequestration in body fat from which the drugs are slowly removed.[21] Intraperitoneal THAM or albumin increases barbiturate removal, but clearances rarely exceed 10 ml/minute, even with these techniques.[13,14,29-31] Polyvinylpyrrolidone has been used as a binding agent in the treatment of experimental barbiturate intoxication in rabbits.[32] Dialysis removes significant quantities of unchanged barbiturates, whereas diuresis may clear metabolites from the circulation.[21,23] Barbiturates may also be removed by concurrent administration of cholestyramine orally[33a] or by hemoperfusion through anion exchange resin columns,[8] or through charcoal.[7,34] Barbitone has been found to accumulate in concentrations of 0.24-1.32 mg % in six patients on chronic dialysis. These patients had taken pentobarbital which has a small contamination of barbitone which apparently binds to albumin and another protein (molecular weight 110,000-140,000) and is retained despite hemodialysis.[35]

Indications for hemodialysis in barbiturate poisoning are:

1. Known ingestion and probable absorption of a potentially fatal dose (3 Gm for short-acting, 5 Gm for long-acting barbiturates).
2. A blood barbiturate level in the potentially fatal range (3.5 mg %, short, 8 mg %, long).
3. Progressive deepening of anesthesia or clinical deterioration.
4. Coexistence of a medical complication delaying elimination of the drug or increasing the hazards of coma.
5. Development of a severe complication such as hyperpyrexia or aspiration pneumonia.

Identification of a drug is not always easy, particularly if multiple drugs were available and the history is unreliable. Serum levels are not always readily available in many hospitals in the evenings or on holidays when ingestion is most likely to occur. It is possible to use the spectrophotometric differences of various barbiturate compounds to approach the problem of identifying a special agent. This is done by comparing the ultraviolet absorption spectrum of the unknown serum with a series of commonly used barbiturates.[3] Thin layer chromatographic techniques are simpler and more rapid and can be helpful in the clinical setting. Gas chromatography is the most accurate method for many organic compounds, but is often less accessible, more expensive and more time consuming. It is important to know which substances potentiate the action of the barbiturates as is the case, for example, with alcohol and a number of tranquilizers.[36]

The placental transfer of barbiturates in epileptic women being treated with these drugs may produce intoxication of newborns. Melchior, *et al.*[37] have shown that the concentration of phenobarbitone in human umbilical cord serum was 95 percent of the material serum concentration. The rate of elimination of the drug from the blood of newborns was slower than adults. With blood concentrations of phenobarbital below 8 mg/L the rate of elimination in four patients was 14 percent/day. In another group of three patients with umbilical cord serum levels up to 25.7 mg/L the highest elimination rate was 20 percent/24 hour. There is considerable intake of phenobarbital through breast milk.[38]

A remarkable recovery was documented where hemodialysis lowered the blood phenobarbital level from over 50 to 9.3 mg % in 13 hours, with recovery of 9.4 Gm in the dialysate.[39] Another patient ingested 20 Gm of amobarbital and recovered when hemodialysis lowered the blood level from 16 mg %.[40] Hemodialysis has caused restoration of electroencephalographic activity[41] and survival after the patient had been pronounced dead.[42]

Several additional reports document clinical improvement in patients with barbiturate poisoning treated by dialysis.[43-50] Hemodialysis improved one patient with a serum level above 20 mg % and removed 2.0 of 12.5 Gm ingested.[44] The blood level of another decreased from 18 to 8.4 mg % as 2.6 of 5.6 Gm ingested was removed by dialysis.[50]

Extended dialysis may be required in the case of short-acting barbiturates. Hudson, *et al.*[51] dialyzed a 21-year-old nurse for 68 hours. She ingested 5.0 Gm secobarbital, 5.0 Gm pentobarbital, 2.5 Gm chlorpromazine, 0.1 Gm perphenazine and 0.6 Gm amitriptyline. The initial serum barbiturate level was 8.3 mg %. The mean rate of removal was 2.7 mg/minute and the clearance was 26.6 ml/minute. The blood concentration declined 0.8 percent/hour for the first 35 hours and 2.7 percent/hour thereafter. The removal was a significant contribution to her recovery.

Wieth[52] recovered 6.2 Gm of pentobarbital in the dialysate of a patient whose blood level decreased from 19.6 to 3.6 mg % in 9.2 hours. For long-acting barbiturates, he measured a serum half-life of 3.6 to 9.7 hours with hemodialysis, which is 3.8 to 27 times faster than the spontaneous half-life (37 to 96 hours) and 2.2 to 10.3 times faster than that due to forced diuresis (21 to 37 hours). Dialysis shortened coma by a factor of 4 to 25. Rosenbaum and Mandanis[53] circulated peritoneal dialysate through an anion exchange resin column for removal of phenobarbital from experimentally intoxicated dogs. Removal by the column was 379 mg in six hours, which increased with the addition to the bath

Table 2. Dialysis for Acute Poisoning. Renal Division, Georgetown University School of Medicine, 1950 - 1970

Barbiturates	88	Diphenylhydantoin	2
Glutethimide	32	Carbon Tetrachloride*	2
Salicylates	10	Methyprylon	1
Bichloride of Mercury*	7	Kanamycin*	1
Ethchlorvynol	3	Aniline	1
Uric Acid	3	Heroin	1
Meprobamate	3	Dextropropoxyphene	1
Methanol	2	Phenformin	1
Ethylene Glycol*	2	Sodium Fluoride	1
Bromide	2	Amanita Phalloides	1
		Total	164

*Dialysis performed within 48 hours of exposure for the removal of nephrotoxin rather than for the treatment of uremia.

of albumin and lipid. Lipid dialysis has been used for the removal of Seconal in both experimental animals and man.[54,55] Linton, Luke and Briggs[53a] showed that the increase in barbiturate clearance with diuresis is independent of the type of diuretic used, except that alkali enhanced phenobarbital excretion. Diuresis was less effective with intermediate-acting drugs than with long-acting barbiturates. Forced diuresis is now being used in many countries in the treatment of barbiturate poisoning.[56-59] Ohlsson in 10 years' experience with "blood lavage" achieved an exceptional overall mortality figure of 2.3 percent.[60] We believe that **phenobarbital** and other long-acting barbiturates readily meet our criteria for the ideal dialyzable poison. Short-acting barbiturates on the other hand have lower plasma values and have a larger distribution space, some of it occasionally in tissues such as the liver. However, they meet the criteria otherwise and in critical cases of severe poisoning, dialysis may be the margin of victory.

The determination of **secobarbital** in a lipid system requires modification, which chiefly involves the use of ethylene dichloride as the organic solvent and sodium chloride to clear the chloroform extract prior to analysis.[61]

Glutethimide (Doriden)

A review of our referral hospitals suggests that cases of minimal **glutethimide** poisoning do not appear in general hospitals or poison control centers with nearly the frequency that obtains with mild cases of barbiturate poisoning. Of those that come, however, the percentage referred to a dialysis center is very much higher. The poisoning is apt to be severe and the mortality rate is considerable. Because of this severity, dialysis therapy has had a substantial clinical trial in both this country[62,63] and abroad.[64] Hickson and Caridis recovered 5.6 Gm of glutethimide in the dialysate from a 48-year-old man with an initial blood level of 4.4 mg %. He recovered in 12 hours. In a 57-year-old male, they recovered 7.0 Gm from a blood level of 3.7 mg % with complete clinical recovery in 48 hours.[64]

Clearance values of glutethimide may reach 90 ml/minute, but clinical results with dialysis are frequently disappointing.[65] Nevertheless, the duration of coma is shortened, blood levels decline more rapidly with dialysis and dialysate recovery represents 30 to 200 times urinary excretion.[62,65-67] Mortality rates are reduced in severe cases from 50 to 18 percent. Removal of glutethimide by dialysis is hampered by protein binding and low circulating blood levels due to 10 to 15-fold concentration in body fat, but can be increased by the use of a lipid dialysate.[39,68,69] King, *et al.*[70] dialyzed a man who ingested 5+ Gm of glutethimide. The blood level of 2.93 mg % was reduced to 2.3 in 1.5 hour, 1.8 in 3.5 hours, 1.0 in 4.5 hours of lipid dialysis and was 0.3 mg % on the following day.

Diuresis and biliary drainage are ineffective.[65] Prevention of continued gastrointestinal absorption by non-absorbable oils is also being studied.[39] Experimentally intoxicated dogs improve clinically with charcoal hemoperfusion which will adsorb about 4.0 Gm of glutethimide per 100 Gm of charcoal.[71] Because of the high mortality rate and the difficulty in removing glutethimide by simpler means, dialysis is recommended for severe intoxication, prolonged coma, a blood level above 3.0 mg % or after ingestion of more than 10 Gm or 0.15 Gm/Kg.

Four additional patients with glutethimide poisoning treated by dialysis have been reported.[72,74,76] DeMyttenaere. Schoenfeld and Maher[72] recovered 1240 mg of glutethimide from the dialysate after eight hours of hemodialysis of their patient, while the concurrent use of peritoneal dialysis removed 580 mg in 48 hours and a simultaneous osmotic diuresis exceeding 3 ml/minute caused excretion of 506 mg in 68 hours. Frey[31] recovered 705 mg in peritoneal dialysate in 72 hours and 130 mg in the urine during the same interval. A significant fraction of the quantity recovered in urine normally represents the metabolite of glutethimide, indicating an even greater relative removal by dialysis. Caplan[74] reported a patient who ingested approximately 10 Gm of glutethimide and became deeply comatose. The serum level decreased from 11.9 to below 1.0 mg % after eight days during which she underwent five hemodialyses, the first two of which removed a total of 1.4 Gm of glutethimide. She awoke after 11 days. Nine months later she ingested an unknown quantity of glutethimide and again became comatose. The serum glutethimide level was 4.1 mg % and she again underwent hemodialysis and recovered. Chazan and Cohen[75] were unable to correlate serum glutethimide levels with the severity of intoxication. Although some of their patients' blood levels were extremely high, they stress that the spectrum of intoxication includes many mild cases. They did not demonstrate a difference in the declining slope of blood levels between patients who underwent dialysis and those who did not. The biologic half-life in each group was in excess of 48 hours. Dialysate recovery in five patients ranged from 950 to 3000 mg. Our studies,[65] however, demonstrate that glutethimide has a high dialysance, a high removal rate by dialysis compared to spontaneous removal and a direct relation between the dose ingested and toxicity. Decker, *et al.*[77] reported two young women who ingested glutethimide, awakened 24 hours after ingestion, returned into coma 12 hours later and woke up again 40 hours later. Blood levels fell, rose and fell again in perfect correlation with consciousness. Patients slept above 2.2 mg %, and awoke below 2 mg %.

Removal of glutethimide is most effective when the patients are seen early. Later it may be limited to some extent by the "virtual" distribution space which exceeds total body water. There is some evidence that the distribution space expands with time and is probably accounted for by the very high concentration which may be reached in body fat. Because of the relatively low arteriovenous differences in small dialyzers, we have followed the practice of connecting a twin coil dialyzer with a pump to a Kiil dialyzer in series, using the pump of the Travenol kidney to circulate the blood. This markedly improves the A-V differences for glutethimide in aqueous dialysis.

Dialysis in glutethimide poisoning should be considered when there has been ingestion of a large dose (6 Gm or more), when blood levels are high (3-8 mg %) and when the patients are unresponsive and have severe hypotension and shock, cerebral or pulmonary edema or neurologic signs, such as fixed, dilated pupils. Aqueous dialysate recovery usually represents about 10 percent of the ingested dose. In severe poisoning, therefore, an extended dialysis or the use of machines in series may be required. The regular removal by hemodialysis is about 20 times faster than by diuresis, and about 12 times faster than peritoneal dialysis. About 4 Gm of glutethimide can be absorbed by 100 Gm of charcoal.

Depressants, Sedatives and Tranquilizers

A major health problem concerning depressants, sedatives and tranquilizers is related to the introduction of larger numbers of new drugs each year, about which little is known of the conditions of absorption and body distribution or the chemical measurement and kinetics of dialysis. Cimino has recently called for federal action to require manufacturers to supply dialysis data on new drugs.[78]

There is good clinical and chemical evidence for the dialytic removal of **diphenylhydantoin** (Dilantin). This synthetic compound has been widely used for more than 25 years as a safe anticonvulsant.[79-81] Severe symptoms following poisoning with this agent include vomiting, difficulty in swallowing, respiratory distress, fatigue, insomnia, irritability, confusion, hallucination and delusions. Adults have recovered after ingestions of 4.5, 8.3 and 21.5 Gm. Dialysis was used in two. A 2¾-year-old child recovered after ingestion of 800 mg. Fatal cases have been reported from ingestion of 2 Gm in a 4½-year-old girl[79] and in a 16-year-old girl from ingestion of an unknown quantity.[82] Tenckhoff, *et al.*[83] and Blair, *et al.*[84] reported effective peritoneal removal in both children and adults.

Clinical improvement and significant lowering of blood levels have also been reported for the anticonvulsant drug **primidone** (Mysoline).[81-84] Peritoneal dialysate concentrations have been reported to be as high as ⅔ of the blood level. There is a dearth of data on other anticonvulsants such as **mephenytoin, ethotoin, trimethadione, paramethadione** or **phenacemide.**

Both peritoneal and hemodialysis have caused clinical improvement in **meprobamate** intoxication.[85-87] Dialysate recovery is substantial and blood levels are decreased by dialysis. Severe intoxication has been reported with blood levels above 12 mg %.

Maddock and Bloomer[88] treated conservatively 10 patients with meprobamate overdosage, one of whom, with a blood meprobamate level of 17.4 mg %, died before effective therapy could be initiated. The severity of coma was directly related to the blood level, deep coma occurring at concentrations about 12 mg %. Dialysis was judged indicated at blood levels approaching 20 mg %. In plasma, 20 percent of the drug was found to be protein bound. Forced diuresis increased renal excretion to a maximum clearance of about one-third of the glomerular filtration rate. In the first 24 hours after ingestion as much as 11 percent appeared in urine. Meprobamate disappears from the plasma at a rate of 8.5 ± 2 percent/hour, mostly due to metabolism. The distribution space equals approximately 75 percent of body weight. In experimentally intoxicated dogs, these authors demonstrated a peritoneal dialysate/plasma ratio of 0.5. Using the standard twin-coil artificial kidney, the dialysance *in vitro* was approximately 100 ml/minute. The patient treated with peritoneal dialysis by Mouton, Cohen and Barrett[89] ingested 20 Gm of meprobamate. The blood meprobamate level decreased from 16 to 10 mg % spontaneously in seven hours and declined to 0.8 mg % after 17 hours, at which time the patient was awake. When the blood level was 4.1 mg %, the patient was responsive. With therapeutic doses the blood meprobamate level is 1.0 to 2.0 mg %. Diuresis achieved a clearance of 7.0 to 8.0 ml/minute and removed 929 mg. The peritoneal clearance exceeded 20 ml/minute and 1375 mg was recovered in the dialysate. The gastric aspirate contained 185 mg. The patient reported by Castell and Sode[90] ingested 30 Gm of meprobamate, had a blood level of 10 mg %, and improved with peritoneal dialysis which removed more than 1 Gm while 900 mg of the drug appeared in the urine. Meprobamate poisoning has recently been reviewed by Gaultier, *et al.*[91] Teehan, *et al.*[92] have reported an experience with six consecutive cases of **ethchlorvynol** (Placidyl) intoxication. They presented with deep coma, hypothermia, apnea and hypotension. Ingestion ranged from 15 to 50 Gm, and plasma concentrations were as high as 16.6 mg %. The distribution space surpassed body water. Mean clearances were 18.5 ml/minute for peritoneal dialysis, 23 ml/minute for forced diuresis (500 ml/hour) and 64 ml/minute for hemodialysis. Hemodialysis shortened serum half-life from 70 to 22 hours. Five patients lived, and one died after 168 hours of coma. Ethchlorvynol intoxication also has been successfully treated in an infant by a combination of exchange transfusion and peritoneal dialysis.[93] Gas-liquid chromatography has been found valuable in the clinical management of adult ethchlorvynol poisoning.[94] A prolonged coma may result from large ingestions of this drug.[95,96] Hemodialysis has been reported to reduce the serum concentration in half by 10 hours. The dialysance is 50-105 ml/minute. Bath recoveries of more than 5 Gm have been noted. Albumin has been used to enhance the removal rate by peritoneal dialysis[97] but since this agent does not ionize, the use of THAM is not recommended.[92] Poisoned patients who have ingested more than 10 Gm or have a blood level above 7.0 mg % should be considered for dialysis. The serum half-life may exceed 72 hours.

Hemodialysis lowered the blood level from 3.0 to 2.0 mg % in a patient with **ethynyl cyclohexyl carbamate** (Valmid) poisoning.[98] **Ethinamate** and its metabolites have been recovered in the dialysate as clinical improvement occurred.[98,99]

Coma, apnea and hypotension due to **methyprylon** (Noludar) are improved rapidly by hemodialysis and more slowly by peritoneal dialysis.[39,100,101] Clearances by hemodialysis are 20 to 50 ml/minute, while forced diuresis may achieve a clearance slightly above 10 ml/minute. The potentially fatal dose is 15 Gm and blood levels of 4 to 11 mg % have been measured during severe intoxication.

The rapid fall in blood methyprylon levels during dialysis has been attributed to metabolism since less than 10 percent of the ingested dose is recovered in the dialysate.[102] Yet there is dramatic clinical improvement during hemodialysis which possibly suggests removal of a toxic metabolite. We have treated by peritoneal dialysis a patient with a serum methyprylon level of 2.9 mg %.[103] Dialysate concentrations were more than 50 percent of the plasma level and clearances were 15 to 20 ml/minute. The renal excretion during mannitol diuresis was 160 mg/hour after which the blood level was 36 mg %.

The **phenothiazines** are not dialyzable. Clearance values of **chlorpromazine** are less than 0.5 mg/minute and insignificant amounts are recovered in dialysate.[104] Clinical trials in chlorpromazine (Thorazine) and **promazine** (Sparine) were unsuccessful.[105,106] **Trifluoperazine** (Stelazine) is not removed by aqueous dialysis, but can be recovered from lipid dialysate.[39] Clinical improvement accompanied hemodialysis for **imipramine** (Tofranil) poisoning, although dialysate recovery was minimal.[107] Fatal poisonings have been reported with imipramine and **dibenzepin** (Noveril) in small children.[206]

Peritoneal clearance was only 1.0 ml/minute and blood levels were 1.7 to 2.5 μg/ml in a fatal case of **amitriptyline** (Elavil) poisoning.[207]

During clinical intoxication and coma due to **chlordiazepoxide** (Librium), blood levels are less than 1.0 μg/ml. Hemodialysis does not significantly decrease the levels of chlordiazepoxide or **diazepam** (Valium) and the drugs are not detectable in dialysate.[100] Chlordiazepoxide intoxication is usually mild, poorly correlated with the ingested dose and frequently occurs as a mixed intoxication where the clinical picture is dominated by the other drug.[208] Cruz, Kramer and Parrish[209] treated by hemodialysis a patient with combined barbiturate and chlordiazepoxide toxicity. She improved as the serum pentobarbital level decreased from 4.5 to 1.6 mg % and the chlordiazepoxide concentration declined from 2.4 to 1.0 mg % during the 10 hour procedure. With therapeutic doses the blood level is less than 0.2 mg %.

Dialysis has also caused clinical improvement in poisoning due to **heroin,**[85] **gallamine triethiodide,**[220] **paraldehyde**[210] and **chloral hydrate.**[211] An infant with **diphenhydramine** (Benadryl) poisoning was successfully treated by exchange transfusion with reduction of the blood level from 0.55 to 0.32 mg %.[212] Two patients have undergone hemodialysis for **paraldehyde** intoxication,[213,214] and one has been reported who was treated by peritoneal dialysis.[215] The metabolic acidosis was corrected in each instance but removal of paraldehyde was not documented.

Another patient with **morphine** intoxication has been treated by dialysis with lowering of the blood level.[216] Several patients have been treated for **opiate** intoxication by dialysis but not reported.[46]

Hemodialysis improved a patient who ingested 5.0 to 7.5 Gm of **methaqualone** and 0.5 to 0.75 Gm of diphenhydramine.[217] The blood methaqualone level decreased from 10.5 to 5.8 mg % and the dialysate concentration was 2.2 mg % after two hours using the twin-coil artificial kidney. Among 87 patients treated by Ibe, *et al.*[218] for methaqualone poisoning, four underwent hemodialysis. These authors used hemodialysis for five of 96 patients with methyprylon poisoning. Proudfoot, *et al.*[219] treated a patient with methaqualone poisoning by both peritoneal dialysis and hemodialysis. There was a decrease in the blood level from an initial 23 mg %, recovery of almost 10 Gm of the drug in dialysate and restoration of some neurologic functions. The clearance values by peritoneal dialysis and hemodialysis averaged 7.5 and 29 ml/minute, respectively.

Recovery has been noted after a massive overdose of diphenhydramine and methaqualone with the use of hemodialysis in an adult.[108]

Many of these drugs are adsorbed by charcoal, which has been used both orally and by hemoperfusion. Decker, Combs and Corby[109] demonstrated that 5.0 Gm of charcoal will adsorb from aqueous solutions more than 80 percent of toxic doses of dextroamphetamine, primaquine, chlorpheniramine, colchicine, diphenylhydantoin, aspirin, iodine, phenol and propoxyphene. Adsorption of other drugs such as quinacrine, meprobamate, quinine, quinidine, chloroquine, glutethimide, methyl salicylate and 2-4 dichlorophenoxyacetic acid is less complete.

Malathion, DDT, ferrous sulfate, N-methylcarbamate and boric acid are poorly adsorbed.

Antidepressants

Amphetamines have become one of the major forms of drug abuse in the United States. It has been the subject of a number of in-depth studies.[110,111] Intravenous amphetamine abuse developed in many addicts. Tolerance for the drug builds rapidly. With larger doses, the individuals may fall into a prolonged semicomatose state. It is estimated that 4,000 individuals in San Francisco regularly take amphetamines.[112] Amphetamine has been removed by peritoneal dialysis[112] and dialysis has ameliorated experimental intoxication.[114] Bath recoveries are small. We have seen a student who took combined amphetamine and barbiturates overdosage and had cyclic coma alternating with muscle twitching and myotonia. He was improved by dialysis.

The **tricyclic antidepressants** include principally the tertiary amines, imipramine hydrochloride (Tofranil), amitriptyline HCl, (Elavil) and doxepin (Sinequan). The secondary amines include desipramine hydrochloride (Pertofrane), nortriptyline hydrochloride (Aventyl HCl) and protriptyline (Vivactil). The side effects include an atropine-like action with dryness of the mouth, constipation and urinary retention for which pyridostigmine may be used. Other drugs may sensitize to seizures and convulsions. The peak action is between three and 24 hours. The drugs are protein bound, disappear from the plasma rapidly[115] and are concentrated in tissues.[116] In spite of minimal dialysate recovery, clinical improvement from hemodialysis has been claimed for imipramine hydrochloride (Tofranil).[117] Hemodialysis was used in a child who recovered.[47]

Another group of antidepressants are the **monoamine oxidase inhibitors.** The principal drugs on the market include isocarboxazid (Marplan), nialamide (Niamid), phenelzine sulfate (Nardil), tranylcypromine (Parnate) and pargyline HCl (Eutonyl). A number of deaths have been reported from these agents. Several of them have been withdrawn from the market. Acute hypertensive crises and cerebral hemorrhage may occur when a MAO inhibitor is taken simultaneously with a sympathomimetic drug such as ephedrine or amphetamines, or with food containing free amines such as cheese. The narcotic effects of meperidine (Demerol) may also be potentiated. The free amine in cheese has been identified as tyramine, which is also contained in certain creams, beers and wines. These are claims of adverse combination effects of MAO inhibitors with alcohol, cocaine, barbiturates, ether, insulin, procaine and opiates. Injection of 5.0 mg of phentolamine (Regitine) is indicated for hypertensive crisis. Primary side effects of the drug include postural hypotension, fainting and bizarre behavior. Although chemical documentation is poor, clinical improvement has been attributed to dialysis in intoxication due to MAO inhibitors.[100,119] A child improved on peritoneal dialysis.[120] The level of 5-hydroxytryptamine was 5 mg/ml (normal 0.1-0.16 mg/ml) pre-dialysis and was undetectable post-dialysis.

Alcohols

Intoxication with **ethanol** and **methanol** represents the almost ideal model for the use of dialysis in drug poisoning. The clearance of both is high and in the case of methanol, there is considerable leverage by virtue of preventing a conversion to its toxic metabolites, formaldehyde and formic acid. Since both ethanol and methanol are converted by the same enzyme for which there is substrate competition, the ideal treatment which has emerged for severe methanol poisoning is the administration of ethanol which slows the metabolic conversion of methanol and the institution of dialysis to remove both simultaneously. We originally demonstrated in our laboratory[121] both the chemical and clinical kinetics of ethanol and methanol intoxication in dogs. The clearance rises directly with blood flow in the artificial kidney and clearances upwards of 200 ml/minute are achievable clinically.

Dialysis is indicated for methanol intoxication to relieve coma and prevent blindness.[121-124] Hemodialysis is more effective than peritoneal dialysis, but the latter can be enhanced with THAM.[125] *In vivo* clearances by hemodialysis are about 100 ml/minute. Dialysate recovery may equal 50 percent of an ingested dose, representing a 70 percent reduction in the fat-immiscible pool. Ethanol should be administered to reach a concentration of 100 mg % to delay methanol metabolism. A definite ingestion history, a blood level above 100 mg %, severe acidosis or visual impairment should be indications for dialysis.

Setter, *et al.*[126] measured an *in vivo* methanol dialysance of 125 ml/minute using the Kiil dialyzer. With the twin-coil artificial kidney, dialysance approached 200 ml/minute. Clearance using peritoneal dialysis was 24 ml/minute at high flow rates and increased to 31 ml/minute with hypertonic dialysate, exceeding urea clearance with each technique. Peritoneal dialysis removed three times as much methanol as renal excretion and hemodialysis increased removal by a factor of 25. The half-life of methanol in the dog treated with both hemodialysis and peritoneal dialysis was two to three hours. With peritoneal dialysis alone it was seven to eight hours, whereas spontaneously the value is 70 hours. Accidental ingestion of methanol in a 10-week-old child with a blood methanol level of 213 mg % and severe acidosis was successfully treated by peritoneal dialysis.[127] Vision was later demonstrated to be normal. Four adults were treated by peritoneal dialysis during a methanol epidemic in Kentucky.[128] The blood levels ranged from 216 to 372 mg %. Three survived. Seven with blood methanol concentrations of 30 to 267 mg % survived with conservative therapy alone and seven others died.

Peritoneal dialysis has been successfully used for the treatment of methanol poisoning in a 10-week-old infant girl, nine hours after ingestion. The blood level was 213 mg %, fell to 120 mg % in 24 hours and 20 mg % in 48 hours. She was given bicarbonate during dialysis and the venous *p*H rose from 7.2 to 7.45. She made a complete recovery without optic atrophy or apparent visual loss.[129,130] Hemodialysis has been used in group methanol poisonings, and artificial kidney centers should be considered a disaster resource.[131]

Hemodialysis has been combined with exchange transfusion in an adult.[132] Dialysis has the additional advantage of correcting the severe acidosis that may be seen in acute chronic methanol poisoning. It also rectifies the hyponatremia, hypokalemia, hypomagnesemia, hypocalcemia and other electrolyte effects, as well as the osmolality defects seen in alcoholic intoxication.[133] Closs and Solberg[134] dialyzed a 63-year-old man 18 hours after drinking suspected methanol. The blood *p*H was 6.95 and CO_2 was 5.7 mM/L. He had increased formaldehyde in the urine and recovered without deficit. Additional dialysis experience with methanol has been reported by Cowen.[135] Dialysis eliminates hangover and in recent studies at the Baltimore City Hospital the theoretically predicted induction of delirium tremens from alcohol removal did not occur. Patients with delirium tremens at the start of dialysis recovered before the end of treatment. Those who did not have delirium tremens failed to develop this syndrome. Chronic alcoholics who previously required four to six days of hospitalization are out of the hospital in 24 hours, remaining sober for an uncharacteristic length of time. Cost of dialysis in the treatment of chronic alcoholism was less than the equivalent cost of hospitalization.

Ethylene glycol intoxication can also be improved by dialysis, preferably with the artificial kidney.[136-138] The results surpass those of alkali therapy alone and include electroencephalographic improvement.

Peritoneal dialysis corrected the metabolic acidosis of ethylene glycol poisoning when used for the therapy of two children.[139]

Freireich, *et al.*[140] treated by hemodialysis a patient who was intoxicated after ingestion of one liter of isopropyl alcohol. Clinical improvement occurred. The blood **isopropanol** level decreased spontaneously in seven hours from 0.346 to 0.212 percent as its metabolite, acetone, increased from 0.117 to 0.188 percent. With hemodialysis the levels decreased from 0.212 to 0.06 percent and 0.188 to 0.150 percent in three hours. A low concentration of each of these volatile compounds was measured in the dialysate and in urine.

King, *et al.*[141] dialyzed a 28-year-old man who ingested 1 L of isopropanol as rubbing alcohol. Dialysis was instituted under ideal circumstances, 4.5 hours after ingestion. The very high blood level of 440 mg % declined to 310 after 1.5 hours, 199 after 3 hours and 100 mg % after 5 hours of dialysis. The initial high acetone level (40 mg %), attesting to the early referral, rose to 100 mg % during dialysis. Although manifesting hypothermia, deep coma, areflexia and hypotension, all potentially fatal complications,[142] the patient became normotensive and responsive after five hours of hemodialysis.

Analgesics

Acetylsalicylic acid (aspirin) is still the leading cause of accidental poisoning in children and a major cause of poisoning deaths in both young and old. Like methanol, there are extremely important side advantages to dialytic therapy. In the early stages of clinical salicylism, there is a respiratory alkalosis, and in the later stage, a severe metabolic acidosis, both of which conditions can be life-threatening and are correctable by dialysis. There are also preventive aspects. Some deaths in severe salicylate intoxication are due to hepatic necrosis or brain destruction from loss of temperature control. Such secondary pathology is preventable by early removal of the salicylate. Acetylsalicylate in high concentrations is a serious nephrotoxin, so that long-term kidney damage may also be prevented by early dialysis. Lawson, *et al.*,[143] drawing on an unusual clinical experience involving 315 patients with salicylate poisoning, concluded that (a) peak plasma salicylate level is the best measure of severity; (b) treatment with oral fluids is inadequate; (c) management of dehydration is essential; and (d) plasma salicylate levels exceeding 60 mg/100 ml should be treated with forced diuresis regardless of symptoms. Our experience closely agrees with theirs, except that we would consider dialysis with a known absorption of more than 0.5 Gm/Kg, or with blood levels above 70-80 mg %. Salicylate absorption may be inhibited in large ingestions by the use of various adsorbents in the GI tract, including cholestyramine resin[144] and activated charcoal. In another study, rats were treated with activated charcoal 30 minutes after sodium salicylate administration. Concentration in the control group ranged from 95-124 mg %. In treated rats, decreases from the control group values averaged 66 percent at 60 minutes, 62 percent at 90 minutes and 62 percent at 120 minutes, thus effectively blocking the progressive rise in serum concentration which occurred in the control group. This method of therapy has also been recommended by Holt and Holtz.[145] Perfusion through a charcoal column also clears salicylate rapidly.[146] Alkaline diuresis has been widely recommended for salicylism. Lawson, *et al.*[113] used a forced cocktail diuresis consisting of 0.5 L of saline (0.9%), 1 L of 5% levulose and 0.5 L of 1.2% sodium bicarbonate with 3 Gm of potassium chloride added. The mixture is administered at the rate of 2 L/hour for three hours. Acetazolamide (Diamox) and sodium bicarbonate have also been used to produce an alkaline bicarbonate Gastric dialysis has also been suggested for both salicylism and aminopyrine and other poisonings.[148]

The dramatic results obtained by dialysis in our original work on salicylism[149] convinced us that dialysis, when available, cannot only prevent mortality but alter morbidity and also at the same time handle most of the electrolyte abnormalities of salicylism. Since that original presentation, hundreds of patients with salicylism have undergone dialysis.[150-156] Patients have survived the ingestion of as much as 210 Gm of salicylate and blood levels in excess of 150 mg %, The dialysance in the average twin coil can be in excess of 100 ml/minute,[157,158] and more than 10 Gm has been removed by hemodialysis. Hemodialysis removes salicylate three to five times faster than diuresis[151] and four times faster than peritoneal dialysis or exchange transfusion.[159] Peritoneal dialysis is also effective for both **acetylsalicylate** and **methylsalicylate**[85,150,153,160,161] and may be enhanced by the addition of albumin or THAM.[14,62,163]

Peritoneal dialysis effected a lowering of the blood salicylate level from 118 to 55 mg % within 24 hours and caused clinical improvement of a child who ingested methyl salicylate.[161] Another child, aged 7 months, recovered after peritoneal dialysis was used for methyl salicylate poisoning with a blood level of 89 mg %.[164]

Although infrequent, **propoxyphene** (Darvon) poisoning may be quite severe. Nalorphine is a specific antidote. Despite adequate diffusion through dialysis membranes, the clinical response is only fair due to the small quantity in circulating blood.[39,165]

Gary, *et al.*[166] studied a patient who ingested 32 mg/Kg of propoxyphene. Hemodialysis lowered the serum level from 3.0 to 0.3 μg/ml in 10 hours. After a secondary increase in the serum propoxyphene level, another hemodialysis decreased the level from 1.2 to 0.6 μg/ml in six hours. Hemodialysis removed 124 mg which equalled 7 percent of the ingested dose. Peritoneal dialysis removed 16 mg in 70 hours and forced diuresis removed 96 mg, of which 40 percent was the dinitrophenol metabolite. Gastric lavage removed 87 mg, more than half of which was recovered in the first few hours. The patient had severe hypoxia when first seen and clinical improvement was minimal. *In vivo* and *in vitro,* the dialysance exceeded 100 ml/minute. It was also demonstrated that 100 Gm of charcoal could absorb 1.8 Gm of propoxyphene. The low blood level in the absence of impaired gastrointestinal absorption was interpreted as sequestration of the drug in tissue and was considered the major impediment to its removal by dialysis. Corby and Decker[167] demonstrated the *in vitro* adsorption of 670 mg of propoxyphene by activated charcoal and recommend its use orally as an adjunct to the therapy of propoxyphene poisoning.

Clinical improvement was attributed to hemodialysis in a patient with acute intoxication due to **acetophenetidin** (phenacetin).[168]

Pimstone and Uys[169] reported a fatal case of **paracetamol** poisoning that was treated by exchange transfusion. They suggested the use of hemodialysis. Peritoneal dialysis was used for one paracetamol intoxicated patient who survived but the peritoneal clearance of this non-salicylate analgesic was less than 3 ml/minute and only 10.2 mg was removed in six hours suggesting that the dialysis was of very limited benefit.[170]

Antibiotics

Dialysis has a place in antibiotic management and can be used for (1) the removal of accidental or deliberate overdoses; (2) removal of toxic materials, *e.g.*, nephrotoxins; (3) removal of the molecule from patients exhibiting serious allergic reaction or side effects (*e.g.*, deafness); and (4) for the administration of antibiotics since significant amounts of most important drugs in this class diffuse through the peritoneum.

Ototoxicity due to **streptomycin** accumulation has been corrected by dialysis, blood levels significantly lowered and streptomycin was demonstrated in dialysate.[171] A 24 percent arteriovenous difference across the dialyzer was reported.[172] Persistence of **kanamycin** in the blood because of renal failure may cause ototoxicity and nephrotoxicity.[173] Passive flow hemodialysis reduces kanamycin levels by about 50 percent.[174] Peritoneal clearance exceeds 5 ml/minute and decreases the prolonged biologic half-life significantly, but not to normal.[175] Retention of **neomycin** because of renal failure also may cause ototoxicity and nephrotoxicity. The blood level has been lowered from 130 to 50 μg/ml and absorption from the peritoneum has been demonstrated.[39,100]

Vancomycin, a penicillinase-resistant antibiotic, is distributed in total body water and after distribution, the serum disappearance rate is dependent upon renal excretion. Lindholm and Murray[176] found measurable serum concentrations after 10-14 days from a single 1 Gm I.V. dose in six oliguric patients. Since 10 percent is protein bound, vancomycin is only slowly dialyzable. Twenty percent of the initial plasma concentration is dialyzed for 24 hours. In batch dialyzer studies, 12 hours of dialysis reduced the serum vancomycin by 10 percent, while serum urea, a molecule with a similar distribution space, was reduced by 60 percent.

Goodwin, Thompson and Friedman[177] measured a mean extraction ratio for streptomycin through the Kiil dialyzer of 17 percent and *in vivo* dialysance of 16.4 ml/minute, and a 66 percent reduction in blood levels in 12 hours. Precht and Briedigkeit[178] measured a biologic half-life of 1.0 hour for streptomycin and 1.9 hour for kanamycin during hemodialysis and considered both drugs readily dialyzable.

Renal failure causes persistence of **penicillin** in the blood. Neuromuscular toxicity or hypersensitivity reactions may be indications for hemodialysis which has been shown to reduce elevated blood penicillin levels. The synthetic penicillins, **oxacillin** and, in particular, **methicillin** are also retained in patients with renal failure.[179] The slow removal by dialysis does not significantly affect blood levels of these drugs.[180] **Ampicillin** is retained in patients with renal failure and blood levels are not substantially affected by peritoneal dialysis, but measurably decrease with hemodialysis.[180,181] Absorption of the synthetic penicillins occurs across the peritoneum.[182]

Dicloxacillin does not accumulate significantly in renal failure and is not removed by hemodialysis.[183,184]

The serum half-life of **carbenicillin** is significantly prolonged by renal failure to 12.5 hours but is reduced by hemodialysis or peritoneal dialysis.[185] A peritoneal clearance of 6.8 ml/minute has peen measured.

Ampicillin is considered easily dialyzable with a biologic half-life of 0.6 hour during hemodialysis whereas oxacillin which is more slowly dialyzed has a half-life of 4.6 hours.[178]

Renal failure causes retention of **cephalothin** which is also absorbed from the peritoneum and **cephaloridine** which has been shown to be dialyzable.[173] Cephalothin is removed slowly by hemodialysis although it is significantly absorbed from the peritoneum.[46]

Dialysis removes **sulfonamides**, lowering blood levels.[186] Toxic hemolytic anemia and nephrotoxicity have been improved by dialysis.

An arteriovenous difference across the dialyzer has been measured for **chloramphenicol.**[187] Peritoneal dialysis does not cause significant removal of chloramphenicol, but it is absorbed from the peritoneum.[175] **Tetracycline** dialysance *in vivo* using the Kiil dialyzer exceeds 20 ml/minute.[158] Peritoneal clearance approximates 5 ml/minute which does not cause significant removal of the drug, although absorption can be demonstrated.[175,188] During hemodialysis the biologic half-life of chloramphenicol is 0.8 hour and oxytetracycline is 2.4 hours.[178] Both are considered dialyzable drugs.

Retention of **nitrofurantoin** in the blood of anuric patients may lead to peripheral neuropathy and an organic acidosis. Nitrofurantoin dialysance equals 70 ml/minute at a blood flow rate of 200 ml/minute.[189]

Polymyxin B and **colistin** are retained in the blood of patients with renal failure.[190] The peritoneal clearance is about 10 ml/minute,[175] but dialysis does not significantly affect blood levels.[174,190] Swick[191] successfully dialyzed a 9-year-old boy who received 20 mg/Kg/day of colistin for a total dose of 1200 mg (1-2 mg/Kg/day is usually well tolerated; 4-5 mg/Kg/day produces nephrotoxity in 30-50 percent of adults). Serum colistin level was 16 μg/ml (1-3 = therapeutic range). After 21 exchanges (1500 ml each) the serum level dropped to 8.0 μg/ml and after 36 exchanges it was 4.0 μg/ml. The patient was anuric for 11+ days and hyposthenuric for 3+ weeks. Similar results were reported by Goodwin and Friedman.[192] The peritoneal clearance exceeds 5 ml/minute, however, averaging 30 percent of the urea clearance.[192] The dialysate/plasma ratio averaged 0.16. Despite a peritoneal clearance of 9.8 ml/minute peritoneal dialysis did not significantly affect blood levels of colistin.[195] Hemodialysis produced an increase in the rate of disappearance of colistin from plasma in the patients studied by Curtis and Eastwood,[195] but Precht and Briedigkeit[178] who measured a biologic half-life of 5.0 hours considered colistin hardly dialyzable.

The serum half-life of **lincomycin** is about doubled by renal failure and this drug is not significantly removed by dialysis.[196] Unpublished studies indicate a peritoneal clearance of 13 and 15 ml/minute for lincomycin.[46]

Isoniazid intoxication improves with dialysis, which reduces blood levels twice as fast as the spontaneous decline.[151,182,197,198] The dialysance of 49 ml/min has been sufficient to decrease blood levels from 14 to 2 mg %. Peritoneal dialysis has effected a decrease in blood levels from 13 to 4 mg % in 24 hours.[199] Using the 2-layer Kiil dialyzer isoniazid blood levels are reduced by 38 percent in 12 hours.[177] The extraction ratio is 18.5 percent and the dialysance 24 ml/minute.

Semicoma due to **cycloserine** intoxication was treated by peritoneal dialysis which lowered the blood level from 91 to 25 μg/ml and removed 520 mg, representing 17 percent of the ingested dose.[200]

Metals

Poisoning by metals remains a major industrial and environmental health hazard. Some metals such as sodium, potassium and magnesium could as readily be considered under the section on endogenous intoxication, since toxic levels often rise in the course of a disease process, such as the hypercalcemia of hyperparathyroidism. However, the extracorporeal behavior of these compounds has much in common. The widespread use of hemodialysis has in itself reawakened interest in both the physical chemistry and epidemiology of metal poisoning. Almost for the first time physicians have had to pay attention to the characteristics of the tap water in their various communities. The occurrence of several accidents and metabolic consequences of altered mineral content of water has focused our attention on the critical aspects of our water supply. Furthermore, the introduction of newer membrane materials has forced us to re-examine some of the unique properties of dialysis membranes which can adsorb, concentrate and perhaps even transport metals. In 1964 we demonstrated that trivalent iron will bind and concentrate on cellophane from an aqueous solution but is removed by blood or protein.[158] Later, we showed that artificial membranes can concentrate calcium from non-electrolyte and, to a lesser extent, from electrolyte solution. Fresh blood clears all bound calcium from membranes.[201] Maher, *et al.*[202] studied the adherence of 17 metals to cellophane and found the highest concentration ratios with silver, zinc, copper, lead and calcium. These metals can be readily removed from cellophane by carriers present in the whole blood. Some peculiarities of metal binding to membranes and to materials forming part of the dialyzer are important not only for potential administration of metals to chronic dialysis patients, but also for calculations of removal rates during *in vivo* and *in vitro* studies extending over short periods of time. They are particularly critical when applied to tracer materials. Metals shall be considered alphabetically in the remainder of this section.

Arsenic. We have treated one patient with arsenic poisoning, jaundice and a hepato-renal syndrome with recovery. Reductions in blood levels and recovery in dialysate have been reported. Peritoneal dialysis has been used in arsine poisoning.[203]

Calcium acute **hypercalcemia** may be treated with either hemodialysis or peritoneal dialysis. We have used chelating agents with peritoneal dialysis to reduce hypercalcemia in a patient with a parathyroid tumor. Distilled or standard concentrates of dialysates may not be used if they contain calcium. Tap water calcium may vary form 0.5 to over 15 mg % and the concentrations are prohibitive in some city water supplies, such as London, England. Distilled or deionized water or special water softeners may be used in these areas. Calcium dialysance may exceed 150 ml/minute.[221] Clinical use has met with variable results.[85,100,222,223]

Eisenberg and Gotch[224] measured a net removal of 150 mEq of calcium in hemodialysate in 8½ hours while forced diuresis removed 35-40 mEq. The serum calcium decreased from 8.8 to 5.95 mEq/L and the patient withstood parathyroid surgery shortly thereafter.

Symptomatic hypercalcemia and hypermagnesemia may be induced by hemodialysis using hard water.[225] The serum calcium may be as high as 9 mEq/L and the serum magnesium 6 mEq/L.

Copper. Since the original report of two fatal cases,[204] there have been a number of reports of acute copper intoxication marked by hemolysis, acidosis, methemoglobinemia, hypoglycemia, vomiting, upper gastric pain, diarrhea, headache and light headedness. These particular acute poisonings have been found related to the use of outdated deionizer cartridges, producing water with a low *p*H which picked up copper from a heat exchanger in the dialysate delivery system. Chronic accumulations may occur from copper plumbing and soft or acidic well water. Lyle[205] found copper concentrations of 175-400 μg/L in soft water. These can be reduced by the use of a water hardener.

Iron. Hemodialysis in combination with alkalinization and chelation has been used to treat acute experimental canine *iron* intoxication.[226] Dialysate recovery of iron was low, however. Dialysance of the Fe^{59} Cl_3-DTPA complex is 50 ml/minute, using the Kiil dialyzer *in vitro*. In experimentally intoxicated dogs, desferrioxamine promoted renal excretion that exceeded the removal by hemodialysis, provided renal function was normal.[227] A patient with ferrous sulfate poisoning improved with peritoneal dialysis where the dialysate concentration of iron increased with the addition of EDTA and the peritoneal clearance was about twice that of the kidneys.[228]

Hemosiderosis complicating chronic hemodialysis has been successfully treated by combined chelation with diethylenetriaminepentaacetic acid (DTPA) and hemodialysis.[229] The quantity of iron removed is directly related to the dose of DTPA. When 4.0 Gm was used, 35 mg was removed during clinical dialysis. Similar doses of chelate given to a patient with iron deficiency did not result in iron removal.

Movassaghi has recently compared the use of exchange transfusion and deferrioxamine in the treatment of acute iron poisoning in dogs.[230] Removal by exchange transfusion was 30 times greater.

Lead. Lead is an increasingly important environmental poison with serious toxic effects on the kidney, hemopoietic system and nervous system. Because of its intercellular concentration it cannot be removed directly. It may be chelated and the dialysance of lead versenate is 30+ ml/minute. Clinical results, however, have been poor.[231] Lead has been recovered in peritoneal dialysate.[100] Mehbod[232] combined the use of edetate calcium disodium and peritoneal dialysis for the therapy of lead intoxication. From four patients he removed 74 to 844 μg of lead per hour by using EDTA and peritoneal dialysis which was more than that removed by dialysis alone (36 to 184 μg/hour) and more than urinary lead after chelate therapy (6 to 35 μg/hour).

Lithium. Outbreaks of lithium poisoning occurred several years ago following its widespread use as a salt substitute (lithium chloride). Recently, the use of lithium carbonate as a psychopharmacologic agent has renewed interest in the subject. It has a very high dialysance and hemodialysis has been used in clinical lithium poisoning.[233] Amdisen dialyzed a 48-year-old man who had taken 1500-2400 mg of lithium carbonate for 10 years and then developed renal failure leading to acute lithium intoxication, with a serum lithium of 3 mEq/L. A 6.5 hour twin coil dialysis lowered serum lithium from 2.8 to 0.7 mEq/L, with a rebound to 1.4 mEq/L. Serum half-life on dialysis was 15 hours, post-dialysis 40-50 hours. Spinal fluid half-life on dialysis was 19 hours. After effects were minimal as previously reported.[234] Hawkins[235] reported a lithium poisoning which ended fatally despite dialysis.

Magnesium. A markedly elevated magnesium concentration above 5 mEq/L can be induced by hemodialysis using hard water or by the excessive ingestion of magnesium containing antacids. Hypermagnesemia is rarely symptomatic clinically, but magnesium is readily dialyzable, with a reported dialysance of 100 ml/minute or greater.[221]

Mercury. Mercury is highly protein bound and adheres to rubber and cellophane with a concentration ratio in excess of 2. It cannot be directly removed, but may be chelated with sulfhydryl groups such as cysteine or BAL. Dialysance of BAL mercury complex is 5 ml/minute.[236]

Potassium. Hyperkalemia is the most lethal of the uremic toxins. Poisoning is usually minimal, below 6.5 mEq/L, moderate between 6.5 and 8 mEq/L and severe above that level. The absolute toxicity is conditioned by both *p*H and associated sodium levels. Hyperkalemic symptoms, and particularly the electrocardiographic effects, may be transiently controlled by calcium gluconate, administration of glucose or glucose and insulin, sodium bicarbonate or hypertonic sodium infusions, cation exchange resins or by hemodialysis and peritoneal dialysis. Caution should be exercised in the dialysis of potassium in patients who are digitalized and who may experience acute digitalis intoxication in the course of potassium removal.

Sodium. Accidental salt poisoning with hypernatremia in excess of 200 mEq/L. has been improved by peritoneal dialysis with restoration of blood levels to normal,[105] and hyponatremia can also be easily corrected by dialysis. Sodium dialysance exceeds 200 ml/minute.

Strontium. Strontium in the form of radio-strontium, and also radio-calcium, has been removed from canine blood *in vivo* and *in vitro,* by hemodialysis and ion exchange resin perfusion.[238] The therapy has interesting potential in the treatment of radioactive fall-out or industrial poisoning associated with the atomic energy industry.

Halides

Dialysis removes **bromide** more rapidly than equilibrium of levels in body fluids occurs and clinical improvement may be dramatic.[150,151,239,240] Dialysance may exceed 200 ml/minute and clearance during hemodialysis approaches 100 ml/minute. Renal clearance, depending on the chloride load and the diuresis achieved, varies from less than 0.5 ml/minute to a maximum of about 14 ml/minute, which is comparable to peritoneal clearance.[240] The serum half-life of bromide is reduced from over 100 hours with no therapy to 5 to 16 hours with diuresis, and to slightly more than one hour with hemodialysis.[240,241] Dialysis may be indicated with a blood level above 20 mEq/L, with intolerance to salt loading, inability to achieve a diuresis or renal failure.

Bromide psychosis may continue beyond the end of dialysis,[150] due to the fact that dialysis from blood is more rapid than the diffusion rate from cerebrospinal fluid and the transport of bromate out of brain tissue. There are a number of reports on the efficacy of an induced diuresis using the newer diuretics, furosemide (Lasix) and ethacrynic acid (Edecrin).[242,243]

Radioiodide has an *in vitro* dialysance as high as 55 ml/minute, but removal at low plasma concentrations is limited by protein binding.[244] Renal failure causes retention of organic **iodide** in the serum, but the iodide can be removed by dialysis.[245]

Fluoride is dialyzable *in vitro* from plasma, but its diffusion is impaired in the presence of other halides. Although clinical improvement has occurred with hemodialysis for fluoride poisoning, the course is usually too rapid to achieve clinical benefit.[85] Fluoride influx occurs during dialysis for chronic uremia from a dialysate concentration of 1.0 mg/L, which is six times the normal level in plasma water.[246]

A recent study by Taves, *et al.*[247] again demonstrated increasing levels of fluoride during hemodialysis. Fluoridated water has a concentration of 53 μM/L while the serum level equals 1.0 μM/L. The fluoride dialysance varied from 44 to 99 ml/minute.

Endogenous Intoxication

Next to uremia the most frequently encountered endogenous intoxication in the general hospital is hepatic coma, which may manifest itself clinically in classical signs of ammonia intoxication or with the pathognomonic pattern involving vasoconstriction, hypovolemia, oliguria and other features which have come to be known as the "hepatorenal syndrome." A significant proportion of such patients do, of course, become azotemic. The long held concept of hepatorenal syndrome as a functional disorder of the kidney, perhaps a transient phase on the way to tubular necrosis, has received great support with recent experience in the transplantation of kidneys from such patients. These kidneys, anuric in the donor, may produce urine within minutes after circulation is established in a uremic recipient without hepatic disease. This has led to a renewed interest in dialysis, exchange transfusion and cross circulation in the management of severe hepatic coma. Saunders, *et al.*[248] used the chimaerized baboon whose blood volume had been replaced with human blood and cross-circulated the baboon with a 29-year-old female in the terminal stages of hepatic coma. After one hour, spontaneous respiration was noted; after four hours the tidal volume was 500 to 600 ml and respiration thereafter normalized. Within 60 hours the patient showed marked clinical improvement and in 72 hours was lucid, oriented and fully conscious. Indications in this case were initial partial response during seven days of deep coma to six exchange blood transfusions with the subsequent development of brain stem dysfunction and extensor, decerebrate spasms. In a similar experience Freeman[248a] noted late hemodynamic changes in the kidney function of the baboon, again suggesting the functional nature of the hepatorenal syndrome, perhaps with a biochemical mediator such as a peptide. Improvement of the "flap" tremor and coma which has been assigned to ammonia intoxication in hepatic coma, has been reported following hemodialysis.[249-252] Keynes[251] reported 4/9 survivors with hemodialysis, 7/19 for exchange transfusion and 2/69 for heterologous liver perfusion. Pig liver perfusion produced neurologic improvement in four patients with hepatic failure.[253] Burnell, *et al.*[254] treated five patients with severe coma, three with cross-circulation, two by exchange transfusion. There was one recovery, but several showed significant clinical improvement. Blumberg and Rohner,[255] however, noted an absolute lack of clinical improvement during and after exchange transfusion in two cases of hepatic dystrophy due to acute hepatitis. **Ammonia** dialysance varies from 50-80 ml/minute[256] and may be reduced by resin column perfusion.[257,258]

Central nervous system changes in patients with a severe burn have been assigned to a protein breakdown product and the prognosis in severe burns has been related to the undetermined nitrogen fraction in burn serum. Dialysis was included in a recent study of burn toxins.[259]

Hyperuricemia complicating leukemia and lymphoma and their treatment can be corrected by dialysis.[260,261] The concurrent use of forced diuresis and allopurinol aid in the restoration of blood **uric acid** levels to normal.[261,262] In chronic tophaceous gout repeated dialysis has removed several grams of uric acid, reduced the miscible pool of urate, improved renal function and restored responsiveness to uricosuric drugs.[263] The use of allopurinol improves control of hyperuricemia in patients with chronic renal failure undergoing maintenance dialysis.[264] Parotid fluid uric acid may also be lowered by hemodialysis.[265]

A patient with hyperuricemia complicating leukemia underwent hemodialysis twice after unsuccessful peritoneal dialysis.[266] The serum uric acid was reduced from 87 to 29 mg % and from 46 to 19 mg % by the two hemodialyses, with removal of 17.9 and 5.7 Gm of uric acid. The latter result followed initiation of allopurinol therapy. Dialysis was followed by diuresis and restoration of normal renal function. Another patient with hyperuricemia complicating leukemia who failed to diurese after mannitol and cystoscopy with alkali lavage underwent peritoneal dialysis.[267] Due to the high catabolic rate following chemotherapy the rising blood urea was only maintained constant by dialysis, whereas the serum uric acid, the synthesis of which was blocked because of allopurinol therapy decreased sharply and diuresis ensued.

Rae and Hopper[268] using peritoneal dialysis induced negative fluid balance of 6.7 to 22.6 L over the course of 41.5 to 114.0 hours in six patients with refractory edema with a resultant weight loss of 4.6 to 24.6 Kg. Three became responsive to thiazide diuretics after dialysis.

Nathan[269] treated four patients with severe hydrops fetalis by peritoneal dialysis. Net fluid loss of 110 to 640 ml was achieved by 9 to 34 hours of dialysis causing clinical improvement. Parkin and Walker[270] showed that in hemolytic disease of the newborn, the mortality is greater in those with edema but in Rh isoimmunization irreparable tissue damage has often occurred before birth and in hydropic infants the results are likely to be disappointing. Two of three edematous infants they treated by peritoneal dialysis died despite the procedure.

A reduction in ascites, weight loss, negative sodium and water balance and increased plasma volume has been achieved in a patient by pumping ascitic fluid through an ultrafiltration dialyzer and reinfusing it into the patient.[271]

Both direct and indirect serum **bilirubin** may decrease during hemodialysis, and a slow rate of removal has been documented.[272] Albumin added to the dialysate enhances removal of bilirubin during peritoneal dialysis.[273] Clearance by this technique increases from 0.5 ml/minute for both bilirubin and its conjugate to about 1.0 ml/minute.[274] Dialysances during hemodialysis are 6.4 and 9.5 ml/minute. Exchange transfusion remains the procedure of choice for neonatal icterus.

Lactic acidosis can be improved by hemodialysis or peritoneal dialysis.[100,275,276] The use of THAM may improve the acidosis. Plasma lactate levels have been lowered from 91 to 54 mg %, pyruvate concentration from 4.8 to 3.0 mg % and blood *p*H increased to normal from levels as low as 6.96. By contrast, metabolic alkalosis improves slowly with dialysis.[277]

Jurgesen[278] treated by peritoneal dialysis using added sodium bicarbonate, a patient with lactic acidosis. Coma, hypotension and oliguria cleared as the *p*H was corrected by dialysis. Another report[279] documents correction of severe metabolic acidosis by peritoneal dialysis in cyanotic babies.

Hemodialysis has been used for the therapy of **schizophrenia** and of **myasthenia gravis** with temporary improvement.[280]

Clinical improvement albeit temporary has also been documented in acute **porphyria** treated by dialysis.[281] *Serotonin* was not measurable in the hemodialysate from a patient with metastatic carcinoid tumor.[85] Despite removal of **cystine** by repeated hemodialysis, tissue accumulation of cystine was not affected in a patient with cystinosis.[282] Improved survival of dogs with endotoxic shock treated by hemodialysis has suggested the presence of a dialyzable vasoactive substance in this syndrome.[283]

Peritoneal dialysis has effected core rewarming in a case of accidental profound hypothermia.[45] Body temperature was increased from 70°F to 97°F in six hours coincident with clinical improvement.

There has been considerable recent activity in the use of hemodialysis in porphyria.[284] Reese, *et al.*[285] dialyzed three patients with severe neurological complications. Dramatic return of a normal mental state was noted in one. The blood urea was 132 mg/100 ml and fell to 42. The uroporphyrin strikingly increased to 860 μg/L (normal 0-40/24 hours) and fell to normal after hemodialysis. Urinary coproporphyrin which was normal before dialysis increased to nearly 800 μg/L three weeks after hemodialysis but the precursors delta aminolevulinic acid were increased more than prophobilinogen and after dialysis both returned to normal.

Last, *et al.*[286] reported on a 22-year-old woman who was able to move a paralyzed ankle four days after hemodialysis but was unaffected in the remaining paralysis of limb and respiratory muscles.

Pringle[287]reported that complete paralysis was unaffected. Eales, *et al.*[288] reported a slight improvement in limb weakness from hemodialysis in a uremic man with acute porphyria variegata. Reese calculated a total removal in 300 L of dialysate of 3.6 mg of prophobilinogen and 11.4 mg of delta aminolevulinic acid. The mechanism of clinical improvement is thus uncertain.

In **hyperosmolar coma** neurologic deficits usually follow hypotension, polyuria (converting to oliguria), stupor and convulsions.[289] The situation occurs predominantly in diabetic patients with extreme hyperglycemia and little or no acidosis and ketosis. The syndrome is often preceded by severe infections, extensive burns or problems involving the pancreas as pancreatitis and carcinoma. Hypernatremia, hyperkalemia and azotemia are usual but variable. Death has ensued in more than half the patients. Rapid improvement may be affected by dialysis plus insulin administration. Most often seen in the diabetic due to glucose, hyperosmolar coma may also be seen from hypernatremia as in childhood diarrhea when oral electrolyte repletion has been used or when errors have been made in infant formula preparation. Mannitol retention has been noted during the diuretic treatment of poisonings.[290]

Tritium dialysance approaches 200 ml/minute,[291] but net water flux is less than 15 ml/minute.[189,292] Ultrafiltration dialysis has been particularly useful in the therapy of **water intoxication** and of intractable heart failure.[293,294] The osmotic attraction of water during peritoneal dialysis can also be of benefit.[94,95] Fluid loss may exceed 7 L, reducing venous pressure and circulation time and restoring responsiveness to diuretics.[295] Fluid loss of 320 ml/hour has been achieved by hemodialysis and 250 ml/hour by peritoneal dialysis.

Miscellaneous Exogenous Poisons and Drugs

Thiocyanate intoxication with blood levels above 20 mg % can be rapidly corrected with hemodialysis which has been reported to remove several grams of the drug. Thiocyanate dialysance approaches 200 ml/minute, while the renal clearance is 2.2 ml/minute.[296,297]

Hemodialysis has been used for **aniline** poisoning and caused clinical improvement, reduction in the blood level from 2.5 to 1.7 mg % and removal of 1300 mg.[182] Clinical improvement has also followed combined exchange transfusion and peritoneal dialysis.[298]

Sodium chlorate poisoning produces profound effects on erythrocyte metabolism[299] with shock, cyanosis, methemoglobinuria and anuria. Varying combinations of hemodialysis, peritoneal dialysis and exchange transfusions have been used in poisoning with **sodium chlorate**[300,301] and **potassium chlorate.**[302] The toxicology of ammonium perchlorate has also been studied.[303]

Hemodialysis and peritoneal dialysis, used to treat a patient with **eucalyptus oil** poisoning, caused clinical improvement, a decline in blood levels from 7.4 μ L % and dialysate recoveries of 7.4 and 0.45 ml by the two procedures.[304]

Several patients with **boric acid** poisoning have been treated by peritoneal dialysis.[85,100,305,306] Blood levels are usually reduced by dialysis to about 65 percent of control values. A dialysate/plasma ratio of 0.75 was reported and dialysate recovery of 3 Gm has been measured. Recently, peritoneal dialysis was successful in treating acute boric acid poisoning in an infant poisoned by skin absorption.[307]

Poisoning with **chromates** is an industrial hazard.[308] Ingestion in children is rare but has occurred from chemistry sets. G.I. symptoms and shock are followed by renal tubular necrosis, hepatic toxicity and CNS damage. Lavage, BAL and dialysis are indicated; 0.5-1.0 Gm may be a lethal dose; 60 percent is excreted in urine within 8 hours. Fritz, *et al.*[309] dialyzed a man poisoned with potassium dichromate and lowered the serum level from 190 to 170 μg %. *In vitro* dialysance was 40 ml/minute, 30 percent of urea. Fristedt[310] had a survival after BAL and three dialyses, lowering the level from 195 to 135 μg %. Kaufman, *et al.*[311] used peritoneal dialysis in a 14-year-old boy ingesting 1.5 Gm of **potassium dichromate.** In 84 hours (126 L) the serum chromium level was lowered from 590 to 90 mg %. The clearance rates were 22.4 mg/24 hours. Hemodialysis has been used in a case of acute renal insufficiency caused by **chromic anhydride** intoxication.[312]

Tritiated **digoxin** is excreted unchanged by the kidney.[313,314] Prolongation of blood levels and reduced excretion have been noted in renal failure[315,316] and in anephric transplantation subjects.[317] There is only 6.4 percent reduction of excretion in unilateral nephrectomy.[318] Digoxin dosage can be related mathematically to the creatinine clearance, as the relationship of digoxin compared to creatinine clearance is near unity.[318] Up to 20 percent of digitalized patients in the hospital suffer from digitalis toxicity. Dialysance of digoxin is usually less than 20 ml/minute. Ackerman, *et al.*[319] reported a peritoneal clearance of 8 ml/minute removing 2 percent of an administered dose and a hemodialysance of 10 ml/minute with 3 percent removal. Removal from an *in vitro* reservoir is much greater, suggesting that binding of digoxin to myocardium, diaphragm and other muscles with a resulting small proportion in the circulating plasma may be the limiting factor in the dialysis of digitalis. Since both the toxic and inotropic action of digitalis are related to potassium concentrations, rapid removal of potassium in a digitalized patient may produce signs of digitalis intoxication, and rapid repletion of potassium by dialysis may reverse an arrhythmia produced by digitalis in the hypokalemic patient.

A dialysance of 75 ml/minute has been measured for **sodium citrate** suggesting its therapeutic use.[272]

A patient who was moribund due to **atropine** poisoning did not respond to hemodialysis.[85]

A patient who ingested 3.8 Gm of **quinine sulfate** was treated by peritoneal dialysis which was associated with a decrease in the blood level from 9.2 to 5.3 mg/L.[320] After 16 hours the dialysate contained 415 mg while 1.22 Gm was recovered from the urine. The peritoneal clearance of quinine is 1 to 8 ml/minute, limited removal being attributed to 70 percent protein binding.[321] *In vitro* removal by the twin-coil hemodialyzer is superior to that achieved by peritoneal dialysis. Renal excretion is increased by mannitol. McKenzie, Mathew and Bailie[322] reported two patients with quinine intoxication occurring after ingestions of 6 and 12 Gm, respectively, who were treated by peritoneal dialysis and recovered. Approximately 640 mg was removed by dialysis in 24 hours from the first and peritoneal clearances were in the range of 6 to 13 ml/minute in the second patient. The toxicology has recently been reviewed.[323]

Thomas[324] used peritoneal dialysis in treating a 62-year-old woman who drank 150 ml **cresol** (Lysol). The dialysate contained 10 mg of free phenol in the first exchange, but only "total phenols" subsequently, while the urine contained 26 times the dialysis yield. Dialysis did prevent the rise in potassium which kills some patients early in the course of cresol poisoning.

The blood level of **dinitro-ortho-cresol** was reported to decline more rapidly from a concentration of 52 mg % when hemodialysis was used than occurs spontaneously.[325]

A **non-halogenated aromatic hydrocarbon** was removed by dialysis from a patient who ingested an unknown solvent.[85] Clinical improvement suggested removal by dialysis of **carbon tetrachloride** from two other patients.[100,326] Gastric lavage with olive oil has also been successfully used to prevent hepatic and renal failure following carbon tetrachloride ingestion.[46] Proudfoot and MacDonald[327] were able to recover only 0.1 mg/100 ml of carbon tetrachloride in peritoneal dialysate whereas urinary and gastric aspirate concentrations were 0.4 and 1.2 mg/100 ml, respectively. It seemed unlikely that the minimal recovery of carbon tetrachloride by peritoneal dialysis reduced the ultimate renal and hepatic damage.

Peritoneal dialysis has been used both in animals and humans in the treatment of **trichlorethylene** poisoning.[328] Clinical improvement following dialysis for trichlorethylene poisoning suggests its removal.[46]

Ginn, *et al.*[329] treated by hemodialysis with a lipid dialysate, a patient who had recurrent seizures following the accidental ingestion of 12 Gm of **camphor.** Clinical improvement occurred within three hours and after 4½ hours 6.6 Gm of camphor was recovered in the lipid.

Transperitoneal diffusion of **THAM** is slow,[14] suggesting that dialysis would not remove this buffer rapidly.

Dialysis can prevent a potentially lethal course in **mushroom** poisoning. It has been noted to remove **Amanita phalloides** toxin.[330] We have recently had an experience dialyzing a young man who ingested a raw fungus mistakenly identified as *Amanita phalloides.* The patient had shock, cyanosis and bradycardia which were very quickly reversed by dialysis. Later correct identification proved the fungus to be of a type producing severe muscarine poisoning.

Hemodialysis was used during the management of a snakebite from *Crotalus rubor rubor* (red diamond rattlesnake).[331]

Laboratory dialysis has recently been used in the isolation of a chromatographically pure toxin of *Clostridium botulinum Type B*[332] and in the isolation of toxic subunits from two murine-toxic proteins from *Pasturella pestis.*[333]

An infant with **ergotamine** poisoning improved with forced diuresis and peritoneal dialysis, which removed 90 μg, representing about 1 percent of the ingested dose.[334]

The cancer chemotherapeutic drugs, **cyclophosphamide, 5-fluorouracil** and **methotrexate,** are removed by hemodialysis.[39,335] Dialysance of methotrexate in a 2 M Klung dialyzer is 64 ml/minute. Methotrexate dialysance exceeds the renal clearance.[46] By employing dialysis of venous blood returning from a site selectively perfused with methotrexate, the blood level can be maintained lower than that of controls.

Rogers[336] demonstrated that by dialysis against **arginase,** serum arginine levels can be drastically reduced to levels well below those reached by standard dialysis and suggested the use of dialysis in the therapy of certain malignancies. Some forms of leukemia are arginine dependent. Galletti[337] is studying the use of cascade dialysis in the management of these conditions.

The behavior of seven plasma enzymes during hemodialysis of four hours' duration in 40 uremic and three intoxicated patients was studied by Kokot, *et al.*[338] Some enzyme activities increase slightly (pyruvic aminotransferase and γ-glutamyl transpeptidase) or significantly (alkaline phosphatase) and others decrease (adenosine deaminase) or do not change at all (aspartic aminotransferase, amylase and acid phosphatase). The mechanism for the changes has not been determined.

Extrarenal hemodialysis has been used in **carbon monoxide** poisoning.[339] The use of diuresis has been reported in acute **diquat** poisoning. Diquat is a widely used contact herbicide which can produce cataracts, delayed wound healing, CNS symptoms and delayed death by an unknown mechanism in rats.[340] Dialysis has been used in a pre-school child poisoned with **orphenadrine**[341] by Stoddart, *et al.* The 2-year-old boy was estimated to have taken 28 tablets or more than 100 mg/Kg. Orphenadrine (Disipal) is used in Parkinsonism and psychiatric disorders, and has a CNS atropine-like action and a weak peripheral sympatholytic action. Fifty percent of ingested dose was found in urine. No drug was identified in the dialysate after seven hours of dialysis, and no obvious clinical improvement resulted.

Acknowledgment

The author acknowledges his gratitude to the many physicians who kindly supplied unpublished information concerning the dialysis of poisons. I wish to thank the National Library of Medicine personnel for their assistance in obtaining complete interval bibliographies through the MEDLARS service.

References

1. Burston, G. R.: Severe self-poisoning in Sunderland, *Brit. Med. J. 1*:679, 1969.
2. Abel, J. I., Rountree, L. G. and Turner, B. B.: On removal of diffusible substances from circulating blood of living animals by dialysis, *J. Pharmacol. Exptl. Therap. 5*:275, 1913.
3. Schreiner, G. E.: The role of hemodialysis (artificial kidney) in acute poisoning, *Arch. Internal Med. 102*:896, 1958.
4. Renkin, E. M.: The relation between dialysance, membrane area, permeability and blood flow in the artificial kidney, *Trans. Am. Soc. Artificial Internal Organs* 2:102, 1956.
5. Maher, John F. and Schreiner, George, E.: The dialysis of poisons and drugs, *Trans. Am. Soc. Artificial Internal Organs 14*:440, 1968.
6. Maher, John F. and Schreiner, George, E.: Current status of dialysis of poisons and drugs. *Trans. Am. Soc. Artificial Internal Organs 15*:461, 1969.
7. Yatzidis, H., Oreopoulos, D., Triantaphyllidis, D., Voudiclari, S., Tsaparas, N., Gavras, C. and Stravroulaki, A.: Treatment of severe barbiturate poisoning, *Lancet* 2:216, 1965.
8. Nealon, Jr., T. F., Sugerman, H., Shea, W. and Fleegler, E.: An extracorporeal device to treat barbiturate poisoning. Use of anion-exchange resins in dogs, *J. Am. Med. Assoc. 197*:118, 1966.
9. Cirksena, W. J., Bastian, R. C., Malloy, J. P. and Barry, K. G.: Use of mannitol in exogenous and endogenous intoxications. *New Engl. J. Med. 270*:161, 1964.
10. Lassen, N. A.: Treatment of severe acute barbiturate poisoning by forced diuresis and alkalinization of the urine, *Lancet* 2:338, 1960.
11. Henderson, L. W.: Enhanced solute transfer using hypertonic peritoneal dialysate, *Clin. Res. 12*:470, 1964.
12. Hare, H. G., Valtin, H. and Gosselin, R. E.: Effect of drugs on peritoneal dialysis in the dog, *J. Pharmacol. Exptl. Therap. 145*:122, 1964.
13. Berman, L. B. and Vogelsang, P.: Removal rates for barbiturates using two types of peritoneal dialysis, *New Engl. J. Med. 270*:77, 1964.
14. Nahas, G. G., Giroux, J. J., Gjessing, J., Verosky, M. and Mark, L. C.: The use of THAM in peritoneal dialysis, *Trans. Am. Soc. Artificial Internal Organs 10*:345, 1964.
15. Shinaberger, J. H., Shear, L., Clayton, L. E., Barry, K. G., Knowlton, M. and Goldbaum, L. R.: Dialysis for intoxication with lipid soluble drugs: enhancement of glutethimide extraction with lipid dialysate, *Trans. Am. Soc. Artificial Internal Organs 11*:173, 1965.
16. McCarthy, M. A.: Selected types of poisoning as causes of accidental death. United States, 1964, *U. S. Public Health Rep. 82*:1025, 1967.
17. Hadden, J., Johnson, K. and Smith, S.: Acute barbiturate intoxication. Concepts of management, *J. Am. Med. Assoc. 209*: 893, 1969.
18. Kennedy, A. C., Briggs, J. D. and Young, N.: Successful treatment of three cases of very severe barbiturate poisoning, *Lancet 1*:995, 1969.
19. Fine, R. N., Stiles, Q. and DePalma, J. R.: Hemodialysis in infants under one year of age for acute poisoning, *Am. J. Diseases Children 116*:657, 1968.
20. Setter, J. G., Maher, J. F. and Schreiner, G. E.: Barbiturate intoxication. Evaluation of therapy including dialysis in a large series selectively referred because of severity, *Arch. Internal Med. 117*:224, 1966.
21. Bloomer, H. A.: The efficacy of alkaline diuresis and peri-

toneal dialysis in pentobarbital intoxication, *New Engl. J. Med.* *272*:1309, 1965.

22. Mysechetsky, A. and Lassen, N. A.: Urea induced osmotic diuresis and alkalinization of urine in acute barbiturate intoxication, *J. Am. Med. Assoc.* *185*:936, 1963.

23. Kyle, L. H., Jeghers, H., Walsh, W. P., Doolan, P. D., Wishinsky, H. and Pallotta, A.: The application of hemodialysis to the treatment of barbiturate poisoning, *J. Clin. Invest.* *32*: 364, 1953.

24. Berman, L. B., Schreiner, G. E., Jeghers, H. and Pallotta, A.: Hemodialysis: An effective therapy for acute barbiturate poisoning, *J. Am. Med. Assoc.* *161*:820, 1956.

25. Kessel, M., Ibe, K., Neuhaus, G., Remmer, H. and Weller, H.: Die extracorporale Dialyse von Luminal, *Klin. Wochschr.* *40*:580, 1962.

26. Linton, A. L., Luke, R. G., Speirs, I. and Kennedy, A. C.: Forced diuresis and haemodialysis in severe barbiturate intoxication, *Lancet* *1*:1008, 1964.

27. Lee, H. A. and Ames, A. C.: Hemodialysis in severe barbiturate poisoning, *Brit. Med. J.* *1*:1217, 1965.

28. Henderson, L. W. and Merrill, J. P.: Treatment of barbiturate intoxication. With a report of recent experience at Peter Bent Brigham Hospital, *Ann. Internal Med.* *64*:876, 1966.

29. Knochel, J. P. and Barry, K. G.: THAM dialysis: An experimental method to study diffusion of certain weak acids in vivo. II. Secobarbital, *J. Lab. Clin. Med.* *65*:361, 1965.

30. Campion, D. S. and North, J. D.: Effect of protein binding of barbiturates on their rate of removal during peritoneal dialysis, *J. Lab. Clin. Med.* *66*:549, 1965.

31. Genefke, I. K.: THAM used in the treatment of barbiturate coma, *Ugeskr. Laeg.* *130*:761, 1968.

32. Ruedy, J. and Chernecki, W.: The use of a binding agent, polyvinylpyrrolidone, in the treatment of experimental barbiturate intoxication in rabbits, *Can. J. Physiol. Pharmacol.* *46*:829, 1968.

33. Bunn, H. F. and Lubash, G. D.: A controlled study of induced diuresis in barbiturate intoxication, *Ann. Internal Med.* *62*:246, 1965.

33a. Edwards, K. D.: Methods of extrarenal removal of drugs, including the use of dialysis and ion exchange resins in barbiturate poisoning, *Bull. Postgrad. Comm. Med. Univ. Sydney* *20*: 89, 1964.

34. Hagstam, K. E., Larsson, L. E. and Thysell, H.: Experimental studies on charcoal hemoperfusion in uremia including histopathologic findings, *Acta Med. Scand.* *180*:593, 1966.

35. Cameron, J. S., Togeland, P. A., Read, J. F., Bewick, M., Ogg, C. S. and Ellis, F. G.: Accumulation of barbitone in patients on regular hemodialysis, *Lancet* *1*:912, 1970.

36. Graham, J. A., Ledingham, I. M. and Gleadle, R. I.: Treatment of intoxication with combinations of drugs and management of the associated shock, *Postgrad. Med.* *45*:697, 1969.

37. Melchior, J. C., Svensmark, O. and Trolle, D.: Placental transfer of phenobarbital in epileptic women and elimination in newborns, *Lancet* *2*:860, 1967.

38. Tyson, R. M., Schrader, E. A. and Perlman, H. H.: Drugs transmitted through breast milk, *J. Pediat.* *11*:824, 1937.

39. Personal communication, 1967.

40. Terplan, M. and Unger, A. M.: Survival following massive barbiturate ingestion, *J. Am. Med. Assoc.* *198*:322, 1966.

41. Doyle, J. E.: *Extracorporeal Hemodialysis Therapy in Blood Chemistry Disorder*, Springfield, Ill. Charles C Thomas, 1962.

42. Mullan, D., Platts, M. and Ridgway, B.: Barbiturate intoxication, *Lancet* *1*:705, 1965.

43. Streicher, E. and Spank, K.: Hämo-und Peritonealdialyse bei akuter Niereninsuffizienz und schweren Vergiftungen, *Deut. Med. Wochschr.* *92*:1619, 1967.

44. Sodi, A., Rizzo, M. and Durval, A.: Considerazioni sull simpiego dell'emodialisi extracorporea nel trattamento dell-'intossicazione da barbiturici, *Minerva Med.* *58*:2093, 1967.

45. Lash, R. F., Burdette, J. A. and Ozdil, T.: Accidental profound hypothermia and barbiturate intoxication. A report of rapid core rewarming by peritoneal dialysis, *J. Am. Med. Assoc.* *201*:269, 1967.

46. Personal communication, 1968.

47. Lee, H. A. and Sharpstone, P.: Haemodialysis in pediatrics, *Acta Pediat. Scand.* *55*:529, 1966.

48. Rosland, G. A.: Hemodialyse ved akutt barbituratforgiftning, *T. Norsk. Laegeforen* *87*:20, 1967.

49. Berg, K. J. and Enger, E.: Behandling av sovemiddelforgiftninger, *T. Norsk. Laegeforen* *87*:941, 1967.

50. Brown, C. R.: Hemodialysis without cutdown, *Penn. Med.* *70*:60, 1967.

51. Hudson, J. B., Dennis, A. J., Jr. and Hobbs, D. R.: Extended hemodialysis in short acting barbiturate poisoning: Case report, *Southern Med. J.* *62*:457, 1969.

52. Wieth, J. O.: Hemodialysis in barbiturate poisoning, *Intern. Anesth. Clin.* *4*:359, 1966.

53. Rosenbaum, J. L. and Mandanis, R.: Treatment of phenobarbital intoxication in dogs with an anion-recirculation peritoneal dialysis technique. *Trans. Am. Soc. Artificial Internal Organs* *13*:183, 1967.

53a. Linton, A. L., Luke, R. G. and Briggs, J. D.: Methods of forced diuresis and its application in barbiturate poisonings, *Lancet* *2*:377, 1967.

54. Mann, J. B., Ginn, H. E., Matter, B. J. and Shinaberger, J. H.: Clinical experience with lipid dialysate, *Clin Res.* *16*:63, 1968.

55. Shinaberger, J. H., Mann, J. B., Matter, B. J. and Ginn, H. E.: Clinical experience with lipid dialysate, *Am. Soc. Nephrol.* *1*:61, 1967.

56. Dos Ramos, Farias, E., Abeijon, B. and Petrolito, J.: Forced diuresis in the treatment of severe barbiturate intoxication, *Prensa Med. Arg.* *56*:1344, 1969.

57. Tass, G., Balogh, G. and Kiss, K.: Comparative study of redimyl therapy and forced diuresis in the treatment of coma caused by barbiturate poisoning, *Orv. Hetilap* *109*:1759, 1968.

58. Warter, J.: Current treatment of barbiturate coma, *Polski Tygod. Lekar.* *23*:1470, 1968.

59. Prieto, M. E., Cohen, A. and Kuhne, W.: Barbiturate poisoning: Its treatment, *Rev. Med. Chile* *96*:734, 1968.

60. Ohlsson, W. T. L.: Forced diuresis after barbiturates, *Lancet* *2*:888, 1967.

61. Brooks, M. H., Knowlton, M. and Barry, K. G.: Determination of secobarbital in a lipid system: An improved technique which permits spectrophotometric analysis, *J. Lab. Clin. Med.* *72*:345, 1968.

62. Schreiner, G. E., Berman, L. B., Kovach, R. and Bloomer, H. A.: Acute glutethimide (Doriden) poisoning: The use of bemigride (Megimide) and hemodialysis, *Arch. Internal Med.* *101*:899, 1958.

63. Chazan, J. A. and Cohen, J. J.: Clinical spectrum of glutethimide intoxication. Hemodialysis reevaluated, *J. Am. Med. Assoc.* *208*:837, 1969.

64. Hickson, B. and Caridis, D. T.: Haemodialysis in glutethimide poisoning, *Brit. Med. J.* *3*:532, 1969.

65. Maher, J. F., Schreiner, G. E. and Westervelt, F. B.: Acute glutethimide intoxication. I. Clinical experience (22 patients) compared to acute barbiturate intoxication (62 patients), *Am. J. Med.* *33*:70, 1962.

66. Kier, L. C., Whitehead, R. W. and White, W. C.: Blood and urine levels in glutethimide (Doriden) intoxication, *J. Am. Med. Assoc.* *166*:1861, 1958.

67. Chandler, B. F., Meroney, W. H., Czarnecki, S. W., Herman, R. H., Cheitlin, M. D., Goldbaum, L. R. and Herndon, E. G.: Artificial hemodialysis in management of glutethimide intoxication, *J. Am. Med. Assoc.* *170*:914, 1959.

68. Shinaberger, J. H., Shear, L., Clayton, L. E., Barry, K. G., Knowlton, M. and Goldbaum, L. R.: Dialysis for intoxication with lipid soluble drugs: Enhancement of glutethimide extraction with lipid dialysate, *Trans. Am. Soc. Artificial Internal Organs* *11*:173, 1965.

69. Shinaberger, J. H., Shear, L., Clayton, L. E., Barry, K. G., Knowlton, M. and Goldbaum, L.: Intraperitoneal lipid: Enhancement of glutethimide extraction during peritoneal dialysis, *Clin. Res.* *13*:54, 1965.

70. King, L. H., Jr., Decherd, J. F. and Newton, J. L.: A clinically efficient and economical lipid dialyzer. Use in treatment of glutethimide intoxication, *J. Am. Med. Assoc.* *211*:652, 1970.

71. DeMyttenaere, M. H., Maher, J. F. and Schreiner, G. E.: Hemoperfusion through a charcoal column for glutethimide poisoning, *Trans. Am. Soc. Artificial Internal Organs* *13*:190, 1967.

72. DeMyttenaere, M., Schoenfeld, L. and Maher, J. F.: Treatment of glutethimide poisoning. A comparison of forced diuresis and dialysis, *J. Am. Med. Assoc.* *203*:855, 1968.

73. Frey, W. G.: Acute glutethimide poisoning managed by peritoneal dialysis, *J. Maine Med. Assoc.* *59*:3, 1968.

74. Caplan, H. L.: Recovery in severe glutethimide poisoning, *Postgrad. Med.* *43*:611, 1967.

75. Chazan, J. A. and Cohen, J. J.: Clinical spectrum of glutethimide intoxication, *J. Am. Med. Assoc.* *208*:837, 1969.

76. Kurtz, G. G., Michael, U. F., Morosi, H. J. and Vaamonde, C. A.: Hemodialysis during pregnancy. Report of a case of glutethimide poisoning complicated by acute renal failure, *Arch. Internal Med.* *118*:30, 1966.

77. Decker, W. J., Thompson, H. L., and Arneson, L. A.: Glutethimide rebound, *Lancet* *1*:778, 1970.

78. Cimino, J. A.: Poison treatment and dialysis information, *New Engl. J. Med.* *282*:1048, 1970.

79. Lubsher, F. A.: Fatal hydantoin poisoning, *J. Am. Med. Assoc.* *198*:1120, 1966.

80. Grosz, H. D.: Dilantin intoxication with report of one case, *Am. Practitioner* *7*:1633, 1956.

81. Kutt, H., Winters, W., Kokenge, R. and McDowell, F.: Diphenylhydantoin metabolism, blood levels and toxicity, *Arch. Neurol.* *11*:642, 1964.

82. Tichner, J. B. and Enselberg, G.: Suicidal Dilantin, sodium-diphenylhydantoin poisoning, *New Engl. J. Med.* *245*:723, 1951.

83. Tenckhoff, H., Sherrard, D. J. and Hickman, R. O.: Acute diphenylhydantoin intoxication, *Am. J. Diseases Children* *116*: 422, 1968.

84. Blair, A. A., Hallpike, J. F. and Lascelles, P. T.: Acute diphenylhydantoin and primidone poisoning treated by peritoneal dialysis, *J. Neurol. Neurosurg. Psychiat.* *31*:520, 1968.

85. Personal communication, 1963.

86. Pogglitsch, H. and Zeichen, R.: Uber die Anwendung der extracorporalen Hämodialyse bei akuten Schlafmittelvergiftungen, *Wien. Med. Wochschr.* *115*:308, 1965.

87. Dyment, P. G., Curtis, D. D. and Gourrich, G. E.: Meprobamate poisoning treated by peritoneal dialysis, *J. Pediat.* *67*:124, 1965.

88. Maddock, R. K. and Bloomer, H. A.: Meprobamate overdosage. Evaluation of its severity and methods of treatment, *J. Am. Med. Assoc. 201*:999, 1967.
89. Mouton, D. E., Cohen, R. J. and Barrett, Jr., O. N.: Meprobamate poisoning: Successful treatment with peritoneal dialysis, *Am. J. Sci. 253*:706, 1967.
90. Castell, D. O. and Sode, J.: Meprobamate intoxication treated with peritoneal dialysis, *Illinois Med. J. 131*:298, 1967.
91. Gaultier, M., Fournier, E. and Bismuth, C.: Acute poisoning by meprobamate. Apropos of 141 cases, *Bull. Soc. Med. Hop. Paris 119*:675, 1968.
92. Teehan, B. P., Maher, J. F., Carey, J. J. H., Flynn, P. D. and Schreiner, G. E.: Acute ethchlorvynol (Placidyl) intoxication. Clinical and therapeutic analysis, *Ann. Internal Med.* In press (June, 1970).
93. Hyde, J. S., Lawrence, A. G. and Moles, J. B.: Ethchlorvynol intoxication. Successful treatment by exchange transfusion and peritoneal dialysis, *Clin. Pediat.* 7:739, 1968.
94. Hedley-White, J. and Laasberg, L. H.: Ethchlorvynol poisoning: Gas liquid chromatography in management, *Anesthesiology 30*:107, 1969.
95. Westervelt, Jr., F. B.: Ethchlorvynol (Placidyl) intoxication. Experience with five patients, including treatment with hemodialysis, *Ann. Internal Med. 64*:1229, 1966.
96. Ogilvie, R. I., Douglas, D. E., Lochead, J. R., Moscovich, M. D. and Raye, M.: Ethchlorvynol (Placidyl) intoxication and its treatment by hemodialysis, *Can. Med. Assoc. J. 95*:954, 1966.
97. Schultz, J. C., Crouder, D. G., and Medart, W. S.: Excretion studies in ethchlorvynol (Placidyl) intoxication, *Arch. Internal Med. 117*:409, 1966.
98. Langecker, H., Neuhaus, G., Ibe, K. and Kessel, M.: Ein Suicid-Versuch mit Valamin mit einem Beitrag zur Elimination und Therapie, *Arch. Toxicol. 19*:293, 1962.
99. Davis, R. P., Blythe, W. B., Newton, M. and Welt, L. G.: The treatment of intoxication with ethynyl cyclohexyl carbamate (Valmid) by extracorporeal hemodialysis: a case report, *Yale J. Biol. Med. 32*:192, 1959.
100. Personal communication, 1965.
101. Xanthaky, G., Freireich, A. W., Matusiak, W., Lukash, L.: Hemodialysis in methyprylon poisoning, *J. Am. Med. Assoc. 198*:1212, 1966.
102. Yudis, M., Swartz, C., Onesti, G., Ramirez, O., Snyder, D. and Brest, A.: Hemodialysis for methyprylon (Noludar) poisoning, *Ann. Internal Med. 68*:1301, 1968.
103. Personal communication, 1969.
104. Avram, M. M. and McGinn, J. T.: Extracorporeal hemodialysis in phenothiazine overdosage, *J. Am. Med. Assoc. 197*:142, 1966.
105. Anderson, J., Lee, H. A. and Stroud, C. E.: Haemodialysis in infants and small children, *Brit. Med. J. 1*:1405, 1965.
106. Grumer, H. A., Stannus, D. G. and Stoddard, G. R.: The feasibility of a hemodialysis unit in a community hospital, *Southern Med. J. 59*:769, 1966.
107. Hawthorne, J. W., Marcus, A. M. and Kaye, M.: Management of massive imipramine overdosage with mannitol and artificial dialysis, *New Engl. J. Med. 228*:33, 1963.
108. Wallace, A. E.: Recovery after massive overdose of diphenhydramine and methaqualone, *Lancet 2*:1247, 1968.
109. Decker, W. J., Combs, H. F. and Corby, D. G.: Adsorption of drugs and poisons by activated charcoal, *Toxicol. Appl. Pharmacol. 13*:454, 1968.
110. Wilke, D.: Addiction to amphetamines, *Brit. Med. J. 2*: 730, 1962.
111. Swanton, C.: The dangerous amphetamines, *Med. J. Australia 1*:795, 1963.
112. Kramer, J. C., Fishman, V. S. and Littlefield, D. C.: Amphetamine abuse, *J. Am. Med. Assoc. 201*:305, 1967.
113. Wallace, H. E., Neumayer, F. and Gutch, C. F.: Amphetamine poisoning and peritoneal dialysis. A case report, *Am. J. Diseases Children 108*:657, 1964.
114. Zalis, E. G., Cohen, R. J. and Lundberg, G. D.: Use of peritoneal dialysis in experimental amphetamine poisoning, *Proc. Soc. Exptl. Biol. Med. 120*:278, 1965.
115. Borden, E. C. and Rostand, S. G.: Recovery from massive amitriptyline overdosage, *Lancet 1*:1256, 1968.
116. Rasmussen, J.: Poisoning by amitriptyline, imipramine and nortriptyline, *Danish Med. Bull. 13*:201, 1966.
117. Hawthorne, J. W., Marcus, A. M. and Kaye, M.: Management of massive imipramine overdosage with mannitol and artificial dialysis, *New Engl. J. Med. 268*:33, 1963.
118. Versaci, A. A., Nakamoto, S. and Kolff, W. J.: Phenelzine intoxication. Report of a case treated by hemodialysis, *Ohio Med. J. 60*:770, 1964.
119. Matter, B. J., Donat, P. E., Brill, M. L. and Ginn, H. E.: Tranylcypromine sulfate poisoning, successful treatment by hemodialysis, *Arch. Internal Med. 116*:18, 1965.
120. Lipkin, D. L. and Kushnick, T.: Pargyline hydrochloride poisoning in a child, *J. Am. Med. Assoc. 201*:57, 1967.
121. Marc-Aurele, J. and Schreiner, G. E.: The dialysance of ethanol and methanol: A proposed method for the treatment of massive intoxication by ethyl or methyl alcohol, *J. Clin. Invest. 39*:892, 1960.
122. Wieth, J. O. and Jørgensen, H. E.: Treatment of methanol and ethanol poisoning by hemodialysis, *Danish Med. Bull. 8*:103, 1961.
123. Felts, J. H., Templeton, T. B., Wolff, W. A., Meredith, J. H. and Hines, J.: Methanol poisoning treated by hemodialysis, *Southern Med. J. 55*:46, 1962.
124. Erlanson, P., Fritz, H., Hagstam, K. E., Liljenberg, B., Tryding, H. and Voigt, G.: Severe methanol intoxication, *Acta Med. Scand. 177*:393, 1965.
125. Gjessing, J.: Peritoneal dialys med THAM vid methanolintoxikation, *Opuscula Med. Bd. 10*:40, 1965.
126. Setter, J. G., Singh, R., Brackett, Jr., N. C. and Randall, Jr., R. E.: Studies on the dialysis of methanol, *Trans. Am. Soc. Artificial Internal Organs 13*:178, 1967.
127. Wenzl, J. E., Mills, S. D. and McCall, J. T.: Methanol poisoning in an infant. Successful treatment with peritoneal dialysis, *Am. J. Diseases Children 116*:445, 1968.
128. Kane, R. L., Talbert, W., Harlan, J., Sizemore, G. and Cataland, S.: A methanol poisoning outbreak in Kentucky. A clinical epidemiologic study, *Arch. Environ. Health 17*:119, 1968.
129. Wenzl, J. E., Mills, S. D. and McCall, J. T.: Methanol poisoning in an infant. Successful treatment with peritoneal dialysis, *Am. J. Diseases Children 116*:445, 1968.
130. Dickerman, J. D., Bishop, W. and Marks, J. F.: Acute ethanol intoxication in a child, *Pediatrics 42*:837, 1968.
131. Salwinska-Cieckiewicz, B. and Grzelec, T.: Group poisoning with methanol, *Polski Tygod. Lekar 23*:1244, 1968.
132. Kirillov, M. M., Staroverov, A. T. and Semenov, V. I.: Extracorporeal hemodialysis and exchange transfusion in methanol poisoning, *Voenno-Med. Zh. 12*:32, 1969.
133. Ogata, M., Mendelson, J. H. and Mello, N. K.: Electrolyte and osmolality in alcoholics during experimentally induced intoxication, *Psychosomat. Med. 30*:463, 1968.
134. Closs, K. and Solberg, C. O.: Methanol poisoning, *J. Am. Med. Assoc. 211*:497, 1970.
135. Cowen, D. L.: Extracorporeal dialysis in methanol poisoning, *Ann. Internal Med. 61*:134, 1964.
136. Schreiner, G. E., Maher, J. F., Marc-Aurele, J., Knowland, D. and Alvo, M.: Ethylene glycol - two indications for hemodialysis, *Trans. Am. Soc. Artificial Internal Organs 5*:81, 1959.
137. Pendras, J.: Ethylene glycol poisoning as an indication for hemodialysis, *Clin. Res. 11*:118, 1963.
138. Hagstam, K. E., Ingvar, D. H., Paatela, M. and Tallqvist, H.: Ethylene-glycol poisoning treated by haemodialysis, *Acta Med. Scand. 178*:599, 1965.
139. Joly, J. B., Huault, G., Frossard, C., Fabiani, P. and Thieffry, S.: Intoxication aiguë par l'ethylene-glycol à propos de quatre cas chez de jeunes enfants, *Bull. Soc. Med. Hôp. Paris 119*:27, 1968.
140. Freireich, A. W., Cinque, T. J., Xanthaky, G. and Landau, D:. Hemodialysis for isopropanol poisoning, *New Engl. J. Med. 277*:699, 1967.
141. King, L. H., Bradley, K. P. and Shires, D. L.: Hemodialysis for isopropyl alcohol poisoning, *J. Am. Med. Assoc. 211*:1855, 1970.
142. Adelson, F.: Fatal intoxication with isopropyl alcohol (rubbing alcohol), *Am. J. Clin. Pathol. 38*:144, 1962.
143. Lawson, A. A., Proudfoot, A. T., and Brown, S. S.: Forced diuresis in the treatment of acute salicylate poisoning in adults, *Quart. J. Med. 38*:31, 1969.
144. Armstrong, C. and Edwards, K. D. G.: Multifactorial design for testing oral ion exchange resins, charcoal and other factors in the treatment of aspirin poisoning in the rat. Effect of cholestyramine, *Med. J. Australia 2*:301, 1967.
145. Holt, L. E., Jr. and Holtz, P. H.: Activated charcoal as an antidote for poisons, Nat. Clearinghouse Poison Control Center, 1-3. (Jan.-Feb.), 1963.
146. Dunea, G. and Kolff, W. J.: Clinical experience with the Yatzidis charcoal artificial kidney, *Trans. Am. Soc. Artificial Internal Organs 11*:178, 1965.
147. Morgan, A. G. and Polak, A.: Acetazolamide and sodium bicarbonate in treatment of salicylate poisoning in adults, *Brit. Med. J. 1*:16, 1969.
148. Hart, L. G., Guarino, A. M. and Schanker, L. S.: Gastric dialysis as a possible antidotal procedure for removal of absorbed drugs, *J. Lab. Clin. Med. 73*:853, 1969.
149. Schreiner, G. E., Berman, L. B., Griffin, J. and Feys, J.: Specific therapy for salicylism, *New Engl. J. Med. 253*:213, 1955.
150. Schreiner, G. E.: The role of hemodialysis (artificial kidney) in acute poisoning, *Arch. Internal Med. 102*:896, 1958.
151. Jorgensen, H. E. and Wieth, J. O.: Dialysable poisons, Hemodialysis in the treatment of acute poisoning, *Lancet 1*:81, 1963.
152. Doolan, P. D., Walsh, W. P., Kyle, L. H. and Wishinsky, H.: Acetylsalicylic acid intoxication. A proposed method of treatment, *J. Am. Med. Assoc. 146*:105, 1951.
153. Kallen, R. J., Zaltzman, S., Coe, F. L. and Metcoff, J.: Hemodialysis in children: Technique, kinetic aspects related to varying body size, and application to salicylate intoxication, acute renal failure and some disorders, *Medicine 45*:1, 1966.
154. Zachau-Christiansen, B.: Three cases of salicylic acid poisoning in infants, *Ugeskr. Laeg. 130*:370, 1968.
155. Anon.: Acute salicylate poisoning, *Lancet 1*:1038, 1969.
156. Anon.: Management of acute salicylate poisoning, *Brit. Med. J. 1*:3, 1969.
157. Schreiner, G. E., Maher, J. F. and Marc-Aurele, J.: The dialysance of exogenous poisons and some common metabolites in the twin-coil artificial kidney, *J. Clin. Invest. 38*:1040, 1959.
158. Maher, J. F., Freeman, R. B., Setter, J. G., Rubin, M. and Schreiner, G. E.: Dialysance studies of varied solutes and bio-

chemical changes during hemodialysis, *Trans. Am. Soc. Artificial Internal Organs 10*:332, 1964.

159. James, J. A., Kimbell, L. and Read, W. T.: Experimental salicylate intoxication. I. Comparison of exchange transfusion, intermittent peritoneal lavage and hemodialysis as means of removing salicylate, *Pediatrics 29*:442, 1962.

160. Cohen, H.: A clinical evaluation of peritoneal dialysis, *Can. Med. Assoc. J. 88*:932, 1963.

161. Kloss, J. L. and Boeckman, C. R.: Methyl salicylate poisoning. A case report and discussion of treatment by peritoneal dialysis, *Ohio Med. J. 63*:1064, 1967.

162. Etteldorf, J. N., Dobbins, W. T., Summitt, R. L., Rainwater, W. T. and Fischer, R. L.: Intermittent peritoneal dialysis using 5% albumin in the treatment of salicylate intoxication in children, *J. Pediat. 58*:226, 1961.

163. Etteldorf, J. N., Montalvo, J. M., Kaplow, S. and Sheffield, J. A.: Intermittent peritoneal dialysis in the treatment of experimental salicylate intoxication, *J. Pediat. 56*:1, 1960.

164. Fine, R. N., Stiles, Q., DePalma, J. R. and Donnell, G. N.: Hemodialysis in infants under 1 year of age for acute poisoning, *Am. J. Diseases Children 116*:657, 1968.

165. Karliner, J. S.: Propoxyphene hydrochloride poisoning. Report of a case treated with peritoneal dialysis, *J. Am. Med. Assoc. 199*:1006, 1967.

166. Gary, N. F., Maher, J. F., DeMyttenaere, M. H., Liggero, S. H., Scott, K. G., Matusiak, W. and Schreiner, G. E.: Acute propoxyphene hydrochloride intoxication, *Arch. Internal Med. 121*:453, 1968.

167. Corby, D. G. and Decker, W. J.: An antidote for propoxyphene HCl, *J. Am. Med. Assoc. 203*:1074, 1968.

168. Fennelly, J. J. and Lasker, N.: Acute renal failure following acetophenetidin ingestion, *J. Med. Soc. New Jersey 61*:115, 1964.

169. Pimstone, B. L. and Uys, C. J.: Liver necrosis and myocardiopathy following paracetamol overdosage, *South African Med. J. 42*:259, 1968.

170. Maclean, D., Peters, T. J., Brown, R. A. G., McCathie, M., Baines, G. F. and Robertson, P. G. C.: Treatment of acute paracetamol poisoning, *Lancet 2*:849, 1968.

171. Edwards, K. D. G. and Whyte, H. M.: Streptomycin poisoning in renal failure. An indication for treatment with an artificial kidney, *Brit. Med. J. 1*:753, 1959.

172. Kunin, C. M. and Finland, M.: Restrictions imposed on antibiotic therapy by renal failure, *Arch. Internal Med. 104*:1030, 1959.

173. Kunin, C. M.: Problems of antimicrobial drug therapy in renal failure, *Proc. 3rd Int. Congr. Nephrol. 3*:193, 1966.

174. Gombos, E. A., Katz, S., Fedorko, J., Allnoch, H. and Lee, T. H.: Dialysis properties of newer antimicrobial agents, *Antimicrobial Agents Chemotherap. 4*:373, 1964.

175. Greenberg, P. A. and Sanford, J. P.: Removal and absorption of antibiotics in patients with renal failure undergoing peritoneal dialysis. Tetracycline, chloramphenicol, kanamycin and colistimethate, *Ann. Internal Med. 66*:465, 1967.

176. Lindholm, D. D. and Murray, J. S.: Persistence of vancomycin in the blood during renal failure and its treatment by hemodialysis, *New Engl. J. Med. 274*:1047, 1966.

177. Goodwin, N. J., Thomson, G. E. and Friedman, E. A.: Antituberculous therapy during maintenance hemodialysis, *Proc. Am. Soc. Nephrol. 1*:25, 1967.

178. Precht, K. and Briedigkeit, H.: Experimentelle Untersuchungen zur Dialysierbarkeit von Antibiotika, *Acta Biol. Med. German 20*:339, 1968.

179. Bulger, R. J., Lindholm, D. D., Murray, J. S. and Kirby, W. W. M.: Effect of uremia on methicillin and oxacillin blood levels, *J. Am. Med. Assoc. 187*:319, 1964.

180. Ruedy, J.: Effects of peritoneal dialysis on physiological disposition of oxacillin, ampicillin and tetracycline in patients with renal disease, *Can. Med. Assoc. J. 94*:257, 1966.

181. Höffler, D., Stegemann, I and Scheler, F.: Ampicillin-Spiegel in Serum und Harn bei eingeschränkter Nierenfunktion, *Deut. Med. Wochschr. 91*:206, 1966.

182. Sitprija, V. and Holmes, J. H.: Isoniazid intoxication. *Am. Rev. Resp. Disease 90*:248, 1964.

183. Williams, Jr., T. W., Lawson, S. A., Brook, M. I., Ory, E. M. and Morgen, R. O.: Effect of hemodialysis on dicloxacillin concentration in plasma, *Antimicrobial Agents Chemotherap. 7*:767, 1967.

184. McCloskey, R. V. and Hayes, Jr., C. P.: Plasma levels of dicloxacillin in oliguric patients and the effect of hemodialysis. *Antimicrobial Agents Chemotherap. 7*:770, 1967.

185. Eastwood, J. B. and Curtis, J. R.: Carbenicillin administration in patients with severe renal failure, *Brit. Med. J. 1*:486, 1968.

186. Skimming, L. H., Knies, P. T., Anthony, M. A., and Melaragno, E. S.: Hemolytic anemia caused by sulfamethoxypyridazine. Report of a case successfully treated with hemodialysis, *Ohio Med. J. 57*:280, 1961.

187. Kunin, C. M., Glazko, A. J. and Finland, M.: Perisistence of antibiotics in blood of patients with acute renal failure. II. Chloramphenicol and its metabolic products in the blood of patients with severe renal disease or hepatic cirrhosis, *J. Clin. Invest. 38*:1498, 1959.

188. Bulger, R. J., Bennett, J. V. and Boen, S. T.: Intraperitoneal administration of broad spectrum antibiotics in patients with renal failure, *J. Am. Med. Assoc. 194*:1198, 1965.

189. Maher, J. F., Schreiner, G. E. and Marc-Aurele, J.: Methodologic problems associated with in vitro measurements of dialysance, *Trans. Am. Soc. Artificial Internal Organs 5*:120, 1959.

190. MacKay, D. N. and Kaye, D.: Serum concentrations of colistin in patients with normal and impaired renal function, *New Engl. J. Med. 270*:394, 1964.

191. Swick, H. M., Maxwell, E. and Charache, P.: Peritoneal dialysis in colistin intoxication: Report of a case, *J. Pediat. 74*:976, 1969.

192. Goodwin, N. J. and Friedman, E. A.: The effects of renal impairment, peritoneal dialysis, and hemodialysis on serum colistimethate levels. *Ann. Internal Med. 68*:984, 1968.

193. Man, P. H.: Urinary excretion of polymyxin B and sodium colistimethate levels, *Ann. Internal Med. 68*:984, 1968.

194. Ito, J.: Colistin nephrotoxicity: report of a case with light and electron microscopic studies, *Acta Pathol. Jap. 19*:55, 1969.

195. Curtis, J. R. and Eastwood, J. B.: Colistin sulfomethate sodium administration in the presence of severe renal failure and during haemodialysis and peritoneal dialysis, *Brit. Med. J. 1*:484, 1968.

196. Reinarz, J. A. and McIntosh, D. A.: Lincomycin excretion in patients with normal renal function, severe azotemia and with hemodialysis and peritoneal dialysis, *Antimicrobial Agents Chemotherap. 5*:232, 1965.

197. Hagstam, K. E. and Lindholm, T.: Treatment of exogenous poisoning with special regard to the need for artificial kidney in severe complicated cases, *Acta Med. Scand. 175*:507, 1964.

198. Durr, F. and Missmahl, H. P.: Extrakorporale hämodialyse bei akuter isoniazid-vergiftung. Zugleich ein beitrag zur dialysierfähigkeit des isoniazid, *Deut. Med. Wochschr. 90*: 1174, 1965.

199. Cocco, A. E. and Pazourek, L. J.: Acute isoniazid intoxication - management by peritoneal dialysis, *New Engl. J. Med. 269*:852, 1963.

200. Atkins, R., Cutting, C. J. and MacKintosh, T. F.: Acute poisoning by cycloserine, *Brit. Med. J. 1*:907, 1965.

201. Freeman, Richard B., Maher, John F. and Schreiner, George E.: The affinity of synthetic membranes for calcium, *Trans. Am. Soc. Artificial Internal Organs 11*:99, 1965.

202. Maher, John F., Freeman, Richard B., Schmitt, Gunther and Schreiner, George E.: Adherence of metals to cellophane membranes and removal by whole blood. A mechanism of solute transport during hemodialysis, *Trans. Am. Soc. Artificial Internal Organs 11*:104, 1965.

203. Hocken, A. G. and Bradshaw, G.: Arsine poisoning, *Brit. J. Ind. Med. 27*:56, 1970.

204. Matter, B. J., Pederson, J., Psimenos, G. and Lindeman, R. D.: Lethal copper intoxication in hemodialysis, *Trans. Am. Soc. Artificial Internal Organs 15*:309, 1969.

205. Lyle, W. H.: Chronic dialysis and copper poisoning, *New Engl. J. Med. 276*:1209, 1967.

206. Vest, M., Hirt, H. R. and Olafsson, A.: Two fatal poisonings with imipramine (Tofranil) and dibenzepin (Noveril) in small children, *Schweiz. Med. Wochschr. 99*:1157, 1969.

207. Sunshine, P. and Yaffe, S. J.: Amitriptyline poisoning. Clinical and pathological findings in a fatal case, *Am. J. Diseases Children 106*:501, 1963.

208. Gjerris, F.: Poisoning with chlordiazepoxide, *Danish Med. Bull. 13*:170, 1966.

209. Cruz, I. A., Kramer, N. C. and Parrish, A. E.: Hemodialysis in chlordiazepoxide toxicity, *J.Am. Med. Assoc. 202*:438, 1967.

210. Maxwell, M. H.: The indications for and the limitations of peritoneal dialysis, *Bull. New Jersey Acad. Med. 6*:341, 1960.

211. Loeser, W. D., Fisher, C. J. and Boulis, G.: Forty-three dialyses in a community hospital, *J. Am. Med. Assoc. 192*:809, 1965.

212. Huxtable, R. F. and Landwirth, J.: Diphenhydramine poisoning treated by exchange transfusion, *Am. J. Diseases Children 106*:496, 1963.

213. Hayward, J. N. and Boshell, B. R.: Paraldehyde intoxication with metabolic acidosis. Report of two cases, experimented data and clinical review of the literature, *Am. J. Med. 23*:965, 1957.

214. Gutman, R. A., Burnell, J. M. and Solak, F.: Paraldehyde acidosis, *Am. J. Med. 42*:435, 1967.

215. Beier, L. W., Pitts, W. H. and Gonick, H. C.: Metabolic acidosis occurring during paraldehyde intoxication, *Ann. Internal Med. 58*:155, 1963.

216. Zabinska, K., Smólenski, O., Hanicki, Z., Bogdal, J., Paczek, Z., Wiernikowski, A. and Hirzel, P.: Ostre zatrucia leczone dialysa, *Przeglad. Lekar. 23*:717, 1967.

217. Cardis, D. T., McAndrew, G. M. and Matheson, N. A.: Hemodialysis in poisoning with methaqualone and diphenhydramine, *Lancet 1*:51, 1967.

218. Ibe, K., Bennhold, I., Burmeister, H. and Kessel, M.: Die extracorporale-Haemodialyse bei schweren Schlafmittelvergiftungen. *Berlin Med. 16*:350, 1965.

219. Proudfoot, A. T., Noble, J., Nimmo, J., Brown, S. S. and Cameron, J. C.: Peritoneal dialysis and hemodialysis in methaqualone (Mandrax) poisoning, *Scot. Med. J. 13*:232, 1968.

220. Feldman, S. A. and Levi, J. A.: Prolonged paresis following gallamine. A case report, *Brit. J. Anaesthesiol. 35*:804, 1963.

221. Wolf, A. V., Remp, D. G., Kiley, J. E. and Currie, G. D.:

Artificial kidney function: kinetics of hemodialysis, *J. Clin. Invest.* *30*:1062, 1951.
222. Maxwell, M. H., Rockney, R. E., Kleeman, C. R. and Twiss, M. R.: Peritoneal dialysis. I. Technique and application, *J. Am. Med. Assoc.* *170*:917, 1959.
223. Rosenbaum, J. L. and Schumacher, O. P.: Hemodialysis in the treatment of hypercalcemia, *Ohio Med. J.* *59*:1208, 1963.
224. Eisenberg, E. and Gotch, F. A.: Normocalcemic hyperparathyroidism culminating in hypercalcemic crisis. Treatment with hemodialysis, *Arch. Internal Med.* *122*:258, 1968.
225. Freeman, R. M., Lawton, R. L. and Chamberlain, M. A.: Hard water syndrome, *New Engl. J. Med.* *276*:1113, 1967.
226. Felts, J. H., Barringer, M. and Meredith, J. H.: Combined chelation, hemodialysis and alkalinization. A possible treatment for iron poisoning, *Trans. Am. Soc. Artificial Internal Organs* *8*:229, 1962.
227. Whitten, C. F., Chen, Y. C. and Gibson, G. W.: Studies in acute iron poisoning. II. Further observations on desferrioxamine in the treatment of acute experimental iron poisoning, *Pediatrics* *38*:102, 1966.
228. Covey, T. J.: Ferrous sulfate poisoning: A review, case summaries and therapeutic regimen, *J. Pediat.* *64*:218, 1964.
229. Tisher, C. C., Barnett, B. M. S., Finch, C. A. and Scribner, B. H.: Treatment of iron overload in patients with renal failure, *Clin. Sci.* *33*:539, 1967.
230. Movassighi, N., Purugganan, G. G. and Leiken, S.: Comparison of exchange tranfusion and desferrioxamine in the treatment of acute iron poisoning, *J. Pediat.* *75*:604, 1969.
231. Smith, H. D., King, L. R. and Margolin, E. G.: Treatment of lead encephalopathy: the combined use of EDTA and hemodialysis, *Am. J. Diseases Children* *109*:332, 1965.
232. Mehbod, H.: Treatment of lead intoxication. Combined use of peritoneal dialysis and edetate calcium disodium, *J. Am. Med. Assoc.* *201*:972, 1967.
233. Amdisen, A. and Skjoldborg, H.: Hemodialysis for lithium poisoning, *Lancet* *2*:213, 1969.
234. Schou, M., Amdisen, A. and Trap-Jensen, J.: Lithium poisoning, *Am. J. Psychiat.* *125*:520, 1968.
235. Hawkins, J. B. and Dorken, P. R.: Lithium, *Lancet* *1*:839, 1969.
236. Maher, J. F. and Schreiner, G. E.: The dialysis of mercury and mercury-BAL complex, *Clin. Res.* 7:298, 1959.
237. Finberg, L., Kiley, J. and Luttrell, C. N.: Mass accidental salt poisoning in infancy. A study of a hospital disaster, *J. Am. Med. Assoc.* *184*:187, 1963.
238. Looney, W. B., Maletskos, C. J., Helmick, M., Reardon, J., Cohen, J. and Guild, W.: The artificial kidney and ion exchange resins as possible methods of removing radioelements from the body, *Radiology* *68*:255, 1957.
239. Merrill, J. P. and Weller, J. M.: Treatment of bromism with the artificial kidney, *Ann. Internal Med.* 37:186, 1952.
240. Schmitt, G. W., Maher, J. F. and Schreiner, G. E.: Ethacrynic acid enhanced bromuresis: A comparison with peritoneal and hemodialysis, *J. Lab. Clin. Med.* *68*:913, 1966.
241. Wieth, J. O. and Funder, J.: Treatment of bromide poisoning: comparison of forced halogen turnover and haemodialysis, *Lancet* *2*:327, 1963.
242. Benke, A.: Two cases of monoureide poisoning, *Wien. Klin. Wochschr.* *80*:715, 1968.
243. Wooster, A. G., Dunlop, M. and Joske, R. A.: Use of an oral diuretic (Doburil) in treatment of bromide intoxication, *Am. J. Med. Sci.* *253*:23, 1967.
244. Maher, J. F., Schreiner, G. E. and Marc-Aurele, J.: Methodologic problems associated with in vitro measurements of dialysance, *Trans. Am. Soc. Artificial Internal Organs* *5*:120, 1959.
245. Hansson, R. and Lindholm, T.: Elimination of hypaque (sodium - 3, 5 diacetamido - 2, 4, 6 - triiodobenzoate) and the effect of hemodialysis in anuria: A clinical study and an experimental investigation on rabbits, *Acta Med. Scand.* *174*:611, 1963.
246. Taves, D. R., Terry, R., Smith, F. A. and Gardner, D. E.: Use of fluoridated water in long term hemodialysis, *Arch. Internal Med.* *115*:167, 1965.
247. Taves, D. R., Freeman, R. B., Kamm, D. E., Ramos, C. P. and Scribner, B. H.: Hemodialysis with fluoridated dialysate, *Trans. Am. Soc. Artificial Internal Organs* *14*:412, 1968
248. Saunders, S. J., Terblanche, J., Bosman, S. C., Harrison, G. G., Biebuyck, J., Dent, D., Pearce, S. and Barnard, C. N.: Acute hepatic coma treated by cross circulation with a baboon and by repeated exchange transfusions, *Lancet* *2*:585, 1968.
248a. Freeman, R. F.: Personal communication, 1970.
249. Kiley, J. E., Pender, J. C., Welch, H. F. and Welch, C. S.: Ammonia intoxication treated by hemodialysis, *New Engl. J. Med.* *259*:1156, 1958.
250. Nienhuis, L. I., Mulmed, E. I. and Kelley, J. W.: Hepatic coma, treatment emphasizing merit of peritoneal dialysis, *Am. J. Surg.* *106*:980, 1963.
251. Keynes, W. M.: Hemodialysis in the treatment of liver failure, *Lancet* *2*:1236, 1968.
252. Powell, E. D. V., Perry, A. W. and Lieth, M. P.: Exchange transfusion and hemodialysis. Management of hepatorenal failure, *Can. Med. Assoc. J.* *100*:129, 1969.
253. Abouna, G. M., Kirkley, J. R., Hull, C. J., Ashcroft, T. and Kerr, D. N. S.: Treatment of hepatic coma by extracorporeal pig liver perfusion, *Lancet* *1*:64, 1969.
254. Burnell, J. M., Dawborn, J. K., Epstein, R. B., Guttman, R. A., Leinbach, M. B., Thomas, E. D. and Volwiler, W.: Acute hepatic coma treated by cross-circulation or exchange transfusion, *New Engl. J. Med.* *276*:935, 1967.
255. Blumburg, A. and Rohner, R.: Exchange transfusion in hepatic coma, *New Engl. J. Med.* *276*:984, 1967.
256. Kiley, J. E., Welch, H. F., Pender, J. C. and Welch, C. S.: Removal of blood ammonia by hemodialysis, *Proc. Soc. Exptl. Biol. Med.* *91*:489, 1956.
257. Schechter, P. C., Nealon, Jr., T. F. and Gibbon, Jr., J. H.: A simple extracorporeal device for reducing elevated blood ammonia levels, *Surgery* *44*:892, 1958.
258. Ritchie, H. D., Davies, D. M., Godfrey, J. M., Fan, P., Johns, R. G. S. and Perrin, J.: Extracorporeal methods for reducing high blood ammonia levels, *Gut* *3*:172, 1962.
259. Allgower, M., Burri, C. and Cueni, L.: Study of burn toxins, *Ann. N. Y. Acad. Sci.* *150*:807, 1968.
260. Firmat, J., Vanamee, P., Klauber, L., Krakoff, I. and Randall, H. T.: The artificial kidney in the treatment of renal failure and hyperuricemia in patients with lymphoma and leukemia, *Cancer* *13*:276, 1960.
261. Barry, K. G., Hunter, R. H., Davis, T. E. and Crosby, W. H.: Acute uric acid nephropathy. Treatment with mannitol diuresis and peritoneal dialysis, *Arch. Internal Med.* *111*:452, 1963.
262. Maher, J. F. and Schreiner, G. E.: The dialysis of poisons and drugs, *Trans. Am. Soc. Artificial Internal Organs* *13*:369, 1967.
263. Duncan, H., Elliott, W., Horn, D. B., Kerr, D. N. S., Pearson, D. T. and Robson, A. M.: Effect of hemodialysis on joint symptoms, urate pool and renal function in familial gout, *Metabolism* *12*:252, 1963.
264. Hayes, Jr., C. P., Metz, E. N., Robinson, R. R. and Rundles, R. W.: The use of allopurinol (HPP) to control hyperuricemia in patients on chronic intermittent hemodialysis, *Trans. Am. Soc. Artificial Internal Organs* *11*:247, 1965.
265. Shannon, I. L. and Freeman, R. M.: Effects of probenecid and haemodialysis on human parotid fluid uric acid, *Arch. Oral Biol.* *12*:291, 1967.
266. Holland, P. and Holland, N. H.: Prevention and management of acute hyperuricemia in childhood leukemia, *J. Pediat.* 72:358, 1968.
267. Maher, J. F., Rath, C. E. and Schreiner, G. E.: Hyperuricemia complicating leukemia: treatment with allopurinol and dialysis, *Arch. Internal Med.* *123*:198, 1969.
268. Rae, A. I. and Hopper, Jr., J.: Removal of refractory oedema fluid by peritoneal dialysis, *Brit. J. Urol.* *40*:336, 1968.
269. Nathan, E.: Severe hydrops foetalis treated with peritoneal dialysis and positive pressure ventilation, *Lancet* *1*:1393, 1968.
270. Parkin, J. M. and Walker, W.: Peritoneal dialysis in severe hydrops foetalis, *Lancet* *2*:283, 1968.
271. Page, P. F., Kallmeyer, J. C. and Malherbe, L. F.: Modification of Britton's technique for the treatment of intractable chronic ascites, *South African Med. J.* *42*:1015, 1968.
272. Doyle, J. E.: *Extracorporeal Hemodialysis Therapy in Blood Chemistry Disorder*, Springfield, Ill. Charles C Thomas, 1962.
273. Weg, J. G., Harris, R. F., Miller, M. B., Wilsie, D. S., McPhaul, J. J. and Finkel, M.: Treatment of hepatic coma by hemodialysis, *Texas J. Med.* *60*:736, 1964.
274. Shoskes, M., Kampel, L. J., Moss, J., Levinstone, B. and Ribot, S.: The use of artificial renal dialysis techniques for the removal of bilirubin in the dog, *J. Newark Beth Israel Hosp.* *14*:95, 1963.
275. Ewy, G. A., Pabico, R. C., Maher, J. F. and Mintz, D. H.: Lactate acidosis associated with phenformin therapy and localized tissue hypoxia. Report of a case treated by hemodialysis, *Ann. Internal Med.* *59*:878, 1963.
276. Westervelt, Jr., F. B., Owen, Jr., J. A., Hornbaker, Jr., J. H. and Gorsuch, T. L.: Lactic acidosis. A case treated with THAM and hemodialysis, *Virginia Med. Monthly* *93*:251, 1966.
277. Jørgensen, H. E.: *Haemodialysis. Experimental and Clinical Studies on the Skeggs-Leonards Haemodialyzer with a Follow-up.* Munksgaard, Copenhagen, 1967, p. 209.
278. Jurgesen, J. C.: Dialysis for lactic acidosis, *New Engl. J. Med.* *278*:1350, 1968.
279. Horiuchi, T., Suzuki, H., Ishitoya, T. and Taguchi, Y.: Correction of severe metabolic acidosis by peritoneal dialysis in cyanotic babies, *Tohoku J. Exptl. Med.* *94*:347, 1968.
280. Thölen, H., Stricker, E., Feer, H., Massini, M. A. and Staub, H.: Über die anwendung der Künstlichen Niere bei Schizophrenie und Myasthenia gravis, *Deut. Med. Wochschr.* *85*:1012, 1960.
281. Jutzler, G. A., Neuheisel, S. and Schmid, P.: Experimental treatment of acute intermittent porphyria by extracorporeal hemodialysis, *German Med. Monthly* *9*:402, 1964.
282. Mahoney, C. P., Manning, G. B. and Hickman, R. O.: Hemodialysis in a patient with cystinosis. Effects on amino acid and bone metabolism, *Am. J. Diseases Children* *112*:65, 1966.
283. Moyo, C. T. B., Dosseter, J. B. and MacLean, L. D.: Hemodialysis in the treatment of shock, *J. Surg. Res.* *4*:380, 1964.
284. Plachecka, M., Gutniak, O., Sawulis, J. and Kopeć, M.: Zastosowanie hemodializy pozaustrojowej w przypadku ostrej porfirii przerywanej, *Polski Arch. Med. Wewnet.* *38*:531, 1967.
285. Reese, H. A., Goldberg, A., Cochran, A. L., Williams, M.

J. and Donald, K. W.: Renal hemodialysis in porphyria, *Lancet 1*:191, 1967.
286. Last, P. M.: Haemodialysis in acute porphyria. *Med. J. Australia 2*:749, 1963.
287. Pringle, A.: Discussion, *Proc. Europ. Dialysis Transplant. Assoc. 1*:45, 1964.
288. Eales, L., Dawdle, E. B., Saunders, S. J. and Sweeney, G. D.: Presentation of patients with porphyria, *S. African J. Lab. Clin. Med. 9*:162, 1963.
289. Tyler, F. H.: Hyperosmolar coma, *Am. J. Med. 45*:485, 1968.
290. Morgan, A. G., Bennett, J. M. and Pollack, A.: Mannitol retention during diuretic treatment of barbiturate and salicylate overdosage, *Quart. J. Med. 37*:589, 1968.
291. Kiley, J. E., Barenberg, R. L. and Conklin, W. H.: Dialysance of tritium with the twin-coil artificial kidney, *Clin. Res. 6*:294, 1958.
292. Jφrgensen, H. E.: *Haemodialysis. Experimental and Clinical Studies on the Skeggs-Leonards Haemodialyzer with a Follow-up.* Munksgaard, Copenhagen, 1967, p. 209.
293. Lemmon, W. M., Hirose, T., O'Connor, R. A. and Bailey, C. P.: Congestive heart failure relief by renal dialysis, *J. Am. Med. Assoc. 174*:2124, 1960.
294. Stewart, J. H. and Neale, F. C.: Dialysis: A comparison of the efficiency of peritoneal dialysis with the artificial kidney, *Med. J. Australia 2*:210, 1966.
295. Mailloux, L. U., Swartz, C. D., Onesti, G., Heider, C., Ramirez, O. and Brest, A. N.: Peritoneal dialysis for refractory congestive heart failure, *J. Am. Med. Assoc. 199*:873, 1967.
296. Danzig, L. E.: Dynamics of thiocyanate dialysis. The artificial kidney in the therapy of thiocyanate intoxication, *New Engl. J. Med. 252*:49, 1955.
297. Hockmuth, R. E., Faber, L. C. and Mason, E. E.: Extracorporeal dialysis in renal failure, *J. Iowa Med. Soc. 52*:199, 1962.
298. Giuliano, H.: Intoxicacao aguda por anilina tratada com exsanguino-transfusao e diályse peritoneal, *Hospital 68*:1377, 1965.
299. Mengele, K., Schwarzmeier, J. and Schmidt, P.: Clinical aspects and studies of erythrocyte metabolism during poisoning with sodium chlorate, *Intern. Z. Klin. Pharmakol. Therapy Toxikol. 2*:120, 1969.
300. Knight, R. K., Trounce, J. R. and Cameron, J. S.: Suicidal chlorate poisoning treated with peritoneal dialysis, *Brit. Med. J. 3*:601, 1967.
301. Klendshoj, N. C., Burke, W. J., Anthone, R. and Anthone, S.: Chlorate poisoning, *J. Am. Med. Assoc. 180*:1133, 1962.
302. Hockmuth, R. E., Faber, L. C. and Mason, E. E.: Extracorporeal dialysis in renal failure, *J. Iowa Med. Soc. 52*:199, 1962.
303. Selivanova, L. N. and Vorob'Eva, E. N.: Toxicology of ammonium perchlorate during repeated action on the organism, *Farmakol. Toksikol. 32*:480, 1969.
304. Gurr, F. W. and Scroggie, J. G.: Eucalyptus oil poisoning treated by dialysis and mannitol infusion, with an appendix on the analysis of biological fluids for alcohol and eucalyptol, *Australasian Ann. Med. 14*:238, 1965.
305. Segar, E.: Peritoneal dialysis in the treatment of boric acid poisoning, *New Engl. J. Med. 262*:798, 1960.
306. Wong, L. C., Heimbach, M. D., Truscott, D. R. and Duncan, D. B.: Boric acid poisoning: Report of 11 cases, *Can. Med. Assoc. J. 90*:1018, 1964.
307. Baliah, T., MacLeish, H. and Drummond, K. N.: Acute boric acid poisoning: Report of an infant successfully treated by peritoneal dialysis, *Can. Med. Assoc. J. 101*:166, 1969.
308. Walsh, E. N.: Chromate hazards in industry, *J. Am. Med. Assoc. 153*:1305, 1953.
309. Fritz, K. W., Böhm, P., Bantru, G. and Lowen, C. H.: Die akute gewerbliche Dichromatvergiftung und ihre Behundlung, *Klin. Wochschr. 38*:856, 1960.
310. Fristedt, B., Lindquist, B., Schütz, A. and Ovrum, P.: Survival in a case of acute oral chronic acid poisoning with acute renal failure, treated by haemodialysis, *Acta Med. Scand. 177*:153, 1965.
311. Kaufman, D. B., DiNicola, W. and McIntosh, R.: Acute potassium dichromate poisoning treated by peritoneal dialysis, *Am. J. Diseases Children 119*:374, 1970.
312. Chiesura, P. and Bonadonna, A.: On a case of acute renal insufficiency caused by chromic anhydride intoxication, *Minerva Nefrol. 15*:152, 1968.
313. Doherty, J. E. and Perkins, W. H.: Studies following intramuscular tritiated digoxin in human subjects, *Am. J. Cardiol. 15*:170, 1965.
314. Marcus, F. I., Kapadia, G. J. and Kapadia, G. G.: The metabolism of digoxin in normal subjects, *J. Pharmacol. Exptl. Therap. 145*:203, 1964.
315. Doherty, J. E., Perkins, W. H. and Wilson, M. C.: Studies with tritiated digoxin in renal failure, *Am. J. Med. 37*:536, 1964.
316. Marcus, F. I., Peterson, A., Sadel, A. F., Scully, J. and Kapadia, G. G.: Metabolism of tritiated digoxin in renal insufficiency in dogs and man, *J. Pharmacol. Exptl. Therap. 152*:372, 1966.
317. Doherty, J. E., Flannigan, W. J., Perkins, W. H. and Ackerman, G. L.: Studies with tritiated digoxin in anephric human subjects, *Circulation 35*:298, 1967.
318. Doherty, J. E., Flannigan, W. J., Patterson, R. M. and Dalrymple, G. V.: The excretion of tritiated digoxin in normal human volunteers before and after unilateral nephrectomy, *Circulation 40*:555, 1969.
319. Ackerman, G. L., Doherty, J. E. and Flannigan, W. J.: Peritoneal dialysis and hemodialysis of tritiated digoxin, *Ann. Internal Med. 67*:718, 1967.
320. Markham, T. N., Dodson, V. N. and Eckberg, D. L.: Peritoneal dialysis in quinine sulfate intoxication, *J. Am. Med. Assoc. 202*:1102, 1967.
321. Donadio, J. V., Whelton, A., Gilliland, P. F. and Cirksena, W. J.: Peritoneal dialysis in quinine intoxication, *J. Am. Med. Assoc. 204*:274, 1968.
322. McKenzie, I. F. C., Mathew, T. H. and Bailie, M. J.: Peritoneal dialysis in the treatment of quinine overdose, *Med. J. Australia 1*:58, 1968.
323. Frisius, H. and Beyer, K. H.: A severe quinine poisoning, Clinic, toxicology and therapy, *Arch. Toxikol. 24*:201, 1969.
324. Thomas, B. B.: Peritoneal dialysis and lysol poisoning, *Brit. Med. J. 3*:720, 1969.
325. Precht, K., Strangfeld, D. and Thielsch, E.: Hämodialyse bei Dinitro-ortho-Kresolvergiftung, *Deut. Gesundheit. 21*:781, 1966.
326. Driessen, W. N., Frederiks, P. W. and Mijdeveld, P. G.: Carbon tetrachloride poisoning, *Nederl. T. Geneesk. 113*:243, 1969.
327. Proudfoot, A. T. and MacDonald, R. H.: Infectious mononucleosis-like syndrome following hemodialysis for carbon tetrachloride poisoning, *Postgrad. Med. 44*:249, 1968.
328. Sukhinin, P. L., Shimanko, I. I. and Dagnev, V. N.: The use of peritoneal dialysis in the treatment of dichlorethane poisoning, *Klin. Med. (Moskva) 45*:65, 1967.
329. Ginn, H. E., Anderson, K. E., Mercier, R. K., Stevens, T. W. and Matter, B. J.: Camphor intoxication treated by lipid dialysis, *J. Am. Med. Assoc. 203*:230, 1968.
330. Thölen, H., Frohlich, T., Huber, F. and Massini, M. A.: Early haemodialysis in poisoning by Amanita phalloides, *German Med. Monthly 11*:89, 1966.
331. Frazier, D. B. and Carter, F. H.: Use of the artificial kidney in snakebite, *Calif. Med. 97*:177, 1962.
332. Dasgupta, B. R., Boroff, D. A. and Cheong, K.: Isolation of chromatographically pure toxin of Clostridium Botulinum Type B, *Biochem. Biophys. Res. Com. 32*:1057, 1930.
333. Montie, T. C., Montie, D. B. and Leon, S. A.: Isolation of toxic subunits from two murine-toxic proteins from Pasturella Pestis, *Biochem. Res. Commun. 33*:423, 1968.
334. Jones, E. M. and Williams, B.: Two cases of ergotamine poisoning in infants, *Brit. Med. J. 1*:466, 1966.
335. Galletti, P. M., Pasqualino, A. and Geering, R. G.: Hemodialysis in cancer chemotherapy, *Trans. Am. Soc. Artificial Internal Organs 12*:20, 1966.
336. Rogers, S.: Significance of dialysis against enzymes to the specific therapy of cancer and genetic deficiency diseases, *Nature, 220*:1321, 1968.
337. Galletti, P.: Personal communication, 1970.
338. Kokot, F., Kuska, J., Koziak, H. and Zazgornik, J.: Behavior of some plasma enzymes during extracorporeal hemodialysis, *Acta Med. Polski 8*:461, 1967.
339. Chukhrienko, D. P. and Liul'Ko, A. V.: Extrarenal hemodialysis in carbon monoxide poisoning, *Vrachebnoe Delo 12*:18, 1968.
340. Oreopoulos, D. G. and McEvoy, J.: Diquat poisoning, *Postgrad. Med. 45*:635, 1969.
341. Stoddart, J. C., Parkin, J. M. and Wynne, N. A.: Orphenadrine poisoning. A case report, *Brit. J. Anaesthesiol. 40*:789, 1968.

From the Renal and Electrolyte Division, Department of Medicine, Georgetown University School of Medicine, Washington, D. C., and the Editorial Office, TRANSACTIONS, American Society for Artificial Internal Organs, c/o Georgetown University School of Medicine, Washington, D. C. Supported in part by grants from the Pharmaceutical Manufacturers Association Foundation, The John A. Hartford Foundation, the Georgetown Kidney Research Fund, and a resolution of support from the membership of the American Society for Artificial Internal Organs.
Dr. John F. Maher has played a major role in the compilation of former reviews. Subsequent to the 1969 edition, Dr. Maher has moved to become Director of the Nephrology Division at the University of Missouri Medical School, Columbia, Missouri. The Editor wishes to express his appreciation to Dr. Maher for past contributions. Miss Joan P. Ryan assisted in the preparation of the current manscript.

23

Drug interference with diagnostic tests

by Vincent E. Bouchard and J. Edward Bell

The various diagnostic tests available to today's medical practitioners represent an important aid in the diagnosis and treatment of many diseases. Indeed, the assessment of treatment including drugs is often measured utilizing one or more laboratory tests. Test results often confirm a physician's impression of a particular diagnosis or they may reveal a disorder which the physician had not considered. Hospitalized patients usually receive a series of routine laboratory tests which include serology and urinalyses. These tests are relatively easy to perform and often uncover common disorders such as diabetes or anemia. Modern laboratory equipment now allows for simultaneous measurements of several tests requiring but one sample from the patient.

Laboratory tests are important tools in the diagnosis of disease; they also serve as useful parameters for monitoring the course of a patient's progress through his hospital stay. Monitoring the effects of drugs on patients has become a responsibility of many pharmacists. With this responsibility comes the necessity for an understanding of laboratory tests, their relationship to a variety of disorders and to drugs being administered to patients. This latter consideration is important since many drugs can affect test results with the possibility of producing an erroneous diagnosis. The problem is complex and represents the main consideration of this chapter.

In general, diagnostic tests are attempts to measure the level or the presence or absence of

CHECK TESTS DESIRED ☒ MERCY HOSPITAL, PITTSBURGH, PA.
DEPARTMENT OF PATHOLOGY–CLINICAL CHEMISTRY

PATIENT IDENTIFICATION

NURSE: DATE: A.M. P.M.

CLINICAL IMPRESSIONS:

Check Test	Result	Check Test	Result	Check Test	Result		Glucose Tolerance Test	Blood	Urine
Acetone		Fibrinogen GM %		Potassium Meq/L.			Fasting		
Acetyl Cholinesterase		Glucose MGM %		Osmolality			½ Hour		
Amylase		GOT		Protein Bound Iodine Microgram %			1 Hour		
Bilirubin Total MGM %		GPT		T_4 by Column Microgram %			2 Hours		
Bilirubin Conj. MGM %		HBD		Prothrombin	Spec.	Control	3 Hours		
BSP Retention (45 min.)		LDH					4 Hours		
Calcium MGM %		Lipase		Time	Sec.	Sec.	5 Hours		
Cephal. Floc.		Magnesium MGM %		pH Arterial			6 Hours		
Chloride Meq/L.		Phosphatase, Alkaline		pCO_2 Arterial mm Hg			OTHER TESTS		
Cholesterol Total MGM %		Phosphatase, Prostatic Acid		pO_2 Arterial mm Hg					
CPK		Phosphorus, Inorganic MGM %		Sodium Meq/L.					
CO_2 Content Meq/L.		Protein, Serum GM %		Triglyceride					
Creatinine MGM %		Albumin GM %		Urea Nitrogen MGM %					
Diastase		Globulin GM %		Uric Acid MGM %					

CLINICAL CHEMISTRY Form No. 205 (Rev. 5-71)

Reported (Date)______at______A.M. P.M.______ Technician

Figure 1. Clinical chemistry form

chemical constituents in the body. Disease states can alter these levels from "normal" or from levels obtained in patients without some disease state. Laboratory "normals," which in most instances are ranges of values, are obtained by measuring a specific chemical in a group of individuals considered to be healthy. Statistical calculations are used to obtain means, standard deviations and boundaries of normality. Since testing procedures may vary from one laboratory to another, normals or ranges of normality may also vary. It becomes important then to know the specific procedure used by a given laboratory and the normals associated with that procedure.

Ordering Tests

One of the more tangible events by which the hospitalized patient assesses his care is the observation that "they are doing tests." In most cases it is the physician who initiates the order for a test. He usually does this by writing a request that the test be performed. He may simply write the request in the order section of the patient's chart or he may complete a laboratory form himself. In most hospitals it is a nurse or clerk who transfers the physician's order from the chart to a laboratory order form. A typical order form is shown in Figure 1. Several copies of the form are sent to the laboratory along with the patient's sample (blood, urine, sputum, feces, etc.). When the test is completed laboratory personnel indicate the results on a copy of the order form and return it to the nursing unit. These forms are placed in the patient's chart and become a permanent part of his medical record. In many hospitals the "normals" for each test are printed on the laboratory forms. This is helpful to those who are initiating a program of clinical practice.

Tests can be grouped in various ways. The physician often groups them mentally by organ or body system or disease process, *e.g.* heart—CPK, LDH, SGOT, SGPT; liver—SGOT, SGPT, BSP, bilirubin, serum alkaline phosphatase; pancreatitis—urine amylase, serum amylase, lipase and trypsin, calcium. Tests can also be grouped by the section or division of the laboratory which performs the test, *e.g.*, microbiology, hematology, serology, clinical chemistry, etc. Laboratory order forms are usually color coded according to the division of the laboratory responsible for performing the test.

It is important to recognize that there are very few test results which, on an individual basis, confirm or rule out the presence of a disease. The usual case is that a pattern of values for several tests will point to a particular diagnosis. The physician must consider a variety of test results, interpret the pattern which he is witnessing and pool this relative data with other patient information in attempting to arrive at a definitive diagnosis. Many physicians who did not "expect" a particular abnormal value are suspicious of the laboratory and will re-order the test. Drug-induced modifications of tests may be the cause of many of these unexpected abnormalities.

For many clinicians, ordering tests becomes a rapid reflex beginning with a few perfunctory observations at the bedside followed by a profound list of entries in the chart. A patient with a "palpable liver" might induce LFTS with BSP, protime, bleed time, clot time, serum electrophoresis, TP with A/G, liver scan, biopsy, SGOT, SGPT, etc.

It is difficult to assess the need for one or several tests in a given situation. Medical authors have, on many occasions, been critical of their colleagues who "shot gun" orders for laboratory tests. The high and increasing costs for performing many of today's sophisticated test procedures must be a consideration important to all who have responsibilities in this area of patient care.

EFFECTS OF DRUGS ON LABORATORY TESTS

Mechanisms by which drugs affect laboratory tests can be considered from either of two viewpoints. A knowledge of the specific mechanism responsible for a particular drug-induced laboratory test modification is essential for assessing the clinical significance of the effect and recommending appropriate action, if any, to be taken. However, a consideration of such particular mechanisms for each reported drug-laboratory test modification is beyond the scope of this chapter (refer to Hansten; Davidsohn and Henry). Mechanisms can, however, be categorized as to type and it is these types which will be considered with reference to specific modification mechanism by way of examples.

As discussed above, clinical laboratory tests are basically an attempt to measure the level (or presence or absence) of some chemical constituent of the body. Drugs, being chemicals with biologic (or pharmacologic) activity, can alter such measurements. A drug, or a metabolite, present in a sample obtained for analysis may be active in or interfere with the procedure used in the laboratory. Modification of this type is termed *chemical interference* and causes a false test result (false positive and false negative). If the circumstances warrant, a way of circumventing the interference may be sought or the drug discontinued and the test repeated.

On the other hand, a drug may, through a biologic effect, alter the level of a constituent to be analyzed. A sample subsequently obtained may contain increased or decreased levels of the substance. Such modification produces a true result (true positive or true negative). The alteration may be due to a *pharmacological* effect of the drug, an *adverse reaction* or an *allergic response.* The common feature is that the test result reported from the laboratory is correct and represents the actual level in that patient. However, the effect is drug-induced rather than disease-related. This is not to imply that the result may then be ignored. Consideration of the mechanism by which the drug produces the abnormal result and its clinical significance may draw attention to an adverse or allergic reaction which might otherwise go undetected for a period of time. A caution common to the use of many drugs is the monitoring of renal, hepatic and/or hemolytic function with common laboratory tests.

In all instances of suspected drug-induced modification, knowledge of the specific mechanism is essential to ascertain whether the result represents a true or false modification and to assess the clinical significance of the laboratory values. Several examples of specific mechanisms are given in the following discussion of the basic types of modification.

Chemical Interference

Chemical interference represents, in a sense, a self-limiting type of drug-induced laboratory test modification. If the interference is marked, it will usually be detected by the laboratory technician as the result will be grossly beyond the "usual" abnormal range and the report returned as "interfering substance" rather than a specific result. For example, such reports are common when, through oversight, measurement of protein-bound iodine (PBI) is attempted a day or two after the administration of iodine containing radiopaque media.

When less obvious interference is present, the fact that tests are generally run as groups or "batteries" prevents a false test result from leading to misdiagnosis. As discussed above, diagnosis of a specific disease is generally based on a pattern of abnormal results rather than a single value. When the modification of a test result is due to chemical interference, the effect is usually specific for one test in the battery. For example, erythromycin estolate causes a false elevation in glutamic-oxalacetic transaminase (SGOT). However, other tests for hepatic disease or cardiac damage will be normal if disease is not present. If, in a set of tests run as an organ or system battery, a single value does not fit the pattern established by the other results and the patient's clinical picture, it is usually not pursued.

If more than one test related to a particular organ or system is falsely abnormal, the pattern may point to a drug effect. For example, in the presence of thyroid disease, PBI and T-3 uptake results deviate from normal in the same direction. Iodine contamination, however, causes an *elevated* PBI and a decrease in T-3 uptake. Thus, a drug effect is readily recognized. (Evaluation of thyroid function in such a situation is discussed below.)

When a falsely abnormal result is obtained on a screening test, the battery associated with that organ or system may be ordered in the belief that disease is present. Essentially normal results will be obtained with the exception of the screening test which is generally repeated as part of the group. It may be argued that time and expense have been wasted. However, even if the clinician is aware of a drug effect, it would be advisable to perform at least one of the other tests, if not the battery, to insure that the abnormal result is due *solely* to drug interference, particularly if there was an initial suspicion of disease in the organ or system associated with that test.

While the foregoing discussion may lead to the conclusion that chemical interference should not be a significant problem, there is another aspect to consider. A falsely abnormal result, not recognized as such, may be diagnostically perplexing to the physician. Depending on the test's potential significance to the patient's condition and the physician's curiosity and diagnostic perseverance, a series of fruitless and unnecessary analyses may be undertaken. If the abnormal result is explained by chemical interference, such information can be of considerable importance to the physician and patient.

When accurate evaluation is necessary, there are several alternatives. Choosing the most appropriate is contingent on an understanding of the specific mechanism responsible for the modification.

It may be possible to measure the same substance using an alternate analytical procedure not affected by the drug. Obviously, knowledge of the chemistry of the procedure and the way in which the drug interferes is necessary.

Many substances can be measured by more than one technique. If the analytical or biochemical bases are different, one procedure may be used when chemical interference occurs with the other.

For example, PBI measures iodine bound to serum proteins. The test is valid only if the assumption that all the iodine so measured is present as endogenous tri-iodothyronine and thyroxine and that thyroxine-binding globulin (TBG) levels are normal. Exogenous iodides and iodine compounds, such as iodine-containing radiopaque media, if present in the patient's blood, will precipitate with the serum protein and be measured in the analytic reaction, giving a false result. Alternately, the quantitation of T-4 (thyroxine) by the Murphy-Patee procedure can be used to evaluate thyroid function. In this test, I-131 labeled T-4 is added to the sample and the amount which is taken up (bound) by the TBG in the sample is measured. The patient's T-4 level may then be calculated. Since the Murphy-Patee procedure is specific for T-4, interference by exogenous iodine compounds is circumvented.

The ability to utilize alternate procedures may be limited by the equipment available in a given laboratory. Additionally, accuracy and reproducibility (usually with standards provided by another laboratory) and, in some instances, range of normal limits for a given procedure should be established independently in each laboratory. Even if this is not required, the necessity of running simultaneous controls or establishing a standard curve may represent more effort than the test is worth to the physician. However, if a laboratory is not able to offer a given procedure, a sample can usually be sent out for analysis by a commercial laboratory.

Where an alternate procedure is not available, consideration can be given to discontinuing the interfering drug and, if necessary, substituting other therapy.

If treatment can be interpreted, knowledge of the time required for clearance of the drug or its metabolites from the body is desirable. Thus, sufficient time between discontinuing the drug and obtaining the sample for analysis can be permitted to elapse.

The specific mechanism of the drug interference should also be considered, in addition to clearance time, when the clinical situation requires continued therapy with an alternate drug. Obviously, the drug substituted should produce the same therapeutic effect as the former. However, potential for causing the same interference must also be evaluated. A drug's ability to react or interfere with a given analytical procedure is usually related to its basic chemical structure or the presence of a functional group in the molecule. In utilizing reference material, a particular drug not mentioned as interfering with a given laboratory procedure does not, in itself, necessarily mean the drug does not interfere. Lacking specific information in the literature, a drug which will produce the same therapeutic effect and is of a different chemical structure represents a reasonable alternative to one that is known to produce chemical interference.

Pharmacologic Effect

The use of the term, pharmacological effect, as a type of drug-induced modification of laboratory test results has several connotations. It implies explanation of the mechanism of the effect by the drug's currently known pharmacology, *i.e.*, consistent occurrence of the effect from patient to patient (magnitude of the effect being dependent on dose and patient variability) and that the result reported by the laboratory is the true value. The clinical significance of a drug induced alteration of the level of a substance in the body is related to the nature of the substance and its significance to the patient's condition. The situation may only require knowledge that the effect is drug- rather than disease-related. If necessary, taking an alternate approach to evaluating function of the organ or system in question can be considered. Third, the fact that the substance is present in abnormal quantities may, in itself, have adverse implications to the patient's condition, requiring substitution of a drug which does not have the pharmacological property responsible for producing the abnormal diagnostic test.

The elevation of PBI by estrogens is an example of a situation not requiring change of therapy. Estrogens cause an increase in TBG and, therefore, an abnormal protein-*bound* iodine level. Since the effect on the T-3 uptake is opposite (decreased), a drug effect is easily recognized. If thyroid function is normal, the quantity of biologically active (unbound) thyroid hormone remains within the normal range and the patient is euthyroid.

On the other hand, diagnosis of thyroid disease may be required in the presence of a drug effect. In this example, T-4 by Murphy-Patee cannot be utilized because TBG levels are altered. However, computation of the Free T-4 Index (FT-4I) gives a reasonably accurate assessment of the thyroid status. The arithmetic involved cancels the opposite deviations of PBI and T-3 uptake, resulting in a correction for the effect of the estrogens.

Hypophosphatemia and hypercalcemia due to intensive antacid therapy represents a situation which calls for change of therapy. Aluminum hydroxide-containing antacids bind dietary phosphorus as insoluble aluminum phosphate. The decreased phosphate absorbtion results in hypophosphatemia which causes a secondary increase in serum calcium. The hypercalcemia can be symptomatic. Substitution of aluminum phosphate gel will alleviate the problem. While this situation is relatively straightforward, it should be noted that proper corrective action is based on recognition of a drug-induced laboratory test modification. Otherwise, significant time and expense may be involved in attempting to elucidate the etiology of the observed hypercalcemia.

Adverse Reactions

The alteration of laboratory parameters as manifestations of adverse reactions is probably the most common type of drug-induced laboratory test modification. These, as well as many of the pharmacological effect type, are properly considered adverse reactions rather than laboratory test modifications. Diagnostically, however, importance must be given to recognition of possible relationships between drugs and the abnormal tests. The association, if established, is generally secondary in that the test results reflect the presence of drug-induced disease. Certainly, a low hemoglobin and hematocrit will be found in anemia secondary to drugs. Drug-induced hepatotoxicity or renal damage will be manifest in abnormal diagnostic tests as well as symptoms and physical signs.

In some instances the drug may be several steps removed from the test result etiologically as, for example, decreased hemoglobin and hematocrit secondary to ulcer disease caused by a drug being administered to the patient.

Prospectively, judicious use of drugs often requires that appropriate laboratory tests be performed periodically to detect incipient adverse reactions. Retrospectively, however, drug therapy is often overlooked as a possible etiology of the disease being evaluated and should certainly be considered when abnormal laboratory results, consistent with an adverse reaction to one of the patient's drugs, are obtained.

In evaluating such a possibility, assumptions based on simple one to one relationships should be avoided. Superficially, a drug may be incriminated. However, the mechanism of the specific abnormality known to be produced by the drug may be inconsistent with the clinical laboratory data regarding the patient's problem.

For example, lists of drugs having the potential for decreasing hemoglobin and/or hematocrit can be found in various references. But the drugs included may cause various anemias such as blood loss, marrow depression, folate deficiency (antagonism) or hemolysis. Furthermore, with blood loss, the route (gastrointestinal ulceration, hematuria) must be considered and with hemolytic anemias, the particular type (G-6-PD deficiency, Coomb's reaction).

Obviously, the details of the suspected drug effect must be consistent with the patient's clinical picture before a causal relationship can be assumed. In addition to mechanism, other available data in the literature (such as dose, duration of therapy and predisposing factors) should be considered, if applicable.

The same reasoning also applies to the evaluation of possible abnormalities mediated by chemical interferences, pharmacologic effect or allergic response. In short, all available data should be considered before a decision is made.

The basis for distinguishing adverse reaction from pharmacological effect is that in a clinical sense, drug-induced diseases represented by the former and the properties of the drug responsible for them are usually considered *adverse reactions* or effects rather than one of the drug's *pharmacological* effects.

Corrective action depends on the clinical significance of the adverse effect. If alternate therapy is indicated, obviously a drug should be selected which has little, if any, potential for producing the same effect. If it has been elucidated, knowledge of the specific mechanism of the adverse reaction may be helpful in this regard. Comparison of this with the known effects of possible alternate drugs may provide a basis for selection. On the other hand, it may be necessary to rely on the fact that the reaction has not been *reported* for a particular drug. This assumption should be made cautiously and be based on an adequate review of the literature.

Allergy

Laboratory test modifications due to drug allergy could be considered a sub-group of the adverse reaction type. However, the theoretical distinction of an antibody-mediated response has additional practical implications both diagnostically and therapeutically.

In some instances, it is possible to demonstrate antibodies to drug *in vitro*. Examples include several of both the hemolytic anemias characterized by a positive Coomb's reaction and the drug-induced thrombocytopenias. If available, such tests can be valuable in evaluating a drug as a possible etiology.

Other allergic reactions may be associated with an elevated eosinophil count. Eosinophilia usually occurs with phenothiazine-induced hepatitis.

Alternate therapy requires selection of an antigenically dissimilar substitute. In patients allergic to it, the substitute again may itself be capable of the same effect. However, this does not contraindicate its use for a given individual if it is unrelated chemically to the offending drug in that patient.

Caution is indicated in the use of pharmacologically different, but chemically similar drugs in a patient who has had such a response. Chemical relationships between drugs of different "groups" are often not considered. For example, Coomb's positive hemolytic anemia has been reported with the antibacterial sulfonamides, the sulfonamide diuretics and the sulfonylureas. Cross-sensitivity to these compounds may be exhibited by the same individual.

Diagnostic Tests and Clinical Pharmacy Practice

It is obvious that a working knowledge of the common diagnostic tests and their relationship to disease states is an important asset to the clinical pharmacy practitioner. Indeed, a meaningful assessment of a patient's clinical situation would be impossible without an understanding of laboratory test data.

The phenomena of drug-induced modifications of test data are complex. The potentialities are legion. The modifications reported in the literature represent an unknown portion of all the possibilities. The magnitude of the problem with respect to data creates an almost impossible task for the physician who is attempting to consider all possibilities which might account for test abnormalities. A pharmacist monitoring a patient's therapy program is faced with this problem.

Given a pharmacist-patient-physician situation where the pharmacist is responsible for monitoring the patient's drug therapy, and where the pharmacist has access to the patient's records, and where the pharmacist and physician work in concert regarding decisions concerning the patient's medication program—what alternatives are available to the pharmacist which would insure that he recognize the potential interference problems in a given patient situation? The following are suggested:

1. From personal knowledge, the pharmacist recognizes a potential interference.
2. The pharmacist suspects a potential interference and confirms the suspicion by recourse to the literature.
3. The pharmacist checks all possibilities on a one-to-one basis—drug and laboratory test, drug and drug—by recourse to the literature.
4. The pharmacist has a record system (manual) which responds to the patient's drug and laboratory test profile and alerts him to potential interferences.
5. The pharmacist has a record system (automated) which responds to the patient's drug and laboratory test profile and alerts him to potential interferences.

Each alternative will be considered briefly.

Personal Knowledge

There is a small group of common interferences which have become the prime examples used to illustrate the importance of the drug-laboratory test and the drug interaction problems, *e.g.*, the potentiation of warfarin by sulfonamide, a positive Coomb's test with cephalothin, the inhibition of tetracycline absorption by antacids or milk.

These examples occur frequently, are often clinically significant and occasionally warrant alteration in drug therapy. However, they represent a very small portion of the potential problems in a typical patient situation. It is clearly impossible for a pharmacist, from personal knowledge, to be informed of all potentialities in a variety of drug-laboratory test profiles.

Suspicion Confirmed in the Literature

This procedure is certainly a sound one and is warranted in any case where uncertainty prevails. The significant limitation is the amount of time required should this procedure be used for comprehensive monitoring. The variety of tables available to us makes this job simpler than reviewing original articles or textbooks.

Checking All Possibilities in the Literature

The time required to check all possibilities in a large number of patient situations by recourse to the literature is clearly impractical.

Manual Record System

There have been several reports of manual record systems (usually card files) which permit a relatively rapid checking procedure for potential interferences. However, this procedure usually requires the written transfer of information from patient's charts to intermediate records for subsequent checking.

Automated Record System

The experiences of the clinical pharmacy staff at Mercy Hospital of Pittsburgh, with the previous alternatives, suggested the development of a system which would require a minimum amount of pharmacist time, little or no written transfer of information and a method which would bring reported interferences to the pharmacist's attention when the interferences were a potentiality in a specific patient situation.

Drug interference with diagnostic tests represents a unique complication of modern drug therapy with which the pharmacist should be identified as the individual with expertise in this area. The clinical significance of many drug-test combinations is widely scattered. The very nature of this randomness demands someone who has access to the reported potentialities and who has the ability to assess a particular patient's situation in light of his entire clinical picture. The decision to alert the physician to a potential or actual problem must be an informed decision. The judgments required of the clinical pharmacy practitioner are highly sophisticated. This is consistent with the levels of sophistication apparent in all facets of modern medical practice.

References

1. Goodale, R. H. and Widman, F. K.: *Clinical Interpretation of Laboratory Tests,* F. A. Davis Co., Philadelphia, Pa., 1970.
2. Hansten, P. D.: *Drug Interactions,* Lea and Febiger, Philadelphia, Pa., 1971.
3. Garb, S.: *Clinical Guide to Undesirable Drug Interactions and Interferences,* Springer Publishing Co., Inc., New York, 1971.
4. Garb, S.: *Laboratory Tests in Common Use,* ed. 5, Springer Publishing Co., Inc., New York, NY, 1971.
5. Collins, R. D.: *Illustrated Manual of Laboratory Diagnosis,* J. B. Lippincott Co., Philadelphia, Pa., 1968.
6. Hartshorn, E. A.: *Handbook of Drug Interactions,* Donald E. Francke, Cincinnati, Ohio, 1970.
7. Davidsohn, I. and Henry, J. B.: *Todd-Sanford Clinical Diagnosis by Laboratory Methods,* W. B. Saunders Co., Philadelphia, Pa., 1969.
8. Wallach, J.: *Interpretation of Diagnostic Tests,* Little, Brown and Co., Boston, Mass., 1970.

24

Significance of selected laboratory tests

by Dorothy L. Smith

Laboratory tests play a significant role in the total therapy of the patient. The physician bases his diagnosis, prognosis and treatment on data collected from the history of the patient, from the physical examination and from laboratory procedures. The following chapter is designed to serve as a brief introduction to the more common laboratory tests performed in a hospital and to assist pharmacists practicing in the clinical area. Only if the pharmacist has an understanding of the significance of the various laboratory procedures can he adequately relate drug therapy to laboratory test results. This chapter presents the significance of common laboratory tests rather than the technical procedures involved in performing them. The material is not proposed to be all-inclusive and the reader should refer to a comprehensive textbook on laboratory examinations in clinical diagnosis when further information is required.

The data are arranged alphabetically under each of the following headings:

1. Tests performed on blood
2. Tests performed on urine
3. Tests performed on cerebrospinal fluid
4. Tests performed on feces
5. Miscellaneous tests

Normal values for each of the tests appear in Table 1 in the middle of the chapter. It must be remembered that the normal value range will vary from one institution to another depending upon the individual differences of the laboratory personnel and the laboratory equipment.

TESTS PERFORMED ON BLOOD

Blood is a fluid which is representative of the whole body and is composed of a fluid portion, the plasma, in which are suspended the formed elements (red cells, platelets, and white cells). The type and number of circulating cells in blood uniquely changes in response to various stimuli. Many of the changes in response to disease are nonspecific; however, there is usually some deviation from normal in one of the measurable constituents in almost all diseases. This explains why most of the diagnostic laboratory tests currently used are entitled "blood tests."

Tests performed on the blood may be divided into three general areas.

1. Clinical chemistry tests
2. Hematologic tests
3. Miscellaneous tests

Clinical Chemistry Tests

The majority of chemical determinations are done on whole blood, plasma or serum. Some of the factors that influence the chemical composition of blood in diseases are alterations of permeability of membranes of the lungs, kidneys, and liver; accumulation of nitrogenous waste products; changes in the rate of formation or metabolism of these constituents; and the administration of certain drugs. One of the most valuable instruments in the clinical laboratory is the 12-channel SMA-12 AutoAnalyzer. This machine analyzes and prints on calibrated paper the levels of twelve blood constituents from a single serum specimen (*i.e.*, glucose, total bilirubin, albumin, alkaline phosphatase, urea nitrogen, uric acid, cholesterol, lactic dehydrogenase, total protein, glutamic oxaloacetic transaminase, calcium and inorganic phosphate).

Albumin Globulin; Total Protein; A/G Ratio. The normal range of albumin is 4-5.5 g %; for globulin, 1.5-3 g %; for total protein 6-8 g %; and the albumin-globulin (A/G) ratio is usually between 1.5:1 and 2.5:1. These tests are usually performed together. They may be useful in the diagnosis of kidney, liver, and some other diseases.

The main function of the serum albumin appears to be the maintenance of osmotic pressure of the blood. One of the functions of serum globulin is to assist in maintaining the osmotic pressure of the blood. Since the globulin molecule is several times as large as the albumin molecule, it is less efficient, gram for gram, in maintaining osmotic pressure. In certain diseases, the albumin may leak out of capillary walls while the larger globulin molecules are retained within the blood stream. The body may then compensate for loss of albumin by producing more globulin so that the globulin becomes responsible for a larger share of the osmotic pressure. Despite normal or even increased total dissolved protein in the serum, osmotic pressure may be less than normal because of the lesser effectiveness of globulin and result in edema.

In hemoconcentration due to dehydration from vomiting or diarrhea, the total protein increases and both the albumin and globulins increase in the same proportions so that the A/G ratio is unchanged. Globulins are increased in severe liver disease, multiple myeloma and certain infectious diseases.

A low albumin level is caused by increased loss of albumin in the urine, decreased formation or decreased protein intake. Severe hemorrhage may cause low serum protein levels because following the hemorrhage, the plasma volume is restored more quickly than the protein level.

Conditions in which the albumin-globulin ratio is lowered are chronic nephritis, lipoid nephrosis, liver disease, amyloid nephrosis and malnutrition.

Acid Phosphatase. This is a test to determine metastasizing carcinomas of the prostate. Normally, small amounts of acid phosphatase are found in the serum. A metastasizing prostate carcinoma releases the enzyme into the serum and increases the serum concentration markedly. Other conditions which produce elevated serum acid phosphatase levels include: Paget's disease, hyperparathyroidism, metastatic mammary carcinoma, multiple myeloma, renal insufficiency, osteogenesis imperfecta, thrombocytosis, arterial embolism, myocardial infarction, thrombophlebitis, pulmonary embolism, and sickle-cell crisis.

Alkaline Phosphatase. Alkaline phosphatase is present in high concentration in bone, and serum levels are elevated in growing children and in diseases associated with increased osteoblastic activity. There is normally a small amount of alkaline phosphatase in the serum. Since alkaline phosphatase is excreted into the bile, serum levels are increased in liver diseases associated with intrahepatic or extrahepatic obstruction of the biliary passages. Alkaline phosphatase elevation precedes bilirubin accumulation in early obstruction. Obstruction of the common duct causes mild elevation, but obstruction of the smaller biliary radicles causes far higher levels. The highest levels of all occur with primary biliary cirrhosis while ascending cholangitis and cholestatic hepatitis cause more moderate changes. Changes are relatively slight in infectious hepatitis and nonbiliary cirrhosis.

The levels are also elevated in hyperparathyroidism, osteitis deformans, osteomalacia, Goucher's disease, rickets, healing fractures, Boeck's sarcoid, hyperthyroidism (Grave's disease), leukemia, after the administration of large amounts of vitamin D and in pregnancy.

Ammonia. Ammonia is normally produced by bacterial action in the intestine and absorbed into the portal venous system. Most of the ammonia is removed from the portal circulation by the liver and converted into urea. As a result, the ammonia levels rise in severe liver disease. Blood ammonia determinations are used for evaluating the progress of severe liver damage.

Bilirubin Partition (Direct and Indirect van den Bergh Test). Bilirubin circulates in the blood in low concentrations. A small amount is directly excreted into the urine. The majority is excreted into the bile by the liver cells and passes into the intestines where it is bacterially reduced to urobilinogen. Urobilinogen is primarily excreted in the feces; however, some is reabsorbed into the blood and re-excreted by the liver as bilirubin or urobilinogen. The kidneys also excrete a small amount of absorbed urobilinogen into the urine.

Bilirubin is formed from hemoglobin of destroyed erythrocytes by the reticuloendothelial system and is normally found enroute to the liver for excretion. When the ability of the liver to excrete bilirubin is impaired by obstruction, it is believed that the excess circulating bilirubin is free of any attached protein: However, when the increase in circulating bilirubin is due to increased destruction of red blood cells (hemolysis), it is believed that the bilirubin is bound to protein. By measuring the amount of free bilirubin (direct) and the amount bound to protein (indirect), there is some indication as to whether the patient's illness is based on obstruction or hemolysis.

If most of the bilirubin is found on the direct test, the patient probably has an obstructive lesion. If most is found on the indirect test, the illness is probably hemolytic.

Bilirubin Total. When the destruction of red blood cells becomes excessive or when the liver is unable to secrete the ordinary quantities of bilirubin produced, the concentration in the serum rises. This test enables one to discover an increased concentration of serum bilirubin before jaundice appears.

Blood Sugar. The concentration of sugar (glucose) in the blood is maintained within a narrow range by four general mechanisms: (1) ability of the intestine to absorb glucose, (2) skeletal muscle mass, (3) ability of the liver to store and metabolize glycogen, and (4) production and release of insulin by the pancreas. Routine blood sugar determinations are performed on whole blood specimens and if plasma or serum is used, values will be higher by approximately 20 mg/100 ml than for whole blood. In evaluating a blood sugar level, it is important to consider whether venous or capillary blood was used because after a glucose load, the capillary blood levels are approximately 40 mg/100 ml higher than those of venous blood. It is also important to consider whether the patient is receiving an intravenous glucose supplement.

Fasting Blood Sugar (FBS). The blood glucose concentration rises following a meal and it is therefore essential that this test be run on fasting blood specimens rather than random samples. The test requires that the patient has not eaten for at least eight hours so that digestion is completed. It is for this reason that the blood specimen is usually drawn in the morning before breakfast. The "fasting state" signifies that the patient has not eaten any food including cream, sugar, tea, cola drinks or drugs that affect the blood glucose level, and has not experienced emotional disturbances that may release glucose into the blood.

Blood glucose levels are elevated in diabetes mellitus; hyperactivity of the thyroid, pituitary, and adrenal glands; pancreatitis; pancreatic carcinoma; meningitis; encephalitis; hemorrhage; and following administration of anesthetics. Blood glucose levels are lowered in hypothyroidism (myxedema and cretinism), hypopituitarism, hypoadrenalism, glycogen storage disease, and overtreatment of diabetes with insulin.

Glucose Tolerance Test. The glucose tolerance test usually gives more information than can be derived from a fasting blood sugar. This test is intended to assist in the diagnosis of doubtful or borderline cases of diabetes, but has no quantitative significance to severity of the diabetes or insulin requirement.

Blood specimens are taken fasting and ½ hour,

2 hours and 3 hours after ingestion of a predetermined amount of glucose. After ingestion and a lag period, the blood sugar curve rises sharply to a peak, usually in 15-60 minutes. The curve then falls steadily, but more slowly, reaching normal levels at 2 hours. It is assumed that the subsequent rise and fall of the blood sugar is due mainly to production of insulin in response to hyperglycemia and that the degree of insulin response is mirrored in the behavior of the blood glucose.

The intravenous test is somewhat more sensitive than the oral since the factor of absorption from the gastrointestinal tract is not involved and is of value in conditions characterized by poor intestinal absorption or vomiting after glucose ingestion.

An increase in the blood level after glucose ingestion (a diminished glucose tolerance) is most commonly seen in diabetes mellitus.

Blood Urea Nitrogen (BUN). Urea is the chief end product of protein metabolism and is the chief component of nonprotein nitrogenous material in the blood. From its hepatic origin, urea travels through the blood to the kidneys for urinary excretion. In certain kidney disorders the ability to excrete urea may be impaired so that the concentration of urea nitrogen in the blood increases. The protein content of the diet will also influence the quantity of urea in the blood since the concentration of urea is directly related to protein metabolism. *Uremia* is the term for the condition in which urea is found in the blood in increased amounts.

The most common cause of elevated BUN values is renal disease, either acute or chronic. Other causes of elevated BUN values include urinary obstruction, intestinal obstruction, lead poisoning, cardiac failure, and conditions characterized by increased protein catabolism (*i.e.*, burns with subsequent fluid loss, massive hemorrhage, infarction, pancreatitis, severe diabetic ketoacidosis and far-advanced carcinoma).

Calcium. Approximately one-half of the serum calcium is combined with proteins in the serum and the remainder is in a diffusible form. Elevated levels of calcium are found in hyperparathyroidism, excessive administration of vitamin D, and multiple myeloma. Low values are found in hypoparathyroidism, rickets, osteomalacia, steatorrhea, and advanced renal failure.

Carbon Dioxide Content and Combining Power. Carbon dioxide may be determined as the *CO_2-content* which is the actual plasma or serum content when analyzed anaerobically, or as the *CO_2-combining power* which is the CO_2 content of the plasma after equilibration with a gas of fixed carbon dioxide partial pressure of 40 mm. These tests estimate the plasma bicarbonate which is used to measure the acid-base balance of the body. Changes in CO_2-combining power do not always represent changes in pH of the blood since the latter depends on the ratio and not on the absolute amounts of basic and acidic substances. Measurement of the CO_2-combining power does not require anaerobic handling of blood specimens; however, the results are less accurate than measurement of total CO_2.

An increase in CO_2-combining power is usually a manifestation of alkalosis while a decrease is usually a manifestation of acidosis. High CO_2-combining power is usually found in excessive vomiting; drainage of the stomach with loss of hydrochloric acid; excessive sodium bicarbonate intake in the presence of poor kidney function; excessive administration of ACTH or cortisone; and hypoventilation. Low CO_2-combining power is usually found in diabetic acidosis, severe diarrhea or drainage of intestinal fluids, certain kidney diseases and hyperventilation.

Chloride. Chloride is an anion of the extracellular fluid and is found in serum plasma, cerebrospinal fluid, tissue fluid, and urine. The test for chloride is routinely performed on plasma or serum and not on the whole blood since two-thirds of the anion is present in the plasma and only one-third in the red blood cells. Chlorides are involved in the maintenance of normal osmotic relationships, acid-base balance, and water balance of the body. There is a reciprocal relationship between the chloride and bicarbonate anions of the extracellular fluid.

A decrease in blood chlorides (hypochloremia) is seen in diabetic acidosis, Addison's disease, heat exhaustion, excessive vomiting and diarrhea and following certain surgical procedures. An elevation in blood chlorides (hyperchloremia) is seen in Cushing's syndrome, complete renal shutdown, hyperventilation and dehydration.

Cholesterol. The liver excretes esterified cholesterol into the plasma. Normally, one-half to three-quarters of the serum cholesterol is present in esterified form and a decline in the percentage of esters signifies hepatocellular disease, notably acute hepatitis and active cirrhosis.

Hypercholesteremia, with a normal percentage of esters accompanies obstructive jaundice, diabetes mellitus, hypothyroidism, and the nephrotic syndrome. Low levels of total cholesterol, with a normal percentage of esters, accompanies hyperthyroidism and chronic malnutrition.

Creatinine. Creatinine is derived from muscle creatinine and phosphocreatine. Creatine in muscle is phosphorylated to phosphocreatine which is an important compound for storing muscular energy. When energy is needed for metabolic processes, phosphocreatine is broken down to creatinine. The quantity of creatine converted to creatinine is related directly to the total body muscle mass and is unaffected by variations in the rate of protein catabolism. Creatinine is excreted primarily by glomerular filtration and when the filtration rate falls, the serum creatinine level rises. An elevated blood creatinine level is usually indicative of depressed renal function.

Fasting Blood Sugar (FBS)—
see Blood Sugar

Globulin—
see Albumin Globulin

Glucose Tolerance Test—
see Blood Sugar

Inorganic Phosphorus—
see Phosphorus, Inorganic

Lactic Dehydrogenase (LDH). This test is used in the diagnosis of myocardial infarction. Lactic hydrogenases are enzymes found in serum and in several organs including the heart. Therefore, an increase in levels of lactic dehydrogenase is not specific but in conjunction with other tests it can help diagnose the presence of myocardial infarction. After an infarction occurs, the serum level rises in 6-12 hours and persists 1-3 weeks.

The lactic dehydrogenase is elevated in myocardial infarction, acute leukemia, malignant lymphoma, megaloblastic anemia, sickle-cell anemia, liver disease and extensive carcinomas.

Magnesium. A magnesium deficiency results in a state of tetany which in appearance is indistinguishable from the tetany of low calcium.

Serum magnesium levels are increased in acute and chronic renal disease, liver disease, and diabetic coma. The levels are decreased in Addison's disease, malabsorption syndrome, diarrhea, chronic alcoholism and occasionally in pancreatitis.

Non-Protein Nitrogen (NPN). This is a kidney function test. Approximately half of the nonprotein nitrogen is usually urea which is normally excreted by the kidney. The remainder consists of amino acids, ammonia, creatine, creatinine and uric acid. When kidney function is markedly diminished, the urea and therefore, the nonprotein nitrogen level in the blood rises. This measurement is less accurate than the urea nitrogen test.

Non-protein nitrogen levels are elevated in conditions of decreased kidney function, eclampsia, and hepatic failure.

pH. The normal blood pH ranges from 7.35-7.45. The blood pH is elevated in hypoventilation, severe diarrhea, Addison's disease, and diabetic acidosis. The blood pH is lowered in Cushing's syndrome, hyperventilation, and excessive vomiting.

Phosphatase, Acid—
see Acid Phosphatase

Phosphatase, Alkaline—
see Alkaline Phosphatase

Phosphorus, Inorganic. Phosphorus in the blood exists as (1) inorganic phosphorus, (2) lipid phosphorus, and (3) organic or ester phosphorus. Determinations are usually made only of inorganic phosphorus and of lipid phosphorus. The concentration of calcium in the serum and body fluids tends to vary inversely with the concentration of inorganic phosphorus.

The inorganic phosphate level is increased in severe kidney disease, hypoparathyroidism, acromegaly, and excessive vitamin D intake. Phosphorus levels are decreased in rickets and hyperparathyroidism.

Potassium. Potassium is essentially an intracellular cation, and the extracellular concentration is approximately the same as that in the blood. The serum potassium concentration is often not an accurate measurement of intracellular potassium and a patient may have a potassium deficiency even when the serum potassium is normal. For practical purposes, potassium depletion may be suspected from an abnormally low serum potassium in combination with characteristic electrocardiogram changes or the presence of alkalosis. A marked decrease in serum potassium may cause cardiac arrythmias and muscle weakness. A marked increase in serum potassium produces a series of electrocardiographic changes and arrythmias. There may also be depression, lethargy and coma.

The only common situation of high potassium values is renal shutdown with failure to produce adequate urine quantities and, therefore, an inability to excrete enough potassium. Increased serum potassium levels may be found in conditions of severe cell damage and destruction, adrenal cortical deficiency and hypoventilation.

Decreased serum potassium levels occur in severe diarrhea, periodic familial paralysis, chronic kidney disease, hyperfunction of the adrenal cortex and following the administration of insulin and glucose in diabetes without supplementary potassium. Besides being produced by alkalosis, hypokalemia can itself lead to or cause a tendency toward alkalosis. Potassium depletion usually caused by the use of diuretic agents or electrolyte manipulations may sensitize the heart to digitalis glycosides and may produce arrythmias.

Serum Transaminases. Transaminases are enzymes that catalyze the transfer of an amino grouping from an amino acid to an alpha keto acid. Organs in which transaminases are normally found are heart, liver, muscle, kidney and pancreas. In certain disease conditions in which cells are damaged, the transaminases leak from the damaged cells and the serum levels are thus elevated.

The most commonly measured transaminases are the serum glutamic oxaloacetic transaminase (SGOT) and the serum glutamic pyruvic transaminase (SGPT).

Elevations of serum transaminase levels are not specific. Because there are several transaminases in each type of cell, there are likely to be serum elevations of more than one type of transaminase when an organ is damaged. To be of value, the levels must be compared with the results of the physical examination and other laboratory tests.

***Serum Glutamic Oxaloacetic Transaminase* (SGOT).** Glutamic oxaloacetic transaminase (GOT) is present in large quantities in the liver, heart, kidney and skeletal muscle. Acute destruction of any of these tissues (especially heart and liver tissues) results in a rise in the serum level of this enzyme.

The test is useful in the diagnosis of myocardial infarction. The peak level is usually reached about 24 hours after infarction and returns to normal by approximately the fifth day. In acute hepatitis, SGOT levels may be elevated 10-100 times normal and remain elevated for relatively long periods of time. In extrahepatic obstruction, there is no elevation unless secondary parenchymal acute damage is present. In cirrhosis, SGOT may or may not be abnormal and depends upon the degree of hepatic decompensation of cell necrosis.

Serum Glutamic Pyruvic Transaminase (SGPT). Glutamic pyruvic transaminase (GPT) is an enzyme found mainly in the liver. It is elevated in liver disease but is less sensitive than the SGOT and apparently requires somewhat more extensive or severe acute parenchymal damage to give abnormal values. It has the advantage of being relatively specific for liver cell damage. It usually returns to normal levels before the SGOT.

In cases of hepatitis, SGPT levels rise higher than SGOT levels and fall slowly reaching normal levels in about 2-3 months, unless complications occur.

The major clinical value of the test appears to be in the differential diagnosis of jaundice. If the jaundice is caused by disease in the liver itself, SGPT levels are likely to be considerably higher than 300 units. If the jaundice results from a condition outside the liver, the SGPT levels are likely to be less than 300 units.

> ***NOTE: Cephalin Flocculation.*** Both the SGOT and SGPT, if elevated, do so before the cephalin flocculation becomes abnormal, but they both return to normal ranges considerably in advance of the cephalin flocculation. This explains why the cephalin flocculation sometimes will be abnormal in the presence of normal enzyme studies, due either to a minimal amount of hepatocellular damage or from obtaining the tests after the enzymes had returned to normal. In general, the cephalin flocculation is less sensitive than the SGOT, but is elevated longer and is more specific for acute hepatic cell destruction.
>
> If the SGOT is normal or only minimally elevated, the cephalin flocculation is valuable as a means to confirm acute liver cell damage. If the SGOT is elevated, there usually is little use in getting a cephalin flocculation. (See Cephalin–Cholesterol Flocculation under Miscellaneous Tests.)

Sodium. Sodium is the chief cation of the plasma and is involved in the maintenance of osmotic pressure and acid-base balance. The sodium concentration of the plasma is maintained within a very narrow range.

Increased serum sodium levels are found in markedly restricted water intake and administration of excessive amounts of sodium. Decreased serum sodium levels are found in pregnancy, pyloric obstruction, severe nephritis, Addison's disease, diarrhea, and heat exhaustion.

Total Protein—see Albumin Globulin

Urea Nitrogen—see Blood Urea Nitrogen

Uric Acid. Uric acid is the end product of purine metabolism and is formed from the breakdown of cell nucleic acids. The main excretory pathway of uric acid is the kidney. Differential micropuncture studies have shown that there is initially total clearance of uric acid at the glomerular level. This is followed by almost total tubular reabsorption through an active transport mechanism. The amount excreted equals the amount filtered. A second route of uric acid excretion is the gastrointestinal mucosa.

Blood uric acid levels are usually increased in conditions characterized by excessive cell breakdown and catabolism of nucleic acids. Blood uric acid levels are elevated in gout, excessive exposure to roentgen rays, multiple myeloma, leukemia, toxemia of pregnancy, chronic glomerulonephritis, and Fanconi syndrome.

Hematologic Tests

Several hematologic tests are required as a part of the physical examinations performed by a physician in either his office or in the hospital. There are two primary sources of blood for laboratory tests: (1) peripheral or capillary blood and (2) venous blood. There is no significant difference between cell counts performed on venous blood or capillary blood as long as the samples are freely flowing. When several hematologic procedures are necessitated, it is more practical to collect the blood from a vein rather than a finger. If the blood sample is collected by venipuncture, an anticoagulant must be added to the specimen to prevent coagulation. Two anticoagulants which prevent coagulation by binding the calcium and which are suitable for most hematologic tests are: (1) balanced oxalate which is a mixture of ammonium and potassium oxalate and (2) Sequestrene which is disodium ethylenediaminetetraacetate or EDTA.

Bleeding Time Tests. The Ivy bleeding time test and the Duke bleeding time test are the two commonly performed bleeding time tests. These tests measure the time necessary for active bleeding to cease from a clean, superficial wound. The main disadvantage in performing these tests is in the production of an adequate and standardized skin puncture. The bleeding time is influenced by the number and functional activity of platelets, ability of tissue constituents to initiate or accelerate clotting, elasticity of the skin and the capillary tonus. Defects in the coagulation process have little effect on the bleeding time and bleeding time is *not* equivalent to coagulation time. The bleeding time is prolonged in conditions characterized by poor capillary retraction and platelet deficiency. The bleeding test is positive in thrombocytopenic purpura, thrombasthenia, von Willebrand's disease, thrombocytopathia and constitutional capillary inferiority. The bleeding time is normal in hemophilia.

Blood Counts. Any blood cell count is done on a small sample of whole blood (generally capillary blood). The procedures used for enumeration of the formed elements of the blood utilize microscopic techniques. The blood sample is first diluted to an appropriate volume and using either an electronic cell counter or a manual method, the various formed elements are counted to obtain the number of cells in 1 mm^3 of whole blood.

Platelet count. Platelets are involved in coagulation of the blood and normal hemostasis. A decrease in the number of platelets may signify a generalized bleeding tendency and a prolonged bleeding time. An increase in the number of platelets may characterize a tendency toward thrombosis.

Thrombocytopenia (a decrease in platelets) occurs in thrombocytopenic purpura, aplastic anemia, Goucher's disease, and septicemia. Thrombocytosis (an increase in platelets) occurs in polycythemia, certain types of anemia, fractures, chronic myelogenous leukemia, rheumatic fever, and with some drug therapies used in the treatment of leukemia.

Red blood cell count. The erythrocytes contain hemoglobin which is the essential oxygen carrier of the blood. The significance of the red-cell count is limited since it may be normal in hypochromic anemias and thalassemia. The hematocrit or hemoglobin should be determined to detect the presence of anemia. If anemia is diagnosed, the red-cell count is valuable in determining the red-cell corpuscular values.

A decrease in red blood cells may result from hemorrhage or one of the anemias. (Anemia can also be caused by decreased blood cell or hemoglobin formation.) An increase in red blood cells may indicate polycythemia or hemoconcentration.

Reticulocyte count. Reticulocytes are immature red blood cells which show basophilic reticulum under vital staining. This test gives some indication of bone marrow activity. If there is red cell loss through bleeding or hemolysis, erythropoiesis becomes more active and the number of circulating reticulocytes increases. In conditions of blood loss, absence of an elevated reticulocyte count indicates bone marrow hypofunction.

This test is often used to evaluate the response to anemia therapy.

White cell differential count. There are several kinds of white blood cells (leukocytes) which can be identified microscopically. The proportions of these various types of cells in the blood may direct attention to a particular group of diseases. The differential count consists of identification and counting of a minimum of 100 white blood cells. The number of different white cells recorded is an estimate of the approximate percentages of white cells comprising the total white blood cell count.

Neutrophils comprise approximately 60 to 70 percent of the total number of leukocytes in adults. The neutrophils (neutral staining multinucleated cells) are increased in most bacterial infections, neoplasms, drug and chemical intoxications (especially in poisonings with liver damage), and acute hemorrhage. Neutrophilia is a term designating an increase in the absolute number of neutrophils. Decreased neutrophil counts accompany vitamin B_{12} and folic acid deficiencies, disseminated lupus erythematosus, anaphylaxis and disorders associated with splenomegaly, bone marrow damage (due to aplastic anemia, irradiation or drug idiosyncrasy).

The *eosinophils* (acid staining multinucleated cells) comprise 2-4 percent of the total number of leukocytes. The eosinophils are increased in parasitic infestations and allergic conditions, and in the Thorn test for studying the adrenal response to ACTH.

The *basophils* (basic staining multinucleated cells) comprise 0-1 percent of the total leukocytes. The basophils may be increased in some blood dyscrasias. Basophil counts are used to study allergic reactions.

The *lymphocytes* comprise 22-30 percent of the total leukocytes. The lymphocytes may be increased (lymphocytosis) in measles, whooping cough, infectious mononucleosis, infectious lymphocytosis, brucellosis, typhoid fever, syphilis, agammaglobulinemia, hepatitis, herpes zoster, herpes simplex, chickenpox, and chronic exposure to irradiation. The lymphocytes may be decreased (lymphopenia) in myelocytic leukemia, Hodgkin's disease, lupus erythematosus, and acute irradiation syndrome.

The *monocytes* comprise 4-8 percent of the total leukocytes and are phagocytic. The monocytes may be increased (monocytosis) during recovery from severe infections, Hodgkin's disease and lipoid storage diseases.

Clotting Time (Coagulation Time). This is a test which measures the length of time required for a sample of venous blood to clot. The whole blood clotting time is a measure of the time required to form intrinsic thromboplastin. Deficiencies of any factor in the intrinsic clotting scheme or in the common phase commencing with Factor X may prolong the clotting time, as may fibrinogen deficiency or presence of a circulating anticoagulant. The clotting time is difficult to standardize and demonstrates only gross abnormalities of hemostasis. A prolonged clotting time indicates that a problem exists, but a normal clotting time does not ensure that hemostasis is normal. The whole blood clotting time is used to control heparin therapy.

Coombs' Test, Direct. This is also known as a direct antiglobulin test. It is an immunologic procedure which reveals antigen-antibody reactions that are incomplete or weak. Coomb's serum is added to a preparation of red blood cells which is coated with antibody. Antibodies to human red cells may damage or increase the fragility of red blood cells without causing visible agglutination. The test is used early in diagnosis of erythroblastosis fetalis, autoimmune hemolytic anemia, and the cross-matching of blood for patients with a high risk of transfusion reaction. A positive test indicates that some antibody is attached to the red cells, but does not indicate the exact nature of the antibody.

Coombs' Test, Indirect. This test is used in the detection of various minor blood-type factors including Rh antibodies. It is thereby possible to eliminate bloods which might cause reactions because of incompatibilities of the minor blood-type factors.

Erythrocyte Sedimentation Rate (ESR). The erythrocyte sedimentation rate is a method of measuring the rate at which red cells settle to the bottom of a glass test tube. When blood is anticoagulated and allowed to settle, sedimentation of the erythrocytes occurs. The rate of sedimentation depends upon the number of erythrocytes, the size of the erythrocytes, and certain technical factors. Fibrinogen and globulin increase the tendency of the red cells to aggregate and to form rouleaux. The increase in the sedimentation rate is primarily a measure of the degree of rouleaux formation.

The test is non-specific but can (1) supply objective evidence of disease at a time when other signs are lacking. This would suggest that more specific information be sought. (2) The ESR can serve as a measure of the intensity of tissue destruction or repair since the rate of sedimentation reflects the degree to which these processes are active.

The ESR is increased in almost all infections, in most cases of carcinoma, severe anemia, active tuberculosis, rheumatoid arthritis, and acute coronary thrombosis. The ESR slowly returns to normal as patients recover from infectious diseases. The ESR is decreased when the plasma fibrinogen level is decreased, *i.e.*, severe liver diseases, polycythemia, sickle cell anemia and congestive heart failure.

Hematocrit (HCT). The hematocrit is the percentage of red-cell mass to original blood volume. After centrifugation of anticoagulated whole blood the percentage of packed red cells gives an indirect estimate of the number of red blood cells per 100 ml of whole blood. This in turn is an indirect estimate of the amount of hemoglobin. The hematocrit is useful in the evaluation and classification of various types of anemia. The Wintrobe test and the microhematocrit method are the two most commonly used procedures. The hematocrit is decreased in anemias and after hemorrhage and is increased in polycythemia and dehydration.

Hemoglobin (HgB). The amount of hemoglobin, the essential oxygen carrier of the blood, per 100 ml can be used as an index of the oxygen-carrying capacity of the blood. Total blood hemoglobin depends on the number of red blood cells and on the amount of hemoglobin in each red blood cell.

The hemoglobin is decreased in polycythemia and in newborn infants. The hemoglobin is decreased in anemia and this test is useful in the differential diagnosis of certain anemias. For example, in iron deficiency anemias, the hemoglobin is decreased more than the red blood cell count whereas the red blood cell count is decreased more than the hemoglobin in pernicious anemia.

Iron-Binding Capacity (Unsaturated). Iron is transported in the serum from the intestines where it is absorbed to the point of use in the erythropoietic system. The iron is combined with a fraction of beta globulins and is available for formation of hemoglobin. The unsaturated iron-binding capacity is the amount of iron that the protein (transferrin) could absorb to be fully saturated. Ordinarily, the actual serum iron is approximately one-third the level of the total iron-binding capacity.

Low values are found in iron-deficiency anemia, acute or chronic blood loss, pregnancy, and hemochromatosis. Elevated values are found in pernicious anemia, hemolytic anemia, cirrhosis, uremia, and some infections.

Lupus Erythematosus (LE) Cell Test. The lupus erythematosus cell test is clinically important in the diagnosis of disseminated lupus erythematosus. The test depends upon the reaction of an abnormal gamma globulin factor in the serum of the patient with the nucleus of a leukocyte. This results in the formation of a swollen homogeneous mass of nuclear material which is phagocytosed by a normal granulocyte to form the LE cell.

Mean Corpuscular Hemoglobin—see Red Blood Cell Indices

Mean Corpuscular Hemoglobin Concentration—see Red Blood Cell Indices

Mean Corpuscular Volume—see Red Blood Cell Indices

Prothrombin Time. Prothrombin is formed in the liver where its production depends on an adequate intake and absorption of vitamin K. Vitamin K is produced by the normal intestinal flora so that a deficiency of the vitamin is unusual in the otherwise healthy adult. Prothrombin is converted to thrombin in the clotting process. A low prothrombin level is usually indicative that the clotting tendency of the blood is diminished.

This test measures the time needed for citrated or oxalated plasma to clot after tissue thromboplastin and calcium chloride have been added.

The prothrombin time is often done during the acute stages of myocardial infarction in order to assist the physician to determine the next dose of anticoagulant. Clotting normally occurs in 11-14 seconds depending upon the control. An abnormal result is not pathognomonic of prothrombin deficiency as any one of the factors necessary for stage II and stage III of the clotting process may be involved.

A lowered plasma prothrombin may mean either dysfunction of the liver or a deficient supply of vitamin K. Since vitamin K is not absorbed from the intestine in the absence of bile salts, biliary obstruction of any type can result in vitamin K deficiency, a lowered prothrombin concentration and a consequent bleeding tendency in the patient. Depressed prothrombin times are also seen in premature and breast-fed infants.

A prothrombin determination without preliminary parenteral administration of vitamin K can be interpreted in terms of a possible bleeding tendency due to lack of this factor in the coagulation mechanism. The plasma prothrombin activity should not be regarded as a test of liver function unless an adequate dose of vitamin K is given parenterally 24 hours before the observation is made.

Red Blood Cell Indices. *Mean corpuscular hemoglobin (MCH).* The mean corpuscular

Table 1. Table of Normal Values

CLINICAL CHEMISTRY

TEST	SPECIMEN	VALUES
A/G ratio	Serum	1.5-2.5
Albumin	Serum	4-5.5 g%
Aldolase	Serum	6.1-21.3 dihydroxyacetone units
Amino acid nitrogen	Plasma	3.5-7 mg%
	Urine	50-200 mg/24 hr
Ammonia	Urine	0.5-1 g/24 hr
Ammonia nitrogen	Whole blood	35-100 μg%
Amylase (diastase)	Serum	60-200 Somogyi units
	Urine	35-260 units/hr
Atherogenic index (AI)	Serum	Below 50 units
BEI	Serum	3.2-6.4 μg%
Bilirubin (all methods)		
Direct	Serum	0.1-0.4 mg%
Total	Serum	0.3-1.3 mg%
Indirect	Serum	0.2-0.8 mg%
BMR		±10% of Dubois standards
Bromsulphalein (BSP)		
2 mg/Kg body weight	Serum	Not more than 15% after 30 min
5 mg/Kg body weight	Serum	0-5% after 45 min
Calcium	Serum	8.5-10.5 mg%
	Urine	50-400 mg/24 hr
Cephalin-cholesterol flocculation	Serum	No flocculation
Ceruloplasmin (copper oxidase)	Serum	35-65 IU (15-35 mg%)
Chloride	Serum	98-110 mEq/L (575-645 mg% as NaCl)
	Whole blood	77-88 mEq/L (450-515 mg% as NaCl)
	Urine	10-15 g/24 hr as NaCl
Cholesterol, total	Serum	150-270 mg%
Cholesterol esters	Serum	68-74% of total cholesterol
Cholinesterase	Serum	40-80 units
Copper	Serum	70-150 μg%
	Urine	Up to 40 μg/day
CO_2-combining power	Plasma	24-34 mM/L (53-76 vol%)
CO_2 content	Plasma	20-25 mM/L (45-55 vol%)
Creatine	Serum	0.5-0.9 mg%
Creatine phosphokinase (CPK)	Serum	0-5 μg/hr/ml
Creatinine	Serum	0.6-1.2 mg%
	Urine	1-1.5 g/24 hr
ET_3	Serum	11-17% after 2 hr of incubation
Fat tolerance	Serum or plasma	Increase to 17.5 mEq/L fatty acids
Fatty acids		
Esterified	Serum	7-14 mEq/L
Free	Serum or plasma	0.35-1.2 mEq/L
Fibrinogen	Plasma	200-400 mg%
Galactose tolerance	Whole blood	Index up to 160 mg%
Globulin	Serum	1.5-3 g%
Glucose		
Folin-Wu method	Whole blood	80-125 mg%
Somogyi method	Whole blood	65-69 mg%
	Serum or plasma	80-115 mg%
Glutamic oxaloacetic transaminase (GOT)	Serum	8-30 Reitman-Frankel units
Using diazonium salt	Serum	8-30 units (same as Reitman-Frankel method)
Glutamic pyruvic transaminase (GPT)	Serum	5-25 Reitman-Frankel units
Using diazonium salt	Serum	5-25 units (same as Reitman-Frankel method)

CLINICAL CHEMISTRY

TEST	SPECIMEN	VALUES
Hippuric acid synthesis		
Intravenous	Urine	0.7-1.6 g/hr
Oral	Urine	3-3.5 g/4 hr
Hydroxybutyrate dehydrogenase (HBD)	Serum	56-125 IU/L
Icterus index	Serum	2-6 units
Iron	Serum	70-150 μg%
Iron-binding capacity, total	Serum	200-400 μg%
Isocitric dehydrogenase (ICD)	Serum	238-686 KGA units/ml
Lactic dehydrogenase (LDH)	Serum	41-98 units
	Urine	550-2050 units in 8 hr specimen
Using tetrazolium salt	Serum	27-77 IU
Leucine aminopeptidase (LAP)		
Adults	Serum	5-20 units
Infants	Serum	5-24 units
Adults	Urine	2-18 units/24 hr
Levulose tolerance	Whole blood	Not more than 26-30 mg% above fasting level
Lipase	Serum	0-1 unit
Magnesium	Serum	1.6-2.1 mEq/L
	Urine	1.1-0.2 g/24 hr
Nonprotein nitrogen (NPN)	Whole blood	25-45 mg%
Oxygen capacity		
Men	Whole blood	20.7 vol% (15.4 g Hb)
Women	Whole blood	19 vol% (14.2 g Hb)
Oxygen saturation	Arterial blood	95-97%
	Venous blood	60-85%
pH	Venous blood	7.32-7.42
	Arterial blood	7.35-7.45
	Urine	4.8-7.6 (average 6)
Phosphatase, acid		
Bessey-Lowry		
Men	Serum	0.13-0.63 B-L unit
Women	Serum	0.01-0.56 B-L unit
Using alpha-naphthylphosphate	Serum	1-1.9 IU/L
Phosphatase, alkaline		
Bessy-Lowry		
Adults	Serum	0.8-2.3 B-L units
Children	Serum	2.8-6.7 B-L units
Using phenolphthalein monophosphate	Serum	9-35 IU
Phospholipids	Serum	150-350 mg% (average 230 mg%); 6-14 mg% lipid phosphorus
Phosphorus, inorganic		
Adults	Serum	2.5-5 mg%
Children	Serum	3.5-6 mg%
Adults	Urine	0.78-1.1 g (1.8-2.5 P_2O_5)
Potassium	Serum	4-5.6 mEq/L (16-22 mg%)
Prostatic acid phosphatase	Serum	Up to 0.15 units
Protein, total	Serum	6-8 g%
Protein-bound iodine (PBI)	Serum	4-8 μg%
Prothrombin time	Serum	70-110% (11-15 sec)
Sodium	Serum	135-145 mEq/L (310-335 mg%)
TBI		
Euthyroid	Serum	0.9-1.1
Hyperthyroid	Serum	Less than 0.9
Hypothyroid	Serum	Greater than 1.1
T_4 by column chromatography	Serum	3.0-6.4 μg%
Thymol turbidity	Serum	0-5 units

CLINICAL CHEMISTRY

TEST	VALUES	SPECIMEN
Thyroxine-binding globulin capacity	Serum	12-20 μg thyroxine-binding capacity/100ml
Total lipids	Serum	400-1000 mg%
Total nitrogen	Urine	10-16 g/24 hr
Triglycerides	Serum	40-145 mg% (1.4-4.9 mEq/L)
Urea	Serum or whole blood	22-40 mg%
	Urine	10-40 g/24 hr
Urea nitrogen	Serum or whole blood	10-18 mg%
Uric acid	Serum	2.5-8 mg%
	Urine	0.4-0.8 g/24 hr
Urobilinogen	Urine	0.4-1 mg/day
	Feces	30-220 mg/100 mg of stool or 40-280 mg/day
Zinc sulfate turbidity	Serum	2-8 units

URINARY HORMONES

Catecholamines	20-180 μg/day
Hydroxyindolacetic acid (HIAA)	2-9 mg/day
Hydroxysteroids	10-15 mg/day
17-Ketosteroids	
Males	10-18 mg/day
Females	6-15 mg/day
Vanillyl mandelic acid (VMA)	2-14 mg/day

KIDNEY FUNCTION TESTS

Creatinine clearance (endogenous)	100-120 ml/min
Concentration test (sp. gr.)	1.030 or more
Dilution test (sp. gr.)	1.002-1.001
Inulin clearance (average)	123 ml/min/1.73 m²
PAH clearance (average)	634 ml/min/1.73 m²
Phenolsulfonphthalein test (PSP)	26% excretion after 15 min
	40% excretion after 30 min
Urea clearance	
Maximal	70-110% of normal (75 ml/min)
Standard	70-110% of normal (54 ml/min)

CEREBROSPINAL FLUID

Cells	1-5/mm³
Chlorides	113-127 mEq/L
Glucose	45-100 mg/100ml
Protein	20-45 mg/100 ml
Urea	8-28 mg/100 ml

HEMATOLOGY

Test	Value
Bleeding time (Ivy)	
Average	4 min
Range	1-7 min
Blood volume	
Males	52-70 ml/kg
Females	53-62 ml/kg
Bone marrow differential count	
Reticuloendothelial cells	0-1%
Myeloblasts	0-2%
Promyelocytes	1-5%
Myelocytes	
Neutrophilic	5-25%
Eosinophilic	0-3%
Basophilic	0-0.5%
Metamyelocytes	10-20%
Band granulocytes	15-30%
Neutrophilic granulocytes	10-25%
Eosinophils	0-5%
Basophils	0-0.5%
Lymphocytes	5-20%
Monocytes	0-3%
Plasma cells	0-5%
Nucleated RBC	
Rubriblasts	1-5/100 WBC
Prorubricytes	1-6/100 WBC
Rubricytes	5-25/100 WBC
Metarubricytes	2-20/100 WBC
Myeloid:erythroid ratio	3-8:1
Megakaryocytes	1-2 or more/ high-power dry field
Clot retraction	
Begin	1 hr
Complete	24 hr
Coagulation time (Lee-White)	10-12 min (8.5-15.5 min)

Differential count				
Adults				
Neutrophils	56-65%			
Band granulocytes	1-5%			
Lymphocytes	25-34%			
Monocytes	4-5%			
Eosinophils	0.5-4%			
Basophils	0-1.5%			
Children	Birth (%)	2 mo - 2 yr (%)	2-8 yr (%)	8-16 yr (%)
Polymorphs (neutrophils)	45-65	30	30-50	50-60
Band granulocytes	6-12	3	3	2-5
Eosinophils	2	2.5	2.5	2.5
Basophils	0.5	0.5	0.5	0.5
Lymphocytes	26-35	59-63	60-39	30-40
Monocytes	5	5	4	5

Test	Value
Eosinophilic count	150-300/mm³
Erythrocytic count	
Males	
Average	4.8 million/mm³
Range	4.4-5.4 million
Females	
Average	4.3 million/mm³
Range	3.8-5 million
Hematocrit	
Males	40-52 vol%/100 ml
Females	38-47 vol%/100 ml
Children	
Birth	45-65 vol%
2 yr	30-40 vol%
8 yr	32-42 vol%
Hemoglobin	
Males	14.9 g% (15.4 ± 1.5)
Females	13.7 g% (14.2 ± 1.5)
Children	
Birth	21.5 g% (23.9 ± 3.0)
4 wk	16 g% (15.3 ± 3.0)
2 mo	13.5 g% (13.1 ± 2.2)
1 yr	12 g% (11.6 ± 1.5)
4 yr	13 g% (12.2 ± 1.5)
Leukocyte count	
Birth	9000-30,000 WBC/mm³
2 mo-2 yr	6000-17,000 WBC/mm³
2-8 yr	6000-13,000 WBC/mm³
8-16 yr	5000-13,000 WBC/mm³
16-21 yr	4500-11,000 WBC/mm³
Mean corpuscular hemoglobin (MCH)	$29 \pm 2 \mu\mu g$
Mean corpuscular hemoglobin concentration (MCHC)	34 ± 2%
Mean corpuscular volume (MCV)	$87 \pm 5 \mu^3$
Methemoglobin	0-3% total hemoglobin (0.03-0.13 g/100 ml)
Osmotic fragility	
0.30% saline solution	100% hemolysis
0.40% saline solution	50-95% hemolysis
0.55% saline solution	0% hemolysis
Partial thromboplastin time (kaolin-activated)	30-45 sec
Platelet count	
Average	260,000/mm³
Range	145,000-350,000/mm³
Prothrombin consumption time	Longer than 21 sec
Prothrombin time	11-12.8 sec
Red cell count	See erythrocyte count
Reticulocyte count	0-2%
Sedimentation rate (Wintrobe)	
Men	0-9 mm
Women	0-15 mm
Children	0-13 mm
White cell count	See leukocyte count

hemoglobin is the amount of hemoglobin by weight in the average red blood cell.

Mean corpuscular hemoglobin concentration (MCHC). The mean corpuscular hemoglobin concentration is an expression of the percent of the average hemoglobin concentration per cell.

Mean corpuscular volume (MCV). The mean corpuscular volume is the volume of the average red blood cell.

Miscellaneous Tests

Amylase. The determination of serum amylase is the most useful single test in the diagnosis of pancreatic disease. The normal range of serum amylase is 60-200 Somogyi units. In acute pancreatitis, it is consistently elevated often to values over 500 Somogyi units. Other conditions which may cause amylase elevation are mumps, perforated peptic ulcer, gallstones, intestinal obstruction, ruptured ectopic pregnancy, renal insufficiency, nonpenetrating abdominal trauma and the administration of morphine and morphine-like drugs. The elevation in these cases is typically transient, lasting a few hours to three days. Tests for urinary amylase add little or nothing to blood amylase determination, although the elevated urinary excretion may sometimes last several days longer. In severe destructive pancreatitis, serum amylase may go down rather than up because of the inability of the pancreas to produce enzymes.

Some surgeons order routine serum amylase tests for the first few days after any operation which might have injured the pancreas. Whenever an elevation in the amylase level occurs, they can institute therapy for pancreatitis early.

Anti-Streptolysin O Titer. This is a test usually used when rheumatic fever is suspected. Since rheumatic fever is related to a recent streptococcal infection, an increase in the titer of the anti-streptolysin is usually found in rheumatic fever. The test is non-specific.

Bromsulphalein Test (BSP). This is a test for liver function and is particularly valuable in the diagnosis of cirrhosis and other diffuse diseases not accompanied by jaundice.

The BSP test is based on the ability of the liver to remove injected sulfobromophthalein sodium from the blood stream. When sulfobromopthalein sodium is injected intravenously, it is rapidly removed from the blood stream by the liver and excreted in the bile. The time required for its removal depends upon the size of the dose and the functional capacity of the liver. Since the dye is removed via the bile flow, it is essential that the bile flow is not obstructed in order to achieve accurate results.

Doses of 5 mg/Kg of body weight are normally completely removed from the blood after 45 minutes. Impairment of liver functions will show a retention of dye from 6-40 percent or more. Since sulfobromophthalein sodium may interfere with the use of phenolsulfonphthalein as a test for kidney function, at least 24 hours should elapse between the two tests.

C-Reactive Protein (CRP). This is a non-specific test for inflammation and tissue breakdown. An abnormal protein (C-reactive protein) has been demonstrated in the blood during the acute phases of many inflammatory disorders. This substance forms a precipitate with the non-type-specific or somatic C polysaccharide of the pneumococcus. An animal antiserum against this protein is used as the test reagent.

The test is non-specific and has the same indications, interpretations and limitations as the erythrocyte sedimentation rate (ESR). The test is useful in following the progress of rheumatic fever.

Cephalin-Cholesterol Flocculation. Properly diluted serum of normal persons will not flocculate a colloidal suspension of cephalin and cholesterol. The serum of persons with damaged liver cells will flocculate the suspension. This test affords a rough quantitative measurement of liver cell function and is sometimes used to follow the course of patients with a known liver disease (*i.e.*, cirrhosis).

The test is sensitive and frequently positive in the early stages of liver disease before jaundice appears. It is negative in acute obstruction of the biliary tract of short duration. If the obstruction persists, secondary damage to the liver cells occurs and the cephalin flocculation test becomes positive.

Congo Red Retention Test. In amyloidosis, deposits of amyloid tissue are laid down in the liver, kidneys and spleen and eventually interfere with proper function. The amyloid material has an affinity for congo red and the dye is removed from the blood more quickly in patients with amyloidosis.

A standard dose of 10 ml of a 1 percent solution of congo red is administered intravenously. If over 80 percent of the dye is removed from the blood within one hour, there is strong presumptive evidence of amyloidosis. A negative test, however, does not rule out the disease.

Icterus Index. Bilirubin is yellow in color. This is a simple test for measuring the approximate amount of bilirubin in the serum by measuring the degree of yellowness of the serum. An increase in the icterus index usually parallels an increase in the serum bilirubin. The test does not differentiate between bilirubin due to excess hemolysis or due to obstruction of the biliary tract.

Latex Slide Agglutination Test. This is a test used in the diagnosis of rheumatoid arthritis. Serum from patients with rheumatoid arthritis will cause small biologically inert particles coated with human gamma globulin to clump together. It is also positive in lupus erythematosus and dermatomyositis.

Protein Bound Iodine (PBI). This is a test of thyroid function. Thyroxine normally contains most of the serum iodine and is mainly bound to certain serum proteins. The protein-bound iodine represents the organic fraction of blood iodine that precipitates with serum proteins. The level of PBI in the serum correlates well with the thyroid status and provides an indirect estimation of thyroxine in the body.

Low serum PBI values are found in hypothyroidism and nephrosis. Serum PBI values are elevated in hyperthyroidism and pregnancy. Since thyroxine is carried to some extent by albumin and prealbumin proteins, any condition (*i.e.*, nephrotic syndrome or severe liver disease) which leads to a marked decrease of these proteins will falsely decrease PBI. Contamination from certain medications and x-ray contrast media is a problem and some of the factors that can falsely influence the PBI are pregnancy, estrogen therapy, thyroid hormone therapy, antithyroid drugs, and adrenocortical steroid therapy. Mercurial diuretics may cause erroneously low results due to the interference of mercury, and drugs containing inorganic iodine will cause false high results. All patients should be questioned about the prior administration of these drugs before determining the protein-bound iodine. In general, all radio-opaque, iodine-containing injectable contrast media are likely to produce falsely elevated protein-bound iodine levels for six months. Some of these contrast media may exert an effect for 20 or more years.

Thymol Turbidity. The thymol turbidity test measures the degree of turbidity produced when blood serum is mixed with a buffered thymol solution. Normal sera produce no or very little turbidity. Sera from patients with liver disease contain altered gamma globulins and phospholipids which cause pronounced turbidity. The turbidity is usually increased in liver conditions where the liver cells are damaged. In biliary obstruction without damage to the liver cells, the turbidity is usually normal.

The thymol turbidity test is a test of liver functon and roughly correlates with the results of the cephalin flocculation test. It seems less sensitive than the cephalin flocculation test and becomes positive later, but tends to remain positive longer. The test is high in infectious hepatitis, cirrhosis, Hodgkin's disease, coccidioidomycosis, disseminated tuberculosis, lobar pneumonia, and bacterial endocarditis.

Zinc Sulfate Turbidity. The zinc sulfate turbidity test depends upon the amount of gamma globulins present in the sera. Since the amount of gamma globulins in the serum is elevated when the liver cells are damaged, the test is useful in evaluating the presence of liver damage. The test is not specific for liver disease because the procedure depends upon an increase in gamma globulins, and conditions in which gamma globulins are increased will give a false positive result, *i.e.*, multiple myeloma.

TESTS PERFORMED ON URINE

The urinalysis, a composite examination on a specimen of urine, is an integral part of the initial examination of patients in all branches of medicine. The urinalysis is composed of four general parts.

1. Physical properties
2. Chemical tests for abnormal constituents
3. Microscopic examination of the urine sediment
4. Special tests

Physical Properties

Urine Color. Normal urine varies in color from faint yellow to amber depending upon the concentration of the urine. Color is not an adequate measurement of concentration, however, and specific gravity or osmolarity values are preferred. The three normal urinary pigments are urochrome, uroerythrin, and urobilin. Clinical conditions which affect the urine color include porphyria (red urine), alcaptonuria (brown/black urine), and extensive melanotic sarcoma (black urine). There are numerous color changes caused by some drugs and foods but these are usually of little clinical significance.

Urine Odor. Normal urine has a characteristic, faintly *aromatic* odor due to presence of certain volatile acids. Upon standing, bacteria in the specimen breakdown urea, ammonia is formed, and the urine acquires a strong *ammoniacal* odor. This odor is an indication that the urine specimen is too old to be worth examining and a fresh specimen should be obtained. Urine heavily infected with bacteria is foul-smelling and in diabetic ketosis, the urine has a characteristic "fruity" or sweet odor.

Urine Transparency. Freshly voided normal urine is usually, but not necessarily, clear and upon standing will become cloudy. When a freshly voided specimen is cloudy, a microscopic analysis of the urinary sediment can usually ascribe the cloudiness to amorphous phosphates, amorphous urates, pus, blood, bacteria or fat.

Specific Gravity. Specific gravity of urine is the ratio of the weight of a given volume of urine to the weight of the same volume of water at a temperature of 4°C. The normal range is 1.010 to 1.030 and the morning specimen shows the greatest concentration with a specific gravity of 1.020 or higher. The specific gravity of urine always should be reported to the third decimal point to have clinical significance and since it is a ratio, there are no units.

The specific gravity of the urine is dependent upon the concentrating ability of the kidneys and the state of hydration of the patient. It is a reflection of the amount of dissolved substances present in the solution and varies inversely with urine volume. The specific gravity is decreased in high fluid intake, low salt intake, diabetes insipidus and chronic nephritis. The specific gravity is increased in diabetes mellitus, acute glomerulonephritis, fever, sweating, vomiting, and diarrhea.

pH. The pH of urine depends greatly upon the acid-base composition of the blood. The kidney maintains the blood at constant pH range by excreting into the urine any excess ions which might alter the pH of the blood. Therefore, the urinary pH varies and changes do not necessarily indicate abnormality. Freshly voided urine usually has a pH value of 5 or 6; however, because of the presence of phosphate salts and other buffers in the glomerular filtrate and of ammonia formed by the tubular cells, the kidney is capable of producing urine ranging from pH 4.5 to 8.0.

The pH of the urine influences the preservation of formed elements in the urine sediment. In renal insufficiency, the ability to excrete acid is reduced owing chiefly to impairment in ammonia excretion. It is not uncommon for urine to be alkaline following a heavy meal or after ingestion of large amounts of alkaline salts. Otherwise, the presence of constantly alkaline urine may be due to the presence of urea-splitting organisms in the urine, a potassium deficiency, primary aldosteronism, after blood transfusions, or frequent vomiting. Strongly acidic urine occurs in acidiosis, diabetes mellitus, gout, and after ingestion of ammonium chloride, ammonium mandelate, or a high protein diet. When it is necessary to control the urinary pH in the management of kidney infections, renal calculi, and in some drug regimens, regulation of the diet is one of the methods of control.

Chemical Tests for Abnormal Constituents

Acetoacetic Acid—see Ketones

Acetone—see Ketones

Albumin. Ordinarily the albumin in the blood does not pass through the glomerulus into the urine. Albuminuria refers to albumin that has passed from the blood into the urine and as the glomerular membrane is progressively damaged, proteins appear in the urine in the order of their molecular size. Albumin has the smallest molecular size and is released first and is followed by the globulins and rarely fibrinogen. The test for urinary protein is probably the most significant single finding in the detection and diagnosis of renal disease. Proteinuria must be correlated with the microscopic examination of the urinary sediment and treatment should be started as soon as possible in order to prevent permanent renal damage.

Slight albuminuria may occur after excessive muscular exertion, exercise, protein ingestion and in late pregnancy. Albuminuria may be caused by (1) increased permeability of the glomerulus and (2) decreased reabsorption of protein by the renal tubular cells. Albuminuria is found in all stages of nephritis, nephrosis and nephrosclerosis. Albuminuria is also common in hypertension, certain infectious processes involving the kidney, (*i.e.*, tuberculosis, pyelonephritis, pyelitis, septic emboli), non-infectious processes (*i.e.*, polycystic disease, hemorrhage, incompatible transfusions, amyloidosis, calculi), and diabetes mellitus. Mercurial compounds and gold salts may produce albuminuria secondary to tubular damage. If venous return from the kidneys to the heart is impaired (*i.e.*, renal vein thrombosis, congestive heart failure, constrictive pericarditis), albuminuria may result.

Beta Hydroxybutyric Acid—see Ketones

Bilirubin. This is a test of liver function. Bilirubin is formed from hemoglobin by the reticuloendothelial system and is normally excreted from the body by the liver through the intestine. Free bilirubin linked to protein is excreted by the liver rather than the kidneys because it cannot pass through the glomerular capsule. The urine normally contains no bilirubin.

Bilirubin which has passed through the liver (posthepatic) diffuses more readily than prehepatic bilirubin. Consequently, the bilirubin of obstructive jaundice is found in the urine earlier than that of hemolytic jaundice. Bilirubin may be absent in patients with hemolytic jaundice with a fairly high icterus index. In infectious or toxic hepatitis, cholangitis, and in partial obstruction of the biliary tract, bilirubin is present because the liver is unable to handle the bilirubin absorbed from the intestinal tract plus the bilirubin formed by the reticuloendothelial system. A less common, but important cause of bilirubin in the urine is an excessive production of bilirubin associated with pathologically increased destruction of erythrocytes.

Chlorides, Quantitative. This test is performed to evaluate the urinary excretion of chlorides. A normal person will excrete extremely small amounts of sodium and chloride in the urine when he is fed a diet low in these elements. The ability of the body to conserve sodium and chloride depends upon the functional integrity of the adrenal cortex.

A decrease in urinary chlorides occurs when there is a decrease in blood chlorides, starvation, excessive sweating, vomiting, pneumonia, ascites, pleuritic effusion, heart failure, nephritis, nephrosis and burns.

In Addison's disease, there is increased urinary excretion of chloride in spite of decreased plasma chloride.

Clearance Tests. Clearance is the volume of blood or plasma that contains the amount of a substance which is excreted in the urine in one minute. Clearance tests allow the physician to evaluate the extent of renal damage and to differentiate between glomerular lesions and tubular lesions.

The three specific functions of the kidney which are commonly measured are:

1. Renal plasma flow
2. Glomerular filtration rate
3. Tubular function

The *renal plasma flow* is commonly determined by using sodium p-aminohippurate (PAH) which, at low blood concentrations, is almost completely removed by tubular excretion in a single circulation through the kidney.

The *glomerular filtration rate* is determined by measuring the clearance of any substance that is filtered at the glomerulus but is not excreted or reabsorbed by the tubules. Inulin clearance, creatinine clearance, and urea clearance are all methods of measuring the glomerular filtration rate.

The *tubular function* may be subdivided into tubular secretion and tubular absorption. Diodrast, para-aminohippuric acid, and phenol red can overload tubular secretory mechanisms and high blood levels of glucose can exceed tubular reabsorption. The clearance rate of these substances (after being corrected for that amount simultaneously filtered by the glomerulus) is an indication of average tubular function (Tm).

Concentration and Dilution. These tests measure the ability of the kidneys to concentrate and dilute urine. The normal kidneys excrete urine that differs markedly in volume and specific gravity at different periods within a 24 hour period. These variations represent an attempt to maintain normal body fluids under conditions of varying fluid intake. Damaged kidneys lose partially or completely this ability to respond to the needs of the body with the result that the urine has almost the same specific gravity throughout the day.

Diacetic Acid—see Ketones

Glomerular Filtration Rate—see Clearance Tests

Hemoglobin. Blood in the urine may appear as intact red blood cells (hematuria) or dissolved hemoglobin derived from destroyed red blood cells (hemoglobinuria). Hematuria is the result of bleeding somewhere along the urinary tract. The site of bleeding is determined by more precise methods. Hemoglobinuria usually results from conditions outside the urinary tract. The red blood cells are hemolyzed and the dissolved hemoglobin in the plasma is excreted by the kidney. This occurs in severe burns, transfusion reactions, severe malaria, poisoning and paroxysmal hemoglobinuria.

Ketones. Ketone bodies are normal products of fat metabolism and include: acetone, diacetic acid, and β-hydroxybutyric acid. They are not normally detectable in blood or urine. The ketone bodies are utilized by muscle tissue as an energy source; however, if an excessive amount of fat is metabolized, the muscles may be unable to utilize all the resulting ketone bodies. Ketosis (increased concentration of ketones in the blood) and ketonuria (increased concentration of ketones in the urine) are the clinical results.

Acetone. This test is important in the diagnosis of ketosis. In diabetes mellitus, sugar is not utilized properly and excessive fat is metabolized. The fatty acids are broken down into acetoacetic acid and β-hydroxybutyric acid which are converted to acetone and excreted by the kidneys. There is normally no acetone in the urine of adults. Acetone in the urine indicates a severe disorder of metabolism and is present in diabetes mellitus, in a certain percentage of small children, and in starvation. It is also increased if the patient received sulfobromophthalein sodium (BSP) or phenolsulfonphthalein in the past 48 hours.

Beta-hydroxybutyric acid. Of the three ketone bodies, β-hydroxybutyric acid is relatively nontoxic. It is excreted in the urine in combination with a fixed base (sodium) and loss of the body cations may lead to acidosis. In uncontrolled diabetes, acetone is the first ketone body to appear, diacetic acid is later excreted and when the situation becomes severe, β-hydroxybutyric acid appears.

Diacetic (aceto-acetic) acid. The test for diacetic acid is used in the diagnosis of metabolic ketosis. Like acetone, diacetic acid is produced when glucose is not properly utilized and excessive fat is metabolized. A positive test for diacetic acid indicates a more severe degree of ketosis than a positive acetone test alone.

Myoglobin. Myoglobin is a normal constituent of muscle and similar in many respects to hemoglobin. Myoglobin appears in the urine after extensive destruction of muscle (*i.e.*, crush injuries or following occlusion of a main limb artery, and in the rare disease termed acute paralytic myoglobinuria or acute recurrent rhabdomyolysis).

Myoglobin has one quarter the molecular weight of hemoglobin and is more rapidly cleared by the kidney. Myoglobin is quite soluble in alkaline urine, but if the urine is acidic, the myoglobin may precipitate in the kidney tubules and cause kidney damage.

Porphyrins. Porphyrins are pigments which are normally contained in red blood cells. Normally, there is an insignificant amount of porphyrin in the urine. In lead poisoning and toxic liver damage, some blood disorders, pellagra, and congenital porphyria, the urinary excretion of porphyrins rises. The Watson-Schwartz test for urinary porphobilinogen is useful in the diagnosis of acute intermittent porphyria in relapse.

Renal Plasma Flow—see Clearance Tests

Sugar. Traces of sugar, particularly glucose, may occur in normal urine. The occurrence of any sugar in the urine is termed glycosuria. Sugars that may be present in the urine are glucose, pentose, galactose, lactose and levulose. All tests for urine sugar may be classified as either nonspecific tests for sugars, which are based on the reducing ability of glucose, or specific tests for glucose, which are based on the enzyme of glucose oxidase.

The renal threshold is the lowest blood glucose concentration that will result in glycosuria, and at this point (usually 170-180 mg %) any additional glucose will not be reabsorbed into the blood but will be excreted in the urine. When glucose is detected in urine, it is important to determine if the underlying cause is benign or pathologic. Benign glycosuria occurs after eating a large quantity of glucose or other carbohydrate or after emotional reactions. Pathologic glycosuria is due chiefly to diabetes mellitus, but may also occur in pregnancy, hyperthyroidism, increased intracranial pressure, hyperpituitarism, chronic liver disease, and acidosis of anesthesia or asphyxia.

Tubular Function—see Clearance Tests

Urobilinogen. When bilirubin enters the intestine, it is acted upon by bacteria which convert it to urobilinogen. This is a test used to differentiate between complete and incomplete obstruction of the biliary tract. Tests for urine urobilinogen are valuable in early detection of liver damage because one of the first mechanisms altered in a damaged liver is the inability to remove urobilinogen from the blood and excrete it via the intestine. As a result, urobilinogen is removed by the kidney.

Increases in urinary urobilinogen occur in many conditions including hemolytic diseases, liver damage, congestive heart failure, and severe infections. However, in complete obstructive jaundice without infection there is ordinarily no excess urobilinogen in the urine.

Microscopic Examination of the Urine Sediment

The centrifuged sediment of the urine contains all the insoluble materials that have accumulated in the urine in the process of glomerular filtration and during passage of the fluid through tubules of the kidneys and lower urinary tract. When renal disease is present, it is often possible to surmise from examination of the urine sediment, the nature of the pathologic process in the kidney and its degree of activity. Localization of disease in the lower urinary tract may be aided by use of fractional urine collection.

Significance of Cells in Urine Sediment. *Leukocytes.* The white blood cells that appear in urine are predominantly polymorphonuclear neutrophils. Pyuria is the condition in which increased numbers of white cells are found in the urine. The presence of increased numbers of leukocytes in the sediment is often indicative of urinary tract infection, especially when clumping occurs. Occasional white cells are frequently found in normal urine sediment. Increased numbers of leukocytes and epithelial cells occur in glomerulonephritis and other diseases not associated with bacterial infection.

Erythrocytes. Erythrocytes, like leukocytes, may enter the urine from any part of the urinary tract. Hematuria is the condition in which red blood cells are found in the urine. In the urine, red blood cells act as osmometers and alter in size and appearance depending on the osmolarity of the urine. In concentrated urine, they lose their usual biconcave contour and become small and crenated. In dilute urine, they may appear large and swollen, or they may rupture leaving only a ring of stroma or "ghost cell."

Increased numbers of red blood cells may appear in the urine during the acute febrile phase of streptococcal infections without significant disease of the kidneys or urinary tract. Hematuria occurs in glomerulonephritis; renal infarction; tuberculosis of kidneys; pyelonephritis; carcinomas of kidneys, ureters and bladder; polycystic kidneys; calculi; and hemorrhagic diseases such as purpura hemorrhagica and hemophilia. Hematuria has occurred following anticoagulant therapy of thrombophlebitis, phlebothrombosis, etc.

Epithelial cells. Cells of the renal tubular epithelium are round, mononuclear and generally larger than leukocytes. Their presence in the urine in elevated numbers signifies degenerative exfoliation of the tubular epithelium and may appear in glomerulonephritis and other vascular nephritides following exposure to nephrotoxic substances or during acute infections involving the renal medulla. When intense degenerative changes occur, whole sheets of epithelial cells may appear in the sediment. Large numbers of renal tubular epithelial cells are usually excreted in the urine of patients with massive proteinuria from any cause.

Significance of Casts in Urine Sediment. Casts are cylindrical structures that form in the kidney tubules by the coagulation of protein. The occurrence of casts is called cylindruria. For casts to form, protein must be present in tubular urine in sufficient concentration and under conditions favorable to coagulation. Within the coagulum may be trapped the cells, bacteria crystals and other debris present at the site of formation. Thus, the cast provides a method of examining the contents of the kidney tubule because anything present within a cast must have been present in the tubule.

Noncellular casts. The noncellular casts are hyaline, granular, waxy and fatty in type.

Hyaline casts result from precipitation of protein within the kidney tubule lumens and are seen in increased numbers when proteinuria is present from any cause. Hyaline casts should be carefully inspected for inclusions since the presence of formed elements within the casts indicates that these are derived from the kidney rather than the lower urinary tract.

Granular casts are thought to represent cellular casts that have undergone degenerative changes after formation. Their presence suggests nephrosis, orthostatic proteinuria or some type of glomerulonephrosis.

Waxy casts may represent the final degenerative end product in the evolution of cellular casts. They do not occur in normal urine and are most often seen in chronic renal disease of long duration.

Fatty casts may appear in the nephrotic syndrome. They consist of lipid droplets in the epithelial cell or granular casts.

Significance of Crystals in Urine Sediment. Crystals can be divided into those that appear in acid urine and those that appear in neutral or alkaline urine. Increased quantities of crystals may occur in patients who tend to form renal stones and there are certain chemicals that may crystallize in the urine (*i.e.*, cystine, leucine, tyrosine) in certain metabolic diseases.

Special Tests

Ferric Chloride Test on Urine—see Phenylketonuria Test

17-Hydroxycorticosteroids. This is primarily a test of adrenal cortex function. The adrenal cortex produces corticosteroids which are altered and then excreted primarily in the urine. The urinary excretion of 17-hydroxycorticosteroids is an indication of the rate at which the adrenals are producing the corticosteroids. In Cushing's syndrome (hyperadrenalism), the urinary levels are higher than normal. However, the reverse is not necessarily true. In cases of adrenal cortical underfunction, the urinary levels may be within the normal range. If adrenal cortical underfunction is suspected, but the urinary 17-hydroxycorticosteroid levels are normal, ACTH may be administered and then the 17-hydroxycorticosteroid excretion levels retested. If adrenal cortical function is normal, the urinary excretion of 17-hydroxycorticosteroids will rise markedly after ACTH. However, if adrenal cortical function is poor, the urinary levels of 17-hydroxycorticosteroids will not rise appreciably.

Immunologic Test for Pregnancy. The immunologic tests rely upon commercially available anti-human chorionic gonadotropin antibody (anti-HCG). After fertilization of the ovum, chorionic gonadotropin is produced. When the test is performed, the patient's serum or urine is incubated with the antibody; HCG, if present, reacts with it and thereby inactivates the antibody. The incubated antibody sample mixture is then added to an indicator. If HCG is present in the sample, the antibody is inactivated and the red cells or particles remain unagglutinated. If the sample does not contain HCG, the antibody remains active, and agglutination occurs. The test has a 95-99 percent accuracy rate.

17-Ketosteroid Excretion. The urinary 17-ketosteroids are metabolites of adrenal cortical steroids, adrenal androgens and gonadal androgens. They represent an index of the activity of the adrenal cortex and the gonads in the male and an approximation of the activity of the adrenal cortex in the female. In normal subjects, there is a moderate variation in the 17-ketosteroid excretion in a 24-hour period. The urinary 17-ketosteroid values for normal subjects are higher in men than in women. In children, the level is normally very low.

Normal levels are found in adrenal benign tumor, menopausal women and thyrotoxicosis. Low levels of 17-ketosteroids are found in adrenal hypofunction (*i.e.*, Addison's disease, myxedema, pituitary hypofunction, primary ovarian agenesis, eunuchoid men, and starvation. High levels of 17-ketosteroids are found in adrenal hyperplasia, adrenal malignant tumor, adrenogenital syndrome and idiopathic hirsutism. Very marked elevations, over 100 mg a day, suggest either carcinoma of the adrenal cortex or the extremely rare interstitial cell tumor of the testis.

Phenolsulfonphthalein (PSP) Test. This test measures the secretory activity of the proximal tubules. In the plasma, phenolsulfonphthalein (PSP) is reversibly bound to the albumin fraction of plasma protein. Because of this binding, very little of the dye is excreted by glomerular filtration and over 90 percent of an administered dose is excreted by the renal tubules.

The PSP test is an empirical measure of the rate of excretion of a standard test dose of the dye over a fixed period of time. The rate of excretion depends chiefly on the renal plasma flow since the test dose produces too low a concentration in the plasma to saturate the tubular excretory mechanism. The dye is given as a single intravenous injection and is most rapidly excreted during the first few minutes after injection when the plasma concentration is high. After the plasma concentration is reduced to low levels, the remainder of the dose is excreted more slowly. In normal kidney function, 30 percent of the dye is excreted after 15 minutes, an additional 15 percent after 30 minutes, and another additional 10 percent after 60 minutes.

In the presence of reduced renal blood flow or inactive renal tubules, the blood must be recirculated through the kidney over a longer period of time to excrete the same amount of dye. If allowed sufficient time, the damaged kidney will excrete the same amount of PSP as the normal kidney and abnormally low excretion may be apparent only during the first 15 or 20 minutes after injection. The cumulative excretion over a period of 2 hours may be the same for normal and damaged kidneys and is usually 70-80 percent of the test dose. Approximately 15-25 percent of the test dose is excreted by the liver and is not recovered in the urine. The test is not reliable in hepatorenal disease. In summary, this test is a crude measure of the integrity of the renal tubules and their rate of perfusion with plasma.

Phenylketonuria Test (Ferric Chloride Test). This test is designed to uncover early cases of phenylketonuria. In this condition, the patient—an infant—is unable to metabolize phenylalanine properly. As a result, pathologic metabolic end products are formed which lead to permanent mental deficiency. If the disorder is recognized early, a phenylalanine deficient diet can be prescribed and the mental deficiency avoided. In many states, the law requires that every infant be tested for phenylketonuria.

TESTS PERFORMED ON CEREBROSPINAL FLUID (CSF)

Cerebrospinal fluid fills the ventricles of the brain and the central canal of the spinal cord. It acts as a fluid buffer which can enlarge or diminish in volume, when necessary, to protect the brain and spinal cord from compression injury when slight changes occur in the volume of space enclosed by the cranium and spinal column. The fluid helps prevent jarring of the brain, supplies oxygen nutrients to the brain and cord and removes waste.

Cerebrospinal fluid is produced from blood by the choroid plexus and has many of the characteristics of an ultrafiltrate of plasma. It differs from blood plasma in that it has no bilirubin, low cholesterol, low protein, less sugar, calcium and nonprotein nitrogen but more chloride. It is in osmotic equilibrium with the blood. Because of its intimate association with the brain and spinal cord, cerebrospinal fluid is a useful indicator of neurologic disorders, inflammatory diseases, and hemorrhage in the meninges.

The cerebrospinal fluid is obtained by lumbar puncture between the third and fourth lumbar vertebrae. Cerebrospinal fluid is examined when there are unexplained signs of cerebral or meningeal irritation; or when there is an unexplained coma or evidence of subarachnoid hemorrhage; or when symptoms of poliomyelitis, syphilis of the central nervous system or bacterial meningitis are present. The more common laboratory tests conducted on a spinal fluid specimen are described below.

Cell Count. *Red blood cell count.* Blood in the cerebrospinal fluid may result from injury to a meningeal vessel during the "tap" or from subarachnoid hemorrhage. With a "bloody tap," the CSF will clot but the supernatant fluid after centrifugation is clear and colorless. In contrast, following a subarachnoid hemorrhage, the blood does not clot because it is defibrinated and the supernatant fluid after centrifugation is xanthochromic.

White blood cell count. The normal number of white cells in cerebrospinal fluid is 0 to 5 per $mm.^3$ The test does not provide specific diagnostic information, but values tend to fall within ranges characteristic of certain diseases. The cell count often indicates infection and is moderately increased ($10\text{-}200/mm^3$) in poliomyelitis, encephalitis, neurosyphilis, chronic degenerative diseases of the central nervous system, epilepsy, and uremia. The cell count is greatly increased (several $1000/mm^3$) in purulent meningitis.

Chlorides. Chloride levels in the cerebrospinal fluid are lowered in all forms of generalized meningitis, except syphilitic disease. The chloride level is not altered in tumors, encephalitis, brain abscess or the chronic degenerative diseases.

Protein. Protein levels are usually elevated in proportion to the degree of leucocytosis in the cerebrospinal fluid. High protein levels accompany acute purulent meningitis and lower levels characterize chronic less virulent diseases. Protein is also elevated by the presence of blood.

Serological Tests. Serological tests are useful in the diagnosis of neurosyphilis.

Sugar. The concentration of glucose in the cerebrospinal fluid depends upon the blood glucose level and the presence of pyogenic organisms or inflammatory cells that utilize sugar in their metabolism. The spinal fluid glucose level is approximately half the blood glucose level. The spinal fluid sugar level is not altered in central nervous system glucose, chronic degenerative and neoplastic diseases. The spinal fluid sugar is moderately decreased in tuberculous meningitis and markedly decreased in pyogenic bacterial infections.

TESTS PERFORMED ON FECES

Blood. In bleeding lesions of the upper intestinal tract, gross blood is not detected macroscopically in the stool because of the effect of digestion. In such cases it is necessary to do a test for occult blood (guaiac test). The test for occult blood may be positive for ruptured varicose veins of the esophagus or stomach; swallowed blood from pulmonary hemorrhage; rupture of aortic aneurysm into the esophagus; carcinoma of the esophagus, stomach or intestine; ulcer of stomach or duodenum; intestinal ulcers due to typhoid fever or tuberculosis; embolism of the superior mesenteric artery; venous thrombosis of mesenteric veins; ulcerative colitis; bacillary and amebic dysentery; hemophilia; hemolytic jaundice; and purpura.

In general, blood originating from a lesion in the lower colon is bright red and hemorrhage from the upper gastrointestinal tract results in a tarry stool. The presence of blood in any tarry or red stool should be confirmed by a chemical test for occult blood. Any degree of positiveness of the guaiac test for occult blood usually signifies bleeding in the gastrointestinal tract and a thorough investigation for the source of bleeding is indicated.

Fat Determination. Very few neutral fat globules are found in the normal stool. The presence of large amounts of neutral fat may suggest that the patient has been taking an oily laxative. This test is used to study any patients with symptoms suggesting intestinal malabsorption and to confirm a diagnosis of steatorrhea (excess fat in the stools). Total fat is increased in the feces in ileitis, extrahepatic obstructive jaundice, pancreatitis, obstruction of the pancreatic duct, sprue, and celiac disease. Some patients with pancreatic insufficiency may have an increase in neutral fat content of the stools. An increase of fat content of the stool does not, however, permit a specific diagnosis of pancreatic deficiency to be made since pancreatic enzymes may be normal in certain instances of steatorrhea.

Guaiac Test—see Blood

Parasites. Examinations of feces for parasites are performed in order to identify the parasites or their eggs. The therapy will usually depend on the type of parasite found so that precise identification is important.

MISCELLANEOUS TESTS

Basal Metabolic Rate (BMR). The oldest and least specific test of thyroid function is the basal metabolic rate (BMR). This measurement of oxygen consumption is expressed as kilocalories expended per square meter of body surface per hour, with the fasted patient in a condition of physical and mental repose.

The BMR may be elevated in hyperthyroidism, anxiety, infection, leukemia, severe pulmonary or cardiovascular disease, acidosis, polycythemia, severe anemia, acromegaly, diabetes insipidus, and Cushing's disease.

The BMR may be decreased in hypothyroidism, hypopituitarism, malnutrition, Addison's disease, anorexia nervosa and nephrotic syndrome.

This test is often replaced by more specific tests of thyroid function.

Chloride in Sweat. This is a test for cystic fibrosis of the pancreas. Children with cystic fibrosis excrete greater quantities of chloride in their perspiration than do normal children.

Radioiodine Uptake. The radioiodine uptake test is used in the diagnosis of certain thyroid conditions. It is based on the fact that the radioactive isotope of iodine, I^{131}, is taken up by the thyroid in the same manner as ordinary iodine. The breakdown of I^{131} to more stable elements results in the release of gamma rays which can be detected and counted by a scintillation counter. The degree of radioactivity is a measure of the degree of iodine uptake. Uptake below normal suggests hypothyroidism and uptake above normal suggests hyperthyroidism.

Thorn Test. The thorn test is a test of adrenal function. It is based on the fact that ACTH produces a decrease of at least 50 percent in four hours in persons with a normally functioning adrenal cortex. Patients with normal adrenal function respond to ACTH injections by a decrease in the circulating eosinphils and an increase in the excretion of uric acid as compared to creatinine. Patients with Addison's disease do not respond to ACTH injections. The thorn test is also a test of adrenal cortical reserve before surgery and a test to differentiate functional hypopituitarism from organic disease of the adrenal cortex.

References

1. Bauer, J. D., Ackerman, P. G. and Toro, G.: *Bray's Clinical Laboratory Methods,* ed. 7, C. V. Mosby Co., St. Louis, 1968.

2. Collens, R. D.: *Illustrated Manual of Laboratory Diagnosis—Indications and Interpretations,* J. B. Lippincott Co., Philadelphia, 1968.

3. Davidsohn, I. and Wells, B. B.: *Clinical Diagnosis by Laboratory Methods,* ed. 13, W. B. Saunders Co., Philadelphia, 1966.

4. Garb, S.: *Laboratory Tests in Common Use,* ed. 5, Springer Publishing Co., Inc., New York, 1971.

5. Linné, J. J. and Ringsrud, K. M.: *Basic Laboratory Techniques for the Medical Laboratory Technician,* McGraw-Hill Book Co., New York, 1970.

6. Page, L. B. and Culver, P. J.: *Syllabus of Laboratory Examinations in Clinical Diagnosis,* ed. 4, Harvard University Press, Massachusetts, 1966.

7. Ravel, R.: *Clinical Laboratory Medicine—Application of Laboratory Data,* Year Book Medical Publishers, Inc., Chicago, 1969.

8. Wells, B. B. and Halsted, J. A.: *Clinical Pathology—Interpretation and Application,* ed. 4, W. B. Saunders Co., Philadelphia, 1967.

25

Principles of experimental design for clinical drug studies

by Charles Ralph Buncher

Although clinical drug trials have been described and studied for decades, and numerous articles have been written on their methodology, it is still not clear just what a clinical trial of drugs is. Some people think of an elaborate trial of two or more drugs which requires the cooperation of physicians, pharmacists, pharmacologists, nurses, statisticians, computer experts and a great array of clerical help. This investigational army must make use of elaborate forms to record responses from the patients, use fancy codes to disguise the identity of their medications, meet and agree upon the definitions of symptoms and responses and they must expend a great effort as measured in time, personnel and money. Other people would say that any time a person consumes even one dose of a drug, there is a clinical trial.

There is a certain truth in each of these extreme positions. The essence of a clinical trial contains these elements: (1) one or more treatments which we shall consider as pharmacologic entities; (2) experimental subjects who are human beings; and (3) a measurement of the change caused by the treatment. Everything else may be considered as accessory. Still, most people think that more information is forthcoming from a bigger study than a smaller one, that a carefully planned and executed study is better than one with less planning and poorer execution and that adherence to certain principles make a study better than one which ignores the principles of good experimentation.

This chapter is an effort to discuss some of the principles of good clinical drug trials from the viewpoint of a pharmacist so that he will know his contribution, so that he can help decide for himself about the quality of the studies that he reads in journals and so that he can advise others on the quality of studies.

INVESTIGATIONAL DRUGS AND PROTOCOLS

Before discussing the various methods of studying drugs, we should first classify drugs from the regulatory standpoint. In accordance with the Federal Food, Drug and Cosmetic Act and various Food and Drug Administration (FDA) regulations, there are two classes of drugs. Drugs are designated as old or new depending upon general acceptance by qualified medical experts as to safety and effectiveness for the specific clinical indication claimed and whether the drug has been used to a material extent and for a material time. An example of an old drug is aspirin which is generally regarded by qualified experts as safe and effective for use as an analgesic in the treatment of temporary pain. Any qualified manufacturer may distribute an old drug without being required to conduct new clinical studies to reestablish its safety and efficacy, although proof of bioavailability may be required.

In the case of a new drug, the manufacturer is required to establish its safety and efficacy for the claimed clinical indication prior to distributing such drug for other than investigational use. Each new drug sponsor is required to have on file with the FDA an approved New Drug Application (NDA). This NDA must contain the results of animal pharmacologic and toxicologic studies, human pharmacology studies, adequate and well-controlled clinical studies, analyses of the drug's efficacy and side effects and various supporting information such as the manufacturing and control methods. The NDA also contains the precise labeling to be used with the drug. It should be noted that once an NDA is approved by the FDA, it may be revoked or suspended for a number of reasons including the event that new knowledge becomes available concerning the lack of safety or efficacy of the new drug.

A new drug does not have to be a newly de-

52

Form FD 1573
Department of Health, Education and Welfare
Food and Drug Administration

STATEMENT OF INVESTIGATOR

Date ______

Name of Investigator ______

Name of Drug ______

To:

Dear Sir:

The undersigned, ______, submits this statement as required by section 505 (i) of the Federal Food, Drug, and Cosmetic Act and § 130.3 of Title 21 of Code of Federal Regulations as a condition for receiving and conducting clinical pharmacology with a new drug limited by Federal law (or United States) to investigational use.

1. Attachment 1. A statement of my education and experience.

2. If any hospital, institutional, and clinical laboratory facilities, etc., are available and will be employed in connection with the investigation, an identification of each follows:

(If this information has previously been submitted to the sponsor, reference to the previous submission will be adequate.)

3. Attachment 2. The investigational drug will be used by the undersigned or under his supervision in accordance with the plan of investigation.

4. The undersigned understands that the following conditions, generally applicable to new drugs for investigational use, govern his receipt and use of this investigational drug:

a. The sponsor is required to supply the investigator with full information concerning the preclinical investigations that justify clinical trials, together with fully informative material describing any prior investigations and experience and any possible hazards, contraindications, side effects, and precautions to be taken into account in the course of the investigation.

b. The investigator is required to maintain adequate records of the disposition of all receipts of the drug, including dates, quantities, and use by subjects, and if the investigation is terminated to return to the sponsor any unused supply of the drug.

c. The investigator is required to prepare and maintain adequate and accurate case histories designed to record all observations and other data pertinent to the investigation on each individual treated with the drug or employed as a control in the investigation.

53

d. The investigator is required to furnish his reports to the sponsor of the drug who is responsible for collecting and evaluating the results obtained by various investigators. The sponsor is required to present progress reports to the Food and Drug Administration at appropriate intervals not exceeding 1 year. Any adverse effect that may reasonably be regarded as caused by, or probably caused by, the new drug shall be reported to the sponsor promptly, and if the adverse effect is alarming, it shall be reported immediately. An adequate report of the investigation should be furnished to the sponsor shortly after completion of the investigation.

e. The investigator shall maintain the records of disposition of the drug and the case histories described above for a period of 2 years following the date a new-drug application is approved for the drug; or if the application is not approved, until 2 years after the investigation is discontinued. Upon the request of a scientifically trained and properly authorized employee of the Department, at reasonable times, the investigator will make such records available for inspection and copying. The subjects' names need not be divulged unless the records of particular individuals require a more detailed study of the cases, or unless there is reason to believe that the records do not represent actual cases studied, or do not represent actual results obtained.

f. The investigator certifies that the drug will be administered only to subjects under his personal supervision or under the supervision of the following investigators responsible to him,

and that the drug will not be supplied to any other investigator or to any clinic for administration to subjects.

g. The investigator certifies that he will inform any subjects, including subjects used as controls, or their representatives, that drugs are being used for investigational purposes, and will obtain the consent of the subjects, or their representatives, except where this is not feasible or, in the investigator's professional judgment, is contrary to the best interests of the subjects.

Very truly yours,

Signed ______

______
(Name of investigator)

______
(Address)

______

(This form should be supplemented or amended from time to time if new subjects are added or if significant changes are made in the plan of investigation.)

veloped compound. An old drug may become a new drug by virtue of a new indication, changes in the formulation, changes in the manufacture, a new combination of drugs, new dosage or a new carrier, coating, excipient or menstruum.

Clearly, one would be able to study for a new indication a compound that has been marketed for some time more easily than a new compound that has never been used in man, but by regulation, each would be considered a new drug and for each a Notice of Claimed Investigation Exemption for a New Drug (IND) must be filed with the FDA. Form FD-1571, which details the attachments necessary to prove a drug is ready for investigational use and includes the prospective plans for clinical pharmacology studies and information about the investigators who will study the drug, is illustrated in Figure 1. Thirty days after submission of the IND, subject to FDA agreement, the supervisor of the intended investigations may begin to study the new drug in humans.[1]

There are many ways in which the pharmacist can and should play a part in preparing for a clinical drug trial. For instance, if there is a drug manufacturer that wishes to have a hospital physician act as an investigator for a new drug, then the pharmacist should help evaluate the information about the new drug supplied by the manufacturer. He may check that the toxicity testing is adequate to indicate that the drug will be safe in the patients and that there is some reason for believing the drug will be efficacious. He will also want to evaluate the pitfalls found in previous studies of the drug.

Occasionally, the pharmacist may wish to call attention to the need for a clinical study as in the case of a drug that is being used for an indication for which it has not been approved.[2,3] An example would be an anti-arrhythmic agent that is being used to prevent attacks of angina pectoris. This problem has been discussed elsewhere and one possible solution is to put the agent under investigational study. In some cases, the pharmacist may wish to recommend use of a drug that is not currently used by the hospital staff. Perhaps he can convince the appropriate hospital committee that a study should be set up to compare his choice with the drug currently being used by the hospital staff or to test his new drug against a placebo.

Animal and Clinical Pharmacology

Before any drug is ready to be given to a human, it should have undergone extensive testing in animals. Animal testing provides a model for the results to be expected when the drug is used in humans. Thus, lack of serious side effects in several species of animals gives a measure of assurance that the drug will be reasonably safe for use in man. Toxicity testing indicates the nature of difficulties that can be expected from overdosing and the most susceptible organs or tissues. Metabolic testing provides information about accumulation of the drug in the bloodstream and tissues and the route of excretion. Finally, animal models provide the indications that certain drugs, *e.g.*, pressor amines, are likely to be efficacious in humans, whereas others, *e.g.*, psychotropic medications, have effects which are much more difficult to extrapolate to humans. Testing in animals also provides insight into the possible therapeutic dosage (mg of drug per Kg of body weight), for its use in humans.

The first clinical trial of a new drug entity is in human volunteers in a rigidly controlled environment. These volunteers are usually normal human subjects not suffering from the disease or condition to be treated, with some exceptions such as in the study of anticancer agents. These first studies, known as Phase I, assure the experimenters that the drug is reasonably well tolerated and sufficiently safe for further clinical testing. Additional information on range of therapeutic dosage is provided by first giving the medication in the range of the lowest possible active dose working up to the range of therapeutic doses, and then continuing on to the production of side effects to discern their expected nature and severity.

During Phase II studies, those persons who are candidates for treatment with the drug are studied so that the emphasis shifts from normal subjects to clinical patients. During this period, the definitive dosage studies are undertaken and completed, and the drug metabolism studies are extended. Decisions concerning the various possible formulations as well as the preferred routes of administration are made. A more complete description of these early clinical pharmacology studies is found in the literature cited.[4]

Throughout these early studies, extensive laboratory testing has been employed to study the effect of the drug, if any, on important constituents of the blood, various enzyme systems and organ function. Any serious effect discovered in one or more of these tests could immediately halt the years of research to provide assurance on any major question of safety. Providing that none of these difficulties has arisen, the drug passes on to Phase III, the clinical drug trials to assess efficacy, safety and usual side effects. Accepting this described background as a minimum for any drug that has passed on to Phase III trials, we can now discuss the principles involved in efficient and effective clinical drug trials.

The Protocol

Creation of the protocol or study design is the first step in any clinical trial. Any human endeavor that involves a number of people from disciplines that have been taught to think differently is bound to involve misunderstanding and disagreement. Does the physician or the nurse fill out the report form? Does the pharmacist or physician give the capsules to the patient? Should one week's medication or two be given to the patient at the first visit? Which standard medication is best for patients after they drop out of the trial? What other medications will be denied to the patient as long as he is in the study?

Most trials require the use of new report forms and/or new procedures by the physician, nurse and pharmacist. A rule of thumb for any trial is to try using all of the new methods and report forms prior to beginning the trial. Are there special times the medication is to be taken? Try it with a standard drug to see that there is no confusion. Is a special form to be filled out by the patient? Try it on comparable patients to see if they understand the instructions. Is the physician going to phone the pharmacy for a special preparation to be ready immediately? Try it a few times to make sure that more routine work will not be obstructed. Are the drugs to be given to the patients in the emergency room? Try it to see if this produces unexpected problems during the emergency situation. Does the nurse have to keep a record of the administration of the drug? Try it to see if this interferes with other work.

A protocol should contain descriptions of each of the following elements: the objective of the study, how patients are diagnosed for the disease being treated, which patients will be included and which excluded from the study, the criteria that will be used to measure efficacy, the study design and the anticipated statistical analysis. Each of these points must be discussed and decided as part of the work necessary prior to beginning a clinical drug trial.

Objective of the Study

A precise statement of the objective of the study is an essential part of the protocol. Occasionally the research will have gone many steps with a vague goal such as investigating the new drug in patients with mammary carcinoma. This is not an adequate statement because a trial must be designed to answer one or more specific questions. Typical examples are as follows: This study will investigate whether the new drug is more efficacious in the treatment of hypertension than is the standard drug in men and in women above the age of child-bearing; this study will investigate whether the new drug causes weight loss in diabetic patients of ages 40 to 60 when compared to an identical appearing placebo; this study will investigate whether 200 mg of the new drug is more efficacious as a hypnotic than 100 mg of the new drug. In order for the objective to be precise, each of the essentials of the objective must be precisely described in the protocol. Thus, the protocol must go on to define "more efficacy," "weight loss" and "more efficacious" in these examples, and to explain fully how each will be measured and how the various diseases will be diagnosed.

Defining the Disease Entity

An agreement on the disease entity involved is a perennial problem, especially in multiclinic studies in which several investigators are involved. Are only patients who have vomited to be included, or also those complaining of dry heaving? Are both squamous cell carcinoma and basal cell carcinoma included, or only one of the two? Is the clinician's diagnosis sufficient, or must it be confirmed by pathologic examination? Does the diagnosis of anxiety have to be made by two completely independent examinations, or can the two clinicians discuss and arrive at a joint diagnosis? What type of pains will be necessary to make the patient eligible for the study? A precise definition of the disease entity can be the most difficult decision in the study. In a case such as lung carcinoma, the definition can be reasonably precise once a tissue specimen is obtained and evaluated by a pathologist. In the case of pains or nausea or depression, the definition of the disease or symptom is quite difficult and subject to a great deal of dispute. Thus, the first rule is to define the disease entity as precisely as possible, and then to be certain that the patients who will take part in the clinical trial have been shown to have the disease. For instance, if a microbiologic cure is to be demonstrated, one must be able to demonstrate that the individual has a given bacteria. If the drug is to prevent a disease, there should be a demonstration that the patients are susceptible.

The pharmacist has several important roles to

FORM FD-1571 (4/67)
DEPARTMENT OF HEALTH, EDUCATION, AND WELFARE
FOOD AND DRUG ADMINISTRATION

50

Form Approved
Budget Bureau No. 57-R0030

NOTICE OF
CLAIMED INVESTIGATIONAL EXEMPTION
FOR A NEW DRUG

Name of Sponsor

Address

Date

Name of Investigational Drug

To the Secretary of Health, Education, and Welfare
For the Commissioner of Food and Drugs
Washington, D.C. 20204

Dear Sir:

The sponsor, ____, submits this notice of claimed investigational exemption for a new drug under the provisions of section 505(i) of the Federal Food, Drug, and Cosmetic Act and §130.3 of Title 21 of the Code of Federal Regulations.

Attached hereto, in triplicate, are:

1. The best available descriptive name of the drug, including to the extent known the chemical name and structure of any new-drug substance, and a statement of how it is to be administered. (If the drug has only a code name, enough information should be supplied to identify the drug.)

2. Complete list of components of the drug, including any reasonable alternates for inactive components.

3. Complete statement of quantitative composition of drug, including reasonable variations that may be expected during the investigational stage.

4. Description of source and preparation of, any new-drug substances used as components, including the name and address of each supplier or processor, other than the sponsor, of each new-drug substance.

5. A statement of the methods, facilities, and controls used for the manufacturing, processing, and packing of the new drug to establish and maintain appropriate standards of identity, strength, quality, and purity as needed for safety and to give significance to clinical investigations made with the drug.

6. A statement covering all information available to the sponsor derived from preclinical investigations and any clinical studies and experience with the drug as follows:

a. Adequate information about the preclinical investigations, including studies made on laboratory animals, on the basis of which the sponsor has concluded that it is reasonably safe to initiate clinical investigations with the drug: Such information should include identification of the person who conducted each investigation; identification and qualifications of the individuals who evaluated the results and concluded that it is reasonably safe to initiate clinical investigations with the drug and a statement of where the investigations were conducted and where the records are available for inspection; and enough details about the investigations to permit scientific review. The preclinical investigations shall not be considered adequate to justify clinical testing unless they give proper attention to the conditions of the proposed clinical testing. When this information, the outline of the plan of clinical pharmacology, or any progress report on the clinical pharmacology, indicates a need for full review of the preclinical data before a clinical trial is undertaken, the Department will notify the sponsor to submit the complete preclinical data and to withhold clinical trials until the review is completed and the sponsor notified. The Food and Drug Administration will be prepared to confer with the sponsor concerning this action.

b. If the drug has been marketed commercially or investigated (e.g. outside the United States), complete information about such distribution or investigation shall be submitted, along with a complete bibliography of any publications about the drug.

c. If the drug is a combination of previously investigated or marketed drugs, an adequate summary of preexisting information from preclinical and clinical investigations and experience with its components, including all reports available to the sponsor suggesting side-effects, contraindications, and ineffectiveness in use of such components: Such summary should include an adequate bibliography of publications about the components and may incorporate by reference any information concerning such components previously submitted by the sponsor to the Food and Drug Administration. Include a statement of the expected pharmacological effects of the combination.

7. A total of five copies of all informational material, including label and labeling, which is to be supplied to each investigator: This shall include an accurate description of the prior investigations and experience and their results pertinent to the safety and possible usefulness of the drug under the conditions of the investigation. It shall not represent that the safety or usefulness of the drug has been established for the purposes to be investigated. It shall describe all relevant hazards, contraindications, side-effects, and precautions suggested by prior investigations and experience with the drug under investigation and related drugs for the information of clinical investigators.

8. The scientific training and experience considered appropriate by the sponsor to qualify the investigators as suitable experts to investigate the safety of the drug, bearing in mind what is known about the pharmacological action of the drug and the phase of the investigational program that is to be undertaken.

51

9. The names and a summary of the training and experience of each investigator and of the individual charged with monitoring the progress of the investigation and evaluating the evidence of safety and effectiveness of the drug as it is received from the investigators, together with a statement that the sponsor has obtained from each investigator a completed and signed form, as provided in subparagraph (12) or (13) of this paragraph, and that the investigator is qualified by scientific training and experience as an appropriate expert to undertake the phase of the investigation outlined in section 10 of the "Notice of claimed investigational exemption for a new drug." (In crucial situations, phase 3 investigators may be added and this form supplemented by rapid communication methods, and the signed form FD 1573 shall be obtained promptly thereafter.)

10. An outline of any phase or phases of the planned investigations, as follows:

a. Clinical pharmacology. This is ordinarily divided into two phases: Phase 1 starts when the new drug is first introduced into man—only animal and in vitro data are available—with the purpose of determining human toxicity, metabolism, absorption, elimination, and other pharmacological action, preferred route of administration, and safe dosage range; phase 2 covers the initial trials on a limited number of patients for specific disease control or prophylaxis purposes. A general outline of these phases shall be submitted, identifying the investigator or investigators, the hospitals or research facilities where the clinical pharmacology will be undertaken, any expert committees or panels to be utilized, the maximum number of subjects to be involved, and the estimated duration of these early phases of investigation. Modification of the experimental design on the basis of experience gained need be reported only in the progress reports on these early phases, or in the development of the plan for the clinical trial, phase 3. The first two phases may overlap and, when indicated, may require additional animal data before these phases can be completed or phase 3 can be undertaken. Such animal tests shall be designed to take into account the expected duration of administration of the drug to human beings, the age groups and physical status, as for example, infants, pregnant women, premenopausal women, of those human beings to whom the drug may be administered, unless this has already been done in the original animal studies.

b. *Clinical trial.* This phase 3 provides the assessment of the drug's safety and effectiveness and optimum dosage schedules in the diagnosis, treatment, or prophylaxis of groups of subjects involving a given disease or condition. A reasonable protocol is developed on the basis of the facts accumulated in the earlier phases, including completed and submitted animal studies. This phase is conducted by separate groups following the same protocol (with reasonable variations and alternatives permitted by the plan) to produce well-controlled clinical data. For this phase, the following data shall be submitted:

i. The names and addresses of the investigators. (Additional investigators may be added.)

ii. The specific nature of the investigations to be conducted, together with information or case report forms to show the scope and detail of the planned clinical observations and the clinical laboratory tests to be made and reported.

iii. The approximate number of subjects (a reasonable range of subjects is permissible and additions may be made), and criteria proposed for subject selection by age, sex, and condition.

iv. The estimated duration of the clinical trial and the intervals, not exceeding 1 year, at which progress reports showing the results of the investigations will be submitted to the Food and Drug Administration.

(The notice of claimed investigational exemption may be limited to any one or more phases, provided the outline of the additional phase or phases is submitted before such additional phases begin. This does not preclude continuing a subject on the drug from phase 2 to phase 3 without interruption while the plan for phase 3 is being developed.)

Ordinarily, a plan for clinical trial will not be regarded as reasonable unless, among other things, it provides for more than one independent competent investigator to maintain adequate case histories of an adequate number of subjects, designed to record observations and permit evaluation of any and all discernible effects attributable to the drug in each individual treated, and comparable records on any individuals employed as controls. These records shall be individual records for each subject maintained to include adequate information pertaining to each, including age, sex, conditions treated, dosage, frequency of administration of the drug, results of all relevant clinical observations and laboratory examinations made, adequate information concerning any other treatment given and a full statement of any adverse effects and useful results observed, together with an opinion as to whether such effects or results are attributable to the drug under investigation.

11. It is understood that the sponsor will notify the Food and Drug Administration if the investigation is discontinued, and the reason therefor.

12. It is understood that the sponsor will notify each investigator if a new-drug application is approved, or if the investigation is discontinued.

13. If the drug is to be sold, a full explanation why sale is required and should not be regarded as the commercialization of a new drug for which an application is not approved.

Very truly yours,

(Sponsor)

Per

(Indicate authority)

s notice may be amended or supplemented from time to time on the basis of the experience gained with the new drug.
ress reports may be used to update the notice.)

ALL NOTICES AND CORRESPONDENCE SHOULD BE SUBMITTED IN TRIPLICATE.

play during the time that the protocol is being written.[5] He must remember that the obligation and responsibility for the drug use remain by law, with the principal investigator who is the physician in charge. Form FD-1573, shown in Figure 2, details the responsibilities of the investigator. Physicians will usually welcome the help of the pharmacist in maintaining the extensive records necessary after receipt of the drug including quantities, dates and use by subjects. At the end of the investigation, the unused supply of the drug is to be returned to the sponsor. Records must be kept for at least two years from the end of the investigation.

The pharmacist, by reason of his training and knowledge, should advise about the role of other drugs, and perhaps even foods, that will be used by the patient during the course of the trial. He can advise about differences in vehicle, particle size, disintegration properties and differences in salt form. He should help decide which other drugs are sufficiently important that they should be incorporated into the study design, which other drugs are not to be used at all during the course of the study and which drugs may be used and their usage recorded on the report forms.[5] Thus, the decision might be in studying an anti-anginal drug that nitroglycerin is important enough that it should be taken into account in the design of the study, other anti-anginal agents should not be used during the study and diuretics are permitted but should be recorded as concomitant therapy on the report form.

In preparing the trial, objective measures of efficacy are preferred to subjective ones since the former usually vary much less from investigation to investigation and are less likely to be influenced by non-drug factors. Thus, a microbiologic culture is preferable to a patient reporting congestion. In many difficult areas of research, the only measures available for use are subjective. Only the patient can report whether the pain is more severe or less severe today than yesterday; it is well known that the patient is not very good in being able to report this fact precisely. By objective, we imply a method that would give the same result for the same stimulus at all times and for all persons.

In actual fact, we know that bacterial cultures will have a certain amount of variable growth even if they started with the same number of organisms in the first place. Likewise, there is a certain amount of variability in serum glucose values because of the sampling problem, because of variation in the electronic or other equipment, because of the technician and so forth. We know that a given pain stimulus may produce a great array of responses in different people from no pain through severe pain. Thus, we are really saying that the variability in objective measurements tends to be small as compared to the variability in subjective measurements, and we prefer measurements with as small as possible variability due to factors that are not under study. There is another important reason for preferring objective measurements to subjective. Subjective measurements are more prone to biases from the surroundings. Thus, if the day is cloudy, patients are likely to report feeling a little worse than if the day is sunny and bright. If the physician is feeling upset because of a fight with the nurse, this attitude can come through in the patients' subjective evaluations. Readings from hemocytometer or auto-analyzer are not so easily biased; they may change by a few points but are not likely to have switched a whole qualitative rating.

It should be noted that one definition of objective as used in medicine is a report by one other than the patient on the patient's condition. Thus, if the nurse reports that the patient looks better today, this can be considered in medicine to be an objective measure. Truly objective measurements, those derived by machines which are not susceptible to subtle biases, are always the goal in clinical drug trials. Third party direct observation is often a useful alternative to subjective reporting by the patient if no other more objective methods are available.

Ethical Considerations

In setting up a clinical drug trial, one must always pay due attention to ethical considerations. The treatment of human patients and the proper place of ethics in this treatment is the province of physicians, but all others involved in the potential trial must also consider this factor. The purpose of a trial is to use information on the patients involved to try to decide what treatment should be given to future patients. It would not be ethical to do anything with the patients under study that is not for their own benefit; judging this benefit is very difficult indeed.[6,7,8]

The consent of the patients is another part of the problem of ethics that is the province of the physician-patient relationship. It is now generally agreed that patients must consent to the clinical trial of a drug being used for investigational purposes, and that they cannot properly consent unless they are fully informed of the risks that are involved, whether the risks are large or small. In practical fact, the patient would have to be as educated as the physician and pharmacist with perhaps a touch of statistician thrown in to evaluate properly the risks in order to make an "informed" decision. Nevertheless, most people do understand the term informed consent to mean that there has been no deliberate hiding of the facts from the patient and to the best of his ability he has understood and decided that he should participate in the trial.

Two principles are sufficient to decide the question of ethics in a trial for the author of this chapter. The trial should be in the best interests of the patients involved, as judged by the physician and the patient's informed consent, and as will be explained later, placebo is the best drug therapy for the patient until some other compound is proven to be superior. The discussion of ethical considerations could be a chapter itself and will not be discussed further here.

The points mentioned are only to give the reader an idea of the many possible problems involved in any clinical drug trial. Other potential problems will no doubt come to mind. Each particular environment, such as the hospital, specialized center, emergency clinic, university training area and private practice, produces its own special problems. Other discussions of this are found in the literature cited.[9,10,11]

Study Design

A balance must be sought between complicated trials and control of anticipated problems. Thus, if a trial was set up to compare two hypnotic drugs in a hospital, the physician could prescribe the first drug to the first patient, the second drug to the second patient, the first drug to the third patient and so on alternately. Then the patient could report how long it took him to get to sleep. This trial would certainly be simple and there would be little problem in bookkeeping or missing observations or nurses being called away when they were supposed to be observing the patients. On the other hand, the study could be very carefully designed so that there is a balance between men and women, between young and old, between chronic users of hypnotics and first time users, between ward patients and private patients, between pre-operative patients and post-operative patients and so forth. Moreover, the patient might report his sleep characteristics for that evening, and in addition the nurse might observe him every 15 minutes, and perhaps the physician would observe him once each evening. In fact, the study could be so carefully controlled because of the anticipated problems that a book of instructions might have to be written.

The point of this example is merely that complicated protocols are frequently necessary in order to control problems that might invalidate the whole study. Contrarily, too much control is impractical since the members of the investigating team usually have other duties and do not have the opportunity to follow a whole book of regulations that has been specially written for this trial, even if they would take time to read it. Thus, one of the basic balances to be achieved is to make the study sufficiently restricted to overcome the most likely and most important problems but at the same time to keep the study sufficiently simple so that it can be carried out as designed.

To understand the modern principles of proper and acceptable and meaningful clinical trials, one should consider the history of the subject. For thousands of years various pharmacologic remedies have been tried in an attempt to cure or to mitigate certain disease entities. The basic trial consisted of a person being given the medication by a testing prescriber of medication, sometimes a physician, sometimes a pharmacist and sometimes a mother. The patient would get better in a great majority of cases, regardless of medication or prescribing person. Therefore, after almost any medication, the majority of patients would be considered "cured." The results of these "experiments" would be in the form of testimonials for the new drug.

The control in this "experimentation" was that the new treatment performed at least as well as some idea of a historical control. Thus, each patient had some expectation of the outcome without the advent of the new drug, and if on the average, patients did not do at least that well, the new drug would be rejected. Furthermore, drugs that worked for only one or two prescribers and not for others were subject to sufficient dispute to prevent widespread use in spite of a small band of ardent and confirmed admirers.

CHARACTERISTICS OF A GOOD CLINICAL TRIAL

Over the years, many principles for carrying out clinical drug trials have evolved. Through the hard lessons of many investigations in the course of time, it was found that certain goals for proper research were necessary.[12] If these goals were reached, there would be no question that the study was valid, informative and a contribution to the pharmaceutical literature. If the goals were not reached, the study might be almost all right with a few nagging questions, or of interest but not necessarily valid or simply not valid, or even completely useless or useless and dangerous to the participants. A set of guidelines describing "adequate and well-controlled" clinical investigations was published by the FDA in the *Federal Register* May 8, 1970.[13] For present purposes the characteristics of a good clinical drug trial have been reduced to the following six points.

1. Controlled comparisons
2. Blind evaluation
3. Randomized allocation
4. Orthogonal contrasts
5. Replicated study
6. Proper administration

Each of these characteristics will be discussed in more detail.

Controlled Comparisons

In order to estimate the effects of the drug, the drug must be compared to something. There are a number of possibilities that can be classified into the four categories described briefly below. A discussion of placebo comparisons will follow because of the particularly important role of placebo in clinical drug trials.

Placebo controlled. The new drug can be compared to an identically appearing preparation which is known to be pharmacologically inert for that indication. Thus, lactose is a usual placebo for analgesics, but mannose, with almost no calories, would be a more appropriate placebo for a study of anorexia. The placebo comparison tests whether the new preparation has effects greater than those due to placebo with the implication that the extra effects found are due to its pharmacologic properties.

Positive drug controlled. The new drug can be compared to an identically appearing medication known to be efficacious for the indication of interest. If there is a drug that is considered standard, for instance isoproterenol for bronchodilation, then it is frequently the ethical thing to do to compare the new drug with this standard. The only point is that whatever placebo effect there might be should work for the new drug as well as for the comparison drug so that the differences will be due to therapeutic differences and not placebo effect differences. Moreover, the new drug should be superior to an accepted standard in terms of efficacy, safety or convenience in some patients or it would not be a pharmaceutical advance.

Historical controlled. If there is a long and consistent history of the outcome of the disease, especially if the outcome is death, then it is possible to compare the new treatment to the historical standard. This type of control is useful if there is a major improvement from the new drug. If 25 percent of the cases are now cured, whereas only 5 percent cures would be expected on a historical basis, then there will be little argument that the new drug therapy is effective. If the improvement is not large, for instance the life of the patient is prolonged by two months on the average, then all of the old problems of proving this contention against a rigid standard will arise again. In those cases in which historical control is used, the search is for a marked improvement over the current therapy.

Uncontrolled. Occasionally the measurements necessary to prove efficacy are sufficiently objective that no control seems necessary. For instance, if a new drug were designed to remove mercury from the blood stream, it might be reasonable merely to make measurements of the serum mercury before the drug treatment and then at successive time intervals during and after the drug treatment. In this experiment, there would be no control group that was receiving placebo or other therapy. Again, if the differences found are large and consistent, there will be convincing evidence of efficacy of the drug; if the differences are small and variable, skeptics will question the validity of the trial.

The third and fourth possibility must be thought of as useful only in certain unusual and carefully chosen situations. Misuse of these two types of controls would turn the clock back to the days when experiments were poorly controlled or uncontrolled.

Use of the placebo. One difficulty with the testimonial type studies is what is known as the placebo effect. Placebo, from the latin for "I shall please," is well known to pharmacists as some chemical entity that has no pharmacologic property that will affect disease or symptoms. Unfortunately this attitude does not do justice to a drug that can practically work miracles.

How do we know the effects of any drug? We must compare the drug with another drug or some other therapy. Therefore, we must compare the effects of placebo to the effects that would occur without placebo. Placebo is well-known to be a good analgesic; it cures or reduces the pain from headaches, backaches, post-operative pain, rheumatoid arthritis, angina pectoris and cardiac pain; it has cured motion sickness, gastric hyperacidity, the symptoms of common cold, clinical cough; and can tranquilize or stimulate.[14] A vast catalogue of effects could be cited, but one interesting case might prove the point. About one-tenth of all women who were anovulatory ovulated following administration of a placebo under study conditions.[15] Moreover, side effects from placebo therapy are even more extensive than the list of conditions that are aided by placebo. Headaches, nausea, vomiting, dizziness, diarrhea, pain, dermatitis, drowsiness, anxiety-nervousness, weakness-fatigue, dry mouth, abdominal pain, insomnia, urinary frequency, urticaria, loss of libido, tinnitis and so forth have all been caused by the administration of placebos. One study reported the following conclusion: "Virtually no toxic effects were reported from 'known' control pills containing lactose, but the exactly similar 'unknown' control pills, which were thought by the subjects to contain iron, produced as many side-effects as the pills which did, in fact, contain it."[16]

Uncertainty is seen to be an important factor in the placebo effect. Virtually no one reacts to a known placebo; virtually everyone reacts at some time to some unknown therapeutic remedy that later turns out to be a placebo. The setting that is implicit in a clinical drug trial is also the setting that is most likely to bring out the placebo reaction: hospital or other medical setting, a prestigious investigator who states that the drug therapy is likely to be beneficial, a pharmacist representing knowledge of the pharmacopeia and some symptom or disease that is likely to disappear with the right drug therapy.

Several suggestions may come to mind. Why not eliminate placebo reactors leaving only the people who will truly react to a therapeutically effective drug? This is much easier to say than to do. One might try to give placebo first to everyone and eliminate those who are cured by placebo from the rest of the trial. Only those patients who have not been cured by placebo will be in the next stage which will be a comparison of the drug and placebo. In studying analgesics, this sort of design has been used to help sharpen the contrast between an active drug and a placebo or between two active drugs. The term "active drug" is used for a chemical entity as long as there is a possibility that it has some therapeutic effect for the given indication, over and above that due to placebo reactions. Penicillin is an active drug for antibiotic uses, but it is just another placebo as an analgesic. Placebos and active drugs may produce an array of side effects so the term placebo is used to mean a chemical entity without pharmacologic efficacy.

Unfortunately for the ease of research, the cases that produce the most placebo response are also likely to produce highly variable placebo response. Thus, a group of people who respond to placebo today for pain relief, may not respond to placebo next week. Moreover, those who are non-responders this week may well turn out to be placebo responders next week. Those who respond to placebo for one indication may not respond for another. With this word of caution, it is again repeated that elimination of "placebo reactors" is an accepted way of reducing the problem of large placebo effects, although it certainly does not solve the problem completely.

Another frequent question is, what is the placebo rate for pain relief? This question has no meaning without attention to the principle already discussed: exact definitions are necessary before we can talk intelligently about any condition. If we ask what proportion of patients is cured of angina pectoris by placebo, the answer is about zero. If we ask what proportion of patients has a reduction in the frequency and severity of attacks, the answer is about 30 to 40 percent. If we ask what proportion of patients has some reduction in number of attacks at some time during a 10 week trial due to placebo, the answer will be close to 100 percent. There is no single placebo response rate for an indication; there must be a careful definition of what is meant by placebo response and then a rate can be found.

The ethics of treating a patient with a placebo have often been confused by those who equate placebo with its pharmacologic properties rather than its therapeutic properties. If a drug has not been proven effective, then it must be equated with a placebo in its therapeutic abilities. A number of drugs have been given for years because they were thought to be effective, but later, when tested in a controlled trial, they were shown to be equivalent to a placebo. Surely administering these drugs which were unproven by scientific experiment was just as unethical as administering a placebo when an alternative is available. Conversely, the statement can be put in the positive sense as follows: placebo is the best drug therapy available until some other drug has been proven superior in a valid controlled clinical trial. Sometimes it has been said that a placebo has no chance of being effective, whereas the active drug has some chance of being effective; therefore, one is more likely to do well on the average with a pharmacologically active agent. This argument is specious and does not take into account the fact that the new drug is quite likely to be harmful, perhaps more likely to be harmful than helpful.

Blinding

The recommended type of experiment is known as double-blind; both the patient and the physician-rater must be unaware of which treatment is being tested and which is the control. Surely, if the patient knows he is getting an inert treatment, he will react differently than if he knows the agent has some potential benefit. If he knows one is the old standard drug and the other is a new untested drug, the patient is going to react differently. The essence of solving the problem of placebo effect is to compare the drug in such a way that we can find out whether the drug produces additional effect above and beyond that produced by the placebo. The second person who must be unaware of the identification of the drug and placebo is the physician, the one who rates the progress of the patient. The physician must remain unaware because almost all humans will rate the improvement of a patient differently if they know the patient is receiving a placebo than if they are not aware of the identity of the drug therapy. In addition, physicians influence the patient and affect the patient's response to the drug. Consider the difference between these two questions the physician might ask: "You look a little tired today, Mrs. Smith; how have you been feeling this past week?" An alternative is, "You certainly look better today, Mrs. Smith; how have you been feeling this past week?" Perhaps the differences are obvious in this example. From numerous studies in which differences were both obvious and more subtle, the method of questioning by the physician, the nurse or any other rater can produce biased rating of patients. Although this problem is clearly more difficult in the subjective rating of pain for instance, it is not difficult to guess that as objective a measure as blood pressure might be influenced by these same two questions.

One of the points often raised by physicians is that they cannot adequately cope with the problems of medication in the case when the patient has some untoward effect during the trial unless they know whether the patient is taking the drug or the placebo. Obviously, the code must be available so that when an unusual effect is noted, the physician can immediately decide whether corrective treatment is necessary. Perhaps more importantly, each administration of a single drug to a single individual must be thought of as an experiment and side effects are always possible.

What is the role of the pharmacist in this blinding procedure, and how can he contribute to the scientific quality of the clinical trial? The pharmacist should see that the medications are to all appearances equivalent and he may administer the coding of drug and placebo to allow the physician to remain blind as to treatment. The implication is that the medications are to be given by the same form of administration; for instance, both must be capsules, or both given intravenously in order for the trial to remain blind. Sometimes the studies are such that the patient cannot remain blind, for example, if the comparison is between two marketed products such as antacids which look different, taste different, require different dosages and are well known to the patients. Blinding is always a goal but sometimes an unobtainable one.

To obtain the goal, first, the appearance of the two treatments must be equal. If one is capsule and the other tablet, this difference would negate any intended blinding. On the other hand, a tablet can often be put in a capsule to make it appear the same as another medication given in capsule form. Certainly, the placebo should be prepared as a capsule to compare with the treatment drug as a capsule, and as a tablet to compare with a treatment drug administered by tablet. Obviously, no markings should be available to differentiate between drug and placebo such as manufacturer's identification, color differences or different shape of the tablets.

The medications must be given in equal frequency, that is, both given b.i.d., t.i.d., q.i.d. or whatever. When comparing a drug to a placebo, this means that the number of placebo tablets must be the same as the number of drug tablets. When comparing a drug to a standard, this means maintaining the same number of tablets even if some of them must be placebos. For instance, in comparing a b.i.d. drug to one given once a day, one should have the drug given once a day paired with one placebo tablet so that the instructions for each treatment will read, take b.i.d.

Another problem is taste of the medication. Sometimes the taste of the drug is very different than that of the placebo. One way to overcome this problem is to add an additional taste, such as that of quinine, to both tablets so that the additional taste masks any taste difference. Another possibility is a sugar coating over both tablets so that the taste is masked on the trip through the oral cavity and remains masked until the tablet begins disintegrating in the gastrointestinal tract.

Incorrect choice of labeling can negate the effect of preparing identical medications. The treatments should be labeled so that one can immediately tell from a code sheet whether the patient has been given drug or placebo. On the other hand, even if one had all of the medication labels lined up in front of him, he should not be able to discern which medication is which from the labeling. Thus an appropriate set of labels will have patient 1, week 1; patient 2, week 1; patient 3, week 1; and so forth, while an inappropriate set of labels would label all of those on drug A-1, A-2, etc. and on placebo, B-1, B-2, etc.

Randomization

One of the great advances in making clinical trials scientific has been the introduction of randomization. Randomization in a trial implies that whether the patient receives investigational drug or placebo will be decided by a chance mechanism. Randomization is usually set up by the statistician in the study. He employs a prepared set of numbers that have the property of being the same as numbers that were generated by perfect coin tossing or dice throwing; these numbers appear in a table of random digits or perhaps a table of random permutations. After the trial is completed, the statistician must check that the random assignment did in fact balance the obvious factors such as age and sex and severity of disease or use some statistical method to mathematically balance these factors.

It is of utmost importance to note that random in the statistical sense is not the same as haphazard. It is not appropriate for the investigator or pharmacist just to scatter the active drug and placebo treatments over the patients. It is necessary that the order be generated originally by some random device such as perfect coin tossing or mathematical analogues of coin tossing. Many tests have shown that human beings cannot generate anything close to random numbers by just acting with no intended pattern. Human beings act in patterns; tables of random digits must be the basis for assigning treatments to patients.

Alternation of treatments is not acceptable,[17] nor is using the letters in the patients names. Letters, for example, produce ethnic biases since persons of the same or similar ethnic groups tend to have the same name. Alternation allows the code to be broken too easily, and may introduce some bias. Certain methods of convenience are possible. For instance, in studies of patients who have a six- or seven-digit hospital number assigned in the order of entry into the hospital, the last digit, *i.e.*, the units place, can often be considered as a random digit for the sake of convenience. The best method is to use a table of random digits.

There are three basic reasons why randomization is necessary and useful in a clinical trial. First, randomization avoids bias in any of the treatment groups. A patient arrives in the doctor's office, and by diagnosis and evaluation, the physician decides whether the patient is suitable for the trial or not. If the patient does not fit the definition of the protocol, then the patient is treated as the physician desires. If, however, the patient fulfills the requirements set forth in the protocol, then the patient becomes a member of the trial. In effect, at that time a coin is tossed to decide whether the patient is to receive the drug or a placebo. Of course, in practice the code already has been established and the patient receives the next package, which may be drug or placebo. Note that when the doctor selects the patient for the trial, he has no way of knowing which treatment the patient will receive and therefore he cannot select consciously or subconsciously a particular type of patient to receive drug or placebo. It has been shown that in some instances, physicians will select the more ill patients to be given the active drug if they have some way of knowing whether the patient will receive drug or placebo, thereby biasing the trial against the drug.

Perhaps more important than conscious biases, if the study is blinded, is the effort to overcome unknown biases. Suppose women react to a drug differently than men. If patients are randomized, then on the average, half of the women will be given the drug and half placebo. At the same time, half of the men will be given the drug and half placebo. The same situation applies if some completely unknown factor such as an unknown enzyme system is involved. By randomization, this factor is balanced between the two treatment groups, on the average.

The second reason for using randomization is that it helps convince others that the trial has been conducted properly. Thus, even though the physician may not be subject to any biases, he is more likely to convince the unknown reader of the validity of his experiment if he has randomized because of the reasons mentioned above.

The third reason for randomization is that the statistical theory upon which the tests of differences between drug and placebo will be based depends upon randomization. Though this point is a topic for a statistical text, the pharmacist should know that the randomization is a requirement for the proper application of the statistical tests.

Orthogonal Contrasts

To understand the characteristic of Orthogonal Contrast, consider a simple drug trial. Suppose 20 patients were to be studied in each of two hospitals. Two obvious ways of doing the experiment would be to give drug A in the first hospital to 20 patients and drug B in the second hospital to 20 patients. Another way of doing the experiment would be to give drug A to 10 patients and drug B to 10 patients in each of the two hospitals. Is there an obvious advantage to one of these designs? Suppose the hospitals are different; in the first design, any differences detected between drug A and drug B are also differences between the two hospitals. In fact, we cannot tell whether an observed difference between the two study groups is due to a difference in treatment or in the hospitals. Since we cannot tell these two apart, we say that they are *confounded*. On the other hand, in the second design, the drugs are compared within hospitals and the study is merely repeated in two locations. Now, if there is a difference between drugs, it should be found in each of the two hospital studies. Alternatively, if there is a difference between the two hospitals, then both drugs should do better in one hospital than in the other. Since we can separate the effects of the drugs and the hospitals, we say that these two factors are Orthogonal.

The characteristic of Orthogonal Contrasts is an important one anytime a study is being designed. One must be careful that the differences between treatments are not confounded with any other differences in such a way that when the experiment is over, a critic could suggest that drug differences were caused by another obvious factor. For example, the cardiologist tells his patient to take this drug three times daily and stop smoking cigarettes. Are improvements in this patient's health due to the drug or the reduction in cigarettes? The two effects have been confounded. Of course, orthogonalization is a goal which can be only approximately achieved in reality. Thus, if there are different people on the two drugs, then whatever differences are observed are differences between the people as well as the drugs. Likewise, if each person takes both drugs, then the differences between the drugs are confounded with whether the person took the drug first or second. Neither of these problems is important in practice if we average the effect over the group of people and compare averages, and if we balance differences such as which drug is taken first by giving drug A first to half of the group and drug B to the other half. On the average, the people in the drug group will be about the same as those in the control group; if any obvious differences are found, they should be balanced by a statistical method such as analysis of covariance.

Giving all of drug A during one time period and then giving all of drug B during a later time period, thus confounding time of administration and drug differences, is a pitfall to be avoided. Also to be avoided are similar cases such as giving drug A to the ward patients and drug B to private patients, thus confounding differences in patients and difference in drugs, or giving drug A to Doctor Smith's patients and drug B to Doctor Johnson's patients, thus confounding differences in doctors and differences in drugs, or giving drug A to patients in City Hospital and drug B to patients in General Hospital, thus confounding differences in hospital and differences in drugs. The rule is to randomize the assignment of treatments in each of the smallest units of the trial.

Replicated Study

When a single patient responds to a new drug, we are often pleased, and begin to believe that the new drug will have some efficacy. Because there may be something special about this patient that has nothing to do with the drug, the experiment should be repeated in other patients. The characteristic of replication merely suggests that before a study is convincing, it must be repeated in different patients and different settings so that one will know whether the original findings are valid in a wider sense. Thus, it takes more than one patient, one physician, one community and if possible, more than one geographic area, and on occasion even more than one culture, before the drug is generally considered efficacious.

A perennial question that is asked is, how many patients are enough? This question, of course, has no practical answer unless one is willing to give a better definition of "enough." If one finishes an experiment and makes some conclusion about the results, he will usually be correct in his conclusion, but there is a chance that he may have made one of two errors. The first type of error, sometimes called the alpha error, is that he may have said the two drugs differ when, in fact, they do not differ; the observations just happened to favor one drug by chance. Conversely, he might make the second type of error, sometimes called the beta error, which is to have said the two drugs do not differ when in fact they do, but by chance the differences were minimized in his experiment. These two types of errors are with us anytime we make a conclusion and are particularly important in clinical drug trials. All of our experience tells us that if one is to make this decision on the basis of four patients, he would tend to make more mistakes of both kinds than if he were to make his conclusions on the basis of 400 patients. This brings us back to the question of how many patients are enough.

The statistician can tell the number of patients that will be enough if he is given the proportion of times that the investigator is willing to be wrong in his conclusions in both type 1 and type 2 errors. Usual levels of error are five out of 100 times, or one out of 100 times. In addition, the statistician must know how much better the new drug is likely to be than the old one in relation to the variation among patients. Thus, for example, if the investigator were to tell the statistician that he would be willing to make type 1 and type 2 errors only five out of 100 times, and that he was studying an antihypertensive drug that he thought would lower the blood pressure by about 10 mm Hg more than the old drug and that the usual variation in his patients was about 15 mm Hg, (by usual variation we mean standard deviation) then the statistician could tell him how many people he would need in order to do a clinical trial of the new antihypertensive agent compared to the old. If the investigator were to say he did not like the idea of having errors five out of 100 times, but would rather expect to make the error one out of 100 times, the statistician would be able to give him a new number which would be about 70 percent larger. The investigator might then decide that the new size of the experiment would be too large to be practical, and then he might have to accept the larger possibility of there being an error in his conclusions.

In fact, the most important reason to consult a statistician before doing a trial is to get some idea of the sample size necessary to find the anticipated difference in the new drug therapy. Quite frequently it is found that the new therapy is likely to produce a difference so small that only a massive trial would demonstrate the efficacy of this new drug. It may turn out that the possible advantages are too small to make it practical to demonstrate them. Many investigators have discovered this principle only upon completion of their study when they consulted a statistician and were told that the study involved too few patients to have discovered convincingly the possible drug effect. In other words, the study was so small it was a waste of effort. Better investigators have consulted the statistician prior to the clinical trial, discovered the futility of the suggested trial, decided against the trial and turned their efforts to more fruitful possibilities.

Occasionally, an investigator even overestimates the number of patients needed.

It is easy to decide, with the aid of statistical hypothesis and models, how large a trial is necessary to produce a statistically significant result. It is an impossible task to decide how large a trial or how many trials will be necessary to convince the appropriate people that the new drug is advantageous. Convincing is an element of philosophy and not science. Clearly, a finding along generally accepted pharmaceutical theory will be more quickly accepted than a finding that breaks tradition. Thus, there is a certain conservative bias operating against radically new drug therapy.

Proper Administration

The last characteristic is proper administration, for even if the other five characteristics are designed into a study, they are wasted unless the study is actually carried out as designed. Thus, it is one thing to design the study to be double-blind and yet another to find out that the patients knew which medication was which because of some characteristic side effect. It is important that some member of the clinical drug trial team monitor the study to see if the design is adequate, and also whether the various team members are fulfilling their tasks as designed. Thus, if some scheduling problem has prevented the physician from asking the patients whether they feel better this week than last, and the answer was to be one measure of efficacy, something must be changed. Perhaps a simple rescheduling would be sufficient; perhaps the nurse can ask the question instead of the physician. It is better to change a study in midstream than to continue on with some defect that would invalidate the results anyway.

Another important reason for a change is because of the suspicion that there is an important finding which was indicated by some bits of data. Thus, after talking with the patients, the pharmacist may hypothesize that the patients who took the medication before meals are getting nauseous while those who took the medication after meals show no side effects. If he is correct, this information should certainly be recorded even though the original protocol missed this point. Moreover, the statistician may be able to randomly select half of the patients to get special instructions to take the medication before meals while the remainder are told to take the medication after meals.

Changes should not be made lightly. Often the problem is a unilateral change by one member of the team. This procedure should be avoided; if a change is necessary, then the whole research team should discuss the change, establish the precise change to be made and agree on how to implement it.

A very important problem is whether the patient has taken the medication as prescribed in the protocol. The pharmacist can make a major contribution by keeping track of the medication that was not used by each of the patients. As is well known, patients do not always follow the recommendations for taking their medication and whether a patient follows instructions or not will certainly have an effect on the efficacy of the medication and the interpretation of that efficacy. If the patient should have consumed all but two of his tablets, and returns 12 as unused, this item of information is important in the analysis of the clinical trial. Equally important would be the fact that the patient has taken all of his tablets when in fact, he should have 10 left over at the end of the trial.

When a study is taking much longer than anticipated, this fact should be considered a sign of some sort of problem. It may be simply that the protocol writers were too optimistic in their predictions for eligible patients, but it may also be that something has changed so that the study is progressing slowly because of lack of interest and lack of care by those who are supposed to be carrying it out.

Another frequent problem is that the dropouts, that is people who have asked to be removed from the study, or are removed by the investigator because they have moved out of town or have been hospitalized or are uncooperative, are more frequent than anticipated. Frequently, the dropouts provide information on the efficacy of the drugs. Thus, if the great majority of the dropout group had been taking placebos and they have dropped out complaining that the unknown medication has not helped them, this tends to support the claim that the new drug is efficacious. If a great majority of the dropouts are on the active drug, and they dropped out of the study because they have been cured or are feeling much better, this tends to support the contention that the drug is effective. These two examples point out the importance of knowing why the patients are dropping out of the study, and of recording the reasons prior to breaking the blind code. If the investigator knows which treatment the patient was on when he became a dropout, some bias, overt or subtle, might creep into the study. Conversely, if the investigator does not know the treatment before he fills out all of the forms, any information that he records must be treated as unbiased with respect to the drug therapy.

Occasionally there have been many dropouts and the trial still has some time to run. The investigator would like to know whether the dropouts have been on the active drug or on placebo. It would be wrong to allow him to break the code at this point and ascertain the treatment at the time of dropout. Instead, the pharmacist or the statistician should ascertain whether a disproportionate share of the dropouts are in one or the other drug category and make recommendations accordingly. This procedure, though thwarting curiosity and ego impulses, and difficult to carry out, also thwarts biasing the study and therefore makes it more likely to be worthwhile.

Occasionally, investigators think that only the patients who completed the study need to be reported in evaluation of the drugs. This is, of course, incorrect, as all persons who started the trial provide some information on the drugs and must be accounted for in the write-up. One must be certain that the dropouts have not reacted differently to the drug than those who have completed the study.

But What If You Cannot Do it?

The discussion in this chapter concerning the characteristics of any proper study must be considered as an attainable utopia. In a great number of studies, all of these considerations can be attained and randomization, double-blind techniques, a control treatment, careful blocking and so forth will contribute to the ability to derive new knowledge and to convince others of the knowledge gained with regard to the drugs tested. Intelligent readers have already considered, however, that in many cases, this utopian solution is not attainable. What if double-blind does not work? How can we blind an efficacy trial of a standard procedure that requires oral drug treatment morning and evening with another standard procedure that requires only one intramuscular injection per day? Certainly, this trial cannot be made double-blind without changing the standard procedures.

Other examples in which double-blind can be a goal, but not attainable, can be easily found. An intramuscular drug with a characteristic side effect such as a rash, when compared to another drug without that side effect or to placebo, will certainly allow many patients to guess which treatment is being administered. Placebo will also cause a rash in some patients so a few people will guess incorrectly. To assume merely because the medications were neatly coded, that the patient is "blind" as to treatment would be foolhardy. Moreover, the patient is likely to discuss his side effects with the rating physician, and inquire whether those side effects are to be expected or are they serious. The physician, then, knowing the expected side effects of the drug, will be called "blind" only by the naive.

To avoid breaking the whole code if the physician needs to know whether drug or placebo was given to a patient, either the pharmacist should tell him the treatment for that one patient, or the containers may be labeled in such a way that drug or placebo is stated, but sealed inside the label. Then the sealed part of the label is available to the physician anytime he needs to break the code for that one person.

Finally, it should be noted that many investigators will not agree to give high doses of new chemical entities to subjects or patients in a blind fashion. They would prefer knowing which patients will be given large doses of the drug to be prepared since some experimental designs would call for the patient to receive, as his first experience with the drug, the highest dose to be used in the study.

From the preceding discussion, it is clear that double-blind cannot always be attained, and we must consider when it should be assumed unattainable. A certain amount of cleverness will help in being able to administer drugs double-blind in a study in cases where the less clever will have given it up. For instance, the physician who rates the patient's progress does not necessarily have to be the physician with whom the patient will discuss his treatment and side effects. It is often possible to have the patient discuss his progress with a non-blind physician who has as his role, patient care. Another physician, whose major role is rating of patient progress, can be completely blind as to treatment, even if one must resort to giving him a set list of written questions that he will ask of the patient. Perhaps the patient may have to be cautioned not to discuss treatment or side effects with the rating physician.

In point of fact, ascertaining the correct answer is the objective of the drug trial. If this goal is accomplished in less than double-blind, controlled fashion, the trial has still produced the correct answer. One should not become so enamoured of methodology that double-blind becomes more important than getting the correct result. The medical history of the 18th and 19th centuries is replete with samples of this form of effective, but less than adequate and well-controlled scientific investigation and conclusion. One has the feeling, however, that most of the easy problems have been solved, leaving only more difficult, more subtle and more confusing issues for current investigators. Therefore, carefully controlled studies not only make it easier to attain the correct answer, but make that correct answer more convincing to those who read the reports of the original investigators.

A proper attitude is that double-blinding and controlled comparisons and randomization are usually attainable goals and that the investigator who forsakes one of these goals should be able to, and be compelled to, document why it was that he forsook his goal. The intelligent reader of the outcome of the study will evaluate for himself whether the investigator has done the best that he could in the given circumstances.

STATISTICAL DESIGN OF EXPERIMENTS

We all recognize that a great deal of careful thought must go into the selection of the number of patients in a clinical drug trial, when each will get the various drugs, whether all drugs will be used on all patients, whether men will be considered differently from women with regard to the treatments, old differently from young, obese differently from thin, hypertensive differently from normotensive, whether laboratory results on Monday will be considered the same as laboratory results on Thursday, whether everyone will take placebo first and then take an unknown medication and a great many other details. The usual formats for various trials are part of the field called the "Design of Experiments" which is a branch of statistics and was originally developed in regard to agricultural experimentation. The study of the design of experiments shows that certain designs have advantages over others such as fewer patients required to draw the same conclusion whereas other designs have the advantage of simplicity.

Clinical drug trials are usually conducted according to certain standard designs. A brief description of these is given below so that the reader may have some feeling for the advantages and disadvantages of each.

Randomized Design

Perhaps the most commonly used design is the simple randomized design. In this design, patients are accepted into the trial in one large group without any distinctions among patients. No subcategories are permitted. Which treatment the patient is given is decided upon on the basis of a randomized code. In other words, patient 1 gets that bottle of medication labeled patient 1, and whether that is drug or placebo has been previously decided by the randomized code. Usually the study is double-blind, but it could be single-blind or even unblinded, depending on the nature of the comparison to be made.

The advantage of a randomized design is its ease of use and lack of any requirement about foreknowledge of important parameters in the study. If we are ignorant of any factors that are associated with the disease, we can still design the trial in the simple randomized pattern.

The analysis of the randomized design looks at two different estimates of variation. The first is the estimate of variation between the treatment group and the placebo group. The second is the estimate of variation within each of the treatment groups. If it is found that the differences between treatment groups are of the same size as the differences within treatment groups, then we conclude that there is no difference in the two treatments. If on the other hand, the differences between treatments are much greater than the differences within treatments, then we conclude that the two treatments are, in fact, different.

The exact analysis of the situation and methods of calculation are given in any standard textbook on experimental design, such as those listed at the conclusion of this chapter, where the reader can also find additional information on the various designs.

As can be seen from the above description of the analysis, anything that can be done to reduce the amount of within-treatment variation will make it easier to detect between treatment variation. The next designs attempt to accomplish that aim by making each of the groups of people who are compared for treatment differences more similar.

Randomized Block

If two or more identifiable subgroups are expected to react differently in a clinical trial, then the proper design may be the Randomized Block design. Essentially, this design is the use of a simple randomized design in each of two or more groups of patients, called blocks, where each block consists of relatively homogenous patients. Thus, if men and women are expected to react differently in the trial, the investigator is said to block on this factor. He has available one random code for the women and one random code for the men.

Frequently, age is an important variable in clinical trials. One way to overcome the problems of age differences would be to block the incoming patients on the basis of age, thus for example, there may be five blocks: all those less than 40 years of age, those 40-50 years of age, those 51-60, 61-70 and those more than 70 years of age.

To test whether a topical drug application causes a rash in a patient, the drug could be applied on one arm and either a comparison treatment or placebo on the other arm. In this case, the patient is the block, and the comparison is within patient. If two or more treatments cannot be given simultaneously, but must be given successively, then there is another form of blocking by patient which will be described below under Crossover Analysis.

Other possible blocking factors include family members, male or female children of the same mother, students in one grade of a school, patients of one private practitioner, ward patients vs. private patients, and patients in one hospital.

The randomized block design thus allows control for one variable, the blocking variable, in that a particular characteristic is specifically fixed in the experimental design. Thus, the design provides certain conceptual gains, and at the same time, certain practical gains. If the experimenter can reduce the variation due to the blocking factor, he will more easily be able to find differences due to the treatment factor. With an efficient blocking design, the experimenter will be able to ascertain the same differences that he might have found using a simple randomized design, but he will need fewer patients. If the blocking factor is useless, the same sample size will be required with the only addition being those extra patients necessary because of the administrative complications of the slightly more complicated design.

In a complete randomized block design, each treatment is used the same number of times in each block, for example.[18] If there are four drugs being compared, then blocks of four patients can be used with one drug randomly assigned to each of the four patients. Suppose that each block consists of three children of the same parents, and there are seven drugs, A, B, C, D, E, F and G, to be compared. Although complete blocks will have to be forsaken, balance can be retained if there are seven carefully chosen blocks, each with three drugs randomly assigned to the three children, *e.g.*, ABC, ADE, AFG, BDG, BEF, CDF, CEG. This design is called a balanced incomplete block design, and is a very convenient alternative to having all drugs used in each block. An example of this type is described at the end of the discussion on crossover designs.

Matched Pairs

A particularly important example of blocking is called the matched pairs design. In this type of trial, the block consists of exactly two persons. The matching is such that the two people resemble each other as closely as possible. The goal is to have identical twins and to give one the test drug and the other the control. The practical solution is to use as a pair, two persons who are as alike as possible within the framework of the study. In the simplest case, a single characteristic is chosen, and the patients are matched for it. For example, women in a study of the nausea and vomiting of pregnancy could be matched on the number of previous pregnancies. Thus, a woman on her first pregnancy would be matched to another woman on first pregnancy, and then one randomly chosen to be given drug A and the other to get drug B or placebo. In this manner, differences between the matching characteristic are eliminated.

This example shows an instance in which matching on one factor tends to match for several factors. Thus, by matching on number of previous pregnancies, there tends to be a match on age of the prospective mother, age of the father and so forth. In case several variables are each of importance, the matching can be more extensive, for instance, there may be a requirement to match on the number of previous pregnancies, and at the same time, social class of the mother as divided into three categories. Then, a middle class woman with two previous pregnancies will be matched with another middle class woman with two previous pregnancies. The number of matching factors can be extended, but it is soon obvious that the more categories there are for matching, the more difficult it will be to find exact matches for the subjects. In fact, in most studies, the matching will be of the most common subjects, and particularly uncommon persons will have no match, or if all persons must be matched, the uncommon persons will be poorly matched. Thus, if there is a woman with 12 previous pregnancies, the necessary match will have to have 12 previous pregnancies also, or the matching will have to be relaxed so that the category is perhaps, seven or more previous pregnancies. Even with relaxed rules, it is often impossible to get a good match for the more unique subjects.

When does the matching occur? If the study

is such that a list of all patients is available prior to beginning the study, then it is most efficient to set up the matched pair before beginning the study. If the investigator has 50 candidates for the study, he will set up the 25 matched pairs, or fewer if he decides that it is better to eliminate some of the unique persons rather than to force a match. He can look at the individual cases and decide who is to be excluded because none has yet taken the drugs, and so no bias is involved. Once pairs have been set up, then which member of each pair is to receive drug A will be randomly chosen. Some investigators have formed two groups of people and then randomly decided that one group will receive Drug A. This practice is not to be recommended since it is subject to unknown biases that are avoided when one randomly assigns the drug pair by pair; the value of random assignment of individuals pairs is negated if groups are established first and one randomization decides all.

Frequently, as for example in studying the nausea and vomiting of pregnancy, the patients arrive sequentially, and matching or pairing is not possible prior to beginning the study. In this case, the investigator will set up his categories beforehand and match as the patients are taken into the study. Thus, the investigator decides he will have five categories as determined by the number of previous pregnancies: no previous pregnancy, one previous pregnancy, two, three or four, and five or more previous pregnancies. Then a random code is set up for each of these categories in the same manner as for other randomized block designs.

Latin Square

Sometimes there are two factors that can be controlled at the same time. If the number of treatments and the number of levels of each of the two factors is the same, then a Latin square design can be used. For example, if there are four patients who are to receive four different drugs on each of four different days, then the Latin square design is an appropriate one. Of course, any multiple of four patients will also do. Since dropouts are a common occurrence in clinical drug trials and the Latin square designs require a level of control beyond the randomized block design, they are frequently started but sometimes found to be impractical in actual use. Sizes up to five treatments are usually successful while those of size seven or larger usually fail. The experimenter should know that the successful completion of a large Latin square is difficult when humans, with all of their idiosyncrasies, are the experimental units. Nevertheless, if there are two factors that should be controlled, the Latin square design is a good one. The reason is, a failure in one of the blocking factors still leaves a randomized block design as the outcome, while if the investigator and his patients are up to the task, an even more meaningful study will have been completed. Again, if the blocking factors are effective, the investigator will be able to obtain more information on treatment differences by eliminating the extra variation due to differences in the blocking factors. Because the Latin square is a somewhat more complicated design than randomized blocks, it has the problem of increased administrative skill required for its successful completion.

Related Designs

It is also possible to control three or more factors at the same time if the number of each of the factors to be controlled is the same, for example, four different drugs to be taken by four patients during one of four weeks and evaluated by one of four physicians. In practice, these designs, called Graeco-Latin Squares, are so difficult to use that they are infrequently, if ever, actually used in clinical drug trials. Other more commonly used designs are Youden Squares, which are incomplete Latin squares, so that the requirement of equal number of each of the blocking factors is unnecessary for one of the factors. Another type of Latin square is that balanced for residual effects. With this type of design, one can test whether each of the drugs has any effects in the succeeding period. The balance that must be struck is to control by some sort of blocking, the most important known factors in order that, for instance, variation between patients does not obscure the variation between treatments within the same patient. This advantage of blocking must be balanced against the additional complications of knowing the factors on which to block, getting the number of each factor to be the same, and then carefully monitoring the study to see that the many requirements of the more precise design are actually employed as designed. A majority of the time the balance found is to use the randomized block design. That the randomized design is probably the next most common design used is more likely due to lack of knowledge about the proper blocking factor or lack of imagination than the fact that it is the appropriate design. Numerous other designs exist if the number of treatments in the blocking factors are not equal. An example is described following the crossover design which is discussed below.

Crossover Designs

A particularly popular design conceptually is the crossover design (sometimes called change-over or switchback) in which each patient is given the two or more treatments that are being studied, and the tendency for patients to improve is taken into account in the analysis. In this type of design, each patient is given both treatments and then the patient is compared with himself.[19] As the name implies, he is crossed over from treatment one to treatment two. However, the danger of bias exists in that the second treatment period may not be the same as the first treatment period, for example, if the patient's condition is improving with time. Therefore, it is clear that one must try to balance the treatment period by having equal numbers of patients in the sequence treatment one to treatment two as in the sequence treatment two to treatment one, or otherwise the treatment differences and period differences would be confounded. The gain is that the same patient is more like himself from one month to the next, or one day to the next, than are two randomly chosen patients; therefore the sample size can be reduced. Randomization enters into this design when it comes time to assign the patient to one sequence or the other.

A vital assumption in using crossover studies is that there is no carryover effect of the drug from one period to the next. This means that the periods of the study must be sufficiently far apart so that the treatment given in the first period is not pharmacologically active in the second period.[20] Thus a drug with a biologic half-life of 3½ days should not be followed one week later by a comparison drug since one-quarter of the original drug will still remain active at the beginning of the second period. It is often thought that the condition being treated ought to remain constant over the duration of the experiment, but in fact, that is not necessary. For example, in comparing postoperative pain, we would expect the pain to be reduced with each day after the operation. The crossover design is still possible because the treatment given first to one patient, and thus to one having more pain to overcome, would be balanced in another patient by being given second. One purpose of the crossover design is to remove this period effect that most patients will tend to get better over the course of the experiment. Another advantage of this design is that temporal effects can be withdrawn as a source of variation by comparing period one and period two and removing this effect from the total variation. As an example, differences in the weather from the beginning to the end of a clinical trial may produce different rates of improvement. It is important to differentiate between period effects which affect both drugs equally, and are permitted in this design, and carryover effects which give a different effect in the two sequences and must be avoided. A frequent method of avoiding the problem of carryover effects would be to give both drug and placebo for, say, eight weeks each in a crossover study, but to analyze only the last four weeks of each period for efficacy.

Since it is true that variation between patients is very large and that a crossover experiment, when the assumptions necessary have been met, eliminates this factor, why doesn't the crossover design receive an unqualified recommendation? The answer is found in several points. First, suppose there is an adverse effect found two weeks after the study. How do you know which drug, if either, should be held responsible? Suppose at the end of the study with a placebo versus a new drug that eight patients have died. The records show that all eight patients took the new drug. What the records do not show because of this design is how many patients would have died if they had taken the placebo alone. If only four patients died in a non-crossover on the new treatment and four more died on the placebo, then one would have a better idea of how to evaluate the result. Likewise, if eight patients had died on the drug, and none on the placebo in a non-crossover design, one would better know how to evaluate the result. Thus, a crossover design makes particularly difficult the evaluation of other events besides those being used for efficacy measurement in the study. Second, suppose the assumption of no carryover effect from period one into period two is not true. After taking the drug in period one, the patient is less likely to be sick in period two when he is taking placebo. On the other hand, after taking placebo in period one, there will be no change in his usual reaction in period two. Thus, we underestimate the treatment effect. In this case, the crossover design will require more patients (patience) to prove efficacy than if there were no carryover effect.

The simple crossover design consists of only two periods and two treatments, and is, in fact, equivalent to a Latin square of size two. If the disease condition warrants, there can be three treatment periods in the order drug, placebo, drug, compared with the sequence placebo, drug, placebo; and by adding a fourth period, drug, placebo, drug, placebo, compared with placebo, drug, placebo, drug. Though there is no theoretical reason why any more periods could not be used, four periods is the usual upper limit in practice. Another extension would be to use three different treatments in three different periods, but this design can also be thought of as a Latin square and other extensions are also variations of a Latin square.

A clinical drug trial that employed many of the principles that have been discussed in this section concerned the use of three analgesics which were self-administered by pregnant women during labor pains.[21] There were three analgesic mixtures, 50 percent nitrous oxide and 50 percent air, 75 percent nitrous oxide and 25 percent oxygen, and 0.5 percent trichlorethylene and the rest air. The usual randomized block experiment would have each patient (the blocking factor) use each analgesic in random order. The constraint was that patients were not expected to be able to use more than two of the analgesic mixtures during their labor pains. The design finally selected was to have each of 150 women use two mixtures so that each of the three pairs of drugs was compared by 50 women randomly selected so that each woman had equal chance of being in any of the three groups. Moreover, the 50 women were subjects in a crossover design so that 25 had one mixture first and the other second while the other 25 had the second mixture first and then the first. Each subject was asked, "Which was more effective in relieving the pain of uterine contraction?" in order to evaluate the pair of analgesics. The clearcut results showed that the 50 percent nitrous oxide mixture was the weakest and the other two were about equally effective. The design can be seen to be an example of a balanced incomplete block design since each block is missing one analgesic and the blocks are balanced for all possible combinations. This example is mentioned to suggest to the reader that the standard designs mentioned above are only the simplest of samples out of a vast design warehouse. The simplest designs have the advantage of being easier to finish successfully, but any time there is a need to overcome some problem, the statistician should be consulted to see if there is an experimental design that will accomplish the desired study within the constraints encountered.

Factorial Designs

One final series of designs will be described because of the importance of these designs in the study of combination drugs. Suppose one is comparing drug A to a placebo in a randomized block design. Perhaps half of the patients in each of these groups may be taking vitamin C, but this factor is ignored and the patients taking drug A are compared with the patients taking the placebo as equals whether they are taking vitamin C or not. The assumption made is that the results of vitamin C consumption are independent of the results of drug A. In the same manner, one can compare drug A to a placebo in the presence of drug B in half of the patients. There are now four groups of patients: Group P, those taking only placebo; Group A, those taking only drug A; Group B, those taking only drug B; and Group AB, those taking both drug A and drug B. The effectiveness of drug A can be found by comparing group P with group A, but its effectiveness also can be found by comparing group B with group AB. In this manner a second factor has been introduced without increasing the size of the experiment. The imaginative person will have already projected on to realize that drug D could be given to half of each of these four groups adding another factor without increasing the size of the experiment, and so forth.

Actually, there are two problems. One is the additional complication and bookkeeping which leads to enough errors to prevent the addition of factors without good reason. The second problem is that the blocks must be enlarged, from four to eight in this example, which prevents the homogeneity that can be gained from smaller blocks. The larger block size prevents an increase in factors without paying the penalty of less precision in the determination of efficacy.

The advantages of factorial designs far outweigh the disadvantages for the study of combination drugs. First there is the determination of the efficacy of drug A and, by looking at B versus P and AB versus A, the simultaneous determination of the efficacy of drug B. Also, it is important to know that drug A works under more than just the condition of being given as a single entity since many patients are taking other drugs concurrently. Moreover, the findings about drug A and drug B are in the same sample of patients and therefore the worry that the results are due to different patient groups is negated.

Finally, the advantage of factorial designs that makes them particularly useful for studying combination drugs is the ability to test the assumption that drug A is independent of drug B. If drug A is a standard bronchodilator, and drug B is a new bronchodilator, then their action may be independent in which case the cumulative effect as measured in the AB group will be simply the addition of the effects measured in the A group and the effects in the B group. Another way of thinking about that additivity is that there are two doses of the same drug so that the effect in the AB group is merely the effect of a larger dose. If the assumption of independence is not true, then the combination will have less effect than the sum of the two drugs (for example, two antagonistic drugs), or there will be more effect from the combination than from the sum of the ingredients (synergism).

The analogous measurements with regard to side effects are as important as the measurement of efficacy and the determination of interaction between the drugs. Perhaps the combination has the simple additive effect of its ingredients but the rate of side effects has been reduced from what would be anticipated by the addition of side effects from each of the two drugs. Again there is support for the use of a combination product. These side effects data should always be recorded and analyzed.

Various extensions of the factorial design from the simple case of two drugs at each of two levels include using more drugs, using more levels, using some fraction of all possible combinations and using some combination of these possibilities.

A word of caution is appropriate at this point in regard to the work of a statistician in a clinical drug trial. It is true that one of the roles of a statistician is to compress a lot of data about many patients taking several drugs into a small amount of easily usable information such as drug A is better than drug B for almost everyone. The comment heard occasionally that a statistician was not needed in this study because there were only ten patients is not true. As shown, some statistical designs will get more information out of ten patients than others and that only one who has mastered this field, be he investigator or statistician, should decide on the best design for a given study. Even a study with a thousand patients can be useless if the drug treatments have been confounded with, for example, hospital differences (drug A given in one hospital and drug B given in another). Thus it is imperative that investigators consider the statistical principles when they set up the experiment and not wait until it is time to analyze the data.

Statistical Analysis

Regardless of the type of study, certain parts of the statistical analysis are essential. Some sort of null-hypothesis must be made; for example, the two drugs are equal or, the larger dose does not produce any greater efficacy than the smaller dose. It is this null-hypothesis that will be tested by the study; the only possible results from the study relate to this null-hypothesis. Prior to the beginning of the study, a set of probabilities of possible outcomes can be generated based on the null-hypothesis, the sample size and the type of investigation. This set of probabilities provides a guideline against which the observations will be compared.

At the end of the study, the observations of the study will be compared to the expectations according to the null-hypothesis and the deviations of reality from theory will be evaluated on a probability basis. If the observations are quite ordinary, that is, the probability of obtaining the results actually found according to the null-hypothesis is large, then there is every reason to believe the null-hypothesis is correct and there is no reason to reject this hypothesis. On the other hand, if the probability of the observations according to the null-hypothesis is very small, then the null-hypothesis is probably incorrect and more likely some event of greater probability according to an alternative hypothesis has occurred. When the report is written this is often summarized as $p < .05$ or $p < .01$ or some other level. This p refers to the probability of observing the sample, if the null-hypothesis were, in fact, true. By custom among investigators, the 0.05 level is often accepted as the borderline separating those results which are likely if the null-hypothesis is true ($p > .05$) and those results which would not have occurred had the null-hypothesis been true ($p < .05$). Statisticians actually think of this 0.05 level as a fuzzy area of indecision with the decision becoming clearer the further one goes in either direction away from the 0.05 level. Thus, most would agree that a probability of 0.50 is very likely to be a case of random variation, while the probability of 0.001 is quite unlikely to have a chance mechanism as its cause.

It is further true that a larger sample size usually makes it easier to discern a difference. Thus, when one finds a result of a trial with probability 0.15, according to the null-hypothesis, this result can be interpreted in two ways: (1) a slightly unusual result has occurred but the null-hypothesis appears to be true or (2) that an unusual event according to the null-hypothesis has occurred, but the sample size is insufficient to characterize this difference at a 0.05 significant level. A careful wording of the results enables the investigator to keep both of these possibilities in mind. Thus, if the null-hypothesis is not rejected, one can write the conclusion that the data are consistent with the null-hypothesis or the null-hypothesis is not rejected by these data. It is incorrect to say the null-hypothesis is accepted because the comparison is only whether the data are consistent or not with the null-hypothesis. When the data produce an unlikely result, this is usually stated by saying the finding is statistically significant which merely means that the investigator has prechosen the level of significance such as 0.05, and that according to the null-hypothesis, the probability of obtaining the results found is less than this prechosen significance level; therefore, the investigator is concluding that a chance variation does not explain the observations but rather that a repeatable difference has been observed. He fully expects that the next time treatment A is compared to treatment B, the finding will again be that A is better than treatment B, and the next time, and the next time. Investigators who have followed the principles for clinical drug studies discussed in this chapter can then conclude that the observed difference is due to a difference between the experimental drug and the control. Other investigators may find that the statistically significant differences are due to biased allocation of patients to some confounded factor, to unblind patients responding to drug and not a known placebo, or to dozens of other possibilities and not because of a drug difference.

Notice that the statistical test just described fixes the number of patients in the trial and then varies the degree of conviction, the p value, depending upon the outcome of the trial. It is also possible to reverse these priorities and fix the degree of conviction that you will accept and vary the number of patients in the trial. This form of decision making is called sequential testing since the statistical test is calculated after each patient is completed rather than at the end of the clinical trial. As soon as the decision is reached, the study is over and the patients will begin using the better drug. One can find a description of these studies in *Sequential Medical Trials*.[22] The chief advantage is, of course, that fewer humans need be exposed to the poorer drug, a great advantage if the outcome of the trial is life or death, but of much less importance if the outcome is lower blood pressure for a week.

A few disadvantages of sequential testing should be noted. The method is only applicable if the patients enter the study sequentially and if the treatment period is relatively short so that the trial can be ended before some of the patients have spent weeks or months on the poorer drug. In actual practice, it is difficult to convince the reader of efficacy since the study may involve very few patients, and the conclusions are just at the 0.05 or 0.01 level. Administrative problems are very different since the analysis must be updated each time a patient completes the study. The balance of advantages and disadvantages is such that sequential testing is not for usual studies, but should definitely be considered in case the outcome may be death in some short period of time as for instance, in the case of premature children. Proper statistical design can save lives.[23]

Concluding Thoughts

It is important to remember that the statistical conclusions are based upon groups of people. Suppose, however, you have been one of the individuals to receive drug B which the investigator says is not as good as drug A. Suppose further that when you received drug B it worked excellently for you. What would you prefer to be your treatment next time? You know two pieces of information: (1) treatment B worked for you in the one time that you have been exposed to either A or B and (2) on the average, treatment A was better than treatment B. Given this information, many an individual would prefer repeating the treatment that worked previously for him as an individual.

The thoughtful investigator will try to look over his results when he is finished to find whether there is some way he can characterize those individuals on each drug for whom the drug worked. Perhaps they have the same blood type, or their level of a particular enzyme is high, or they are the younger people in the study, or they are the ones with higher blood pressure.

One source of scientific progress is this final look at the data to find out whether there is some subtle characterization within the population that was not considered prior to the investigation. Perhaps drug A is better than drug B on the average, but drug B is better for those people who are blood type P. These are the type of clues that a good investigator will look for and, if successful, find in his data.

The final evaluation is the comparison of the efficacy rating with the side effect rating. A drug that is very efficacious is useless if it causes too many side effects. A new drug may be no more efficacious than the old, or even slightly worse, but the side effects may have been reduced greatly so that the new drug must be rated as the drug of choice. Finally, that which is a side effect of the drug for the indication under study may turn out to be a new indication for the drug; for example, the thiazides, which were first developed as diuretic agents, were observed to reduce blood pressure. This observation was capitalized upon when this class of drugs was developed into one of the mainstays of antihypertensive therapy.

In pharmacologic terms, this chapter is intended to be an analgesic and not a panacea. Hopefully, careful reading and thinking over the points raised will help remove some of the pain involved in setting up a proper clinical trial. Much more extensive reading, starting with the references and suggested readings found at the end of the chapter, and considerable experience are required before the reader will be ready to cure all of the problems in a drug trial. By that time the reader will understand that there can be no perfect trial and no one should expect to see perfection. What we should all expect and require is that any trial be free from obvious defect that would have been easily corrected if properly considered before the trial began. This is the goal to which we should all strive in planning and conducting clinical drug trials.

References

1. Finkel, M. J. and Zatman, J.: Investigational and New Drugs, *FDA Papers 4*:31-33 (Nov.) 1970.
2. Provost, G. P.: "Homeless" or "Orphan" Drugs (editorial), *Am. J. Hosp. Pharm. 25*:609 (Nov.) 1968.
3. Unfug, H. V., Anderson, B. J. and Hayes, T. H.: Nonapproved Uses of FDA-Approved Drugs (Question and Answers), *J. Am. Med. Assoc. 211*:1705 (Mar. 9) 1970.
4. Dollery, C. T. and Davies, D. S.: The Conduct of Initial Drug Studies in Man, *Brit. Med. Bull. 26*:233-236 (Sept.) 1970.
5. Canada, A. T., Jr. and McHale, M. K.: A Pharmacy's Vital Role in Clinical Drug Evaluations, *Hosp. Pharm. 5*:7-9 (Jan.) 1970.
6. Beecher, H. K.: Ethics and Clinical Research, *New Engl. J. Med. 274*:1354-1360 (June 16) 1966.
7. Melmon, K. L., Grossman, M., and Morris, R. C., Jr.: Emerging Assets and Liabilities of a Committee on Human Welfare and Experimentation, *New Engl. J. Med. 282*:427-431 (Feb. 19) 1970.
8. Hill, A. B.: Medical Ethics and Controlled Trials, *Brit. Med. J. 1*:1043-1049 (Apr. 20) 1963.
9. Mainland, D.: The Clinical Trial - Some Difficulties and Suggestions, *J. Chronic Diseases 11*:484-496 (May) 1960.
10. Hill, A. B.: The Clinical Trial, *New Engl. J. Med. 247*:113-119 (July 24) 1952.
11. Lasagna, L.: The Controlled Clinical Trial: Theory and Practice, *J. Chronic Diseases 1*:353-367 (Apr.) 1955.
12. Lionel, N. D. W. and Herxheimer, A.: Assessing Reports of Therapeutic Trials, *Brit. Med. J. 3*:637-640 (Sept. 12) 1970.
13. Anello, C.: FDA Principles on Clinical Investigations, *FDA Papers 4*:14-15, 23-24 (June) 1970.
14. Roueche, B.: *A Man Named Hoffman*, Berkley Medallion Books, S1259, New York, 1966, pp 68-82.
15. Johnson, J. E., Jr. *et al.*: The Efficacy of Clomiphene Citrate for Induction of Ovulation, *Intern. J. Fertility 11*: 265-270 (July-Sept.) 1966.
16. Kerr, D. N. S. and Davidson, S.: Gastrointestinal Intolerance to Oral Iron Preparations, *Lancet 2*:489-492 (Sept. 6) 1958.
17. Greenberg, B. G.: Why Randomize?, *Biometrics 7*: 309-322 (Dec.) 1951.
18. Sevelius, H. and Colmore, J. P.: Objective Assessment of Antitussive Agents in Patients with Chronic Cough, *J. Clin. Pharmacol. J. New Drugs 6*:216-223 (July-Aug.) 1966.
19. Parker, C. E., Edwards, A. E. and Cohen, S.: The Effect of Bamethan on Cardiovascular Response, *J. Clin. Pharmacol. J. New Drugs 6*:55-61 (Jan.-Feb.) 1966.
20. Kantor, T. G. *et al.*: Oral Analgesic Studies—Pentazocine Hydrochloride, Codeine, Aspirin, and Placebo and Their Influence on Response to Placebo, *Clin. Pharmacol. Therap. 7*:447-454 (July-Aug.) 1966.
21. Stewart, E. H.: Self-Administered Analgesia in Labour with Special Reference to Trichlorethylene, *Lancet 2*:781-783 (Oct. 29) 1949.
22. Armitage, P.: *Sequential Medical Trials*, Blackwell Scientific Publications, Oxford, 1960.
23. Silverman, W. A., Fertig, J. W. and Berger, A. P.: The Influence of the Thermal Environment Upon the Survival of Newly Born Premature Infants, *Pediatrics 22*:876-886 (Nov.) 1958.

Additional Readings

Blackwell, B. and Ayd, F. J., Jr.: Problems in the Evaluation of a New Antidepressant Drug in Prison Volunteers, *J. Clin. Pharmacol. J. New Drugs 11*:19-26 (Jan.-Feb.) 1971.

Cochran, W. G. and Cox, G. M.: *Experimental Designs*, ed. 2, John Wiley and Sons, Inc., New York, 1957.

Cronheim, G. E.: Theoretical and Practical Approach to Drug Research Analysis, *Military Med. 135*:1021-1027 (Nov.) 1970.

Hicks, C. R.: *Fundamental Concepts in the Design of Experiments*, Holt, Rinehart and Winston, New York, 1964.

Hill, A. B.: *Principles of Medical Statistics*, ed. 8, Oxford University Press, New York, 1966. (Chapter 20, Clinical Trials.)

Li, C. C.: *Introduction to Experimental Statistics*, McGraw-Hill Book Company, New York, 1964.

Oliver, J. E.: Distortions in a Psychiatric Double-blind Trial—Comparing Chlordiazepoxide with Placebo-with-side-effects, *Clin. Trials J. 5*:991-995 (May) 1968.

Wilson, G. M.: The Experimental Trial of New Drugs in Man, *Proc. Roy. Soc. Med. 63*:986-990 (Oct.) 1970.

PERSPECTIVES IN CLINICAL PHARMACY

Subject Index

D

M

N

O

Q

R

S